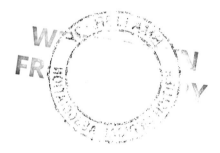

Endocrine and Metabolic Medical Emergencies

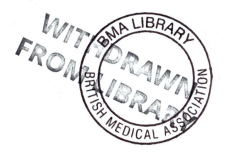

I dedicate this book to all people living with endocrine and metabolic problems and the healthcare professionals who look after them. I also dedicate this book to my family, especially wife Marcia and parents Enid and Sid, without whose continued support and encouragement the book would never have been started never mind finished!

Endocrine and Metabolic Medical Emergencies

A Clinician's Guide

Edited by

Glenn Matfin, BSc (Hons), MSc (Oxon), MB BCh, DGM, FACE, FACP, FRCP

Consultant in Acute and General Medicine, Diabetes and Endocrinology
Honorary Professor of Medicine
National Health Service, UK

Professor of Medicine
MBRU College of Medicine
Dubai Healthcare City
Dubai, UAE

Second Edition

This Work is a co-publication between the Endocrine Society and John Wiley & Sons, Ltd.

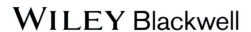

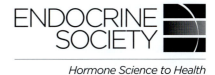

Registered Office(s)
John Wiley & Sons, Inc., 111 River Street, Hoboken, NJ 07030, USA
John Wiley & Sons Ltd, The Atrium, Southern Gate, Chichester, West Sussex, PO19 8SQ, UK

Editorial Office
9600 Garsington Road, Oxford, OX4 2DQ, UK

For details of our global editorial offices, customer services, and more information about Wiley products visit us at www.wiley.com.

Wiley also publishes its books in a variety of electronic formats and by print-on-demand. Some content that appears in standard print versions of this book may not be available in other formats.

Library of Congress Cataloging-in-Publication Data

Names: Matfin, Glenn, editor.
Title: Endocrine and metabolic medical emergencies : a clinician's guide / [edited] by Glenn Matfin.
Description: Second edition. | Hoboken, NJ : Wiley, 2018. | Includes bibliographical references and index. |
Identifiers: LCCN 2017049999 (print) | LCCN 2017050741 (ebook) | ISBN 9781119374763 (pdf) | ISBN 9781119374756 (epub) | ISBN 9781119374732 (cloth)
Subjects: | MESH: Endocrine System Diseases | Metabolic Diseases | Emergency Treatment
Classification: LCC RC649 (ebook) | LCC RC649 (print) | NLM WK 140 | DDC 616.4–dc23
LC record available at https://lccn.loc.gov/2017049999

Cover images: ©donskarpo / Getty Images-Thyroid level conceptual meter
©shansekala / Getty Images-Stethoscope on cardiogram concept for heart care
©juststock / Getty Images-Hypoglycemia Printed Diagnosis Medical Concept
Cover design by Wiley

Set in 10/12pt WarnockPro by Aptara Inc., New Delhi, India
Printed and bound in Singapore by Markono Print Media Pte Ltd

1   2018

Contents

Notes on Contributors

Angela M. Abbatecola
Azienda Sanitaria Locale (ASL) Districts
B,C,D
Frosinone, Italy

Krystallenia I. Alexandraki
National University of Athens
Athens, Greece

Rebecca S. Bahn
Mayo Clinic
Rochester, USA

Anita Banerjee
Guy's and St Thomas' Hospital
London, UK

Luigi Bartalena
University of Insubria
Varese, Italy

John P. Bilezikian
Columbia University
New York, USA

Fausto Bogazzi
University of Pisa
Pisa, Italy

Eva Boonen
KU Leuven
Leuven, Belgium

Claire Briet
Centre hospitalier universitaire d'Angers
Angers, France

Henry B. Burch
Walter Reed National Military Medical
Center
Bethesda, USA

Philippe Chanson
Bicêtre University Hospital
Paris, France

Curtiss B. Cook
Mayo Clinic Arizona
Scottsdale, USA

David S. Cooper
Johns Hopkins University School of
Medicine
Baltimore, USA

Stephen N. Davis
University of Maryland School of Medicine
Baltimore, USA

Ketan Dhatariya
Norfolk and Norwich University Hospitals
NHS Foundation Trust
Norwich, UK

Dima L. Diab
University of Cincinnati Bone Health and
Osteoporosis Center
Cincinnati, USA

Robert H. Eckel
University of Colorado
Denver, USA

Graeme Eisenhofer
University Hospital Carl Gustav Carus
Dresden, Germany

Nuha El Sayed
Joslin Diabetes Center
Boston, USA

Kate Evans
Derriford Hospital
Plymouth, UK

Hasan Fattah
NYU Langone Medical Center
New York, USA

Dorothy A. Fink
Hospital for Special Surgery
New York, USA

Miles Fisher
Glasgow Royal Infirmary
Glasgow, UK

Paul J. Frost
University Hospital of Wales
Cardiff, UK

Rodolfo J. Galindo
Emory University School of Medicine
Atlanta, USA

Aoife Garrahy
Beaumont Hospital/RCSI Medical School
Dublin, Ireland

James A. Garrity
Mayo Clinic
Rochester, USA

Hossein Gharib
Mayo Clinic
Rochester, USA

Helena Gleeson
University Hospitals Birmingham NHS
Foundation Trust
Birmingham, UK

David S. Goldfarb
NYU Langone Medical Center
New York, USA

Anda R. Gonciulea
Johns Hopkins University School of
Medicine
Baltimore, USA

Aidar R. Gosmanov
Albany Medical College
Albany, USA

Niyaz R. Gosmanov
University of Oklahoma Health Sciences
Center
Oklahoma City, USA

Ashley B. Grossman
Oxford Centre for Diabetes, Endocrinology
and Metabolism
Oxford, UK

Jan Gunst
KU Leuven
Leuven, Belgium

James V. Hennessey
Beth Israel Deaconess Medical Center
Boston, USA

Suzanne M. Jan de Beur
Johns Hopkins University School of
Medicine
Baltimore, USA

Andrzej Januszewicz
Institute of Cardiology
Warsaw, Poland

Ursula B. Kaiser
Brigham and Women's Hospital
Boston, USA

Gregory Kaltsas
National University of Athens
Athens, Greece

Natasha Kasid
Joslin Diabetes Center,
Boston, USA

Han Na Kim
Johns Hopkins University School of
Medicine
Baltimore, USA

Anne Klibanski
Massachusetts General Hospital
Boston, USA

Robin H. Lachmann
National Hospital for Neurology and
Neurosurgery
London, UK

Elizabeth M. Lamos
University of Maryland School of Medicine
Baltimore, USA

Edward R. Laws
Brigham and Women's Hospital
Boston, USA

Jacques W.M. Lenders
Radboud University Medical Centre
Nijmegen, The Netherlands

Patricia A. Mackey
Mayo Clinic Arizona
Phoenix, USA

Enio Martino
University of Pisa
Pisa, Italy

Glenn Matfin
National Health Service
London, UK; MBRU College of Medicine
Dubai, UAE

Nestoras Mathioudakis
Johns Hopkins University School of
Medicine
Baltimore, USA

Jeffrey I. Mechanick
Marie-Josee and Henry R. Kravis Center for
Cardiovascular Health at Mount Sinai Heart
New York, USA

Mark E. Molitch
Northwestern University Feinberg School of
Medicine
Chicago, USA

John E. Morley
St Louis University School of Medicine
St. Louis, USA

Reza Morovat
John Radcliffe Hospital
Oxford, UK

Elaine Murphy
National Hospital for Neurology and
Neurosurgery
London, UK

Connie B. Newman
NYU School of Medicine
New York, USA

Kjell Oberg
Uppsala University Hospital
Uppsala, Sweden

David R. Owens
Institute of Life Sciences College of
Medicine
Swansea, UK

Christina Pamporaki
University Hospital Carl Gustav Carus
Dresden, Germany

Gerry Rayman
Ipswich Hospitals NHS Trust
Ipswich, UK

Megan J. Ritter
Joslin Diabetes Center
Boston, USA

David B. Sacks
National Institutes of Health
Bethesda, USA

Katherine Samaras
St Vincent's Hospital
Darlinghurst, Australia

Alissa R. Segal
Joslin Diabetes Center
Boston, USA

Pankaj Shah
Mayo Clinic
Rochester, USA

Ethel S. Siris
Columbia University Medical Center
New York, USA

Mark A. Sperling
Icahn School of Medicine at Mount Sinai
New York, USA

Richard H. Sterns
University of Rochester
Rochester, USA

Bithika M. Thompson
Mayo Clinic Arizona
Scottsdale, USA

Christopher Thompson
Beaumont Hospital/RCSI Medical School
Dublin, Ireland

Jonathan A. Tobert
University of Oxford
Oxford, UK

Luca Tomisti
University of Pisa
Pisa, Italy

Andrew Toogood
University Hospitals Birmingham NHS
Foundation Trust
Birmingham, UK

Nicholas A. Tritos
Massachusetts General Hospital
Boston, USA

Guillermo E. Umpierrez
Emory University School of Medicine
Atlanta, USA

Anand Vaidya
Brigham and Women's Hospital
Boston, USA

Greet Van den Berghe
KU Leuven
Leuven, Belgium

Mark Vanderpump
The Physicians' Clinic
London, UK

Joseph G. Verbalis
Georgetown University School of
Medicine
Washington, USA

Michael A. Via
Icahn School of Medicine at Mount Sinai
New York, USA

Alicia L. Warnock
Walter Reed National Military Medical
Center
Bethesda, USA

Nelson B. Watts
Mercy Health Osteoporosis and Bone
Health Services
Cincinnati, USA

Jianping Weng
The Third Affiliated Hospital of Sun
Yat-sen University
Guangdong Province, China

Robert A. Wermers
Mayo Clinic
Rochester, USA

Anthony S. Wierzbicki
Guy's & St Thomas' Hospitals
London, UK

Catherine Williamson
King's College London
London, UK

Matt P. Wise
University Hospital of Wales
Cardiff, UK

Wen Xu
The Third Affiliated Hospital of Sun
Yat-sen University
Guangdong Province, China

Mabel Yau
Icahn School of Medicine at Mount Sinai
New York, USA

Lisa M. Younk
University of Maryland School of
Medicine
Baltimore, USA

Foreword

The field of endocrinology is in constant evolution, reflecting the rapid pace of change in medicine and science more generally. In its earliest stages, endocrinology defined the clinical features of acromegaly, Graves' disease, myxedema, Cushing's syndrome, and diabetes mellitus. This era was followed by the discovery of hormones and a renaissance catalyzed by radioimmunoassays (RIAs). These measurements allowed rigorous determinations of circulating hormones and an understanding of complex hormonal feedback mechanisms. The last few decades have witnessed a more sophisticated understanding of perturbations of homeostasis in which we better diagnose disorders such as primary hyperparathyroidism, subclinical hyperthyroidism, and subclinical hypercortisolism.

Endocrine and Metabolic Medical Emergencies was conceived by Glenn Matfin, an endocrinologist with extensive clinical experience in several countries and in areas relevant to the topics covered in the text. He and his co-authors recognized a paradigm shift in the field of endocrinology and metabolism. Namely, our patients rarely present with endocrine disease in isolation. Rather, hormonal disorders occur in combination with other conditions such as critical illness, or HIV/AIDS, which directly or through their treatments precipitate endocrine disease or illicit physiologic responses that alter hormonal pathways. Hospitalized patients are also increasingly complex and critically ill. This setting is rife with stress-related hormonal responses and is rarely appropriate for the methodical evaluation of endocrine conditions. Consequently, in the hospital setting, the emphasis has shifted to acute management of endocrine emergencies such as hypoglycemia, hyponatremia, hypercalcemia, adrenal insufficiency, thyroid storm, and pituitary apoplexy.

The essence of medical textbooks is to transfer knowledge and improve clinical care. The second edition of this book expands the repertoire of traditional endocrine emergencies to myriad other conditions that require urgent attention to optimize clinical outcomes. It contains more than a dozen new chapters by internationally renowned experts. *Endocrine and Metabolic Medical Emergencies* is a timely resource for managing today's complex inpatients with endocrine abnormalities. Each chapter addresses a common situation encountered by the practicing endocrinologist. Thanks to this book, we are now armed with innovative chapters such as "Endocrine and Metabolic Emergencies in Transplantation" and "Management of Concentrated Insulins in Acute Care Settings." We are indebted to these authors for an innovative contribution to the medical literature.

J. Larry Jameson
Philadelphia, PA

Preface

The specialty of endocrinology and metabolism is no longer at the fringes of medicine, and now includes some of the most common conditions and serious public health challenges facing high-, middle-, and low-income countries alike. Prevalent endocrine and metabolic conditions include obesity and diabetes, thyroid disorders, and metabolic bone diseases. The associated human, financial, and societal costs incurred by people with these and other endocrine and metabolic disorders are sobering.

Acute medical care is a major focus for many healthcare providers and funders, and patients with endocrine and metabolic emergencies constitute a large proportion of this workload. In addition, many patients are not ideally managed (including safety issues) due to the lack of excellent, up-to-date, and practical guidance. There is therefore an unmet need for a comprehensive clinician resource covering acute endocrine and metabolic emergencies. As the Endocrine Society is a world-leader in education and translation of clinical endocrinology, it is understandable that this unmet need be addressed by the Endocrine Society. The purpose of this updated book, *Endocrine and Metabolic Medical Emergencies* (second edition), is to help fill this gap by updating and collating existing knowledge on the management of numerous everyday endocrine and metabolic emergencies facing clinicians everywhere. This expanded edition has been updated completely and also has several new features including key points; case studies, and many new figures.

We believe that this new edition will bring the topic areas up-to-date, set a standard for diagnosis and treatment in each category, blending the most current medical science knowledge with clinical and practical advice using the best international guidance. The authors of each chapter are acknowledged experts in their respective areas and were specifically chosen for their recognized clinical skills. This book provides a highly practical and useful reference compendium of the experts' personal approaches to each problem. Some topics (e.g., pituitary apoplexy) are covered in several different chapters, and give different perspectives on management. The contents (while not fully inclusive of all possible disorders) cover many of the common (and not so common) endocrine and metabolic emergencies. In addition, some of the thorny issues which are especially taxing to the clinician or areas not often addressed in publications (such as the management of insulin pumps or concentrated insulins in the inpatient setting) are covered. Each chapter is written to stand alone and the chapters can be read at any time and in any sequence.

This book is divided into eleven Parts. Most of these Parts have an Introduction which sets the scene for the specific section. Part I covers acute medical care. This starts with an updated Introduction originally written by Sir Richard Thompson (Past-President of the Royal College of Physicians), and the distinguished endocrinologist, John Wass, of the challenges and opportunities of delivering acute medical care in the current healthcare environment. This provides the context within which endocrine and metabolic emergency care occurs. In addition, all clinicians need to be familiar with the basic management of acute medical illnesses (especially when covering the inpatient service intermittently), and this is outlined next. Part II focuses on the effects of acute medical and critical illness on the endocrine and metabolic systems, and the impact of these changes and other factors on endocrine investigations in this setting. Several special populations of patients are then discussed in Part III, including the unique impact of aging, pregnancy, and HIV/AIDS on emergency endocrine and metabolic disorders presentation and management. For the second edition, this special populations section now includes new chapters on endocrine and metabolic emergencies in transitional care; perioperative; late-effects; inherited metabolic diseases; and transplantation patients. The remaining Parts cover various different endocrine and metabolic systems including pituitary; thyroid; adrenal; calcium, phosphate, and metabolic bone diseases; neuroendocrine tumors; glucose; sodium; and obesity and clinical lipidology.

I would like to thank Larry Jameson for again writing the Foreword. In his current and previous multifaceted roles, Dr. Jameson truly understands the complex challenges faced by endocrinologists and other clinicians in delivering high-quality, patient-centered, cost-effective care for all patients including those presenting with endocrine and metabolic emergencies. I would also like to acknowledge the tremendous effort by the authors. Despite very tight deadlines and having numerous other commitments, they generously shared their time and expertise in writing the excellent chapters. In the second edition, we have a number of new authors so I would also like to thank previous authors for their input. I owe special thanks to the Endocrine Society/Wiley Health Sciences publishing alliance for agreeing to publish this book. Publishing books was a defining moment in the advancement of humanity. This is no less true in the 21st Century, although this now involves multinational resources and collaboration. I personally thank all the persons involved for bringing this superb volume to fruition. It is certain to prove a valuable resource that will benefit endocrinologists and other clinicians (including acute medicine, internists, critical care, and hospitalists), as well as their patients for years to come.

Last but not least, I owe special thanks to the reader. Your commitment to delivering excellent patient care, while maintaining (and even expanding) your knowledge using resources like this book are to be applauded – it's not easy! Your feedback is always welcome.

Glenn Matfin
Editor
February 2018

List of Abbreviations

5-HIAA	5-hydroxyindoleacetic acid	ATC	anaplastic thyroid cancer
βHBA	3-beta-hydroxybutyrate	ATD	antithyroid drugs
A1C	HbA1c	AVP	arginine vasopressin
AACE	American Association of Clinical Endocrinologists	AVPU	Alert, Voice, Pain, Unresponsive
ABCDE	Airway, Breathing, Circulation, Disability, and Exposure	BG	blood glucose
		bid/BID	twice a day
		BMD	bone mineral density
ABG	arterial blood gas	BMI	body mass index
ABI	ankle brachial index	BP	blood pressure
ac	pre-meals	BPD	biliopancreatic diversion
ACa	adjusted calcium	BPDDS	biliopancreatic diversion with duodenal switch
ACE	angiotensin-converting enzyme	BUN	blood urea nitrogen
ACR	albumin/creatinine ratio	CAH	congenital adrenal hyperplasia
ACS	acute coronary syndromes	cART	combined antiretroviral therapy
ACTH	adrenocorticotrophic hormone	CaSR	calcium-sensing receptor
ACU	ambulatory care unit	CBG	capillary blood glucose
ADA	American Diabetes Association	CGM	continuous glucose monitoring
ADH	antidiuretic hormone	CHF	congestive heart failure
AF	atrial fibrillation	CII	continuous insulin infusion
AFF	atypical femur fractures	CK	creatine kinase
AG	anion gap	CKD	chronic kidney disease
AIDS	acquired immune deficiency syndrome	CN	Charcot neuroarthropathy
		COPD	chronic obstructive pulmonary disease
AIRE	autoimmune regulator gene		
AKI	acute kidney injury	CPAP	continuous positive airway pressure
AMU	acute medical unit		
APACHE II	acute physiology and chronic health evaluation II	CPOE	computerized physician order entry
APS	autoimmune polyglandular syndrome	CRH	corticotropin-releasing hormone
ARB	angiotensin receptor blocker	CRP	C-reactive protein
ARDS	adult respiratory distress syndrome	CRRT	continuous renal replacement therapy

CSF	cerebrospinal fluid	GvHD	graft versus host disease
CSII	continuous subcutaneous insulin infusion	HAAF	hypoglycemia-associated autonomic failure
CT	computed tomography	HAART	highly active antiretroviral therapy
CVD	cardiovascular disease		
CYP3A4	cytochrome P450 3A4	HbA1c	glycated (glycosylated) hemoglobin
DDAVP	desmopressin		
DCCT	Diabetes Care and Complications Trial	HBO	hyperbaric oxygen
		HDL-C	high-density lipoprotein cholesterol
DFI	diabetic foot infection		
DFU	diabetic foot ulcer	HDU	high dependency unit
DI	diabetes insipidus	HHM	humoral hypercalcemia of malignancy
DIDMOAD	DI, Diabetes Mellitus, Optic Atrophy, and Deafness		
		HHS	hyperglycemic hyperosmolar state
DKA	diabetic ketoacidosis		
DPP4	dipeptidyl peptidase 4	HIV	human immunodeficiency virus
DVT	deep vein thrombosis		
EASD	European Association for the Study of Diabetes	HMG CoA	3-hydroxy-3-methylglutaryl-coenzyme A
ECF	extracellular fluid	HPA	hypothalamic-pituitary adrenal
ECG	electrocardiograph		
ED	emergency department	HPG	hypothalamic-pituitary gonadal
eGFR	estimated glomerular filtration rate		
		HPT	hypothalamic-pituitary thyroid
EMA	European Medicines Agency		
EN	enteral nutrition	ICF	intracellular fluid
ENETS	European Neuroendocrine Tumor Society	ICU	intensive care unit
		IFCC	International Federation of Clinical Chemistry
ESRD	end-stage renal disease		
FBC	full (complete) blood count	IGF-1	insulin-like growth factor-1
FDA	Food and Drug Administration	IGF-2	insulin-like growth factor-2
		IGFBP	IGF-binding proteins
FFA	free fatty acids	IIT	intensive insulin therapy
FGF23	fibroblast growth factor 23	IM	intramuscular
FNA	fine-needle aspiration	IMD	inherited metabolic disease
FPG	fasting plasma glucose	ISPAD	International Society for Pediatric and Adolescent Diabetes
FRIII	fixed rate intravenous insulin infusion		
FSH	follicle-stimulating hormone	IST	insulin stress test
FT3	free triiodothyronine	ITT	insulin tolerance test
FT4	free thyroxine	IU	international units
GCS	Glasgow Coma Scale (Score)	IV	intravenous
GH	growth hormone	IWGDF	International Working Group on the Diabetic Foot
GHRH	growth hormone-releasing hormone		
		JBDS	Joint British Diabetes Societies
GKI	glucose-potassium-insulin	JTA	Japanese Thyroid Association
GLP-1	glucagon-like peptide-1	LAGB	laparoscopic adjustable gastric banding
GnRH	gonadotropin-releasing hormone		
		LDL-C	low-density lipoprotein cholesterol
GSD	glycogen storage disorder		

LFT	liver function tests	PCSK9	proprotein convertase subtilisin/kexin type 9
LH	luteinizing hormone	PE	pulmonary embolism
LMWH	low molecular weight heparin	PEDIS	Perfusion, Extent, Depth, Infection and Sensation
LOPS	loss of protective sensation		
LSG	laparoscopic sleeve gastrectomy	PN	parenteral nutrition
MACE	major adverse cardiovascular events	pNETS	pancreatic NETs
		PO	by mouth
MALA	metformin-associated lactic acidosis	POC	point of care
		PRIDE	Planning Research in In-patient Diabetes
MAP	mean arterial pressure		
MDT	multidisciplinary team	PRL	prolactin
MELAS	mitochondrial encephalomyopathy, lactic acidosis, and stroke-like episodes	PRRT	peptide receptor radionuclide therapy
		PTH	parathyroid hormone
		PTHrP	parathyroid hormone-related peptide
MEN 1	multiple endocrine neoplasia syndrome 1	qid/QDS	four times a day
MI	myocardial infarction	QTc	corrected QT interval duration
MIBG	I^{123}-metaiodobenzylguanidine		
MRI	magnetic resonance imaging	RAI	radioactive iodine
MRSA	methicillin-resistant *Staphylococcus aureus*	RAIU	radioactive iodine uptake
		RANK	receptor activator of nuclear factor–κB
NaDIA	National Diabetes Inpatient Audit		
		RANKL	RANK ligand
NBM	nil-by-mouth	RCT	randomized controlled trial
NEC	neuroendocrine carcinoma	RR	respiratory rate
NEN	neuroendocrine neoplasm	Rx	treatment
NET	neuroendocrine tumor	RYGB	Roux-en-Y gastric bypass
NEWS	National Early Warning Score	SBAR	situation, background, assessment, and recommendation
NHS	National Health Service		
NICE	National Institute for Health and Care Excellence		
		SBP	systolic blood pressure
NIV	non-invasive ventilation	SC	subcutaneous
NPO	nil per oral	SGLT-2	sodium glucose co-transporter 2
NSAID	non-steroidal anti-inflammatory drug		
		SI	Système International
NSTEMI	non-ST-elevation myocardial infarction	SIADH	syndrome of inappropriate antidiuretic hormone
NTI	non-thyroidal illness	SIRS	systemic inflammatory response syndrome
ODS	osmotic demyelination syndrome		
		SMBG	self-monitoring of blood glucose
ONJ	osteonecrosis of the jaw		
OSA	obstructive sleep apnea	STEMI	ST-elevation myocardial infarction
PAD	peripheral arterial disease		
PAS	Pituitary Apoplexy Score	T1DM	type 1 diabetes mellitus
PCI	percutaneous coronary interventions	T2DM	type 2 diabetes mellitus
		T_3	triiodothyronine
PCP	pneumocystis pneumonia	T_4	thyroxine

TBG	thyroxine-binding globulin	UAO	upper airway obstruction
TCC	total contact cast	UKPDS	United Kingdom Prospective
TDD	total daily dose		Diabetes Study
TFT	thyroid function test	ULN	upper limit of normal
TG	thyroglobulin	UTI	urinary tract infection
TIA	transient ischemic attack	VBG	venous blood gas
tid/TDS	three times a day	VF	visual field
TPN	total parenteral nutrition	VRIII	variable rate intravenous
TPO	thyroid peroxidase		insulin infusion
TPP	thyrotoxic periodic paralysis	VTE	venous thromboembolism
TRH	thyrotropin-releasing	WDHA	watery diarrhea, hypokalemia,
	hormone		achlorhydria
TSH	thyroid-stimulating hormone	WHO	World Health Organization
U and E	urea and electrolytes	ZES	Zollinger-Ellison syndrome

Part I

General Aspects of Acute Medical Emergencies

Introduction

Acute Medical Care: A Crisis with Solutions

Glenn Matfin

Key Points

- There is a crisis in acute medical care for multifarious reasons.
- These include rising acute medical admissions with increased bed occupancy levels; increasingly older and frailer patients with complex, high-acuity illnesses and multimorbidities; systemic failures of care; poor patient experience; existence of healthcare disparities; multi-ethnic populations; medical and nursing workforce crisis; social and primary care crisis; constant reconfiguration in health and social care delivery and legislation; and ever increasing costs of health and social care in a time of austerity and/or financial instability. There is also a lack of candor when things go wrong.
- A new model of care for hospitals of the future has been proposed and the first principle is that of putting patients first (i.e., patient-centred). Patients should be treated with compassion and dignity. They should be involved in decisions on their condition and treatment (i.e., shared-decision making). Teams should work together towards common goals and in the best interest of patients. Patient safety is critical, and having an open culture of providing safe care and utilizing tools such as electronic prescribing can help. A duty of candor when problems arise is needed.
- Seven-day care is important too and there should be cover 24 hours a day, 7 days a week. Patient care should cross the boundaries of primary, secondary, post-acute and social care with care pathways designed for each of the morbidities that a patient experiences. In this regard, as in all, effective communication is key.
- There are important consequences of this and that is that there needs to be more doctors trained and engaged in generalist medicine. This does not mean that specialist care (such as diabetes and endocrinology) is less important or less prioritized. This will remain essential and indeed the degree of expertise available in the specialties is ever increasing. On-going postgraduate training requirements as well as maintenance/assessment of competencies and other professional attributes is expensive, complicated, and time-consuming. However, it is critical if we want a medical workforce that is up-to-date and fit-to-practice; and can also train the next and future generations of clinicians.
- The challenges and opportunities involved in delivering safe, timely, high-quality, patient-centred, holistic, cost-effective acute medical care, will resonate with all stakeholders globally involved with this complex, expensive, yet essential undertaking.

Endocrine and Metabolic Medical Emergencies: A Clinician's Guide, Second Edition. Edited by Glenn Matfin.
© 2018 John Wiley & Sons Ltd. Published 2018 by John Wiley & Sons Ltd.

Introduction

There is a crisis in acute medical care for multifarious reasons. We are all living in increasingly "graying" societies due to increasing numbers of the older population. In the USA alone, this population (defined as persons 65 years or older) numbered 41.4 million in 2011 (or one in every eight Americans). By 2025, this number is expected to increase to 62.5 million people (or almost one in every five Americans) according to the Endocrine Society's workforce analysis (1). This has important implications for healthcare. For example, the life expectancy at birth in the UK is now 12 years longer than what it was at the inception of the National Health Service (NHS) in 1948; and people aged over 60 now make up nearly a quarter of Britain's population. Half of these have a chronic illness and this proportion will increase as the number of people aged 85 or older doubles in the next 20 years. Nearly two-thirds of patients admitted to hospital are over 65 years old and around 25% of these patients have a diagnosis of dementia (with more than a third of people living in care homes having this diagnosis). Diabetes and endocrine problems are also common in this population, with almost one-quarter US older adults having diabetes (1,2). Approximately half of those persons with diabetes are undiagnosed and an additional one-half of older adults have prediabetes (2). The frail elderly in particular make up a large proportion of patients presenting for acute medical care, including endocrine and metabolic emergencies (e.g., hypoglycemia, hyperglycemia, hyponatremia, and hypercalcemia) (3).

There are increased numbers of acute medical admissions with higher inpatient bed occupancy levels. Pressure on beds in the NHS (and elsewhere) results in increased waiting times in emergency departments (so-called "trolley waits"). This crowding in the emergency departments (and other parts of the hospital) can lead to patient safety concerns (including maintaining cleanliness and controlling infections), is stressful for the patient (especially as these patients tend to get moved around to accommodate others) and also staff. As the various assessment units (e.g., medical admissions unit or equivalent) also become fuller due to increased admissions and an inability to "push" patients to the most suitable wards (i.e., specialist or general medical beds), this increases the likelihood that the patient will end up on the "wrong" ward such as medical outlier wards (i.e., medical patients within the surgical or non-medical bed base). The additional burden of staffing these non-medical wards with appropriately skilled medical, nursing and other relevant healthcare professionals (e.g., physiotherapists, occupational therapists) is a major daily challenge. All of these (and many other) issues can further delay timely access to the right specialty, and discharge-dependent investigative and/or therapeutic procedures. In addition, the inability to discharge patients who are "medically fit" but who have onward community care needs (i.e., post-acute care such as rehabilitation, or social care) is also concerning, due to significant issues in post-acute and social care delivery (including chronic underfunding and lack of staff). The number of patients stuck in hospital in the UK because of delays in discharge has increased 80% in the past 5 years (4). Consequently, the average length of stay in acute care in the UK in 2010 was 7.7 days which is significantly higher than Australia (5.1), the Netherlands (5.8) and the USA (4.9). Most recent figures (2017) for average length of medical stay from the author's facility are 7.95 days (for patients staying more than 24 hours).

There is also an increase in mortality of around 10% among patients admitted at weekends. Although the reasons are complex, there is an association between the presence of senior doctors and improved clinical outcome for patients. There are other problems as well. Junior doctors are working shorter hours (due in part to safety concerns and consequent limits on work hours) and there is often a lack of communication at handover. Due to an increase in demand for medical care and other reasons (including not training enough "home-grown" doctors or being able to retain them), medical trainees are under increased pressure and there is evidence that they do not get the mentorship or training that they deserve because of increasing demands on senior staff.

Ongoing postgraduate training needs as well as maintenance/assessment of competencies or certification and other professional attributes are expensive, complicated, time-consuming and do not always translate into improved patient care (5). The last two decades have witnessed a multitude of changes in postgraduate medical education. These changes are in part a response to the changing environment which doctors practice medicine. These drivers for change are related to both patients and doctors. Patient-related drivers include changes in patient demographics (an increase in older population as noted above), higher patient expectations both in terms of their own health status and the public's expectations of better services from the medical profession. Doctor-related drivers includes improvements in medical technology (e.g., influence of information technology [IT]) and advances in therapy, complexities of multiprofessional healthcare delivery, greater emphasis on patient safety, and the expectations of the medical professionals themselves in terms of a better work-life balance (6).

Health workers are the cornerstone of health systems. Jobs in the health and social care sector accounted for more than 10% of total employment in most OECD countries in 2016 (7). The current health workforce is suffering from growing pressures (with increased risk of clinician burnout leading to physical and emotional exhaustion and drop in productivity). In addition, the medical workforce is ageing rapidly (i.e., babyboomers) with almost third doctors aged 55 or older in USA and the OECD countries (7). Manpower issues in healthcare provision are significant with a lack of workforce planning and/or expenditure resulting in inadequate numbers of medical, nursing, and other healthcare professionals. This has resulted in migration of healthcare professionals from many other potentially more needy populations around the world (especially Asia, Central/South America, and Eastern Europe) to more affluent societies; with detrimental effects on the local healthcare delivery needs and workforce planning of the migrants' country of origin. The USA is by far the main destination country of foreign-trained health workers in absolute numbers, with more than 200,000 doctors (25% of total) and almost 250,000 nurses trained abroad in 2013 (7). The UK is the second main country of destination in absolute numbers, with more than 48,000 foreign-trained doctors and 86,000 foreign-trained nurses in 2014 (7).

What Is the Impact of the Acute Medical Crisis on Diabetes and Endocrinology Speciality Delivery?

Acute medical care is a major focus for many clinicians, including specialist diabetologists and endocrinologists. These generalist commitments can cannibalize on specialty roles and negatively impact on both inpatient and outpatient services. However, there is also an opportunity to positively impact on patients with endocrine and metabolic issues/emergencies which constitute a large proportion of the acute medical care workload. For example, the proportion of inpatients with diabetes continues to grow (e.g., 17% of inpatients in the UK; and more than 20% in the USA) (8). The UK's National Diabetes Inpatient Audit (NaDIA) projects that the numbers of hospital beds occupied by persons with diabetes will increase to nearly 20% by 2020; in many hospitals it already exceeds 30% (9). This high prevalence of inpatients with diabetes can lead to a number of issues, including the safe use of in-hospital insulin therapy throughout all areas of this care setting. Almost half (46%) of inpatients treated with insulin therapy had a prescription or medication management error in the NaDIA (9). NaDIA also showed that almost 1 in 10 inpatients (9%) with diabetes had active foot disease on admission, with almost 1 in 20 inpatients directly admitted for this problem (4%). Worryingly, 1 in 75 patients with diabetes developed a new foot lesion during their in-hospital stay (1.4%). In defiance of UK National Institute for Health and Care Excellence (NICE) guidelines on diabetic foot clinical care pathway (10), less than one-third (30%) of inpatients with diabetes had a specific diabetic foot exam within 24 hours (9).

Hyponatremia is the most common electrolyte abnormality, affecting up to 30–42% of hospitalized patients and is associated with increased morbidity and mortality (11). In a large in-hospital registry of the current state and management of hyponatremia (focused on syndrome of inappropriate antidiuretic hormone [SIADH]), it was shown that ineffectual therapies were commonly used. The most commonly chosen monotherapy treatments, fluid restriction and isotonic saline, failed to increase the serum sodium concentration by ≥ 5 mmol/L in 55% and 64% monotherapy treatments respectively (10). In addition, fluid restriction or isotonic saline only increased the serum sodium concentration ≥ 130 mmol/L in 28% and 18% monotherapy treatments respectively. Appropriate laboratory tests to diagnose SIADH (12) were obtained in <50% patients (11).

Many patients with diabetes and endocrine issues/emergencies are not ideally managed in the acute care setting leading to unwarranted clinical variation. This can be due to many factors including lack of time, training and/or expertise among healthcare providers. For example, many clinicians (especially junior doctors and non-endocrine specialists) believe that patients presenting with various emergency endocrine and metabolic disorders with abnormal values (e.g., level of glucose, sodium, osmolality, anion gap ["closing the gap"], and blood pressure) must be corrected to "normal" as quickly as possible (3). This practice can lead to increased morbidity and mortality (e.g., osmotic demyelination syndrome with over-rapid correction of hyponatremia) (12). Preventing rapid- and over-correction by appropriate education, guidelines, care pathways, audit, and other resources (such as this book) may reduce unnecessary suffering and potentially save lives.

Solutions/Opportunities

These various issues together with the UK Francis Enquiry on the Mid Staffordshire NHS Foundation Trust (13) highlighting, among other things, that patients were not at the center of care showed that fundamental change was necessary in the running of the NHS (14) and in particular the organization of medical care in hospitals.

Against this background (i.e., rising acute medical admissions with increased bed occupancy; increasingly older and frailer patients with complex, high-acuity illnesses and multimorbidities; systemic failures of care; underfunding; poor patient experience; constant changes in healthcare delivery and legislation; social and primary care crisis; and a medical and other healthcare professionals workforce crisis), the Future Hospital Commission (14) was set up by the Royal College of Physicians under the chairmanship of Sir Michael Rawlins. In September 2013, it set out 11 core principles for hospitals of the future (Table I-1). The first principle is that of putting patients first (i.e., patient-centered). Patients should be treated with compassion and dignity. They should be involved in decisions on their condition (i.e., shared-decision making) including taking into account social and cultural norms especially for multi-ethnic populations (i.e., cultural distinction). A new model of care is needed and the suggestion (already taken up by many Trusts in the UK) is that there should be a medical division led by a chief of medicine (similar to the current practice in the USA) as the senior doctor responsible for making sure working practices facilitate collaborative, patient-centered working and that teams work together toward common goals and in the best interest of patients. Therefore effective leadership is essential.

Seven-day care is important too and there should be cover 24 hours a day, 7 days a week. This is particularly because, as above, patients often present with multiple morbidities requiring a range of support. This aspect

Table I-1 Core principles of patient care (15)

1. Fundamental standards of care must always be met.
2. Patient experience is valued as much as clinical effectiveness.
3. Responsibility for each patient's care is clear and communicated.
4. Patients have effective and timely access to care, including appointments, tests, treatment and moves out of hospital.
5. Patients do not move wards unless this is necessary for their clinical care.
6. Robust arrangements for the transfer of care are in place.
7. Good communication with and about patients is the norm.
8. Care is designed to facilitate self-care and health promotion.
9. Services are tailored to meet the needs of individual patients, including vulnerable patients.
10. All patients have a care plan that reflects their individual clinical and support needs.
11. Staff are supported to deliver safe, compassionate care, and committed to improving quality.

too has being taken up in many hospitals in the UK, but there are often problems (especially with the smaller hospitals and certain specialities) being able to provide 24/7 coverage.

There is an important consequence of this and that is that there needs to be more doctors trained in generalist medicine (including acute medicine, internal medicine, hospitalists, enhanced and intensive care). This does not mean that specialist care is less important or less prioritized. This will remain essential and, indeed, the degree of expertise available in the specialties is ever increasing. Accredited training in aspects of super specialist care should be available and will further enhance the quality of specialist input. This will be time-consuming and expensive to do but is important to maintain and grow generalist and specialist expertise. Postgraduate medical education in the UK (i.e., "shape of training") and the USA (i.e., "next accreditation system"), among others, are trying to re-focus toward generalist outcomes-based training, as well as addressing other important generic competencies/behaviors

such as medical professionalism, leadership and team working, communication and interpersonal skills, duty hours and fatigue management, care transitions, health promotion and illness prevention, safeguarding vulnerable groups, and integrating junior doctors into patient safety and health care quality improvement (6,16,17). It is also important to increase the number of medical and nursing students. Undergraduate medical education is also evolving with greater focus on generalist training.

It is imperative to explore ways of incentivizing doctors to work in the most challenging and in-demand areas of medicine (and also in the more remote/rural areas) (4). For example, in the USA, only 12% of all doctors are general/family practitioners with 88% specialists; whilst in the UK, 29% of all doctors are general/family practitioners with 71% specialists (7). The rapid growth of hospitalists in the USA is a good example of attracting clinicians to an area of unmet clinical need. Hospitalists now number more than 50,000 in the USA and are larger than any subspecialty of internal medicine (the largest of which is cardiology with 22,000 physicians) (18). Promoting innovative models of medical staffing including nurse practitioners, physician associates and other mid-level clinicians is important. Our trainees are important and should, as far as possible, work in stable medical teams which educate and mentor the next generation of senior clinicians.

It is essential to find innovative ways of avoiding hospital admission ("front-door") by best practice streaming, such as improving prehospital care (e.g., paramedic glucagon administration to treat severe hypoglycemia is underutilized in many parts of the USA) and patient triage from primary care; earlier speciality review and treatment for patients who may otherwise decompensate via virtual- or rapid-access clinics; and earlier generalist review and treatment in an ambulatory care unit environment (or similar), which can safely and effectively treat various conditions without admission, such as deep vein thrombosis, as well as early diabetic ketoacidosis. Once the patient is admitted, improving patient-flow throughout the hospital such as early senior review of patients in the emergency department; "pushing" and "pulling" speciality patients to speciality wards from the assessment or general medical/outlier wards earlier in the day; and having daily ward and/or board rounds all help. "Front-door" reconfiguration measures and effective discharge planning by multidisciplinary interactions with post-acute, social and primary care providers can facilitate timely discharge from hospital ("back-door") to the most appropriate setting, and hopefully will prevent readmission.

Patient safety is key (with recent data suggesting that medical errors are the third-leading cause of death in the USA) and the Royal College of Physicians and many other national and international organizations are looking at ways of improving patient safety. Why can't the medical profession have the success that airlines do? Having a culture of providing safe care with senior leadership endorsement and utilizing tools such as electronic prescribing can help. The recent UK Wachter Report (chaired by Professor Robert Wachter) outlined various recommendations to further implement IT in healthcare (19), especially the use of electronic health records and other digital tools (including artificial intelligence) which can further enhance safer patient care. However, adopting over-complex, slow, non-integrated IT systems and the recent NHS cyber attack demonstrate the potential risks of over-reliance on IT in healthcare (20). Increased education is also important to improve safety, such as insulin prescribing and administration, and should be mandatory for all healthcare providers involved with patients with diabetes across the acute care setting. Having real-time "root cause analysis" when things do go wrong is desirable to prevent further occurrences. A duty of candor when problems arise is needed.

Patient care should cross the boundaries of primary, secondary, post-acute and social care with care pathways designed for each of the morbidities that a patient experiences. Regrettably, the NHS at the moment has walls between primary and secondary care which actively need to be broken down and

this is already happening in many specialties (although the situation in the USA can be even worse with more fragmented and less integrated patient care). In this regard, as in all, effective communication is key.

Increasing healthcare funding and wiser spending is critical to meet ever increasing demand for health services, reduce healthcare disparities and to fund projects that can transform and sustain healthcare delivery. Investing in prevention is also important to try and decrease future healthcare demands (e.g., iodine deficiency disorders, smoking cessation, diabetes, obesity, and hypertension); as well as universal access to critical therapies (e.g., insulin); and eliminating food insecurity.

There are many challenges for the future of care of medical patients and these have never been so great (e.g., on 2nd January 2018, NHS England postponed all non-urgent inpatient operations [such as elective hip replacements] and canceled routine outpatient appointments [e.g., diabetes and endocrine clinics] until February 2018 due to winter "crisis" and opioid crisis in the USA), but there are solutions and we as a profession need to lead, like Henry V, from the front. The medical profession must not be contumacious and reactionary as it can be. While written predominantly from a UK perspective, the challenges and opportunities outlined will resonate with all stakeholders involved in delivering safe, timely, high-quality, patient-centred, holistic, cost-effective acute medical care globally. If acute medical care is not delivered optimally, this can have a detrimental impact on the management of other conditions such as endocrine and metabolic emergencies, which also occurs in this complex setting.

Acknowledgments

The current author wishes to acknowledge the contributions to the previous edition by the Past-President of the Royal College of Physicians, Sir Richard Thompson, and the distinguished endocrinologist, Professor John Wass, upon which portions of this introduction are based.

References

1 Vigersky RA, Fish L, Hogan P, et al. The clinical endocrinology workforce: current status and future projections of supply and demand. *J Clin Endocrinol Metab.* 2014;99:3112–3121.

2 Kalyani RR, Golden SH, Cefalu WT. Diabetes and aging: unique considerations and goals of care. *Diabetes Care.* 2017;40:440-443.

3 Matfin G. Preparing for a growing caseload of endocrine emergencies. 2014. http://www.kevinmd.com/blog/2014/11/preparing-growing-caseload-endocrine-emergencies.html (accessed April 24, 2017).

4 Royal College of Physicians London. Underfunded, underdoctored, overstretched: the NHS in 2016. 2016. www.rcplodon.ac.uk/missionhealth (accessed April 24 2017).

5 Welcher CM, Kirk LM, Hawkins RE. Alternative pathways to Board Recertification. To what end? *JAMA.* 2017;317:2279–2280.

6 Patel M. Changes to postgraduate medical education in the 21st century. *Clin Med.* 2016;16:311–314.

7 OECD. Health workforce policies in OECD countries: right jobs, right skills, right places. 2016. http://dx.doi.org/10.1787/9789264239517-en (accessed May 2017).

8 Anonymous. Inpatient care and diabetes: putting poor glycaemic control to bed. *Lancet Diabetes and Endocrinology* 2017;5:770.

9 Health and Social Care Information Centre. *National Diabetes Inpatient audit (NaDIA), Open Data 2016,* 2017. www.digital.nhs.uk/pubs/nadia2016

10 National Institute for Health and Care Excellence. *Diabetic Foot Problems: Prevention and Management. NICE Guideline NG19,* 2016. https://www.nice.org.uk/guidance/ng19 (accessed April 24, 2017).

11 Verbalis JG, Greenberg A, Burst V, et al. Diagnosing and treating the syndrome of inappropriate antidiuretic hormone secretion. *Am J Med.* 2016;129:537.e9–537.e23.

12 Ball S, Barth J, Levy M, the Society for Endocrinology Clinical Committee. Emergency management of severe symptomatic hyponatraemia in adult patients (2016). DOI: 10.1530/EC-16-0058/

13 *Report of the Mid Staffordshire NHS Foundation Trust Public Enquiry chaired by Robert Francis QC,* London, Stationery Office; 2013.

14 Black N. Can England's NHS survive? *N Eng J Med.* 2013;369:1–3.

15 Future Hospital Commission. *Caring for Medical Patients.* London: Royal College of Physicians; 2013.

16 Nasca TJ, Philibert I, Brigham T. The next GME Accreditation system – rationale and benefits. *NEJM.* 2012;366:1051–1056.

17 General Medical Council. Generic professional capabilities framework. 2017. http://www.gmc-uk.org/Generic_professional_capabilities_framework_0517.pdf_70417127.pdf (accessed June 2017).

18 Wachter RM, Goldman, L. Zero to 50,000 — The 20th Anniversary of the Hospitalist. *N Eng J Med.* 2016;375: 1009–1011.

19 Wachter review. *Using Information Technology to Improve the NHS.* 2016. https://www.england.nhs.uk/digital technology/info-revolution/wachter-review (accessed 24th April 2017).

20 Martin G, Kinross J, Hankin C. Effective cybersecurity is fundamental to patient safety. *BMJ.* 2017;357:j2375.

1

Early Management of Acute Medical Emergencies

Paul J. Frost and Matt P. Wise

Key Points

- Acute medical emergencies are those illnesses that can cause organ failures and death within minutes to hours of their presentation.
- These illnesses present with little warning, and affected patients are usually distressed, frightened, and often uncooperative.
- These episodes can occur in any hospital location, and the ability of available staff to deal with them may vary considerably. Given these circumstances, it is unsurprising that management errors occur, resulting in failures of care and poor outcomes.

- Effective, early management of acute medical emergencies requires prompt recognition, immediate correction of life-threatening physiological abnormalities, the methodical application of the Airway, Breathing, Circulation, Disability, and Exposure (ABCDE) approach, and rapid diagnosis and treatment of the underlying condition.
- Endocrine and metabolic disorders are common causes of acute medical emergencies.

Introduction

Acute medical emergencies are those illnesses that can cause organ failures and death within minutes to hours of their presentation. These illnesses may present with little warning, and affected patients are usually distressed, frightened, and often uncooperative. These episodes can occur in any hospital location, and the ability of available staff to deal with them may vary considerably. Given these circumstances, it is unsurprising that management errors can occur, resulting in failures of care and poor outcomes (1). Effective, early management of acute medical emergencies requires

prompt recognition, immediate correction of life-threatening physiological abnormalities and rapid diagnosis and treatment of the underlying condition. Endocrine and metabolic disorders are common causes of acute medical emergencies.

Recognition of Medical Emergencies

Medical emergencies are usually recognized by clinical signs of severe cardiorespiratory or neurological insufficiency. In a large, multinational, observational study, serious physiological deterioration, most frequently

---

Table 1-1 Medical emergency: possible clinical signs

Skin: mottled; sweaty: cyanosis; warm and vasodilated or cold peripheries.

Neurological: agitation; confusion; depressed level of consciousness; seizures; localizing signs.

Respiratory: stridor; grunting; drooling; use of accessory muscles; tracheal tug; intercostal in-drawing; nasal flaring; respiratory rate (RR) >25 breaths/min. or <8 breaths/min.; audible wheeze or silent chest.

Cardiovascular: capillary refill time >2 seconds; pulse >150 beats/min. or <50 beats/min.; low volume pulse; absent peripheral pulses; systolic blood pressure <90 mmHg; mean arterial pressure (MAP) <70 mmHg; postural hypotension; urine output <0.5 ml/kg/hour or anuria.

hypotension and a fall in the Glasgow Coma Scale (GCS) score, was documented in 60% of patients prior to cardiac arrest, death, or intensive care unit (ICU) admission (2). Although the underlying diagnosis may initially be elusive, the clinical signs that accompany a medical emergency are readily identified, and include: tachycardia or bradycardia; hypotension; cold peripheries; oliguria; cyanosis; tachypnea or bradypnea; seizures; agitation; confusion; and coma (Table 1-1). These signs are usually detected by simple, bedside observations, such as pulse, blood pressure, respiratory rate, peripheral oxygen saturations, temperature, and conscious level. In the UK, these bedside observations have been used to develop a National Early Warning Score (NEWS). NEWS is derived by aggregating points assigned to increasing deviations from the normal range, in each observation (3). This score is linked to a graded response strategy, such that acutely ill patients who score highly are immediately reviewed by an appropriately trained, rapid-response-team (3). Although intuitively sensible, convincing evidence that rapid response systems like NEWS are effective in preventing adverse outcomes, such as death or intensive care admission is currently lacking (4–6). Deficiencies in rapid response systems include

the facts that observations may not be reliably taken and scores miscalculated (7,8). Moreover, the sensitivity and specificity of the NEWS as a test for acute illness will be affected by patient-specific factors such as age, drug therapy, and comorbidity. For example, a severe gastrointestinal bleed may not cause a high NEWS in a previously hypertensive patient, treated with beta blockers because blood pressure and pulse rate may remain in the "normal range" despite significant hypovolemia. Recognition of the emergency nature of these sorts of presentations remains dependent on a high degree of clinical suspicion informed by clinical experience. Nonetheless, over recent years rapid response-systems have been adopted by hospitals worldwide as the default mechanism for the recognition and immediate management of deteriorating patients and medical emergencies (9). Recently, the Third International Consensus Definitions for Sepsis Taskforce have redefined sepsis as "life-threatening organ dysfunction due to a dysregulated host response to infection." The taskforce recommended the quick-Sepsis-related Organ Failure Assessment (qSOFA) as a bedside prompt to identify patients with suspected infection who may have sepsis or septic shock (10). The qSOFA assigns one point for an altered mental status (GCS <15), a respiratory rate of ≥22 breaths per minute, and a systolic blood pressure of ≤100 mmHg. The score ranges from 0–3 points, and in a large, retrospective analysis of electronic health record encounters a qSOFA of ≥2 was associated with a greater risk of death or prolonged intensive care unit stay (11). Despite the taskforce's recommendation, early evidence suggests that qSOFA may be inferior to the NEWS as a means of identifying patients at risk of deterioration (12).

Once alerted to a medical emergency, the challenge to the responsible clinician is to make the diagnosis while providing supportive care, so that effective treatment can be administered. While most clinicians are familiar with the Airway, Breathing, and Circulation (ABC) approach, these activities may best be coordinated using an Airway,

Breathing, Circulation, Disability, and Exposure (ABCDE) approach. Application of this approach at the bedside requires that the attending clinician organizes available staff into an effective team. This leadership role is largely understated in widely publicized resuscitation guidelines and yet is crucial to achieving good outcomes. Crisis resource management (CRM) has been defined as: "the ability to translate the knowledge of what needs to be done into effective treatment activity in the complex and real world of medical treatment" (13). It is important that clinicians managing medical emergencies are familiar with CRM principles and adhere to them whenever possible.

The ABCDE Approach

It is axiomatic that outcomes from medical emergencies are improved by early diagnosis and treatment. For example, prompt reperfusion can reduce infarct size and prolong life in myocardial infarction and stroke, while early, effective antibiotics improve survival in septic shock (14–16). However, before a diagnosis is reached, these patients may die from severe physiological disturbances, such as hypoxemia and shock (17). The ABCDE approach can be seen as a mechanism to preserve life, while a diagnosis is sought so that definitive treatment can be administered (18). The process starts at the bedside with a preliminary assessment of the patient's general condition; this swift assessment focuses on the presence of clinical signs associated with life-threatening cardiorespiratory and/or neurological insufficiency (Table 1-1).

Much of this preliminary assessment can be completed by observation of the patient, inspection of the clinical observation charts, and brief discussion with the bedside nurse. At the conclusion of this assessment, it may be obvious that the patient is moribund or "peri-arrest" and that the "cardiac arrest" or the "rapid-response team" should be called. In the UK, the National Health Service (NHS) Institute for Innovation and Improvement has recommended the situation, background,

Table 1-2 Situation, background, assessment, and recommendation (SBAR) communication tool

---

Situation: Identify yourself (name, role, location); person you are speaking to and patient. State reason for call and urgency:

Example: My name is Dr Frost, I am the House officer (Resident) on Ward 6. Are you the on-call critical care clinician?
I am with Mrs Smith, a 65-year-old lady, who is in extremis with oxygen saturations of 78%.

Background: Briefly relate history – date of admission, diagnosis and current management:

Example: Mrs Smith is a previously well lady who was admitted 1 week ago, following a stroke, for which she is undergoing rehabilitation.

Assessment: State your working diagnosis:

Example: I think Mrs Smith has respiratory failure secondary to a severe hospital-acquired-pneumonia.

Recommendation: State the request:

Example: I think Mrs Smith is likely to need endotracheal intubation and mechanical ventilation. Please attend the ward immediately.

---

assessment, and recommendation (SBAR) method for referring acutely ill patients (Table 1-2) (19). Regardless of the hospital system in place, once an emergency is recognized, assistance should be requested immediately. It is rarely the case that these situations can be effectively managed by a single practitioner. At this juncture, the team (or individual clinician awaiting the arrival of assistance) should establish basic monitoring (e.g., electrocardiography [ECG], pulse oximetry, and blood pressure), and calmly and methodically work through the ABCDE approach, correcting life-threatening physiological disturbances as they are discovered. Other measures, such as point-of-care blood glucose testing, should also be performed as clinically indicated.

Airway Assessment and Management

Upper airway obstruction (UAO) must be diagnosed and treated quickly; complete obstruction will lead to cardiac arrest within minutes, while partial obstruction can impair ventilation and cause hypoxemia. UAO may be recognized by impaired or absent speech; stridor; grunting; drooling; severe respiratory distress; paradoxical chest wall movement ("see-saw" movements); prominent neck veins; facial swelling, and absent breath sounds. In general terms, the aim of management is to provide a secure, patent airway but specific therapy will be determined by the underlying cause.

When the diagnosis is obvious, interventions to clear and support the airway can proceed immediately. For example, oral-pharyngeal inspection and removal of an easily accessible foreign body or application of simple, airway-opening-manoeuvres, such as a chin-lift or jaw-thrust, for coma. When the diagnosis is unclear, manipulation of the airway and insertion of airway adjuncts should be avoided as these interventions may precipitate complete UAO, for example, in the setting of epiglottitis. Generally, if conscious, patients with UAO should be allowed to assume the position that they find most comfortable to breathe in. Forcing these patients into the recovery or supine position can precipitate cardiac arrest. All patients with UAO should be assessed by an anaesthetist as endotracheal intubation is frequently required to definitively secure the airway. Occasionally the airway can only be secured by a surgical technique such as cricothyroidotomy or tracheostomy. Computed tomography (CT) of the neck and chest and/or flexible bronchoscopy may be required for diagnosis of the underlying cause of the UAO, but for safety, the airway should be secured prior to these investigations being undertaken.

Breathing Assessment and Management

Once the airway is deemed to be safe or secured, then breathing should be assessed for signs of respiratory insufficiency (Table 1-1). Auscultation is important both diagnostically and as a means to assess response to treatment; bronchial breath sounds may help confirm the diagnosis of pneumonia, while the detection of breath sounds, following drainage of a pneumothorax suggests that the lung has re-inflated.

Peripheral oxygen saturations should be routinely measured in all patients with respiratory distress and hypoxemia rapidly corrected. A wide variety of oxygen delivery devices are available, but in the setting of acute illness the most appropriate device to use is a non-rebreathing face mask with reservoir and one-way valve. When connected to wall oxygen at a flow rate of 15 L/minute, this device may provide an inspired oxygen concentration (FiO2) of up to 90%. High-flow nasal oxygen therapy is increasingly being used postoperatively and in both ward-based and critical care areas. A number of commercial devices are available and provide high gas flow rates (up to 60 L/minute) of blended gas up to 100% oxygen (20). Gases are warmed and humidified increasing patient comfort and compliance, and the high flow rates generate a small degree of continuous positive airway pressure (CPAP). Expert consensus guidance suggests that in the setting of critical illness, oxygen saturation targets should generally be 94–98% (21). In some patients with chronic obstructive pulmonary disease (COPD) and carbon dioxide retention, supplemental oxygen therapy is associated with worsening hypercapnia and respiratory failure (22). In these patients, inspired oxygen should be titrated to achieve saturations of 88–92%, and non-invasive ventilation (NIV) considered (23).

Mechanical ventilation should be considered for those patients with reversible disease and persistent failure of oxygenation and/or ventilation (i.e., carbon dioxide clearance). NIV is particularly indicated in patients with COPD and respiratory acidosis (pH 7.25–7.35) and hypercapnic respiratory failure secondary to chest wall deformity or neuromuscular disease. It is important to recognize when a patient is failing on NIV and requires intubation and invasive mechanical ventilation, as delayed intubation in this setting is associated with worse outcomes (24,25). Generally, invasive ventilation (i.e., tracheal intubation), is indicated in those patients with respiratory failure and impaired consciousness or copious pulmonary secretions (23).

Circulatory Assessment and Management

Once appropriate steps have been taken to address any breathing difficulties, attention should be directed to the assessment and management of circulatory insufficiency (Table 1-1). Acute or chronic fluid loss is usually followed by peripheral vasoconstriction and a compensatory tachycardia in order to preserve perfusion of vital organs. There is a wide spectrum in the ability of patients to compensate for fluid loss; unsurprisingly, young, fit patients can compensate for greater fluid losses than older patients, particularly those with significant cardiovascular comorbidity. Typically, after 30–40% of circulating volume has been lost, decompensation occurs, manifested by marked hypotension and multi-organ dysfunction, characteristic of shock (17). Treatment of shock requires the restoration of an effective circulating blood volume to reverse decompensation and restore organ perfusion. This process depends on the diagnosis of the underlying condition so that specific therapies can be administered. A useful aide-memoire for the differential diagnosis of shock is to classify this condition into four groups according to the main mechanism of decompensation: (a) hypovolemia; (b) cardiogenic; (c) obstructive (e.g., pulmonary embolism, cardiac tamponade); or (d) distributive (e.g., sepsis, anaphylaxis) (17). In the setting of infection, patients with septic shock can be clinically identified by a vasopressor requirement to maintain a mean arterial pressure of 65 mmHg or greater and serum lactate level greater than 2 mmol/L in the absence of hypovolemia (10).

As always, accurate history is the most important determinant of the diagnosis, physical examination, aside from confirming the presence of a shock state, may be less rewarding; particularly in advanced disease. Patients with shock require urgent resuscitation, a useful mnemonic to describe the important components is the **VIP** rule: **v**entilate (oxygen administration), **i**nfuse (fluid resuscitation), and **p**ump (administration of vasoactive agents) (17). Generally, patients with shock require intravenous (IV) fluid resuscitation; a caveat to this are those patients with pulmonary oedema as gas exchange may deteriorate in these individuals. If there is diagnostic uncertainty, a fluid challenge can be helpful in identifying those patients who are likely to be fluid-responsive. A fluid challenge can be delivered by administering 250 ml of IV fluid over 2 minutes; hypovolemic patients will show an improvement in their blood pressure and pulse rate (26).

There has been considerable debate in the literature as to the optimal resuscitation fluid – over the years, a variety of fluids, including crystalloids, colloids, and human albumin solutions, have been used and a number of problems identified. Current evidence would seem to support the use of balanced electrolyte solutions, such as Ringer's lactate or Hartmann's solution as appropriate first line resuscitation fluids. Regardless of the type of resuscitation fluid selected, frequent patient reassessment against relevant clinical end-points such as peripheral perfusion, pulse, blood pressure and urine output is essential so that therapy can be titrated and inadvertent fluid and electrolyte overload can be averted (27). Hyperlactatemia (>1.5 mmol/L) is also typically present in acute circulatory failure and can be monitored (17). Vasoactive drugs may be necessary if blood pressure and cardiac output remain low, these patients need to be transferred to the ICU for further management.

Disability Assessment and Management

Neurological dysfunction is frequently implicated in medical emergencies and is due either to primary neurological disease or arises as a consequence of non-neurological illnesses. For example, coma may arise as a consequence of an intracerebral hemorrhage, severe hypoglycemia, severe hyponatremia, or severe circulatory shock. Disability refers to emergency neurological assessment and management and starts with a basic assessment of level of consciousness. AVPU and the GCS are two systems that standardize the assessment of consciousness. AVPU is simple to remember and apply: A = the patient is alert; V = the patient only responds to voice; P = the patient only responds to pain; and U = the patient is unresponsive. The Glasgow Coma Scale provides a more detailed description of consciousness in terms of eye opening, verbal response, and motor response and can be summarized using an aggregate numerical score ranging from 3, deeply unconscious, to 15, alert and cooperative. An individual patient is best described using the Glasgow Coma Scale rather than the score, which was originally designed for audit and research purposes (28). On the Glasgow Coma Scale, a patient is arbitrarily defined as being in a coma if they can perform no better than eye opening to pain (E2), incomprehensible sounds (V2), and withdraw to a painful stimulus (M4). Generally, if the GCS score is <8/15, or if the patient only responds to pain, or is unresponsive on the AVPU scale, the ability of the patient to maintain a patent airway might be impaired. This can cause partial airway obstruction, reduced ventilation, and an increased vulnerability to pulmonary aspiration. Adherence to the ABCDE approach should ensure that the airway is secured in these patients (see section on Airway above). There is a wide differential diagnosis for coma and its evaluation requires a comprehensive history, general physical examination, and neurological assessment (Table 1-3).

Exposure

The ABCDE approach concludes with E = exposure, which is a prompt to complete a full physical examination. At this stage, life-threatening abnormalities have been addressed and the patient is better able to tolerate and cooperate with the demands of the examination.

Table 1-3 Causes of coma; aide-memoire IF SOMNOLENT

IF SOMNOLENT
Infection
Fits
Stroke
Overdose: alcohol, tri-cyclic antidepressants, benzodiazepines, etc.
Metabolic: uremia, hepatic encephalopathy, hyponatremia, hypernatremia
Neoplasm: primary or secondary brain tumors
Oxygen deficiency: post-cardiac arrest, near drowning
Low temperature; low blood pressure
Endocrine: hypoglycemia, hyperglycemia, hypopituitarism, hypothyroidism, hypercalcemia, Addison's disease
Narcotics
Trauma

Definitive Diagnosis and Treatment

For medical emergencies, the traditional path to diagnosis (i.e., history, physical examination and investigation) is modified and integrated with the ABCDE approach. Diagnostic synthesis and the ABCDE approach should be viewed as complementary and simultaneous processes (Figure 1-1).

History

The patient should not be needlessly exhausted by detailed interrogation; much of the relevant history can be gleaned from medical records, nursing staff, or relatives. However, it is important to enquire as to the presence and characteristics of any pain, not only is this a cardinal diagnostic symptom but it will need to be relieved. It is likely that clinicians will use both non-analytical (pattern recognition) and analytical methods in formulating a diagnosis. This process has been termed iterative diagnosis and is prone to well-recognized cognitive errors

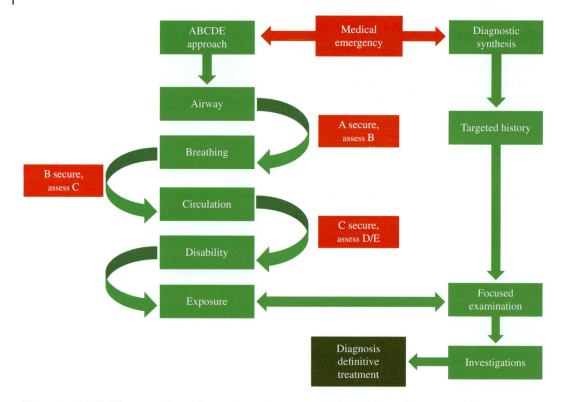

Figure 1-1 The ABCDE approach and diagnostic synthesis are complementary and simultaneous processes.

(29). Diagnostic errors usually arise because of over-reliance on pattern recognition and intuition rather than analytical reasoning. Diagnostic uncertainty should be managed by mental reversion to a highly analytical approach, rigorously analyzing available data against diagnostic hypotheses. In the setting of severe shock, the aide-memoire (i.e., hypovolemia; cardiogenic; obstructive; or distributive) provides the full range of diagnostic possibilities against which available clinical data can be analyzed.

Physical Examination

Physical examination is completed at the conclusion of the ABCDE approach, and is focused on those systems which are likely to be diagnostically helpful. For example, a comprehensive abdominal examination is essential in a patient with peritonitis and shock but not immediately required in a patient with an acute myocardial infarction. The physical examination should be modified to minimize patient exertion and the deleterious effects of re-positioning. It is important to note that breathing difficulties and hypoxemia are exacerbated by movement from the semi-recumbent to supine position, particularly in obese patients (30).

Investigations

These are guided by diagnostic impressions but basic blood tests such as arterial or venous blood gases, complete (full) blood counts, blood urea nitrogen (BUN) or urea, electrolytes, blood glucose, and blood cultures are usually helpful.

Illness severity can be assessed with a blood lactate; one prospective study reported an 83% mortality in patients with a blood lactate of >5 mmol/L (31); while bedside investigations such as ECG, plain radiology, ultrasound, and echocardiography may be diagnostic.

It may be necessary to transfer patients for other tests such as CT. In these circumstances patients should be stabilized (as much as possible), and the transfers undertaken by suitably trained personnel. It is important to consider the risks and benefits of all investigations, as over-investigation may delay definitive treatment.

Treatment

Generally medical emergencies will be managed in an emergency department, acute medical unit (AMU) or equivalent, as well as more advanced step-up facilities such as high dependency unit (HDU), or ICU. Many therapies, such as blood and blood products, drugs (e.g., antimicrobials; antiplatelet agents, analgesics, diuretics), and, of course, oxygen and IV fluid, should be given at the bedside prior to transfer to HDU or ICU if required. International guidelines have recommended the administration of broad-spectrum antibiotics within one hour of recognizing sepsis or septic shock (32). Definitive management of this condition may require surgical, source control (e.g., drainage of an abscess or resection of ischemic bowel).

ICU admission is indicated for patients who require organ support, most commonly mechanical ventilation and close nursing observation. The decision to admit a patient to the ICU is informed primarily by clinical factors, such the potential reversibility of the illness, and the wishes of the patient or their surrogates. Old age in itself is not a reason to refuse ICU admission but old age undoubtedly reduces physiological reserve and is more likely to be accompanied by serious comorbidity. Severity of illness scoring systems such as the acute physiology and chronic health evaluation II (APACHE II) and the simplified acute physiology score (SAPS) are used to estimate hospital mortality for groups of patients and cannot be used to predict individual outcomes. Moreover, these systems do not provide any information about longer-term survival, for example, 6–12 months following critical illness, or quality of life or functional status. Frailty is a multifaceted syndrome characterized by a demise in physical and cognitive reserves and increasing vulnerability (33). Although yet to be evaluated in critically ill patients, it has been suggested that clinical measures of frailty, may help identify those elderly patients who would most benefit from ICU admission (34).

Medical emergencies should not be confused with the natural process of dying, the distinction is not always straightforward, but where there is clear evidence of terminal illness, such as advanced cancer, the treatment imperatives are comfort and dignity not aggressive resuscitation.

Conclusions

Acute medical emergencies can arise at any time and effective early management depends on prompt recognition, good team work, and the methodical application of the ABCDE approach.

References

1 National Confidential Enquiry into Patient Outcome and Death. An acute problem? 2005. www.ncepod.org.uk/2005report/index.html (accessed December 1, 2013).
2 Kause J, Smith G, Prytherch D, et al. A comparison of antecedents to cardiac arrests, deaths and emergency intensive care admissions in Australia, New Zealand and the United Kingdom – the ACADEMIA study. *Resuscitation*. 2004; 62:275–282.
3 Royal College of Physicians. National early warning score (NEWS). www.rcplondon.ac.uk/resources/national-early-warning-score-news(accessed December 1, 2013).

4 McGaughey J, Alderdice F, Fowler R, Kapila A, Mayhew A, Moutray M. Outreach and Early Warning Systems (EWS) for the prevention of intensive care admission and death of critically ill adult patients on general hospital wards. *Cochrane Database Syst Rev*. 2007;18(3):CD005529.

5 Chan PS, Jain R, Nallmothu BK, Berg RA, Sasson C. Rapid response teams: a systematic review and meta-analysis. *Arch Intern Med*. 2010;170(1):18–26.

6 McNeill G, Bryden D. Resuscitation: do either early warning systems or emergency response teams improve hospital patient survival? A systematic review. *Resuscitation*. 2013;84(12):1652–1667.

7 Gordon CF, Beckett DJ. Significant deficiencies in the overnight use of a Standardised Early Warning Scoring system in a teaching hospital. *Scott Med J*. 2011;56:15–18.

8 Smith T, Den Hartog D, Moerman T, Patka P, Van Lieshout EM, Schep NW. Accuracy of an expanded early warning score for patients in general and trauma surgery wards. *Br J Surg*. 2012;99:192–197.

9 Litvak E, Pronovost PJ. Rethinking rapid response teams. *JAMA*. 2010;304(12):1375–1376.

10 Singer M, Deutschman CS, Seymour CW, et al. The Third International Consensus Definitions for Sepsis and Septic Shock (Sepsis-3). *JAMA*. 2016;315(8):801–810. doi: 10.1001/jama.2016.0287.

11 Seymour CW, Liu VX, Iwashyna TJ, et al. Assessment of clinical criteria for sepsis: For the Third International Consensus Definition for Sepsis and Septic Shock (Sepsis-3). *JAMA*. 2016;315(8):762–764. doi: 10.1001/jama.2016.0288. Erratum in: *JAMA*. 2016;315(20):2237.

12 Churpek MM, Snyder A, Han X, et al. Quick sepsis-related organ failure assessment, systemic inflammatory response syndrome, and early warning scores for detecting clinical deterioration in infected patients outside the intensive care unit. *Am J Respir Crit Care Med*.

2017;195(7):906–911. doi: 10.1164/rccm. 201604-0854OC.

13 Rall M, Gaba D. Human performance and patient safety. In: Miller R, ed. *Miller's Anesthesia*. 6th ed. Philadelphia, PA: Elsevier Churchill Livingstone; 2005: 3021–3072.

14 Vemulapalli S, Zhou Y, Gutberlet M, et al. Importance of total ischemic time and pre-procedural infarct-related artery blood flow in predicting infarct size in patients with anterior wall myocardial infarction (from the CRISP-AMI Trial). *Am J Cardiol*. 2013112(7):911–917.

15 Wardlaw JM, Murray V, Berge E, Del Zoppo GJ. Thrombolysis for acute ischaemic stroke. *Cochrane Database Syst Rev*. 2009;(4):CD000213.

16 Kumar A, Roberts D, Wood KE, et al. Duration of hypotension before initiation of effective antimicrobial therapy is the critical determinant of survival in human septic shock. *Crit Care Med*. 2006;34: 1589–1596.

17 Vincent J-L, De Backer D. Circulatory shock. *N Engl J Med*. 2013;369:1726–1734.

18 Frost PJ, Wise MP. Early management of acutely ill ward patients. *BMJ*. 2012;345: e5677.

19 NHS Institute for Innovation and Improvement. SBAR: Situation, background, assessment, recommendation. http://www.institute.nhs.uk/qualityandser viceimprovementtools/qualityandservice improvementtools/sbar-situation-background-assessment-recommen dation.html (accessed December 1 2013).

20 Nishimura N. High-flow nasal cannula oxygen therapy in adults: physiological benefits, indication, clinical benefits, and adverse effects. *Respiratory Care*. 2016; 61(4):529–541.

21 O'Driscoll BR, Howard LS, Davison AG; British Thoracic Society. BTS guideline for emergency oxygen use in adult patients. *Thorax*. 2008;63,Suppl 6:vii–68.

22 Abdo WF. Heunks LMA. Oxygen-induced hypercapnia in COPD: myths and facts. *Crit Care*. 2012;16(5):323.

23 British Thoracic Society Standards of Care Committee. Non-invasive ventilation in acute respiratory failure. *Thorax*. 2002; 57(3):192–211.

24 Gristina, G.R., Antonelli, M., Conti, G., GiVi-TI (Italian Group for the Evaluation of Interventions in Intensive Care Medicine), et al. Noninvasive versus invasive ventilation for acute respiratory failure in patients with hematologic malignancies: a 5-year multicenter observational survey. *Crit Care Med*. 2011;39(10):2232–2239. doi:10.1097/CCM.0b013e3182227a27.

25 Molina R, Bernal T, Borges M, et al. EMEHU study investigators: ventilatory support in critically ill hematology patients with respiratory failure. *Crit Care*. 2012;16(4):R133. doi: 10.1186/cc11438.

26 Cecconi M, Parsons AK, Rhodes A. What is a fluid challenge? *Curr Opin Crit Care*. 2011;17(3):290–295.

27 Frost P. Intravenous fluid therapy in adult inpatients. *BMJ*. 2015;350:g7620 doi: 10.1136/bmj.g7620 T.

28 Barlow P. A practical review of the Glasgow Coma Scale and Score. *Surgeon*. 2012;10(2):114–119.

29 Norman G, Barraclough K, Dolovich L, Price D. Iterative diagnosis. *BMJ*. 2009;339:b3490. doi: 10.1136/bmj.b3490.

30 Altermatt FR, Muñoz HR, Delfino AE, Cortínez LI. Pre-oxygenation in the obese patient: effects of position on tolerance to apnea. *Br J Anaesth*. 2005;95(5):706–709.

31 Stacpoole PW, Wright EC, Baumgartner TG, et al. Natural history and course of acquired lactic acidosis in adults. DCA-Lactic Acidosis Study Group. *Am J Med*. 1994;97(1):47–54.

32 Dellinger RP, Levy MM, Rhodes A, et al., Surviving Sepsis Campaign Guidelines Committee including The Pediatric Subgroup. Surviving Sepsis Campaign: international guidelines for management of severe sepsis and septic shock, 2012. *Intensive Care Med*. 2013;39(2):165–228.

33 Rockwood K, Song X, MacKnight C, et al. A global clinical measure of fitness and frailty in elderly people. *CMAJ*. 2005; 173(5):489–495.

34 McDermid RC, Stelfox HT, Bagshaw SM. Frailty in the critically ill: a novel concept. *Crit Care*. 2011;15(1):301.

Part II

General Endocrine and Metabolic Aspects of Acute and Critical Illness

Introduction

Endocrine Testing and Responses in Acute and Critical Illness

David B. Sacks

Key Points

- The clinical laboratory has an integral role in the management of patients with acute and critical illness.
- This group of patients has diverse presentations, multi-organ dysfunction is frequent and some of the life-threatening pathophysiologic disruptions may be occult. The laboratory is necessary to detect many of these conditions and is essential for both monitoring responses to treatment and detecting or avoiding deleterious consequences of therapy.
- Critically ill patients are prone to metabolic derangements and alterations to endocrine systems that are unique. Several factors contribute to these changes, including: (a) the stress of acute illness may augment (e.g., hypothalamic-pituitary-adrenal) or attenuate (e.g., hypothalamic-pituitary-gonadal) the activity of hormone axes; (b) in addition to changes in hormone secretion, hormone metabolism and clearance can be altered by reduced circulation, inflammation, hypoxia or other insults; (c) the normal diurnal variation that occurs with a number of hormones is also disrupted; (d) acute and critically ill patients usually receive numerous therapeutic agents, some of which may alter endocrine homeostasis; (e) during acute and critical illness the amount of binding protein may change considerably, and the direction of the change (increase or decrease) is dependent on the underlying condition(s). In addition, the amount of binding of hormone to carrier protein can be affected by numerous factors.
- Thus, an endocrine evaluation of an acute or critically ill patient requires consideration of numerous elements.

The clinical laboratory has an integral role in the management of patients with acute medical and critical illness. This group of patients has diverse presentations, multi-organ dysfunction is frequent and some of the life-threatening pathophysiologic disruptions may be occult. The laboratory is necessary to detect many of these conditions and is essential for both monitoring responses to treatment and detecting or avoiding deleterious consequences of therapy. For example, during treatment of hyperglycemia with insulin, blood glucose concentrations need to be measured frequently to avoid hypoglycemia and serum potassium must be monitored to prevent hypokalemia, which may occur due to the stimulation of potassium uptake into cells by insulin.

Endocrine and Metabolic Medical Emergencies: A Clinician's Guide, Second Edition. Edited by Glenn Matfin.
© 2018 John Wiley & Sons Ltd. Published 2018 by John Wiley & Sons Ltd.

Critically ill patients are prone to metabolic derangements and alterations to endocrine systems that are unique. Several factors contribute (1). The stress of acute illness may augment (e.g., hypothalamic-pituitary-adrenal) or attenuate (e.g., hypothalamic-pituitary-gonadal) the activity of hormone axes. In addition to changes in hormone secretion, hormone metabolism and clearance can be altered by reduced circulation, inflammation, hypoxia or other insults. The normal diurnal variation that occurs with a number of hormones is also disrupted. Moreover, acute and critically ill patients usually receive numerous therapeutic agents, some of which may alter endocrine homeostasis. Thus, endocrine evaluation of an acutely ill patient requires the consideration of numerous elements.

Another aspect that needs to be contemplated is hormone binding proteins. Several hormones, including thyroid hormones (triiodothyronine [T_3] and thyroxine [T_4]), cortisol and testosterone, are transported in the circulation by carrier proteins. During acute illness, the amount of binding protein may change considerably and the direction of the change (increase or decrease) is dependent on the underlying condition(s). In addition, the binding of hormone to carrier protein may be altered by medication, renal failure, pH change, or other conditions common to critical illness. It is generally believed that only the free hormone is biologically active. Importantly, the free hormone comprises a small fraction (e.g. $\sim$0.1% and 5% for T_3 and cortisol, respectively) of the total circulating hormone. Most assays measure the total hormone concentration, which may not correlate with the biologically active moiety, especially when amounts or binding affinities of carrier proteins are altered. Attempts to overcome this limitation with equations to calculate the free hormone have met with limited success. Several techniques, including equilibrium dialysis and ultrafiltration, have been used to separate free from bound hormone, followed by measurement of the free fraction. These approaches require rigorous attention to detail, as temperature,

pH, leakage or adsorption can substantially influence the results. The overwhelming majority of endocrine analyses are performed using antibodies (termed immunoassays). These assays frequently have inadequate sensitivity to accurately quantify the low concentrations of free hormone. Moreover, immunoassays suffer from inaccuracy, a lack of specificity, and often are not standardized, so the results can vary widely among different laboratories and different instruments. The implementation in clinical laboratories of mass spectrometry has the potential to address many of these problems. A considerable advantage of mass spectrometry is the exquisite sensitivity which enables measurement of very low concentrations of substances, yielding accurate results for both total and free hormones. Nevertheless, progress to standardize mass spectrometry analyses remains slow and considerable differences are found among laboratories.

While a lack of standardization limits most hormone assays, this problem has essentially been resolved for hemoglobin A1c (HbA1c), a ubiquitous test in patients with diabetes. Although early methods to measure HbA1c were not standardized, the establishment in 1995 of the NGSP (previously known as the National Glycohemoglobin Standardization Program) has resulted in significantly reduced variability among methods and laboratories (2). This improvement led to the adoption over the last few years of HbA1c as a criterion for diagnosis of diabetes. HbA1c, which reflects long-term blood glucose concentration, is not altered by stress, food ingestion, diurnal variation or other factors that modulate glucose in critically ill patients (3). Nevertheless, it may be influenced by certain conditions in the critically ill, e.g., blood loss, hemolysis, or blood transfusion.

Until recently, HbA1c was reported throughout the world as a percentage of total hemoglobin. The development by the International Federation of Clinical Chemistry (IFCC) of a reference method employing mass spectrometry yields values lower than NGSP standardized results by 1.5–2.0% HbA1c (4). To avoid confusion, a decision was reached to report IFCC values in Système International (SI) units as mmol HbA1c per mol Hb. For example, HbA1c of 6.5 and 7% correspond to 48 and 53 mmol/mol, respectively. A linear equation is required to convert between the two sets of units (5) (see http://www.ngsp.orgs/convert1.asp for a conversion table and convenient calculator). Several countries, predominantly in Europe, have elected to report HbA1c exclusively in SI units (5). Many journals now require that both sets of HbA1c units be used in publications.

Measuring patient samples at the bedside (termed point-of-care [POC]), usually performed on a blood or urine sample using a small hand-held device, has several appealing features. Advantages include eliminating transport of the sample to the central laboratory, no or minimal sample processing (analysis is usually conducted with whole blood, obviating the need for centrifugation), simple analytic process, minimal sample requirement (e.g. only a drop of blood), and very rapid availability of results (1–2 min). By contrast, POC test results are generally less accurate than those obtained from laboratory analyzers, usually cost substantially more and, in general, are more prone to interference from drugs and other substances. While several different analytes can be measured with POC devices, glucose is by far the most common substance measured in patients' blood at the bedside.

A highly contentious subject is the use of POC glucose meters in critically ill patients. Several published studies document increased mortality in hospitalized patients who have hyperglycemia or hypoglycemia. Compelling evidence revealed that intensive insulin therapy to maintain blood glucose concentrations at 80–110 mg/dL (4.4–6.1 mmol/L) significantly reduced the morbidity and mortality of patients in a surgical intensive care unit (ICU) (6). This approach, termed "tight glucose control," was rapidly and widely adopted in hospital ICUs. The publication 8 years later of the Normoglycemia in Intensive Care Evaluation-Survival Using Glucose Algorithm Regulation (NICE-SUGAR) trial (7) considerably dampened enthusiasm for tight glucose control protocols. The latter study observed that the intensive-control group had significantly higher mortality than the conventional-control group. Multiple other studies have been performed and these have variably reported that tight glucose control protocols in ICU patients result in better, equivalent or worse outcomes than standard glucose control. Reasons for the discrepancies in the published literature include variations in insulin protocols, patient populations, mortality rates, glucose targets, and parenteral nutrition. The methods and samples used for glucose analysis are likely to contribute substantially (8). The initial study by Van den Berge et al. (6) measured glucose in arterial blood using an accurate arterial blood gas analyzer. Many of the subsequent studies used capillary blood and measured glucose with POC meters (the sample and/or method of analysis is not mentioned in many publications). The different glucose results that are produced by the diverse methods and samples will lead to different insulin doses, with potentially wide variations in the true glucose concentrations among patients.

In the USA, the Food and Drug Administration (FDA) has not approved the use of glucose meters for tight glucose control protocols in ICUs. Glucose meters are considerably less accurate than blood gas or central laboratory analyzers. For many years, the most widely accepted criteria for meter performance were that 95% of the time the result should be ±20% of the "true" glucose value at ≥75 mg/dL (4.2 mmol/L) and ±15 mg/dL (0.83 mmol/L) at glucose concentrations <75 mg/dL (4.2 mmol/L). Guidelines published in 2013 advocate tighter acceptance criteria requiring 95% of results to be within ± 12.5% of the "true" glucose value at ≥100 mg/dL (5.6 mmol/L) and ±12 mg/dL (0.67 mmol/L) at glucose concentrations <100 mg/dL (5.6 mmol/L). Note that the vast majority of published studies that have evaluated glucose meters used the old criteria. In addition, patient factors, especially in critically ill subjects, contribute to inaccurate results with meters. Some glucose meters are affected by pO_2, pH, hypothermia, drugs or hematocrit (9). The reduced tissue perfusion in hypotensive patients creates large differences between glucose concentrations in capillary and arterial blood samples. It is important to be aware that postprandial capillary glucose values are 20–25 mg/dL (1.1–1.4 mmol/L) higher than those in venous blood.

As mentioned above, critically ill patients pose multiple challenges for laboratory analysis. These range from alteration of circulating concentrations of hormones and electrolytes to interferences in the assays. The myriad underlying conditions can exert diverse effects on hormone secretion, elimination, and function. Thus, the "normal" concentration of many hormones in acutely ill patients is different to those in other patient populations. Interference in laboratory analysis is also common in critical illness. For example, parenteral nutrition can markedly increase serum lipids, which can artefactually alter several measurement procedures. The severe nature of the condition often requires frequent and rapid modifications of therapy. The need for virtually immediate availability of laboratory results (short turnaround time) creates problems. POC testing is a solution that provides rapid results, but the compromise is often considerably reduced accuracy.

Notwithstanding these issues, advances in technology are likely to alleviate or even resolve many of these concerns in the future. A number of approaches can reduce turnaround time for critically ill patients. Some can be adopted now, e.g., using whole blood in the central laboratory to measure glucose electrolytes and creatinine, thereby shortening turnaround time to minutes (analogous to current blood gas analysis).

Alternatively, small, tabletop analyzers can be set up in ICUs and operating rooms with assays performed by trained medical technologists. Improvements in indwelling devices with continuous – and accurate – measurement of glucose and electrolytes have the promise to substantially improve tight glucose control protocols. Considerable effort is being invested in developing closed-loop systems with automated, accurate continuous blood measurement and computer-controlled insulin delivery. The successful development of such a system should improve tight glucose control in ICUs. Current mass spectrometers are expensive, labor-intensive, require considerable technical expertise to operate and have limited throughput. Therefore, they are predominantly confined to large-scale reference laboratories and university-based medical centers. In the future, user-friendly, relatively inexpensive, high-throughput, automated mass spectrometers are likely to become available and be widely adopted by clinical laboratories. In addition, analysis by mass spectrometry of panels of multiple different steroids for endocrine evaluation using only a few microliters of blood should become widespread. In the longer term, the introduction into the clinical laboratory of metabolomics, while challenging in many respects, may yield considerable insight into both our comprehension and management of acutely ill patients.

Acknowledgments

Work in the author's laboratory is funded by the Intramural Research Program of the National Institutes of Health.

References

1 Hassan-Smith Z, Cooper MS. Overview of the endocrine response to critical illness: how to measure it and when to treat. *Best Pract Res Clin Endocrinol Metab.* 2011;25:705–717.

2 Little RR, Rohlfing CL, Sacks DB. Status of hemoglobin A1c measurement and goals for improvement: from chaos to order for improving diabetes care. *Clin Chem.* 2011;57:205–214.

3 Sacks DB. A1C versus glucose testing: a comparison. *Diabetes Care.* 2011;34:518–523.

4 Hoelzel W, Weykamp C, Jeppsson JO, et al. IFCC reference system for measurement of hemoglobin A1c in human blood and the national standardization schemes in the United States, Japan, and Sweden: a method-comparison study. *Clin Chem.* 2004;50:166–174.

5 Sacks DB. Measurement of hemoglobin A(1c): a new twist on the path to harmony. *Diabetes Care.* 2012;35:2674–2680.

6 van den Berghe G, Wouters P, Weekers F, Verwaest C, Bruyninckx F, Schetz M, et al. Intensive insulin therapy in the critically ill patients. *N Engl J Med.* 2001;345:1359–1367.

7 Finfer S, Chittock DR, Su SY, Blair D, Foster D, Dhingra V, et al. Intensive versus conventional glucose control in critically ill patients. *N Engl J Med.* 2009;360:1283–1297.

8 Scott MG, Bruns DE, Boyd JC, Sacks DB. Tight glucose control in the intensive care unit: are glucose meters up to the task? *Clin Chem.* 2009;55:18–20.

9 Dungan K, Chapman J, Braithwaite SS, Buse J. Glucose measurement: confounding issues in setting targets for inpatient management. *Diabetes Care.* 2007;30:403–409.

2

Endocrine Testing in Acute and Critical Illness

Reza Morovat

Key Points

- Many factors combine to increase the complexity of endocrine testing in the acute and critically ill patient, not only in terms of laboratory service provision but particularly in the interpretation of results.
- The endocrine changes in the acute and critically ill patient involve most systems; they vary with primary pathology and with time. The changes are further complicated by changes in hormone binding proteins and by drug therapy.
- Therefore, when considering illness, consideration needs to be given to the fact that a host of disparate etiologies can bring about changes in the endocrine system through distinct or shared mechanisms, such that two patients with the same severe illness may display differences in some of their circulating hormones depending on

whether or not, for example, they are fed well. In other scenarios, such as active inflammatory bowel disease, a multitude of pathological, nutritional, and pharmacological factors operate to influence various endocrine systems, and the final endocrine response would depend on the balance of the effects of these factors.
- Interference in hormone assays can be difficult to identify, and differences in assay bias and difficulties with standardization determine that local assay-specific reference ranges must be applied.
- It cannot be over-emphasized that laboratory results should be reviewed critically and any discordance with the patient's condition, or with previous results considered with suspicion and discussed with the laboratory.

Introduction

A plethora of endocrine systems and their functions are affected by acute and chronic illness. Depending on the physiological insult, endocrine responses may vary, but they often show significant overlap. The pathological states that influence endocrine function are not limited to systemic illness, but also encompass a host of physiological and psychological stressors. For example, malnutrition triggers changes in the thyroid system that is not very dissimilar to those found in chronic illness. Despite receiving adequate nutrition, children with emotional stress tend not to grow well, mainly due to an impaired somatotropic axis. Individuals with psychological stress

Endocrine and Metabolic Medical Emergencies: A Clinician's Guide, Second Edition. Edited by Glenn Matfin.

may also exhibit a deficit in their immune function due to excessive activation of the hypothalamic-pituitary adrenal (HPA) axis, as well as impairments of other axes such as hypothalamic-pituitary-gonadal (HPG). The HPG axis is also adversely affected both by malnutrition or prolonged periods of vigorous exercise in otherwise super-fit individuals. Therefore, when considering illness, consideration needs to be given to the fact that a host of disparate etiologies can bring about changes in the endocrine system through distinct or shared mechanisms, such that two patients with the same severe illness may display differences in some of their circulating hormones depending on whether or not, for example, they are fed well. In other scenarios, such as active inflammatory bowel disease, a multitude of pathological, nutritional and pharmacological factors operate to influence various endocrine systems, and the final endocrine response would depend on the balance of the effects of these factors.

Many factors combine to increase the complexity of endocrine testing in the acute and critically ill, not only in terms of laboratory service provision but particularly in the interpretation of results. The aim of this chapter is to highlight some of the pitfalls to be avoided by both the clinician and the laboratory.

Factors Influencing Laboratory Hormone Results or Their Interpretation in Acute Illness

Physiological Changes

Throughout the endocrine systems there are some common changes found in acute illness which impact on investigations and their interpretation (Table 2-1). For the evaluation of plasma hormone concentrations during illness, a number of crucial physiological factors that influence hormone activity need to be considered:

- Illness may affect the manufacture and release of hormones from glands or tissues through stimulatory or inhibitory extra- and intra-cellular signals that are not measured in the laboratory.
- Hormone-binding proteins are generally negative acute phase reactants, in the sense that their concentrations fall during illness. This decrease can affect total (bound plus free) and bioavailable free plasma hormone concentration in opposite directions, but very often only the total hormone is measured.
- Illness may bring about changes in the uptake or clearance of hormones, and modify their half-lives significantly.
- The sensitivity of target tissues to hormones may be modified by changes in the binding capacity and the affinity of cellular hormone receptors.
- The activity of a number of hormones in target tissues is regulated by the conversion of a relatively inactive hormone into the active form, and, separately, by the deactivation of the active hormone. Enzymes that activate or deactivate hormones are usually influenced by illness.

For these reasons, hormone concentrations that are obtained during illness may not correlate well with cellular hormone activity. Furthermore, the use of reference intervals derived from healthy populations are often inappropriate for interpreting hormone results during illness. It is also important to recognize that laboratory methods that are used for measuring hormones may be adversely affected by conditions brought about by illness or therapies. This is particularly the case when measuring free hormone concentrations.

In addition, the use of dynamic function tests in the critically ill patient may well be contraindicated and in practice, other than the short adrenocorticotropic hormone (ACTH) stimulation test, are rarely performed in this setting. It should be noted that the effect of pharmacological stimulation in addition to the physiological stimulation of the stress response may be difficult to assess and may not accurately reflect endocrine status.

Table 2-1 Effects of critical illness on specific hormones

Hormone	Effects of illness on test results	Mechanisms of change
Thyroid function tests	Acute: $\leftrightarrow\uparrow$TSH; $\uparrow$FT$_4$; $\downarrow$FT$_3$ Chronic: $\downarrow$TSH; $\downarrow$FT$_4$; $\downarrow\downarrow$FT$_3$	$\downarrow$D1 activity (periphery) $\uparrow$D2 (tanycytes and periphery) $\uparrow$D3 (periphery) $\downarrow$TRH by $\uparrow$CRH, $\downarrow$leptin $\uparrow$ILs-1,2&6, $\uparrow$TNFα
Cortisol and ACTH	Acute: $\uparrow\uparrow$cortisol $\leftrightarrow\uparrow$ ACTH Chronic: $\uparrow$cortisol $\leftrightarrow\downarrow$ACTH	$\uparrow$CRH by $\uparrow$NPY, $\uparrow$catecholamines, $\uparrow$cytokines, $\uparrow$GLP-1 $\downarrow$Cortisol clearance $\downarrow$CBG, reducing total cortisol
Catecholamines	Acute: $\uparrow\uparrow$catecholamines and metabolites Chronic: $\uparrow$ catecholamines and metabolites	Stress response
Gonadal function tests	<u>Men</u> Acute (secondary hypogonadism): $\downarrow$Testosterone; $\downarrow$LH; $\leftrightarrow\downarrow$FSH Chronic (primary hypogonadism): $\downarrow$Testosterone; $\uparrow$LH; $\leftrightarrow\uparrow$FSH <u>Women</u> $\downarrow$LH; $\downarrow$FSH ($\uparrow$LH & $\leftrightarrow$FSH in CKD)	Distinction between acute and chronic phase mechanisms is difficult. In general, GnRH affected by noradrenaline, CRH, POMC products, cortisol, leptin and cytokines $\downarrow$SHBG, except in chronic liver disease ($\uparrow$) LH retention in CKD
Growth hormone and IGF-1	Acute: $\uparrow$GH; $\downarrow$IGF-1 Chronic: $\leftrightarrow\downarrow$GH; $\downarrow\downarrow$IGF-1	Interplay of GHRH, somatostatin, catecholamines, ghrelin, cortistatin. In chronic illness, somatotrophs remains responsive. $\downarrow$IGF-1 by $\downarrow$nutrition, $\downarrow$thyroid hormones, $\uparrow$IGFBP-2, $\downarrow$IGFBP-3, $\uparrow$cytokines
Vitamin D	$\downarrow$	$\downarrow$Binding protein, especially in tissue damage
Prolactin	$\uparrow$	Stress response

ACTH = adrenocorticotropic hormone; CKD = chronic kidney disease; CRH = corticotropin-releasing hormone; FSH = follicle stimulating hormone; GH = growth hormone; GLP-1 = glucagon-like peptide-1; IGF-1 = insulin-like growth factor-1; IL = interleukin; LH = luteinizing hormone; NPY = neuropeptide Y; D = deiodinase; T3 = triiodothyronine; T4 = thyroxine; TNFα = tumor-necrosis factor-α; TSH = thyroid stimulating hormone; $\leftrightarrow$ = no change

Pharmacological Influences

Pharmacological effects on endocrine systems may be due to either direct effect(s) on hormone secretion and metabolism or to interferences in the hormone assays. There are limitations in our understanding of these effects in the acutely ill, where many drugs are given simultaneously and where drug pharmacokinetics and metabolite concentrations are more variable.

Examples of Endocrine System Testing in Acute and Critical Illness

Hypothalamic-Pituitary Axis

Patients with acute and critical illness can have significant changes in pituitary hormone levels. In addition, the cause of the acute admission (e.g., traumatic brain injury or subarachnoid hemorrhage) may result in direct (and indirect) damage to the hypothalamic-pituitary axis. In terms of laboratory investigations in this setting, an illustrative example highlights this complexity: a patient with severe acute headache is found to have an unsuspected pituitary tumor on imaging. Measurement of serum prolactin, along with other pituitary hormones at baseline is suggested. However, the interpretation of the prolactin result is complicated by the fact that there may be significant overlap in serum prolactin concentrations found due to stress of acute illness and those due to a microprolactinoma. In addition, the presence of macroprolactin (immunoglobulin bound prolactin which is biologically inactive) as a cause of elevated serum prolactin must be excluded (Figure 2-1). This can be detected with polyethylene glycol (PEG) precipitation followed by analysis of the supernatant for monomeric prolactin. Reference intervals for PEG-treated samples should be used. In addition, very high concentrations of a hormone (e.g., severe hyperprolactinemia) may "swamp" the reagent antibodies used in an immunoassay leading to falsely low results and is termed the "hook effect" (Figure 2-1). Laboratories should have procedures in place to identify this effect (e.g., prolactin levels should be run at 1:100 v/v dilution in patients with large [>3 cm] pituitary macroadenomas or incidentalomas).

Hypothalamic-Pituitary-Thyroid (HPT) Axis

Regulatory Mechanisms

The thyroid gland's activity is controlled by pulsatile release of thyroid-stimulating

hormone (TSH) from the pituitary thyrotrophs, which are stimulated by thyroid-releasing hormone (TRH) release from hypothalamic paraventricular nucleus (PVN), and inhibited by thyroid hormones (1). By activating the phosphatidylinositol-protein kinase C pathway, TRH is a stimulator of TSHα and especially TSHβ gene expression, increases TSH glycosylation that is crucial for optimal TSH activity, and causes the release of TSH. The active thyroid hormone, 3,5,3'-triiodothyronine (T_3), inhibits the TSHβ gene expression and the TSH synthesis by binding thyrotroph nuclear T_3 receptors (TR) $\beta2$ in particular, but also TR-$\alpha1$. These receptors act as transcription factors, modulating the expression of TSH genes. The inhibitory effects of thyroxine (T_4) on TSH secretion are mediated by its conversion to T_3 within thyrotrophs by selenium containing deiodinase (D) type-2 (D2), which exerts an important level of control on thyrotroph responsiveness (Figure 2-2). TSH synthesis and secretion are also modulated by changes in the binding capacity of T_3 receptors for their ligand (2). T_3 also inhibits TRH secretion by its binding to TR-$\beta2$ in the hypothalamus, with D2 in tanycytes regulating the conversion of T_4 to T_3 and thereby the amount of T_3 that reaches TRH-secreting neurons (3). Importantly, hypothalamic TRH secretion is also under the control of neuronal signals that include α-adrenergic pathways, leptin, as well as glucocorticoids (4–6).

The thyroid gland secretes predominantly T_4. The molar ratio for the amount of T_4 to T_3 on thyroglobulin is 13:1 (7,8), with an estimate of secreted T_3 to be around 11–12% of the total thyroid hormone secretion (9). Thyrocytes also possess D2, and modify the ratio of the secreted hormones. However, most of the T_3 in circulation is derived from the peripheral conversion of T_4 to the active hormone by D1, present in the liver and kidney, and D2 that occurs in myocytes and adipocytes (Figure 2-2). These organs are therefore capable of adjusting their intracellular T_3 concentrations according to their needs. D1 is also capable of deactivating

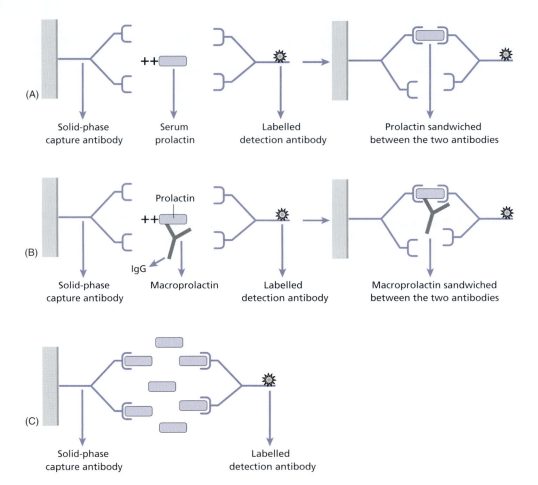

Figure 2-1 (A) A two-site immunometric assay for the measurement of serum prolactin uses two antibodies that are specific for different epitopes of prolactin. Prolactin is sandwiched between a capture antibody attached to a solid-phase matrix and a labeled detection antibody; (B) Circulating macroprolactin (complexes of immunoglobulin G [IgG] and prolactin) is detected but is not bioactive. Thus, the result is a false positive and clinically misleading; (C) The "hook effect": very high serum prolactin levels simultaneously saturate both the capture and detection antibodies, preventing "sandwich formation" and the detection of prolactin. This will result in a falsely low measurement. Reproduced with permission of John Wiley & Sons Ltd.

T_4 and T_3 by converting them to 3,3′,5′-triiodothyronine (reverse T_3; rT_3) and 3,3′ T2, a feat that is also achieved by D3, which prevails in brain tissues other than the pituitary, and also in fetal tissues and the placenta.

In the circulation, thyroid hormones are bound to three binding proteins (BPs): thyroxine-binding globulin (TBG), transthyretin and albumin. Of the three BPs, TBG has the highest affinity and the lowest capacity for thyroid hormones, whereas albumin possesses the lowest affinity and the highest capacity. Normally around 99.7% of T_3 and 99.97% of T_4 are in bound states. However, the degree of binding is affected not only by changes in the concentrations of the individual BPs, but also by the presence of molecules that displace thyroid hormones from these proteins. These compounds may be metabolites, especially free fatty acids liberated during catabolic states, or medications that display protein binding, and thereby compete with thyroid hormones for binding to their BPs, particularly albumin.

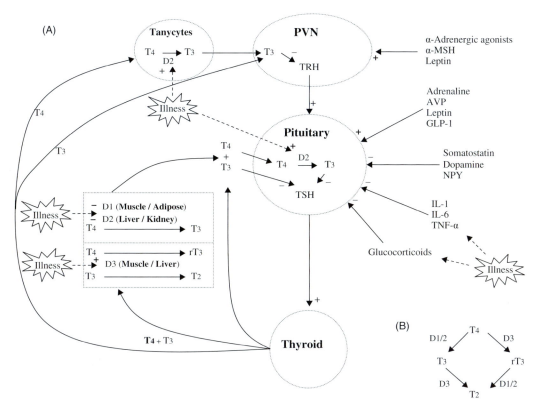

Figure 2-2 Influence of illness on the HPT axis: (A) Many of the effects are mediated through modulation of deiodinases (D) enzymes; (B) Whereas D1 and D2 have half-lives of around 12 h, D3 has a short half-life of only about 20 min., and therefore offers a rapid adaptable response in the pituitary thyrotrophs and tanycytes, with the latter supplying inhibitory T_3 to the paraventricular nucleus (PVN) TRH-secreting neurons that lack deiodinases. Many of the effects of cytokines on the thyrotrophs are mediated through simulation of D2 enzyme. D2 has a greater affinity for T_4 than for rT_3, whereas D3 has a greater affinity for T_3 than T_4. α-MSH = α-melanocyte stimulating hormone; AVP = arginine vasopressin; GLP-1 = glucagon-like peptide-1; NPY = neuropeptide Y; IL-1/6 = interleukin 1/6; TNF-α = tumor necrosis factor-α.

Effects of Illness on the HPT Axis

Mechanisms by which illness results in changes in TSH and free thyroid hormones may be crudely grouped into those involving neuroendocrine hormones and signals that act at the hypothalamic-pituitary level; proteins and messengers released as part of the immune response to infections; and changes in the deiodination of thyroid hormones in the pituitary, the thyroid, and/or the target tissues (Figure 2-2).

Thyrotrophs are modulated by dopamine, α-adrenergic agonists, opioids and other agents through either direct neural inputs or indirectly through its portal blood (10).

Influential hormones include corticotropin-releasing hormone (CRH) and glucocorticoids that have inhibitory effects on the TRH-TSH axis (5,11,12). Increases in the circulating cortisol, for example, during surgical procedures, precede changes in T_3 and rT_3 (13,14). Leptin, the reduction of which during illness and calorie deprivation permits a greater inhibition of the TRH-secreting neurons, also has a significant regulatory role (15). Plasma total T_4, free T_4 (FT_4) and free T_3 (FT_3), but not TSH, show associations with interleukin-6 (IL-6) concentrations (16–18). Also FT_3 correlates negatively, and rT_3 positively, with IL-2 in patients with chronic disease (19), whereas IL-1β and tumor necrosis factor (TNF)-α inhibit TSH release in a manner that appears to be independent of TRH and the effects on thyroid hormones (20,21).

Thyroid hormone deiodination pathways also play a crucial role in modulating intracellular hormone concentrations and thereby the HPT axis (Figure 2-2). Changes in deiododinases in tanycytes and thyrotrophs result in the tuning of the TRH-TSH axis, whereas modifications of hepatic and myocyte deiodinases influence circulating thyroid hormones. The activity of liver and muscle D1, which converts T_4 to T_3 and also deactivates rT_3, was shown to decrease in tissues obtained from critically ill patients (22). In such patients, there is a significant increase in the conversion of T_4 to inactive rT_3 by an increase in liver and muscle expression of D3, which is normally absent from these tissues (23). Additionally, the pool of T_4 and T_3 is reduced in illness by a paradoxical increase in D2 that converts T_4 to T_3, only for the latter to be deactivated to T2 by the D3 enzyme (24).

The induction of D3 in myocytes and hepatocytes is also responsible for the "consumptive hypothyroidism" that has been shown in many cases with vascular tumors that express D3 (25,26). Also, tanycytes and pituitary thyrotrophs possess D2 that generates T_3 from T_4, but do not harbor either D1 or D3, an increase in the activity of D2 enzyme in these cells results in an increase in their T_3. The T_3 released from tanycytes inhibits adjacent TRH-secreting neurons, and the increase in thyrotroph T_3 inhibits TSH production, further reducing circulating thyroid hormones as seen in prolonged non-thyroidal illness (NTI). Finally, but importantly, factors such as cytokines play a significant role in modulating thyroid hormone deiododinases (27).

Effects of Critical Illness on Thyroid Function Test Results

Laboratory assessments of the HPT axis usually comprise measuring TSH and FT_4, and,

depending on the findings, FT_3. The effects of critical illness on thyroid hormones have been studied over the course of the past four decades, during which different generations of TSH and, importantly, free hormone assays have appeared. As will be described below, some free hormone assays have been particularly prone to changes in circulating BPs. This needs to be considered when faced with some discrepancies in free hormone results obtained by different assays in different assay era.

In critical illness, endocrine adaptations, especially those that involve anterior pituitary hormones, tend to display a bi-phasic response (28). Critical illness initially evokes a mild increase in the pituitary TSH secretion. This increase is usually within the reference interval, and if increased, is rarely above 10 mIU/L (normal 0.5–5.0). There is also an increase in circulating FT_4, with concentrations that are often above the upper limit of the reference interval. These are accompanied by both a decrease in the plasma concentration of FT_3 and an increase in rT_3 (29). Contrary to FT_4, total T_4 (TT_4), if measured, shows a decrease, and this is concordant with a decrease in plasma BPs, especially TBG, that occurs in the early phase of acute illness (30,31). Increased free fatty acids secondary to illness-associated lipolysis also displace T_4 from its BPs, and contribute to a high FT_4. The reduction in FT_3 occurs fairly rapidly. Studies have shown that induction of anesthesia and surgery can rapidly decrease circulating FT_3 and increase rT_3 (14). The decrease can reduce FT_3 to below the lower limit of the reference interval, but is more often within but toward the lower end of it. The free hormone concentrations normalize during recovery when patients resume normal food intake. With a normal or high to normal TSH and with the help of FT_3 measurements, thyroid function test (TFT) results during the acute phase of an illness are easily distinguishable from those found in primary or secondary thyroid dysfunction. When only TSH and FT_4 are measured and these are both increased, some clinicians may wrongly assume the possibility of a very rare

TSH-secreting tumor or resistance to thyroid hormones. FT_3 measurements that show low values discard both these diagnostic possibilities. The clinical history and previous TFT results are always very informative and should alert the physician or the laboratorian that they are dealing with changes due to NTI, and usually a repeat thyroid function testing some time after recovery is all that is required as assurance. However, when dealing with a set of thyroid hormone results in which there are discrepancies, a possibility of interference in one of the assays should also be considered.

In severe, protracted illness, TSH and T_4 begin to fall, and T_3 tends to decrease further (32). Occasionally, TSH may be undetectable, particularly in the elderly and especially in those who are in a poor nutritional state. This may partly be due to the fact that TSH tends to decline with advanced age (33,34), and the elderly also tend to be more predisposed to poor nutrition. As illness prolongs, FT_3 decreases even further and is usually below the lower limit of the reference interval. The magnitude of the decrease of T_3 bears a relationship with the disease outcome (35).

In practice, TFT results in patients with severe NTI may cause interpretation issues. A significant number of patients with NTI display a low or suppressed TSH, but with FT_4 values that may be either normal or low. FT_3 results are valuable in NTI, and are usually below the lower limit of the reference interval in chronic, severe illness. Notwithstanding the fact that TFT results on specimens collected during severe illness do not reliably serve in excluding primary or secondary thyroid disease (especially if mild to moderate), distinctions need to be made between abnormal findings in critical illness and specific thyroid pathologies. In one study of hospitalized patients, 3.1% were found to show undetectable TSH. On the follow-up of these patients, the low TSH of 40% was attributable to NTI, with glucocorticoid being responsible for 36% of low TSH cases, and the remaining 24% deemed to have thyroid disease (39). On the other hand, a high TSH concentration of >20 mIU/l was seen in

1.6%, and of these half were found on follow-up to have hypothyroidism (36).

In co-existing hyperthyroidism, a reduction in circulating thyroid hormones, due partly to their increased peripheral catabolism, may mask the condition by virtue of FT_4 and FT_3 concentrations being within their reference intervals. Although thyroid hormone concentrations may not be helpful, and a suppressed TSH has no diagnostic power in this setting, a detectable TSH usually rules out hyperthyroidism even in the setting of NTI. However, a repeat analysis after recovery is always recommended. A TRH stimulation test is unhelpful in this setting, as the TSH response to TRH is blunted in chronic illness and starvation (10).

A more common and important condition that should be considered with either normal or low thyroid hormones, whenever TSH is also low or suppressed, is secondary hypothyroidism due to pituitary failure. In the assessment of these patients, measurement of cortisol, with considerations for a short ACTH stimulation test if cortisol is subnormal, should be standard practice. As part of the pituitary assessments, gonadotropins should also be measured, and an isolated follicle-stimulating hormone (FSH) measurement is particularly valuable when dealing with a post-menopausal female patient (FSH should be high). An illness-related fall in TSH may also mask primary hypothyroidism. Normally, the ratio of T_3 to T_4 is increased in primary hypothyroidism, but is rather insensitive in NTI. Anti-thyroid antibody measurements may be helpful, but repeat TFT after recovery is recommended.

Thyroid Status in Malnutrition

Changes in TFT results in chronic calorie deficiency and starvation bear resemblance to those seen in NTI. However, whereas food deprivation decreases FT_3 and increases rT_3, there appears to be some discrepancies between changes in TSH and FT_4 as observed in different studies. These anomalies may relate to the underlying pathophysiology, as food deprivation studies have been carried out on either normal or obese individuals, and separately on those with conditions such as anorexia nervosa. In food-deprived obese individuals, total T_4 tends to falls, but TSH and FT_4 show little change, although FT_4 may actually show an increase similar to that seen in the acute phase of illness (37–39). On the other hand, chronically malnourished patients with anorexia show a pattern of laboratory results that resembles those seen in chronic illness, with findings that are akin to those found in central hypothyroidism (40).

Technical Aspects of Thyroid Function Testing

Influence of Low Plasma Binding Proteins in Illness

Depending on the extent of TRH stimulation, thyrotrophs can secrete TSH molecules with different degrees of glycosylation, which affects the activity of the hormone. TSH with a higher glycosylation index has a greater activity. Although TSH assays are standardized, assay antibodies can cross-react with TSH to different extents according to it glycosylation, such that there may be a poor correlation between antibody cross-reactivity and TSH bioactivity (41). This may hamper the ability of TSH assays to accurately assess both the hormone's concentrations and its bioactivity.

Total thyroid hormones concentrations are greatly influenced by the concentrations of BPs, which are reduced in NTI. In that respect, measurements of free thyroid hormones have made huge improvements over total hormone assays in the interpretation of thyroid results. However, accurate measurements of free thyroid hormones by immunoassay have offered serious challenges, mainly because separating and/or measuring the free hormone fraction without disturbing the equilibrium between bound and free fractions (42,43) is difficult. Furthermore, since binding of hormones to binding proteins are temperature-dependent,

assays carried out at a temperature other than that of the body have the potential to produce biased results when binding protein concentrations in the specimen are very different from those in the assay calibrants (44,45). Most automated laboratories employ one-step, analog, free-hormone immunoassay methods to measure free thyroid hormones. These have the advantage of being faster, but even a small degree of binding of the analog to thyroid hormone-binding proteins can produce erroneous results. They also have a number of disadvantages, mainly related to variations in BPs concentrations in studied samples (43). Such assays have been validated mainly based on hormone-binding to albumin at physiological or near-physiological albumin concentrations, and tend not to perform well when binding protein concentrations deviate from normal or when other compounds that displace thyroid hormones from their BPs are present (42,46–48). Therefore, caution should be taken in interpreting results of these assays in samples from ill patients, who can have grossly-abnormal thyroid hormone-BPs.

Assay Interference

When dealing with a set of discrepant thyroid hormone results, as is often seen in patients with NTI, it is important to consider the possibility of interference in one of the assays. In order to decide whether assay interference is a possibility, a careful assessment of previous results, time course of changes and, very importantly, the clinical history should be made. The problem of assay interference arises when found present in the sample are antibodies against antigens from the animal species that is the source of the antibodies used in that assay. These antibodies can be present in serum of individuals who, for example, have kept rodents or rabbits as pets. Such human antibodies can form an anchor for particular assay's antibodies, causing usually an over-estimation, but also occasionally an under-estimation of TSH or, less frequently, thyroid hormones. It is the role of the laboratory to investigate discrepant thyroid function results by dilution or precipitation studies for TSH, and assay by two-step methods, assessment of TBG or measurement of total hormones to assess free hormone results.

The Hypothalamic-Pituitary-Adrenal (HPA) Axis

Regulatory Mechanisms

Similar to thyroid hormones, glucocorticoids influence a vast array of cellular activities in different cell types. They orchestrate responses to stress, and are key mediators of physiological and behavioral adaptations against injury and illness. They mobilize stored fuel to meet demand, regulate the inflammatory response, and have direct and indirect effects on various tissues. Cortisol is the major glucocorticoid secreted by the adrenal cortex in man. Its secretion is under the influence of ACTH, which, through G-coupled melanocortin receptor-2 in the adrenal cortex, increases cholesterol delivery and expression of steroidogenic enzymes, particularly corticosteroid 11β-hydroxylase. ACTH is released in a pulsatile fashion from the pituitary corticotrophs, which are regulated by a multitude of neuroendocrine signals, but mostly by CRH from the hypothalamic PVN. Cortisol is also released in pulses, and this pulsatile nature of production for both ACTH and cortisol is maintained in stress and illness. Both ACTH and cortisol displays a circadian variation, with peaks before awakening in the morning, and troughs late at night. The amplitude of the circadian variation in cortisol is about twice that of ACTH. These oscillations are governed by CRH and arginine vasopressin (AVP) released from PVN, but are principally under the control of the suprachiasmatic nucleus (SCN) that regulates the body's circadian rhythms and has neural projections that reach PVN. The circadian rhythm is also influenced by the spanchnic nervous stimulation of the adrenals (49).

Cortisol suppresses both CRH and ACTH through a feedback mechanism operating at various levels of the HPA axis (50,51). In the circulation, about 80% of cortisol is bound to cortisol-binding globulin (CBG), nearly 15% to albumin, with only around 5% being free and bioavailable. CBG is more than a reservoir for cortisol, and serves an important role in the targeted delivery of cortisol to tissues and its bioavailability. Tissue-specific cleavage of CBG can enable the release of bound cortisol for targeted, local activity (52). CBG is also nearly fully saturated, and an increase in cortisol or a decrease in CBG concentrations can increase the free, bioavailable cortisol fraction significantly. Cortisol acts by binding to both glucocorticoid and mineralocorticoid receptors (GR and MR, respectively), which act as ligand-gated transcription factors (53). Cortisol has a several-fold higher affinity for MR than for GR (54). Beside their effects on DNA transcription, glucocorticoids also exert non-genomic effects, which are rapid and may be in part mediated through low-affinity cellular receptors (55–57). Cortisol receptors display a tissue-specificity, with GR present in the brain and peripheral tissues, while MR occurs in the corticolimbic region of the brain, the cardiovascular, liver, and kidney tissues (2). A complex control of glucocorticoid bioactivity in different tissues is made possible by different ratios of MR to GR in various organs and cell types, different receptor capacities and affinities resulting in different receptor occupancies, as well as fluctuations in cortisol that can differentially change the occupancy of the non-genomic and the two genomic receptors (58). Furthermore, in tissues such as the kidneys, upon which mineralocorticoids act, 11β-hydroxysteroid dehydrogenase type 2 deactivates cortisol and allows aldosterone to bind to the MR. In other tissues such as the brain and fat, the type 1 isoenzyme can work in the opposite direction, forming cortisol and increasing its action locally (59).

Effects of Stress and Illness on the HPA Axis

The HPA axis stimulation is largely driven by neuronal activity (Figure 2-3). Noradrenergic

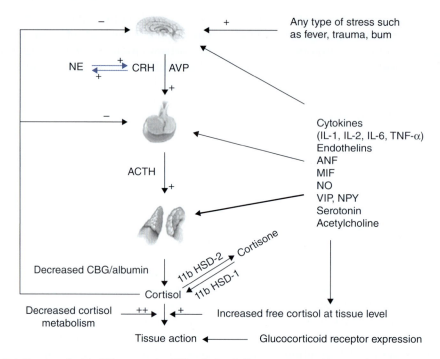

Figure 2-3 Influence of critical illness on the HPA axis. Pro-inflammatory cytokines such as IL-1, IL-6, and TNF have been recognized as important modulators of the HPA axis in critically ill patients. In addition, they may increase free cortisol release from bound cortisol by promoting the action of neutrophil elastase. Recent data suggest that reduced cortisol metabolism rather than increased cortisol production is the main contributor to the elevated cortisol levels during critical illness. The intracellular cortisol generation may be altered by the action of 11-beta HSD (51).

ACTH = adrenocorticotrophic hormone; ANF = atrial natriuretic factor; AVP = vasopressin; CBG = cortisol binding globulin; CRH = corticotropin-releasing hormone; 11-beta HSD-2 = 11-beta hydroxysteroid dehydrogenase type 2; 11-beta HSD-1 = 11-beta hydroxysteroid dehydrogenase type 1; MIF = macrophage-migration inhibitory factor; NE = norepinephrine; NO = nitric oxide; NPY = neuropeptide Y; TNF-α = tumor necrosis factor-α; VIP = vasoactive intestinal peptide

neuronal activity is required for the response of the HPA axis to a variety of homeostatic stimuli, inflammatory signals, and psychological distress (60) Neuropeptidergic signals, such as angiotensin-II, glucagon-like peptide-1 and neuropeptide Y (NPY) also act upon PVN to stimulate CRH secretion, which is also modulated by catecholamines, glutamate and GABA neurotransmitters (61). The neuronal control of the HPA axis enables a very rapid stress response within minutes, and may be turned off similarly quickly. There appear to be distinct time-course-related responses to stress. In acute stress, CRH stimulates arcuate nucleus neurons that secrete pro-opiomelanocortin (POMC), and, through α-melanocyte-stimulating hormone

(α-MSH) secretion and possibly inhibition of NPY, elicit signals that suppress appetite. Inhibition of the HPA axis may be achieved through agents such as enkephalin, GABA and somatostatin. In chronic psychological stress, increased cortisol suppresses CRH, and any earlier energy deficit is addressed with what appears to be a cortisol-promoted increase in NPY that stimulates appetite, particularly for palatable food that contributes to visceral obesity (62). Cytokines also act on PVN, although they can also influence pituitary corticotrophs (63,64).

In chronic illness, cortisol secretion and its baseline plasma concentrations are usually increased (65,66), although low cortisol may also be found in a significant portion of patients (67). The cortisol rise may not be entirely due to stimulated ACTH secretion, as the latter may not show an increase in some patients, suggesting the involvement of other neuroendocrine modulators (68,69). A suppressed ACTH in patients receiving intensive care, and the observations of reduced cortisol metabolizing enzymes in severe illness have raised the notion that a reduction in the metabolism of cortisol may explain at least part of high plasma cortisol concentrations in such patients (Figure 2-3) (70,71). Nevertheless, ICU patients appear to be able to show an ACTH and cortisol response to exogenous CRH (66). Also, whereas stimulation of the adrenals may result in a degree of adrenal hypertrophy, which may be at least partly due to an increased ACTH and sympathetic stimulation of the adrenals (72), adrenal insufficiency appears to occur in severe chronic illness with a much higher prevalence than expected, suggesting that short- and long-term effects on the adrenals may be different (73).

Effects of Illness on Laboratory HPA Testing

The laboratory assessment of the HPA axis in the acute setting is generally limited to measuring cortisol and ACTH. A CBG assay, which would be very useful for assessing free cortisol index, is not routinely available in clinical settings. A random cortisol is generally unhelpful unless significantly elevated. A morning (8 or 9 a.m.) cortisol of >500 nmol/L (18 µg/dL) in an unstressed person excludes HPA pathology, and one of >400 nmol/L (14.5 µg/dL) is usually associated with adequate ACTH reserve. Much more preferably, a stimulated cortisol is evaluated for investigation of adrenal hypofunction. For this, an insulin stress (tolerance) test (IST [ITT]), a CRH test, or a short corticotopin (250 µg synthetic ACTH [cosyntropin or synacthen]) stimulation test is used to assess the HPA axis, the PA axis or only the adrenal response, respectively. The short ACTH stimulation test is the most commonly used test, and also shows good correlation with IST (ITT), since chronic ACTH deficiency leads to adrenal atrophy and an abnormal cortisol response to short ACTH stimulation testing. A cortisol of >500 nmol/L (18 µg/dL) 30 or 60 minutes after short ACTH stimulation testing excludes adrenal insufficiency, and <500 nmol/L (18 µg/dL) may suggest a need for steroid replacement during illness. However, assays cross-react differently with cortisol, and the target and threshold values are assay-dependent and local reference ranges used.

The increased requirement for cortisol during physiological stress makes it important not to miss a diagnosis of adrenal insufficiency in acute and critically ill patients. In severe illness, cortisol is expected to be increased, but there is currently no consensus as to what the magnitude of the stimulated cortisol should be. The uncertainty stems partly from the variable cortisol response that appears to be somewhat dependent upon the severity of the disease in some, but not in all, studies (67,74,75), and partly from a lack of knowledge about the extent of influence of the type of critical illness on the cortisol response, given that most studies have been carried out on patients with sepsis. A recommendation was made for a short ACTH test to be used in critically ill patients, except those with either septic shock or acute respiratory distress syndrome, since these patients benefit from receiving glucocorticoids anyway (76). In patients with septic shock, the short ACTH test also shows irreproducibility (77). According to the recommendations, an increment of <250 nmol/L (9 µg/dL) in cortisol at 30 min. was deemed abnormal, carrying a poor chance of survival (78), independent of baseline cortisol concentration (79). However, this has been questioned (51), as it takes no account of the absolute cortisol values, and also in a large study by a group of authors of the recommendation, it was found that 46.7% of patients with septic shock failed to respond adequately according to the criterion, with no difference in outcomes at 28 days between responders and non-responders (80). Others have corroborated the high positive test rates in septic shock patients, reviewed in (81). An inverse relationship between baseline cortisol and the increment in its value in ill patients has been reported (82,83), and the significance of a high baseline cortisol and a suboptimal increase post-stimulation is unclear. One study of ill patients undergoing coronary artery bypass grafting has shown significant changes in the response of cortisol to ACTH stimulation over the course of days from the immediate pre-operative period (84). Finally, it should be considered that patients with a high body mass index (BMI) due to fat mass elicit a higher 30-min. cortisol response.

Despite being used to differentiate primary versus secondary adrenal insufficiency, ACTH levels may also be unhelpful in critical illness, since its concentrations may not be increased in chronic illness. It is still unclear whether there may be longitudinal changes in ACTH that are dependent on the type of illness and whether the relation between ACTH and cortisol changes over time (85,86). Assessing pituitary dysfunction may therefore prove difficult. A CRH or an IST (ITT) is required for the purpose, but since patients with critical illness may show an exaggerated ACTH response to CRH despite having higher plasma cortisol (66), it is unclear whether what would otherwise be a normal ACTH response may be adequate in critical illness.

Patients with Cushing's syndrome display an increased secretion of cortisol, and a loss of its normal circadian rhythm and amplitude. The laboratory diagnosis of Cushing's syndrome is often challenging and relies on the results from a few lines of investigation. These comprise increased urine excretions of free cortisol (UFC) over 24-hr periods, loss of circulating cortisol's normal circadian rhythm, failure of overnight dexamethasone to suppress the morning increase in plasma cortisol, and an abnormal ACTH response to a CRH stimulation test (87). Some of these findings can be mimicked in patients with critical illness or in those with depression and emotional disorders. Severely ill patients and those with depression display both an increased baseline cortisol and a loss of normal circadian rhythm that are often indistinguishable from patients with Cushing's syndrome. Patients with depressive disorders, obesity, and alcoholism may have UFC excretions that overlap with those found in Cushing's syndrome (88, 89), with the problem of differentiating increased UFC excretion in depressive illness and Cushing's syndrome being compounded by the fact that depression is common among patients with Cushing's syndrome (90). Low-dose, overnight dexamethasone suppression test results may give false positive results in patients with critical illness or depression (66,87). Drug or hormonal treatments, such as estrogens, that cause an increase in plasma CBG and therefore total cortisol may also lead to such false positive results. Midnight plasma cortisol concentration, which is normally low (especially when sleeping), is often increased to > 50 nmol/L (1.8 µg/dL) in severe illness and in depression (91,92). For these reasons, a greater reliance is placed on CRH stimulation or occasionally an IST (ITT) to distinguish hypercotisolemia of depression from that of Cushing's syndrome. Unlike patients with Cushing's syndrome, those with depression tend to elicit normal cortisol responses to CRH stimulation test, albeit with a lower-than-normal increase in ACTH, and also display a normal response to insulin-induced hypoglycemia (92,93). As described above, an exaggerated ACTH response to CRH in critical illness also makes the test unsuitable for diagnosing Cushing's syndrome in severe illness.

Laboratory Limitations for the Assessment of HPA Axis

There are also serious limitations imposed by laboratory assays on the interpretation of post-ACTH stimulation cortisol results. During illness, low BPs cause a reduction of the plasma-bound cortisol fraction, and can mask the magnitude of increase in cortisol at a time when low CBG (and often low albumin) actually increase plasma-free, bioavailable cortisol (94). Therefore, by measuring total cortisol, laboratories under-estimate cortisol bioavailability during illness, and may also under-estimate the increment in the measured cortisol, with a risk of false positive results (95). Consideration should also be given to conditions, such as hepatic disease, in which the CBG-synthesizing capacity of the liver is reduced (96).

Furthermore, assays cross-react differently with cortisol, and results are not transferable from one laboratory to another (97). In one study, the variation in the 5th centile of 30-min. post-ACTH cortisol value in normal individuals was found to vary from 510 to 626 nmol/L (18.5–22.7 µg/dL) (98). Furthermore, in a study of critically ill patients assessed, based on the criterion of the recommended increment in plasma cortisol, variation in assay results would misclassify 27% of the patients (99). Therefore, laboratories should establish and employ appropriate assay-specific increments in cortisol to interpret the short ACTH stimulation test results. An assessment of the recent medications is also necessary, since cortisol assays have a 30–40% cross-reactivity with exogenous prednisolone, which is also generated from prednisone.

Catecholamines

Catecholamine and Laboratory Assessment of Related Tumors

Physiological stress from illness elicits a neuroendocrine response, whereby the sympathetic nervous system and the adrenal medulla are stimulated to release catecholamines. This homeostatic response is essential for maintaining blood pressure, organ perfusion, fuel substrate availability, and enabling survival in a "fight or flight" scenario. Synaptic nerve clefts secrete noradrenaline (NA), also termed norepinephrine which serves as a neurotransmitter, but a portion of it ultimately finds its way into the circulation. Mesenteric tissues also synthesize NA, and their production accounts for just over one-third of the NA formed in the body. Most of circulating adrenaline (AD), also termed epinephrine, is of adrenal origin, and unlike NA, serves as a systemic hormone. Half of the body's dopamine (DA) is also produced by the mesentery.

Almost all adrenal pheochromocytomas and extra-adrenal paragangliomas (which also tend to be called pheochromocytomas) secrete catecholamines. Adrenal tumors have a propensity to secrete AD or NA, whereas NA alone or both NA and AD tend to be secreted by paragangliomas. Some pheochromocytomas produce DA with or without NA. These three neurotransmittrs are metabolized by o-methylation to metadrenaline (MA) (metanephrine), normetadrenaline (NMA) (normetanephrine) and 3-methoxytyramine (3MT), cumulatively termed metadrenalines (metanephrines). These may be measured in urine and plasma, and their combination, particularly free metadrenalines (metanephrines) in plasma, may have the highest diagnostic power (100). Plasma-free metadrenalines (metanephrines) also seem to offer further advantages, such as a greater stability of concentrations in the face of fluctuating secretions from tumors, as well as a better correlation with the tumor mass (101). Plasma measurements are not available in many laboratories, but their diagnostic performance are very closely matched by urine fractionated metadrenalines (metanephrines) (102). In fact, some studies suggest that the urine assay may offer a better specificity, unless plasma specimens are collected in a seated position, and the results are adjusted for BMI (103). Fasting is also important for plasma sampling (104). It is worth noting that the urine vanilyl mandelic acid (VMA) measurement has long been outdated, does not offer the sensitivity required, and is also prone to interference.

Catecholamines During Critical Illness Versus Pheochromocytoma

Unsurprisingly, patients with critical illness show significantly increased catecholamine metabolites, and these metabolites correlate with β-endorphins (105). An inverse relationship between the Glasgow Coma Scale (GCS) score and AD and NA metabolites can be observed in trauma and brain injury patients, but dopamine metabolites may not be increased (106). Pain from procedures carried out on cardiac surgical patients under intensive care do not seem to elicit (further) increases in catecholamine metabolites (107), whereas sedation was found to reduce the metabolites in ventilated patients (108).

Pheochromocytomas may present with cardiovascular complications. In patients with pheochromocytoma, supraphysiological amounts of catecholamines result in down-regulation of myocardial β-adrenergic receptors, adversely affecting myofibrils and contractility of myocytes (109). Catecholamine metabolites can also increase the permeability of sarcolemmal membrane, increasing intracellular calcium entry (110), with resulting myocarditis, diffuse interstitial inflammatory infiltrates, myocellular necrosis, and cardiac failure. In the presence of hypovolemia, decreased cardiac output may culminate in cardiogenic shock (110,111). Tumors may remain undiagnosed until patients present with complications (112). Since such complications of pheochromocytomas can carry a poor prognosis, clinical history and manifestations that may suggest the presence of a pheochromocytoma should prompt laboratory and radiological investigations.

Although patients with pheochromocytomas have much greater increases in catecholamines and metabolites than those with critical illness, there is an overlap between the ranges of values. In a study that compared pheochromocytoma patients who presented with or without crisis (113), 25 who were in crisis had ranges of maximum catecholamines that were 3.5- to 646-times the upper limit of normal (ULN) (median 22.8-times) compared with 112 non-crisis patients, whose catecholamines were from within the reference interval to 54-times the ULN (median 3.7-times); not significantly different. Catecholamine metabolites had a better discriminatory power, such that

in-crisis patients' maximum results range was 1.9–511 times the ULN (median 11.6 times), while non-crisis patients' range of maximum results was from within the reference interval to 90-times the ULN (median 6.3-times); (p = 0.007). With an obvious inability to describe what the upper limit of concentrations should be in patients who have different acute or chronic illnesses, the only means of identifying pheochromocytomas in those who present unwell is vigilance and reliance on imaging.

Hypothalamic-Pituitary Gonadal (HPG) Axis

Regulation of the HPG Axis and Effects of Illness and Stress Signals

The HPG axis comprises a sparse number of hypothalamic arcuate nucleus neurons that release gonadotropin-releasing hormone (GnRH) in a pulsatile fashion, the pituitary gonadotrophs that secrete the luteinizing and follicle-stimulating hormones (LH and FSH) also in pulses, and the gonads that generate sex hormones and gametes. The release of GnRH is stimulated by leptin and a number of neurotransmitters, including GABA, dynorphin and RF-related peptides. Depending on the stage of the cycle in females, the hypothalamic cells are also under a positive feed-forward influence of estradiol and progesterone. However, the same gonadal hormones, as well as inhibin and testosterone, inhibit GnRH, as do a number of neurotransmitters, such as kisspeptin, glutamate, NA, and neurokinin-B. Around 45% of testosterone and estradiol bind to the sex-hormone binding globulin (SHBG), and about half to albumin, so that only up to 3% of testosterone in men and around 1% in women is in a free state.

Systemic and psychological illnesses and stress have profound suppressive influences on the HPG axis. The stress response affecting the HPG axis mainly involves an interplay of CRH and NA that act, both directly and indirectly, to inhibit GnRH release. These effects are modulated by the products of the POMC molecule, including β-endorphin and α-MSH. Glucocorticoids also inhibit the release of GnRH, FSH and particularly LH, and also reduce the sensitivity of target tissues to sex hormones (114). The pulsatile nature of GnRH, as well as gonadal hormone synthesis, may be directly inhibited by cytokines, especially IL-6 and TNF-α, with indirect effects brought through activation of the HPA axis (115). Additionally, changes in SHBG and albumin influence circulating free, bioavailable, gonadal hormone concentrations. SHBG has a direct relationship with thyroid hormones and estrogens (and therefore elevated thyroid hormones in the post-menopausal state when estrogen is low, is significant and unlikely to be BP-related), whereas it is inversely correlated with androgens, insulin, and glucocorticoids, with thyroid hormones and insulin being the only modulators of hepatic SHBG gene transcription.

Nutrition, probably mostly through adipose tissue, influences the HPG axis. The influence of adipocytes on the HPG is on at least three levels. They secrete leptin, which decreases NPY, stimulates POMC and CRH neurons, and also has a stimulatory effect on the pituitary gonadotrophs (116,117). Adipocytes also contribute significantly to the aromatization of androgens, thereby increasing estrogens in men (118–120). Furthermore, adipocytes secrete pro-inflammatory adipokines, including TNF-α and IL-6 that are released from macrophages that infiltrate hypertrophic adipose tissue. Beside contributing to the metabolic syndrome, these cytokines directly depress the HPG axis, or may do so indirectly through stimulating the HPA axis (121–123).

Effects of Illness on Laboratory Indices of Gonadal Function

Sex hormones are the major contributors to bone mineral density. Also, plasma HDL-C correlates directly with testosterone, which increases apolipoprotein A1, HDL's major component (124,125). Therefore, gonadal dysfunction is important to identify particularly in chronically ill individuals, such as those with chronic kidney disease (CKD) or diabetes. However, with illness suppressing the gonadal function, assessing whether or not related HPG hormonal derangements are due to illness is extremely difficult, and reassessments would be necessary when a patient's condition changes over time.

In men, acute illness often affects hypothalamic and pituitary secretions, resulting in low gonadotropins and secondary gonadal failure. On the other hand, in most chronic systemic illnesses, there is primary hypogonadism, with increased gonadotropins and inhibin B. The end results are testicular Leydig cell dysfunction, reduced testosterone, and/or spermatogenesis. Identifying secondary testicular dysfunction is not always easy because of the wide inter-individual variation in normal testosterone values. However, primary testicular failure is less difficult to diagnose because of the associated increase in gonadoropins. Testosterone should always be measured in the morning, when there is a circadian increase in the plasma concentrations.

Men with severe acute-onset conditions, such as myocardial infarction, severe burns or surgery, display a decrease in plasma total testosterone, and despite a significant reduction in circulating SHBG, free testosterone is also decreased (126). On the other hand, men with chronic liver disease and cirrhosis display an increase in SHBG, which in combination with a decrease in gonadal androgen production leads to a significant reduction in free testosterone, even though this is somewhat mitigated by their low plasma albumin concentrations. As a result, around half of men with CKD have sexual dysfunction (127), with a low testosterone, and a secondary increase in LH that may also be partly related to the retention of LH by the kidneys (128). In CKD, there may be factors retained in plasma that render some refractoriness of Leydig cells to LH, since human chorionic gonadotropin (hCG) administration is unable to elicit the normal response in these cells (129).

Similarly, approximately half of patients with diabetes have sexual dysfunction. A reduction in testosterone, testicular volume, reduced motile sperm, and increased gonadotropins have been found in diabetic men, with gonadotropin levels correlating with glycemic control (130–132). Circulating insulin and testosterone correlated with one another in patients with type 2 diabetes (133). This association may be partly due to the decrease in SHBG that occurs in obesity and hyperinsulinemia, and decreases measured total testosterone concentrations.

In order to address the effects of low BPs on laboratory testosterone results, some laboratories calculate either free testosterone index based on SHBG concentration, or bioavailable testosterone that also takes weakly albumin-bound testosterone into account. These give better assessments of testosterone during illness, and there are online calculators of these indices available (134). However, the calculated values are very much assay method-dependent, and for this important reason, laboratories that use such indices ought to have established their own reference intervals for the calculated values.

Gender-related differences in HPG axis stress response may at least in part be explained by the sensitivity of the HPA axis to estrogens, which stimulate CRH gene transcription and reduce catecholamine catabolism, and these changes are related to the stage of the menstrual cycle (135–137). In post-pubertal, pre-menopausal females, oligomenorrhea or amenorrhea highlights a problem with the HPG axis, prompting laboratory investigations. However, the interpretation of the findings is fraught with difficulties because of uncertainties related to the stage of the menstrual cycle, which may be absent. Systemic illness, psychological stress, and weight loss impose disturbances in the female HPG axis, with reductions in LH secretion frequency and amplitude (138). Prolactin should be measured, but the interpretation should take into account that stress and CKD increase prolactin, which also shows a circadian peak in the early morning. In women with CKD, FSH is usually normal, and there is an increase in LH/FSH ratio. The pulsatility of LH is hampered, but its response to GnRH seems to be preserved. Estradiol, progesterone, and testosterone are decreased (139).

Chronic strenuous physical exercise can lead to a suppression of the HPG axis, particularly in women. This is mediated through a combination of HPA axis effects and nutritional signals, resulting in reduced gonadotropins and gonadal hormones (140, 141). In severe nutritional disorders, there is usually amenorrhea, and gonadotropins are very low and lack pulsatility. In this respect, leptin plays a significant role in the modification of the HPG axis, and is a predictor or amenorrhea (142,143). However, normalization of leptin after eating may not result in a resumption of normal HPG axis activity until insulin-like growth factor-1 (IGF-1) levels have normalized (144). In patients with depression, the pathophysiology of the HPG axis is similar to that seen in patients with eating disorders, with low gonadotropins associated with suppression of the hypothalamic-pituitary activity in both women and men, and lack of a positive estradiol feed-forward stimulatory mechanism in females (145). In such pituitary suppression scenarios, a laboratory re-evaluation of male patients after the condition has resolved may be recommended, with assessments also necessary in females if normal menstruation does not return.

Growth Hormone and Insulin-Like Growth Factor-1

Physiological Considerations

Growth hormone (GH) modifies aspects of glucose, lipid, and protein metabolism, either directly or indirectly, and promotes somatic and linear growth. It stimulates lipolysis, promotes muscle uptake and oxidation of free fatty acids, and reduces muscle and liver glucose uptake and insulin sensitivity (146).

Pulsatile pituitary GH secretion is under the regulation of a number of hormones and neurotransmitters (147). Hypothalamic GH-releasing hormone (GHRH) from arcuate nucleus neurons is a major stimulant of somatotroph GH synthesis and release through a G protein-coupled receptor and cAMP-mediated increase in intracellular calcium. Ghrelin, an orexigenic hormone that is released mainly by the oxyntic mucosa cells of the stomach, also promotes GH release by stimulating GHRH neurons and somatotrophs, an effect that is brought about by a G protein-coupled receptor-mediated increase in calcium via inositol triphosphate (148). An important inhibitory effect on both GHRH and GH release is mediated by somatostatin (SS), also released by hypothalamic neurons. Furthermore, cortistatin, a neuropeptide with homology to SS and released by the brain cortex, also acts at high concentrations to inhibit somatotropic GH release (149). SS-releasing neurons that innervate GHRH cells are stimulated by NPY and CRH, and inhibited by serotonin and acetylcholine. GH's feedback inhibitory effects on the hypothalamic-pituitary axis are mainly by the stimulation of hypothalamic SS- and NPY-secreting neurons, rather than by direct inhibitory effects on GHRH cells and somatotrophs. However, inhibition of somatotrophs by IGF-1 allows GH to exert an indirect hormonal regulation of the pituitary. Cortisol also has significant effects on GH secretion, with a stimulatory effect in the short term, but suppression of GH secretion when there is chronic exposure to high cortisol concentrations (150).

Binding of GH to its receptor ultimately leads to tyrosine kinase-related phosphorylation of signal transducers and activators of transcription that dimerize, translocate to the nucleus, and regulate expression of target genes, including IGF-1. The effects of GH on the synthesis of IGF-1 depend on both the concentration and the pulsatility of GH (151). In plasma, 40–50% of GH is bound to a GH-binding protein, which is also involved in regulating GH receptor expression (152,153). In the post-absorptive state, GH reduces amino acid oxidation and increases protein synthesis (154,155). These anabolic effects are mediated largely through a GH-stimulated increased in IGF-1 (156,157). In the fasted state, the increased release of GH results in a metabolic switch and the utilization of fat as energy source, sparing muscle protein catabolism for gluconeogenesis (146). The mechanisms for GH-induced insulin insensitivity in the fasted state are not entirely understood, but increased free fatty acids appear to play a role. In the fasted state, there is both a decrease in liver GH receptors and an inhibition of post-GH-receptor events (158). These impose a refractoriness to GH, reducing IGF-1 production. IGF-1 synthesis is also dependent upon amino acid availability. When protein is restricted in the diet, although hepatic GH receptors are maintained, GH does not elicit an IGF-1 response, and the plasma half-life of IGF-1 is also reduced (159).

Whereas IGF-1 is produced in virtually all tissues and acts locally in an autocrine/paracrine fashion, its circulating concentrations are derived almost entirely from hepatocytes. IGF-1 functions principally through activation of its transmembrane tyrosine kinase receptor, which is structurally related to the insulin receptor. Insulin is the major stimulator of hepatic IGF-1 synthesis (160), and also to a great extent mediates the positive influence that nutritional state has on plasma IGF-1 concentrations (161). Thyroid hormones also have a permissive role in GH-mediated IGF-1 increase (162,163). In that respect, the reduction in thyroid hormones in chronic illness or in starvation may be responsible for breaking the direct relationship between GH and IGF-1.

In plasma, 99% of IGF-1 binds to six plasma IGF-binding proteins (IGFBP), of which, IGFBP-3 carries around 90% of the circulating hormone. IGF-BP3 and IGF-BP5 increase in response to GH, but their magnitude of change in response to GH is less than that of IGF-1, because the two BPs are also regulated by IGF-2, which is not particularly influenced by GH. IGF-1 activity is dependent upon a ternary complex of IGF-1, IGFBP-3, and an acid-labile subunit (ALS).

The hepatic production of ALS is also stimulated by GH, and the ternary complex has a prolonged half-life. IGFBP-2 has the second highest concentration among IGFBPs, and since it is far from being saturated, it acts as a reservoir for IGF-1. Fluctuations in its concentrations can therefore have a significant influence on total and free IGF-1 concentrations.

Effects of Acute and Critical Illness on GH and IGF-1

Although there may initially be a short period of preservation of body proteins after the onset of illness, the body ultimately enters a catabolic state, in which breakdown of muscle protein enables the supply of amino acids necessary for the manufacture of a vast array of proteins needed for inflammatory, immune, and other physiologic responses, and also to meet increased energy demands for various metabolic activities. As with some other anterior pituitary cells, somatotrophs show a biphasic pattern of response to illness, with an increase in GH secretion during the acute phase, and a suppressed GH production as the illness prolongs (164).

In acute illness, GH production is increased in a way similar to that found during starvation. There is an incr1ase in both baseline GH and its pulse peaks in plasma (164,165). Despite this, IGF-1 decreases and remains refractory to GH, and this is at least partly mediated by a decrease in GH receptors (91,166,167). In conjunction with low IGF-1, plasma IGFBP-3 and ALS also decrease in response to reduced GH effects (166), with an increase in the activity of a protease that degrades IGFBP-3 (168). Discrepancies do, however, exist. For example, patients with burns show a reduction in IGF-1, but no decrease in IGFBP-3 (169). During recovery from acute illness, there is a rapid restoration of these parameters (168).

When critical illness is prolonged, GH displays reduced pulse amplitude, although the pulse frequency and baseline GH may be normal (170,171). Stimulation of GH secretion by GHRH or ghrelin agonists elicit a response, suggesting that the effects of illness are through modulation of hypothalamic and other signals, rather than a refractoriness of the somatotrophs (171). IGF-1 remains low (171), and its concentrations may be particularly affected by the increase in IGFBP-1 and IGFBP-2 that occurs in severe illness, also resulting in a reduction in plasma free IGF-1. The plasma concentrations of these two IGF-BPs show some correlation with the severity of the disease, clinical outcomes, and/or survival (169,172–174).

Post-mortem studies of ill patients have revealed an increased number of GHRH-secreting neurons, suggesting that the hypothalamus remains responsive to stimuli (175). During illness, cytokines also have an influence on GH secretion. Thus, whereas IL-6 increases GH secretion (176), IL-1 can promote GH resistance and protein catabolism (177).

Laboratory Assessments of GH and IGF-1 During Illness

The pulsatile nature of GH precludes its random measurement for the laboratory investigation of GH deficiency or excess in any patient. Rather, dynamic function tests, in which GH is either stimulated or suppressed, are required. IGF-1 measurements are diagnostically valuable, especially for the investigation of GH-secreting adenomas, although their power for diagnosing GH-deficiency is not as high as GH-stimulation tests. Alternatively, repeated overnight sampling takes advantage of the increased GH secretion during stages 3, 4, and REM sleep.

During both acute and chronic illness, the only consistent change in the GH-IGF-1 axis is a reduction in IGF-1. Unsurprisingly, the magnitude of decrease in IGF-1 is dependent on the category of illness, with intensive care patients, for example, having a greater reduction in IGF-1 than that seen in trauma patients (178). GH concentrations are variable, and a decrease in GH also seems illness-dependent. Thus, sepsis, burns, and surgical patients may show no reduction in plasma GH (179,180). It is therefore very difficult, if not impossible, to study an underlying pathology related to GH-IGF-1 axis in critical illness, and there is no evidence that assessing GH secretion in critical care is of any benefit.

Plasma GH in patients with critical illness responds to GHRH and other secretagogues, such as ghrelin agonists (171). IGF-1 remains low (171,181), but the value of such provocative tests during critical illness remains uncertain, especially given that GH deficiency is prevalent in older age. Administration of GH to critically ill patients carries a increased risk of adverse outcome (182). It may be only presumed that a critically ill patient with a GH-secreting adenoma would have a high plasma GH pattern with a normal IGF-1 (based on the normalization of IGF-1 in GH-treatment during illness), but whether such investigation of critically ill patients with a suspected adenoma as such is fruitful and the test results interpretable is very much uncertain.

Vitamin D

Over the past two decades, there has been an increasing recognition of the importance of vitamin D (vit D) in a number of physiological processes beyond those involving calcium and phosphate metabolism. Epidemiological and clinical evidence have accumulated to show an involvement of vitamin D in modulating the immune, renin-angiotensin, as well as glucose homeostatic systems (183–185). There have also been suggestions that vitamin D deficiency may have a significant role in the pathogenesis of some chronic diseases, and may also be associated with an increased susceptibility to cardiovascular disease, neuropathology, cancer and mortality (186–190).

Laboratory assessment of vitamin D status is performed by measuring its 25-hydroxylated form, 25(OH)-vit D, produced in the liver. Its 1-hydroxylation in the kidneys converts 25(OH)-vit D into the active 1,25(OH)2-vit D, but usually other than in enzyme or receptor defects, this is rarely measured, as it has very limited value. Active vitamin D metabolites bind to receptors that belong to the superfamily of nuclear receptors and act as transcription factors when ligand-bound. Plasma 25(OH)-vit D has a half-life of 2–3 weeks, but it can increase significantly over a short period of time after exposure of warm skin to sunshine. Vitamin D is stored in the liver and the fatty tissue. Many hospitalized patient populations have low 25(OH)-vit D, but assessing whether a low vitamin D status in patients is related to illness is difficult, since, aside from the seasonal variation of its plasma metabolites, significant portions of screened healthy general populations, particularly those living in high latitudes, have deficient circulating 25(OH)-vitamin D concentrations (191,192).

In the circulation, around 90% and 85% of 25(OH)- and 1,25(OH)2-vit D are bound, respectively, to group-specific component globulin (Gc-globulin), commonly known as vitamin D-binding protein, which is synthesized by the liver. The main role of Gc-globulin is thought to be its involvement in the actin-scavenging system, which also has indirect, but important, implications for circulating 25(OH)-vit D concentrations. Actin, released from damaged tissues can polymerize and form filaments that complex with Factor Va. These complexes can form capillary plugs that impede microvascular blood flow, causing organ damage (193). Assisted by gelsolin protein, Gc-globulin functions by binding monomeric actin, and presents it to the hepato-reticuloendothelial system for uptake (194). As a result of the actin-scavenging process and the removal of the actin-bound Gc-globulin complexes from the circulation, the concentrations of Gc-globulin and its associated 25(OH)-vit D in plasma decrease significantly after tissue damage.

Hardly any studies have addressed changes in vitamin D related to acute tissue injury or illness. In one study, knee arthroplasty resulted in a 40% decrease in plasma vit D in a population with an already low vit status, and the decreased values persisted for three months post-operatively (195). In another similar study, there was around a 20% decrease in circulating 25(OH)-vit D and Gc-globulin after orthopedic surgery (196). Such a fall in circulating 25(OH)-vit D confounds assessment of vit D status in ill patients, particularly those with tissue injury. For example, in one study, virtually all patients admitted with myocardial infarction had deficient levels of 25(OH)-vit (197), and it is not known to what extent a low value in such patients is the result of tissue damage as opposed to lifestyle. Nevertheless, for either reason and/or insufficient vitamin D replacement, it appears that low vitamin D persists in such groups of patients, and may be assumed to reflect a new vitamin D steady-state (198).

Low 25(OH)-vit D concentrations have also been described in many cohorts of hospital inpatients, as well as those admitted to acute or intensive care units. Severely ill patients with sepsis were found to have low 25(OH)-vit D (199), as did the majority of one study's critically ill pediatric patients, in whom pediatric mortality risk score was associated with low plasma 25(OH)-vit D concentrations (200,201). Indeed, low vitamin D status has been associated with a high risk of adverse events and outcomes in patients with myocardial infarctions and acute coronary syndromes (202,203). However, in other ICU settings, vit D status had no prognostic value (204). Furthermore, either no benefit or mixed outcomes were found when vit D deficiency was treated in acute care settings (205,206).

Although decreases in 25(OH)-vit D are associated with illness in some studies, changes in plasma Gc-globulin may prove to have a more direct association with the course of illness and to be a predictor of clinical outcomes. The magnitude of the decrease in plasma Gc-globulin has been shown to be of prognostic value in patients with acute and severe organ damage, particularly hepatic injury (207–209). With only 5% of Gc-globulin occupied by active vitamin D metabolites, the exact relationship between changes in plasma 25(OH)-vit D and Gc-globulin is unclear, especially when concentrations may be governed by a number of factors, including the magnitude of decrease in Gc-globulin.

Conclusions

The endocrine changes in the acute and critically ill patient involve most systems, and vary with primary pathology and with time. These changes are further complicated by effects on hormone-binding proteins and by drug therapy. Interference in hormone assays can be difficult to identify, and differences in assay bias and difficulties with standardization determine that local assay-specific reference ranges must be applied. It cannot be over-emphasized that laboratory results should be reviewed critically and any discordance with the patient's condition, or with previous results considered with suspicion and discussed with the laboratory.

References

1 Reichlin, S, Utiger, RD. Regulation of the pituitary-thyroid axis in man: relationship of TSH concentration to concentration of free and total thyroxine in plasma. *J Clin Endocrinol Metab*. 1967;27:251–255.

2 Silva JE, Larsen PR. Peripheral metabolism of homologous thyrotropin in euthyroid and hypothyroid rats: acute effects of thyrotropin-releasing hormone, triiodothyronine, and thyroxine. *Endocrinology*. 1978;102:1783–1796.

3 Fekete C, Lechan RM. Negative feedback regulation of hypophysiotropic thyrotropin-releasing hormone (TRH) synthesizing neurons: role of neuronal afferents and type 2 deiodinase. *Front Neuroendocrinol*. 2007;28:97–114.

4 Lechan RM, Fekete C. Role of thyroid hormone deiodination in the hypothalamus. *Thyroid*. 2005;15:883–897.

5 Jackson IM. Thyrotropin-releasing hormone and corticotropin-releasing

hormone: what's the message? *Endocrinology*. 1995;136:2793–2794.

6 Luo LG, Bruhn T, Jackson IM. Glucocorticoids stimulate thyrotropin-releasing hormone gene expression in cultured hypothalamic neurons. *Endocrinology*. 1995;136: 4945–4950.

7 Laurberg P. Thyroxine and 3,5,3'-triiodothyronine content of thyroglobulin in thyroid needle aspirates in hyperthyroidism and hypothyroidism. *J Clin Endocrinol Metab*. 1987;64: 969–974.

8 Izumi M, Larsen PR. Triiodothyronine, thyroxine, and iodine in purified thyroglobulin from patients with Graves' disease. *J Clin Invest*. 1977;59:1105–1112.

9 Fisher DA, Oddie TH, Thompson CS. Thyroidal thyronine and non-thyronine iodine secretion in euthyroid subjects. *J Clin Endocrinol Metab*. 1971;33:647–652.

10 Mariotti S, Beck-Peccoz P. Physiology of the hypothalamic-pituitary-thyroid axis. 2016. In: De Groot LJ, Chrousos G, Dungan K, et al., eds. *Endotext [Internet]*. South Dartmouth, MA: MDText.com, Inc.; 2000-. http://www.ncbi.nlm.nih. gov/books/NBK278958/

11 Re RN, Kourides IA, Ridgway EC, Weintraub BD, Maloof F. The effect of glucocorticoid administration on human pituitary secretion of thyrotropin and prolactin. *J Clin Endocrinol Metab*. 1976;43:338–346.

12 Smallridge RC, Wartofsky L, Dimond RC. Inappropriate secretion of thyrotropin: discordance between the suppressive effects of corticosteroids and thyroid hormone. *J Clin Endocrinol Metab*. 1979;48:700–705.

13 Hagenfeldt I, Melander A, Thorell J, et al. Active and inactive thyroid hormone levels in elective and acute surgery. *Acta Chirurgica Scandinavica*. 1979;145:77–82.

14 Adami HO, Johansson H, Thoren L, et al. Serum levels of TSH, T3, rT3, T4 and T3-resin uptake in surgical trauma. *Acta Endocrinologica*. 1978;88:482–489.

15 Nillni EA, Vaslet C, Harris M, Hollenberg A, Bjorbak C, Flier JS. Leptin regulates prothyrotropin-releasing hormone biosynthesis. Evidence for direct and indirect pathways. *J Biol Chem*. 2000;275: 36124–36133.

16 Boelen A, Platvoet-ter Schiphorst MC, Wiersinga WM. Association between serum interleukin-6 and serum 3,5,3'-triiodothyronine in nonthyroidal illness. *J Clin Endocrinol Metab*. 1993; 77:1695–1699.

17 Abozenah H, Shoeb S, Sabry A, Ismail H. Relation between thyroid hormone concentration and serum levels of interleukin-6 and interleukin-10 in patients with nonthyroidal illness including chronic kidney disease. *Iran J Kidney Dis*. 2008;2:16–23.

18 Davies P, Black EG, Sheppard MC, Franklin JA. Relation between serum interleukin-6 and thyroid hormone concentration in 270 hospital in-patients with non-thyroidal illness. *Clin Endocrinol*. 1996;44:199–205.

19 Allegra A, Corica F, Buemi M, et al. Plasma interleukin-2 levels and thyroid function in elderly patients with nonthyroidal illness. *Arch Gerontol Geriatr*. 1998;26: 275–282.

20 van der Poll, T, Romijn JA, Wiersinga, WM, Sauerwein HP. Tumor necrosis factor: a putative mediator of the sick euthyroid syndrome in man. *J Clin Endocrinol Metab*. 1990;71:1567–1572.

21 Wassen FW, Moerings EP, Van Toor H, De Vrey EA, Hennemann G, Everts ME. Effects of interleukin-1 beta on thyrotropin secretion and thyroid hormone uptake in cultured rat anterior pituitary cells. *Endocrinology*. 1996;137: 1591–1598.

22 Peeters RP, van der Geyten S, Wouters PJ, et al. Tissue thyroid hormone levels in critical illness. *J Clin Endocrinol Metab*. 2005;90:6498–6507.

23 Peeters RP, Wouters PJ, Kaptein E„ van Toor H, Visser TJ, Van den Berghe G. Reduced activation and increased inactivation of thyroid hormone in tissues of critically ill patients. *J Clin Endocrinol Metab*. 2003;88:3202–3211.

24 Mebis L, Langouche L, Visser TJ, Van den Berghe G. The type II iodothyronine deiodinase is up-regulated in skeletal muscle during prolonged critical illness. *J Clin Endocrinol Metab*. 2007;92: 3330–3333.

25 Huang SA, Fish SA, Dorfman DM, et al. A 21-year-old woman with consumptive hypothyroidism due to a vascular tumor expressing type 3 iodothyronine deiodinase. *J Clin Endocrinol Metab*. 2002;87:4457–4461.

26 Huang SA, Tu HM, Harney JW, et al. Severe hypothyroidism caused by type 3 iodothyronine deiodinase in infantile hemangiomas. *N Engl J Med*. 2000;343: 185–189.

27 Gereben B, Zavacki AM, Ribich S, et al. Cellular and molecular basis of deiodinase-regulated thyroid hormone signaling. *Endocr Rev*. 2008;29:898-938.

28 Van den Berghe G, de Zegher F, Bouillon R. Acute and prolonged critical illness as different neuroendocrine paradigms. *J Clin Endocrinol Metab*. 1998;83: 1827–1834.

29 Wartofsky L, Burman KD. Alterations in thyroid function in patients with systemic illness: the "euthyroid sick syndrome." *Endocr Rev* 1982;3:164–217.

30 Afandi B, Vera R, Schussler GC, et al. Concordant decreases of thyroxine and thyroxine binding protein concentrations during sepsis. *Metabolism*. 2000;49: 753–754.

31 den Brinker M, Joosten KF, Visser TJ, et al. Euthyroid sick syndrome in meningococcal sepsis: the impact of peripheral thyroid hormone metabolism and binding proteins. *J Clin Endocrinol Metab*. 2005;90:5613–5620.

32 Van den Berghe G, de Zegher F, Veldhuis JD, et al. Thyrotropin and prolactin release in prolonged critical illness: dynamics of spontaneous secretion and effects of growth hormone-secretagogues. *Clin Endocrinol*. 1997;47:599–612.

33 Surks MI, Boucai L. Age- and race-based serum thyrotropin reference limits. *J Clin Endocrinol Metab*. 2010;95:496–502.

34 Sawin CT, Geller A, Kaplan MM, et al. Low serum thyrotropin (thyroid-stimulating hormone) in older persons without hyperthyroidism. *Arch Intern Med*. 1991;151:165–168.

35 Maldonado LS, Murata GH, Hershman JM et al. Do thyroid function tests independently predict survival in the critically ill? *Thyroid*. 1992;2:119–23.

36 Spencer CA, Eigen A, Shen D, et al. Specificity of sensitive assays of thyrotropin (TSH) used to screen for thyroid disease in hospitalized patients. *Clin Chem*. 1987;33:1391–1396.

37 Carlson HE, Drenick EJ, Chopra IJ, Hershman JM. Alterations in basal and TRH-stimulated serum levels of thyrotropin, prolactin, and thyroid hormones in starved obese men. *J Clin Endocrinol Metab*. 1977;45:707–713.

38 Spencer CA, Lum SM, Wilber JF, Kaptein EM, Nicoloff JT. Dynamics of serum thyrotropin and thyroid hormone changes in fasting. *J Clin Endocrinol Metab*. 1983; 56:883–888.

39 Komaki G, Tamai H, Kiyohara K, Fukino O, et al. Changes in the hypothalamic-pituitary-thyroid axis during acute starvation in non-obese patients. *Endocrinol Jpn*. 1986;33: 303–308.

40 Douyon L, Schteingart DE. Effect of obesity and starvation on thyroid hormone, growth hormone, and cortisol secretion. *Endocrinol Metab Clin North Am*. 2002;31:173–189.

41 Donadio S, Morelle W, Pascual A, Romi-Lebrun R, Michalski JC, Ronin C. Both core and terminal glycosylation alter epitope expression in thyrotropin and introduce discordances in hormone measurements. *Clin Chem Lab Med*. 2005;43:519–530.

42 Ekins R. Measurements of free hormones in blood. *Endocr Rev*. 1990;11:5–46.

43 Ekins R. The free hormone hypothesis and measurement of free hormones. *Clin Chem*. 1992;38:1289–1293.

44 Csako G, Zweig MH, Glickman J, Kestner J, Ruddel M. Direct and indirect

techniques for free thyroxin compared in patients with nonthyroidal illness. I. Effect of free fatty acids. *Clin Chem*. 1989;35: 102–109.

45 Ross HA, Bernard TJ. Is free thyroxine accurately measurable at room temperature? *Clin Chem*. 1992;38: 880–887.

46 van der Sluijs Veer G, Vermes I, Bonte HA, Hoorn RKJ. Temperature effects on free thyroxine measurements: analytical and clinical consequences. *Clin Chem*. 1992;38:1327–1331.

47 Csako G, Zwieg MH, Glickman J, Ruddel M, Kestner J. Direct and indirect techniques for free thyroxin compared in patients with nonthyroidal illness. II. Effect of prealbumin, albumin and thyroxin-binding globulin. *Clin Chem*.1989;35:1655–1662.

48 Stockigt JR, Lim CF. Medications that distort in vitro tests of thyroid function, with particular reference to estimates of serum free thyroxine. *Best Pract Res Clin Endocrinol Metab*. 2009;23:753–767.

49 Nicolaides NC, Charmandari E, Chrousos GP, Kino T. Circadian endocrine rhythms: the hypothalamic-pituitary-adrenal axis and its actions. *Ann N Y Acad Sci*. 2014;1318:71–80.

50 Myers B, McKlveen JM, Herman JP. Neural regulation of the stress response: the many faces of feedback. *Cell Mol Neurobiol*. 2012;352:683–696.

51 Hamrahian AH, Fleseriu M, Committee AAS. Evaluation and management of adrenal insufficiency in critically ill patients: disease state review. *Endocr Pract*. 2017. DOI:10.4158/EP161720.RA.

52 Meyer EJ, Nenke MA, Rankin W, Lewis JG, Torpy DJ. Corticosteroid-Binding globulin: a review of basic and clinical advances. *Horm Metab Res*. 2016;48: 359–371.

53 De Kloet ER, Vreugdenhil E, Oitzl MS, Joëls M. Brain corticosteroid receptor balance in health and disease. *Endocr Rev*. 1998;19:269–301.

54 McEwen BS, De Kloet ER, Rostene W. Adrenal steroid receptors and actions in the nervous system. *Physiol Rev*. 1986;66: 1121–1188.

55 Haller J, Mikics E, Makara GB. The effects of non-genomic glucocorticoid mechanisms on bodily functions and the central neural system: a critical evaluation of findings. *Front Neuroendocrinol*. 2008; 29:273–291.

56 Mitre-Aguilar IB, Cabrera-Quintero AJ, Zentella-Dehesa A. Genomic and non-genomic effects of glucocorticoids: implications for breast cancer. *Int J Clin Exp Pathol*. 2015;8:1–10.

57 Lee SR, Kim HK, Youm JB, et al. Non-genomic effect of glucocorticoids on cardiovascular system. *Pflügers Arch*. 2012;464:549–559.

58 Joels M, Karst H, DeRijk R, de Kloet ER. The coming out of the brain mineralocorticoid receptor. *Trends Neurosci*. 2008;31:1–7.

59 Seckl JR, Walker BR. Minireview: 11beta-hydroxysteroid dehydrogenase type 1- a tissue-specific amplifier of glucocorticoid action. *Endocrinology*. 2001;142:1371–1376.

60 Ulrich-Lai YM, Herman JP. Neural regulation of endocrine and autonomic stress responses. *Nat Rev Neurosci*. 2009;10:397–409.

61 Herman, JP, Figueiredo HF, Mueller NK, et al. Neurochemical systems regulating the hypothalamo-pituitary-adrenocortical axis. In: Blaustein J, Lajtha A, eds. *Handbook of Neurochemistry and Molecular Neurobiology: Behavioral Neurochemistry, Neuroendocrinology, and Molecular Neurobiology*. New York: Springer; 2007.

62 Cavagnini F, Croci M, Putignano P, Petroni ML, Invitti C. Glucocorticoids and neuroendocrine function. *Int J Obes Relat Metab Disord*. 2000;24:Suppl. 2:77–79.

63 Melmed, S, gp130-related cytokines and their receptors in the pituitary. *TEM*. 1998; 9:155.

64 Rettori V, Dees WL, Hiney JK, Lyson K, McCann SM. An interleukin-1-alpha-like neuronal system in the preoptic-hypothalamic region and its

induction by bacterial lipopolysaccharide in concentrations which alter pituitary hormone release. *Neuroimmunomodulation*. 1994;1: 251–258.

65 Herman JP, Adams D, Prewitt C. Regulatory changes in neuroendocrine stress-integrative circuitry produced by a variable stress paradigm. *Neuroendocrinology*. 1995;61:180–190.

66 Reincke M, Allolio B, Würth G, Winkelmann W. The hypothalamic-pituitary-adrenal axis in critical illness: response to dexamethasone and corticotropin-releasing hormone. *J Clin Endocrinol Metab*. 1993;77:151–156.

67 Rydvall A, Brändström AK, Banga R, Asplund K, Bäcklund U, Stegmayr BG. Plasma cortisol is often decreased in patients treated in an intensive care unit. *Intensive Care Med*. 2000;26:545–551.

68 Vermes I, Beishuizen A, Hampsink RM, Haanen C. Dissociation of plasma adrenocorticotropin and cortisol levels in critically ill patients: possible role of endothelin and atrial natriuretic hormone. *J Clin Endocrinol Metab*. 1995;80:1238–1242.

69 Bornstein SR, Engeland WC, Ehrhart-Bornstein M, Herman JP. Dissociation of ACTH and glucocorticoids. *Trends Endocrinol Metab*. 2008;19:175–180.

70 Boonen E, Vervenne H, Meersseman P, et al. Reduced cortisol metabolism during critical illness. *N Engl J Med*. 2013;368: 1477–1488.

71 Boonen E, Van den Berghe G. Cortisol metabolism in critical illness: implications for clinical care. *Curr Opin Endocrinol Diabetes Obes*. 2014;21:185–192.

72 Ulrich-Lai YM, Figueiredo HF, Ostrander MM, Choi DC, Engeland WC, Herman JP. Chronic stress induces adrenal hyperplasia and hypertrophy in a subregion-specific manner. *Am J Physiol Endocrinol Metab*. 2006;291:E965–E973.

73 Barquist E, Kirton O. Adrenal insufficiency in the surgical intensive care unit patient. *J Trauma*. 1997;42: 27–31.

74 de Jong MF, Beishuizen A, Spijkstra JJ, Groeneveld AB. Relative adrenal insufficiency as a predictor of disease severity, mortality, and beneficial effects of corticosteroid treatment in septic shock. *Crit Care Med*. 2007;35: 1896–1903.

75 Bouachour G, Tirot P, Gouello JP, Mathieu E, Vincent JF, Alquier P. Adrenocortical function during septic shock. *Intensive Care Med*. 1995;21: 57–62.

76 Marik PE, Pastores SM, Annane D, et al., American College of Critical Care Medicine. Recommendations for the diagnosis and management of corticosteroid insufficiency in critically ill adult patients: consensus statements from an international task force by the American College of Critical Care Medicine. *Crit Care Med*. 2008;36: 1937–1949.

77 Loisa P, Uusaro A, Ruokonen E. A single adrenocorticotropic hormone stimulation test does not reveal adrenal insufficiency in septic shock. *Anesthesia Analgesia*. 2005;101:1792–1798.

78 Annane D, Sébille V, Troché G, Raphaël, Gajdos P, Bellissant E. A 3-level prognostic classification in septic shock based on cortisol levels and cortisol response to corticotrophin. *J Am Med Assoc*. 2000;283:1038–1045.

79 Yang Y, Liu L, Jiang D, et al. Critical illness-related corticosteroid insufficiency after multiple traumas: a multicenter, prospective cohort study. *J Trauma Acute Care Surg*. 2014;76:1391–1396.

80 Sprung CL, Annane D, Keh D, et al. Hydrocortisone therapy for patients with septic shock. *N Engl J Med*. 2008;358: 111–112.

81 Venkatesh B, Cohen J. The utility of the corticotropin test to diagnose adrenal insufficiency in critical illness: an update. *Clin Endocrinol*. 2015;83:289–297.

82 Bruno JJ, Hernandez M, Ghosh S, Pravinkumar SE. Critical illness-related corticosteroid insufficiency in cancer patients. *Support Care Cancer.* 2012;20: 1159–1167.

83 Menon K, Ward RE, Lawson ML, et al., Canadian Critical Care Trials Group. A prospective multicenter study of adrenal function in critically ill children. *Am J Respir Crit Care Med.* 2010;15; 182:246–251.

84 Henzen C, Kobza R, Schwaller-Protzmann B, Stulz P, Briner VA. Adrenal function during coronary artery bypass grafting. *Eur J Endocrinol.* 2003;148:663–668.

85 Vassiliadi DA, Dimopoulou I, Tzanela M, et al. Longitudinal assessment of adrenal function in the early and prolonged phases of critical illness in septic patients: relations to cytokine levels and outcome. *J Clin Endocrinol Metab.* 2014;99: 4471–4480.

86 de Jong MF, Beishuizen A, van Schijndel RJ, Girbes AR, Groeneveld AB. Risk factors and outcome of changes in adrenal response to ACTH in the course of critical illness. *J Intensive Care Med.* 2012;27:37–44.

87 Perry LA, Grossman AB. The role of the laboratory in the diagnosis of Cushing's syndrome. *Ann Clin Biochem.* 1997;34:345–359.

88 Trainer PJ, Grossman AB. The diagnosis and differential diagnosis of Cushing's syndrome. *Clin Endocrinol.* 1991;34:317–330.

89 Aron DC, Tyrell, LB, Fitzgerald PA, Findling JW, Forsham PH Cushing's syndrome, problems in diagnosis. *Medicine.* 1981;60:25–35.

90 von Werder K, Muller OA. Cushing's syndrome. In: Grossman A, ed. *Clinical Endocrinology, 1st ed.* Oxford: Blackwell Scientific Publications; 1992: 445.

91 Ross RJM, Miell JP, Holly JMP, et al. Levels of GH binding activity, IGFBP-I, insulin, blood glucose and cortisol in intensive care patients. *Clin Endocrinol.* 1991;35:361–367.

92 Besser GM, Edwards CRW. Cushing's syndrome. *Clin Endocrinol Metab.* 1972;1:451–490.

93 James VHT, Landon JL, Wynn V, Greenwood FE. A fundamental defect of adrenocortical control in Cushing's disease. *J Endocrinol.* 1968;40:15–28.

94 Hamrahian AH, Oseni TS, Arafah BM. Measurements of serum free cortisol in critically ill patients. *N Engl J Med.* 2004;350:1629–1638.

95 Moisey R, Wright D, Aye M, Murphy E, Peacey SR. Interpretation of the short Synacthen test in the presence of low cortisol-binding globulin: two case reports. *Ann Clin Biochem.* 2006;43: 416–419.

96 Fede G, Spadaro L, Tomaselli T. Adrenocortical dysfunction in liver disease: a systematic review. *Hepatology.* 2012;55:1282–1291.

97 El-Farhan N, Pickett A, Ducroq D, et al. Method-specific serum cortisol responses to the adrenocorticotrophin test: comparison of gas chromatography-mass spectrometry and five automated immunoassays. *Clin Endocrinol.* 2013;78: 673–680.

98 Clark PM, Neylon I, Raggatt PR, Sheppard MC, Stewart PM. Defining the normal cortisol response to the short Synacthen test: implications for the investigation of hypothalamic-pituitary disorders. *Clin Endocrinol.* 1998;49:287–292.

99 Briegel J, Sprung CL, Annane D, et al. Multicenter comparison of cortisol as measured by different methods in samples of patients with septic shock. *Intensive Care Med.* 2009;35:2151–2156.

100 Pacak K. Phaeochromocytoma: a catecholamine and oxidative stress disorder. *Endocr Regul.* 2011;45:65–90.

101 Roden M. How to detect pheochromocytomas? The diagnostic relevance of plasma free metanephrines. *Wien Klin Wochenschr.* 2002;114: 246–251.

102 Grouzmann E, Drouard-Troalen L, Baudin E, et al. Diagnostic accuracy of free and total metanephrines in plasma

and fractionated metanephrines in urine of patients with pheochromocytoma. *Eur J Endocrinol*. 2010;162:951–960.

103 Kim HJ, Lee JI, Cho YY, et al. Diagnostic accuracy of plasma free metanephrines in a seated position compared with 24-hour urinary metanephrines in the investigation of pheochromocytoma. *Endocr J*. 2015; 62:243–250.

104 Därr R, Pamporaki C, Peitzsch M, et al. Biochemical diagnosis of phaeochromocytoma using plasma-free normetanephrine, metanephrine and methoxytyramine: importance of supine sampling under fasting conditions. *Clin Endocrinol*. 2014;80:478–486.

105 Schmidt C, Kraft K. Beta-endorphin and catecholamine concentrations during chronic and acute stress in intensive care patients. *Eur J Med Res*. 1996;1:528–532.

106 Woolf PD, Hamill RW, Lee LA, McDonald JV. Free and total catecholamines in critical illness. *Am J Physiol*. 1988;254:E287–E291.

107 van Gulik L, Ahlers S, van Dijk M, et al. Procedural pain does not raise plasma levels of cortisol or catecholamines in adult intensive care patients after cardiac surgery. *Anaesth Intensive Care*. 2016; 44:52–56.

108 Kong KL, Willatts SM, Prys-Roberts C, Harvey JT, Gorman S. Plasma catecholamine concentration during sedation in ventilated patients requiring intensive therapy. *Intensive Care Med*. 1990;16:171–174.

109 Kassim TA, Clarke DD, Mai VQ, Clyde PW, Mohamed Shakir KM. Catecholamine-induced cardiomyopathy. *Endocrine Pract*. 2008;14:1137–1149.

110 Schifferdecker B, Kodali D, Hausner E, Aragam J. Adrenergic shock—an overlooked clinical entity? *Cardiology Rev*. 2005;13:69–72.

111 Steppan J, Shields J, Lebron R. Pheochromocytoma presenting as acute heart failure leading to cardiogenic shock and multiorgan failure. *Case Rep Med*. 2011; 2011:596354.

112 Prejbisz A, Lenders JW, Eisenhofer G, Januszewicz A. Cardiovascular manifestations of phaeochromocytoma. *J Hypertens*. 2011;29:2049–2060.

113 Scholten A, Cisco RM, Vriens MR, et al. 2013 Pheochromocytoma crisis is not a surgical emergency. *J Clin Endocrinol Metab*. 2013;98:581–591.

114 Rivier C, Rivier J, Vale W. Stress-induced inhibition of reproductive functions: role of endogenous corticotropin-releasing factor. *Science*. 1986;231:607–609.

115 Tsigos C, Papanicolaou DA, Kyrou I, Raptis SA, Chrousos GP. Dose-dependent effects of recombinant human interleukin-6 on the pituitary-testicular axis. *J Interferon Cytokine Res*. 1999;19: 1271–1276.

116 Mitchell M, Armstrong DT, Robker RL, Norman RJ. Adipokines: implications for female fertility and obesity. *Reproduction*. 2005;130:583–597.

117 Pasquali R, Vicennati V, Gambineri A. Adrenal and gonadal function in obesity. *J Endocrinol Invest*. 2002;25:893–898.

118 Fischer-Posovszky P, Wabitsch M, Hochberg Z. Endocrinology of adipose tissue: an update. *Horm Metab Res*. 2007;39:314–321.

119 Haffner SM. Sex hormones, obesity, fat distribution, type 2 diabetes and insulin resistance: epidemiological and clinical correlation. *Int J Obes Relat Metab Disord*. 2000;24,Suppl. 2:56–58.

120 Tchernof A, Després JP. Sex steroid hormones, sex hormone-binding globulin, and obesity in men and women. *Horm Metab Res*. 2000;32:526–536.

121 Dupont J, Pollet-Villard X, Reverchon M, Mellouk N, Levy R. Adipokines in human reproduction. *Horm Mol Biol Clin Invest*. 2015;24:11–24.

122 Yudkin JS. Inflammation, obesity, and the metabolic syndrome. *Horm Metab Res* 2007;39:707–709.

123 Goulis DG, Tarlatzis BC. Metabolic syndrome and reproduction: I. testicular function. *Gynecol Endocrinol*. 2008;24: 33–39.

124 Freedman DS, O'Brien TR, Flanbers WD, DeStefano F & Barboriak JJ. Relation of serum testosterone levels to high density lipoprotein cholesterol and other characteristics in men. *Arter Thromb Vasc Biol*. 1991;11:307–315.

125 Van Pottelbergh I, Braeckman L, De Bacquer D, De Backer G & Kaufman JM. Differential contribution of testosterone and estradiol in the determination of cholesterol and lipoprotein profile in healthy middle-aged men. *Atherosclerosis*. 2003;166:95–102.

126 Baker HW. Reproductive effects of nontesticular illness. *Endocrinol Metab Clin North Am*. 1998;27:831–850.

127 Toorians AW, Janssen E, Laan E, et al. Chronic renal failure and sexual functioning: clinical status versus objectively assessed sexual response. *Nephrol Dial Transp*. 1997;12:2654–2663.

128 Schaefer F, Veldhuis JD, Robertson WR, Dunger D, Schärer K, Cooperative Study Group on Pubertal Development in Chronic Renal Failure. Immunoreactive and bioactive luteinizing hormone in pubertal patients with chronic renal failure. *Kidney Intl*. 1994;45:1465–1476.

129 Dunkel L, Raivio T, Laine J, Holmberg C. Circulating luteinizing hormone receptor inhibitor(s) in boys with chronic renal failure. *Kidney Int*. 1997;51:777–784.

130 Ali ST, Shaikh RN, Ashfaqsiddiqi N, Siddiqi PQR. Serum and urinary levels of pituitary-gonadam hormones in insulin-dependent and non-insulin-dependent diabetic males with and without neuropathy. *Arch Androl*. 1993;30:117–123.

131 Handelsman Dj, Dong Q. Hypothalamo-pituitary gonadal axis in chronic renal failure. *Endocrinol Metab Clin N Am*. 1995;43:331–337.

132 Semple CG, Gray CE, Beastall GH. Androgen levels in men with diabetes mellitus. *Diab Med*. 1988;5:122–125.

133 Andersson B, Marin P, Lissner L, Vermeulen A, Björntorp P. Testosterone concentrations in women and men with NIDDM. *Diab Care*. 1994;17:405–411.

134 http://www.issam.ch/freetesto.htm

135 Vamvakopoulos NC, Chrousos GP. Evidence of direct estrogenic regulation of human corticotropin-releasing hormone gene expression: potential implications for the sexual dimophism of the stress response and immune/inflammatory reaction. *J Clin Invest*. 1993;92:1896–1902.

136 Vamvakopoulos NC, Chrousos GP. Hormonal regulation of human corticotropin-releasing hormone gene expression: implications for the stress response and immune/inflammatory reaction. *Endocr Rev*. 1994;15:409–420.

137 Chrousos GP, Torpy DJ, Gold PW. Interactions between the hypothalamic-pituitary-adrenal axis and the female reproductive system: clinical implications. *Ann Intern Med*. 1998;129:229–240.

138 Reame NE, Sauder SE, Case GD, Kelch RP, Marshall JC. Pulsatile gonadotropin secretion in women with hypothalamic amenorrhea: evidence that reduced frequency of gonadotropinreleasing hormone secretion is the mechanism of persistent anovulation. *J Clin Endocrinol Metab*. 1985;61:851–858.

139 Handelsman DJ. Hypothalamic-pituitary-gonadal dysfunction in renal failure, dialysis and renal transplantation. *Endocr Rev*. 1985;6:151–182.

140 Cano Sokoloff N, Misra M, Ackerman KE. Exercise, training, and the hypothalamic-pituitary-gonadal axis in men and women. *Front Horm Res*. 2016;47:27–43.

141 MacConnie SE, Barkan A, Lampman RM, Schork MA, Beitins IZ. Decreased hypothalamic gonadotropinreleasing hormone secretion in male marathon runners. *N Engl J Med*. 1986; 15:411–417.

142 Mantzoros C, Flier JS, Lesem MD, Brewerton TD, Jimerson DC. Cerebrospinal fluid leptin in anorexia nervosa: correlation with nutritional status and potential role in resistance to weight gain. *J Clin Endocrinol Metab*. 1997;82:1845–1851.

143 Kopp W, Blum WF, von Prittwitz S, et al. Low leptin levels predict amenorrhea in underweight and eating disordered females. *Molec Psych*. 1997;2:335–340.

144 Audi L, Mantzoros CS, Vidal-Puig A, Vargas D, Gussinye M, Carrascosa A. Leptin in relation to resumption of menses in women with anorexia nervosa. *Molec Psych*. 1998;3:544–547.

145 Young EA, Korszun A. The hypothalamic-pituitary-gonadal axis in mood disorders. *Endocrinol Metab Clin North Am*. 2002;31 63–78.

146 Jørgensen JO, Møller L, Krag M, Billestrup N, Christiansen JS. Effects of growth hormone on glucose and fat metabolism in human subjects. *Endocrinol Metab Clin. North Am*. 2007;36:75–87.

147 Steyn FJ, Tolle V, Chen C, Epelbaum J. Neuroendocrine Regulation of Growth Hormone Secretion. *Compr Physiol*. 2016;6:687–735.

148 Khatib N, Gaidhane S, Gaidhane AM, et al. Ghrelin: ghrelin as a regulatory Peptide in growth hormone secretion. *J Clin Diagn Res*. 2014;8:MC13–MC17.

149 Ibáñez-Costa A, Luque RM, Castaño JP. Cortistatin: a new link between the growth hormone/prolactin axis, stress, and metabolism. *Growth Horm IGF Res*. 2017;33: 23–27.

150 Mazziotti G, Giustina A. Glucocorticoids and the regulation of growth hormone secretion. *Nat Rev Endocrinol*. 2013;9: 265–276.

151 Jørgensen JO, Møller N, Lauritzen T, Christiansen JS. Pulsatile versus continuous intravenous administration of growth hormone (GH) in GH-deficient patients: effects on circulating insulin-like growth factor-I and metabolic indices. *J Clin Endocrinol Metab*. 1990;70:1618–1623.

152 Schilbach K, Bidlingmaier M. Growth hormone binding protein – physiological and analytical aspects. *Best Pract Res Clin Endocrinol Metab*. 2015;29:671–683.

153 Mullis PE, Wagner JK, Eblé A, Nuoffer JM, Postel-Vinay MC. Regulation of human growth hormone receptor gene transcription by human growth hormone binding protein. *Mol Cell Endocrinol*. 1997;131:89–96.

154 Fryburg DA, Barrett EJ. Growth hormone acutely stimulates skeletal muscle but not whole-body protein synthesis in humans. *Metabolism*. 1993;42:1223–1227.

155 Buijs MM, Romijn JA, Burggraaf J, et al. Growth hormone blunts protein oxidation and promotes protein turnover to a similar extent in abdominally obese and normal-weight women. *J Clin Endocrinol Metab*. 2002;87:5668–5674.

156 Fryburg DA. Insulin-like growth factor I exerts growth hormone- and insulin-like actions on human muscle protein metabolism. *Am J Physiol*. 1994;267: E331–E336.

157 Sjögren K, Leung KC, Kaplan W, Gardiner-Garden M, Gibney J, Ho KK. Growth hormone regulation of metabolic gene expression in muscle: a microarray study in hypopituitary men. *Am J Physiol Endocrinol Metab*. 2007;293:E364–E371.

158 Thissen JP, Underwood LE, Ketelslegers JM. Regulation of insulin-like growth factor-I in starvation and injury. *Nutr Rev*. 1999;57(6):167–176.

159 Ketelslegers JM, Maiter D, Maes M, Underwood LE, Thissen JP. Nutritional regulation of insulin-like growth factor-I. *Metabolism*. 1995;44;Suppl 4:50–57.

160 Kaytor EN, Zhu JL, Pao CI, Phillips LS. Insulin-responsive nuclear proteins facilitate Sp1 interactions with the insulin-like growth factor-I gene. *J Biol Chem*. 2001;276: 36896–36901.

161 Merimee TJ, Zapf J, Froesch ER. Insulin-like growth factors in the fed and fasted states. *J Clin Endocrinol Metab*. 1982;55:999–1002.

162 Miell JP, Taylor AM, Zini M, Maheshwari HG, Ross RJ, Valcavi R. Effects of hypothyroidism and hyperthyroidism on insulin-like growth factors (IGFs) and growth hormone- and IGF-binding proteins. *J Clin Endocrinol Metab*. 1993;76:950–955.

163 Westermark K, Alm J, Skottner A, Karlsson A. Growth factors and the

thyroid: effects of treatment for hyper- and hypothyroidism on serum IGF-I and urinary epidermal growth factor concentrations. *Acta Endocrinol*. 1988; 118:415–421.

164 Ross R, Miell J, Freeman E, et al. Critically ill patients have high basal growth hormone levels with attenuated oscillatory activity associated with low levels of insulin-like growth factor-I. *Clin Endocrinol*. 1991;35:47–54.

165 Hartman ML, Veldhuis JD, Johnson ML, et al. Augmented growth hormone (GH) secretory burst frequency and amplitude mediate enhanced GH secretion during a two-day fast in normal men. *J Clin Endocrinol Metab*. 1992;74:757–765.

166 Baxter RC, Hawker FH, To C, Stewart PM, Holman SR. Thirty-day monitoring of insulin-like growth factors and their binding proteins in intensive care unit patients. *Growth Horm IGF Res*. 1998; 8:455–463.

167 Hermansson M, Wickelgren RB, Hammarqvist F, et al. Measurement of human growth hormone receptor messenger ribonucleic acid by a quantitative polymerase chain reaction-based assay: demonstration of reduced expression after elective surgery. *J Clin Endocrinol Metab*. 1997;82: 421–428.

168 Timmins AC, Cotterill AM, Hughes et al. Critical illness is associated with low circulating concentrations of insulin-like growth factors-I and -II, alterations in insulin-like growth factor binding proteins, and induction of an insulin-like growth factor binding protein 3 protease. *Crit Care Med*. 1996;24:1460–1466.

169 Nedelec B, de Oliveira A, Garrel DR. Acute phase modulation of systemic insulin-like growth factor-1 and its binding proteins after major burn injuries. *Crit Care Med*. 2003;31:1794–1801.

170 Van den Berghe G, de Zegher F, Lauwers P, Veldhuis JD. Growth hormone secretion in critical illness: effect of dopamine. *J Clin Endocrinol Metab*. 1994;79:1141–1146.

171 Van den Berghe G, de Zegher F, Veldhuis JD, et al. The somatotropic axis in critical illness: effect of continuous growth hormone (GH)-releasing hormone and GH-releasing peptide-2 infusion. *J Clin Endocrinol Metab*. 1997;82:590–599.

172 Baxter RC. Changes in the IGF-I/GFBP axis in critical illness. *Best Pract Res Clin Endocrinol Metab*. 2001;15:421–434.

173 Ding H, Kharboutli M, Saxena R, Wu T. Insulin-like growth factor binding protein-2 as a novel biomarker for disease activity and renal pathology changes in lupus nephritis. *Clin Exp Immunol*. 2016;184:11–18.

174 van den Beld AW, Blum WF, Brugts MP, Janssen JA, Grobbee DE, Lamberts SW. High IGFBP2 levels are not only associated with a better metabolic risk profile but also with increased mortality in elderly men. *Eur J Endocrinol*. 2012; 167:111–117.

175 Goldstone AP, Unmehopa UA, Swaab DF. Hypothalamic growth hormone-releasing hormone (GHRH) cell number is increased in human illness, but is not reduced in Prader-Willi syndrome or obesity. *Clin Endocrinol*. 2003;58: 743–755. Erratum in *Clin Endocrinol*. 2003;59:266.

176 Papanicolaou DA, Wilder RL, Manolagas SC, Chrousos GP. The pathophysiologic roles of interleukin-6 in human disease. *Ann Intern Med*. 1998;15;128: 127–137.

177 Cooney RN, Shumate M. The inhibitory effects of interleukin-1 on growth hormone action during catabolic illness. *Vitam Horm*. 2006;74:317–340.

178 Pittoni G, Gallioi G, Zanello M, et al. Activity of GH/IGF-I axis in trauma and septic patients during artificial nutrition: different behavior patterns? *J Endocrinol Invest*. 2002;25:214–223.

179 Gianotti L, Broglio F, Aimaretti G, et al. Low IGF-I levels are often uncoupled with elevated GH levels in catabolic conditions. *J Endocrinol Invest*. 1998;21:115–121.

180 Baue AE, Günther B, Hartl W, Ackenheil M, Heberer G. Altered hormonal activity

in severely ill patients after injury or sepsis. *Arch Surg.* 1984;119:1125–1132.

181 Van den Berghe G, Baxter RC, Weekers F, Wouters P, Bowers CY, Veldhuis JD. A paradoxical gender dissociation within the growth hormone/insulin-like growth factor I axis during protracted critical illness. *J Clin Endocrinol Metab.* 2000;85: 183–192.

182 Takala J, Ruokonen E, Webster NR, et al. Increased mortality associated with growth hormone treatment in critically ill adults. *N Engl J Med.* 1999;341:785–792.

183 Moro JR, Iwata M, von Andriano UH. Vitamin effects on the immune system: vitamins A and D take centre stage. *Nat Rev Immunol.* 2008;8:685–698.

184 Rammos G, Tseke P, Ziakka S. Vitamin D, the renin-angiotensin system, and insulin resistance. *Int Urol Nephrol.* 2008;40: 419–426.

185 Danescu LG, Levy S, Levy J. Vitamin D and diabetes mellitus. *Endocrine.* 2009;35: 11–17.

186 Artaza JN, Mehrotra R, Norris KC. Vitamin D and the cardiovascular system. *Clin J Am Soc Nephrol.* 2009;4:1515–1522.

187 Tuohimaa P, et al. Vitamin D, nervous system and aging. *Psychoneuroendocrinology.* 2009;34(Suppl 1):S278–S286.

188 Peterlik M, Grant WB, Cross HS. Calcium, vitamin D and cancer. *Anticancer Res.* 2009;29:3687–3698.

189 Zittermann A, Gummert JF. Borgermann J. Vitamin D deficiency and mortality. *Curr Opin Clin Nutr Metab Care.* 2009; 12:634–639.

190 Lee P, Eisman JA, Center JR. Vitamin D deficiency in critically ill patients. *N Engl J Med.* 2009;360:1912–1914.

191 Ford L, Graham V, Wall A, Berg J. Vitamin D concentrations in an UK inner-city multicultural outpatient population. *Ann Clin Biochem.* 2006;43:468–473.

192 MacFarlane GD, Sackrison JL Jr, Body JJ, Ersfeld DL, Fenske JS, Miller ABHypovitaminosis D in a normal,

apparently healthy urban European population. *J Steroid Biochem Mol Biol.* 2004;89–90:621–622.

193 Furmaniak-Kazmierczak E, Nesheim ME, Côté GP. Coagulation factor Va is an actin filament binding and cross-linking protein. *Biochem Cell Biol.* 1995;73: 105–112.

194 Lee WM, Galbraith RM. The extracellular actin-scavenger system and actin toxicity. *N Engl J Med.* 1992;326:1335–1341.

195 Meier U, Gressner O, Lammert F, Gressner AM. Gc-globulin: Roles in response to injury. *Clin Chem.* 2006;52: 1247–1253.

196 Reid D, Toole BJ, Knox S, et al. The relation between acute changes in the systemic inflammatory response and plasma 25-hydroxyvitamin D concentrations after elective knee arthroplasty. *Am J Clin Nutr.* 2011;93: 1006–1111.

197 Waldron JL, Ashby HL, Cornes MP, et al. Vitamin D: a negative acute phase reactant. *J Clin Path.* 2013:66:620–622.

198 Lee JH, Gadi R, Spertus JA, Tang F, O'Keefe JH. Prevalence of vitamin D deficiency in patients with acute myocardial infarction. *Am J Cardiol.* 2011;107:1636–1638.

199 Barth JH, Field HP, Mather AN, Plein S. Serum 25 hydroxy-vitamin D does not exhibit an acute phase reaction after acute myocardial infarction. *Ann Clin Biochem.* 2012;49:399–401.

200 Jeng L, Yamshchikov AV, Judd SE, et al. Alterations in vitamin D status and anti-microbial peptide levels in patients in intensive care unit with sepsis. *J Transl Med.* 2009;7:28–36.

201 Prasad S, Raj D, Warsi S, Chowdhary S. Vitamin D deficiency and critical illness. *Indian J Pediatr.* 2015;82:991–995.

202 Milazzo V, De Metrio M, Cosentino N, Marenzi G, Tremoli E. Vitamin D and acute myocardial infarction. *World J Cardiol.* 2017;9:14–20.

203 Naesgaard PA, León de la Fuente RA, et al. Suggested cut-off values for vitamin

d as a risk marker for total and cardiac death in patients with suspected acute coronary syndrome. *Front Cardiovasc Med.* 2016;3:4.

204 Cecchi A, Bonizzoli M, Douar S, et al. Vitamin D deficiency in septic patients at ICU admission is not a mortality predictor. *Minerva Anestesiol.* 2011;77: 1184–1189.

205 Grädel L, Merker M, Mueller B, Schuetz P. Screening and treatment of vitamin D deficiency on hospital admission: is there a benefit for medical inpatients? *Am J Med.* 2016;129:116.e1–116.e34.

206 Christopher KB. Vitamin D and critical illness outcomes. *Curr Opin Crit Care.* 2016;22:332–338.

207 Dahl B, Schiodt FV, Nielsen M, Kiaer T, Williams JG, Ott P. Admission levels of Gc-globulin predicts outcome after multiple trauma. *Injury.* 1999;30:275–281.

208 Schiodt FV, Bangert K, Shakil AO, et al., the Acute Liver Failure Study Group. Predictive value of actin-free Gc-globulin in acute liver failure. *Liver Transpl.* 2007;13:1324–1329.

209 Schiødt FV. Gc-globulin in liver disease. *Dan Med Bul.* 2008:55:131–146

3

Endocrine Responses to Critical Illness

Novel Insights and Therapeutic Implications

Jan Gunst, Eva Boonen, and Greet Van den Berghe

Key Points

- Critical illness is defined as any life-threatening condition requiring support of vital organ functions to prevent imminent death. This condition can be evoked by a variety of insults such as multiple trauma, complicated surgery, and severe medical illnesses.
- Critical illness, an extreme form of severe physical stress, is characterized by important endocrine and metabolic changes.
- The role of these endocrine and metabolic responses to acute and prolonged critical

  illness in mediating or hampering recovery remains highly debated.
- In recent years, important novel insights in the pathophysiology and the consequences of these endocrine responses to acute and chronic critical illness have been generated. Any therapeutic implications of these novel insights have important implications for the patient, and also for clinicians who are faced with many difficult challenges in this highly fluid clinical environment.

Introduction

Critical illness is defined as any life-threatening condition requiring support of vital organ functions to prevent imminent death. This condition can be evoked by a variety of insults, such as multiple trauma, complicated surgery, and severe medical illnesses. Without modern critical care medicine, critically ill patients would not survive. Critical illness is thus the ultimate form of severe physical stress and all the immediate biological responses that are evoked are expected to be of greater magnitude in critically ill patients. These immediate stress responses comprise many orchestrated endocrine adaptations that are presumably directed toward providing the required energy for the "fight or flight" response in a context of exogenous substrate deprivation. Indeed, alterations within the different hypothalamic-pituitary axes bring about lipolysis, proteolysis, and gluconeogenesis and redirect energy consumption toward those processes that mediate acute survival, while anabolism is postponed to more prosperous times.

Although survival from previously lethal conditions is nowadays possible, often recovery does not swiftly follow and patients enter a chronic phase of critical illness during which they continue to depend upon vital

---

organ support for weeks, while the original trigger of the critical illness has long been resolved. This stage is characterized by distinct endocrine and metabolic alterations, which may no longer be solely beneficial as they may hamper recovery. An example is the relative maintenance of fat stores, while large amounts of proteins continue to be wasted from skeletal muscle and organs (1). This response may impair recovery of vital organ functions, extend weakness and hamper rehabilitation (2) and expose patients to severe, often infectious, complications (3). The understanding of the mechanisms determining why certain patients recover and others do not remains very limited, but recent studies point to variable abilities to remove cell damage as playing a key role (4,5). When patients remain dependent upon critical care support, it is ultimately decided to withdraw care because of futility. Hence, further understanding of the underlying pathways of recovery and investigation of whether these pathways can be beneficially affected by treatment are of high clinical relevance.

In recent years, important novel insights in the pathophysiology and the consequences of these endocrine responses to critical illness have been generated. This chapter summarizes these insights with a specific focus on the hypothalamic-pituitary-thyroid axis, the hypothalamic-pituitary-adrenal axis, and on the impact of the hyperglycemic response on recovery from critical illness. The therapeutic implications of these novel insights are critically analyzed.

Hypothalamic-Pituitary-Thyroid Axis

Responses within the Hypothalamic-Pituitary-Thyroid Axis during Acute Critical Illness

It has long been known that both fasting and acute illnesses immediately affect the circulating levels of thyroid hormones. Most typically, plasma concentrations of triiodothyronine (T_3) decrease and plasma concentrations of reverse T_3 (rT_3) rise, suggesting an immediate inactivation of thyroid hormone in peripheral tissues such as the liver, likely mediated by a suppressed activity of the type-1 deiodinase (D1) and/or an activated type-3 deiodinase (D3) (6,7). Concentrations of thyroxine (T_4) and thyroid-stimulating hormone (TSH) have been shown to be briefly increased immediately after surgery (7). Thereafter, plasma TSH and T_4 concentrations often return to "normal," although a normal nocturnal TSH surge is absent (8,9). This constellation of low plasma T_3 concentrations and elevated rT_3 is generally referred to as the *acute low-T_3 syndrome*, the *euthyroid-sick syndrome* or the *non-thyroidal illness syndrome* (Figure 3-1).

Several possible mediators of the acute fall in plasma T_3 concentrations in critically ill patients include the lack of nutrients or the release of cytokines or hypoxia (10–12). Tumor necrosis factor-alpha, interleukin-1, and interleukin-6 are capable of mimicking the acute stress-induced alterations within the thyroid axis. However, neutralizing antibodies to these cytokines in a human experiment of LPS-induced inflammation failed to restore normal thyroid hormone concentrations (13). Acute decreases in plasma concentrations of thyroid hormone binding proteins and the inhibition of hormone binding, transport and metabolism by elevated levels of free fatty acids and bilirubin may also play a role (14).

The low T_3 concentrations that occur with fasting have been shown to be adaptive, as they appear to protect the organism against the deleterious catabolic consequences of lack of macronutrients (15,16). In critical illness, it was suggested that the low T_3 concentrations could be maladaptive, since the magnitude of the acute T_3 decrease was associated with the severity of illness and with the risk of death (17,18). However, the acute fall in circulating levels of thyroid hormone in response to illness could also be an adaptive attempt to reduce energy expenditure, as happens with fasting in healthy subjects, in which case, it should be left untreated (15). Improved postoperative cardiac function

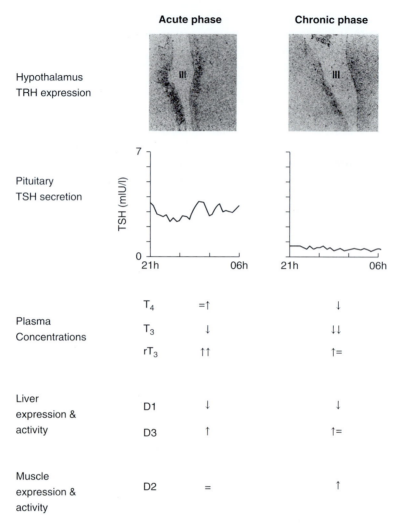

Figure 3-1 Changes in the central and peripheral thyroid axis in acute versus prolonged critical illness. The upper panel shows reduced TRH gene expression in the hypothalamus of prolonged ill patients. The central panel illustrates adaptations in nocturnal TSH secretion with a loss of pulsatility during prolonged critical illness. The bottom panel summarizes schematically the changes in circulating thyroid hormone concentrations and changes in peripheral deiodinase enzyme activity levels. Adapted from (26,47,143,144). D1 = type-1 deiodinase, D2 = type-2 deiodinase, D3 = type-3 deiodinase.

was observed after short-term intravenous (IV) administration of T_3 to patients during elective cardiac surgery (19,20). However, supranormal plasma T_3 concentrations were evoked, and thus it is uncertain whether these findings were merely due to a pharmacological effect. More recently, the results of a large randomized controlled trial (RCT), investigating the impact of early parenteral nutrition as compared with tolerating pronounced caloric deficit in critically ill patients, provided indirect evidence for an adaptive nature of the low T_3 levels (21,22). This study revealed that providing nutrition in the acute phase of critical illness impaired rather than improved outcome. The provision of macronutrients partially prevented the acute thyroid hormone changes, which was also observed in a rabbit model of critical illness (23). In the clinical study, specifically the rise in T_3 and in the ratio of T_3 over rT_3 with early forceful feeding statistically explained the worsening of the outcome (22). These data therefore suggest that at least part of the acute fall in T_3 concentrations during critical illness is related to the concomitant fasting and that this part of the response is likely adaptive. Presumed benefits include the expected reduction in energy expenditure with low T_3 levels, or a direct effect of increased D3 activity locally in granulocytes which could optimize bacterial killing capacity (12,24).

Responses within the Hypothalamic-Pituitary-Thyroid Axis during Prolonged Critical Illness

However, when patients are treated in intensive care units (ICU) for several weeks, receiving full enteral and/or parenteral nutrition, the alterations within the thyroid axis appear different. In this phase of critical illness, low plasma T_3 concentrations now coincide with low T_4 concentrations and low-normal TSH concentrations in a single morning sample (25). Moreover, overnight repeated sampling revealed that the pulsatility of TSH secretion is virtually lost, which relates to low plasma thyroid hormone levels, a presentation resembling central hypothyroidism (Figure 3-1) (25). In line with this interpretation, Fliers and colleagues (26) demonstrated in postmortem brain samples of chronic critically ill patients, that the gene expression of thyrotropin releasing hormone (TRH) in the hypothalamic paraventricular nuclei was much lower than in patients who died after acute insults (Figure 3-1). Furthermore, a positive correlation was observed between the TRH mRNA expression and the plasma concentrations of TSH and T_3. Together, these data indicate that production and/or release of thyroid hormones is reduced in prolonged critical illness due to reduced hypothalamic stimulation of

the thyrotropes, in turn leading to reduced stimulation of the thyroid gland. The observation that a rise in TSH levels precedes the onset of recovery from severe illness further supports this interpretation (27).

The factors triggering hypothalamic suppression during prolonged critical illness are unknown. Since plasma cytokine concentrations are usually much lower in the prolonged phase of critical illness (28), other mechanisms likely play a role, such as endogenous dopamine or elevated cortisol levels in the hypothalamus, as exogenous dopamine and hydrocortisone are known to provoke or aggravate hypothyroidism in critical illness (29–31). A local increase in type-2 deiodinase (D2) activity in the hypothalamus could elevate local thyroid hormone levels, whereby the set point for feedback inhibition could be altered (32). Indeed, in a rabbit model of prolonged critical illness and low thyroid hormone plasma concentrations, hypothalamic TRH mRNA was low and D2 mRNA was high. However, the hypothalamic T_4 and T_3 concentrations were not increased (33). Increased pituitary D2 could also play a role in suppressing local TSH mRNA (34), although this was not confirmed in an animal model of prolonged critical illness (35).

During prolonged critical illness, peripheral tissues seem to respond to low T_3 levels to increase local hormone availability and effects. For example, in skeletal muscle and liver biopsies from prolonged critically ill patients, the monocarboxylate transporter MCT-8 was over-expressed (Figure 3-2) (36). This was confirmed in an animal model, where the upregulation of the monocarboxylate transporters in liver and kidney was reversable by treatment with thyroid hormones (36,37). Also, in skeletal muscle biopsies from prolonged critically ill patients, D2 expression and activity were upregulated as compared with healthy controls and with acutely ill patients (Figure 3-1) (37). Upregulation of D2 in lungs was found to be adaptive in sepsis and acute lung injury, further accentuated by the observation that a D2 polymorphism was associated with less sepsis

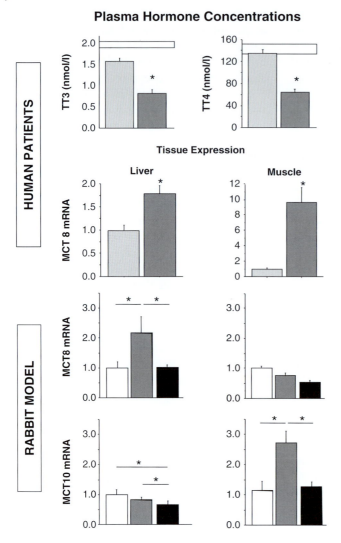

Figure 3-2 The upper panel represents the circulating thyroid hormone parameters in acutely stressed (light gray bars, n = 22) and chronically ill patients (dark gray bars, n = 64). The white bars designate the normal ranges. The central panel shows the relative *MCT8* mRNA expression levels measured in liver and skeletal muscle of acutely stressed (light gray) and chronically ill (dark gray) patients. The lower panels represents the relative expression levels of *MCT8* and *MCT10* in liver and muscle of healthy control rabbits (white bar), saline-treated prolonged ill rabbits (dark gray), and $T_3 + T_4$ treated (black bar) ill rabbits. Data are expressed as mean $\pm$ SEM. *$P < 0.05$ versus acute values. Adapted from (36). Reproduced with permission of European Society of Endocrinology.

susceptibility (38). At the level of the thyroid hormone receptor (TR), an inverse correlation was observed between the active TR-1/inactiveTR-2 ratio, a surrogate marker of thyroid hormone sensitivity, and the ratio of T_3/rT_3 in liver biopsies of prolonged critically ill patients (39). Together, the data suggest that when the production of thyroid hormones falls in prolonged critical illness, peripheral tissues adapt by increasing thyroid hormone transporters, local activation of thyroid hormone and gene expression of the active receptor isoform.

In protracted critical illness, low T_3 levels were found to correlate inversely with markers of muscle breakdown and of bone loss, which could indicate either an adaptive and protective response against catabolism or a causal maladaptive relationship (40). As the cause of the low thyroid hormone levels during prolonged critical illness appears to be a suppressed TRH expression, whereby reduced thyroid hormone production, the question could be addressed by assessing the effect of TRH treatment. When patients were given a TRH-infusion, plasma T_3 and

T_4 could be increased, but also rT_3 concentrations rose (41). However, when TRH was combined with a growth hormone (GH)-secretagogue, this rise in rT_3 was prevented, explained by a GH-mediated effect on the inactivating D3 (42). This treatment also induced an anabolic response which suggested a causal relationship between low thyroid hormone levels and the impaired anabolism during prolonged critical illness (40). Furthermore, the negative feedback exerted by thyroid hormones on the thyrotropes was found to be maintained during TRH-infusion, a self-limitation which precludes overstimulation of the thyroid axis (41,43).

Diagnostic Implications

Taken the nature of the changes within the thyroid axis evoked by critical illness, the diagnosis of pre-existing thyroid disease during critical illness is very difficult. Patients with preexisting primary hypothyroidism are expected to reveal low serum levels of T_4 and T_3 in combination with high TSH concentrations. However, when primary hypothyroidism and severe non-thyroidal critical illness coincide, TSH levels may be lower than anticipated. Moreover, serum TSH may be paradoxically low because of iatrogenic factors such as iodine wound dressings, iodine-containing contrast agents and drugs such as high-dose corticosteroids, dopamine, somatostatin analogues, and amiodarone (30,44). So, a normal or low TSH during critical illness does not exclude primary hypothyroidism. Also, the low T_4 and T_3 levels in patients with severe hypothyroidism can be indistinguishable from those values observed in prolonged nonthyroidal critical illness. A high ratio of T_3/T_4 in serum, a low thyroid hormone-binding ratio, and a low serum rT_3 may favor the presence of primary hypothyroidism. However, the diagnostic accuracy is limited. In these patients, history, physical examination, and the possible presence of thyroid auto-antibodies may give further clues to the presence of thyroid disease. Repeated thyroid function tests after improvement of the non-thyroidal illness are required to confirm the diagnosis.

Elevated plasma T4 and T3 concentrations are so unusual during critical illness that they should always raise concern of pre-existing hyperthyroidism. However, undetectable TSH has no diagnostic value for hyperthyroidism during critical illness.

Therapeutic Implications

As the available evidence now indicates that the acute "low T_3 syndrome" appears to be an adaptive response partially explained by fasting, treatment is likely not indicated (22,23). In contrast, the low T_4 and T_3 levels during the prolonged phase of critical illness could be maladaptive. Experimental studies showed that in animal models of prolonged critical illness and in prolonged critically ill patients who are receiving nutrition, the syndrome can be reversed via hypothalamic-releasing factors, with an anabolic response at the tissue level (40). However, the effect on clinical outcome of such a treatment remains to be investigated, so therapeutic implications are currently lacking. A theoretical advantage of such treatment is the lack of suppression of negative feedback inhibition on the pituitary gland by thyroid hormones, which may prevent overstimulation of the pituitary-thyroid axis.

An alternative option for treatment could be the administration of thyroid hormones T_4 or T_3 or the combination to normalize the plasma concentrations. In animal studies, substitution doses of T_4, T_3 or their combination were unable to alter circulating levels of thyroid hormones, likely explained by the increased metabolism of thyroid hormones during critical illness, perhaps in part mediated by sulfoconjugation as was also shown in patients (45–48). Three times the substitution dose of T_4 normalized plasma T_3 concentrations in this model but resulted in supranormal T_4 levels and a rise in rT_3. A dose of T_3 that was able to normalize the plasma T_3 concentrations, five times the substitution dose, suppressed TSH and T_4 to subnormal levels via negative feedback inhibition. A combination of these doses of T_4 and T_3 resulted in dramatic overtreatment. Similar dosing issues were present in the few available small randomized studies in critically ill patients, which also did not show outcome benefits (49–52).

It also remains controversial when and how to treat primary hypothyroidism during critical illness. When patients were receiving active treatment for hypothyroidism before critical illness, it seems wise to continue their usual dose of thyroid hormone. For myxedema coma, it is generally accepted that patients should be treated with parenteral infusion of thyroid hormones. However, the proper initiation of replacement therapy during other types of critical illnesses remains controversial. There is no consensus on the type of thyroid hormone nor on the optimal initial dose for replacement therapy. Many clinicians prefer a high IV loading dose of 300–500 µg of T_4 to reach quickly 50% of the euthyroid value of T_4 (53–55), followed by 50–100 µg of IV T_4 daily until oral medication can be given. Some authors have suggested the use of a co-infusion of the biologically active form T_3 and T_4. Morreale de Escobar and colleagues (56) showed in an animal study that T_4 alone did not ensure euthyroidism in all tissues, which was achieved by combined treatment with T_4 and T_3. An experimental protocol for thyroid hormone therapy during prolonged intensive care of presumed hypothyroidism advises administering a 100–200 µg bolus of IV T_4 per 24 hours alone or, when required to also increase plasma T_3, combined with T_3 at 0.6 µg/kg ideal body weight per 24 hours in a continuous IV infusion, targeting serum thyroid hormone levels in the low-normal range (57). When the patients start to recover, the prompt tapering of this dose may be required.

The treatment for primary hyperthyroidism is less affected by concomitant critical illness, except that treatment requirements could be lower in the presence of increased thyroid hormone metabolism. Furthermore, when patients were receiving active treatment for hyperthyroidism, they should be monitored because of potential toxicity of the medication and the impact of other frequently used medication on thyroid hormone levels.

Hypothalamic-Pituitary-Adrenal Axis

Responses within the Hypothalamic-Pituitary-Adrenal Axis during Acute and Prolonged Critical Illness

The stress hormone cortisol is an essential component of the "fight or flight" reaction to the stress of illness and trauma, and both very high and low cortisol levels have been associated with risk of death in such patients (58). Whenever the brain senses a stressful event, activation of the hypothalamic-pituitary-adrenal (HPA) axis initiates the release of the corticotropin-releasing hormone (CRH) and arginine vasopressin (AVP) from the hypothalamus which stimulates the anterior pituitary corticotrophs to secrete adrenocorticotropic hormone (ACTH). High cortisol levels during critical illness likely contribute to the provision of extra energy to vital organs by acutely shifting carbohydrate, fat and protein metabolism and by delaying anabolism. Moreover, cortisol likely affects the hemodynamic system by intravascular fluid retention and by enhancing inotropic and vasopressor responses to respectively catecholamines and angiotensin II. In addition, the anti-inflammatory effects of cortisol can be interpreted as an attempt to prevent over-activation of the inflammatory cascade (59,60).

During critical illness, plasma cortisol concentrations are substantially elevated, traditionally explained by several-fold elevated cortisol production in the adrenal cortex driven by ACTH. However, Vermes et al. reported only transiently elevated ACTH concentrations in patients with multiple trauma or sepsis, whereas cortisol concentrations remained high (61). This was confirmed in a more heterogeneous critically ill patient population. In this study, plasma ACTH concentrations were found to be suppressed already from admission to the ICU onward and stayed below the lower limit of normality throughout the first week of critical illness (62). Whether the expected initial ACTH rise in response to stress was missed in this study and had already occurred before ICU admission, for example, in the operating room or emergency department, remains unknown.

Low plasma ACTH in the presence of high plasma cortisol concentrations has been interpreted as non-ACTH-driven cortisol production, among which cytokines could play a role (61,63). Alternatively, this constellation could be caused by reduced cortisol breakdown suppressing the production of adrenocortical hormones via feedback inhibition. In fact, direct evidence of increased cortisol production during critical illness has been lacking. Recent work that used a state-of-the-art cortisol-tracer technique showed that daytime cortisol production during critical illness was only slightly higher than in healthy subjects. Furthermore, cortisol production was only increased in patients with excessive inflammation while it was unaltered in other critically ill patients (Figure 3-3) (62). Cortisol breakdown, on the other hand, was substantially reduced, irrespective of the inflammatory status, attributable to suppressed expression and activity of A-ring reductases in the liver and by suppressed activity of 11β-hydroxysteroid

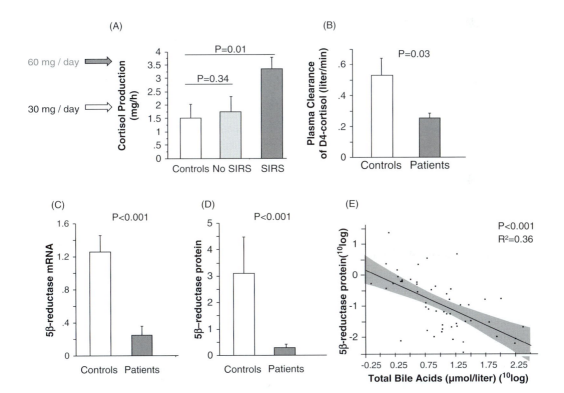

Figure 3-3 Panel A depicts cortisol production in critically ill patients with the systemic inflammatory response syndrome (SIRS) (n = 7; dark gray bar) and no systemic inflammatory response syndrome (n = 4; light gray bar) compared to controls (n = 9; white bar) Based on these results, 24h cortisol production was estimated and depicted with the arrows. Panel B depicts cortisol plasma clearance as assessed with a small dose of deuterated-cortisol tracer. Bar charts represent means and standard errors. Panel C-E show mRNA and protein expression of 5β-reductase in liver of 20 controls (white bar) and 44 patients (gray bar) and the relation to plasma total bile acid concentrations. Bar charts represent means and standard errors. The mRNA data are expressed, normalized to GAPDH, as a fold difference from the mean of the controls. Protein data are expressed normalized for CK-18 protein expression, as a fold difference from the mean of the controls. Adapted from (62).

dehydrogenase type 2 in kidney (62). It remains unclear, however, what is driving the suppression of these enzymes, but an inverse correlation between elevated plasma concentrations of bile acids and the expression level of the A-ring reductases could point to bile acids playing a role (Figure 3-3) (62,64). Indeed, bile acids are potent inhibitors of the cortisol metabolizing enzymes, both via competitive inhibition and by suppression of gene and protein expression (65–67).

The concept of increasing the bioavailability of cortisol levels primarily in tissues that produce these enzymes and to a lesser extent in the circulation could be interpreted as a highly economic way to keep cortisol levels high without spending too much energy producing it. This concept is further supported by low plasma cortisol binding globulin levels in critical illness, causing increased levels of free cortisol, the biologically active form. Furthermore, as such cortisol is elevated locally in liver and kidney, where it is needed for an optimal fight or flight response, without an undue exposure of immune cells and vulnerable target tissues such as skeletal muscle or brain to the deleterious side effects of hypercortisolism. The local effects of cortisol appear to be further regulated at the level of glucocorticoid receptor (GR) expression. Previous work indeed showed suppressed expression of GR in white blood cells of critically ill children, which could be a way to allow the innate immune response to effectively protect the host against infections in the presence of hypercortisolism (68). Clearly, this novel concept of tissue-specific regulation of glucocorticoid activity during critical illness requires further investigation.

The new insight that during critical illness cortisol metabolism is suppressed, contributing to hypercortisolism, could also explain the concomitantly low plasma ACTH concentrations, via negative feedback inhibition at the level of the pituitary gland and/or the hypothalamus. This is supported by a detailed study of nocturnal ACTH and cortisol secretory profiles, which revealed a suppressed nocturnal pulsatile ACTH and cortisol secretion in the presence of hypercortisolemia, albeit with an unaltered cortisol secretory response to any given ACTH concentration (69). Such sustained suppressed ACTH secretion could cause adrenal atrophy in the prolonged phase of critical illness. Recently, a study of adrenal cortex biopsies revealed a profound depletion of cholesterol esters and a suppression of ACTH-regulated steroidogenic genes (70). Such risk of adrenal atrophy could explain the reported 20-fold higher incidence of symptomatic adrenal insufficiency in critically ill patients being treated in the ICU for more than 14 days (71). Other factors contributing to adrenal failure are also possible, such as endothelial dysfunction (72,73), although confirmatory human studies are lacking.

Diagnostic Implications

Since the last decade, reference has been made to "relative adrenal insufficiency" in the context of critical illness (74–76). It refers to the condition in which, despite a maximally ACTH-activated adrenal cortex in response to critical illness, the cortisol production is still insufficient to generate enough glucocorticoid and mineralocorticoid receptor activation to maintain hemodynamic stability. From large association studies, such a condition is thought to be identifiable by an insufficient rise (< 9 µg/dL [250 nmol/L]) in plasma cortisol in response to a 250 µg ACTH bolus, irrespective of the baseline plasma cortisol concentration, which is usually much higher than in healthy humans (74). In such a condition of insufficiently increased cortisol production, a very high plasma ACTH concentration would be expected. However, the recent robust findings that ACTH plasma concentrations are suppressed, that cortisol production is not much elevated, if at all, and that instead reduced cortisol breakdown plays a major role during critical illness, further complicate the issue of diagnostic criteria for adrenal failure in that setting. Moreover, it was recently shown that cortisol responses to ACTH stimulation in critically ill patients correlated positively with both cortisol production rate and cortisol plasma clearance, but patients who revealed the lowest response to ACTH, to the extent of absolute adrenal failure, were the ones with the most suppressed cortisol breakdown, while their cortisol production was similar to healthy subjects (62). These findings hint that a low cortisol response to an ACTH injection reflects the degree of negative feedback inhibition exerted by the high levels of circulating cortisol, a situation similar to patients treated with exogenous glucocorticoids for an extended time, who also reveal a suppressed response to ACTH injection. Whether this low response during critical illness indicates that cortisol availability would be "insufficient" to cope with the stress of illness remains unclear.

Alternatively, a random total cortisol of < 10 µg/dL (275 nmol/L) during critical illness has been suggested for the diagnosis of "relative adrenal insufficiency" (77). However, total plasma cortisol concentration is the net effect of adrenal production and secretion, distribution, binding, and elimination of cortisol. Judging the adequacy of the adrenal cortisol production in response to critical illness based on a single measurement of total plasma cortisol is merely indicative. Furthermore, circulating total cortisol concentrations do not reveal the glucocorticoid effect. Since only free cortisol can pass the cell membrane to bind to GR and suppressed circulating levels of the binding proteins, cortisol-binding globulin (CBG) and albumin, as well as decreased CBG binding affinity via increased cleavage from CBG at inflammatory loci or by increased temperature, were established (78–81), plasma-free cortisol may be more appropriate to assess the HPA-axis function. However, more research is needed as plasma-free cortisol assays are not readily available and the normal ranges for plasma-free cortisol during critical illness have not been defined. Additionally, increasing evidence from both animal and human experiments suggests altered GR regulation during critical illness (68,82–86), precluding conclusions about the "adequacy" of cortisol availability

and function during illness. Finally, assays to quantify plasma cortisol concentrations are often inaccurate and vary substantially (87), making it impossible to identify one cut-off value for clinical practice. Recently, the Adrenal Scientific Committee of the American Association of Clinical Endocrinologists (AACE) proposed a diagnostic algorithm to diagnose adrenal insufficiency in critically ill patients, with different cut-offs depending on the blood albumin concentration and the presence or absence of septic shock (88). However, like other algorithms, this algorithm is insufficiently supported by clinical studies. Hopefully, ongoing studies will provide more answers (89).

Recently, measuring interstitial cortisol levels was introduced to assess the amount of active tissue cortisol levels in critically ill patients (90,91). Therefore, a microdialysis catheter is inserted into the subcutaneous adipose tissue. However, critical illness presents frequently with edema and regional blood flow is variable. Furthermore, the subcutaneous adipose tissue is not the main target tissue for cortisol, nor is it the main cortisol metabolizing organ during critical illness (62).

Therapeutic Implications

It is generally accepted that patients with an established diagnosis of primary or central adrenal failure or patients on chronic treatment with systemic glucocorticoids prior to critical illness, should receive additional coverage to cope with the acute stress (53,92). Also, patients who are diagnosed with an acute Addisonian crisis in the ICU are typically treated with high doses of glucocorticoids. This therapeutic strategy is based on the assumption that cortisol production is several-fold increased in critical illness. The conventional treatment proposes the administration of a bolus of 100 mg of hydrocortisone followed by 50–100 mg every 6 hours on the first day, 50 mg every 6 hours on the second day, and 25 mg every 6 hours on the third day, tapering to a maintenance dose by the fourth to fifth day (53,92). Currently, the

Endocrine Society Clinical Practice Guideline still recommends a high loading dose on the first day, but more rapid tapering. Initially, a bolus of 100 mg of hydrocortisone is recommended, followed by 200 mg/d for the first 24 hours and reduced to 100 mg/d on the following day (93).

The doses of hydrocortisone advised for treatment of "relative adrenal failure" is another controversial issue. The proposed dose of 200–300 mg of hydrocortisone per day, referred to as "low dose" in the literature, is approximately 6–10 times higher than the normal amount of daily cortisol production in healthy humans (94–97) and between 2- to 6-fold higher than the production which has been quantified in critically ill patients (Figure 3-3). In view of the substantially reduced cortisol breakdown during critical illness, the currently proposed doses for adrenal failure during critical illness may be too high. This may further explain why the multi-center RCTs which assessed the effect of hydrocortisone treatment during severe sepsis/septic shock could not confirm the benefit that was originally observed in the pilot study (94,97,98).

Also the duration of treatment is under debate. Treating critically ill patients with glucocorticoids in a too high dose for too long a time could inferentially aggravate the loss of lean tissue, increase the risk of myopathy and prolong the ICU dependence, which could increase the susceptibility to potentially lethal complications (99,100).

Finally, since glucocorticoid sensitivity likely varies among individuals (101) and among cell types in critically ill patients (68,83,85) and glucocorticoid treatment may downregulate GR-α via induction of miR-124, the dosing issue is further complicated (102). Moreover, single nucleotide polymorphisms in the GR gene, with an altered response to glucocorticoids, have been identified (103). However, it remains a challenge to identify specific clinical biomarkers of glucocorticoid receptor activation to guide optimal glucocorticoid therapy for individual patients and illnesses (i.e., precision or personalized medicine).

Based on the results of stable isotope studies (62), a dose of $+/-60$ mg of hydrocortisone, equivalent to about a doubling of the normal daily cortisol production, may be interesting to further investigate when patients at risk can be identified. A fast tapering down to the lowest effective dose should limit the adverse effects of excessive amounts of glucocorticoids during critical illness.

The Hyperglycemic Response to Critical Illness: To Treat or Not to Treat?

Blood Glucose and Critical Illness: Robust Associative Data

In humans, the natural endocrine and immunological responses to stress provoke hyperglycemia by activating gluconeogenesis and by reducing the sensitivity to insulin. Traditionally, this was considered to be an adaptive response, in order to increase glucose availability for organs and tissues that predominantly rely upon glucose as metabolic substrate, such as the brain and the blood cells. Numerous observational studies, however, have found a significant J-shaped association between blood glucose concentrations of critically ill patients and the risk of death (104–107). Repeatedly, in both critically ill children and adults, it was shown that the lowest mortality risk was associated with normal fasting blood glucose concentrations (Figure 3-4). In critically ill patients with established diabetes mellitus, the J-shaped curve is significantly blunted in the hyperglycemic zone and the nadir is slightly shifted to higher blood glucose concentrations (104–107).

Hyperglycemia and Adverse Outcome: Cause or Consequence?

An associational relationship, however, does not imply causality. Alternatively, high blood glucose concentrations could merely be a marker of illness severity, in itself harmless.

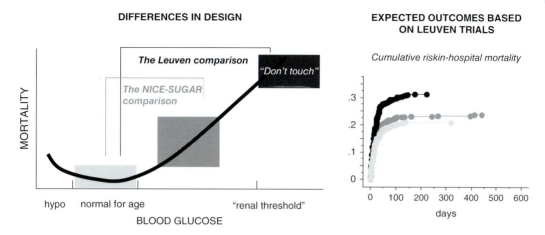

Figure 3-4 Different designs of key intervention trials and expected outcome benefits. The left panel shows J-shaped association curve between blood glucose and risk of death. The NICE–SUGAR trial was executed in the flatter part of the J-shaped curve. A very small benefit from aiming at lowering blood glucose further down from an intermediate level to strict normoglycemia was hereby traded off against a similar risk of harm by hypoglycemia, particularly when using inaccurate tools. The right panel shows the dose response in the two adult Leuven Trials compared to the NICE-SUGAR trial. Black circles represent blood glucose > 150 mg/dL (8.4 mmol/L), dark gray circles represent blood glucose 110–150 mg/dL (6–8.3 mmol/l) and light gray circles represent blood glucose < 110 mg/dL (< 6 mmol/L). The maximal benefit that could be expected from lowering blood glucose from an intermediate level to normoglycemia is < 1%, provided blood glucose could be perfectly separated between the two study arms. In order to confidently conclude that such a small benefit is not present, 70,000 patients should have been included. Hence, NICE-SUGAR, with 6100 patients, was in fact underpowered to address this hypothesis. Reproduced with permission from (145).

Three single-center RCTs conducted in Leuven challenged the classical dogma of hyperglycemia being an adaptive phenomenon and provided proof that hyperglycemia can contribute to a worse outcome (108–110). The Leuven studies randomized critically ill patients to controlling blood glucose concentrations within the normal fasting range (80–110 mg/dL [4.4–6.0 mmol/L] for adults; 60–100 mg/dL [3.3–5.6 mmol/L] for children older than 1 year and 50–80 mg/dL [2.8–4.4 mmol/L] for infants) with insulin therapy, or to tolerating hyperglycemia up to the renal threshold (215 mg/dL [11.9 mmol/L]). The three studies, conducted in the adult surgical ICU (108), adult medical ICU (109), and pediatric ICU (110) respectively, all revealed a significant clinical benefit. Indeed, targeting normal fasting blood glucose concentrations with insulin significantly lowered short-term mortality and improved morbidity by preventing organ failure, reflected in a shorter duration of mechanical ventilation,

a decreased incidence of acute kidney injury and critical illness polyneuropathy. Importantly, the clinical benefit was maintained up to four years after randomization with, in critically ill children, a beneficial effect on neurocognitive development (111,112). In addition, the intervention was shown to be cost-effective (113). The study was highly standardized, resulting in a strong internal validity. Frequent blood glucose measurements (interval 0.5h–4h) on whole arterial blood by an accurate blood gas analyzer were done by well-trained nurses, and insulin was continuously infused exclusively via a dedicated lumen of a central venous line with an accurate syringe pump (108–110). However, all patients included in the Leuven trials received early parenteral nutrition as part of standard care, as recommended by European guidelines at that time (114). Recently, this feeding strategy, which iatrogenically increases the risk of hyperglycemia, was shown to be harmful in two large multicenter RCTs, even in a context of strictly controlling blood glucose levels (21,115). The underlying mechanisms of hyperglycemia-induced toxicity were identified to involve cellular damage occurring in those cells that do not require insulin for glucose uptake, such as hepatocytes, renal tubular cells, the endothelium, immune cells and neurons (99,116–120).

Soon after the first Leuven study was published, the intervention was swiftly implemented in clinical practice worldwide, with several studies confirming benefit after local implementation of a glucose control strategy (27,121,122). Subsequent RCTs were neutral or only confirmed a morbidity benefit (123–129). However, several RCTs were relatively small (123–125) and the larger, multicenter RCTs had a smaller difference in glucose concentrations between the study groups than the Leuven studies, in part explained by a lower blood glucose target in the control group (126–129). Hence, these studies were underpowered to detect a difference in mortality.

The NICE-SUGAR multicenter trial (Normoglycemia in Intensive Care Evaluation and Survival Using Glucose Algorithm Regulation) was designed to be the definitive study to answer the question whether lowering glucose levels to strict normal values improves survival of adult critically ill patients (130). The study compared tight blood glucose control to healthy fasting concentrations (80–110 mg/dL [4.4–6.0 mmol/L]) in the intervention group with an intermediate target of 140–180 mg/dL (8–10 mmol/L) in the control group (130). The study revealed that tight glucose control increased mortality as compared with intermediate glucose control in the control group (130), which was subsequently attributed to a 13-fold increase in hypoglycemia (131). As this study was designed for a high external validity, the first conclusion is that very tight blood glucose control is not readily applicable in general daily clinical practice. However, the usual care had already evolved significantly between the first Leuven study and the start of NICE-SUGAR: at that time, tolerating

excessive hyperglycemia was deemed a no-go zone, compared to the higher (215 mg/dL [11.9 mmol/L]) tolerance threshold five years earlier (i.e., the first Leuven study did not treat blood glucose ["don't touch" in Figure 3-4] in the control group unless hyperglycemia was >215 mg/dL [11.9 mmol/L], higher than the renal threshold for glycosuria). Second, due to its pragmatic nature, there was no emphasis on standardization in NICE-SUGAR. All sorts of glucose measurement methodologies were allowed and practitioners were not specifically trained to perform the complex treatment. In addition, a very strict and unvalidated insulin infusion protocol was used, which included the use of insulin boli and which did not correct for changes in feeding intake. Now it has become clear that tight blood glucose control requires accurate blood gas analyzers, such as those used in the Leuven studies, to target a narrow range of blood glucose (132). In addition, capillary glucose measurements, as allowed in NICE-SUGAR, need to be avoided in critically ill patients, especially in patients with shock (133). It is also clear that extensive experience is crucial to avoid undetected episodes of hypoglycemia and to treat hypoglycemia when it occurs. Certainly profound, prolonged/undetected hypoglycemia can have grave consequences and may even result in death. Moreover, spontaneous hypoglycemia is a strong predictor of outcome (134). Hence, hypoglycemia should be avoided as much as possible. Nevertheless, several studies suggest that a brief episode of iatrogenic hypoglycemia may not by itself affect the outcome of critically ill patients (112,134–136). Furthermore, adequate treatment of hypoglycemia, which includes prevention of overtreatment, is essential, as rebound hyperglycemia may also cause brain damage (137). Detailed protocols for prompt and gentle correction of hypoglycemia were often not in place in subsequent RCTs, which again contrasts with the Leuven studies (130). Finally, however, in contrast to the Leuven studies, patients in the NICE-SUGAR study received less parenteral nutrition in the acute phase of critical illness. Patients in the Leuven studies all received early parenteral nutrition, a feeding strategy that was subsequently shown to be harmful (21,115). Due to the lack of adequately powered RCTs, it remains unclear whether tight blood glucose control, when used with accurate tools to prevent hypoglycemia, is still effective and safe in the context of withholding early parenteral nutrition. A meta-analysis has suggested that the benefit of tight blood glucose control may depend on the amount of parenteral calories administered (138). However, this meta-analysis did not correct for other methodological differences between the trials apart from the feeding regimen. Moreover, post hoc analyses of the Leuven studies and mechanistic animal studies suggest that tight blood glucose control is also beneficial in the absence of early parenteral feeding (135,139,140).

Therapeutic Implications: How to Translate This into General Clinical Practice?

What could then be a sensible approach for daily practice? The optimal blood glucose target remains to be defined and may depend on the available logistics, the patient population, and the feeding regimen. As clearly demonstrated by NICE-SUGAR, safe implementation of tight blood glucose control requires accurate glucose measurements and a validated glucose control algorithm. Post-hoc analyses of the Leuven clinical trials revealed that the bulk of the beneficial effects of blood glucose control lay in bringing overt hyperglycemia to moderate levels (Figure 3-4) (135,141). More can be gained by further tightening the blood glucose control, but this requires a substantial investment in training and technology to do this safely. Hence, targeting blood glucose below 145 mg/dL (~8 mmol/L) seems a reasonable compromise. Critically ill diabetic patients may benefit from treatment to somewhat higher glycemic targets, depending on their premorbid levels (135). The impact of tight blood glucose control, applied with accurate tools but in the absence of early parenteral

nutrition, remains to be studied in an adequately powered RCT. Irrespective of the chosen target level, several methodological aspects ought to be taken into account to assure patient safety whenever insulin treatment is used. These include frequent blood glucose measurements, the use of on-site blood gas analyzers as the preferred measurement tool and the avoidance of capillary blood samples, the continuous infusion of insulin with accurate syringe pumps through a dedicated lumen of a central venous catheter. Finally, insulin dosing decisions should not be based on a sliding scale system but on a (computerized) algorithm which was clinically validated for critically ill patients, especially when stricter blood glucose concentrations are targeted (142).

Conclusions

Recent studies have generated important novel insights in the endocrine and metabolic responses to critical illness (Table 3-1). Although many aspects remain unresolved, an important recent insight with therapeutic implications is that most of the acute

Table 3-1 Novel insights into endocrine changes in critical illness

- Part of the acute fall in T_3 plasma concentrations during critical illness is related to the concomitant fasting and this part of the response seems adaptive.
- Cortisol production during critical illness is only moderately increased, and only in patients suffering from systemic inflammatory response syndrome (SIRS), while unaltered in patients without SIRS, in the face of several-fold higher plasma cortisol in all patients.
- Cortisol plasma clearance is substantially reduced in all critically ill patients and contributes substantially to hypercortisolism during critical illness, irrespective of type and severity of illness and irrespective of the inflammation status.
- The optimal blood glucose target in critically ill patients remains to be defined and may depend on the available logistics, the patient population, and the feeding regimen.

endocrine responses are likely adaptive and thus should probably not be treated. Nevertheless, many patients who survived the initial phase of critical illness still remain in the ICU for a long time and face a risk of death that increases steadily with every day that recovery does not set in. Hence, more work is required to find better treatments to further prevent protracted critical illness, to enhance recovery from organ failure and to optimize rehabilitation.

Acknowledgments

The work summarized in this review has been supported by research grants from the Research Foundation, Flanders, by the Methusalem Program funded by the Flemish Government (METH/14/06), and by the European Research Council under the European Union's Seventh Framework Program (FP7/2013-2018 ERC Advanced Grant Agreement n° 321670).

References

1 Casaer MP, Langouche L, Coudyzer W, et al. Impact of early parenteral nutrition on muscle and adipose tissue compartments during critical illness. *Crit Care Med*. 2013;41(10):2298–2309.

2 Puthucheary ZA, Rawal J, McPhail M, Connolly B, et al. Acute skeletal muscle wasting in critical illness. *JAMA*. 2013; 310(15):1591–1600.

3 Villet S, Chiolero RL, Bollmann MD, et al. Negative impact of hypocaloric feeding and energy balance on clinical outcome in ICU patients. *Clin Nutr*. 2005;24(4): 502–509.

4 Hermans G, Casaer MP, Clerckx B, et al. Effect of tolerating macronutrient deficit on the development of intensive-care unit acquired weakness: a subanalysis of the EPaNIC trial. *Lancet Respir Med*. 2013; 1(8):621–629.

5 Vanhorebeek I, Gunst J, Derde S, et al. Insufficient activation of autophagy allows cellular damage to accumulate in critically ill patients. *J Clin Endocrinol Metab*. 2011;96(4):E633-E45.

6 Chopra IJ, Huang TS, Beredo A, Solomon DH, Chua Teco GN, Mead JF. Evidence for an inhibitor of extrathyroidal conversion of thyroxine to 3,5,3′-triiodothyronine in sera of patients with nonthyroidal illnesses. *J Clin Endocrinol Metab*. 1985;60(4):666–672.

7 Michalaki M, Vagenakis AG, Makri M, Kalfarentzos F, Kyriazopoulou V. Dissociation of the early decline in serum T(3) concentration and serum IL-6 rise and TNFalpha in nonthyroidal illness syndrome induced by abdominal surgery. *J Clin Endocrinol Metab*. 2001;86(9): 4198–4205.

8 Bartalena L, Martino E, Brandi LS, et al. Lack of nocturnal serum thyrotropin surge after surgery. *J Clin Endocrinol Metab*. 1990;70(1):293–296.

9 Romijn JA, Wiersinga WM. Decreased nocturnal surge of thyrotropin in nonthyroidal illness. *J Clin Endocrinol Metab*. 1990;70(1):35–42.

10 Redout EM, van der Toorn A, Zuidwijk MJ, et al. Antioxidant treatment attenuates pulmonary arterial hypertension-induced heart failure. *Am J Physiol Heart Circ Physiol*. 2010;298(3): H1038–H1047.

11 Wajner SM, Goemann IM, Bueno AL, Larsen PR, Maia AL IL-6 promotes nonthyroidal illness syndrome by blocking thyroxine activation while promoting thyroid hormone inactivation in human cells. *J Clin Invest*. 2011;121(5): 1834–1845.

12 Boelen A, Kwakkel J, Fliers E. Beyond low plasma T3: local thyroid hormone metabolism during inflammation and infection. *Endocr Rev*. 2011;32(5): 670–693.

13 Van der Poll T, Van Zee KJ, Endert E, et al. Interleukin-1 receptor blockade does not

affect endotoxin-induced changes in plasma thyroid hormone and thyrotropin concentrations in man. *J Clin Endocrinol Metab*. 1995;80(4):1341–1346.

14 Lim CF, Docter R, Visser TJ, et al. Inhibition of thyroxine transport into cultured rat hepatocytes by serum of nonuremic critically ill patients: effects of bilirubin and nonesterified fatty acids. *J Clin Endocrinol Metab*. 1993;76(5): 1165–1172.

15 Gardner DF, Kaplan MM, Stanley CA, Utiger RD. Effect of tri-iodothyronine replacement on the metabolic and pituitary responses to starvation. *N Engl J Med*. 1979;300(11):579–584.

16 Moshang T, Parks JS, Baker L, et al. Low serum triiodothyronine in patients with anorexia nervosa. *J Clin Endocrinol Metab*. 1975;40(3):470–473.

17 Peeters RP, Wouters PJ, van Toor H, Kaptein E, Visser TJ, Van den Berghe G. Serum 3,3′,5′-triiodothyronine (rT3) and 3,5,3′-triiodothyronine/rT3 are prognostic markers in critically ill patients and are associated with postmortem tissue deiodinase activities. *J Clin Endocrinol Metab*. 2005;90(8):4559–4565.

18 Rothwell PM, Lawler PG. Prediction of outcome in intensive care patients using endocrine parameters. *Crit Care Med*. 1995;23(1):78–83.

19 Klemperer JD, Klein I, Gomez M, et al. Thyroid hormone treatment after coronary-artery bypass surgery. *N Engl J Med*. 1995;333(23):1522–1527.

20 Mullis-Jansson SL, Argenziano M, Corwin S, et al. A randomized double-blind study of the effect of triiodothyronine on cardiac function and morbidity after coronary bypass surgery. *J Thorac Cardiovasc Surg*. 1999;117(6):1128–1134.

21 Casaer MP, Mesotten D, Hermans G, et al. Early versus late parenteral nutrition in critically ill adults. *N Engl J Med*. 2011; 365(6):506–517.

22 Langouche L, Vander Perre S, Marques M, et al. Impact of early nutrient restriction during critical illness on the nonthyroidal illness syndrome and its relation with

outcome: a randomized, controlled clinical study. *J Clin Endocrinol Metab*. 2013;98(3):1006–1013.

23 Mebis L, Eerdekens A, Güiza F, Princen L, et al. Contribution of nutritional deficit to the pathogenesis of the nonthyroidal illness syndrome in critical illness: a rabbit model study. *Endocrinology*. 2012; 153(2):973–984.

24 Boelen A, Boorsma J, Kwakkel J, et al. Type 3 deiodinase is highly expressed in infiltrating neutrophilic granulocytes in response to acute bacterial infection. *Thyroid*. 2008;18(10):1095–1103.

25 Van den Berghe G, de Zegher F, Veldhuis JD, et al. Thyrotrophin and prolactin release in prolonged critical illness: dynamics of spontaneous secretion and effects of growth hormone-secretagogues. *Clin Endocrinol (Oxf)*. 1997;47(5): 599–612.

26 Fliers E, Guldenaar SE, Wiersinga WM, Swaab DF. Decreased hypothalamic thyrotropin-releasing hormone gene expression in patients with nonthyroidal illness. *J Clin Endocrinol Metab*. 1997; 82(12):4032–4036.

27 Bacci V, Schussler GC, Kaplan TB. The relationship between serum triiodothyronine and thyrotropin during systemic illness. *J Clin Endocrinol Metab*. 1982; 54(6):1229–1235.

28 Damas P, Reuter A, Gysen P, Demonty J, Lamy M, Franchimont P. Tumor necrosis factor and interleukin-1 serum levels during severe sepsis in humans. *Crit Care Med*. 1989;17(10):975–978.

29 Faglia G, Ferrari C, Beck-Peccoz P, Spada A, Travaglini P, Ambrosi B. Reduced plasma thyrotropin response to thyrotropin releasing hormone after dexamethasone administration in normal subjects. *Horm Metab Res*. 1973;5(4): 289–292.

30 Van den Berghe G, de Zegher F, Lauwers P. Dopamine and the sick euthyroid syndrome in critical illness. *Clin Endocrinol (Oxf)*. 1994;41(6):731–737.

31 Van den Berghe G, de Zegher F, Lauwers P. Dopamine suppresses pituitary

function in infants and children. *Crit Care Med*. 1994;22(11):1747–1753.

32 Boelen A, Kwakkel J, Thijssen-Timmer DC, Alkemade A, Fliers E, Wiersinga WM. Simultaneous changes in central and peripheral components of the hypothalamus-pituitary-thyroid axis in lipopolysaccharide-induced acute illness in mice. *J Endocrinol*. 2004;182(2): 315–323.

33 Mebis L, Debaveye Y, Ellger B, et al. Changes in the central component of the hypothalamus-pituitary-thyroid axis in a rabbit model of prolonged critical illness. *Crit Care*. 2009;13(5):R147.

34 Alkemade A, Friesema EC, Kuiper GG, et al. Novel neuroanatomical pathways for thyroid hormone action in the human anterior pituitary. *Eur J Endocrinol*. 2006; 154(3):491–500.

35 Langouche L, Princen L, Gunst J, Güiza F, Derde S, Van den Berghe G. Anterior pituitary morphology and hormone production during sustained critical illness in a rabbit model. *Horm Metab Res*. 2013;45(4):277–282.

36 Mebis L, Paletta D, Debaveye Y, et al. Expression of thyroid hormone transporters during critical illness. *Eur J Endocrinol*. 2009;161(2):243–250.

37 Mebis L, Langouche L, Visser TJ, Van den Berghe G. The type II iodothyronine deiodinase is up-regulated in skeletal muscle during prolonged critical illness. *J Clin Endocrinol Metab*. 2007;92(8): 3330–3333.

38 Ma SF, Xie L, Pino-Yanes M, et al. Type 2 deiodinase and host responses of sepsis and acute lung injury. *Am J Respir Cell Mol Biol*. 2011;45(6):1203–1211.

39 Thijssen-Timmer DC, Peeters RP, et al. Thyroid hormone receptor isoform expression in livers of critically ill patients. *Thyroid*. 2007;17(2):105–112.

40 Van den Berghe G, Wouters P, Weekers F, et al. Reactivation of pituitary hormone release and metabolic improvement by infusion of growth hormone-releasing peptide and thyrotropin-releasing hormone in patients with protracted

critical illness. *J Clin Endocrinol Metab*. 1999;84(4):1311–1323.

41 Van den Berghe G, de Zegher F, Baxter RC, et al. Neuroendocrinology of prolonged critical illness: effects of exogenous thyrotropin-releasing hormone and its combination with growth hormone secretagogues. *J Clin Endocrinol Metab*. 1998;83(2):309–319.

42 Weekers F, Michalaki M, Coopmans W, et al. Endocrine and metabolic effects of growth hormone (GH) compared with GH-releasing peptide, thyrotropin-releasing hormone, and insulin infusion in a rabbit model of prolonged critical illness. *Endocrinology*. 2004;145(1):205–213.

43 Van den Berghe G, Baxter RC, Weekers F, et al. The combined administration of GH-releasing peptide-2 (GHRP-2), TRH and GnRH to men with prolonged critical illness evokes superior endocrine and metabolic effects compared to treatment with GHRP-2 alone. *Clin Endocrinol (Oxf)*. 2002;56(5):655–669.

44 Mebis L, van den Berghe G. The hypothalamus-pituitary-thyroid axis in critical illness. *Neth J Med*. 2009;67(10): 332–340.

45 Debaveye Y, Ellger B, Mebis L, et al. Tissue deiodinase activity during prolonged critical illness: effects of exogenous thyrotropin-releasing hormone and its combination with growth hormone-releasing peptide-2. *Endocrinology*. 2005;146(12):5604–5611.

46 Debaveye Y, Ellger B, Mebis L, Visser TJ, Darras VM, Van den Berghe G. Effects of substitution and high-dose thyroid hormone therapy on deiodination, sulfoconjugation, and tissue thyroid hormone levels in prolonged critically ill rabbits. *Endocrinology*. 2008;149(8): 4218–4228.

47 Debaveye Y, Ellger B, Mebis L, Darras VM, Van den Berghe G. Regulation of tissue iodothyronine deiodinase activity in a model of prolonged critical illness. *Thyroid*. 2008;18(5):551–560.

48 Peeters RP, van der Geyten S, Wouters PJ, et al. Tissue thyroid hormone levels in critical illness. *J Clin Endocrinol Metab.* 2005;90(12):6498–6507.

49 Acker CG, Singh AR, Flick RP, Bernardini J, Greenberg A, Johnson JP. A trial of thyroxine in acute renal failure. *Kidney Int.* 2000;57(1):293–298.

50 Becker RA, Vaughan GM, Ziegler MG, et al. Hypermetabolic low triiodothyronine syndrome of burn injury. *Crit Care Med.* 1982;10(12):870–875.

51 Brent GA, Hershman JM. Thyroxine therapy in patients with severe nonthyroidal illnesses and low serum thyroxine concentration. *J Clin Endocrinol Metab.* 1986;63(1):1–8.

52 Sirlak M, Yazicioglu L, Inan MB, et al. Oral thyroid hormone pretreatment in left ventricular dysfunction. *Eur J Cardiothorac Surg.* 2004;26(4):720–725.

53 Debaveye Y, Vandenbrande J, Van den Berghe G. Endocrine emergencies. In: Tubaro M, Danchin N, Filippatos G, Goldstein P, Vranckx P, Zahger B, eds. *The ESC Textbook of Intensive and Acute Cardiac Care.* New York: Oxford University Press; 2011: 709–717.

54 Nicoloff JT. Thyroid storm and myxedema coma. *Med Clin North Am.* 1985;69(5):1005–1017.

55 Ringel MD. Management of hypothyroidism and hyperthyroidism in the intensive care unit. *Crit Care Clin.* 2001;17(1):59–74.

56 Escobar-Morreale HF, Obregón MJ, Escobar del Rey F, Morreale de Escobar G. Replacement therapy for hypothyroidism with thyroxine alone does not ensure euthyroidism in all tissues, as studied in thyroidectomized rats. *J Clin Invest.* 1995;96(6):2828–2838.

57 Van den Berghe G. Endocrine aspects of critical care medicine. In: Jameson J, De Groot L, eds. *Endocrinology: Adult and Pediatric.* St Louis, MO: WB Saunders; 2010: 2084–2085.

58 Finlay WE, McKee JI. Serum cortisol levels in severely stressed patients. *Lancet.* 1982;1(8286):1414–1415.

59 Munck A, Guyre PM, Holbrook NJ. Physiological functions of glucocorticoids in stress and their relation to pharmacological actions. *Endocr Rev.* 1984;5(1):25–44.

60 Starling EH. The wisdom of the body: The Harveian Oration, delivered before The Royal College of Physicians of London on St. Luke's Day, 1923. *Br Med J.* 1923;2(3277):685–690.

61 Vermes I, Beishuizen A, Hampsink RM, Haanen C. Dissociation of plasma adrenocorticotropin and cortisol levels in critically ill patients: possible role of endothelin and atrial natriuretic hormone. *J Clin Endocrinol Metab.* 1995;80(4):1238–1242.

62 Boonen E, Vervenne H, Meersseman P, et al. Reduced cortisol metabolism during critical illness. *N Engl J Med.* 2013;368(16): 1477–1488.

63 Bornstein SR, Engeland WC, Ehrhart-Bornstein M, Herman JP. Dissociation of ACTH and glucocorticoids. *Trends Endocrinol Metab.* 2008;19(5):175–180.

64 Vanwijngaerden YM, Wauters J, Langouche L, et al. Critical illness evokes elevated circulating bile acids related to altered hepatic transporter and nuclear receptor expression. *Hepatology.* 2011;54(5):1741–1752.

65 Ackermann D, Vogt B, Escher G, et al. Inhibition of 11beta-hydroxysteroid dehydrogenase by bile acids in rats with cirrhosis. *Hepatology.* 1999;30(3): 623–629.

66 McNeilly AD, Macfarlane DP, O'Flaherty E, et al. Bile acids modulate glucocorticoid metabolism and the hypothalamic-pituitary-adrenal axis in obstructive jaundice. *J Hepatol.* 2010;52(5):705–711.

67 Stauffer AT, Rochat MK, Dick B, Frey FJ, Odermatt A Chenodeoxycholic acid and deoxycholic acid inhibit 11 beta-hydroxysteroid dehydrogenase type 2 and cause cortisol-induced transcriptional activation of the mineralocorticoid receptor. *J Biol Chem.* 2002;277(29):26286–26292.

68 Van den Akker EL, Koper JW, Joosten K, et al. Glucocorticoid receptor mRNA levels are selectively decreased in neutrophils of children with sepsis. *Intensive Care Med*. 2009;35(7): 1247–1254.

69 Boonen E, Meersseman P, Vervenne H, et al. Reduced nocturnal ACTH-driven cortisol secretion during critical illness. *Am J Physiol Endocrinol Metab*. 2014; 306(8):E883–E892.

70 Boonen E, Langouche L, Janssens T, et al. Impact of duration of critical illness on the adrenal glands of human intensive care patients. *J Clin Endocrinol Metab*. 2014;99(11):4214–4222.

71 Barquist E, Kirton O. Adrenal insufficiency in the surgical intensive care unit patient. *J Trauma*. 1997;42(1):27–31.

72 Kanczkowski W, Chatzigeorgiou A, Grossklaus S, Sprott D, Bornstein SR, Chavakis T. Role of the endothelial-derived endogenous anti-inflammatory factor Del-1 in inflammation-mediated adrenal gland dysfunction. *Endocrinology*. 2013;154(3): 1181–1189.

73 Prigent H, Maxime V, Annane D. Science review: mechanisms of impaired adrenal function in sepsis and molecular actions of glucocorticoids. *Crit Care*. 2004; 8(4):243–252.

74 Annane D, Sébille V, Troché G, Raphaël JC, Gajdos P, Bellissant E. A 3-level prognostic classification in septic shock based on cortisol levels and cortisol response to corticotropin. *JAMA*. 2000;283(8):1038–1045.

75 Beishuizen A, Vermes I, Hylkema BS, Haanen C. Relative eosinophilia and functional adrenal insufficiency in critically ill patients. *Lancet*. 1999; 353(9165):1675–1676.

76 Richards ML, Caplan RH, Wickus GG, Lambert PJ, Kisken WA The rapid low-dose (1 microgram) cosyntropin test in the immediate postoperative period: results in elderly subjects after major abdominal surgery. *Surgery*. 1999;125(4): 431–440.

77 Annane D, Pastores SM, Rochwerg B, et al. Recommendations for the diagnosis and management of corticosteroid insufficiency in critically ill adult patients. (Part I): Society of Critical Care Medicine (SCCM) and European Society of Intensive Care Medicine (ESICM) 2017. *Intensive Care Med*. 2017;43:1751–1763.

78 Chan WL, Carrell RW, Zhou A, Read RJ. How changes in affinity of corticosteroid-binding globulin modulate free cortisol concentration. *J Clin Endocrinol Metab*. 2013;98(8):3315–3322.

79 Hamrahian AH, Oseni TS, Arafah BM. Measurements of serum free cortisol in critically ill patients. *N Engl J Med*. 2004; 350(16):1629–1638.

80 Holland PC, Hancock SW, Hodge D, Thompson D, Shires S, Evans S. Degradation of albumin in meningococcal sepsis. *Lancet*. 2001;357(9274): 2102–2104.

81 Pugeat M, Bonneton A, Perrot D, et al. Decreased immunoreactivity and binding activity of corticosteroid-binding globulin in serum in septic shock. *Clin Chem*. 1989;35(8):1675–1659.

82 Bergquist M, Nurkkala M, Rylander C, Kristiansson E, Hedenstierna G, Lindholm C. Expression of the glucocorticoid receptor is decreased in experimental Staphylococcus aureus sepsis. *J Infect*. 2013;67(6):574–583.

83 Guerrero J, Gatica HA, Rodríguez M, Estay R, Goecke IA. Septic serum induces glucocorticoid resistance and modifies the expression of glucocorticoid isoforms receptors: a prospective cohort study and in vitro experimental assay. *Crit Care*. 2013;17(3):R107.

84 Indyk JA, Candido-Vitto C, Wolf IM, et al. Reduced glucocorticoid receptor protein expression in children with critical illness. *Horm Res Paediatr*. 2013;79:169–178.

85 Peeters RP, Hagendorf A, Vanhorebeek I, et al. Tissue mRNA expression of the glucocorticoid receptor and its splice variants in fatal critical illness. *Clin Endocrinol (Oxf)*. 2009;71(1):145–153.

86 Siebig S, Meinel A, Rogler G, et al. Decreased cytosolic glucocorticoid receptor levels in critically ill patients. *Anaesth Intensive Care*. 2010;38(1): 133–140.

87 Cohen J, Ward G, Prins J, Jones M, Venkatesh B. Variability of cortisol assays can confound the diagnosis of adrenal insufficiency in the critically ill population. *Intensive Care. Med* 2006;32(11):1901–1905.

88 Hamrahian AH, Fleseriu M, Committee AAS. Evaluation and management of adrenal insufficiency in critically ill patients - disease state review. *Endocr Pract*. 2017 doi:10.4158/EP161720.RA.

89 Research project: HPA axis in critical illness: cause and consequence of altered cortisol metabolism (3M140210). Available from: https://www.kuleuven.be/onderzoek/portaal/#/projecten/3M140210?hl=en⟨=en.

90 Vassiliadi DA, Ilias I, Tzanela M, et al. Interstitial cortisol obtained by microdialysis in mechanically ventilated septic patients: correlations with total and free serum cortisol. *J Crit Care*. 2013; 28(2):158–165.

91 Venkatesh B, Morgan TJ, Cohen J. Interstitium: the next diagnostic and therapeutic platform in critical illness. *Crit Care Med*. 2010;38(10 Suppl):S630–S636.

92 Chung T, Grossman A, Clark A. Adrenal insufficiency. In Jameson J, De Groot L, eds. *Endocrinology: Adult and Pediatric*. St Louis, MO: WB Saunders; 2010: pp. 1853–1863.

93 Bornstein SR, Allolio B, Arlt W, et al. Diagnosis and treatment of primary adrenal insufficiency: an Endocrine Society Clinical Practice Guideline. *J Clin Endocrinol Metab*. 2016;101(2):364–389.

94 Annane D, Sébille V, Charpentier C, et al. Effect of treatment with low doses of hydrocortisone and fludrocortisone on mortality in patients with septic shock. *JAMA*. 2002;288(7):862–871.

95 Bollaert PE, Charpentier C, Levy B, Debouverie M, Audibert G, Larcan A. Reversal of late septic shock with supraphysiologic doses of hydrocortisone. *Crit Care Med*. 1998;26(4):645–650.

96 Briegel J, Forst H, Haller M, et al. Stress doses of hydrocortisone reverse hyperdynamic septic shock: a prospective, randomized, double-blind, single-center study. *Crit Care Med*. 1999;27(4): 723–732.

97 Sprung CL, Annane D, Keh D, et al. Hydrocortisone therapy for patients with septic shock. *N Engl J Med*. 2008; 358(2):111–124.

98 Keh D, Trips E, Marx G, Wirtz SP, et al. Effect of hydrocortisone on development of shock among patients with severe sepsis: The HYPRESS randomized clinical trial. *JAMA*. 2016;316(17):1775–1785.

99 Hermans G, Wilmer A, Meersseman W, et al. Impact of intensive insulin therapy on neuromuscular complications and ventilator dependency in the medical intensive care unit. *Am J Respir Crit Care Med*. 2007;175(5):480–489.

100 Hermans G, De Jonghe B, Bruyninckx F, Van den Berghe G. Clinical review: Critical illness polyneuropathy and myopathy. *Crit Care*. 2008;12(6):238.

101 Hauer D, Weis F, Papassotiropoulos A, et al. Relationship of a common polymorphism of the glucocorticoid receptor gene to traumatic memories and posttraumatic stress disorder in patients after intensive care therapy. *Crit Care Med*. 2011;39(4):643–650.

102 Ledderose C, Möhnle P, Limbeck E, et al. Corticosteroid resistance in sepsis is influenced by microRNA-124–induced downregulation of glucocorticoid receptor-α. *Crit Care Med*. 2012;40(10): 2745–2753.

103 Baker AC, Chew VW, Green TL, et al. Single nucleotide polymorphisms and type of steroid impact the functional response of the human glucocorticoid receptor. *J Surg Res*. 2013;180(1):27–34.

104 Falciglia M, Freyberg RW, Almenoff PL, D'Alessio DA, Render MLHyperglycemia-related mortality in critically ill patients varies with admission

diagnosis. *Crit Care Med.* 2009;37(12): 3001–3009.

105 Wintergerst KA, Buckingham B, Gandrud L, Wong BJ, Kache S, Wilson DM. Association of hypoglycemia, hyperglycemia, and glucose variability with morbidity and death in the pediatric intensive care unit. *Pediatrics.* 2006; 118(1):173–179.

106 Kosiborod M, Rathore SS, Inzucchi SE, et al. Admission glucose and mortality in elderly patients hospitalized with acute myocardial infarction: implications for patients with and without recognized diabetes. *Circulation.* 2005;111(23): 3078–3086.

107 Krinsley JS, Egi M, Kiss A, et al. Diabetic status and the relation of the three domains of glycemic control to mortality in critically ill patients: an international multicenter cohort study. *Crit Care.* 2013;17(2).

108 Van den Berghe G, Wouters P, Weekers F, et al. Intensive insulin therapy in critically ill patients. *N Engl J Med.* 2001;345(19): 1359–1367.

109 Van den Berghe G, Wilmer A, Hermans G, et al. Intensive insulin therapy in the medical ICU. *N Engl J Med.* 2006;354(5): 449–461.

110 Vlasselaers D, Milants I, Desmet L, et al. Intensive insulin therapy for patients in paediatric intensive care: a prospective, randomised controlled study. *Lancet.* 2009;373(9663):547–556.

111 Ingels C, Debaveye Y, Milants I, et al. Strict blood glucose control with insulin during intensive care after cardiac surgery: impact on 4-years survival, dependency on medical care, and quality-of-life. *Eur Heart J.* 2006;27(22): 2716–2724.

112 Mesotten D, Gielen M, Sterken C, et al. Neurocognitive development of children 4 years after critical illness and treatment with tight glucose control: a randomized controlled trial. *JAMA.* 2012;308(16):1641–1650.

113 Van den Berghe G, Wouters PJ, Kesteloot K, Hilleman DE. Analysis of healthcare resource utilization with intensive insulin therapy in critically ill patients. *Crit Care Med.* 2006;34(3):612–616.

114 Singer P, Berger MM, Van den Berghe G, et al. ESPEN guidelines on parenteral nutrition: intensive care. *Clin Nutr.* 2009;28(4):387–400.

115 Fivez T, Kerklaan D, Mesotten D, et al. Early versus late parenteral nutrition in critically ill children. *N Engl J Med.* 2016;374(12):1111–1122.

116 Ellger B, Debaveye Y, Vanhorebeek I, et al. Survival benefits of intensive insulin therapy in critical illness: impact of maintaining normoglycemia versus glycemia-independent actions of insulin. *Diabetes.* 2006;55(4):1096–1105.

117 Vanhorebeek I, Gunst J, Ellger B, et al. Hyperglycemic kidney damage in an animal model of prolonged critical illness. *Kidney Int.* 2009;76(5):512–520.

118 Vanhorebeek I, Ellger B, De Vos R, et al. Tissue-specific glucose toxicity induces mitochondrial damage in a burn injury model of critical illness. *Crit Care Med.* 2009;37(4):1355–1364.

119 Weekers F, Giulietti AP, Michalaki M, et al. Metabolic, endocrine, and immune effects of stress hyperglycemia in a rabbit model of prolonged critical illness. *Endocrinology.* 2003;144(12):5329–5338.

120 Ellger B, Langouche L, Richir M, et al. Modulation of regional nitric oxide metabolism: blood glucose control or insulin? *Intensive Care Med.* 2008;34(8): 1525–1533.

121 Krinsley JS. Effect of an intensive glucose management protocol on the mortality of critically ill adult patients. *Mayo Clin Proc.* 2004;79(8):992–1000.

122 Krinsley JS, Jones RL. Cost analysis of intensive glycemic control in critically ill adult patients. *Chest.* 2006;129(3): 644–650.

123 Jeschke MG, Kulp GA, Kraft R, et al. Intensive insulin therapy in severely burned pediatric patients: a prospective randomized trial. *Am J Respir Crit Care Med.* 2010;182(3):351–359.

124 Bilotta F, Spinelli A, Giovannini F, Doronzio A, Delfini R, Rosa G. The effect of intensive insulin therapy on infection rate, vasospasm, neurologic outcome, and mortality in neurointensive care unit after intracranial aneurysm clipping in patients with acute subarachnoid hemorrhage: a randomized prospective pilot trial. *J Neurosurg Anesthesiol*. 2007;19(3): 156–160.

125 Bilotta F, Caramia R, Paoloni FP, Delfini R, Rosa G. Safety and efficacy of intensive insulin therapy in critical neurosurgical patients. *Anesthesiology*. 2009;110(3): 611–619.

126 Preiser JC, Devos P, Ruiz-Santana S, et al. A prospective randomised multi-centre controlled trial on tight glucose control by intensive insulin therapy in adult intensive care units: the Glucontrol study. *Intensive Care Med*. 2009;35(10):1738–1748.

127 Kalfon P, Giraudeau B, Ichai C, et al. Tight computerized versus conventional glucose control in the ICU: a randomized controlled trial. *Intensive Care Med*. 2014;40(2):171–181.

128 Annane D, Cariou A, Maxime V, et al. Corticosteroid treatment and intensive insulin therapy for septic shock in adults: a randomized controlled trial. *JAMA*. 2010;303(4):341–348.

129 Agus MS, Wypij D, Hirshberg EL, et al. Tight glycemic control in critically ill children. *N Engl J Med* 2017;376(8): 729–741.

130 Finfer S, Blair D, Bellomo R, et al. Intensive versus conventional glucose control in critically ill patients. *N Engl J Med*. 2009;360(13):1283–1297.

131 Finfer S, Liu B, Chittock DR, et al. Hypoglycemia and risk of death in critically ill patients. *N Engl J Med*. 2012;367(12):1108–1118.

132 Scott MG, Bruns DE, Boyd JC, Sacks DB. Tight glucose control in the intensive care unit: are glucose meters up to the task? *Clin Chem* 2009;55(1):18–20.

133 Finfer S, Wernerman J, Preiser J-C, et al. Clinical review: consensus recommendations on measurement of blood glucose and reporting glycemic control in critically ill adults. *Crit Care*. 2013;17(3).

134 Kosiborod M, Inzucchi SE, Goyal A, et al. Relationship between spontaneous and iatrogenic hypoglycemia and mortality in patients hospitalized with acute myocardial infarction. *JAMA*. 2009; 301(15):1556–1564.

135 Van den Berghe G, Wilmer A, Milants I, et al. Intensive insulin therapy in mixed medical/surgical intensive care units: benefit versus harm. *Diabetes*. 2006; 55(11):3151–3159.

136 Vanhorebeek I, Gielen M, Boussemaere M, et al. Glucose dysregulation and neurological injury biomarkers in critically ill children. *J Clin Endocrinol Metab*. 2010;95(10):4669–4679.

137 Suh SW, Gum ET, Hamby AM, Chan PH, Swanson RA. Hypoglycemic neuronal death is triggered by glucose reperfusion and activation of neuronal NADPH oxidase. *J Clin Invest*. 2007;117(4):910–918.

138 Marik PE, Preiser JC. Toward understanding tight glycemic control in the ICU: a systematic review and metaanalysis. *Chest*. 2010;137(3):544–551.

139 Derde S, Vanhorebeek I, Ververs E-J, et al. Increasing intravenous glucose load in the presence of normoglycemia: Effect on outcome and metabolism in critically ill rabbits. *Crit Care Med*. 2010;38(2): 602–611.

140 Sonneville R, den Hertog HM, Derde S, et al. Increasing glucose load while maintaining normoglycemia does not evoke neuronal damage in prolonged critically ill rabbits. *Clin Nutr*. 2013;32(6): 1077–1080.

141 Van den Berghe G, Wouters PJ, Bouillon R, et al. Outcome benefit of intensive insulin therapy in the critically ill: Insulin dose versus glycemic control. *Crit Care Med*. 2003;31(2):359–366.

142 Van Herpe T, Mesotten D, Wouters PJ, et al. LOGIC-Insulin algorithm-guided versus nurse-directed blood glucose

control during critical illness: the LOGIC-1 single-center, randomized, controlled clinical trial. *Diabetes Care.* 2013;36(2):188–194.

143 Vanhorebeek I, Langouche L, Van den Berghe G. Endocrine aspects of acute and prolonged critical illness. *Nat Clin Pract Endocrinol Metab.* 2006;2(1):20–31.

144 Mebis L, Van den Berghe G. Thyroid axis function and dysfunction in critical illness. *Best Pract Res Clin Endocrinol Metab.* 2011;25(5):745–57.

145 Van den Berghe G. Intensive insulin therapy in the ICU: reconciling the evidence. *Nat Rev Endocrinol.* 2012;8(6): 374–378.

Part III

Special Populations

4

Endocrine and Metabolic Emergencies in Pregnancy

Anita Banerjee and Catherine Williamson

Key Points

- Endocrine disease may present for the first time as an emergency during pregnancy or endocrine emergencies can occur in pregnant women with pre-existing endocrine conditions.
- Pre-pregnancy counseling should be offered to all women with pre-existing endocrine disease to ensure stability of the disease prior to conception and to discuss the safety profile of medication(s) during pregnancy.
- As with all comorbid conditions in pregnancy, multidisciplinary team (MDT) management is critical; it is important to be aware that at least two lives are involved; prompt senior review should be available at all times; and many standard of care investigations (e.g., nuclear scans) and drugs (e.g., bisphosphonates) may be contraindicated or need to be modified or have not been tested in the pregnant setting.
- Diabetes mellitus is the commonest endocrine disorder in pregnant women and despite goals targeting near normal glycemia in pregnancies complicated by pre-existing or newly diagnosed diabetes, pregnant women with diabetes may present with urgent challenges. Suboptimal outpatient glycemic control in the woman who presents with a newly diagnosed unplanned pregnancy; extremes of blood glucose levels as with diabetic ketoacidosis and severe

hypoglycemia; iatrogenic hyperglycemia from treatment with glucocorticoids to promote fetal lung maturity; and rapidly changing insulin requirements during the peripartum period present unique and emergent challenges to the healthcare provider.
- Maternal obesity is increasing in number and is associated with adverse outcomes including gestational diabetes, pre-eclampsia, instrumental and cesarean births, infections, and post-partum hemorrhage.
- In women with pituitary tumors, an acute presentation due to pressure effects or excessive secretion of a specific hormone can occur. Pituitary apoplexy is rarely reported in pregnancy. Sheehan's syndrome (i.e., hypopituitarism) may occur after post-partum hemorrhage.
- Hypothalamic or posterior pituitary disorders are more commonly complicated by emergencies because of inadequate treatment or overtreatment (e.g., resulting in electrolyte imbalance in diabetes insipidus or development of hypoadrenalism in women with adrenocorticotropic hormone [ACTH] deficiency).
- Most adrenal adenomas are pre-existing during pregnancy, but the first presentation of a pheochromocytoma may occur.

Endocrine and Metabolic Medical Emergencies: A Clinician's Guide, Second Edition. Edited by Glenn Matfin.

- Thyroid diseases are common in pregnancy, but, if adequately treated, hypothyroidism and hyperthyroidism are rarely complicated by medical emergencies. However, thyroid storm may occur and it is important to distinguish between gestational thyrotoxicosis and thyrotoxicosis.

- Severe hypercalcemia can occur during pregnancy and may be a consequence of hyperparathyroidism. As with parathyroid tumors in non-pregnant individuals, excessive parathyroid hormone secretion is associated with hypertension and pregnant women with hyperparathyroidism may present with pre-eclampsia.

Introduction

Most endocrine disorders have a good prognosis if diagnosed and treated prior to pregnancy. Emergencies may be the consequence of a new diagnosis in pregnancy or due to women avoiding treatment when they conceive, often due to an incorrect assumption that the drugs used to treat an endocrine disorder will harm the fetus. It may be difficult to establish the underlying etiology in women presenting with gestational endocrine emergencies as the normal ranges for many endocrine tests change in normal pregnancy. The influence of pregnancy on hormones that are used for diagnostic tests in endocrinology is summarized in Table 4-1.

Diabetes Mellitus

Carbohydrate metabolism is adapted during pregnancy, to maintain glucose homeostasis and ensure that energy is available to the fetus during the maternal fasting state. The management of diabetes during pregnancy is described in detail in the 2013 Endocrine Society Clinical Practice Guidelines (1).

Diabetic Ketoacidosis

Diabetic ketoacidosis (DKA) is a medical emergency during pregnancy and can be complicated by fetal loss rates as high as 10–25% (2). The incidence is 1–3%. During pregnancy, there is an accelerated maternal response to starvation and this predisposes women with diabetes mellitus to DKA.

Common precipitants during pregnancy include urinary tract infections, hyperemesis gravidarum, and insulin "pump failure" in women using CSII (continuous subcutaneous insulin infusion). The diagnosis and treatment algorithm of DKA in pregnancy is like the non-pregnant case (although euglycemic DKA can occur resulting in early addition of dextrose to insulin to reduce ketone levels). The management of DKA requires close maternal and fetal monitoring. Prompt management and adherence to standard guidelines are essential (3).

Hypoglycemia during Pregnancy

Hypoglycemia is common during pregnancy (4). Insulin sensitivity increases during the first trimester and insulin requirements may fall at this stage of pregnancy. Therefore, it is not surprising that women with Type I diabetes mellitus are reported to have severe hypoglycemia (i.e., requiring third party assistance) occurring 3–5 times more frequently in the first trimester (5). Associated risk factors for severe hypoglycemia in pregnancy include duration of diabetes (i.e., >10 years increased risk), a history of severe hypoglycemia in the preceding year, women with impaired hypoglycemia awareness, and tight glycemic control in early pregnancy. Insulin doses should be reduced within the first trimester of pregnancy, and women encouraged to increase the frequency of self-monitoring of blood glucose. If hypoglycemia awareness is blunted, patients are encouraged to use continuous glucose monitoring if the resources are available.

Table 4-1 Effects of pregnancy on specific hormones

Hormone	Effect of pregnancy	Explanation
LH and FSH	• Undetectable during pregnancy	• Suppressed by high circulating levels of estrogen and progesterone
GH	• Total GH concentration increases	• Placental GH production (assays cannot distinguish this from pituitary GH)
ACTH	• Total ACTH level increases approximately two-fold after the first trimester	• Placental production of cortisol releasing factor and ACTH, however pituitary ACTH secretion is unchanged
IGF-1	• Increases in normal pregnancy	• IGF-1 production stimulated by human placental lactogen
ADH	• Reduction in circulating ADH	• Placental vasopressinase production
Prolactin	• Progressive increase throughout pregnancy	• Increased estrogen stimulates pituitary prolactin release • Prolactin synthesized by decidual tissue but only small amounts enter fetal or maternal circulation
Renin	• Increase up to four-fold by 20 weeks of gestation then plateaus	• Renin aldosterone system activation results from the fall in total peripheral resistance and resulting afterload reduction, and therefore allows the expansion of plasma volume
Aldosterone	• Levels increase up to three-fold in the first trimester and ten-fold in the third trimester	• Response to increase renin and angiotensin II
Angiotensin II	• Increased three-fold	• Increased renin and angiotensinogen
Thyroid hormones	• 50% more thyroid hormone required • Increased iodine requirement • Increased T_4 production and subsequent TSH suppression, particularly in first trimester • Upper end of normal range for free T_3 and T_4 reduced in later pregnancy • Higher levels of total T_3 and T_4	• De-iodination in placenta and increase in TBG • Increased renal iodine clearance and fetal iodine uptake • Structural similarity of TSH and hCG leading to hCG mediated stimulation of TSH receptors in thyroid tissue • Hemodilution • Increase in TBG
Cortisol	• Serum cortisol (reflecting total cortisol) increases up to three-fold • Urinary 24-h free cortisol (reflecting free cortisol only) increases • Suppression by exogenous corticosteroid is blunted	• Increase in CBG, corticotropin releasing hormone and progesterone
PTH	• No known change in reference range	
Vitamin D	• Reference ranges for normal pregnancy not established	
Catecholamines	• No known change in reference range	

ACTH = adrenocorticotropic hormone; ADH = antidiuretic hormone; CBG = cortisol binding globulin; FSH = follicle-stimulating hormone; GH = growth hormone; hCG = human chorionic gonadotropin; IGF-1 = insulin growth factor-1; LH = Luteinizing hormone; PTH = parathyroid hormone; T_3 = triiodothyronine; T_4 = thyroxine; TBG = thyroid binding globulin; TSH = thyroid stimulating hormone

The confidential enquiries into maternal and child health (CEMACH) study in the UK described recurrent hypoglycemia in 61% of type 1 diabetes patients, and 25% experienced severe hypoglycemia (6). Reassuringly, there has been no evidence of teratogenicity associated with hypoglycemia.

Non-Diabetic Starvation Ketoacidosis

In the third trimester of pregnancy, ketoacidosis develops more rapidly than in non-pregnant individuals following episodes of starvation or protracted vomiting. This can result in metabolic acidosis that has similar risks of fetal mortality to DKA (7). This condition responds well to an infusion of 10% dextrose and it is possible that emergency delivery may be avoided with rapid diagnosis and treatment.

Pituitary Disease

Pregnant women with pituitary disease most commonly have tumors of the anterior pituitary gland. Non-functioning tumors are likely to be the most common pituitary tumor as they have been reported in approximately 10% of individuals at autopsy. However, prolactinoma is the commonest pituitary tumor in women of reproductive age, followed by growth hormone (GH) and adrenocorticotrophic hormone (ACTH)-secreting tumors. Pituitary tumors may cause an acute presentation due to pressure effects or excessive secretion of a specific hormone. Pituitary apoplexy is a rare complication of pituitary tumors in pregnancy, and can occur in women in whom the tumor had not been diagnosed.

Prolactinomas

The management of hyperprolactinemia in the non-pregnant and pregnant state is described in detail in the 2011 Endocrine Society Clinical Practice Guidelines (8). Hyperprolactinemia is a common cause of infertility in women as it inhibits pulsatile gonadotrophin releasing hormone from the hypothalamus, and treatment with a dopamine agonist can result in a rapid return of fertility, and therefore conception. If, a pregnant woman has a microprolactinoma, it is unlikely to enlarge in a clinically relevant manner in pregnancy. In contrast, women with macroprolactinomas have a 14–46% chance of symptomatic expansion in pregnancy (9–11). Formal visual field testing should be performed every 6–8 weeks in women with macroprolactinoma. Pituitary imaging is required if tumor enlargement is suspected due to changes in visual fields or if there are new symptoms of headache, nausea or diabetes insipidus (DI). Figure 4-1 demonstrates a pituitary macroadenoma with suprasellar extension but no chiasmal compression. As the pregnancy progresses, Figure 4-1 demonstrates the macroadenoma with chiasmal compression causing a bilateral superior temporal field defect. Magnetic resonance imaging (MRI) with contrast is safe in pregnancy, and can be performed in the first trimester if required (12).

Dopamine receptor agonists are usually discontinued in early pregnancy, but can be continued in cases of macroprolactinoma at risk of symptomatic tumor expansion. If there is confirmed evidence of tumor enlargement, they should be restarted. Bromocriptine and cabergoline are not associated with increased rates of congenital malformation, nor adverse pregnancy outcome (e.g., preterm labour, intrauterine growth restriction [IUGR] or pre-eclampsia) (9,10, 13). It is important to be aware that the UK Medicine and Healthcare Products Regulatory Authority has advised that pregnancy should be excluded before using ergot derivatives (cabergoline and bromocriptine), due to a theoretical risk of maternal or fetal cardiac valve fibrosis. However, at present, there are no studies that report these complications in women treated with dopamine agonists in pregnancy, and bromocriptine or cabergoline should be used if a pregnant woman has symptomatic enlargement of a pituitary tumor.

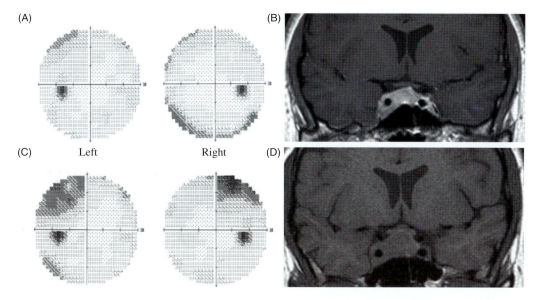

Figure 4-1 (A) Normal visual fields assessed using Humphrey's perimetry; (B) T1-weighted MRI (coronal view) showing a pituitary macroadenoma with suprasellar extension but no chiasmal compression; (C) Perimetry demonstrating a bilateral superior temporal field defect; (D) T1-weighted MRI (coronal view) showing a pituitary macroadenoma with chiasmal compression (48). Reproduced with permission from John Wiley & Sons Ltd.

Non-Functioning Pituitary Tumors

A recent UK cohort study of pituitary tumors in pregnancy demonstrated that non-functioning pituitary tumors are almost as common as macroprolactinoma in pregnancy and that they can present with symptomatic tumor enlargement (9). This is likely to relate to enlargement of adjacent pituitary tissue and can be treated in the same way as when this occurs in women with macroprolactinoma. Non-functioning tumors may be complicated by pituitary apoplexy.

Acromegaly

Pregnancy in patients with acromegaly is uncommon, because the majority of affected women have reduced fertility due to hyperprolactinemia from pituitary stalk compression. They also have increased rates of polycystic ovary syndrome and may have reduced secretion of gonadotropins. Most diagnostic assays cannot distinguish between pituitary and placental GH (Table 4-1) so confirmation of the diagnosis may have to wait until after delivery when the placental GH falls rapidly. Macroadenomas are relatively common in acromegaly and enlargement of normal adjacent pituitary tissue can cause an emergency presentation with visual symptoms, as with non-functioning pituitary tumors. Acromegaly can increase the risk of gestational diabetes, pregnancy-induced hypertension and pre-eclampsia, and these complications occur more commonly in women with high levels of GH and insulin-like growth factor-1 (IGF-1) before pregnancy (14,15). Acromegaly-associated cardiac disease, including coronary artery disease and cardiomyopathy, can manifest for the first time in pregnancy as cardiac emergencies.

Medical treatment is usually interrupted at the time of pregnancy (16). Dopamine receptor agonists are normally stopped early in pregnancy and somatostatin analogs withheld due to a lack of clear safety data surrounding their use, and there are some data implicating them in IUGR (14,15). Interruption for the duration of pregnancy will not usually affect the course of the condition but should be decided on a case-by-case basis. If the clinical team believe it is appropriate to continue both classes of drugs due to headache or tumor extension, it is a reasonable approach if the benefits of treatment are thought to outweigh the potential risks. Only a small number of women with acromegaly have been reported to have deteriorated in pregnancy, with tumor growth and one case of pituitary apoplexy. Therefore, the same advice as for prolactinomas should be followed with respect to tumor size and monitoring.

Pituitary Apoplexy

Pituitary apoplexy has been reported in association with prolatinoma, ACTH-secreting and non-functioning pituitary tumors. In a series of seven cases, all presented with severe headache and visual symptoms, and some had co-existing vomiting or altered consciousness (17). Investigation and treatment should be the same as for non-pregnant women. Computed tomography (CT) and MRI scans can be used, and there is no contraindication to treatment with glucocorticoids.

Pituitary Insufficiency

This can result from previous pituitary surgery or radiotherapy, lesions such as adenomas, infarction or lymphocytic hypophysitis, and may lead to subfertility as the gonadotropin stimulus to ovulation may be absent. Hence, ovulation induction therapies may be required. If adequate hormonal replacement has been achieved prior to pregnancy, there is no effect of this condition on maternal outcome. If the condition is not diagnosed or is inadequately treated, it can be associated with miscarriage and stillbirth (18). Also, women with hypopituitarism requiring ovulation induction have increased rates of IUGR and fetal loss, including mid-trimester fetal death, so they should be managed as high-risk pregnancies (18). The principal emergencies associated with

pituitary insufficiency are hypoadrenalism and severe DI.

Lymphocytic Hypophysitis

Lymphocytic hypophysitis occurs at increased frequency in late pregnancy and postpartum, and it can cause isolated ACTH deficiency. Diagnosis in the acute setting is challenging as the hormone levels used to diagnose pituitary insufficiency are affected by pregnancy. Luteinizing hormone (LH) and follicle-stimulating hormone (FSH) are suppressed, so the diagnosis is limited to assessment of the thyroid and hypothalamic-pituitary-adrenal (HPA) axis. Thyroid function may be normal initially due to the long half-life of thyroxine (T_4) so repeated measurements are important. HPA axis assessment relies on ACTH and cortisol levels. The adrenal response to ACTH will remain normal in acute pituitary insufficiency so a short ACTH stimulation test is not diagnostically useful initially. Prolactin can be useful as the level may be abnormally low. Plasma sodium levels do not usually change significantly in pregnancy, although there is a slight reduction in the normal reference range due to a "reset osmostat" mechanism (see below). However, in most cases, hyponatremia can be diagnosed using normal laboratory reference ranges. Hormone replacement should be given in the same way as for non-pregnant individuals. There is no evidence that replacement levels of glucocorticoids cause risks for the mother or fetus (although dexamethasone should not be used for routine glucocorticoid replacement in pregnancy).

Diabetes Insipidus

The symptoms of DI can worsen in pregnancy because of placental vasopressinase production and an associated reduction in antidiuretic hormone (ADH) levels. ADH analogs such as desmopressin can be continued and no adverse effects have been reported, but a higher dose may be required. It is important to reduce the dose rapidly to pre-pregnancy levels after delivery as otherwise hyponatremia may occur. Transient DI can occur in pregnancy secondary to placental vasopressinase production. This may be a feature of significant hepatic pathology (e.g., acute fatty liver of pregnancy). In this condition the hepatic breakdown of placental vasopressinase is reduced. It is therefore important to exclude liver disease in addition to other pituitary disorders that may cause *de novo* DI in pregnancy. Polyuria and polydipsia are included in the "Swansea criteria" that are valuable in the diagnosis of acute fatty liver of pregnancy (19).

As DI is a disorder of the posterior pituitary, it can be associated with reduced oxytocin production. This can have important consequences at delivery, as labor may not progress and there is an increased rate of uterine atony.

SIADH and Hyponatremia

In normal pregnancy, there is altered sensitivity to ADH, resulting in a "reset osmostat" phenomenon. This correlates to raised levels of human chorionic gonadotropin (hCG), although the underlying mechanism is not fully understood. Pregnant women typically develop thirst at a plasma osmolality that is 5–10 mOsm/kg lower than non-pregnant individuals, and the sodium concentration is 5 mmol/L lower (20). It is important to be aware of this when women present with hyponatremia in pregnancy. Conditions that may be complicated by maternal hyponatremia include hyperemesis gravidarum, hypoadrenalism, drug reactions (e.g., carbamazepine), fluid overload, aggressive oxytocin therapy and syndrome of inappropriate ADH (SIADH).

Hyponatremia rarely occurs because of SIADH in pregnant women. Approximately 50% of cases have pre-eclampsia and most other cases have recognized associated disorders (21). It is important to be aware of the normal gestational alterations in ADH secretion and plasma osmolality when assessing these cases. If clinicians attempt to raise the plasma sodium inappropriately in women with hyponatremia that is not due to SIADH, they will cause thirst and polydipsia.

Adrenal Disease

Pregnant women may present with endocrine emergencies as a result of adrenal tumors or insufficiency.

Pheochromocytoma

The incidence of pheochromocytoma in pregnancy is estimated to be 1 in 50,000 (22). The maternal and fetal mortality rates have fallen considerably over the years, declining to 17% and 20% respectively in the 1980s, and to 4% and 11% in 1988–1997. More recent studies have reported low maternal mortality if the diagnosis is made during the antenatal period, but the risk of fetal death remains relatively high at 15% (23). A high mortality rate is associated with the presence of an unanticipated pheochromocytoma. A low threshold for investigation of hypertension presenting in the first half of pregnancy is likely to explain the increasing number of cases that are diagnosed in the antenatal period. Management should be undertaken through a multidisciplinary approach. Figure 4-2 depicts a left adrenal mass (pheochromocytoma) and a fetus *in utero*. The aim should

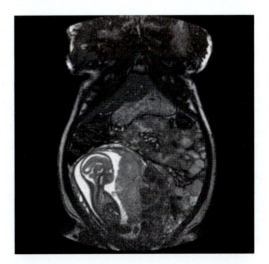

Figure 4-2 T1-weighted MRI (coronal view) showing a pheochromocytoma and fetus *in utero*.

be to treat blood pressure appropriately with initial use of an alpha-blocker and review for hyperglycemia. Phenoxybenzamine should be used during pregnancy as the safety data are reassuring (24,25). If pheochromocytoma is diagnosed in the first half of pregnancy, it is reasonable to consider laparoscopic removal during the second trimester.

Conn's Syndrome

This in uncommon during pregnancy and there are very few cases described in the literature. There is a rise in aldosterone levels and plasma renin activity during pregnancy and this can pose challenge for diagnosis of the condition (Table 4-1). Conn's syndrome may present with hypokalemia and hypertension in pregnancy, and when this occurs, it is important to correct blood pressure and the electrolyte imbalance. Spironolactone is the treatment of choice outside of pregnancy, but it is rarely used to treat Conn's syndrome in pregnant women due to theoretical concerns about anti-androgenic effects causing ambiguous genitalia in a male fetus. Alternative anti-hypertensive drugs include eplerenone and amiloride, both of which have been reported in single cases (26,27). Reported maternal and fetal complications of Conn's syndrome include placental abruption, intrauterine death and fetal distress (28,29).

Adrenal Insufficiency

In the developed world, Addison's disease is the most common cause of hypoadrenalism in fertile women. One large population cohort study demonstrated all pregnancies complicated by Addison's disease have increased maternal and fetal risks (30). Newly diagnosed Addison's disease is very uncommon during pregnancy. It may be challenging to recognize the symptoms during pregnancy. Non-specific symptoms include nausea, fatigue, and anorexia and are all common in pregnant women. During pregnancy, there is a rise in total plasma cortisol, cortisol binding globulin, and

24-hour urinary cortisol. During the third trimester, there is a 3- to 10-fold rise in cortisol levels (31). There is also a rise in aldosterone levels and plasma renin activity during pregnancy (Table 4-1). A morning cortisol and short ACTH stimulation test are safe during pregnancy. Trimester-specific cortisol levels should be used to interpret these results. A morning cortisol level of less than 11 μg/dL (300 nmol/L), 16.3 μg/dL (450 nmol/L) and 21.7 μg/dL (600 nmol/L) in the 1st, 2nd and 3rd trimester respectively raises the suspicion of hypocortisolism. The optimal cut off for the 30- or 60-minute cortisol level as part of the short ACTH stimulation test should be greater than 25.3 μg/dL (700 nmol/L), 29 μg/dL (800 nmol/L) and 32.6 μg/dL (900 nmol/L) in the 1st, 2nd and 3rd trimester respectively (32). Maternal and fetal risks of inadequately treated adrenal insufficiency include preterm delivery, IUGR, and adrenal crisis. An acute adrenal crisis may occur due to hyperemesis gravidarum or intercurrent illness. Most women with pre-existing Addison's disease require a 30–40% rise in their hydrocortisone dose during the third trimester. Fludrocortisone doses are not usually affected during pregnancy due to the anti-mineralocorticoid effects of progesterone. Hydrocortisone is the drug of choice for this condition. All women require intrapartum hydrocortisone regardless of mode of delivery. Hydrocortisone doses of 50 mg– 100 mg three to four times a day are usually administered intra-muscularly or intravenously. Immediately postpartum, women should remain on twice their pre-delivery dose for the first 24–48 hours and then be rapidly tapered back to maintenance dose.

Thyroid Disease in Pregnancy

Thyroid disease is common during pregnancy and, if treated appropriately, medical emergencies are rare. Trimester-specific thyroid-stimulating hormone (TSH) and T_4 ranges are important to account for the pregnancy effects on the hypothalamic-pituitary-thyroid axis. An underactive thyroid is more common during pregnancy with a prevalence of 2–5%, while overt hypothyroidism is seen in 0.3–0.5% of pregnancies. An overactive thyroid during pregnancy has a prevalence of 0.1–0.4%, and Graves' disease accounts for 85% of all cases. Distinguishing between hyperthyroidism and gestational thyrotoxicosis is important and can be challenging.

Hypothyroidism

Hypothyroidism is common in women of child-bearing age (33). It is recognized either by the clinical presentation of classic symptoms or incidentally during the work-up of infertility. If inadequately treated, there is an increased risk of gestational hypertension, placental abruption, and postpartum hemorrhage. If untreated, there is a risk of low birth weight, preterm delivery, and neonatal respiratory distress. Ideally thyroid disease should be stable prior to conception. The TSH value during pregnancy should be maintained within population-specific and gestation-specific normal ranges (34). During pregnancy, some women with known hypothyroidism may require an increase in their thyroxine dose (34–36). This may be due to increased levels of thyroid-binding globulin, or because they were inadequately treated prior to conception. Once the thyroid function tests are stable, pregnant women only require surveillance each trimester and 6–8 weeks postpartum, unless they become symptomatic. If symptomatic or first diagnosed during pregnancy the thyroid function tests may be measured more frequently until stable. Hypothyroidism is rarely associated with medical emergencies in pregnancy.

Hyperthyroidism

The symptoms of hyperthyroidism usually predate pregnancy. If inadequately treated, there is a risk of IUGR, low birth weight, pre-eclampsia, preterm delivery, stillbirth, and miscarriage. The symptoms of Graves' disease tend to worsen in the first trimester and improve in the latter half of pregnancy.

When diagnosed before pregnancy, the disease should be stabilized prior to conception. Definitive treatments such as radioactive iodine (RAI) are contraindicated during pregnancy and women considering pregnancy are counseled to wait at least 6 months after RAI treatment to conceive. Surgical interventions should only be considered during pregnancy if medical treatment cannot be tolerated. The optimal time to perform surgery is the second trimester.

During pregnancy, anti-thyroid medication is first line treatment for thyrotoxicosis (34). Options include methimazole (MMI), carbimazole (CBM), and propylthiouracil (PTU). All have similar transplacental transfer kinetics. Anti-thyroid medication is associated with a 0.3–0.5% risk of aganulocytosis. PTU in adults can lead to hepatoxicity in 1 in 10,000. Both MMI and CBM are associated with increased risk of congenital anomalies. The congenital anomalies seen include aplasia cutis, choanal atresia and intestinal anomalies (37–39). Due to these effects, current guidelines advocate the use of PTU in the first trimester and MMI/CBM in the second and third trimester (34). However, a recent Danish cohort study of 817,093 children, including 1820 exposed to PTU or MMI/CBM, demonstrated congenital malformations in 8% of children exposed to PTU, 9% of those taking MMI/CBM and 10% of children treated with both drugs (40). Thus, clinicians should individualize decisions about treatment with anti-thyroid drugs in pregnancy, with cognizance of the need to maintain good maternal control while minimizing the risk to the fetus. Consensus statements have proposed that, "practitioners should use their clinical judgment in choosing the anti-thyroid medication, including the potential difficulties in switching from one drug to another" (34). Thyroid function tests should be measured every 4–6 weeks with the aim of maintaining the T_4 in the upper limits of the non-pregnant normal range. If the TSH becomes detectable, the anti-thyroid medication should be reduced further. MMI, CBM and PTU are all safe during breast feeding, although in the context of high maternal doses, it is advisable to ensure the neonate remains euthyroid. Antenatal management of thyrotoxicosis may include symptomatic treatment with ß-blockers. They are safe during pregnancy, and short-acting ß-blockers such as propranolol and metoprolol are effective. After delivery, hyperthyroidism may relapse or worsen.

TSH receptor antibodies should be measured at 22–26 weeks gestation. These antibodies cross the placenta. If raised more than 2- to 3-fold, there is an increased risk of fetal thyrotoxicosis. Management includes fetal surveillance and treatment with anti-thyroid drugs *in utero*.

Gestational Thyrotoxicosis

Gestational thyrotoxicosis is usually limited to the first half of pregnancy and associated with hyperemesis gravidarum in 5–10 cases per 1000 pregnancies. Biochemically there is a raised T_4 and suppressed TSH. The condition is thought to be caused by elevated hCG in the first trimester, and the homology with TSH leads to these biochemical findings. It occurs in the absence of thyroid antibodies. Other causes of this clinical picture include multiple gestation, hydatidiform mole, hyperreactio luteinalis and hyperplacentosis.

It is important to distinguish between gestational thyrotoxicosis and Graves' disease because the conditions are managed differently. With gestational thyrotoxicosis the symptoms only occur during pregnancy, the nausea and vomiting are profound and usually the main symptom. Rehydration, appropriate anti-emetic medication and reassurance are necessary. With Graves' disease, the symptoms often predate the pregnancy and can be associated with the usual clinical features (e.g., Graves' opthalmopathy).

Thyroid Storm

This is an uncommon event in pregnancy, but may be life-threatening. It can be precipitated by infection, pre-eclampsia and during the intrapartum period either by labor or cesarean-section (41). It can also occur in women with severe hyperemesis gravidarum in whom severe vomiting prevents ingestion of anti-thyroid medication. Symptoms are similar to non-pregnant individuals. The management is supportive in an intensive care unit setting with a multidisciplinary approach. Anti-thyroid medication should be commenced immediately. PTU is preferred due to its ability to block conversion of T_4 to triiodothyronine (T_3) (42). Tachyarrhythmias may be managed with ß-blocking medication. Other additional medications include high dose glucocorticoids and oral potassium iodide (43).

Parathyroid Disease in Pregnancy

Primary hyperparathyroidism in pregnancy is rare with a reported annual incidence of 8 cases per 100,000 women of childbearing age. The actual incidence in pregnancy is unknown, due to likely under-reporting and there are fewer than 250 cases in the peer-reviewed literature to date. Primary hyperparathyroidism causes hypercalcemia as a consequence of excessive secretion of parathyroid hormone (PTH), usually due to an adenoma of the parathyroid gland. Maternal complications are reported in approximately 65% of cases. These include hyperemesis gravidarum, nephrolithiasis, peptic ulcer disease, and pancreatitis. Hypertension or pre-eclampsia occurs in up to 25% of cases (44). Primary hyperparathyroidism can occasionally precipitate a life-threatening hypercalcemic crisis. The incidence of fetal complications is approximately 50%, and these include miscarriage, IUGR, stillbirth, neonatal tetany and neonatal death (45).

Hyperparathyroidism is diagnosed by identifying a high plasma calcium concentration with a corresponding high or inappropriately normal PTH concentration and high urinary calcium levels. Identification of hypercalcemia in pregnancy can be difficult as the total calcium concentration can appear normal as a result of the lower albumin concentration. Isotope studies are contraindicated in pregnancy, but ultrasound or arterial phase CT scan can be used to identify adenomas. Most pregnant women with hypercalcemia respond well to admission and hydration. However, many cannot maintain normocalcemia without ongoing administration of intravenous fluids. Furthermore, the increased risk of adverse pregnancy outcome, including stillbirth, is of concern in women with hypercalcemia secondary to hyperparathyroidism, and therefore parathyroidectomy is the treatment of choice in the majority of cases. Ideally parathyroidectomy should be performed at the end of the first trimester or in the second trimester, but it can be performed in pregnancy at most gestational ages. If surgery is not performed, management involves maintaining hydration and administering oral phosphates. In addition to the increased risk of pre-eclampsia in women with primary hyperparathyroidism in pregnancy, those with a history of parathyroidectomy more than two years

prior to pregnancy also have increased rates of hypertensive disease in pregnancy (46).

Conclusions

Pre-pregnancy counseling should be offered to all women with pre-existing endocrine disease to ensure stability of the disease prior to conception and to discuss the safety profile of medication(s) during pregnancy. Endocrine and metabolic emergencies in pregnancy should be managed by a multidisciplinary team that includes endocrinologists, obstetricians, obstetric anesthetists, and neonatologists. As with all comorbid conditions in pregnancy, it is important to be aware that at least two lives are involved; prompt senior review should be available at all times; and many standard of care investigations (e.g., nuclear scans) and drugs (e.g., bisphosphonate in hypercalcemia) may be contraindicated or need to be modified or have not been tested in the pregnant setting.

References

1 Blumer I, Hadar E, Hadden DR, et al. Diabetes and pregnancy: an endocrine society clinical practice guideline. *J Clin Endocrinol Metab*. 2013;98(11):4227–4249.

2 De Veciana M. Diabetes ketoacidosis in pregnancy. *Semin Perinatol*. 2013;37(4): 267–273.

3 Dhatariya K, Savage M, Claydon A, et al. Joint British Diabetes Societies Inpatient Care Group. The management of diabetic ketoacidosis in adults. September 2013. https://www.diabetes.org.uk/Documents/About%20Us/What%20we%20say/Management-of-DKA-241013.pdf. (accessed May 30, 2017).

4 Seaquist ER, Anderson J, Childs B, et al. Hypoglycemia and diabetes: a report of a workgroup of the American Diabetes Association and the Endocrine Society. *J Clin Endocrinol Metab*. 2013;98(5): 1845–1859.

5 Ringholm L, Pedersen-Bjergaard U, Thorsteinsson B, Damm P, Mathiesen ER. Hypoglycaemia during pregnancy in women with Type 1 diabetes. *Diabet Med*. 2012;29(5):558–566.

6 Modder J, ed. *Confidential Enquiry into Maternal and Child Health. Pregnancy in Women with Type 1 and Type 2 Diabetes in 2002–03, England, Wales and Northern Ireland*. London: CEMCH; 2005.

7 Frise CJ, Mackillop L, Joash K, Williamson C. Starvation ketoacidosis in pregnancy. *Eur J Obstet Gynecol Reprod Biol*. 2013; 167(1):1–7.

8 Melmed S, Casanueva FF, Hoffman AR, et al. Diagnosis and treatment of hyperprolactinemia: an Endocrine Society clinical practice guideline. *J Clin Endocrinol Metab*. 2011;96(2):273–288.

9 Lambert K, Rees K, Seed PT, et al. Macroprolactinomas and nonfunctioning

pituitary adenomas and pregnancy outcomes. *Obstet Gynecol.* 2017;129(1): 185–194.

10 Lebbe M, Hubinont C, Bernard P, Maiter D. Outcome of 100 pregnancies initiated under treatment with cabergoline in hyperprolactinaemic women. *Clin Endocrinol (Oxf).* 2010;73(2):236–242.

11 Bronstein MD, Paraiba DB, Jallad RS. Management of pituitary tumors in pregnancy. *Nat Rev Endocrinol.* 2011;7(5): 301–310.

12 Kanal E, Barkovich AJ, Bell C, et al. ACR guidance document for safe MR practices: 2007. *AJR Am J Roentgenol.* 2007;188(6): 1447–1474.

13 Raymond JP, Goldstein E, Konopka P, Leleu MF, Merceron RE, Loria Y. Follow-up of children born of bromocriptine-treated mothers. *Horm Res.* 1985;22(3):239–246.

14 Caron P, Broussaud S, Bertherat J, et al. Acromegaly and pregnancy: a retrospective multicenter study of 59 pregnancies in 46 women. *J Clin Endocrinol Metab.* 2010; 95(10):4680–4687.

15 Cheng S, Grasso L, Martinez-Orozco JA, et al. Pregnancy in acromegaly: experience from two referral centers and systematic review of the literature. *Clin Endocrinol (Oxf).* 2012;76(2):264–271.

16 Katznelson L, Laws ER, Jr, Melmed S, et al. Acromegaly: an endocrine society clinical practice guideline. *J Clin Endocrinol Metab.* 2014;99(11):3933–3951.

17 de Heide LJ, van Tol KM, Doorenbos B. Pituitary apoplexy presenting during pregnancy. *Neth J Med.* 2004;62(10): 393–396.

18 Overton CE, Davis CJ, West C, Davies MC, Conway GS. High risk pregnancies in hypopituitary women. *Hum Reprod.* 2002;17(6):1464–1467.

19 Ch'ng CL, Morgan M, Hainsworth I, Kingham JG. Prospective study of liver dysfunction in pregnancy in Southwest Wales. *Gut.* 2002;51(6):876–880.

20 Harris K, Shankar R, Black K, Rochelson B. Reset osmostat in pregnancy: a case report. *J Matern Fetal Neonatal Med.* 2014;27(5): 530–533.

21 Nawathe A, Govind A. Pregnancy with known syndrome of inappropriate antidiuretic hormone. *J Obstet Gynaecol.* 2013;33(1):9–13.

22 Ahlawat SK, Jain S, Kumari S, Varma S, Sharma BK. Pheochromocytoma associated with pregnancy: case report and review of the literature. *Obstet Gynecol Surv.* 1999;54(11):728–737.

23 van der Weerd K, van Noord C, Loeve M, et al. Endocrinology in pregnancY: Case series and review of literature: pheochromocytoma in pregnancy. *Eur J Endocrinol.* 2017 Apr. 5.

24 Darr R, Lenders JW, Hofbauer LC, Naumann B, Bornstein SR, Eisenhofer G. Pheochromocytoma - update on disease management. *Ther Adv Endocrinol Metab.* 2012;3(1):11–26.

25 Oliva R, Angelos P, Kaplan E, Bakris G. Pheochromocytoma in pregnancy: a case series and review. *Hypertension.* 2010; 55(3):600–606.

26 Al-Ali NA, El-Sandabesee D, Steel SA, Roland JM. Conn's syndrome in pregnancy successfully treated with amiloride. *J Obstet Gynaecol.* 2007;27(7):730–731.

27 Cabassi A, Rocco R, Berretta R, Regolisti G, Bacchi-Modena A. Eplerenone use in primary aldosteronism during pregnancy. *Hypertension.* 2012;59(2): e18–e19.

28 Lu W, Zheng F, Li H, Ruan L. Primary aldosteronism and pregnancy: a case report. *Aust N Z J Obstet Gynaecol.* 2009;49(5):558.

29 Ronconi V, Turchi F, Zennaro MC, Boscaro M, Giacchetti G. Progesterone increase counteracts aldosterone action in a pregnant woman with primary aldosteronism. *Clin Endocrinol (Oxf).* 2011;74(2):278–279.

30 Schneiderman M, Czuzoj-Shulman N, Spence AR, Abenhaim HA. Maternal and neonatal outcomes of pregnancies in women with Addison's disease: a population-based cohort study on 7.7 million births. *BJOG.* 2016;15.

31 Jung C, Ho JT, Torpy DJ, et al. A longitudinal study of plasma and urinary cortisol in pregnancy and postpartum. *J Clin Endocrinol Metab*. 2011;96(5):1533–1540.

32 Lebbe M, Arlt W. What is the best diagnostic and therapeutic management strategy for an Addison patient during pregnancy? *Clin Endocrinol (Oxf)*. 2013;78(4):497–502.

33 Teng W, Shan Z, Patil-Sisodia K, Cooper DS. Hypothyroidism in pregnancy. *Lancet Diabetes Endocrinol*. 2013;1(3):228–237.

34 Alexander EK, Pearce EN, Brent GA, et al. 2017 Guidelines of the American Thyroid Association for the Diagnosis and Management of Thyroid Disease During Pregnancy and the Postpartum. *Thyroid*. 2017;27(3):315–389.

35 Alexander EK, Marqusee E, Lawrence J, Jarolim P, Fischer GA, Larsen PR. Timing and magnitude of increases in levothyroxine requirements during pregnancy in women with hypothyroidism. *N Engl J Med*. 2004;351(3):241–249.

36 Reid SM, Middleton P, Cossich MC, Crowther CA, Bain E. Interventions for clinical and subclinical hypothyroidism pre-pregnancy and during pregnancy. *Cochrane Database Syst Rev*. 2013;(5):CD007752. doi: (5):CD007752.

37 Clementi M, Di Gianantonio E, Cassina M, et al. Treatment of hyperthyroidism in pregnancy and birth defects. *J Clin Endocrinol Metab*. 2010;95(11):E337–E341.

38 Cooper DS, Laurberg P. Hyperthyroidism in pregnancy. *Lancet Diabetes Endocrinol*. 2013;1(3):238–249.

39 Yoshihara A, Noh J, Yamaguchi T, et al. Treatment of Graves' disease with antithyroid drugs in the first trimester of pregnancy and the prevalence of congenital malformation. *J Clin Endocrinol Metab*. 2012;97(7):2396–2403.

40 Andersen SL, Olsen J, Wu CS, Laurberg P. Birth defects after early pregnancy use of antithyroid drugs: a Danish nationwide study. *J Clin Endocrinol Metab*. 2013;98(11):4373–4381.

41 Chan GW, Mandel SJ. Therapy insight: management of Graves' disease during pregnancy. *Nat Clin Pract Endocrinol Metab*. 2007;3(6):470–478.

42 Cooper DS. Antithyroid drugs. *N Engl J Med*. 2005;3;352(9):905–917.

43 Mestman JH. Hyperthyroidism in pregnancy. *Best Pract Res Clin. Endocrinol Metab*. 2004;18(2):267–288.

44 Schnatz PF, Thaxton S. Parathyroidectomy in the third trimester of pregnancy. *Obstet Gynecol Surv*. 2005;60(10):672–682.

45 Norman J, Politz D, Politz L. Hyperparathyroidism during pregnancy and the effect of rising calcium on pregnancy loss: a call for earlier intervention. *Clin Endocrinol (Oxf)*. 2009;71(1):104–109.

46 Hultin H, Hellman P, Lundgren E, et al. Association of parathyroid adenoma and pregnancy with preeclampsia. *J Clin Endocrinol Metab*. 2009;94(9):3394–3399.

47 Frise CJ, Williamson C. Endocrine disease in pregnancy. *Clin Med*. 2013;13:176–181.

48 Banerjee A, et al. High dose cabergoline therapy for a resistant macroprolactinoma during pregnancy. *Clin Endocrinol (Oxf)*. 2009;70:812–813.

5

Endocrine and Metabolic Emergencies in Inherited Metabolic Diseases

Acute Presentations in Adulthood

Elaine Murphy and Robin H. Lachmann

Key Points

- Inherited metabolic diseases (IMDs) are clinically heterogeneous, individually rare disorders that can present at any age, and typically, but not always, are associated with abnormal biochemical tests (usually specialist rather than routine laboratory testing).
- Broadly speaking, IMDs can be divided into three groups: (a) disorders of intoxication give rise to an acute or progressive intoxication secondary to the accumulation of toxic compounds proximal to a metabolic block; (b) disorders of energy metabolism resulting in an energy deficiency in tissues such as liver, muscle, brain, or heart; and (c) disorders of complex molecules causing disturbance in the synthesis or catabolism of complex molecules. Symptoms tend to be progressive and not dependent on dietary/energy intake.
- The majority of adults with an IMD will already have a known diagnosis, usually made in childhood. They may bring with them specific guidelines for emergency management of their condition.
- However, affected adult individuals can also present for the first time. It is important for clinicians to be aware of these disorders, not only to manage survivors of

childhood but also to recognize patients presenting in adulthood.
- The possibility of an underlying IMD should always be considered in patients presenting with encephalopathy, disturbances of acid-base balance, atypical stroke, psychiatric features, or rhabdomyolysis, particularly if these episodes are recurrent and there is no other obvious underlying cause.
- Hypoglycemia is a fairly unusual initial presentation in adulthood. Adults can maintain their blood glucose levels despite significant metabolic disturbance and thus presentation with hypoglycemia often represents a late event in a severe metabolic decompensation.
- IMD should also be considered if events are recurrent and where acute decompensations are triggered by metabolic "stress."
- As they are genetic diseases, missing the diagnosis may have implications both for the affected individuals and for their families.
- Not all diagnostic tests are readily available in the emergency setting, so appropriate samples should be collected during the acute event.

Endocrine and Metabolic Medical Emergencies: A Clinician's Guide, Second Edition. Edited by Glenn Matfin.
© 2018 John Wiley & Sons Ltd. Published 2018 by John Wiley & Sons Ltd.

Introduction

Inherited metabolic diseases (IMDs) are clinically heterogeneous, individually rare disorders that can present at any age, and typically, but not always, are associated with abnormal biochemical tests (usually specialist rather than routine laboratory testing).

Broadly speaking, IMDs can be divided into three groups: (a) disorders of intoxication give rise to an acute or progressive intoxication secondary to the accumulation of toxic compounds proximal to a metabolic block, for example, disorders of amino acid metabolism such as phenylketonuria (PKU), the organic acidurias, and the urea cycle defects such as ornithine transcarbamylase (OTC) deficiency; (b) disorders of energy metabolism resulting in an energy deficiency in tissues such as liver, muscle, brain, or heart, for example, mitochondrial respiratory chain defects, fatty acid oxidation defects, and glycogen storage disorders (GSDs); and (c) disorders of complex molecules causing disturbance in the synthesis or catabolism of complex molecules. Symptoms tend to be progressive and not dependent on dietary/energy intake, for example, the lysosomal storage disorders and the peroxisomal disorders.

The majority of adults with an IMD arriving at emergency services will already have a known diagnosis, usually made when they were children. Ideally they will carry some sort of information or even bring guidelines for emergency management of their condition (in some countries nationally agreed guidelines are accessible via the internet (e.g., the British Inherited Metabolic Disease Group Guidelines, www.BIMDG.org.uk)), but often their medical condition may prevent them giving an accurate history. Other patients may present for the first time in adulthood.

In the pediatric setting, the possibility of an acutely sick child having an IMD is well recognized but in the adult emergency department the emphasis is, quite correctly, on diagnosing acquired conditions such as infection or intoxication. Nonetheless, the possibility of an underlying IMD should always be considered in patients presenting with encephalopathy (which can be a psychiatric presentation in adults), disturbances of acid-base balance, atypical stroke, psychiatric features, or rhabdomyolysis – particularly if these episodes are recurrent and there is no other obvious underlying cause. Hypoglycemia, which is a frequent presentation of a number of IMDs in children, is a fairly unusual initial presentation in adulthood. Due to compensatory mechanisms adults can maintain their blood glucose levels despite significant metabolic disturbance and thus presentation with hypoglycemia often represents a late event in a severe metabolic decompensation (e.g., in fatty acid oxidation disorders or organic acidemias).

IMD should also be considered if events are recurrent and where acute decompensations are triggered by metabolic "stress," such as fasting, intercurrent infection, major surgery, gastrointestinal illness, and excessive alcohol or exercise. However, it is not always possible to identify a precise precipitating factor.

This chapter deals with some of the more frequent acute presentations of adults with IMDs and their emergency management (Table 5-1). It is important for adult clinicians to be aware of these disorders as effective treatments are available for many, and, as the disorders are genetic, making the diagnosis has implications both for the affected patient and their relatives. Not all diagnostic tests are readily available in the emergency setting, or even outside specialist laboratories, so appropriate samples (ideally including deoxyribonucleic acid [DNA]) should be collected and stored in the acute setting.

Rhabdomyolysis

Muscle has high energy requirements, particularly during exercise. These are supplied by metabolism of carbohydrate and of lipids. Stored glycogen is metabolized to pyruvate, which enters the mitochondria. Long-chain fatty acids are transported across the

Table 5-1 Summary of potential inherited metabolic diseases presenting as an emergency in adulthood

Disorder	Emergency presentation	Useful laboratory tests	Treatment options
Glycogen storage disorders	Rhabdomyolysis Cardiomyopathy	Creatine kinase	Modified diet Exercise advice
Fatty acid oxidation disorders	Rhabdomyolysis Cardiomyopathy	Creatine kinase Acylcarnitine profile Urine organic acids Fibroblast FAO studies Plasma ketones	iv dextrose Modified diet Exercise advice Bezafibrate L-carnitine
Urea cycle defects	Encephalopathy Stroke-like episode Psychiatric features	Ammonia Plasma amino acids Urine orotic acid	iv dextrose Hemofiltration Arginine Sodium benzoate Sodium phenylbutyrate
Organic acidemias	Encephalopathy Cardiac disease Renal impairment Metabolic acidosis	Blood gases Ammonia Acylcarnitine profile Urine organic acids	iv dextrose Hemofiltration L-carnitine
Homocystinuria	Thrombosis Lens dislocation Psychiatric features	Plasma amino acids	Pyridoxine Folate B12 Betaine
Lysosomal storage disorders	Cardiomyopathy Psychiatric features Stroke	White cell enzyme activities Filipin staining of fibroblasts	Enzyme replacement therapy Substrate reduction therapy
Adrenoleukodystrophy	Adrenal insufficiency Spastic paraparesis	Very long chain fatty acid levels Short ACTH stimulation test	Adrenal replacement Consider bone marrow transplant
Mitochondrial disease	Cardiomyopathy Stroke-like episode Lactic acidosis	See text	See text
Acute porphyrias	Abdominal pain Psychiatric features Neuropathy	Urine porphobilinogen	Heme arginate infusion
Hereditary fructose intolerance	Hypoglycemia Liver/renal impairment Metabolic acidosis	Liver function tests & coagulation Blood gases Assess renal tubular function	Eliminate all sources of fructose Organ support (HDU/ITU)

mitochondrial membrane by a process mediated by acylcarnitinetranslocase and carnitine palmitoyltransferases (CPT) 1 and 2. In the mitochondria, these substrates are then used to generate acetyl CoA, which feeds into the Kreb's cycle, ultimately delivering electrons to the mitochondrial respiratory chain to produce energy in the form of adenosine triphosphate (ATP). Inherited defects of glycogen metabolism or fatty acid oxidation are therefore frequently associated with muscle pathology.

In the acute setting, the most common metabolic causes of exercise-induced rhabdomyolysis in adulthood are GSDs types V and VII and the fatty acid oxidation disorders CPT2 and very long chain acyl-CoA dehydrogenase (VLCAD) deficiencies. At presentation, patients may give a history of previous episodes of less severe muscle pain precipitated by exercise or illness, or a family history of others with muscle pain.

GSD V (McArdle Disease)

GSD V (McArdle disease) is characterized by muscle pain that typically comes on within a few minutes of starting exercise (1). GSD V is characterized by a second-wind phenomenon: if aerobic exercise (e.g., jogging, cycling) is continued but at a slower, gentler pace, after several minutes exercise tolerance improves (evidenced by a reduction in heart rate) and patients can continue to exercise for long periods. This happens with the switch from glycolysis to fatty acid beta oxidation as the main source of energy for exercising muscle.

Static or isometric exercise (e.g., bench press, shoulder raises, carrying heavy shopping) is poorly tolerated in GSD V, as is sprinting. Some older patients may have evidence of a fixed proximal myopathy with wasting.

Diagnosis

Laboratory tests will show elevated creatine kinase (CK), urate and myoglobinuria and, in severe cases, renal impairment. In up to 85% of patients from Northern Europe, a common mutation, R50X, can be detected, and so, in patients with a typical clinical history, genetic mutation analysis may be used as a first line diagnostic test. GSD V can also be confirmed by a muscle biopsy which shows an excess of glycogen and absence of muscle phosphorylase (2). The ischemic forearm exercise test, measuring lactate and ammonia, the traditional screening test for muscle disorders of carbohydrate metabolism, is less often performed now as it is painful for the patient, not specifically diagnostic for GSD V, and has been largely superseded by genetic testing. A more modern functional test involves exercising the patient and demonstrating the "second wind" phenomenon (i.e., denotes a sudden, marked improvement in the tolerance to exercise such as walking or cycling after about 10 min, that is, disappearance of the excessive fatigue, breathlessness and tachycardia that were triggered by the start of exertion).

Management

Acute severe rhabdomyolysis should be treated with prompt fluid (normal saline) replacement and renal support as required. Intravenous (IV) dextrose during acute crises and oral sucrose prior to exercise may also be helpful. Patients should be given advice on safe forms of exercise and how to achieve the "second wind" phenomenon.

Fatty Acid Oxidation Disorders

Fatty acid oxidation disorders, such as CPT2 or VLCAD deficiencies often present for the first time in adolescence/adulthood (3). Patients typically develop myalgia/muscle stiffness/rhabdomyolysis after more prolonged exercise, for example, playing sport or marathon running. Prolonged fasting, cold exposure, intercurrent infection or even emotional stress are other well-recognized precipitants. Symptoms may last for a number of weeks following an acute attack, but patients may be completely asymptomatic, with normal muscle strength on examination, between attacks.

Diagnosis

If there is a strong suspicion of a fatty acid oxidation disorder, then a muscle biopsy may be avoided. Instead an acylcarnitine profile (plasma or blood spot) may suggest the condition which can then be confirmed by measurements of fatty acid oxidation and/or CPT2 enzyme activity in skin fibroblasts (grown from a punch skin biopsy) (2). Genetic testing allows screening of other potentially affected family members.

Management

Acute severe rhabdomyolysis should be treated with prompt fluid (saline) replacement, IV dextrose and renal support as required. Other measures that may be helpful in preventing recurrent symptoms include restriction of dietary long-chain fat, with substitution by medium-chain triglyceride (MCT) and carbohydrate. Note that patients with fatty acid oxidation disorders cannot achieve the "second wind" phenomenon.

Encephalopathy

Acute encephalopathy is a rapid decrease in conscious level (over hours or days), not secondary to ictal or syncopal episodes. In adult patients with IMDs, encephalopathy may be intermittent, fluctuating, or rapid and fulminant, progressing to coma (see case study). Patients may present with a change in personality (often agitated/aggressive), confusion, lethargy, drowsiness or coma. Vomiting is often a feature. Neurological findings may include secondary seizures, abnormal posturing, abnormal gait and poor coordination. These symptoms are due to brain swelling and, if treatment is not instituted promptly, permanent neurological damage can occur. A metabolic cause is a possibility in any adult who presents with encephalopathy: consideration should be given to hyperammonemia, hypoglycemia, and metabolic acidosis.

In late-onset, "attenuated," forms of IMD in adults, metabolic decompensation can often be precipitated by intercurrent infection, alcohol or drug (mis)use: clinicians should be wary of attributing all encephalopathic symptoms to these intoxicants, particularly if patients are not responding as expected to standard treatments. A history of previous unexplained episodes of confusion or agitation, or unusual dietary habits such as protein aversion, should be sought from family and friends.

All adults who present with acute or acute-on-chronic encephalopathy in whom there is no obvious cause (e.g., recent trauma, infection, a cerebrovascular event or hypoxia) should have a plasma ammonia level measured promptly.

By far the most common cause of hyperammonemia in adults is hepatic disease, often associated with portosystemic shunting. Once this has been excluded as a cause, then consideration should be given to other causes, and defects of the urea cycle are important among these (4). Hyperammonemia can also occur in fatty acid oxidation disorders or organic acidemias (5), but in these conditions first presentation usually occurs in infancy/childhood rather than in adulthood. Another important secondary cause of elevated ammonia is valproate therapy. Valproate is an organic acid and can inhibit the urea cycle, precipitating hyperammonemia. Valproate therapy can be the trigger for metabolic decompensation in individuals with a previously unknown urea cycle defect.

In the emergency setting, the vast majority of cases of metabolic acidosis are due to lactic acidosis secondary to hypoxia and tissue hypoperfusion, or diabetic ketoacidosis. When the anion gap is not accounted for by lactic acid or ketone bodies, consideration should be given to the presence of other organic acids. Most often these will be drugs or poisons, but if the event has been triggered by metabolic stress rather than toxin ingestion, an underlying organic acidemia is a possibility.

Diagnosis

Definitive diagnosis should not delay immediate treatment but appropriate samples should be taken, preferably during the acute presentation, in order that chronic management can be tailored and genetic counseling can be given to both the index patient and other potentially affected family members.

The following tests should be taken as a minimum, but others may be required depending on the specific presentation:

Routine Chemistry
- Liver function tests
- Complete (full) blood count
- Lactate, glucose, CK
- Blood gas analysis,
- Blood and urine cultures
- Toxicology

Specialist Chemistry
- Plasma amino acids
- Urine amino acids
- Urine organic acids (specifically for orotic acid)
- Acylcarnitine profile
- Store DNA for future mutation analysis

These tests should be discussed with your local specialist laboratory to ensure the correct sample conditions and transport. It is very important to avoid hemolysis and delayed separation of samples.

Management

While the precise underlying cause of hyperammonemia may take some time to elucidate, it is essential to start treatment immediately in order to avoid long-term neurological damage or death. The aims of treatment are to reduce catabolism and ammonia production and to lower plasma ammonia before cerebral edema develops.

In severe hyperammonemia with marked encephalopathy, seizures or coma, hemofiltration is the most efficient way to reduce plasma ammonia (peritoneal dialysis is not as efficient and should be avoided). Vascular access should be secured and continuous hemofiltration started as soon as possible in the high dependency unit (HDU) or intensive care unit (ICU) setting.

Protein intake should be stopped for 24–48 hours, and a hypercaloric solution (IV 10% dextrose; Intralipid) started, with insulin if needed to enhance anabolism. Intravenous arginine and ammonia scavengers (sodium benzoate and sodium phenylbutyrate) will promote the excretion of non-urea nitrogen-containing metabolites in the urine.

Long-term management will require input from a specialist center to ensure appropriate dietary advice (including supplementation of vitamins and minerals in those on a restricted diet) and titration of oral medications to ensure optimal metabolic control.

In organic acidemias, treatment is also based on prevention of catabolism, restriction of protein and removal of toxic metabolites (6). Intravenous carnitine is used to conjugate toxic fatty acid derivatives and metronidazole can reduce propionate production by gut microbiota. Hyperammonemia should be treated with sodium benzoate. In severe cases, hemofiltration will remove organic acids efficiently.

Case Study

A 28-year-old woman attended her local emergency department three times over the course of a week. The week before she had had what appeared to be a viral illness with "flu-like" symptoms, headache, and ear pain. She then started to behave oddly, staring blankly and not responding to questions. Her partner brought her to the hospital and a diagnosis of ear infection was made. She was admitted overnight. The next day she was reviewed by the Infectious Disease service. A CT head was normal and, as she was clinically improving, she was discharged home. She then developed abdominal pain and nausea. She became confused and returned to the emergency department. She was reviewed by psychiatry. It was felt her symptoms were secondary to an infection and she was again discharged. The next day she was sleepy and confused. She returned to the hospital and was seen by the neurologists. The possibility of encephalitis was raised and she was admitted. She had a higher degree from her home country and was studying English and working as a waitress. She had had surgery as a child for cleft palate. This operation was uneventful, but after further surgery on her ear she developed impaired balance and vomiting in the postoperative period, accompanied by strange behavior: she was found showering in her clothes. She was otherwise fit and well. She took no regular medication. She was a non-smoker and did not drink alcohol. She was an only child and there was no significant family history. She followed a vegetarian diet because she did not like meat and she also avoided dairy products. Since arriving in the UK, she had lost considerable weight as she did not like British food!

On examination, she weighed 40 kg. Her Glasgow Coma Score (GCS) was 15. However, she had no recall of recent events or of her arrival in the hospital. There was no rash or neck stiffness. Neurological examination showed generalized hyperreflexia and cerebellar ataxia. Initial investigations included normal blood count, renal and liver function tests, thyroid function, and C-reactive protein. ECG was normal. MRI brain was normal and a lumbar puncture showed normal opening pressure and cell counts. Viral PCR was negative. An EEG was reported as showing generalized encephalopathy with no seizure activity.

As viral encephalitis had been excluded, other causes of encephalopathy were considered. The concurrence of gastrointestinal symptoms and behavioral/psychiatric features raise the possibility of acute porphyria or hyperammonemia. A urine porphyrin screen was negative. Plasma ammonia was 293 μmol/L (0–40). Treatment for hyperammonemia was started with IV sodium benzoate and sodium phenylbutyrate. The ammonia levels started to come down and her mental state returned to normal. Urine organic acids, taken during the acute phase of her illness, came back a week later showing an orotate/creatinine ratio of 31 μmol/mmol (0–5), consistent with a diagnosis of ornithine transcarbamylase deficiency. This was confirmed by mutation analysis.

The key learning point is all adults who present with acute or acute-on-chronic encephalopathy in whom there is no obvious cause (e.g., recent trauma, infection, a cerebrovascular event or hypoxia) should have a plasma ammonia level measured promptly.

Acute Adrenal Crisis

Rarely, this may be the first presentation in a male patient with an *ABCD1* gene mutation (adrenomyeloneuropathy/adrenoleukodystrophy) (7). This is an X-linked disorder, so all male patients presenting in adrenal crisis should be asked about a family history of leukodystrophy and/or spastic paraparesis.

Diagnosis and Management
Diagnosis is made by measuring a very long chain fatty acid profile, and confirmed by mutation analysis of the ABCD1 gene. This should be done in all boys presenting with adrenal insufficiency and also needs to be considered in men if a more common cause cannot be confirmed (i.e. no evidence of autoimmunity or another secondary cause) or if there are neurological signs. Immediate management of the adrenal crisis as per standard guidelines.

Stroke

Stroke or stroke-like events can occur in a number of metabolic disorders, including Fabry disease, homocystinuria, mitochondrial disorders, organic acidemias, and urea cycle defects. In some of these conditions, stroke is due to cerebrovascular events, but in others cerebral infarction is secondary to energy deficiency and/or toxic effects of metabolites, so-called metabolic stroke.

Fabry Disease

Fabry disease is an X-linked disorder caused by deficiency of the enzyme alpha-galactosidaseA (α-Gal A). Pain in the extremities (acroparasthesiae), typically associated with pyrexia, angiokeratomas in the bathing trunk area and cornea verticillata are characteristic. Renal, cardiac, and cerebrovascular diseases are the major sources of morbidity and mortality. Male patients typically have more severe symptoms at an earlier age then heterozygote females, who may remain asymptomatic.

Strokes or transient ischemic attacks (TIA) have been reported to occur in approximately 6.9% of men and 4.3% of women with Fabry (8). Some 87% of stroke in this population was ischemic and 13% hemorrhagic. Males with Fabry who are aged between 35 and 45 have a 12-fold higher risk of stroke than men without Fabry. Nonetheless, the prevalence of Fabry disease in populations of patients presenting with stroke is low. Initial data suggested a prevalence of about 4%, but this has not been borne out by subsequent studies and currently there is no evidence to support unselected screening of stroke patients for Fabry.

Diagnosis

If there are clinical features or a family history suggestive of Fabry, diagnosis in males is made by measuring α-Gal A enzyme activity in plasma, isolated leukocytes, and/or cultured cells. In heterozygote females, enzyme activity is unreliable and the diagnosis must be confirmed by finding a pathogenic mutation in the *GLA* gene: sequence variants in the *GLA* gene are common and great care needs to be taken in interpreting molecular genetic results (9).

Management

Enzyme replacement therapy is available and an oral chaperone therapy has recently been licensed in Europe. Patients should be strongly encouraged to stop smoking. Symptomatic parasthesiae, renal and cardiac disease are treated as per standard guidelines.

Homocystinuria

Homocystinuria is an autosomal recessive condition caused by deficiency of the enzyme cystathione β-synthase (CBS). Classical clinical manifestations involve the eye, skeleton, central nervous and vascular systems, but the age of onset, severity, and type of clinical involvement can vary widely among affected individuals.

In a large study of the natural history of 629 individuals with homocystinuria, just over a third had suffered a thromboembolic event, with cerebrovascular accidents accounting for a third of these (10). The chance of having any thromboembolic event was about 50% by age 29 years, and was a significant causative or contributory factor to death in nearly 80% of the 64 patients who had died. Pregnancy is a particular risk factor for cerebral thrombosis in women with homocystinuria.

In patients with milder mutations, causing pyridoxine responsive homocystinuria, thromboembolism may be the first and only manifestation. Consideration of homocystinuria should therefore be part of any prothrombotic screen.

Diagnosis

Diagnosis is made biochemically on a plasma amino acid profile (increased total homocysteine and free homocystine, increased methionine, decreased cysteine). Confirmation is by demonstration of reduced cystathione β-synthase activity in skin fibroblasts and/or mutation analysis of the *CBS* gene (11). In practice, the biochemical profile is characteristic and merits a therapeutic trial of pyridoxine.

Management

Anticoagulation as per local guidelines. Ensure adequate vitamin B12 and folate status. Test for pyridoxine responsiveness (11): pyridoxine is a co-factor for the CBS enzyme and in many patients, particularly those presenting for the first time with a vascular event, will enhance enzyme activity and normalize the biochemistry. Evidence suggests that reducing the plasma total homocysteine level to below 100 μmol/L (>15 is usually considered high) normalizes the risk of thrombosis. If a patient is not pyridoxine-responsive, then consider using betaine, to enhance remethylation of homocysteine, and a low-protein, methionine-restricted diet.

Mitochondrial Disorders

Mitochondrial disorders should be considered as a possible cause of stroke in a patient who presents with a stroke or encephalopathy and involvement of two additional systems (e.g., eye, ear, cardiac, renal, endocrine, gastrointestinal). These disorders are caused by a disruption in the generation of energy by oxidative phosphorylation. There is considerable overlap in the clinical presentation of different mitochondrial disorders.

Diagnosis

There is no single diagnostic test for mitochondrial disease, so the clinical features and biochemical assays are used to direct genetic testing. Input from a specialist centre is advised to direct testing. Tests may include measurement of:

- complete (full) blood count
- tests of endocrine function
- lactic acid (plasma and CSF)
- lactate:pyruvate ratio
- plasma amino acid profile
- acylcarnitine profile
- biotinidase activity
- mononuclear coenzyme Q_{10} level
- plasma/urine thymidine and deoxyuridine
- urine organic acids
- CSF amino acids, protein and neurotransmitters
- muscle biopsy for histology, respiratory chain enzyme analysis and molecular genetic testing.

Management

Management is largely supportive, apart from a small number of potentially treatable conditions caused by specific deficiencies (e.g., of coenzyme Q_{10} or riboflavin). Citrulline and arginine have been suggested as possible useful therapies in the management

Table 5-2 Metabolic disorders associated with cardiac diseases

Arrhythmias, conduction defects
Fatty acid oxidation defects
Congenital disorder of glycosylation
Fabry disease
Cardiomyopathy
Fabry disease
Fatty acid oxidation defects
Glycogen storage disorders (AGL, PRKAG2, LAMP2, RBCK1 mutations)
Organic acidemias (methylmalonic and propionic)
Mucopolysaccharidoses
Mitochondrial disorders (e.g., Barth syndrome)
Refsum disease
Valvular disease
Mucopolysaccharidoses
Mucolipidoses

of mitochondrial encephalomyopathy, lactic acidosis, and stroke-like episodes (MELAS) syndrome (12).

Cardiac Disease

Acute presentations of cardiac disease (cardiomyopathy, arrhythmias, sudden death) secondary to an underlying metabolic disorder can occur in a number of conditions and may be the first presenting feature in adulthood (Table 5-2) (13,14).

Diagnosis

Depends on the clinical features (note that the cardiac disease may be isolated) and family history, which will direct the biochemical and/or genetic testing.

If a cardiac biopsy is taken, then histological analysis should include assessment of glycogen storage – *PRKAG2* gene mutations can cause isolated cardiomyopathy with glycogen storage.

Management

Management is largely as for standard cardiac disease. Patients may require a cardiac

Table 5-3 Metabolic disorders associated with psychiatric features

---

Urea cycle defects

Disorders of B12/folate /homocysteine metabolism
Methylene tetrahydrofolate reductase deficiency
Intracellular cobalamin (B12) processing defects
Homocystinuria

Lysosomal storage disorders
Metachromatic leukodystrophy
Krabbe disease
Niemann Pick C disease

Acute porphyria

Wilson disease

Cerebral adrenoleukodystrophy (ABCD1 gene mutation)

---

pacemaker or an implantable cardioverter defibrillator (ICD). Dietary manipulation and treatment of acute metabolic decompensation may be helpful in the management of the cardiomyopathy of glycogen storage disease type III, fatty acid oxidation disorders, and the organic acidemias. Carnitine supplementation is recommended in carnitine transporter deficiency.

Psychiatric Presentations

Table 5-3 lists IMDs that can potentially present with psychiatric features or behavioral/personality changes. Psychiatric features may be isolated for some time before other organ involvement is noted, particularly if the possibility of organic disease is not considered during the initial presentation (15).

Nonetheless, when the family history is suggestive of recessive or X-linked inheritance; or when the clinical signs are triggered by situations such as intercurrent infection, surgery or prolonged fasting; or when neurological signs such as cognitive or motor dysfunction, or other organ involvement, is present, then an IMD should be considered.

Treatment can be very effective, particularly for the urea cycle defects, disorders of B12/folate and homocysteine metabolism, Wilson disease, and the acute porphyrias. Hence any patient in whom an underlying metabolic cause is suspected should have the following measured as a minimum:

- plasma amino acid profile;
- serum copper and ceruloplasmin;
- urine organic acids, copper and porphobilinogen.

More specialist investigations, depending on the family history, clinical picture (and brain magnetic resonance imaging [MRI] findings) should include:

- very long chain fatty acid levels;
- white cell enzyme activities (for metachromatic leukodystrophy and Krabbe disease);
- filipin staining of fibroblasts (for Niemann-Pick disease type C).

Pregnancy

Pregnancy is not in itself an acute emergency. However, women with certain metabolic conditions may be at increased risk of metabolic decompensation during pregnancy and the puerperium (16). Early pregnancy, if complicated by morning sickness, can be a difficult time for women with inherited disorders of energy metabolism, for example, fatty acid oxidation disorders, glycogen storage diseases, urea cycle defects, and disorders of ketone body metabolism. Nausea and vomiting lead to problems in taking supplements and medications, which may result in episodes of metabolic decompensation.

Pregnancy is also a prothrombotic period and presentation of hypercoagulable conditions, including homocystinuria, during pregnancy, often with cerebral venous sinus thrombus, is well described. In all conditions with a known thrombotic risk, anticoagulation (usually with subcutaneous heparin) during pregnancy and the post-partum period needs to be considered.

Labor and delivery are times of increased energy requirement and women may require additional energy supplementation (usually

IV dextrose) during this time. Following delivery, there is a well-recognized risk period for acute decompensation of some disorders, particularly those of protein metabolism (e.g., the urea cycle defects). Classically this decompensation occurs between day 3–14 post-partum. The reasons for this are not entirely clear but are thought to relate to the relative metabolic stress of the changes of the puerperium and an increased protein load for catabolism following involution of the uterus. Care must be taken not to confuse the behavioral changes of hyperammonemia for symptoms of post-partum psychosis or depression.

Risks to the Fetus

Aside from the risks secondary to acute maternal decompensation, a number of inherited metabolic conditions are thought to be directly teratogenic to the developing fetus. The best-described of these is the maternal PKU syndrome (17). Children exposed to high levels of maternal phenylalanine *in utero* are at risk of developmental delay, microcephaly, cardiac defects, and dysmorphic features. With good maternal control of phenylalanine levels this syndrome can be prevented (18). Hence, women with PKU (19), who present as pregnant/planning pregnancy need to be referred for specialist counseling and management as a matter of urgency.

Conclusions

Inherited metabolic diseases can present acutely to a number of different specialities. While individually these conditions are rare, if not considered in the differential diagnosis, then a potentially treatable condition can be missed, with devastating consequences for the individual and their family.

Any patient identified as being at risk of acute decompensation should be advised to wear a medical alert bracelet, and to carry information with contact details of their treating medical team and an emergency treatment guideline. This should include information on who to contact for advice in the event of emergency, elective surgery, or pregnancy.

References

1 Godfrey R, Quinlivan R. Skeletal muscle disorders of glycogenolysis and glycolysis. *Nat Rev Neurol*. 2016;12(7): 393–402.

2 Olpin SE, Murphy E, Kirk RJ, Taylor RW, Quinlivan R. The investigation and management of metabolic myopathies. *J Clin Pathol*. 2015;68(6):413–417.

3 Spiekerkoetter U, Lindner M, Santer R, et al. Treatment recommendations in long-chain fatty acid oxidation defects: consensus from a workshop. *J Inherit Metab Dis*. 2009;32(4):498–505.

4 Walker V. Severe hyperammonaemia in adults not explained by liver disease. *Ann Clin Biochem*. 2012;49(Pt 3):214–228.

5 Häberle J. Clinical and biochemical aspects of primary and secondary hyperammonemic disorders. *Arch Biochem Biophys*. 2013;15;536(2):101–108.

6 Baumgartner MR, Hörster F, Dionisi-Vici C, et al. Proposed guidelines for the diagnosis and management of methylmalonic and propionic acidemia. *Orphanet J Rare Dis*. 2014;9:130.

7 Kemp S, Huffnagel IC, Linthorst GE, Wanders RJ, Engelen M. Adrenoleukodystrophy – neuroendocrine pathogenesis and redefinition of natural history. *Nat Rev Endocrinol*. 2016;12(10): 606–615.

8 Kolodny E, Fellgiebel A, Hilz MJ, et al. Cerebrovascular involvement in Fabry disease: current status of knowledge. *Stroke*. 2015;46(1):302–313.

9 Linthorst GE, Bouwman MG, Wijburg FA, Aerts JM, Poorthuis BJ, Hollak CE.

Screening for Fabry disease in high-risk populations: a systematic review. *J Med Genet*. 2010 Apr;47(4):217–222.

10 Mudd SH, Skovby F, Levy HL et al. The natural history of homocystinuria due to cystathionine beta-synthase deficiency. *Am J Hum Genet*. 1985;37(1):1–31.

11 Morris AA, Kožich V, Santra S, et al. Guidelines for the diagnosis and management of cystathionine beta-synthase deficiency. *J Inherit Metab Dis*. 2017;40(1):49–74.

12 El-Hattab AW, Adesina AM, Jones J, Scaglia F. MELAS syndrome: Clinical manifestations, pathogenesis, and treatment options. *Mol Genet Metab*. 2015;116(1–2):4–12.

13 O'Mahony C, Elliott P. Anderson-Fabry disease and the heart. *Prog Cardiovasc Dis*. 2010;52(4):326–335.

14 Elliott P, Limongelli G. Cardiac aspects of inherited metabolic diseases. In: Hollak CEM, Lachmann RH, eds. *Inherited Metabolic Disease in Adults: A Clinical Guide*. Oxford: Oxford University Press; 2016.

15 Sedel S, Nadjar Y. Neurological and psychiatric symptoms. In: Hollak CEM, Lachmann RH, eds. *Inherited Metabolic Disease in Adults: A Clinical Guide*. Oxford: Oxford University Press; 2016.

16 Murphy E. Pregnancy in women with inherited metabolic disease. *Obstet Med*. 2015;8(2):61–67.

17 Mabry CC, Denniston JC, Nelson TL, Son CD. Maternal phenylketonuria. a cause of mental retardation in children without the metabolic defect. *N Engl J Med*. 1963;269:1404–1408.

18 Lenke RR, Levy HL. Maternal phenylketonuria and hyperphenylalaninemia: An international survey of the outcome of untreated and treated pregnancies. *N Engl J Med*. 1980;303(21):1202–1208.

19 Van Spronsen FJ, van Wegberg AMJ, Ahring K, et al. Key European guidelines for the diagnosis and management of patients with phenylketonuria. *Lancet Diabetes Endocrinol* 2017. http://dx.doi.org/10.1016/S2213-8587(16)30320-5 (accessed April 28, 2017).

6

Endocrine and Metabolic Emergencies in Transitional Care

Mabel Yau and Mark A. Sperling

Key Points

- The transition of care for adolescents and young adults from a pediatric, family-centered model to an adult, patient-centered model marks an important milestone in the lives of patients with chronic disorders.
- The timing and tempo of transitional care require special consideration to physical, psychological, and social changes occurring during young adulthood.
- Poor glycemic control is a common finding among adolescents with type 1 diabetes and places these young adults at increased risk of diabetic ketoacidosis.
- Other chronic endocrine disorders such as primary adrenal deficiency, congenital or autoimmune hypothyroidism and hyperthyroidism, and hypopituitarism may follow a similar model of care.
- In addition to continued management of existing defects, patients with disorders such as autoimmune polyglandular syndromes will require continued surveillance for manifestations of new endocrinopathies.

- Onset of adrenal insufficiency with adrenoleukodystrophy, X-linked adrenal hypoplasia, and triple A syndrome is variable and patients may present in adrenal crisis as the initial manifestation of adrenal insufficiency during an acute illness.
- Endocrine causes account for a high proportion of cases of secondary hypertension, including acute onset of hypertension due to hyperaldosteronism, pheochromocytomas, ganglioneuromas, Cushing's syndrome, acromegaly, and hyperthyroidism.
- Head trauma is common in young adults associated with risky behaviors and motor vehicle accidents. Patients with traumatic brain injuries are at risk for developing anterior and posterior pituitary defects.
- In the emergency setting, adult healthcare providers should be cognizant of the unique types, presenting features, and approaches to management of diabetes and endocrine conditions in these young adults.

Introduction

The transition of care for adolescents and young adults from a pediatric, family-centered model to an adult, patient-centered model marks an important milestone in the lives of patients with chronic disorders managed from a young age. Transitional care is complex. The timing and tempo of transition require special consideration to physical, psychological, and social changes occurring during young adulthood. Key points in the transition to adult diabetes and endocrine care include: (a) starting the process at least one year before the anticipated transition; (b) assessing individual patients' readiness and preparedness for adult care; (c) providing guidance and education to the patient and family; (d) using transition guides and resources; and (e) maintaining open lines of communication between the pediatric and adult providers. No current single approach is effective for all patients.

Poor glycemic control is a common finding among adolescents with type 1 diabetes. Based on data from the Type 1 Diabetes Exchange, the mean HbA1C peaks at age 19 years with a slow decline until 30 years old (1). The average HbA1C from 18–25 years old was 8.7% (72 mmol/mol). This poor baseline control places these young adults at increased risk of diabetic ketoacidosis (DKA), knowledge that should alert clinicians to carefully manage diabetes during concurrent acute illnesses. Other chronic endocrine disorders, such as primary adrenal deficiency, congenital or autoimmune hypothyroidism and hyperthyroidism, and hypopituitarism may follow a similar model of care.

In addition to continued management of existing defects, patients with the environmental triggers disorders such as autoimmune polyglandular syndromes (APS) will require continued surveillance for manifestations of new endocrinopathies through adulthood. Onset of adrenal insufficiency with adrenoleukodystrophy, X-linked adrenal hypoplasia and triple A syndrome is variable and patients may present in adrenal crisis as the initial manifestation of adrenal insufficiency during an acute illness.

Endocrine causes account for a high proportion of cases of secondary hypertension. Conditions that present with acute onset of hypertension include hyperaldosteronism, pheochromocytomas, ganglioneuromas, Cushing's syndrome, acromegaly, and hyperthyroidism. Endocrine hypertension may also be clinically silent until recognized and evaluated.

Head trauma is common in young adults associated with risky behaviors and motor vehicle accidents. Patients with traumatic brain injuries are at risk for developing anterior and posterior pituitary defects.

This chapter discusses transitional care of diabetes and chronic and evolving endocrine disorders, as well as the management (including emergency care) of endocrine disorders that commonly present in young adulthood.

Type 1 Diabetes Mellitus

Type 1 diabetes mellitus (T1DM) is a state of disordered metabolism that results from severe insulin deficiency brought about by progressive destruction of pancreatic beta cells by autoimmune processes triggered by the interaction of an environmental insult in a genetically predisposed host (2,3). Genes predisposing to T1DM are predominantly those involved in immune regulation, and other autoimmune endocrinopathies such as Hashimoto thyroiditis/hypothyroidism, hyperthyroidism, adrenal insufficiency, and Celiac disease are frequently associated, requiring regular surveillance as part of routine care (2,3). The environmental triggers implicated include viral or other infections, and dietary components that may be reflected in the composition of the gut microbiome (2–4). Markers of autoimmunity such as circulating antibodies to various islet cell components (GAD65, IA2, ZnT8, insulin) may be present for months to years before clinical onset, and are considered the hallmark of T1DM. However, unlike other classical autoimmune diseases, such as systemic lupus, rheumatoid arthritis or Graves' disease, which show a marked sexual dimorphism with female predominance, T1DM affects both sexes equally. This and other disparities, including the failure of immune interventions that are effective in preventing or arresting progressive pancreatic beta cell destruction in animal models but not in humans, have raised questions regarding the currently accepted model of autoimmunity as the sole mechanism (5–7), though the existence of autoimmunity as a major component is indisputable. The

Table 6-1 Clinical and biochemical manifestations of diabetic ketoacidosis (DKA)

Clinical	Biochemical
• Dehydration • Rapid, deep, sighing (Kussmaul) respiration • Nausea, vomiting, and abdominal pain mimicking an acute abdomen • Progressive obtundation and loss of consciousness • Fever only when infection is present	• Hyperglycemia (200–900 mg/dL; 11–50 mmol/L) • Variable degrees of acidosis (pH <7.3; HCO3 <15 mmol/L) • Ketosis (serum betahydroxybutyrate [BOHB] >3 mmol/L) • Elevation of BUN and Creatinine • Increased leukocyte count with left shift • Non-specific elevation of serum amylase

incidence of T1DM is increasing by 1.4–3% per year world-wide, suggesting that environmental factors are likely responsible, since our genomes could not have so dramatically been altered in the past 50 years (8).

At initial diagnosis, about 30–40% of cases of T1DM are in diabetic ketoacidosis (DKA), a potentially life-threatening state of metabolic decompensation characterized by dehydration, hyperglycemia, metabolic acidosis, and ketonemia (9,10). Symptoms of excessive urination, excessive thirst, weight loss, weakness-lethargy, and deep sighing respirations (Kussmaul breathing) are universally present when sought; variable degrees of clouding of consciousness including frank coma are late manifestations (Table 6-1). The severity of illness is defined by the degree of acidosis: pH 7.2–7.3 is considered mild; pH 7.1–7.2 moderate and pH <7.1 considered severe. Corresponding bicarbonate concentrations (HCO3) are 10–15 mmol/L mild, 5–10 mmol/L moderate and <5 mmol/L severe. Disparities between the degree of acidosis as judged by pH and HCO3 may occur because of the effectiveness of breathing to lower pCO2, thereby compensating for the metabolic acidosis with a degree of respiratory alkalosis. The degree of hyperglycemia is generally in the range of 200–900 mg/dL

(11–50 mmol/L); hyperglycemia exceeding 1000 mg/dL (56 mmol/L) is unusual and more commonly observed in the hyperglycemic hyperosmolar state (HHS) and dehydration with milder ketosis in patients with Type 2 diabetes mellitus (T2DM). The pathophysiology of DKA and its management in adolescents are extensively discussed in consensus guidelines published by various associations including the American Diabetes Association (ADA) (9) and the International Society for Pediatric and Adolescent Diabetes (ISPAD) (10). In the simplest terms, the biochemical changes that lead to DKA are absolute insulin deficiency compounded by the synergistic actions of the four counter-regulatory hormones, glucagon, cortisol, growth hormone (GH) and epinephrine, which, sensing intracellular starvation because glucose cannot enter cells in critical tissues (intracellular glucopenia), raise glucose concentrations via glycogen breakdown and gluconeogenesis, induce lipolysis, and turn on ketogenesis. The resulting hyperglycemia leads to osmotic diuresis, dehydration, depletion of electrolytes, and acidosis from the accumulation of lactic acid as well as the keto acids aceto-acetic and β-hydroxy butyric acid (BOHB), which overwhelms buffering capacity. If left untreated, these processes continue until coma and death ensue. Because this entity is considered a medical emergency, there is wide agreement that the required intensive monitoring of electrolyte and pH status, as well as cardiac, respiratory, and neurological status, is best managed in an intensive care unit or equivalent setting, and essential for moderate or severe cases (10). Table 6-1 summarizes the clinical findings in DKA.

Management of DKA

The principles of management are to correct dehydration and electrolyte losses with crystalloid fluids, provide insulin to enable metabolism of glucose and ketones while shutting down ketogenesis, and to monitor the patients' cardiac, renal, respiratory, and cerebral functions (10,11). The keys to successful outcome are medical and nursing staff trained and skilled in the management of diabetes and its complications, and reliable accurate laboratory results of the biochemical changes occurring during treatment. Estimates of the degree of dehydration are based largely on clinical judgment and are notoriously unreliable, resulting in underestimates or overestimates of required fluid replacement; knowledge of recent measurement of body weight or correction for the degree of elevated hematocrit are useful for more accurate estimates of dehydration. A common estimate of moderate to severe dehydration is 10% of body weight in kg; this amount as liters of fluid together with estimated daily maintenance requirement is infused intravenously (IV) over 36–48 h. In a large recent series of 1800 episodes of DKA managed in a single academic center over six years, the type of fluid administered, standard normal 0.9% saline for the first 4–6 h followed by 0.45% saline with added potassium and phosphate, or modified to use lactated Ringer's solution, did not affect outcome or frequency of cerebral edema (12). The recommended therapy is to correct dehydration over 48 h, but in practice this is achieved much sooner. Insulin (and potassium) can be deferred for 1–2 h after starting fluid in order to achieve some correction of volume depletion, and decline in degree of acidosis; fluids alone achieve considerable correction of the metabolic disturbance, and insulin is more effective when acidosis is less severe due to the dissociation of hormones binding from their cognate receptors under conditions of low pH. Indeed, bolus insulin given early in the course of acidosis may be harmful and therefore a bolus of insulin should not be given when insulin treatment is begun. In moderate to severe cases of DKA, recommended insulin dosage is 0.1 U/kg/hr; if response to this dose is rapid and glucose approaches 300 mg/dL (16.5 mmol/L), the dose may be reduced to 0.05 U/kg/hr, but the infusion of insulin should not be discontinued until acidosis is corrected and the pH is ≥ 7.3. Potassium supplementation IV may be begun as soon as urinary output is established, since total body potassium depletion is substantial when serum potassium values are normal

in the context of acidosis. A commonly recommended dose of potassium is 40 mmol/L, added to the fluid infusate, adjusted to allow serum K concentration to remain at 3.5–5 mmol/L; the potassium may be half in the form of K chloride, and half as K phosphate, which serves to limit the amount of chloride infused and thereby limit hyperchloremic acidosis, while providing phosphate to facilitate energy production (ATP). The details of infusing potassium, phosphate and monitoring of the patient are extensively discussed in the ADA and ISPAD guidelines (9,10).

Caveats

1. Ketone bodies as measured in urine grossly underestimate the degree of ketosis, because the common method uses sodium nitroprusside, which reacts strongly with aceto-acetate, weakly with acetone, *and not at all with βOHB*. Yet the actual amount of βOHB may be five times or more that of aceto-acetate, especially in the presence of acidosis. As acidosis is corrected and more of the βOHB is converted to aceto-acetate, it *appears* that the ketosis is getting worse, when in fact acidosis and clinical parameters are improving. Measurements of βOHB via bedside meters or formal laboratory methods are better means to monitor "ketone" status (10).

2. Acidosis may appear to worsen initially for three reasons. First, dilution of the total bicarbonate in the expanding fluid volume lowers the apparent bicarbonate concentration because the HCO3 is expressed as mmol/L, and while the total mmol may not yet have changed, they are distributed in a greater volume (10). Second, with initially rapid rehydration, accumulated lactic acid enters into the circulation. Third, the βOHB acid is excreted in urine after it is converted to Na Butyrate; the Na derives from NaHCO3, leaving bicarbonate, which combines with H⁺ to yield CO_2 and H_2O and permits loss of the CO_2 in respiration. In these processes, HCO3 and Na are lost, further depleting the bicarbonate content of plasma (11). With rehydration and insulin, which together

curtail ketogenesis, the acid base balance gradually returns to normal.

3. The use of phosphate as potassium phosphate, rather than K chloride, may reduce the large amount of chloride used and hence reduce hyperchloremic acidosis, as well as improving oxygen dissociation to enable lactate to be converted to pyruvate. However, this is not accepted by all authorities and some claim no additional benefit from using phosphate. In addition, the use of phosphate may result in hypocalcemia. However, with severe phosphate depletion, the use of phosphate is likely to be beneficial.

4. The use of bicarbonate infusion as a means to more rapidly correct acidosis and restore acid-base balance should be avoided unless pH is <7.0 and cardiac function appears impaired. In adults, studies have not shown a beneficial effect of bicarbonate infusion in DKA; replenishment of fluid and restoration of normal metabolism with curtailment of the production of ketones via insulin are associated with steady recovery of acid-base balance. Indeed, bicarbonate infusion may be harmful because HCO3 combines with H ion to yield H2CO3 that dissociates to H_2O and CO_2; whereas HCO3 does not cross the blood-brain barrier, CO_2 does and may result in worsening of cerebral acidosis. If deemed necessary, the bicarbonate should not be given as a bolus; an infusion of 1 mmol/kg over 2–4 hours is recommended (10).

5. Signs and symptoms of cerebral edema include: headache and slowing of heart rate; change in neurological status (restlessness, irritability, increased drowsiness, and incontinence); specific neurological signs (e.g., cranial nerve palsies, papilledema); rising blood pressure; and decreased O_2 saturation. It is imperative to initiate treatment of cerebral edema as soon as the condition is suspected (10).

Next Steps

As the acute metabolic disturbances resolve, the patient is conscious and able to swallow, transition to routine diabetes care using basal-bolus regimens of insulin and age-appropriate meal plans consistent with the age of the patient, stage of puberty, and cultural preferences may be initiated. Assuming an insulin requirement of 1 U/kg/day, the initial dose of basal insulin is recommended as 0.2 U/kg, while the dose of IV infused insulin is reduced to 0.025–0.05 U/kg/hr. and discontinued before a regularly scheduled meal at which 0.1–0.2 U/kg is given as bolus. This phase is performed after the patient has been transferred out of the ICU (or similar setting) into a regular hospital bed, a process that should involve the diabetes management team to be responsible for the education and subsequent management of the patient. The entire family must be educated in the principles of diabetes care, injection techniques, monitoring of glucose, recognition of hypoglycemia, and management of sick days. A team consisting of diabetes specialists, educators, nutritionists, and social workers work in unison to educate the patient and family, and set mutually agreed-upon goals which may depend on the socio-economic, motivational and educational levels of the family. These steps may define appropriate expectations for the degree of metabolic control. A stable home environment, parental participation, and a supportive trusting relationship between the patient, family, and treating team are generally predictive of better long-term adherence to recommended regimens and attainment of the recommended goal of a HbA1c of $\leq 7.5\%$ (58 mmol/mol). However, as noted in our introductory comments, the age group of 15–25 years is notoriously difficult to attain these goals. *The harmful consequences of smoking, alcohol or other substance abuse, sexually transmitted diseases (STD), and the effects of poorly controlled diabetes in pregnancy on fetal well-being should be discussed with each patient* (12). Before discharge from this initial hospitalization, we recommend screening laboratory tests for thyroid function, lipid profile, and celiac disease to establish a baseline and to treat as appropriate; some recommend that this screening be performed at an initial follow-up visit when acute metabolic changes have returned to normal baseline.

Recurrent Episodes of DKA

Informed about the symptomology of evolving DKA and its causes, chastened by the experience of a life-threatening episode of metabolic decompensation, advised about the importance of monitoring for urinary or serum ketones with vomiting and whom to call for immediate help with emergencies, most adolescents and young persons do not experience repeat episodes. A small subset of patients do experience repeat episodes, and with each episode the prognosis for short-term and long-term outcome worsens (13). In a retrospective survey of 628 admissions to a University Medical Center for DKA involving a cohort of 298 patients over a five-year period between 2007–2012 with follow-up to the end of 2014, the authors report that a single episode of DKA was associated with a 5.2% risk of death within an average of 4.2 years (range 2.8–6 years) of follow-up, compared to 23.4% risk of death in those with multiple admissions ($\geq$5) for DKA within 2.4 years of follow-up (range 2.0–3.8 years of follow-up), $p < 0.001$ (14). Possibly only one death occurred during the actual admission for DKA consistent with experience in many medical centers where management of an acute episode of DKA now results in successful outcomes (13). Those with recurrent DKA were younger at the time of initial diagnosis (14 versus 24 years), had higher levels of HbA1c (11.6% vs 9.4% [103 mmol/mol vs 79 mmol/mol]), had higher levels of social deprivation, were more likely to have been prescribed anti-depressants (47.5% vs 12.6%) (all $p < 0.01$), and tended to be younger (average 25 yrs (22–36) vs 31 yrs (23–42). Thus, recurrent DKA in young socially disadvantaged adults is associated with worse control as reflected in HbA1c and with increased risk of death in the ensuing years from a variety of causes. Over one half of the deaths (52.3%) occurred at home at a median age of 38 years; "psychological issues, neuropathy, previous cardiovascular disease, excess alcohol intake and a longer length of stay during the last hospital admission" were each associated with the increased mortality rates (14). These disheartening findings emphasize the importance of striving for successful transition to adult care of young adolescents from socio-economic deprived backgrounds (13–15).

Other Conditions Leading to ICU Admissions in Patients with T1DM

Other reasons why an adolescent/young person with T1DM may be admitted to an adult ICU include hypoglycemia, preoperative and postoperative management of acute abdominal conditions such as appendicitis, intestinal obstruction or perforation, and management of injuries resulting from accidental trauma, such as motor vehicle accidents. In cases of severe hypoglycemia with coma, the possible causes of hypoglycemia in a person with diabetes should be evaluated; inappropriate insulin with exercise, adrenal insufficiency, hypothyroidism, and celiac disease should be considered and excluded by laboratory testing. Before embarking on surgery, blood glucose and acid base status should be managed via infusion of insulin and correction of fluid deficits. A critical question in the perioperative phase is the degree of glycemic control; does "tight control" with blood glucose maintained close to the normal physiological range of 80–140 mg/dL (4.4–7.8 mmol/L) result in better outcomes or more rapid healing than more lax ranges of 100–180 mg/dL (5.6–10 mmol/L)? This issue has been explored in a number of studies, not all of which have shown a better outcome with tight control whereas hypoglycemia is more frequent and severe with the stricter criteria (16,17). Supplemental GH to aid in protein retention is contraindicated as it was shown to be associated with greater mortality (18).

Hyperglycemic Hyperosmolar State (HHS)

The hyperglycemic hyperosmolar state (HHS) is characterized by blood glucose concentrations >600 mg/dL (>33.3 mmol/L), serum hyperosmolality >320 mmol/L, and minimal acidosis and ketosis; serum bicarbonate remains >15 mmol/L and urinary "ketones" (aceto-acetate) are usually negative or only trace on testing urine via dipstick. Serum ketones are <3 mmol/L. Although there are similarities to DKA, the fundamental difference is a greater degree of dehydration and less acidosis, so that treatment should focus on fluid and electrolyte replacement, and less on provision of insulin; indeed, insulin should be withheld initially to prevent a too rapid fall in serum glucose and lowering of serum osmolality which might result in fluid shifts into the cerebral compartment and cerebral edema (10,19). However, cerebral edema is rarer in HHS than in DKA. The degree of insulin deficiency and the magnitude of counter-regulatory response appear to be less severe, so that the symptoms and signs of DKA are absent or less pronounced; abdominal pain and Kussmaul respiration are absent, and vomiting less severe. These milder features also lead to greater time in evolution, greater degrees of dehydration and electrolyte losses resulting from the polyuria, and are often compounded by intake of highly glucose-enriched carbonated soft drinks. Glucose concentrations commonly exceed 1000 mg/dL (56 mmol/L), dehydration may be as much as twice that occurring in DKA and may be difficult to estimate due to co-existing obesity and hypertonicity which retains fluid in the intra-vascular compartment. Persistence of the polyuria due to the persistence of glucose concentrations exceeding the renal threshold of ~200 mg/dL (11 mmol/L) during treatment, requires careful monitoring of the clinical status and fluid replacement to avoid dehydration and vascular collapse. The risk of thrombosis is greater in HHS than in DKA, possibly as a result of osmotic disruption of endothelial cells, with release of thromboplastins facilitating coagulation.

Treatment should assume dehydration of 10–15% and initially isotonic (normal) 0.9% saline should be provided at 20 ml/kg bolus infusions to restore fluid deficits and

Table 6-2 Monitoring of patients with HHS in the ICU. Modified from (18).

- Continuous cardiac, respiratory and blood pressure monitoring
- Hourly glucose and clinical assessment
- 2–4 hourly assessment of fluid balance(input/output); serum electrolytes, BUN, creatinine, CK (creatine kinase)
- 4–6 hourly calcium, phosphate, magnesium
- Be alert to complications - thrombosis, rhabdomyolosis, hyperpyrexia, cerebral edema

maintain vascular volume with the assessment of serum chemistries every 1–2 hours; subsequently, 0.45–0.75% saline, with added electrolytes should be infused to replace calculated losses over 24–48 hours, guided by laboratory chemistry every 2–4 hours and ongoing clinical monitoring performed in an ICU or equivalent setting. The aim should be to control the decline in blood glucose to 100 mg/dL (5.6 mmol/L) per hour; if glucose is not declining at a rate of at least 50 mg/dL (3 mmol/L), or ketosis is more than mild, insulin at a rate of only 0.025–0.05 U/kg/hour may be used with caution and careful clinical and laboratory monitoring. Potassium, phosphate, and magnesium losses may be considerable; potassium should be infused at 40 mmol/L added to each liter of saline, with balanced mixtures of potassium chloride and potassium phosphate, the latter to replete phosphate depletion which may predispose to rhabdomyolysis and hemolytic anemia. As in DKA, use of bicarbonate is not recommended. Magnesium also may be severely depleted in HHS and predispose to hypocalcemia; the recommended doses of magnesium replacement are 25–50 mg/kg/dose given every 4–6 hours at a maximum infusion rate of 150 mg/min (2 gm/hr) for 3–4 doses (10,19). In addition to cerebral edema, thrombosis, and rhabdomyolysis, malignant hyperthermia is reported as a complication (Table 6-2). Monitoring for these complications is based in part on clinical anticipation and examination, supplemented by appropriate biochemical testing (e.g., serum creatine kinase for presence of muscle damage) and availability of Dantrolene for treatment of malignant hyperthermia.

Some patients have features that combine DKA and HHS that reflect the degree of insulin deficiency; clinical acumen, earlier use of insulin, and careful monitoring of the patient's vital signs and chemistries should guide treatment, especially the earlier use of insulin in appropriate doses. "Classical" HHS in adolescents and young adults is a feature of T2DM, an entity that is increasing at an annual rate of 4.8% in the obese population of the USA (8). Hence the frequency of HHS as a presenting feature is also likely to increase and physicians caring for these patients in an ICU or equivalent setting must be alert to the differences in management with the greater focus on fluid and electrolyte replacement in HHS, rather than the use of insulin as in DKA.

Autoimmune Polyglandular Syndromes (APS)

The autoimmune polyglandular syndromes are clusters of endocrine abnormalities occurring in discrete patterns that permit treatment and anticipation of associated hormonal deficiencies (20–24).

APS1-APECED

APS1 is characterized by hypoparathyroidism, muco-cutaneous candidiasis, and Addison's disease with cortisol deficiency and marked elevations in ACTH, which clinically manifest as hyperpigmentation and hypoglycemia with fasting. In addition to this triad, other manifestations include periodic rash with fever, kerato-conjunctivitis, chronic diarrhea, primary gonadal failure occurring pre- or post-puberty, Hashimoto thyroiditis with hypothyroidism, vitamin B12 deficiency, chronic active hepatitis, T1DM, and ectodermal dystrophy. Hence, the term APECED (**A**utoimmune **P**olyendocrinopathy, **C**andidiasis, **E**ctodermal **D**ystrophy). The causes of this autoimmunity are inactivating mutations in the autoimmune regulator gene (AIRE) on chromosome 21, which normally acts to permit ectopic expression of hormonal and other peripheral antigens in the thymus, so that developing T-cells that acquire receptors for these antigens are eliminated and do not enter the periphery to cause autoimmunity. The peri-post pubertal period is a common time for presentation of some manifestations, although initial presentation may occur as early as the first year of life; surprisingly, T1DM is uncommon in this condition (22). Treatment is based on hormonal and vitamin replacement as well as anti-candida drugs such as ketoconazole and related agents that are themselves known to interfere with cortisol synthesis and hence worsen manifestations of adrenal deficiency. Cortisol should be given in stress dosage, commonly 2–3 times daily maintenance of $\sim$10 mg/m^2/d; consideration should be given to parenteral replacement of steroids or vitamin D agents while in the ICU, because oral medication may be less absorbed due to candidiasis of the esophagus and lower gastrointestinal tract. There is evidence that the predilection for autoimmunity in persons with trisomy 21 (Down's syndrome) may also be due to abnormality in the AIRE gene (25). It is likely that, absent the classic triad of hypoparathyroidism, chronic muco-cutaneous candidiasis, and primary adrenal insufficiency, or two of these three manifestations, many cases are missed; the wide spectrum of potential presentations suggest that genetic testing via AIRE mutational analysis be considered in patients with hepatitis, chronic diarrhea, and periodic rash with fever (20).

APS2-Schmidt Syndrome

APS2 is characterized by the triad of T1DM, Addison's disease, and thyroid autoimmunity with hypothyroidism, hyperthyroidism, or Hashimoto thyroiditis. T1DM and Addison's disease are obligatory components, but thyroid autoimmunity is not and a host of other autoimmune entities can also be associated. These entities include celiac disease, vitiligo, alopecia, myasthenia gravis, pernicious anemia, IgA deficiency, hepatitis, and hypogonadism. Peak prevalence is in the range of 20–40 years of age, and hence an important consideration in those admitted to an ICU during the transitional age range. In keeping with an autoimmune basis, the syndrome is more prevalent in females and associated with specific HLA DR3 and DR4 haplotypes and with the class II HLA alleles DQ2 and DQ8, also strongly linked to celiac disease. Autoantibodies to islet cell components (GAD65, IA2, ZnT8), anti-thyroid (anti-thyroglobulin [TG], anti-thyroid peroxidase [TPO]), anti-21-hydroxylase (Addison's disease), and celiac disease (tissue transglutaminase) are commonly present and should be periodically sought in those with Addison's disease and T1DM. Specific treatment for each entity should be continued in the ICU, with cortisol dosage adjusted for stress (24). A mechanism by which viral disease may trigger autoimmunity in the gut leading to celiac disease has recently been proposed and may have relevance to the other autoimmune diseases that form this entity (26).

APS3

APS3 has the same array of endocrine tissue autoimmune abnormalities as APS2, but without Addison's disease. Almost 20% of patients with T1DM have thyroglobulin (TG) and thyroid peroxidase (TPO) antibodies, but only a minority progress to clinical or biochemical hypothyroidism, so APS3 could be considered as a relatively common disorder (25).

Adrenal Insufficiency

During stress, cortisol produced by the zona fasciculata of the adrenal gland is required to maintain normoglycemia and hemodynamic stability. Cortisol regulates carbohydrate metabolism to maintain normoglycemia, decreases capillary permeability

to maintain a normal blood pressure, and is required for enzymatic activity to convert norepinephrine to epinephrine. Cortisol production is under the regulation of the hypothalamus and pituitary. The hypothalamic-pituitary-adrenal (HPA) axis is mediated through the circulating level of plasma cortisol by negative feedback of cortisol on the corticotropin releasing factor (CRF) and adrenocorticotropic hormone (ACTH) secretion. Aldosterone produced by the zona glomerulosa is predominantly regulated by the renin-angiotensin system. Aldosterone stimulates the kidneys to reabsorb sodium and water and excrete potassium. At high concentrations, cortisol can also act on the mineralocorticoid receptor to increase sodium and water retention, as the activity of 11β-hydroxysteroid-dehydrogenase type 2 (11β-HSD2), which inactivates cortisol to cortisone, is overwhelmed. Presentation of adrenal insufficiency is often chronic, presenting with fatigue, anorexia and weight loss; hyperpigmentation of the buccal mucosa and skin creases or generalized tanning of the skin occur with primary adrenal insufficiency from the excess of melanocyte-stimulating hormone (MSH) or associated factor produced as a by-product in the formation of excess ACTH.

Adrenal insufficiency can be caused by primary adrenal disease or dysfunction of the HPA axis (secondary adrenal insufficiency). The most common etiologies of primary adrenal disease in adolescents and young adults include autoimmune disease and retroperitoneal trauma. Rarely, the genetic syndromes described below can have their initial presentation later in life, unmasked by the requirement for higher secretion during a physiological stress situation such as sepsis or trauma; more commonly, acute episodes of adrenal insufficiency are induced by poor compliance or an inciting event. Secondary adrenal insufficiency is most commonly caused by damage to the hypothalamus or pituitary gland by trauma or neurological surgery or impingement on these structures by a tumor or mass. Suppression of the HPA axis can occur in patients chronically treated with potent glucocorticoid steroids.

Patients with adrenal insufficiency can present acutely in a severe life-threatening event called adrenal crisis, particularly if there is an inciting event such as a septic illness, surgical procedure, anesthesia, or trauma. These patients have symptoms of nausea, vomiting, abdominal pain, dehydration, altered mental status, hypotension, hypoglycemia or shock (27). Hypotension may be unresponsive to fluid resuscitation alone due to deficiency of cortisol required to activate β-adrenergic receptors and vascular tone. Salt-wasting (hyponatremia, hyperkalemia) results from aldosterone deficiency. A cardinal feature of primary adrenal insufficiency is hyperpigmentation owing to concurrent rise in MSH associated with elevated ACTH production. Darkening of the skin is most prominent at the axillae, palmer creases, areolae, genitalia, and pigmentary lines of the gums. This hyperpigmentation does not occur in secondary adrenal insufficiency as there is no rise in ACTH. Secondary adrenal insufficiency and certain forms of primary insufficiency without defect in aldosterone production do not present with salt-wasting.

Because of circadian rhythm and diurnal variation in ACTH and cortisol production, early morning serum cortisol and ACTH concentrations provide the best assessment of endogenous adrenal function. An early morning serum cortisol of <10 µg/dL (278 nmol/L) is suspicious for adrenal insufficiency. The corresponding ACTH concentration is elevated in primary adrenal insufficiency; a low ACTH concentration is suspicious for secondary adrenal insufficiency. However, a randomly timed cortisol measurement of <15 µg/dL (414 nmol/L), in the setting of an acute illness has been proposed as concerning for adrenal insufficiency in adults (27).

ACTH stimulation testing is the best diagnostic test for identifying those with primary adrenal insufficiency. At baseline, ACTH and cortisol blood levels are obtained and 250 µg of synthetic ACTH (cosyntropin or synacthen) is administered either via IV or intramuscular (IM) route. The test is considered diagnostic of adrenal insufficiency if the peak cortisol level is less than 18 µg/dL (500 nmol/L), 30 or 60 minutes following corticotropin administration. (28). Such a supraphysiologic dose of ACTH may overcome a defect in the HPA axis to produce the rise in serum cortisol. If there is a high suspicion of secondary adrenal insufficiency in the face of a normal cortisol response to high dose ACTH, early morning serum cortisol and ACTH concentrations may be more informative, or other tests such as insulin stress (tolerance) test (IST [ITT]) may be warranted.

Congenital Adrenal Hyperplasia (CAH)

Congenital adrenal hyperplasia (CAH) is a group of autosomal recessive disorders that arise from defective steroidogenesis. The most common enzyme deficiency that accounts for more than 90% of all CAH cases is 21-hydroxylase deficiency (21OHD). This section focuses on CAH owing to 21OHD. Data from close to 6.5 million newborn screenings worldwide indicate that classical CAH occurs in 1:13,000 to 1:15,000 live births (29). CAH is classified into two forms: classical and non-classical CAH. The classical form is further subdivided into salt-wasting (SW) CAH and simple-virilizing CAH. Mineralocorticoid deficiency is a feature of SW-CAH, the most severe form of CAH. Females with classical 21OHD CAH generally present at birth with virilization of their genitalia, while affected males may be detected by the newborn screening program or present with adrenal crisis in the newborn period.

Nonclassical CAH (NC-CAH) is an important and frequently unrecognized form of 21OHD. This milder form causes postnatal symptoms of hyperandrogenism and has a variable presentation from premature adrenarche in young children to infertility in adults. The enzyme defect in NC-CAH is only partial and thus, it is not associated with glucocorticoid or mineralocorticoid deficiency in its untreated state. It may, however, lead to an Addisonian crisis during stress, and thus is considered as an entity that may be unmasked or under-treated during a stay in the ICU.

Adrenoleukodystrophy (ALD)

Adrenoleukodystrophy (ALD) is the most common metabolic disorder causing adrenal failure with a worldwide prevalence of 1 in 20,000 to 50,000 (30) It is caused by mutations in the ATP-binding cassette transporter gene (ABCD1) located on the long arm of the X chromosome (Xq28). The ABCD1 gene encodes the adrenoleukodystrophy protein, involved in transporting very long chain fatty acids (VLCFA) into peroxisomes. Progressive demyelination of the central nervous system and adrenal insufficiency result from defective β-oxidation and accumulation of VLCFA (30). The earliest report of an episode of adrenal insufficiency is in a 5-months-old infant. Some carriers for the mutation take decades to develop adrenal insufficiency with a lifetime risk of approximately 90%. Presentation of adrenal insufficiency is variable and can be insidious. Salt-wasting is less common with X-linked ALD, as aldosterone production is not as frequently affected.

The US Department of Health and Human Services recommended in February 2016 that ALD be added to the uniform panel for state newborn screening programs. As of March 2017, only four US states were screening for ALD in newborns (New York, Connecticut, California, and Minnesota). With the widespread adoption of newborn screening for ALD, adrenal insufficiency in these patients will be detected early and the frequency of presentation in adrenal crisis should decrease.

X-Linked Congenital Adrenal Hypoplasia

X-linked congenital adrenal hypoplasia is caused by mutations of the DAX1 gene located on chromosome Xp21. The DAX1 gene encodes a nuclear transcription factor involved in adrenal and testicular development and differentiation (31). The majority of boys are diagnosed with adrenal insufficiency in early infancy with a few patients diagnosed

with AI in later childhood (2–9 years old) (30). Failure to enter pubertal development owing to hypogonadotropic hypogonadism (HH) is a later presenting symptom.

Rarely, X-linked AHC is first diagnosed in young adulthood presenting with progressive or mild adrenal insufficiency and partial HH is diagnosed on further examination (32,33) or arrested pubertal development (34).

Triple A syndrome

Triple A syndrome is an autosomal recessive disorder characterized by ACTH-resistant adrenal insufficiency, achalasia and alacrima (lacrimal secretory disorders); salt-wasting is rare. Alacrima and achalasia are often the earliest symptoms. Autonomic dysfunction and progressive neurodegeneration also occur. It is caused by mutations of the AAAS gene on chromosome 12q13. The AAAS gene encodes ALADIN, an amino acid protein of the nuclear pore complex integral for cellular structural scaffolding (35).

The majority of patients with triple A syndrome present with adrenal insufficiency during childhood (35) with the rare case presenting in adolescence (36). In a majority of patients, there is an inadequate rise in the serum cortisol concentration to ACTH stimulation with a high dose of corticotropin (250 μg). However, occasionally, a normal cortisol response to high dose ACTH stimulation has been reported (37).

Management of Adrenal Insufficiency

The goal of treatment is to replace glucocorticoid and mineralocorticoid deficiencies concurrent with hemodynamic stabilization. Hydrocortisone is the preferred steroid for treatment of adrenal crisis as it is most physiologic and has a rapid onset of action. Stress dose coverage requires doses of hydrocortisone up to 50–100 mg/m^2/day divided into four doses at least every 6 h. Hydrocortisone can be administered IV or IM. Continuous IV infusion of hydrocortisone can be used in patients with recurrent hypoglycemia and hypotension while in the ICU.

At such high doses of hydrocortisone (50–100 mg/m^2/day), hydrocortisone has mineralocorticoid activity and additional mineralocorticoid replacement is not needed.

For patients who are in shock, IV resuscitation with 5% dextrose in normal saline should be given (27). Hypoglycemia owing to glucocorticoid deficiency and electrolyte abnormalities associated with salt-wasting should be corrected acutely.

In non-life-threatening periods of illness or physiologic stress, the oral corticosteroid dose should be increased to two or three times the normal physiologic dose of 10 mg/m^2/day (i.e., 20–30 mg/m^2/day) for the duration of that period, divided into at least three daily doses.

In the event of a surgical procedure, 5–10 times the daily physiologic dose of hydrocortisone is needed. We recommend administration of 50–100 mg hydrocortisone IM/IV at induction of anesthesia, followed by 10 mg/m^2/hour during the surgical procedure, followed by high doses of hydrocortisone during the first 24–48 postoperative hours (20–30 mg/m^2/day).

When the acute illness has resolved, the hydrocortisone dose may be lowered to physiologic dosing. The recommended physiologic hydrocortisone dose is 8–12 mg/m^2/day divided into three doses. The greatest proportion of the daily dose is administered at awakening to most closely mimic the natural circadian rhythm of cortisol, since the endogenous cortisol peak starts with the onset of rapid eye movement sleep in early hours of the morning. Prior to the first dose, a transient early morning adrenal insufficiency can account for the symptoms of fatigue, lassitude, mild nausea, or headache that are often present on awakening (38). Patients with salt-wasting require treatment with the salt-retaining 9α-fludrocortisone acetate. The average dose is 0.1 mg daily (0.05–0.2 mg daily).

Caveat

Untreated patients with NC-CAH may mount an appropriate cortisol surge in the setting of mild illness. Nonetheless, stress dose coverage with hydrocortisone in such patients is recommended during surgery and childbirth and should be considered if symptoms are suspicious for adrenal crisis. In patients with NC-CAH treated with glucocorticoids, there is suppression of the HPA axis. Thus, treated patients with NC-CAH must be managed with stress dose coverage.

Endocrine Hypertension

Hypertension is defined by a systolic blood pressure (BP) and/or diastolic BP ≥95th percentile for gender, age, and height on ≥3 separate readings. When evaluating a suspected hypertensive patient, it is essential that proper tools and technique are used to measure BP. The preferred screening method is auscultation using a mercury sphygmomanometer. Systolic BP is determined by the onset of the "tapping" Korotkoff sounds (K1) while diastolic DBP is defined as the fifth Korotkoff sound (K5), or the disappearance of Korotkoff sounds. The BP cuff should have a width ≥40% of the arm circumference and a length ≥80% of the arm circumference. A small cuff size can falsely elevate the BP reading. An elevated BP reading obtained with an oscillometric device should be confirmed by auscultation. To determine the percentile of BP, the values are compared to standard BP data in children and adults adjusted for age, sex, and height (39).

Hypertensive crises are life-threatening elevations of BP and should be identified and treated promptly to prevent end-organ damage. For the purposes of this section, adolescents will be assumed to have completed growth and thus BP can be interpreted based on adult standards. In adults, BP exceeding 180/120 mmHg constitutes a hypertensive crisis (40). No such cut-off has been defined for growing children. Patients can present with headache, visual changes, dizziness, nausea, or vomiting. Dyspnea, chest pain, and edema are symptoms concerning for heart or renal failure. The leading causes of hypertensive crises include essential hypertension and renal disease followed by endocrine disease.

In most adults, hypertension is primary (essential or idiopathic), but a subgroup of approximately 15% has secondary hypertension. More than 50% of children who present with hypertension have a secondary cause. In young adults (<40 years old), the prevalence of secondary hypertension is approximately 30%. The secondary causes of hypertension include renal causes (e.g., renal parenchymal disease) and endocrine causes. A recent Endocrine Society Scientific Statement suggested that hypertension may be the initial clinical presentation for at least 15 endocrine disorders (41). An accurate diagnosis of endocrine hypertension provides clinicians with the opportunity to render a surgical cure or to achieve an optimal clinical response with specific pharmacologic therapy. Endocrine hypertension typically refers to hypertensive disorders owing to adrenal gland hyperfunction and is usually mediated by the mineralocorticoid activities of cortisol, aldosterone or adrenal steroidogenic precursors with mineralocorticoid activity. Frequently in these cases, elevated BP is associated with suppressed renin activity, indicating a form of hypertension associated with volume-overload and salt-sensitivity. Other endocrine causes of secondary hypertension include pheochromocytoma, hyperthyroidism, and growth hormone excess (41).

Physical findings can provide clues as to the underlying etiology. For example, thyromegaly with bruit and exophthalmos are features of hyperthyroidism. Moon facies, posterior neck fat pad, and violaceous striae are seen in patients with Cushing's syndrome. Initial laboratory evaluation for endocrine etiologies should include thyroid function tests, plasma renin activity, cortisol, aldosterone, fractionated plasma or urinary metanephrines (41).

Hyperaldosteronism

Primary aldosteronism (PA) is a group of disorders in which there is a non-suppressible secretion of aldosterone. At presentation, hypertension is frequently associated with hypokalemia. PA accounts for approximately 10% of cases of hypertension in adults. Although it is considered rare in children, the high prevalence in the general adult population suggests that the disease may develop in the pediatric population prior to its presentation of hypertension and vascular damage in adulthood. Moderate to severe hypertension that does not respond to medication(s), spontaneous or diuretic-induced hypokalemia, and the presence of adrenal mass provide clues to diagnosis.

The major causes of PA are aldosterone-producing adenomas (often small tumors of less than 4 cm in diameter), bilateral or unilateral adrenal hyperplasia and rarely adrenal carcinoma. Plasma aldosterone-renin ratio (ARR) may be used as an initial screening test and should be repeated if the results are not conclusive or are difficult to interpret. Established ARR cut-offs in adults range between 20–40. Further testing through suppressing aldosterone by oral sodium loading, saline infusion, and/or a challenge with either fludrocortisone or captopril can be used for diagnosis confirmation; however, cut-off values and interpretation have only been established in adults. Adrenal CT or MRI scan are used to identify and localize the mass (41).

Definitive treatment with unilateral adrenalectomy for localized masses found on adrenal vein sampling is recommended. A mineralocorticoid antagonist such as spironolactone or eplerenone can be used while awaiting surgery. Hormonal levels rapidly return to baseline once tumors are removed.

Cushing's Syndrome

Hypercortisolemia is associated with hypertension in approximately 80% of adult cases and half of children. In Cushing's syndrome, there is increased hepatic production of angiotensinogen and increased cardiac output stimulated by cortisol, reduced production of prostaglandins via inhibition of phospholipase A, overwhelming of 11β-HSD2 enzymatic activity with increased mineralocorticoid effect through stimulation of the mineralocorticoid receptor by cortisol leading to hypertension. The etiologies of Cushing's syndrome are divided by their dependence on ACTH. ACTH-dependent causes of hypercortisolemia include pituitary adenomas (Cushing's disease) and ectopic tumors. These ACTH-producing ectopic tumors are most commonly localized to the chest. ACTH independent of Cushing's syndrome is usually caused by an adrenal tumor. Rarely, syndromes of micronodular and macronodular adrenal dysplasia affecting both adrenal glands are found. The most common cause of hypercortisolemia in older children and young adults is Cushing's disease.

The recommended biochemical tests include 24-hour urinary free cortisol, plasma ACTH, and plasma cortisol measurements. Urinary free cortisol excretion is the test that confirms the clinical diagnosis of Cushing's syndrome. If plasma ACTH is measurable in the setting of hypercortisolemia, the cause is ACTH-dependent. If plasma ACTH is undetectable, the cause is ACTH-independent. Imaging studies are dictated by the suspected etiology. The dexamethasone-suppression test with a 1 mg oral dexamethasone dose at midnight is a poor screening test with a low positive predictive value. Its use as a screening test for Cushing's syndrome is being challenged (42).

Pheochromocytoma

Pheochromocytoma is a rare cause of hypertension with an incidence of 2–8 cases per million annually. These catecholamine-producing tumors arise from the chromaffin cells of the adrenal medulla and the sympathetic ganglia. Catecholamine production is variable and depends on the activity of the enzymes required for catecholamine synthesis. Thus, episodes of hypertension associated with symptoms of palpitations, sweating, pallor, and headache may vary in duration and frequency.

Plasma-free metanephrines and urine-fractionated metanephrines are the preferred screening tests (41). Plasma catecholamine levels can be normal between episodes and should ideally be measured during an episode of hypertension. A 4-fold elevation of plasma metanephrines above the upper limit of normal is seen in 80% of patients with pheochromocytoma and is diagnostic (43). Measurement of 24-hour urine-fractionated metanephrines is less sensitive and specific. False positive results can be caused by catecholamine-containing foods (coffee, processed meat, fermented foods), certain antipsychotics, selective α-adrenergic blockers, and β-adrenergic receptor blockers (44). The initial imaging studies to localize the lesion include CT and MRI scans. If these studies are equivocal or extra-adrenal disease is suspected, functional imaging using I^{123}-metaiodobenzylguanidine (MIBG) is recommended (44). Hypertension rapidly remits after resection of the pheochromocytoma. The goal of pre-operative management is to maintain a normal BP and avoid intraoperative hypertensive crisis. Alpha-adrenergic blockers that antagonize catecholamine-stimulated vasoconstriction are the agents of choice. A recommended perioperative management protocol of pheochromocytomas has been described (44).

Approximately 35% of cases are associated with germ line or somatic mutations (45). Physical examination along with personal and family history may elucidate clues to inherited disorders. A personal or family history of retinal and CNS hemangiomas or clear cell renal carcinoma suggests Von Hippel-Landau syndrome. Along with pheochromocytomas, patients with Multiple Endocrine Neoplasia (MEN) Type 2 may present with medullary thyroid carcinoma and hyperparathyroidism. On examination, patients with MEN Type 2B have a Marfanoid habitus and mucosal ganglioneuromas. The physical finds of café-au-lait spots and neurofibromas suggest Neurofibromatosis Type 1.

Hyperthyroidism

Thyroid storm is an exaggerated manifestation of hyperthyroidism or thyrotoxicosis. The most common underlying causes are

Graves' disease and toxic multinodular goiter. An inciting event such as surgery, infection or the administration of iodinated contrast dyes, iodine or lithium precipitates thyroid storm (46). Thyrotoxic periodic paralysis is a rare complication of thyrotoxicosis that can be potentially fatal when there is weakness of the respiratory muscles and cardiac arrhythmias due to hypokalemia. This condition is most common in young adult males (20–40 years of age) of Asian descent (47).

Propylthiouracil at a loading dose of 500–1000 mg followed by 250 mg every 4 hours or methimazole (carbimazole) at a daily dose of 60–80 mg is recommended to inhibit new synthesis of thyroid hormones in thyroid storm (48). In addition to inhibiting thyroid hormone production, propylthiouracil inhibits the conversion of T_4 to T_3. Glucocorticoids also inhibit peripheral conversion of T_4 to T_3 and can be used as an adjunct therapy. Propranolol is used to normalize the heart rate and BP and theoretically decreases the conversion of T_4 to T_3.

Growth Hormone Excess

Growth hormone excess causes gigantism while the epiphyseal growth plates are open during childhood. In adolescence and young adulthood in which the growth plates are closed, this disorder leads to acromegaly and coarsening of the facial features. Hypertension is associated with fluid retention and edema. Genetic conditions associated with GH excess include McCune Albright syndrome, Carney complex, and MEN Type 1 (49).

The preferred screening test is an insulin-like growth factor-1 (IGF1) level. The gold standard for diagnosis is a failure to suppress serum GH levels on oral glucose tolerance testing (49). Treatment options for pituitary gigantism include surgery, radiation, and medical therapy (octreotide, bromocriptine, pegvisomant) based on circumstances and availability (49).

Management

Evaluation to determine the etiology of hypertension should occur concurrently and not delay treatment of hypertension. BP reduction in hypertensive crises should occur over 48 hours with a 25% reduction in the first 8–12 hours followed by another 25% reduction in the next 8–12 hours (50,51). Intravenous access for the administration of antihypertensive medications and intra-arterial monitoring of BP are recommended. For the initial management of these crises, IV antihypertensive medications such as hydralazine, labetalol, nicardipine, and sodium nitroprusside are recommended owing to their rapid onset of action and ability to be titrated (51). In the setting of less severe elevations, oral agents can be considered for initial management.

Traumatic Brain Injury (TBI)

Traumatic brain injury (TBI) affects a large number of children and adolescents with an incidence of 180–250 per 100,000 children per year with a bimodal peak at 0–4 years and 15–17 years (52). The severity of TBI is not well correlated to the degree of pituitary dysfunction. GH deficiency and hypogonadism are the most common pituitary dysfunctions but children can also experience ACTH deficiency, diabetes insipidus, central hypothyroidism, and hyperprolactinemia (53). Symptomatic patients should be treated. Acutely after injury, 80% of adults had gonadotropin deficiency, 18% GH deficiency (GHD), 6% ACTH deficiency, 40% abnormalities in antidiuretic hormone (ADH) production (54). Retrospective studies in children show 29–30.3% prevalence of hypopituitarism at 1 year following TBI (55,56). In a prospective study of 31 children and adolescents, three children had transient water imbalance, 8 had hyperprolactinemia, and 1 had adrenal insufficiency but all resolved. Of the 4 children with GHD, one persisted beyond 12 months. One of each of the 13 children with central hypothyroidism and 4 children with GHD persisted beyond 12 months (55).

Since spontaneous recovery of hypothalamic-pituitary axes shortly after TBI occurs frequently, routine surveillance to ensure early detection of hormonal deficiencies should be performed starting 1 year after injury.

Growth Hormone Deficiency (GHD)

Growth hormone deficiency (GHD) is a heterogeneous disorder which often presents in childhood with growth failure, commonly resulting from a variety of etiologies including congenital structural anomalies, genetic abnormalities, and acquired pituitary gland dysfunction owing to infiltrative disease, surgery, and cranial irradiation.

Upon completion of growth, re-evaluation of the somatotropic axis should be performed in patients with isolated GHD (57). A serum IGF1 concentration is the recommended screening test. Those with multiple pituitary deficiencies should be continued on GH therapy without re-testing. If IGF1 is less than mean for age, GH stimulation testing is recommended. Growth hormone therapy should be offered to those with persistent GHD in the transition period. GHD in the transition period and adulthood is characterized by altered fat distribution, glucose intolerance, abnormal lipid profiles, premature atherosclerosis, and osteoporosis (58).

Management

During prolonged hospitalization for critical illness, GH therapy should be discontinued. In two prospective, multi-center, double-blinded, randomized, placebo-controlled trials evaluating the effect of GH treatment on clinical outcomes in critically ill adults receiving prolonged intensive care, the in-hospital mortality rate was higher in the GH treated group (39–44%) compared to the placebo group (18–20%) (18). Further, the GH-treated survivors had longer lengths of stay. Postulated reasons for the increased mortality associated with GH include modulation of the immune system, insulin resistance, inhibition of mobilization of glutamine for rapidly dividing cells, and interference with thyroid or adrenocortical function.

Diabetes Insipidus (DI)

In diabetes insipidus (DI), excessive urinary free water loss is due to vasopressin (AVP, also termed ADH) deficiency. AVP is produced by the posterior pituitary gland. DI is divided into two subtypes: cranial DI and nephrogenic DI. Molecular defects have been described (59). Fluid resuscitation should be initiated with the aim of lowering serum sodium slowly to avoid osmotic demyelination syndrome. Central DI is responsive to vasopressin and desmopressin therapy; whereas nephrogenic DI is not. Treatment options for nephrogenic DI include increased fluid intake, hydrochlorothiazide, and indomethacin.

Hypothyroidism

The most severe presentation of hypothyroidism is myxedema coma. This condition typically occurs in patients with undiagnosed chronic hypothyroidism presenting with an acute systemic illness. Hypothermia (body temperature <80°F) is seen in the majority of patients and can be the first diagnostic clue. Other clinical features include periorbital edema, non-pitting edema, dry skin, macroglossia, and delayed deep tendon reflexes. A surgical scar on the neck indicating prior thyroidectomy or a goiter may be noted on examination of the thyroid.

Thyroid hormone replacement should be initiated immediately. However, there is controversy over the preferred thyroid replacement with T_4 versus T_3 (60). An initial IV bolus of T_4 at a dose of 300–600 mcg followed by a maintenance dose of 50–100 mcg daily has been used clinically in adults (60). Treatment of hypothyroidism can unmask adrenal insufficiency. Hypothyroidism and adrenal insufficiency often coincide with each other, either as primary deficiencies associated with autoimmune syndromes or secondary deficiencies associated with hypopituitarism. Thus, it is important to identify and treat adrenal insufficiency *prior to* initiation of thyroid replacement. Warming of the body temperature with blankets or increased room temperature should be done with caution so as not to cause peripheral vasodilation leading to hypotension.

Sick Euthyroid Syndrome

Sick euthyroid syndrome must be differentiated from true cases of hypothyroidism. In critically ill patients, serum T_3 levels may be unusually low with reduced pituitary TSH secretion (60). Thyroid hormone levels can be low but are often normal. The pattern of low or normal thyroid hormone with low TSH mimics central hypothyroidism. This condition does not require thyroid replacement and thyroid hormone levels normalize with improved clinical condition.

Conclusions

This chapter discusses the transitional care of diabetes and chronic and evolving endocrine disorders, as well as the management (including emergency care) of endocrine disorders that commonly present in young adulthood. Transitional care is complex. Open communication among pediatric and adult clinicians, patient, and family is recommended to facilitate a coordinated seamless shift from pediatric to adult healthcare. However, in the emergency setting, adult providers should be cognizant of the unique types, presenting features, and approaches to management of diabetes and endocrine conditions in these young adults.

References

1 Miller KM, et al. Current state of type 1 diabetes treatment in the U.S.: updated data from the T1D Exchange clinic registry. *Diabetes Care*. 2015;38(6):971–978.

2 Atkinson MA, Eisenbarth GS, Michels AW. Type 1 diabetes. *Lancet*. 2014;383(9911):69–82.

3 Cameron FJ, Wherrett DK. Care of diabetes in children and adolescents: controversies, changes, and consensus. *Lancet*. 2015;385(9982):2096–2106.

4 Paun A, Danska JS. Modulation of type 1 and type 2 diabetes risk by the intestinal microbiome. *Pediatr Diabetes*. 2016;17(7):469–477.

5 Soleimanpour SA, Stoffers DA. The pancreatic beta cell and type 1 diabetes: innocent bystander or active participant?*Trends Endocrinol Metab*. 2013;24(7):324–331.

6 Atkinson MA, et al. How does type 1 diabetes develop?: The notion of homicide or beta-cell suicide revisited. *Diabetes*. 2011;60(5):1370–1379.

7 Greenbaum CJ, et al. Through the fog: recent clinical trials to preserve beta-cell function in type 1 diabetes. *Diabetes*. 2012;61(6):1323–1330.

8 Mayer-Davis EJ, et al. Incidence trends of Type 1 and Type 2 diabetes among youths, 2002–2012. *N Engl J Med*. 2017;376(15):1419–1429.

9 Wolfsdorf J, et al. Diabetic ketoacidosis in infants, children, and adolescents: a consensus statement from the American Diabetes Association. *Diabetes Care*, 2006;29(5):1150–1159.

10 Wolfsdorf JI. The International Society of Pediatric and Adolescent Diabetes guidelines for management of diabetic ketoacidosis: do the guidelines need to be modified? *Pediatr Diabetes*. 2014;15(4):277–286.

11 Kamel KS, Halperin ML. Acid-base problems in diabetic ketoacidosis. *N Engl J Med*. 2015;372(20):1969–1970.

12 White PC. Optimizing fluid management of diabetic ketoacidosis. *Pediatr Diabetes*. 2015;16(5):317–319.

13 Sperling MA, Diabetes: recurrent DKA – for whom the bell tolls. *Nat Rev Endocrinol*. 2016;12(10):562–564.

14 Gibb FW, et al. Risk of death following admission to a UK hospital with diabetic ketoacidosis. *Diabetologia*. 2016;59(10):2082–2087.

15 Lyons SK, Libman IM, Sperling MA, Clinical review: diabetes in the adolescent: transitional issues. *J Clin Endocrinol Metab*. 2013;98(12):4639–4645.

16 De Block CE, et al. A comparison of two insulin infusion protocols in the medical intensive care unit by continuous glucose monitoring. *Ann Intensive Care*. 2016;6(1):115.

17 Van den Berghe G. Intensive insulin therapy in the ICU: reconciling the evidence. *Nat Rev Endocrinol*. 2012;8(6):374–378.

18 Takala J, et al. Increased mortality associated with growth hormone treatment in critically ill adults. *N Engl J Med*. 1999;341(11):785–792.

19 Zeitler P, et al. Hyperglycemic hyperosmolar syndrome in children: pathophysiological considerations and suggested guidelines for treatment. *J Pediatr*. 2011;158(1):9–14, 14 e1–e2.

20 Perheentupa J, Autoimmune polyendocrinopathy-candidiasis-ectodermal dystrophy. *J Clin Endocrinol Metab*. 2006;91(8):2843–2850.

21 Anderson MS, Su MA. AIRE expands: new roles in immune tolerance and beyond. *Nat Rev Immunol*. 2016;16(4):247–258.

22 Fierabracci A. Type 1 diabetes in Autoimmune Polyendocrinopathy-Candidiasis-Ectodermal Dystrophy Syndrome (APECED): a "rare" manifestation in a "rare" disease. *Int J Mol Sci*. 2016;17(7).

23 Kisand K, Peterson P. Autoimmune polyendocrinopathy candidiasis ectodermal dystrophy. *J Clin Immunol*. 2015;35(5):463–478.

24 Kakleas K, et al. Associated autoimmune diseases in children and adolescents with type 1 diabetes mellitus (T1DM). *Autoimmun Rev*. 201514(9):781–797.

25 Gimenez-Barcons M, et al. Autoimmune predisposition in Down syndrome may result from a partial central tolerance failure due to insufficient intrathymic expression of AIRE and peripheral antigens. *J Immunol*. 2014;193(8):3872–3879.

26 Verdu EF, Caminero A. How infection can incite sensitivity to food. *Science*. 2017;356(6333):29–30.

27 Cooper MS, Stewart PM. Corticosteroid insufficiency in acutely ill patients. *N Engl J Med*. 2003;348(8):727–734.

28 Bornstein SR, et al. Diagnosis and treatment of primary adrenal insufficiency: an Endocrine Society Clinical Practice Guideline. *J Clin Endocrinol Metab*. 2016;101(2):364–389.

29 Pang SY, et al. Worldwide experience in newborn screening for classical congenital adrenal hyperplasia due to 21-hydroxylase deficiency. *Pediatrics*. 1988;81(6):866–874.

30 Burtman E, Regelmann MO. Endocrine dysfunction in X-linked adrenoleukodystrophy. *Endocrinol Metab Clin North Am*. 2016;45(2):295–309.

31 Suntharalingham JP, et al. DAX-1 (NR0B1) and steroidogenic factor-1 (SF-1, NR5A1) in human disease. *Best Pract Res Clin Endocrinol Metab*. 2015;29(4):607–619.

32 Tabarin A, et al. A novel mutation in DAX1 causes delayed-onset adrenal insufficiency and incomplete hypogonadotropic hypogonadism. *J Clin Invest*. 2000;105(3):321–328.

33 Ozisik G, et al. An alternate translation initiation site circumvents an amino-terminal DAX1 nonsense mutation leading to a mild form of X-linked adrenal hypoplasia congenita. *J Clin Endocrinol Metab*. 2003;88(1):417–423.

34 Mantovani G, et al. Hypogonadotropic hypogonadism as a presenting feature of late-onset X-linked adrenal hypoplasia congenita. *J Clin Endocrinol Metab*. 2002;87(1):44–48.

35 Milenkovic T, et al. Triple A syndrome: 32 years experience of a single centre (1977–2008). *Eur J Pediatr*. 2010;169(11):1323–1328.

36 Dumic M, et al. Long-term clinical follow-up and molecular genetic findings in eight patients with triple A syndrome. *Eur J Pediatr*. 2012;171(10):1453–1459.

37 Salehi M, et al. The diagnosis of adrenal insufficiency in a patient with Allgrove syndrome and a novel mutation in the

ALADIN gene. *Metabolism*. 2005;54(2):200–205.

38 Tache Y. Cyclic vomiting syndrome: the corticotropin-releasing-factor hypothesis. *Dig Dis Sci*. 1999;44(8 Suppl):79S–86S.

39 National High Blood Pressure Education Program Working Group on High Blood Pressure in, Children and Adolescents. The fourth report on the diagnosis, evaluation, and treatment of high blood pressure in children and adolescents. *Pediatrics*. 2004;114(2 Suppl. 4th Report):555–576.

40 Chobanian AV, et al. The Seventh Report of the Joint National Committee on Prevention, Detection, Evaluation, and Treatment of High Blood Pressure: the JNC 7 report. *JAMA*. 2003;289(19):2560–2572.

41 Young WF, Calhour DA, Lenders JWM, Stowasser M, Textor SC. Screening for endocrine hypertension: an Endocrine Society Scientific Statement. *Endocr Rev*. 2017;38(2):103–122. doi: 10.1210/er.2017-00054.

42 Loriaux DL. Diagnosis and differential diagnosis of Cushing's syndrome. *N Engl J Med*. 2017;376(15):1451–1459.

43 Eisenhofer G, et al. Biochemical diagnosis of pheochromocytoma: how to distinguish true- from false-positive test results. *J Clin Endocrinol Metab*. 2003;88(6):2656–2666.

44 Galati SJ, et al. The Mount Sinai clinical pathway for the management of pheochromocytoma. *Endocr Pract*. 2015;21(4):368–382.

45 Pacak K, Wimalawansa SJ. Pheochromocytoma and paraganglioma. *Endocr Pract*. 2015;21(4):406–412.

46 Klubo-Gwiezdzinska J, Wartofsky L. Thyroid emergencies. *Med Clin North Am*. 2012.;96(2):385–403.

47 Li J, Yang XB, Zhao Y, Thyrotoxic periodic paralysis in the Chinese population: clinical features in 45 cases. *Exp Clin Endocrinol Diabetes*. 2010;118(1):22–26.

48 Bahn RS, et al. Hyperthyroidism and other causes of thyrotoxicosis: management guidelines of the American Thyroid Association and American Association of Clinical Endocrinologists. *Thyroid*. 2011;21(6):593–646.

49 Lodish MB, Trivellin G, Stratakis CA. Pituitary gigantism: update on molecular biology and management. *Curr Opin Endocrinol Diabetes Obes*. 2016;23(1):72–80.

50 Flynn JT, Tullus K. Severe hypertension in children and adolescents: pathophysiology and treatment. *Pediatr Nephrol*. 2009;24(6):1101–1112.

51 Stein DR, Ferguson MA. Evaluation and treatment of hypertensive crises in children. *Integr Blood Press Control*. 2016;9:49–58.

52 Schneier AJ, et al. Incidence of pediatric traumatic brain injury and associated hospital resource utilization in the United States. *Pediatrics*. 2006;118(2):483–492.

53 Rose SR, Auble BA. Endocrine changes after pediatric traumatic brain injury. *Pituitary*. 2012;15(3):267–275.

54 Behan LA, et al. Neuroendocrine disorders after traumatic brain injury. *J Neurol Neurosurg Psychiatry*. 2008;79(7):753–759.

55 Kaulfers AM, et al. Endocrine dysfunction following traumatic brain injury in children. *J Pediatr*. 2010;157(6):894–899.

56 Aimaretti G, et al. Hypopituitarism induced by traumatic brain injury in the transition phase. *J Endocrinol Invest*. 2005;28(11):984–989.

57 Grimberg A, et al. Guidelines for growth hormone and insulin-like growth factor-i treatment in children and adolescents: growth hormone deficiency, idiopathic short stature, and primary insulin-like growth factor-I deficiency. *Horm Res Paediatr*. 2016;86(6):361–397.

58 Yuen KC, et al. American Association of Clinical Endocrinologists and American College of Endocrinology Disease State Clinical Review: update on growth hormone stimulation testing and proposed revised cut-point for the glucagon stimulation test in the diagnosis of adult growth hormone deficiency. *Endocr Pract*. 2016;22(10):1235–1244.

59 Knepper MA, Kwon TH, Nielsen S. Molecular physiology of water balance. *N Engl J Med*. 2015;373(2):196.

60 Wartofsky L. Myxedema coma. *Endocrinol Metab Clin North Am*. 2006;35(4):687–698,vii–viii.

7

Emergency Perioperative Diabetes and Endocrine Management

Glenn Matfin, Kate Evans, and Ketan Dhatariya

Key Points

- The aim of perioperative medicine is to deliver the best possible care for patients before, during, and after surgery.
- Perioperative medicine multidisciplinary teams (MDT) lead the assessment and preparation of patients for surgery to optimize the treatment of co-existing medical disease including diabetes, and/or endocrine and metabolic disorders.
- The number of inpatients with diabetes continues to increase (e.g., 17% of inpatients in the UK have diabetes; and more than 20% in the USA).
- Persons with diabetes require surgical procedures at a higher rate and have longer hospital stays than those without diabetes.
- The presence of diabetes and/or hyperglycemia in surgical patients also leads to increased morbidity and mortality, with perioperative mortality rates up to 50% higher than the non-diabetes population. The reasons for these adverse outcomes are multifactorial.
- Several studies have shown that high preoperative and perioperative glucose and glycosylated hemoglobin (HbA1c) levels lead to poor surgical outcomes. In view of these findings, elective surgery with acceptable glycemic control (e.g., HbA1c <8.5% [<69 mmol/mol] and ambient glycemic

- levels within ranges defined by local guidelines) and no evidence of diabetes-related acute decompensation (e.g., hypoglycemia, diabetic ketoacidosis [DKA], hyperglycemic hyperosmolar state [HHS], or electrolyte disturbance) would be the preferred option for diabetes patients requiring surgery.
- Unfortunately, it is estimated that 5% of persons with diabetes will require emergency surgery (i.e., patients who have an acute condition that threatens life, limb, or the integrity of a body structure) over their lifetime. These operations are time-critical and need to be performed immediately (day or night).
- The actual perioperative glycemic treatment recommendations for a given patient should be individualized based on factors such as current glycemic control, type of diabetes, nature and extent of surgical procedure, and antecedent diabetes therapy.
- The management goal is to optimize metabolic control through close monitoring, adequate fluid and caloric repletion, and judicious use of insulin (usually intravenous in this setting, but subcutaneous route including insulin pumps are also used). Avoiding pressure damage to the feet during surgery and recovery is also critical.

Endocrine and Metabolic Medical Emergencies: A Clinician's Guide, Second Edition. Edited by Glenn Matfin.
© 2018 John Wiley & Sons Ltd. Published 2018 by John Wiley & Sons Ltd.

- Unfortunately, levels of knowledge among healthcare staff regarding diabetes or hyperglycemia management remain poor; and levels of satisfaction among inpatients with diabetes remains low.
- Other endocrine and metabolic derangements (e.g., adrenal insufficiency; hypothyroidism and hyperthyroidism; carcinoid crisis; hyponatremia; hypercalcemia) are also common in the emergency perioperative setting and warrant prompt MDT review and appropriate management.

Introduction

Perioperative generally refers to the three phases of surgery: pre-, intra-, and postoperative. Subsequently the aim of perioperative medicine is to deliver the best possible care for patients before, during, and after surgery. Perioperative medicine multidisciplinary teams (MDT) lead the assessment and preparation of patients for surgery to optimize the treatment of co-existing medical disease including diabetes, and/or endocrine and metabolic disorders.

Emergency Perioperative Diabetes and/or Hyperglycemia Management

The proportion of inpatients with diabetes continues to grow (e.g., 17% in the UK; and more than 20% in the USA) (1). The UK's National Diabetes Inpatient Audit (NaDIA) projects that the numbers of hospital beds occupied by persons with diabetes will increase to nearly 20% by 2020; in many hospitals it already exceeds 30% (2). In addition to people who are known to have diabetes prior to acute inpatient admission, a number of patients with hyperglycemia will be diagnosed with diabetes for the first time during admission (i.e., HbA1c on admission will be increased). In comparison, other patients may develop transient hyperglycemia detected during admission that normalizes after discharge, so-called "stress hyperglycemia" (i.e., HbA1c on admission will be normal or in the pre-diabetes range) (3). Taken together, the numbers of people

in hospital with either diabetes or transient hyperglycemia is large with a prevalence of between 32–38% on general wards; and between 28–80% of patients with critical illness or undergoing cardiac surgery.

Persons with diabetes require surgical procedures at a higher rate and have longer hospital stays than those without diabetes (4). In particular, diabetes patients admitted for general and orthopedic surgery have some of the longest overall lengths of hospital stay (5). The presence of diabetes and/or hyperglycemia in surgical patients also leads to increased morbidity and mortality, with perioperative mortality rates up to 50% higher than the non-diabetes population (6). The reasons for these adverse outcomes are multifactorial, but include failure to identify patients with diabetes and/or hyperglycemia (2); multiple comorbidities including microvascular and macrovascular complications (7–10); complex polypharmacy and insulin-prescribing errors (11), with greater likelihood of insulin prescription and medication management errors if the insulin-treated patient is managed on a surgical compared with a medical ward (2); increased perioperative and postoperative infections (6); associated hypoglycemia and hyperglycemia (6); lack of or inadequate institutional guidelines for management of inpatient diabetes and/or hyperglycemia (6,12); and inadequate knowledge of diabetes and hyperglycemia management among staff delivering care (2).

Several studies have shown that high preoperative and perioperative glucose and glycosylated hemoglobin (HbA1c) levels lead to poor surgical outcomes. These findings occur in both elective and emergency surgery, and include various types of surgery including spinal (13), vascular (14), colorectal (15), cardiac (16,17), trauma-related (18), breast (19), foot and ankle (20), neurosurgery, and hepatobiliary surgery (21). Adverse outcomes related to increased morbidity and mortality include increased wound infection rates, urinary tract infections (UTI), lower respiratory tract infections, admission and time in intensive care, development of acute kidney injury (AKI), or acute coronary syndromes. However, there are data to show that the outcomes of persons with diabetes may not be different – or may indeed be better – than those without diabetes if the diagnosis

is known prior to surgery (22,23). The reasons for this are unknown but may be due to increased vigilance surrounding glucose control given to those with a prior diagnosis of diabetes.

In view of these findings, elective surgery with acceptable glycemic control (e.g., HbA1c <8.5% [<69 mmol/mol] and ambient glycemic levels within ranges defined by local guidelines) and no evidence of diabetes-related acute decompensation (e.g., hypoglycemia, diabetic ketoacidosis [DKA], hyperglycemic hyperosmolar state [HHS], or electrolyte disturbance) would be the preferred option for diabetes patients requiring surgery (Figure 7-1) (24,25).

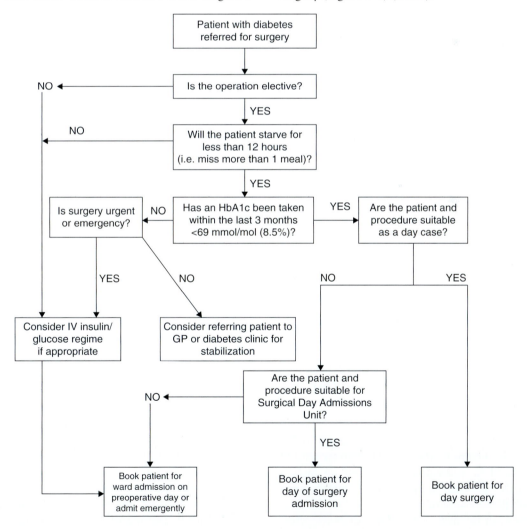

Figure 7-1 Suitability of patients with diabetes for day surgery (24).

However, approximately 5% of persons with diabetes will require emergency surgery over their lifetime (26). About 100,000 emergency surgical procedures are performed per annum in the UK on patients with diabetes. Emergency surgery is performed on patients who have an acute condition that threatens life, limb or the integrity of a body structure. Some emergency operations are time-critical and need to be performed immediately (day or night). Emergency surgical care comprises 40–50% of the workload of most surgical specialties, and can result in additional complications, higher mortality (25%), increased costs, and is disruptive to elective surgery planning and implementation. By definition, the time of occurrence of these emergencies cannot be predicted, and appropriate surgical care must not be unduly delayed. Nonetheless, particular care must be taken in persons with diabetes who are being considered for emergency surgery to exclude DKA (including measuring serum and urine ketones if patient is taking sodium-glucose co-transporter-2 [SGLT2] inhibitors as risk of DKA even with normal blood glucose (BG) levels [i.e., euglycemic DKA]) (27); and other conditions (e.g., vomiting related to undiagnosed or poorly controlled gastroparesis or glucagon-like peptide-1 [GLP-1] agonist adverse effect) that may be mistaken for surgical emergencies. Many patients with DKA and prominent abdominal symptoms have undergone needless surgical exploration for a nonexistent acute abdominal emergency (26).

Approaches to Management of Perioperative Diabetes and/or Hyperglycemia

The actual perioperative glycemic treatment recommendations for a given patient should be individualized, based on factors such as current glycemic control, type of diabetes, nature and extent of surgical procedure, and antecedent diabetes therapy (3,28). Unfortunately, many patients who require emergency surgery will have suboptimal glycemic control. However, this is not necessarily a contraindication to the timely performance of potentially life-saving surgery. An intravenous (IV) access should be secured and immediate blood specimens should be sent for glucose, electrolyte, and acid-base assessment. Gross derangements of volume and electrolytes (e.g., hypokalemia, hypernatremia) should be corrected. Surgery should be delayed (must discuss with the surgeon planned timing of surgery), whenever feasible, in patients with DKA, so that the underlying acid-base disorder can be corrected or, at least, ameliorated. Patients with HHS are markedly dehydrated and should be restored to good volume and improved metabolic status before surgery.

Individuals who develop transient hyperglycemia (i.e., "stress" hyperglycemia) should be treated just as aggressively as people with known diabetes because their risk of postoperative complications is as high (if not higher) than those with prior diagnosis.

For those having emergency surgery, aiming for pragmatic BG values of between 110–180 mg/dL (6–10 mmol/L), with an acceptable range of 72–216 mg/dL (4–12 mmol/L) should be the target (24). The lower limit can be increased (i.e., 108–216 mg/dL [6–12 mmol/L]) in surgical patients who are asleep, unconscious, or unable to communicate because of increased risk of hypoglycemia. A glycemic target range of 140–180 mg/dL (7.8–10 mmol/L) is preferred in the USA for the majority of critically ill and noncritically ill patients according to the American Diabetes Association (ADA) (3). In agreement with this, the GLUCO-CABG trial reported no significant differences in the composite end points of complications and death between an intensive glucose target of 100–140 mg/dL (5.6–7.7 mmol/L) and a conservative target of 141–180 mg/dL (7.8–10 mmol/L) after cardiac surgery (29). However, despite this evidence, the ADA perioperative target glucose range remains broader at 80–180 mg/dL (4.4–10 mmol/L) if the lower level can be achieved safely (3).

Blood glucose monitoring should be at least hourly during the procedure and in the immediate postoperative period using an appropriate point-of-care (POC) measure to allow early detection of any alterations in metabolic control. Continuous glucose monitoring (CGM) provides continuous estimates, direction, and magnitude of glucose trends, which may have an advantage over POC glucose testing in detecting and reducing the incidence of hypoglycemia (3). However, several studies have shown that CGM use did not improve glucose control, but detected a greater number of hypoglycemic events than POC testing. A recent review has recommended against the routine use of CGM in adults in the in-hospital setting until more safety and efficacy data become available (30). In comparison, a number of pilot studies have shown that CGM works well as part of a closed-loop ("artificial pancreas") system in both type 1 and type 2 diabetes patients in the inpatient setting (31).

All patients receiving insulin before admission require insulin during the perioperative period (32,33). In the emergency setting, this is best achieved with an IV continuous insulin infusion (CII, also known as variable rate intravenous insulin infusion [VRIII]), using an effective and safe protocol (preferably using validated written or computerized physician order entry [CPOE]) (Figure 7-2) (3). The short half-life of IV insulin (<15 minutes) allows flexibility in adjusting the infusion rate in the event of unpredicted changes in nutrition or the patient's health. It is expected that if the patient was taking long- or ultra-long-acting basal insulin (human or analog) prior to admission, then this should be continued. Continuation of the background insulin prevents rebound hyperglycemia when the IV insulin is stopped. Other patients not previously on insulin therapy should be reviewed on an individualized basis to determine the appropriate therapy.

Patients not expected to miss more than one meal (i.e., short starvation period) might be candidates for alternative glucose-lowering therapies without the need for CII (VRIII) (24). However, several glucose-lowering therapies are best avoided in the perioperative setting such as GLP-1 agonists (i.e., adverse events include nausea, vomiting, AKI, and pancreatitis); SGLT2 inhibitors (i.e., adverse events include dehydration, AKI, UTI, DKA [including euglycemic], and increased risk of lower limb amputation mostly affecting the mid-foot and toes) (3,27); and metformin (i.e., adverse events include nausea, vomiting, diarrhea, lactic acidosis [especially with eGFR <30 ml/min and severe cardiorespiratory issues], and contrast-related complications). SGLT2 inhibitors should be avoided in severe illness when ketone bodies are present and during prolonged fasting and surgical procedures. Until safety and effectiveness are established, SGLT2 inhibitors are not recommended for routine in-hospital use (3,27). Dipeptidyl peptidase-4 (DPP-4) inhibitors, which enhance circulating concentrations of active GLP-1, are used in the in-hospital setting. Sitagliptin has shown efficacy and safety in both a pilot and more definitive study of patients with mild-moderately severe type 2 diabetes in the inpatient setting. Sitagliptin (using renal dosing) in combination with basal insulin was non-inferior in controlling glycemia versus basal-bolus insulin regimen in medical and surgical patients (34). Sitagliptin (+/− basal insulin) may be especially useful for elderly inpatients. In comparison, saxagliptin and alogliptin have not been widely studied in the in-hospital setting. They should also be discontinued in patients who develop heart failure on starting either of these two agents (more common in patients with established heart or kidney disease) or are contraindicated with existing heart failure.

Patients expected to miss more than one meal should generally have a CII (VRIII). In addition, if BG concentration rises above 180 mg/dL (10 mmol/L), a CII (VRIII) should be considered and continued until the patient is eating and drinking (3,32). Alternatively, an insulin regimen including subcutaneous (SC) basal and correction components might be an option in some patients instead of CII (VRIII)

Variable rate intravenous insulin infusion (VRIII)
Managing blood glucose in adults with
PERIOPERATIVE/Nil By Mouth /
UNSTABLE DIABETES

BEFORE YOU START

- This chart is NOT for DKA or HHS diabetes emergencies - use correct charts
- This chart is NOT applicable for patients who are eating and drinking normally
- CHECK electrolytes 12 HOURLY (at least) be vigilant to prevent hyponatremia and hypokalemia
- For patients on subcutaneous insulin pumps, stop their pump at least 1 hour <u>after</u> VRIII has started, not before
- For further advice contact Medical/Diabetes team on call if out of hours
- Target range 6–10 mmol/L (110–180 mg/dL) unless indicated by Clinician

Perioperative patients	CKD5/eGFR<15ml/min/dialysis patients	Parenteral-fed patients
• Need VRIII if missing 2 or more meals, whether Type 1 or 2 • Aim first on theatre list • After major surgery, likely need additional IV fluids to meet fluid & electrolyte requirements • When transporting to theatre, continue both insulin & fluid infusion pumps. If either fails, stop both - but RESTART as matter of urgency	• MUST discuss IV fluids with Renal team first • Omit IV fluids in anuric patients, give insulin only • Do not add potassium unless <3.5 mmol/L. If given, check electrolytes 4 HOURLY • No potassium if >4.5 mmol/L	• IV fluids NOT routinely required, unless going to surgery, when feed would be stopped and IV fluids started • Must discuss IV fluids with Nutritional Support Team (or similar)

INTRAVENOUS FLUIDS (IV)

Points to consider:
- Rate of IV fluids MUST take into account patient's condition and clinical requirements, caution advised especially in heart failure, renal or liver impairment - seek cardiology/nephrology/hepatology opinion, if needed
- Some patients require additional IV fluids alongside above recommendations
- Aim to maintain serum potassium between 4-5 mmol/L
- Always infuse IV fluids via volumetric pump

<u>Weight</u>

_____ Kg

Selecting your IV fluids:

- If **blood glucose <15 mmol/L (270 mg/dL)**
  500 ml 10% glucose with 10 mmol potassium chloride at 1ml/kg/hour (maximum rate 100 ml/hour)
- If **blood glucose ≥15 mmol/L (270 mg/dL)**
  1000 ml 0.9% normal saline with 20 mmol potassium chloride at 1ml/kg/hour (max rate 100 ml/hour)
  For further advice contact Medical/Diabetes on call if out of hours

SETTING UP INSULIN INFUSION

Points to consider:
- DO NOT give other IV drugs through the peripheral cannula without discussing with pharmacist first, to check compatibility
- Connect IV fluids to the Y connector of the insulin administration set
- The insulin administration set MUST have anti-reflux and anti-syphon valves
- Infuse insulin via syringe driver & IV fluids via volumetric pump

Insulin (Please circle)	Dose	Volume	Prescriber signature	Date & time	Syringe preparation			
					Batch number & expiry insulin	Batch number & expiry saline	Signature	Witness
Actrapid Humulin S	50 units	Made up to 50ml with sodium chloride 0.9% (1 unit per 1 ml)						

CONTINUE the following insulin (State concentration e.g. U100; U200, etc):
Detemir, Glargine, Degludec; or NPH insulins: INSULATARD, HUMULIN I, INSUMAN BASAL

STOP rapid-acting and mixed insulin(s), plus diabetes tablets whilst on VRIII

Figure 7-2 Generic UK example of variable rate intravenous insulin infusion (VRIII). Use in perioperative; unstable diabetes; and nil-by-mouth (NBM) patients.
DKA = diabetic ketoacidosis; HHS = hyperglycemic hyperosmolar state; CBG = Capillary blood glucose; eGFR = estimated glomerular filtration rate.

in the appropriate setting (3). CII (VRIII) are often poorly managed in the perioperative setting and thus require explicit guidelines including how to transition safely and effectively from IV to SC insulin (i.e., it is important to administer the short-, rapid-, or fast-acting insulin at least 30 minutes prior to stopping IV insulin; and the basal insulin component at least 2 h before stopping insulin infusion; 6 hours is preferred for U300 insulin glargine; and 2–4 h for U100/U200 insulin degludec) or non-insulin therapies. Basal insulin or basal plus correction SC insulin regimen may be used during this transition period for non-critically ill patients with poor oral intake or those taking "nil by mouth" (3). Alternatively, an insulin regimen including SC basal, nutritional, and correction components might be the preferred option for non-critically ill patients with good nutritional intake (3,32). As noted above, sitagliptin in combination with basal insulin (+/− correction insulin) was non-inferior in controlling glycemia compared to basal-bolus insulin regimen in surgical patients but needs further evaluation in this population (34). The sole use of SC "sliding scale" insulin (i.e., short-, rapid-, or fast-acting insulin correction coverage only with no basal dosing) in the in-hospital setting is strongly discouraged (3,28).

Other important factors include optimizing and maintaining volume status, electrolyte balance, avoidance of pressure damage to the feet during surgery and recovery, and prevention and optimal treatment of hypoglycemia (episodes of hypoglycemia should be documented and tracked). If hypoglycemia does occur (i.e., <70 mg/dL [3.9 mmol/L]), the treatment regimen must be reviewed and changed to prevent further episodes. Early involvement of the critical care and diabetes specialist teams is recommended in the management of any high-risk surgical patient with diabetes and/or hyperglycemia.

There are several factors that influence glycemic control in the postoperative period, including a variation in nutritional intake, the discontinuation of the usual glucose-lowering medications, the decrease in physical activity, the increase in stress hormones, and the presence of infection or pain. It is therefore important that glycemic control is maintained in addition to fluid and electrolyte imbalance and that pain and postoperative nausea and vomiting are controlled (using multi-modal analgesia combined with appropriate anti-emetics) to permit an early return to a normal diet, and the usual diabetes regimen is paramount.

There should be a structured discharge plan tailored to the individual patient with diabetes and/or hyperglycemia (3,27). Prior to hospital discharge, the patient should be made aware that the metabolic and endocrine effects of surgery may last for several days because of ongoing changes in the amount that they eat, their activity levels, and the levels of stress hormones. The patient should be advised that their BG management may need to change for some time postoperatively. The diabetes specialist team or the patient's usual provider should be involved in this discussion.

Unfortunately levels of knowledge among healthcare staff regarding diabetes and/or hyperglycemia management remain poor; and levels of satisfaction among inpatients with diabetes remains low (2).

Continuous Subcutaneous Insulin Infusion Therapy (CSII), "Insulin Pumps" during the Perioperative Period

Insulin pump therapy, also known as continuous subcutaneous insulin infusion therapy (CSII), was first introduced over 30 years ago; early models were bulky and prone to technical problems. Modern insulin pumps are portable and discreet, and use smart technologies, such as bluetooth transmission of capillary glucose level from glucometer to pump, and the ability to download pump data for analysis. However, contrary to the hopes of many individuals with type 1 diabetes, the pump is not a fully automatic "artificial pancreas," requiring a high level of user involvement.

CSII is used in patients with type 1 diabetes to improve glycemic control and/or reduce the risk of hypoglycemia. CSII is also being studied and used in poorly controlled type 2 diabetes patients on basal-bolus insulin regimens, including during pregnancy. The role of insulin pumps and/or CGM in persons with type 1 or type 2 diabetes (including in-hospital use) was recently comprehensively reviewed in an Endocrine Society 2016 guideline (35).

Pump therapy typically entails infusion of rapid- (or fast-)acting insulin from a reservoir via plastic tubing into a fine-bore cannula placed in the SC tissue. Some newer pumps such as "patch pumps" (e.g., omnipod) have no connecting tubing but just an insulin reservoir and connecting cannula. The cannula is often sited on the abdominal wall although other areas can also be used, and needs to be changed on a regular basis. CSII delivers insulin in two patterns: a pre-programmed continuous background insulin infusion (the rate usually varies over the 24-h period), with additional insulin boluses for food or to correct hyperglycemia. Boluses are delivered under the patient's direction, to cover carbohydrate intake and to correct for high BG levels. Most pump users make use of an in-built "bolus calculator," which uses known variables for that individual (insulin:carbohydrate ratio, insulin sensitivity and target BG range) in conjunction with situation-specific data (current capillary glucose level, estimated carbohydrate intake, and time since last insulin bolus). The basal rates can be temporarily increased/decreased to accommodate fluctuations in BG levels (e.g., as a consequence of increased activity, or ill health). People using CSII do not usually take any additional long-acting insulin so if there is any interruption to insulin delivery (e.g., if the cannula is blocked or dislodged), hyperglycemia and then DKA can develop very quickly, unless the problem is identified (i.e., pump "troubleshooting") and rectified (e.g., by re-siting the cannula; changing the tubing; or starting alternative insulin such as CII [VRIII]). Some insulin pumps work in conjunction with CGM to temporarily suspend insulin delivery if hypoglycemia is developing.

Successful management of inpatient diabetes with the continuation of CSII has been previously demonstrated in select patients (35,36). Clear hospital policies, procedures, and clinicians' orders with specifics on the type of diet, frequency of POC glucose testing, and insulin doses (i.e., basal rates, carbohydrate ratios, and correction formulas) should be in place (35). An inpatient diabetes specialist should assist with the assessment and management of a patient with a CSII. If pump use is contraindicated (e.g., patient is unconscious or incapacitated) or if inpatient diabetes resources are not available, discontinuation of insulin pump and transition to a basal-bolus insulin regimen ("pump holiday") or starting CII (VRIII) is the safest and most appropriate step (Figure 7-3). Most patients knowledgeable in insulin pump therapy are able to display on their pump screen the average total daily insulin used for the past few days. Based on this, safe estimations of basal, nutritional and correction insulin can be calculated (32). To avoid severe hyperglycemia or DKA from lack of basal insulin, it is important to administer the SC basal insulin component at least 2 hours before disconnecting the insulin pump. Insulin pumps are expensive and steps should be taken to ensure they are not lost when a patient is admitted to hospital (35). If a patient is unconscious or incapacitated, ask a relative to look after the pump, alternatively store the pump in the patient's medication locker if this is not possible. Document the location of the pump in the medical notes.

Inpatient management of CSII in an emergency (or elective) perioperative setting depends on the length of surgery and the duration of starvation (Figure 7-4). Fasting is not usually a problem when on CSII; therefore, being "nil by mouth" does not necessarily mean removal of the pump or the need for IV insulin. If the starvation period is likely to be short (i.e., not more than one missed meal), the pump therapy can usually be continued, with the patient remaining on their usual basal rate without needing

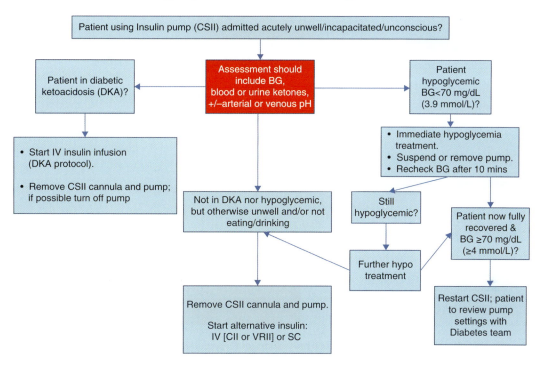

Figure 7-3 Pump management in the acutely unwell patient. If pump is removed, it must be stored appropriately.
BG = blood glucose; CSII = continuous subcutaneous insulin infusion therapy; CII = continuous insulin infusion; VRIII = variable rate intravenous insulin infusion

any bolus doses, until they are eating and drinking normally again. Most patients will be able to manage their pump post-sedation or post-anesthesia just as safely as any patient using standard SC multiple daily injection (MDI) insulin therapy, in fact, a pump user may be more likely to achieve stable BG control. However, some patients will feel unable to self-manage following the procedure and require alternative management, such as conversion to SC basal-bolus MDI insulin or IV insulin.

For minor procedures (i.e., expected to eat and/or drink within 2–3 h) under general anesthetic or sedation, the pump can remain *in situ* (Figure 7-3). Pre-procedure, the patient should ensure that: their cannula is sited away from the operative site and is accessible to the healthcare team; the pump ideally contains new batteries; the

insulin reservoir is full; and capillary BG is in the acceptable range pre-procedure (i.e., 110–180 mg/dL [6–10 mmol/L]). The theater team must monitor the patient's capillary BG levels at least hourly, and start CII (VRIII) if any reading is greater than 180 mg/dL (10 mmol/L). Post-procedure, a correction dose might be required, and possibly a temporary increase in basal rates to counteract the stress response to surgery. If the pump alarms during the procedure, it is advised that the theater staff do not attempt to rectify; change to BG monitoring every 30 mins and start IV insulin if >180 mg/dL (>10 mmol/L). If the pump alarm becomes intrusive, remove pump plus cannula, allow pump to continue to run (the amount of insulin "lost" is minimal) and store safely in a suitable receptacle (do not misplace the pump). For any major surgical procedure (i.e., >2 hours

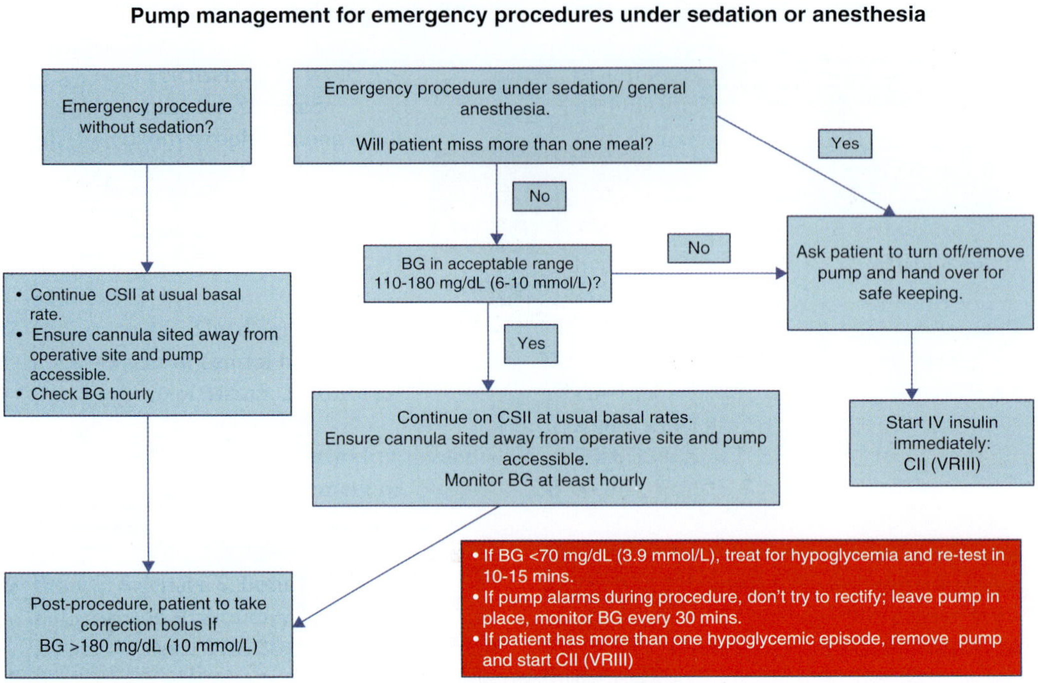

Pump management for emergency procedures under sedation or anesthesia

Figure 7-4 Pump management for emergency procedures under sedation or anesthesia. If pump is removed, it must be stored appropriately.
BG = blood glucose; CSII = continuous subcutaneous insulin infusion therapy; CII = continuous insulin infusion; VRIII = variable rate intravenous insulin infusion

duration and/or unlikely to eat/drink within 2–3 h post-op), CSII should be stopped and replaced by CII (VRIII) until the patient is sufficiently recovered and eating again.

If there is a period of perioperative hypotension, then peripheral skin perfusion may be compromised, thus reducing the absorption of insulin given SC and may necessitate treatment with CII (VRIII), especially if the patient is unable to self-manage.

For CSII patients undergoing radiological investigations, special precautions need to be taken (35). The pump must be suspended and removed prior to magnetic resonance imaging (MRI) scanning, and should not be taken into the scanning room. Pump manufacturers also advise removing the pump prior to computed tomography (CT) scan. For plain x-rays, there is no need to remove the pump, unless its position obscures the area of interest. The patient should reconnect the pump immediately following any radiological investigation. Pumps can be safely suspended/removed for up to an hour at a time without needing alternative insulin. A correction bolus may be needed on reconnecting the pump.

As noted before, a number of pilot studies have shown that CGM and CSII work well as part of a fully automated closed-loop ("artificial pancreas") system in both type 1 and type 2 diabetes patients in the inpatient setting. This led to significantly increased glycemic "time in range." However, much work remains to be done before this system can be rolled out to non-specialist inpatient teams and especially in the emergency setting (32).

Variant "pumps" are also available, such as V-Go, which is a disposable, mechanical device containing rapid-acting insulin and is used (where approved) in poorly controlled type 2 diabetes patients. However, it should not be used in inpatients or during surgery as it has not been studied in these settings.

Emergency Perioperative Endocrine and Metabolic Management

Patients with various endocrine and metabolic issues pose challenges during the perioperative period. As such, a MDT approach is preferred for achieving better patient outcomes in the perioperative period. Unfortunately this is more challenging for acute surgical presentations that are unlikely to be directly related to the coexistent endocrine condition and therefore adequate specific endocrine preparation/investigations/treatment may not have occurred. However, some endocrine and metabolic disorders are associated with surgical emergencies either causally, such as pituitary apoplexy, or bowel obstruction directly by local neuroendocrine tumor (NET), or indirectly due to large desmoplastic fibrotic reaction of the peritoneum usually around the involved lymph nodes in carcinoid syndrome that may cause obstructive symptoms. Alternatively, endocrine and metabolic derangement can occur as a consequence of the systemic illness (e.g., thyroid storm; myxedema coma; DKA or HHS; adrenal insufficiency; hyponatremia) and will result in extreme clinical challenges during emergency surgery and critical care management.

Many endocrine and metabolic disorders significantly affect surgical outcomes and anesthesia strategies and some examples will be outlined.

Airway Management

If a patient needing emergency surgery for a related or unrelated disorder has newly recognized or poorly controlled acromegaly, these patients pose a problem during airway management due to macroglossia, hypertrophy of soft tissues of oropharynx and enlargement of the soft palate, epiglottis, and ariepiglottic fold. This may require preoperative fiberoptic intubation or tracheostomy and careful perioperative airway management is essential (37).

Anatomic airway problems may also be caused by an enlarged thyroid gland (goiter) or by complications of thyroid surgery. Tracheal deviation or narrowing may be caused by compression from goiter. Subsequently the approach to induction and intubation may need to be altered. Surgical airway complications may manifest in the postoperative period as critical emergencies necessitating emergent reintubation. Injury to the nerves innervating the larynx may result in the patient's inability to maintain the airway after extubation. Neck hematomas caused by bleeding from the surgical site may cause airway compression requiring urgent surgical decompression. Rarely, long-standing tracheomalacia may cause collapse of the tracheal wall with airway obstruction.

While most individuals who develop thyroid malignancy can anticipate an excellent chance for cure, patients with anaplastic thyroid cancer (ATC) have an ominous prognosis, even when detected early. The 2012 American Thyroid Association guidelines for management of patients with ATC discussed many detailed recommendations for this condition, including airway management (38). Patients with ATC are at risk for airway obstruction due to local progression of the primary tumor; accordingly, a tracheostomy may be required to avoid asphyxia. Airway obstruction may occur as a direct consequence of a large, obstructing mass, tracheal compression, direct infiltration of the tumor through the tracheal wall, or from massive hemorrhage into the trachea. The benefits of preserving the airway have to be weighed against the overall prognosis of the patient. Palliative interventions with good intent, such as tracheostomy, may ultimately result not only in the prolongation of life, but also prolongation of the anguish the patient may be experiencing. Therefore, the advantages and disadvantages of tracheostomy tube placement need to be weighed carefully. Accordingly, in most circumstances, a surgical airway can be avoided in the management of patients with advanced, unresectable disease. Exceptions to this general principle include the presence of stridor or other acute airway distress, particularly if they are the presenting signs or symptoms of ATC.

Pituitary

Pituitary Apoplexy, Pituitary Surgery, and Neurosurgical Patients

Pituitary apoplexy is an endocrine emergency resulting from catastrophic hemorrhage or infarct of the pituitary gland that typically manifests with headache, nausea and vomiting, visual impairment, and reduced consciousness (39,40). In most cases, apoplexy occurs in an undiagnosed, pre-existing pituitary adenoma (41). Patients with suspected pituitary apoplexy require detailed visual field, visual acuity, and oculomotor nerve examination, pituitary hormone profile assessment, and emergency glucocorticoid treatment. Extensive or deteriorating visual field or visual acuity deficits, or reduced consciousness, necessitate urgent/emergency surgical intervention.

Acute secondary adrenal insufficiency is seen in two-thirds of patients with pituitary tumor apoplexy and is a major source of morbidity and rarely mortality associated with the condition (42). Indications for empirical glucocorticoid treatment in perioperative patients with pituitary apoplexy are hemodynamic instability, altered consciousness level, reduced visual acuity, or severe visual field defects. Steroid replacement is potentially life-saving in these patients. Glucocorticoids are given, most often IV with a stat dose of IV hydrocortisone 100–200 mg, followed by a hydrocortisone IV infusion at a rate of 2–4 mg/hour; or 50–100 mg intramuscular (IM) hydrocortisone every 6 hours. If the patient is hypotensive, resuscitation with IV hydration is indicated.

One of the most common complications after pituitary surgery (which is usually transsphenoidal) is hypopituitarism. This can be partial or total; transient or permanent; and affecting anterior or posterior pituitary, or both (42,43). Cerebrospinal fluid leaks, damage to neurological structures such as the optic chiasm, and vascular complications can also worsen the postoperative course.

Neurosurgical patients (e.g., post-pituitary surgery, pituitary apoplexy, aneurysms, traumatic brain injury) can also be affected by fluid and electrolyte disturbances manifest as either central diabetes insipidus (DI) or, occasionally, syndrome of inappropriate antidiuretic hormone production (SIADH). DI occurs in ~10–30% of patients undergoing pituitary surgery, but persists long-term in only 2–7%. DI is best managed acutely by vasopressin (shorter-acting) rather than desmopressin (longer-acting), as SIADH can quickly follow (as part of the "triple response") (Figure 7-5) (43,44). If DI is permanent, desmopressin is the preferred therapy. SIADH is characterized by euvolemic hyponatremia. In comparison, cerebral salt wasting (which can also occur in the perioperative setting) is characterized by brain natriuretic peptide-mediated hypovolemic hyponatremia. Careful management of fluid and electrolyte balance is essential in the neurosurgical perioperative setting (42–44).

Thyroid

If emergency surgery is required, patients with severe hypothyroidism or hyperthyroidism should receive treatment of their disease prior to surgery, as time allows, in order minimize complications.

Severe Hypothyroidism and Myxedema Coma

For severe hypothyroidism in the emergency perioperative setting, oral or nasogastric administration of thyroxine (T_4) and/or liothyronine (T_3) may be preferred to IV but this depends on the functionality of the gastrointestinal tract (e.g., paralytic ileus or bowel perforation present).

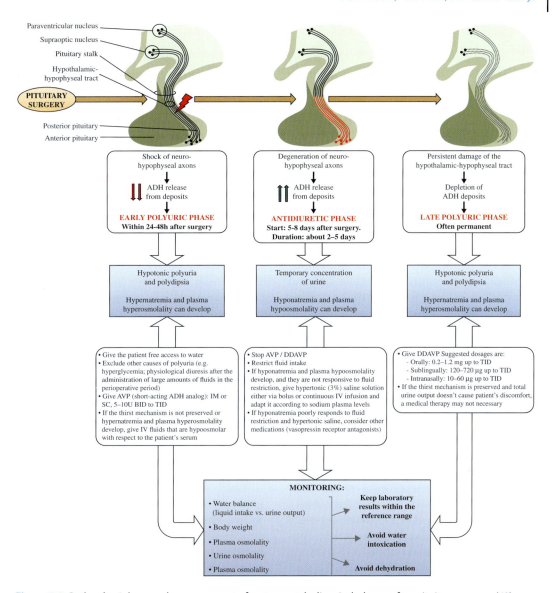

Figure 7-5 Pathophysiology and management of water metabolism imbalance after pituitary surgery (43). Reproduced with permission from SAGE.
ADH, antidiuretic hormone (vasopressin); AVP, arginine vasopressin; bid, twice a day; DDAVP, desmopressin; IM, intramuscular injection; SC, subcutaneous injection; SIADH, syndrome of inappropriate ADH secretion; tid, three times a day.

Myxedema coma is a decompensated state of hypothyroidism resulting from severe and prolonged depletion of thyroid hormones leading to altered mental status and other clinical features related to widespread multi-organ dysfunction. Surgical emergencies can be a precipitating factor (e.g., intrabdominal collection) or a consequence of myxedema coma (e.g., ischemic bowel). Therefore, it is important to promptly recognize and treat myxedema coma in an attempt to improve perioperative outcomes. Hypoventilation and hypercapnia may be managed initially with non-invasive ventilation (NIV).

However, if NIV is ineffective or airway protection is required (e.g., in the setting of a reduced Glasgow Coma Scale [GCS]), these are indications for immediate intubation (associated macroglossia can cause airway management issues) and ventilator support. As hypotension and hemodynamic strain may be present, careful volume resuscitation with normal saline is recommended while balancing considerations for the management of concomitant hyponatremia. Additionally, the presence of refractory hypotension may also be due to adrenal insufficiency. Hydrocortisone should be administered for up to 7–10 days or until hemodynamically stable. For hypothermia, it is recommended to provide gentle warming with blankets, but to avoid excessive rapid external warming as this may lead to peripheral vasodilatation and potentially cardiovascular collapse. It is important to seek and actively treat other precipitants (i.e., in addition to the emergency surgical presentation).

In an acute setting, such as emergency surgery, an IV bolus of thyroxine (T_4) 300–600 mcg (4 mcg/kg lean body weight) should be considered (45). Subsequently, 50–100 mcg oral (or nasogastric) or IV should be given daily. If T_3 therapy is chosen (shorter-acting and therefore less longevity versus T_4 if adverse effect of acute replacement occurs), 5–10 mcg orally or via nasogastric tube is a good initial dose and can be uptitrated as tolerated. IV T_3 is also an option in this setting (45).

Severe Hyperthyroidism and Thyroid Storm

The spectrum of thyrotoxicosis ranges from asymptomatic subclinical disease to a life-threatening metabolic crisis characterized by multisystem dysfunction and high mortality. Thyroid storm is a critical presentation of severe thyrotoxicosis, requiring urgent antithyroid (e.g., propylthiouracil [PTU] preferred) and supportive therapy (including iodine; beta-blockers; glucocorticoids; active cooling; sedatives; seek and treat precipitants). Many cases of thyroid storm occur after a precipitating event (including thyroid surgery, especially if inadequately rendered euthyroid preoperatively), intercurrent illness, or discontinuation of antithyroid drug therapy.

Emergency thyroidectomy is occasionally used to treat thyroid storm, particularly in chronically ill elderly patients with concurrent cardiopulmonary and renal failure, who fail to respond to the standard intensive multifaceted therapy for thyroid storm. Urgent or emergency thyroidectomy may also be required in patients with amiodarone-induced thyrotoxicosis (AIT). AIT is a dangerous condition for the patient because of the additional risk posed by thyrotoxicosis to the underlying cardiac abnormalities. Indeed, AIT has been associated with increased morbidity and mortality, especially in older patients with impaired left ventricular function. Hence, in selected categories of patients, emergency management of AIT including total thyroidectomy should be considered in order to obtain a rapid resolution of thyrotoxicosis (46). If total thyroidectomy is considered, an MDT evaluation of the AIT patient involving cardiologists, endocrinologists, surgeons, and anesthesiologists is warranted.

Rapid preoperative thyroid preparation is occasionally needed for patients with severe thyrotoxicosis requiring urgent or emergency surgery. These patients either have insufficient time to be rendered euthyroid by anti-thyroid drugs (i.e., thionamides) before surgery or have contraindications to their use. Safe and effective therapy with the following (or similar) inpatient regimen of β-blockers (e.g., propranolol 60 mg orally every 12 hours); high dose glucocorticoids (e.g., dexamethasone 2 mg IV every 6 hours), which decrease T_4-to-T_3 conversion; cholestyramine (e.g., 4 g orally every 6 hours), which blocks enterohepatic circulation; and iodine (e.g., SSKI 2 drops orally every 8 hours), which blocks thyroid hormone synthesis; has successfully resulted in rapid correction of thyrotoxicosis when given for 5–10 days before thyroidectomy. Challenges arise in the optimal preparation for total thyroidectomy in AIT patients. This is because the high iodine content of amiodarone limits the ability of additional iodine therapy (e.g., Lugol's, SSKI) to block thyroid hormone synthesis; and also because antithyroid drugs may not work in destructive thyroiditis (i.e., type 2 AIT). Glucocorticoids and beta-blockers may reduce the surgical risk in AIT patients in this setting. Thus, in AIT patients who are candidates for total thyroidectomy, a short course with glucocorticoids is mandatory, irrespective of the AIT type. Plasmapheresis may also be an adjunctive tool to prepare AIT patients for surgery. More important, MDT interaction of an experienced team is fundamental.

Adrenal Crisis

Acute adrenal insufficiency, also termed adrenal crisis, is a life-threatening endocrine emergency brought about by a lack of production of the adrenal hormone cortisol, the major glucocorticoid. Primary adrenal insufficiency is caused by loss of function of the adrenal gland itself, for example, due to autoimmune-mediated destruction of adrenocortical tissue or surgical removal of the adrenal glands. Secondary adrenal insufficiency is caused if the regulation of adrenal cortisol production by the pituitary is compromised (termed hypopituitarism) (42, 43). However, pituitary regulation of cortisol production is also switched off in patients who receive chronic exogenous glucocorticoid treatment (i.e., doses ≥5 mg prednisolone equivalent for more than 4 weeks) or have Cushing's syndrome due to endogenous production (43,47,48). Treatment of adrenal crisis requires immediate bolus injection of 100 mg hydrocortisone IV or IM followed by continuous IV infusion of 200 mg hydrocortisone per 24 hrs (alternatively 50 mg hydrocortisone IM injection every 6 hrs) (47,48). Rehydration with rapid IV isotonic saline infusion followed by further IV rehydration as required (usually 4–6 L in 24 hrs; monitor for fluid overload). It is always important to consider adrenal insufficiency when signs or symptoms potentially suggestive of acute adrenal insufficiency are present, including atypical abdominal pain which may be masquerading as a surgical abdomen. Glucose monitoring is also required as hypoglycemia is common. Check for any medic alert jewellery (or tattoos!) or steroid cards.

Sodium Level

Abnormal serum sodium levels (dysnatremias) are common in patients presenting for surgery. Both hyponatremia (<135 mmol/L) and hypernatremia (>150 mmol/L) are associated with increased morbidity and mortality in the perioperative setting. Preoperative hyponatremia is a prognostic marker for perioperative 30-day morbidity and mortality (49). Hypernatremia has also been associated with a doubling of mortality and prolonged length of stay in the intensive care unit following cardiac surgery (50).

Hyponatremia

Hyponatremia is the most common electrolyte abnormality, affecting up to 30–42% of hospitalized patients, and approximately 1–3% are severe (<125 mmol/L). Acute hyponatremia is classified as <48 h duration (and can be treated rapidly as the brain as not yet adapted); and chronic hyponatremia >48 hrs (correction rate must be controlled in these patients due to brain adaptation which can predispose to osmotic demyelination syndrome [ODS] if corrected too rapidly) (51, 52). Clinical status depends on the balance of several factors including degree of hyponatremia; rate of development (i.e., acute or chronic); ability of the brain to adapt to osmolar stress; and presence of comorbidities (52).

Severe symptoms associated with hyponatremia include vomiting, cardiorespiratory arrest, seizures, and reduced consciousness/coma (GCS score ≤8) (52). These patients must be treated with IV hypertonic (1.8% or 3%) saline with the aim of increasing serum sodium by 5 mmol/L in the first hour or until symptoms abate (52). Acute hyponatremia especially when there is a clear timeline of development of hyponatremia, such as excess hypotonic perioperative fluids, can be rapidly corrected. In comparison, chronic hyponatremia (or when the timeline for development is unclear) must be corrected in a controlled fashion. This is sometimes referred to as the "rule of sixes," i.e., increase serum [Na+] concentration by 6 mmol/L (+/- 2 mmol/L) during first 24 h; but if the patient has severe symptoms/signs, this timing can be pre-loaded to the first 6 h of the first day of correction.

The treatment of choice for depletional hyponatremia (i.e., hypovolemic hyponatremia) is isotonic (0.9%) saline to restore extracellular fluid volume and ensure adequate organ perfusion. This initial therapy is appropriate for patients who either have clinical signs of hypovolemia, or in whom a spot urine [Na$^+$] concentration is <20–30 mmol/L (51).

Active treatment with hypertonic (1.8% or 3% or equivalent) saline or isotonic (0.9%) saline in chronic hyponatremia should be stopped when the patient's symptoms are no longer present, a safe serum [Na$^+$] (usually >120 mmol/L) has been achieved, or the rate of correction has reached maximum limits of 12 mmol/L within 24 h; or 18 mmol/L within 48 hours to avoid precipitating ODS; or 8 mmol/L over any 24-h period in patients at high risk of ODS (51).

Hypernatremia

Hypernatremia is common in the emergency setting and is associated with significant morbidity and mortality (50), primarily caused by cell shrinkage due to extracellular movement of water. Acute hypernatremia usually occurs due to inadequate water intake and/or excessive water loss, leading to inappropriate plasma hyperosmolality. The mainstay of management of acute hypernatremia is rehydration with hypotonic fluids such as 0.45% saline or 5% dextrose, used for their high free water content when compared with isotonic saline (44). However, if the patient is hemodynamically unstable, isotonic saline should be used initially. Acute symptomatic hypernatremia may be corrected rapidly with normalization of plasma sodium within 24 hours of commencement of therapy. Chronic hypernatremia should be corrected more gradually as cerebral edema may develop if the correction is over-rapid; the rate of correction can reach a maximum of 1 mmol/L/hr to a maximum of 10–12 mmol/L/day. In patients at risk of thrombotic episodes, prophylactic anticoagulation should also be considered even in the perioperative setting if can be achieved safely (alternatively use mechanical antithrombotic prevention if the risk of perioperative bleeding contraindicates anticoagulation).

Calcium

Hypocalcemia

Low total plasma calcium (hypocalcemia) may be due to a reduction in albumin-bound calcium, the free fraction of calcium, or both. Hypocalcemia is a common electrolyte disturbance complicating approximately 15–26% of hospital admissions and up to 88% of patients admitted to an intensive care unit (53,54). There are a large number of recognized causes in the perioperative setting, including thyroid and parathyroid surgery, acute pancreatitis, blood transfusions, and numerous medications. Hypocalcemia with neurological, muscular, or cardiac dysfunction is associated with significant morbidity and mortality and should be managed as a medical emergency. Symptomatic patients (e.g., tetany, seizures, laryngospasm or cardiac arrhythmias or dysfunction) or those with adjusted calcium (ACa) (i.e., corrected for albumin concentration) <8 mg/dL (2 mmol/L); or free (ionized) calcium <4 mg/dL (1 mmol/L) should prompt emergency intervention with IV calcium replacement (54,55). It is important to evaluate and treat the underlying cause(s). In postoperative parathyroid-related hypocalcemia (e.g., total thyroidectomy, parathyroid surgery, or anterior neck surgery for cancer) and other cases of hypoparathyroidism, undetectable or inappropriately low parathyroid hormone (PTH) levels in the context of hypocalcemia are consistent with the diagnosis (PTH levels usually checked 4–24 hours post-thyroid surgery to assess risk of permanent hypoparathyroidism developing). Treatment consists of calcium and vitamin D analogs (e.g., alfacalcidol or calcitriol) acutely. Hypomagnesemia should always be corrected as it causes inhibition of PTH secretion as well as resistance to its action; correction of hypocalcemia may be difficult with uncorrected hypomagnesemia. The underlying cause(s) of hypomagnesemia should also be diagnosed and treated.

Hypercalcemia

Hypercalcemia is commonly seen in the context of parathyroid dysfunction and malignancy, and when severe, can be life-threatening (56). The differential diagnosis of hypercalcemia can be broadly categorized based on PTH measurement. Adjusted calcium (ACa) > 12 mg/dL (3.0 mmol/L) is associated with nephrogenic DI, increasingly severe volume contraction, neurological, cardiac, and gastrointestinal dysfunction, and requires urgent treatment to prevent life-threatening consequences. The term "hypercalcemic crisis" is frequently used to describe the severely compromised patient with profound volume depletion, altered sensorium which may be manifest as coma, cardiac decompensation, and abdominal pain that may mimic an acute surgical abdomen. Hypercalcemia of malignancy is the commonest cause of inpatient hypercalcemic crises (>50%) and complicates 10–30% of malignancies. Primary and metastatic cancer associated with hypercalcemia may also result in a surgical emergency (e.g., bowel obstruction or bleeding secondary to local tumor; spinal cord compression; or pathological fracture).

For treatment of severe hypercalcemia, where possible, the cause should be identified, multiple therapies should be started as soon as possible (56). Rapid-acting (hours) approaches including rehydration; short-term calcitonin; and longer-term the most effective antiresorptive agents (e.g., bisphosphonates, denosumab) should be considered (unless imminent parathyroid surgery is planned when increased risk of postoperative hypocalcemia due to "hungry bones" syndrome). If the diagnosis is primary hyperparathyroidism, then surgical removal of parathyroid adenoma(s) should be planned, ideally when the patient is stabilized although occasionally this may warrant emergency surgery. An urgent parathyroidectomy can be considered in all patients with hypertensive crises as a result of hyperparathyroidism, but is more safely performed in the stabilized elective patient. However, initial curative success rates differ only marginally between elective and urgent cases, and long-term outcomes appear similar (57).

Neuroendocrine Tumors (NETs)

Neuroendocrine tumors (NETs) constitute a heterogeneous group of malignant solid tumors that arise in the hormone-secreting tissues of the diffuse neuroendocrine system (58). Consequently, they can have various clinical presentations and courses. Prior to elective and emergency surgery or other interventional treatment in patients with NETs, the tumor type and hormone production must be assessed in order to provide appropriate treatments and also to avoid life-threatening crises that may occur due to the presence of hormonal syndromes associated with some of these tumors (59). In addition, the presence of any triggering factors should also be determined.

Metastatic NETs of the distal small intestine and cecum are often associated with the carcinoid syndrome, which consists of flushing, diarrhea (leading to dehydration, electrolyte abnormalities, and hypoproteinemia), bronchoconstriction, and right-sided valvular heart disease (i.e., carcinoid heart disease). Carcinoid syndrome occurs primarily in metastatic NETs that secrete serotonin directly into the systemic, and not portal, circulation (58). The most significant life-threatening emergency associated with carcinoid syndrome is carcinoid crisis. The term carcinoid crisis describes an episode of acute circulatory collapse caused by the massive release of serotonin and other vasoactive substances into the circulation. This event tends to occur in the perioperative setting, with triggers including general anesthesia, epinephrine, and physical manipulation of tumors. Carcinoid crisis can lead to complete vasomotor collapse, coma, and death. Standard practice has been to administer prophylactic doses of IV or SC octreotide (somatostatin analog) 250–500 mcg to carcinoid syndrome patients prior to an invasive procedure. If periprocedure hypotension develops, the patient should be given IV boluses of 500–1000 mcg until blood pressure normalizes. Perioperative treatment is recommended with continuous IV infusion of 50–200 mcg/h and should be continued at least 48 h after the operation with dose titration (doses up to 500 mcg/h may be needed). With acute operations, IV octreotide is beneficial even if given for only 12 h before anesthesia, since this may achieve adequate suppression of basal amine and peptide levels.

It is important for the medical and anesthetic team to be aware that carcinoid heart disease occurs in more than half of the patients with the carcinoid syndrome. Carcinoid heart disease signposts two distinct challenges for the anesthesiologist: carcinoid crisis and low cardiac output syndrome secondary to right ventricular failure. Patients with carcinoid heart disease who need to undergo surgery (including emergency) should ideally undergo at least limited preoperative evaluation by an expert cardiologist if available and time allows. However,

the anesthetist can use various monitoring tools (including invasive) and avoid certain medications and anesthetic agents to minimize the risk and consequence of carcinoid crisis and also carcinoid heart disease perioperatively (59).

Among patients with rarer NETs: prolonged perioperative treatment with adequately high-dosed proton pump inhibitor (PPIs) is needed for patients with gastrinomas, mainly to prevent gastro-jejunal bleeding; and perioperative IV glucose infusion and monitoring are used to avoid hypoglycemia in patients with insulinoma (59). Patients with glucagonoma require somatostatin analog treatment; and as these patients have a particular predisposition for thromboembolism, prophylactic high-dose low weight molecular heparin should also be administered.

Intravenous fluids and correction of electrolyte disorders are also important in the treatment of dehydration and electrolyte and metabolic imbalances associated with NETs. Effective cytoreductive therapy (including elective and emergency surgery), and medical management of the underlying NETs are important for long-term syndrome control.

Conclusions

There is a wealth of evidence to show that poor perioperative glycemic control is associated with poor surgical outcomes. Despite the lack of robust data to confirm this, most clinicians agree that controlling glucose levels to an acceptable range is likely to reduce the risk of developing complications. The management goal is to optimize metabolic control through close monitoring, adequate fluid and caloric repletion, and judicious use of insulin. The management of perioperative glucose control in the emergency setting usually requires the use of a CII (VRIII). However, where opportunities arise to optimize glycemic control preoperatively (especially to allow the stabilization of patients with diabetes-related crises), then these should be undertaken (it is important to discuss with surgeon timing of surgery).

Other endocrine and metabolic derangements (e.g., adrenal insufficiency, hypothyroidism and hyperthyroidism, carcinoid crisis, hyponatremia, hypercalcemia) are also common in the emergency perioperative setting and warrant prompt MDT review and appropriate management.

References

1 Anonymous. Inpatient care and diabetes: putting poor glycaemic control to bed. *Lancet Diabetes and Endocrinology.* 2017;5:770.

2 Health and Social Care Information Centre. *National Diabetes Inpatient Audit (Nadia), Open Data 2016,* 2017. www.digital.nhs.uk/pubs/nadia2016

3 American Diabetes Association. Diabetes care in the hospital. *Diabetes Care.* 2018;40(Suppl.1):S144–S151.

4 Daultrey H, Gooday C, Dhatariya K. Increased length of inpatient stay and poor clinical coding: audit of patients with diabetes. *J R Soc Med Sh Rep.* 2011;2(11):83.

5 Sampson MJ, Dozio N, Ferguson B, Dhatariya K. Total and excess bed occupancy by age, speciality and insulin use for nearly one million diabetes patients discharged from all English Acute Hospitals. *Diabetes Res Clin Pract.* 2007;77(1):92–98.

6 Frisch A, Chandra P, Smiley D, et al. Prevalence and clinical outcome of hyperglycemia in the perioperative period in noncardiac surgery. *Diabetes Care.* 2010; 33(8):1783–1788.

7 Cullinane M, Gray AJ, Hargraves CM, Lansdown M, Martin IC, Schubert M. Who operates when? II The 2003 report of the national confidential enquiry into perioperative deaths. http://www.ncepod. Org.uk/pdf/2003/03full.pdf. 2003.

8 O'Brien MM, Gonzales R, Shroyer AL, et al. Modest serum creatinine elevation affects adverse outcome after general surgery. *Kidney Int.* 2010;62(2):585–592.

9 Lee TH, Marcantonia ER, Mangione EJ, et al. Derivation and prospective validation of a simple index for prediction of cardiac risk of major noncardiac surgery. *Circulation.* 1999;100(10):1043–1049.

10 Gordois A, Scuffham P, Shearer A, Oglesby A, Tobian JA. The health care costs of diabetic peripheral neuropathy in the U.S. *Diabetes Care.* 2003;26(6):1790–1795.

11 National Patient Safety Agency. Insulin safety. Reducing harm associated with the unsafe use of insulin products. http://www. patientsafetyfirst.nhs.uk/Content.aspx? path=/interventions/relatedprogrammes/ medicationsafety/insulin/. 2010

12 Sampson MJ, Brennan C, Dhatariya K, Jones C, Walden E. A national survey of in-patient diabetes services in the United Kingdom. *Diabetic Med.* 2007;24(6): 643–649.

13 Walid MS, Newman BF, Yelverton JC, Nutter JP, Ajjan M, Robinson JS. Prevalence of previously unknown elevation of glycosylated hemoglobin in spine surgery patients and impact on length of stay and total cost. *J Hosp Med.* 2010;5(1):E10–E14.

14 O'Sullivan CJ, Hynes N, Mahendran B, et al. Haemoglobin A1c (HbA1C) in non-diabetic and diabetic vascular patients: is HbA1C an independent risk factor and predictor of adverse outcome? *Eur J Vasc Endovasc Surg.* 2006;32(2): 188–197.

15 Gustafsson UO, Thorell A, Soop M, Ljungqvist O, Nygren J. Haemoglobin A1c as a predictor of postoperative hyperglycaemia and complications after major colorectal surgery. *Br J Surg.* 2009;96(11):1358–1364.

16 Halkos ME, Lattouf OM, Puskas JD, et al. Elevated preoperative hemoglobin A1c level is associated with reduced long-term survival after coronary artery bypass

surgery. *Ann Thorac Surg*. 2008;86(5): 1431–1437.

17 Alserius T, Anderson RE, Hammar N, Nordqvist T, Ivert T. Elevated glycosylated haemoglobin (HbA1c) is a risk marker in coronary artery bypass surgery. *Scand Cardiovasc J*. 2008; 42(6):392–398.

18 Kreutziger J, Schlaepfer J, Wenzel V, Constantinescu MA. The role of admission blood glucose in outcome prediction of surviving patients with multiple injuries. *J Trauma*. 2010;67(4):704–708.

19 Vilar-Compte D, Alvarez de Iturbe I, Martin-Onraet A, Perez-Amador M, Sanchez-Hernandez C, Volkow P. Hyperglycemia as a risk factor for surgical site infections in patients undergoing mastectomy. *Am J Infect Control*. 2008;36(3):192–198.

20 Shibuya N, Humphers JM, Fluhman BL, Jupiter DC. Factors associated with nonunion, delayed union, and malunion in foot and ankle surgery in diabetic patients. *J Foot Ankle Surg*. 2013;52(2):207–211.

21 Ambiru S, Kato A, Kimura F, et al. Poor postoperative blood glucose control increases surgical site infections after surgery for hepato-biliary-pancreatic cancer: a prospective study in a high-volume institute in Japan. *J Hosp Infect*. 2008;68(3):230–233.

22 Kwon S, Thompson R, Dellinger P, Yanez D, Farrohki E, Flum D. Importance of perioperative glycemic control in general surgery: a report from the surgical care and outcomes assessment program. *Ann Surg*. 2013;257(1):8–14.

23 Fortington LV, Geertzen JH, van Netten JJ, Postema K, Rommers GM, Dijkstra PU. Short and long term mortality rates after a lower limb amputation. *Eur J Vasc Endovasc Surg*. 2013;46(1):124–131.

24 Dhatariya K, Levy K, Flanagan D, et al. for the Joint British Diabetes Societies. Diabetes UK Position Statements and Care Recommendations. NHS Diabetes guideline for the perioperative management of the adult patient with diabetes (2016). http://www.diabetologists-

abcd.org.uk/JBDS/Surgical_guidelines_2015_full_FINAL_amended_Mar_2016.pdf

25 Dinardo M, Donihi AC, Forte P, et al. Standardized glycemic management and perioperative glycemic outcomes in patients with diabetes who undergo same-day surgery. *Endocr Pract*. 2011;17: 404–411.

26 Dagogo-Jack S, Alberti K. Management of diabetes mellitus in surgical patients. *Diabetes Spectr*. 2002;15(1):44–48.

27 Dashora U, Gallagher A, Dhatariya K, et al. Association of British Clinical Diabetologists (ABCD) position statement on the risk of diabetic ketoacidosis associated with the use of sodium-glucose cotransporter-2 inhibitors. *Br J Diabetes*. 2016;16: 206–209.

28 Umpierrez GE, Hellman R, Korytkowski MT, et al. Management of hyperglycemia in hospitalized patients in non-critical care setting: An Endocrine Society Clinical Practice Guideline. *J Clin Endocrinol Metab*. 2012;97(1):16–38.

29 Umpierrez G, Cardona S, Pasquel F, et al. Randomized controlled trial of intensive versus conservative glucose control in patients undergoing coronary artery bypass graft surgery: GLUCO-CABG Trial. *Diabetes Care*. 2015;38:1665–1672.

30 Wallia A, Umpierrez GE, Nasraway SA, Klonoff DC; PRIDE Investigators. Round table discussion on inpatient use of continuous glucose monitoring at the International Hospital Diabetes Meeting. *J Diabetes Sci Technol*. 2016;10: 1174–1181.

31 Rayman G. Closer to closing the loop on inpatient glycaemia. *Lancet Diabetes and Endocrinology*. 2017;5:81–83.

32 Lansang MC, Umpierrez G. Inpatient hyperglycemia management: a practical review for primary medical and surgical teams. *Cleveland Clinic J Med*. 2016;83(Suppl 1):S34–S43.

33 Dobri GA, Lansong MC. How should we manage insulin therapy before surgery? *Cleve Clin*. 2013;80:702–704.

34 Nauck MA, Meier JJ. Sitagliptin plus basal insulin: simplifying in-hospital diabetes

treatment. *Lancet Diabetes Endocrinology*. 2017;5:83–85.

35 Peters AL, Ahmann AJ, Battelino T, et al. Diabetes technology – continuous subcutaneous insulin infusion therapy and continuous glucose monitoring in adults: an Endocrine Society Clinical Practice Guideline. *J Clin Endocrinol Metab*. 2016;101:3922–3937.

36 Evans K. Insulin pumps in hospital: a guide for the generalist physician. *Clin Med (Lond)*. 2013;13:244–247.

37 Katznelson L, Laws, Jr ER, Melmed S, et al. Acromegaly: An Endocrine Society Clinical Practice Guideline. *JCEM*. 2014;99: 3933–3951.

38 Smallridge RC, Ain KB, Asa SL, et al., American Thyroid Association Anaplastic Thyroid Cancer Guidelines Taskforce. American Thyroid Association guidelines for management of patients with anaplastic thyroid cancer. *Thyroid*. 2012; 22: 1104–1139.

39 Baldeweg SE, Vanderpump M, Drake W, the Society for Endocrinology Clinical Committee. Emergency management of pituitary apoplexy in adult patients. (2016). DOI: 10.1530/EC-16-0057.

40 Briet C, Salenave S, Bonneville J-F, Laws ER, Chanson P. Pituitary apoplexy. *Endocrine Rev*. 2015;36:622–645.

41 Molitch ME. Diagnosis and treatment of pituitary adenomas. *JAMA*. 2017;317: 516–524.

42 Fleseriu, M., Hashim, I. A., Karavitaki, N., et al. Hormonal replacement in hypopituitarism in adults: an Endocrine Society Clinical Practice Guideline. *J Clin Endocrinol Metab*. 2016;101:3888–3921.

43 Prete A, Corsello SM, Salvatori R. Current best practice in the management of patients after pituitary surgery. *Ther Adv Endocrinol Metab*. 2017;8:33–48.

44 Hannon MJ, Finucane FM, Sherlock M, Agha A, Thompson CJ. Clinical review: disorders of water homeostasis in neurosurgical patients. *J Clin Endocrinol Metab*. 2012;97:1423–1433.

45 Jonklass J, Bianco AC, Bauer AJ, et al. American Thyroid Association guidelines

46 for the treatment of hypothyroidism. *Thyroid*. 2014;24:1670–1751.

46 Kaderli RM, Fahrner R, Christ ER, et al. Total thyroidectomy for amiodarone-induced thyrotoxicosis in the hyperthyroid state. *Exp Clin Endocrinol Diabetes*. 2016;124:45–48.

47 Arlt W, the Society for Endocrinology Clinical Committee. Emergency management of acute adrenal insufficiency (adrenal crisis) in adult. 2016. DOI: 10.1530/EC-16-0054.

48 Bornstein SR, Allolio B, Arlt W, et al. Diagnosis and treatment of primary adrenal insufficiency: an Endocrine Society Clinical Practice Guideline. *J Clin Endocrinol Metab*. 2016;101:364–389.

49 Leung AA, McAlister FA, Rogers Jr SO, et al. Preoperative hyponatremia and perioperative complications. *Arch Intern Med*. 2012;172:1474–1481.

50 Lindner G, Funk GC, Lassnigg A, et al. Intensive care-acquired hypernatremia after major cardiothoracic surgery is associated with increased mortality. *Intensive Care Med*. 2010;36(10): 1718–1723.

51 Verbalis JG, Goldsmith SR, Greenberg A, et al. Diagnosis, evaluation, and treatment of hyponatremia: expert panel recommendations. *Am J Med*. 2013;126(10 Suppl. 1):S1–S42.

52 Ball S, Barth J, Levy M, the Society for Endocrinology Clinical Committee. Emergency management of severe symptomatic hyponatraemia in adult patients (2016). DOI: 10.1530/EC-16-0058.

53 Zivin J, Gooley T, Zager R, Ryan M. Hypocalcemia: a pervasive metabolic abnormality in the critically ill. *Am J Kidney Dis*. 2001;37:689–698.

54 Brandi ML, Bilezikian JP, Shoback D, et al. Management of hypoparathyroidism: summary statement and guidelines. *J Clin Endocrinol Metab*. 2016;101: 2273–2283.

55 Turner J, Gittoes N, Selby P, the Society for Endocrinology Clinical Committee (2016). Emergency management of acute hypocalcaemia in adult patients. *Endocr*

Connect. 2016;5:G7–G8. DOI: 10.1530/EC-16-0056.

56 Walsh J, Gittoes N, Selby P, the Society for Endocrinology Clinical Committee. Emergency management of acute hypercalcaemia in adult patients. *Endocr Connect*. 2016;(5):G9–G11. DOI: 10.1530/EC-16-0055.

57 Cannon J, Lew J, Solorzano J. Parathyroidectomy for hypercalcemic crisis: 40 years' experience and long-term outcomes. *Surgery*. 2010;148; 807–813.

58 Dimitriadis GK, Weickert MO, Randeva HS, Kaltsas G, Grossman A. Medical management of secretory syndromes related to gastroenteropancreatic neuroendocrine tumours. *Endocr Relat Cancer*. 2016;23(9):R423–436.

59 Kaltsas G, Caplin M, Davies P, et al., all other Antibes Consensus Conference participants. ENETS Consensus Guidelines for the Standards of care in neuroendocrine tumors: pre- and perioperative therapy in patients with neuroendocrine tumors. *Neuroendocrinology*. (2017). DOI: 10.1159/000461583.

8

Endocrine and Metabolic Emergencies in HIV/AIDS

Katherine Samaras

Key Points

- Human immunodeficiency virus (HIV)-1 infection and acquired immune deficiency syndrome (AIDS) are a spectrum of conditions caused by infection with HIV-1.
- United Nations data show that 36.7 million people worldwide were living with HIV-1 infection in 2016.
- The widespread use of combined antiretroviral therapy (cART) has dramatically improved the life expectancy of people living with HIV infection.
- Endocrine and metabolic disorders are frequent in people with HIV infection. They can

arise as a consequence of: (a) opportunistic infections and infiltration processes associated with untreated HIV infection or disease progression; (b) immune reconstitution occurring after cART initiation (early or late); or (c) as complications of cART.
- Some of these disorders can present as emergencies that are potentially life-threatening, including adrenal crisis, Cushing's syndrome. lactic acidosis, diabetic ketoacidosis, hyperglycemic hyperosmolar state, hypertriglyceridemia, thyrotoxicosis, and hypercalcemia.

Introduction

Human immunodeficiency virus (HIV)-1 infection and acquired immune deficiency syndrome (AIDS) form a spectrum of conditions caused by infection with HIV-1. UN data show that 36.7 million people worldwide were living with HIV-1 infection in 2016, the majority aged 15 years and over (www.unaids.org). The natural history of HIV infection has been transformed since the advent of combined antiretroviral therapy (cART), from the high AIDS- and HIV-related morbidity and mortality to dramatically improved life expectancy and quality of life. AIDS is no longer the dominant health issue in HIV infection, in countries where cART is available and accessible. Disparities

in cART access exist internationally, particularly in resource-limited settings.

The care of people living with treated HIV-infection now focuses primarily on suppression of replication of HIV, restoration of the immune system, and management of the chronic health issues that can be associated with treated HIV infection. The latter include cART toxicities, which can vary substantially between different antiretroviral medications, medication classes, and individual patient susceptibility. Endocrine and metabolic disorders are frequent in people with HIV infection (Table 8-1) and can arise as a consequence of: (1) opportunistic infections and infiltration processes associated with untreated HIV infection or disease progression; (2) immune reconstitution

Endocrine and Metabolic Medical Emergencies: A Clinician's Guide, Second Edition. Edited by Glenn Matfin.
© 2018 John Wiley & Sons Ltd. Published 2018 by John Wiley & Sons Ltd.

Table 8-1 Endocrine and metabolic emergencies in HIV infection

	Cause	Explanation
Lactic acidosis	NRTIs	Treatment-associated: • mitochondrial toxicity (NRTIs) • metformin-dolutegravir drug interaction
Diabetic ketoacidosis (DKA)	Insulin deficiency	Immune reconstitution Drug-associated: • pentamidine (beta-cell toxic) • protease inhibitors (acute)
Hyperglycemic hyperosmolar state (HHS)	Relative insulin deficiency	Drug-associated: • pentamidine (beta-cell toxic) • protease inhibitors (acute)
Hypertriglyeridemia		Drug-induced: • protease inhibitor (especially tipranavir, lopinavir, fosamprenavir and ritonavir) • NRTI (e.g., stavudine, didanosine, zidovudine) • NNRTI (e.g., efavirenz)
Hypercalcemia		Drug-induced Immune reconstitution Lymphoma Granulomatous disorders Parathyroid disorders

Adrenal failure/ Addisonian crisis	Primary	Adrenalitis (infectious)
		Iatrogenic suppression:
		• azole antifungals
		• protease inhibitor and CYP3A4 interactions
		  • inhaled glucocorticoids and other synthetic glucocorticoids (e.g., intra-articular triamcinolone)
		  • megesterol
		  • rifampicin

	Secondary	Hypophysitis • autoimmune • HIV-associated
Thyrotoxicosis	Autoimmune	Graves' disease • immune reconstitution • interferon therapy Hashimoto's thyroiditis • immune reconstitution

CYP3A4 = cytochrome P450 3A4; NRTI = nucleoside reverse transcriptase inhibitor; NNRTI = non-nucleoside reverse transcriptase inhibitor

occurring after cART initiation (early or late); and/or (3) as complications of cART. Endocrinologists play an integral role in managing hormonal and metabolic conditions in HIV and its treatment. This chapter will focus on the endocrine and metabolic emergencies that can arise in people living with HIV/AIDS.

Hypoadrenalism

Adrenal dysfunction is common in both treated and untreated HIV infection, due to multiple etiologies (1). Unrecognized, hypoadrenalism is associated with significant morbidity and mortality risk. Clinical attention to the heightened risk of adrenal dysfunction in HIV infection is essential, with evaluation of the hypothalamic-pituitary-adrenal (HPA) axis necessary in all symptomatic patients. Prior to the introduction of cART, infection and infiltration were the most common causes of adrenal abnormalities.

Cytomegalovirus (CMV) infection is the most common infective cause of adrenal failure and is known to affect both the adrenal medulla and the cortex. There is often bilateral adrenal gland involvement and the spectrum of severity can range widely, from mild adrenalitis to necrosis with severe, generalized systemic infection (2). Other infectious agents can cause adrenalitis, including *Mycobacterium tuberculosis* (3), cryptococcal infection (4), *Nocardia* (5), *Mycobacterium avium* complex (4) and *Histoplasma capsulatum* (6). In addition, the HIV virus itself may cause adrenalitis (7). HIV-specific infiltrative processes that can result in primary adrenal insufficiency include lymphoma, malignancy and Kaposi sarcoma, all reported in advanced HIV infection or AIDS (8,9).

Since the advent of cART, the most common form of adrenal failure appears to be medication-induced (iatrogenic) adrenal suppression, including cART-corticosteroid interactions and cytokine-induced complications affecting the HPA axis function. For example, the azole antifungal agents, such as ketaconazole and itraconazole, impair and inhibit adrenal steroidogenesis. The antibiotic rifampicin increases hepatic cortisol metabolism and degradation. The progestin megestrol acetate non-specifically binds the glucocorticoid receptor and can suppress the HPA axis. Care should be undertaken when prescribing these medications to people living with HIV infection, monitoring for changes in physical well-being is recommended, with testing of adrenal function as indicated by symptomatic and clinical status.

Further, the medication class of protease inhibitors, a frequent component of cART, inhibit hepatic cytochrome P450 (CYP) 3A4 drug metabolic pathways. This will potentiate the half-life of medications that can affect adrenal steroidogenesis, particularly synthetic steroids. This can result in iatrogenic Cushing's syndrome (which can be florid) and adrenal suppression. Iatrogenic Cushing's syndrome in HIV-infected patients receiving ritonavir and inhaled fluticasone has been reported (10). The degree of adrenal suppression in these cases can be substantial, leading to adrenal failure and Addisonian crisis if the inhaled steroids are ceased without corticosteroid support (10).

The HPA axis requires evaluation in HIV-infected individuals symptomatic of fatigue, weight loss, nausea, postural presyncope or with hypoglycemia or hyponatremia, especially those with risk factors mentioned above. The approach is the same as in seronegative patients, with the appropriate first step being a short adrenocorticotropic hormone (ACTH) stimulation test. If insufficiency is demonstrated, the clinician should proceed to ACTH levels and imaging to locate the cause of adrenal insufficiency (11).

In protease inhibitor-recipients also treated with inhaled corticosteroids, care should be taken in abruptly ceasing any steroid-containing medications (even if inhaled), due to the risk of precipitating an adrenal crisis, as has been described (10). Patients with evidence of hypocortisolism, regardless of the etiology, should be treated with physiological replacement doses of corticosteroids (with fludrocortisone if there is evidence of mineralocorticoid deficiency) and have regular clinical and biochemical monitoring to avoid over-replacement.

Case Study

A 28-year-old woman with HIV/AIDS was admitted emergently from outpatients with a recent history of polydipsia, polyuria, and profound weight gain. On examination, she was markedly Cushingoid with extensive pathological purple striae on abdomen and back, moon facies, and central obesity. She had a history of moderate asthma and was on inhaled corticosteroids (fluticasone). In view of her HIV/AIDS, she was also on ritonavir and other HIV therapies. She was currently incarcerated in prison and hence her adherence to inhaled fluticasone and other therapies had improved dramatically. Investigations showed high blood glucose 756 mg/dL (42 mmol/L) with no increase in serum ketones. Morning cortisol was 0.18 µg/dL (5 nmol/L) with suppressed ACTH; adrenal magnetic resonance imaging (MRI) showed "normal-"sized adrenal with no abnormalities.

Her Cushing's syndrome was thought to be iatrogenic due to a drug-drug interaction between the synthetic glucocorticoid (fluticasone) and ritonavir (10). As her adherence had improved, she quickly developed this interaction. The ritonavir inhibits CYP3A4, leading to decreased metabolism of the fluticasone which then accumulates and can lead to excessive glucocorticoid exposure. This patient was treated with IV insulin and fluid resuscitation. The fluticasone was switched to a less potent inhaled steroid, and she was also started on oral prednisolone to cover the gradual decrease in glucocorticoid dose which is needed to prevent secondary adrenal insufficiency. The cortisol level was low because the synthetic glucocorticoid was excessive, leading to suppressed ACTH and decreased endogenous cortisol production.

Lactic Acidosis and Mitochondrial Toxicity

Hyperlactinemia is the most significant manifestation arising from the medication class of nucleoside reverse transcriptase inhibitors (NRTI). Use of this medication class is associated with mitochondrial toxicity. In resource-unconstrained countries, the use of older NRTIs associated with the worse mitochondrial toxicity has decreased, however, these are still in use in resource-limited countries. NRTIs exert their action by inhibiting the enzyme HIV reverse transcriptase, which is critical to viral replication. However, they also inhibit mitochondrial DNA polymerase γ, an enzyme responsible for DNA replication (12). This results in the production of dysfunctional mitochondrial proteins, which accumulate and impair crucial aspects of the mitochondrial metabolic function, such as oxidative phosphorylation. With insufficient oxidative phosphorylation, pyruvate is metabolized to lactate rather than acetyl CoA and lactate accumulates. The propensity for lactate accumulation is further exacerbated by concomitant impaired hepatic dysfunction with reduced lactate clearance (12) and renal dysfunction. Therefore, caution should be used in dosing metformin in those patients with renal impairment receiving NRTI-containing cART and metformin. Lactate (and if available) metformin levels are useful in monitoring safety in this specific patient group.

Furthermore, a relatively new cART agent, the integrase inhibitor dolutegravir, can markedly increase circulating metformin levels. Metformin is eliminated by the renal tubules, via active renal tubular secretion through the organic cation transporter molecules. Dolutegravir is a potent inhibitor of these transporter molecules and increases post-dose metformin levels substantially. Therefore, the maximal recommended metformin dose in people receiving dolutegravir is 1000 mg daily (13). In patients receiving dolutegravir and metformin, the risk of lactic acidosis exists, particularly where there is renal impairment, but also in states of dehydration.

The clinical manifestations of hyperlactinemia are broad and non-specific and diagnosis may be delayed by the unpredictability of the onset of mitochondrial toxicity. Signs and symptoms may include abdominal pain, nausea, vomiting, weight loss, fatigue, tachypnea, dyspnea, seizures, impaired cognition, arrhythmias, and heart failure. Blood investigations may reveal anemia and leukopenia as well as elevation in aminotransferases, lipase, and creatine phosphokinase. Hepatic steatosis may be evident on abdominal imaging. All NRTIs may cause hyperlactinemia, however, some drugs are more problematic than others. Zidovudine, lamivduine, stavudine, and didanosine have been most often reported.

In a patient who develops lactic acidosis, the NRTI medication or dolutegravir should be ceased immediately. Supportive care is the mainstay of treatment, aiming to optimize tissue oxygen delivery by cardiopulmonary support. This includes fluid resuscitation and mechanical ventilation, if required. The use of alkali therapy is controversial and may actually worsen the intracellular acidosis. There is limited evidence for the use of metabolic cofactors such as riboflavin, carnitine, and thiamine, however, some authors support their use (14). Resolution of hyperlactinemia requires replenishment of mitochondrial DNA which may take 4–28 weeks to recover (15). After the normalization of lactate levels, a new antiretroviral regimen should be considered, with non-nucleoside reverse-transcriptase inhibitors (NNRTI) and protease inhibitors being a safer regimen for these patients. In those patients on dolutegravir plus metformin, an alternative glucose-lowering medication should be considered.

Hyperglycemia

Diabetes in HIV infection was uncommon in the era prior to highly active antiretroviral therapy (HAART), with early studies suggesting diabetes rates of around 2.0% in treatment-naïve HIV-infected subjects (16,17). Since cART became the treatment standard in HIV infection, the prevalence of diabetes has increased substantially due to the impact on adipocyte and lipid metabolism (18–20). Initially, the development of insulin resistance and diabetes were considered a consequence of protease inhibitors, but certain NRTIs are also implicated (21) and it has become apparent that individual genetic susceptibility to antiretroviral medications exists (22). Duration of antiretroviral medication exposure is also associated with an increased risk of incident diabetes (23) with the D:A:D study showing cumulative antiretroviral exposure was independently associated with incident diabetes (24). In addition, the HIV-infected population are also affected by the traditional diabetes risk factors including family history, inactivity, abdominal obesity, increasing age, and gender (25,26). Primary prevention of prediabetes and diabetes with lifestyle modification is important as weight gain occurs frequently following treatment of HIV. For example, the D:A:D study found an 11% increased risk of diabetes for each one-unit increase in body mass index (BMI) in HIV-infected patients (24).

The exact prevalence and incidence of diabetes in treated HIV infection are difficult to establish due to multiple confounders, not limited to diverse ethnic susceptibilities and medication regimens. Prevalence has been quoted to range from 7–13% in individuals treated with protease inhibitors (19,27,28).

The recognition of hyperglycemia is important because of the long-term consequences of diabetes mellitus (i.e., multiorgan macro- and microvascular disease) and also the potentially severe adverse effects of rapid onset hyperglycemia, as has been described with some protease inhibitors. Diabetic ketoacidosis (DKA), a potentially fatal metabolic complication of diabetes, has been reported in patients commencing protease inhibitor therapy with no other diabetes risk factors (29–31). Patients present with the biochemical triad of hyperglycemia, ketonemia, and anion gap metabolic acidosis which often develops rapidly following a precipitating event. Hyperglycemic hyperosmolar syndrome (HHS), the prototype of hyperglycemic crises in type 2 diabetes, often has a more insidious onset over days or weeks with more profound symptoms including sensorial clouding which may progress to seizure, focal neurology, and coma. The common clinical picture of both conditions include symptoms of hyperglycemia (e.g., polyuria, polydipsia, polyphagia, and weight loss), in addition to physical signs of dehydration. Treatment involves fluid resuscitation, correction of electrolyte disturbances, and a gradual reduction in serum glucose with insulin therapy and correction of plasma osmolality. The underlying precipitating cause requires identification and treatment.

Hypertriglyceridemia

Lipid disorders are highly prevalent in both treated and untreated HIV-infection (32,33). With the introduction of cART and the subsequent improvement in long-term survival, individuals with HIV infection face the same causes of major morbidity and mortality as the uninfected population, increasing the importance of appropriate intervention for lipid disorders and cardiovascular risk reduction.

In untreated HIV infection, multiple lipid disorders are reported, including increased serum triglycerides and reduced total, low-density lipoprotein (LDL) and high-density lipoprotein (HDL) cholesterol (33). Hypertriglyceridemia is associated with greater immune system activation (34). In addition, some antiretroviral medications can also cause lipid abnormalities and each medication can have its own unique effect, making it difficult to assign a "class effect" to any particular drug class (32). Hypertriglyceridemia is common with certain protease inhibitors, in particular those where ritonavir is used to boost other protease inhibitors, such as tipranavir (35), lopinavir, and fosamprenavir (36). In these regimens, ritonavir is used at low dose to boost circulating levels of these other protease inhibitors, due to its efficiency in blocking CYP3A4 metabolism of these other medications. The incidence of hypertriglyceridemic pancreatitis is higher in cohorts of patients with HIV infection, compared to seronegative populations (37). The pathophysiology is not well understood, however, and there is no overall clear evidence supporting an increased risk of pancreatitis associated with protease inhibitor use (37–39).

The management of hypertriglyceridemia should follow established general guidelines. Careful consideration must be given to the potential for adverse drug interactions between lipid-lowering drugs and the agents used to treat HIV infection (32). In cases of hypertriglyceridemic pancreatitis, the severity should be determined (using various scoring systems) and, if severe, intensive care admission is warranted. Initial management is identical to that for other causes of acute pancreatitis (i.e., analgesia, intravenous fluids, and nil-by-mouth). Decreasing the serum triglyceride concentration is a priority and may be achieved by using multifaceted treatment. However, as the patient begins oral intake (usually after pain is controlled), hypertriglyceridemia-associated pancreatitis patients need to avoid oral fat intake. In addition, IV hyperalimentation with fat emulsions is contraindicated. If hyperglycemia is present, an insulin infusion (often combined with heparin) can reduce free fatty acid release from tissues, decrease the glucose substrate for hepatic triglyceride synthesis, and enhance lipoprotein lipase (LPL) activity. Secondary causes of hypertriglyceridemia should be addressed and precipitating drugs (e.g., protease inhibitors) should be reviewed.

Thyrotoxicosis

Prior to the introduction of cART, overt thyroid dysfunction occurred at similar rates to the seronegative population (40). The use of antiretroviral medications, however, can result in thyrotoxicosis through drug interactions or the immune reconstitution inflammatory syndrome (IRIS).

Graves' disease in HIV-infected individuals may be seen as a late complication after initiation of cART and is thought to occur as part of IRIS (41). It may also occur in HIV infection with hepatitis C co-infection as a result of interferon-alpha therapy (42, 43).

The therapeutic options include antithyroid medications (i.e., methimazole, carbimazole, and propylthiouracil), or definitive treatment with radioactive iodine or total thyroidectomy. Interferon therapy may need to be ceased if the thyrotoxicosis is severe. Beta blockers may be used for symptomatic relief of the associated adrenergic symptoms and may be stopped once thyroid function has normalized, as would be treatment standard.

Hypercalcemia

Hypercalcemic crisis carries a high risk of mortality and may be complicated by metabolic encephalopathy, renal failure, and cardiac arrhythmias. Successful management of hypercalcemia depends on identifying and treating its cause. The causes of hypercalcemia are numerous, including abnormal parathyroid function, malignancy, granulomatous disorders, multiple myeloma, iatrogenic and renal failure.

In HIV-infected individuals, hypercalcemia may occur as a result of IRIS. Case reports of hypercalcemia associated with immune reconstitution-related sarcoidosis (44) and tuberculosis (45) have been reported.

Conclusions

Endocrine and metabolic disorders (Table 8-1) are well-recognized complications or accompaniments of HIV infection. With the introduction of cART to treat HIV infection, there has been a paradigm shift from infectious and infiltrative causes to complications associated with cART and IRIS. Endocrine and metabolic disorders contribute to increased morbidity and mortality in people living with HIV infection, highlighting the importance of the endocrinologist in supporting their overall care. Awareness of the endocrine emergencies that can occur and their unique pathophysiology in the setting of HIV infection is critical.

References

1 Lo J, Grinspoon SK. Adrenal function in HIV infection. *Curr Opin Endocrinol Diabetes Obes.* 2010;17(3):205–209.

2 Marks JB. Endocrine manifestations of human immunodeficiency virus (HIV) infection. *Am J Med Sci.* 1991;302(2): 110–117.

3 Baker R, Rook GA, Zumla A. Adrenal function and the hypothalamo-pituitary adrenal axis in immunodeficiency virus-associated tuberculosis. *Int J Tuberc Lung Dis.* 1997;1(3):289–290.

4 Glasgow BJ, et al. Adrenal pathology in the acquired immune deficiency syndrome. *Am J Clin Pathol.* 1985;84(5):594–597.

5 Arabi Y, et al. Adrenal insufficiency, recurrent bacteremia, and disseminated abscesses caused by Nocardia asteroides in a patient with acquired immunodeficiency syndrome. *Diagn Microbiol Infect Dis.* 1996;24(1):47–51.

6 Baraia-Etxaburu Artetxe J, et al. Primary adrenal failure and AIDS: report of 11 cases and review of the literature. *Rev Clin Esp.* 1998;198(2):74–79.

7 Freda PU, et al. Primary adrenal insufficiency in patients with the acquired immunodeficiency syndrome: a report of five cases. *J Clin Endocrinol Metab.* 1994;79(6):1540–1545.

8 Radin DR, et al. AIDS-related non-Hodgkin's lymphoma: abdominal CT findings in 112 patients. *AJR Am J Roentgenol.* 1993;160(5):1133–1139.

9 Tappero JW, et al. Kaposi's sarcoma: epidemiology, pathogenesis, histology, clinical spectrum, staging criteria and therapy. *J Am Acad Dermatol.* 1993;28(3): 371–395.

10 Samaras K, et al. Iatrogenic Cushing's syndrome with osteoporosis and secondary adrenal failure in human immunodeficiency virus-infected patients receiving inhaled corticosteroids and ritonavir-boosted protease inhibitors: six cases. *J Clin Endocrinol Metab.* 2005;90(7): 4394–4398.

11 Bornstein SR, Allolio B, Arlt W, et al. Diagnosis and treatment of primary adrenal insufficiency: an Endocrine Society Clinical Practice Guideline. *J Clin Endocrinol Metab.* 2016;101:364–389.

12 Kakuda TN, Pharmacology of nucleoside and nucleotide reverse transcriptase inhibitor-induced mitochondrial toxicity. *Clin Ther.* 2000;22(6):685–708.

13 Song IH, Zong J, Borland J, et al. The effect of dolutegravir on the pharmacokinetics of metformin in healthy subjects. *J Acquir Immune Defic Syndr.* 2016;72:400–407.

14 Falco V, et al. Severe nucleoside-associated lactic acidosis in human immunodeficiency virus-infected patients: report of 12 cases and review of the literature. *Clin Infect Dis.* 2002;34(6):838–846.

15 Cote HC, et al. Changes in mitochondrial DNA as a marker of nucleoside toxicity in HIV-infected patients. *N Engl J Med.* 2002;346(11):811–820.

16 Kilby JM, Tabereaux PB. Severe hyperglycemia in an HIV clinic: preexisting versus drug-associated diabetes mellitus. *J Acquir Immune Defic Syndr Hum Retrovirol.* 1998;17(1):46–50.

17 El-Sadr WM, et al. Effects of HIV disease on lipid, glucose and insulin levels: results from a large antiretroviral-naive cohort. *HIV Med.* 2005;6(2):114–121.

18 Bradbury RA, Samaras K. Antiretroviral therapy and the human immunodeficiency virus: improved survival but at what cost? *Diabetes Obes Metab.* 2008; 10(6):441–450.

19 Eastone JA, Decker CF. New-onset diabetes mellitus associated with use of protease inhibitor. *Ann Intern Med.* 1997;127(10):948.

20 Dube MP, et al. Protease inhibitor-associated hyperglycaemia. *Lancet.* 1997;350(9079):713–714.

21 Brinkman K, et al. Mitochondrial toxicity induced by nucleoside-analogue reverse-transcriptase inhibitors is a key factor in the pathogenesis of antiretroviral-therapy-related lipodystrophy. *Lancet.* 1999;354(9184):1112–1115.

22 Ranade K, et al. Genetic analysis implicates resistin in HIV lipodystrophy. *AIDS.* 2008; 22(13):1561–1568.

23 Samaras K. The burden of diabetes and hyperlipidemia in treated HIV infection and approaches for cardiometabolic care. *Curr HIV/AIDS Rep.* 2012;9(3):206–217.

24 De Wit S, et al. Incidence and risk factors for new-onset diabetes in HIV-infected patients: the Data Collection on Adverse Events of Anti-HIV Drugs (D:A:D) study. *Diabetes Care.* 2008;31(6):1224–1229.

25 Wohl DA, et al. Current concepts in the diagnosis and management of metabolic complications of HIV infection and its therapy. *Clin Infect Dis.* 2006;43(5):645–653.

26 Quin J. Diabetes and HIV. *Clinical Med.* 2014;14:667–669.

27 Carr A, et al. Diagnosis, prediction, and natural course of HIV-1 protease-inhibitor-associated lipodystrophy, hyperlipidaemia, and diabetes mellitus: a cohort study. *Lancet.* 1999;353(9170):2093–2099.

28 Gelato MC. Insulin and carbohydrate dysregulation. *Clin Infect Dis.* 2003;36 (Suppl 2):S91–S95.

29 Besson C, et al. Ketoacidosis associated with protease inhibitor therapy. *AIDS.* 1998;12(11):1399–1400.

30 Kan VL, Nylen ES, Diabetic ketoacidosis in an HIV patient: a new mechanism of HIV protease inhibitor-induced glucose intolerance. *AIDS.* 1999;13(14):1987–1989.

31 Hughes, CA, Taylor GD. Metformin in an HIV-infected patient with protease inhibitor-induced diabetic ketoacidosis. *Ann Pharmacother.* 2001;35(7–8):877–880.

32 Dube MP, Cadden JJ. Lipid metabolism in treated HIV Infection. *Best Pract Res Clin Endocrinol Metab.* 2011;25(3):429–442.

33 Myerson M. Lipid management in Human Immunodeficiency Virus. *Endocrinol Metab Clin N Am.* 2016;45:141–169.

34 Grunfeld C, et al. Lipids, lipoproteins, triglyceride clearance, and cytokines in human immunodeficiency virus infection and the acquired immunodeficiency syndrome. *J Clin Endocrinol Metab.* 1992;74(5):1045–1052.

35 Hicks, CB, et al. Durable efficacy of tipranavir-ritonavir in combination with an optimised background regimen of antiretroviral drugs for treatment-experienced HIV-1-infected patients at 48 weeks in the Randomized Evaluation of Strategic Intervention in multi-drug reSistant patients with Tipranavir (RESIST) studies: an analysis of

combined data from two randomised open-label trials. *Lancet*. 2006;368(9534): 466–475.

36 Eron J, Jr., et al. The KLEAN study of fosamprenavir-ritonavir versus lopinavir-ritonavir, each in combination with abacavir-lamivudine, for initial treatment of HIV infection over 48 weeks: a randomised non-inferiority trial. *Lancet*. 2006;368(9534):476–482.

37 Riedel DJ, et al. A ten-year analysis of the incidence and risk factors for acute pancreatitis requiring hospitalization in an urban HIV clinical cohort. *AIDS Patient Care STDS*. 2008;22(2):113–121.

38 Reisler RB, et al. Incidence of pancreatitis in HIV-1-infected individuals enrolled in 20 adult AIDS clinical trials group studies: lessons learned. *J Acquir Immune Defic Syndr*. 2005;39(2):159–166.

39 Bush ZM, Kosmiski LA. Acute pancreatitis in HIV-infected patients: are etiologies changing since the introduction of protease inhibitor therapy? *Pancreas*, 2003;27(1): e1–e5.

40 Parsa AA, Bhangoo A. HIV and thyroid dysfunction. *Rev Endocr Metab Disord*. 2013;14(2):127–131.

41 Rasul S, et al. Graves' disease as a manifestation of immune reconstitution in HIV-infected individuals after initiation of highly active antiretroviral therapy. *AIDS Res Treat*. 2011:743597.

42 Prummel MF, Laurberg P. Interferon-alpha and autoimmune thyroid disease. *Thyroid*. 2003;13(6):547–551.

43 Koh L.K., Greenspan F.S., Yeo P.P. Interferon-alpha induced thyroid dysfunction: three clinical presentations and a review of the literature. *Thyroid*. 1997;7(6):891–896.

44 Ferrand RA, et al. Immune reconstitution sarcoidosis presenting with hypercalcaemia and renal failure in HIV infection. *Int J STD AIDS*. 2007;18(2):138–139.

45 Tsao YT, Wu CC, Chu P. Immune reconstitution syndrome-induced hypercalcemic crisis. *Am J Emerg Med*. 2010;29(2):244 e3–e6.

9

Endocrine and Metabolic Emergencies in Late-Effects Patients

Consequences of Cancer Therapy

Helena Gleeson and Andrew Toogood

Key Points

- The past 40 years have seen a great improvement in survival of children and young adults treated for cancer.
- However, the quality of survival is affected by the "consequences of cancer therapy," which develop continually and cumulatively over a number of years after treatment and lead to a multitude of secondary health complications.
- Based on data from childhood cancer survivors in the USA, it has been estimated that nine out of ten survivors will acquire a chronic health disorder by the age of 45, and a quarter will develop a chronic health disorder that is severe and may be life-threatening or disabling.
- Any of the systems in the body may be affected but it is the treatment of some cancer diagnoses, particularly patients treated for a brain or head and neck tumor and hematological malignancies requiring stem cell transplantation, in which endocrine and metabolic consequences occur frequently. They may present soon after completion of cancer therapy or many years after, therefore, if adequate screening is not employed, patients may present as an endocrine or metabolic emergency.
- The acute presentation of a cancer survivor regardless of time since treatment should prompt the treating clinician to consider the potential implication of previous cancer therapy when formulating diagnoses, not only from the perspective of endocrine and metabolic consequences but also other systems as they are at risk of second primary neoplasms and cardiovascular disease and early recognition and treatment may reduce morbidity and mortality.

Introduction

In the UK, there are currently over two million cancer survivors (1) which is predicted to rise to 5.3 million by 2040 (2). Although prognosis varies by the type of cancer and age at diagnosis, treatments in the past four decades have improved drastically, such that half of all people diagnosed with cancer in 2010–2011 in England and Wales are expected to survive for more than 10 years, compared with just a quarter of people diagnosed in 1971–1972 (3). However, the quality of survival is affected by the "consequences of cancer therapy" which develop continually and cumulatively over a number of years after treatment and lead to secondary health complications (4,5). Based on data from childhood cancer survivors in the USA, it has been estimated that nine out of ten survivors will acquire a chronic health disorder by the age of 45 (6), and a quarter will develop a chronic health disorder that is severe and may be life-threatening or disabling (7).

Any of the systems in the body may be affected, but it is the treatment of some cancer diagnoses, particularly patients treated for a brain or head and neck tumor and those requiring stem cell transplantation for hematological malignancies, in which endocrine and metabolic consequences occur frequently (8). They may present soon after completion of cancer therapy or many years later, therefore, if adequate screening is not employed, patients may present as an endocrine or metabolic emergency.

Cancer therapy is continually evolving. Within immunotherapy, in particular the increasing use of immune checkpoint inhibitors and the associated endocrine dysfunction (9), there is now the need for endocrinologists to be involved in the care of increasing numbers of patients undergoing cancer therapy.

The acute presentation of a cancer survivor regardless of time since treatment should prompt the treating physician to consider the potential implication of previous cancer therapy when formulating diagnoses, not only from the perspective of endocrine and metabolic consequences but also other systems as they are at risk of among other health conditions, second primary neoplasms and cardiovascular disease (10), and early recognition and treatment may reduce morbidity and mortality.

This chapter sets out the scenarios that place survivors at risk of presenting as an endocrine and metabolic emergency as well as a recommended approach to care.

Organization of Care for Cancer Survivors

While all cancer survivors should be offered long-term follow-up, this should be stratified to allow for effective use of resources. The National Cancer Survivor Initiative adopted three levels of cancer survivorship (11)

predicting their likelihood of developing consequences of cancer therapy both in terms of prevalence and severity and therefore optimizing their level of care:

Level 1: patients may have had surgery alone and/or low risk chemotherapy and are considered suitable for postal or phone follow-up. Their prevalence of "late effects" was 11.6% with only very occasional patients experiencing life-changing (grade 3 or above) toxicity (12).

Level 2: patients treated with standard risk chemotherapy, such as survivors of acute lymphoblastic leukemia (ALL) or lymphoma, who are considered to be at moderate risk of developing "late effects," for example, anthracycline-induced cardiotoxicity, and could be followed up by an appropriately trained individual, such as a nurse specialist. Their prevalence of "late effects" was 35.8%, of whom 9.3%, 58.8%, 18.5%, 10.3% and 3% had grades 1, 2, 3, 4 and 5 toxicity (12).

Level 3: patients who would require medically supervised follow-up within a multidisciplinary team, that is, those patients that have had a brain tumor (treated with chemotherapy and/or radiotherapy), bone marrow transplants, stage 4 disease, any radiotherapy except low-dose cranial radiotherapy and those who have had intensive therapy. Their prevalence of "late effects" was 65.2%, of whom 5.5%, 34.4%, 36.2%, 22.1% and 1.8% had grades 1, 2, 3, 4 and 5 toxicity, respectively (12).

The majority of patients at risk of endocrine and metabolic consequences are level 3 patients.

Adrenal Insufficiency

Adrenal insufficiency is a life-threatening condition which requires immediate recognition (13) and management. It is therefore important to understand the impact of cancer treatment on adrenal function.

Secondary adrenal insufficiency is more likely in cancer survivors and occurs as a consequence of cranial irradiation (14), secondary to high dose glucocorticoids causing adrenocorticotropic hormone (ACTH) suppression (15) and following the development of hypophysitis with the use of immune checkpoint inhibitors (9). It has not been described as a consequence of other chemotherapeutic agents. Primary adrenal insufficiency is less frequent in cancer survivors, and it has not been described as a consequence of radiotherapy or chemotherapy, but adrenalitis can occur with the use of immune checkpoint inhibitors (9), otherwise it is likely to be secondary to adrenal lymphoma or metastases (16).

Primary adrenal insufficiency resulting in the loss of glucocorticoid and mineralocorticoid production leads to a more acute presentation with dehydration, hypotension, and the typical picture of hyponatremia and hyperkalemia. Patients with secondary adrenal insufficiency retain the majority of their mineralocorticoid function, so the presentation can be more insidious, although decompensation during an intercurrent illness can precipitate an acute Addisonian crisis.

Radiation Affecting the Hypothalamic Pituitary Axis

The hypothalamic pituitary axis is frequently included within the radiation field used for treatment of nonpituitary tumors, including brain tumors, nasopharyngeal tumors, tumors of the skull base, central nervous system prophylaxis in patients with acute lymphoblastic leukemia, and total body irradiation before bone marrow transplantation (14). Radiation-induced hypopituitarism is a well-recognized complication of cranial radiotherapy, which clinically presents insidiously (Figure 9-1), and is often late to be recognized without routine screening.

The presence and severity of hypopituitarism following radiation depend on the total radiation dose delivered to the hypothalamic pituitary axis (Table 9-1), fraction size, total duration of the radiotherapy scheme, and duration of follow-up post-radiation (14). The frequency of deficits in individual anterior pituitary hormone axes is greatest in the growth hormone axis, followed by gonadotropin, ACTH and TSH axes.

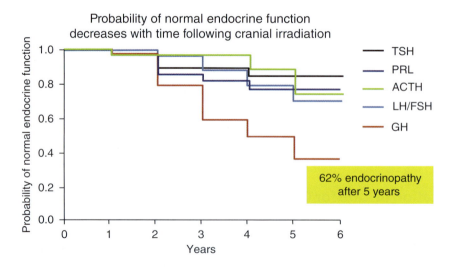

Figure 9-1 The effects of cranial irradiation on hypothalamic-pituitary function were studied over a 5-year period in 31 patients with nasopharyngeal carcinoma. Within 2 years of radiotherapy, significant impairment in the secretion of GH, gonadotropins, corticotropin and thyrotropin were observed. The cumulative probability of endocrine dysfunction was 62% after 5 years. Adapted from (55).

Table 9-1 Effects of cranial irradiation on hypothalamic-pituitary function in children and adolescents. The effect of cranial irradiation dose can be compounded by previous surgery or chemotherapy. Adapted from (14).

Mean dose to hypothalamus	Time to development of GH deficiency	Effect on LH and FSH	TSH deficiency	ACTH deficiency
10–15 Gy	Unknown			
15–20 Gy	60 months	Precocious puberty, in girls more than boys	Rare	Rare
25–30 Gy	36 months	Precocious puberty, equally in girl and boys		
30 Gy		LH and FSH deficiency possible with CRI	Possible	Possible in brain tumor survivors especially, or in
42–60 Gy		doses > 30 Gy		patients with other pituitary hormone deficiencies
> 60 Gy	12 months		Very likely	

CRI = cranial irradiation.

The hypothalamic pituitary axis is believed to be more radiosensitive in childhood compared with adulthood. In support of this, a higher frequency of GH deficiency (GHD) is observed in children who received TBI (9–15 Gy) (17), whereas in adulthood this dose of radiation has not been shown to cause hypopituitarism (18). Following irradiation of childhood brain tumors, the long-term prevalence of GHD has been reported to be almost 100%, when the HP axis is exposed to doses greater than 30 Gy (19). A systematic review of 18 studies included 813 patients with head and neck tumors (n = 608) or non-pituitary brain tumors (n = 205) treated with radiation doses between 46–83 Gy and 25–97 Gy respectively in adulthood (20). The prevalence of hypopituitarism varied from 25–100% in nasopharyngeal cancer patients (Figure 9-1) and from 37–77% in those with non-pituitary brain tumors.

There is no evidence that the hypothalamic pituitary axis is affected by chemotherapy, there is some evidence that it may enhance the effect of radiotherapy on the hypothalamic pituitary axis, especially in the treatment of medulloblastoma (21).

Hypothalamic pituitary dysfunction as a consequence of cranial irradiation has lifelong implications, in childhood, poor growth as well as either early or delayed pubertal development, and in adulthood, including reduced quality of life. There is evidence of benefit from growth hormone replacement in cancer survivors in childhood and adulthood from the perspective of growth and quality of life respectively (22,23).

Unrecognized ACTH deficiency is the most important pituitary hormone deficiency in respect to endocrine emergencies. In childhood cancer survivors treated with cranial irradiation, the estimated point prevalence was 9–24% for ACTH deficiency depending on underlying diagnosis and radiation dose (24). In adult patients, ACTH deficiency was diagnosed in 0–50% of patients with nasopharyngeal tumors and in 3–62% of the patients with non-pituitary brain tumors (20). The approximate onset of ACTH insufficiency in one study following treatment for head and neck tumors was 6 yrs (25) and 3.9 years (range 2.5 years to 5.7 years) in a study following patients treated for non pituitary brain tumors (26).

Due to the impact of cranial radiation on hypothalamic pituitary function as well as hearing loss and severe global cognitive deficiencies, there has been a move to reduce its use (27). For example, it is no longer the norm for prophylactic cranial radiation to be used against CNS relapse in the treatment of children with standard acute lymphoblastic leukemia and in younger children with brain tumors, cranial radiation is often delayed until they are older. In the future the consequence of radiotherapy is also likely to be redefined as proton beam therapy becomes increasingly available, further reducing exposure of normal tissue to the effects of irradiation. Early studies suggest lower rates of endocrine dysfunction in pediatric patients treated for medulloblastoma, particularly in relation to thyroid gland damage and gonadal damage but similar rates of GHD and ACTH deficiency (28).

Recommendations

All patients who have received radiation affecting their hypothalamic pituitary axis require endocrine screening a year after completion of radiotherapy, regardless of life expectancy, and annually for the first 10 years or more frequently if they have symptoms, and should continue to have less frequent surveillance thereafter.

Secondary adrenal insufficiency should be considered in any patient admitted acutely with a history of radiation affecting their hypothalamic pituitary axis. Treatment with parenteral or oral hydrocortisone as appropriate should be instigated immediately, before the results of investigations are available.

Adrenal Suppression Following Glucocorticoids

Prolonged exogenous glucocorticoid treatment can lead to suppression of ACTH and secondary adrenal insufficiency. Studies in children and adults have shown that following high dose glucocorticoid, ACTH suppression occurs. A systematic review of children treated with glucocorticoids for ALL demonstrated that adrenal insufficiency occurs in nearly all children in the first days after cessation of glucocorticoid treatment for childhood ALL (29). The majority of children recovered within a few weeks, but a small

number of children had ongoing adrenal insufficiency lasting up to 34 weeks. There were no apparent differences in the likelihood of adrenal suppression between prednisone and dexamethasone arms. In one study, it appeared that treatment with fluconazole prolonged the duration of adrenal insufficiency (30). The percentage of adult cancer survivors experiencing ACTH suppression following the use of dexamethasone as an antiemetic varies from 16–44% up to 6 months off glucocorticoids with improvements in symptoms in 73% when prednisolone was introduced (31,32). Recovery of the axis will mostly occur, but it can take as long as two years.

Recommendations

All patients treated with glucocorticoids for longer than three months, typically prednisolone or dexamethasone, should be considered at risk of secondary adrenal insufficiency. Reduction in steroid dose with assessment of hypothalamic pituitary adrenal axis is recommended and conversion to hydrocortisone may be required.

Secondary adrenal insufficiency should be considered in any patient admitted acutely who has recently completed a course in the last 6 months or is on reducing doses of glucocorticoids. Treatment with parenteral or oral hydrocortisone as appropriate should be instigated immediately, before the results of investigations are available.

Immune Checkpoint Inhibitors and Endocrine Dysfunction

Immune checkpoint inhibitors are a new and effective class of cancer therapy, Ipilimumab being the most established drug in this category. Ipilimumab blocks the CTLA-4 receptor, causing a reduction in the immune tolerance of the tumor and effectively inducing an autoimmune response which reduces disease volume. There is evidence to suggest that CTLA-4 is expressed in endocrine tissues, explaining why autoimmune endocrinopathy is a common side effect of these agents, including hypophysitis (up to 17%) (9). The main symptom of hypophysitis was headache and fatigue. The mean onset of endocrine side effects is 9 weeks after initiation (range 5–36 weeks). Some recovery of pituitary function can occur at a year but ACTH deficiency often persists. There is no evidence that treatment with high doses of glucocorticoid changes the outcome. In addition to hypophysitis, there have been rare reports of adrenalitis (1%), thyroid dysfunction is more common (up to 15% and 22% when combination therapy used) (9).

Recommendations

All patients who are receiving immune checkpoint inhibitors require endocrine screening prior to each course of therapy, and if symptoms of headache and fatigue develop, with involvement of an endocrinologist if abnormalities develop.

Any patient being admitted acutely who is receiving treatment with immune checkpoint inhibitors with signs and symptoms suggestive of adrenal insufficiency should be immediately treated with parenteral or oral hydrocortisone as appropriate, before the results of investigations are available, and screened for other endocrine abnormalities and other autoimmune consequences.

Thyroid Dysfunction

Thyroid dysfunction is common among patients treated for cancer. Patients may present acutely with symptoms of thyrotoxicosis that may mimic the potential effects of recurrent cancer, particularly weight loss and anxiety.

Childhood cancer survivors experienced steadily increasing cumulative incidence with age for all thyroid disorders. Multivariable analysis confirmed an increased risk for an underactive or overactive thyroid, thyroid nodules, and thyroid cancer in survivors overall as well as for survivors exposed to thyroid and/or hypothalamic pituitary irradiation compared with siblings (33).

Following allogeneic stem cell transplant, three patterns of thyroid dysfunction occur: subclinical and overt hypothyroidism and autoimmune thyroid disease, including thyrotoxicosis secondary to Graves' disease, and is presumably mediated by the transfer of immunocompetent donor lymphocytes to the recipient (34).

Monoclonal antibodies have also been associated thyroid dysfunction. Alemtuzumab, also known as Campath, is used in the management of hematological malignancies, and has been associated with thyrotoxicosis (35). Monoclonal antibodies which act as immune checkpoint inhibitors can also cause thyrotoxicosis as the result of thyroiditis, which can be relatively asymptomatic (9).

Recommendations

Routine thyroid function screening is recommended in patients who have received radiation affecting the thyroid gland, and who have undergone a stem cell transplant or are receiving immune checkpoint inhibitors. Those who have had radiation should also undergo a thyroid examination with ultrasound with or without fine-needle aspiration (FNA) if a nodule is identified.

In at-risk patients presenting with symptoms of thyrotoxicosis, a simple blood test may confirm the diagnosis and prevent unnecessary investigations searching for recurrent disease or a second primary neoplasm.

Diabetes Insipidus

Diabetes insipidus has not been reported in patients as a consequence of having received either cranial irradiation or chemotherapy. A recent case report has implicated temozolomide, used to treat primary brain tumors, in the development of diabetes insipidus which resolves when the treatment is discontinued (36).

Diabetes insipidus can, however, be a presenting feature in patients with germinoma and other suprasellar tumors (37) or as a consequence of surgical intervention or secondary to leukemic infiltration or metastatic disease. The presence of diabetes insipidus can complicate ongoing cancer treatment, particularly if the chemotherapy agents require accompanying hyperhydration as some protocols dictate in the treatment of germinomas. In one retrospective study, a third of chemotherapy cycles required a prolonged admission and 6 out of 21 patients developed serious consequences from fluid and electrolyte imbalance (37). The management of diabetes insipidus is made more complicated if more extensive hypothalamic damage results in adipsia, placing the patient at higher risk of morbidity and mortality (38,39).

Recommendations

Management of patients with proven diabetes insipidus depends on the presence of normal thirst. Standard treatment with desmopressin should control polyuria and polydipsia and maintain euvolemia in those with normal thirst. In those without normal thirst, strict fluid balance with daily weights taken and frequent monitoring of sodium are required.

All patients with diabetes insipidus who are admitted to hospital are at risk of hypo and hypernatremia, particularly if nil by mouth, requiring large volumes of intravenous fluid, or are unable to communicate requirements. This is exacerbated further if the patient has adipsia. Careful patient safety measures are required to protect such individuals.

Metabolic Disorders

Cardiovascular disease (CVD) is the leading non-malignant cause of death in survivors of cancer. The increase in morbidity and mortality from CVD affects childhood cancer survivors (10) and groups of survivors of adult cancer (4,5). Much of the CVD is from direct toxicity from cancer therapy, anthracycline chemotherapy or radiotherapy, either to the heart or arteries, and guidelines

are available to guide monitoring of patients who have had anthracyclines or cardiac irradiation (40). Certain hormone replacements and pregnancy may precipitate silent or worsen known cardiac dysfunction.

Cancer survivors are also at an increased risk of developing diabetes and other adverse cardiovascular risk factors, in particular, clustering of factors resulting in metabolic syndrome. The metabolic syndrome is a set of preventable and reversible risk factors which have been shown to increase the risk of CVD by 2- to 3-fold in the general population (41). In survivors of childhood cancer, metabolic disorders have been shown to occur more frequently than in non-cancer individuals with three times greater risk for hyperinsulinemia, four and a half times for obesity and almost eight times for reduced HDL-cholesterol levels compared with age- and sex-matched controls (42). A study following survivors for 3–18 years (median age 20 years) after bone marrow transplant found the prevalence of metabolic syndrome was 39% in transplant survivors compared with, 8% leukemia patients without a transplant and none in non-cancer controls (43). More recently, a study conducted by the European Group for Blood and Marrow Transplantation (EBMT) of cancer survivors (age at diagnosis 42 years and at follow-up 52 years) in Europe has shown that 37% have metabolic syndrome using International Diabetes Federation (IDF) criteria (44). Similarly, metabolic syndrome based on Adult Treatment Program (ATP)-III criteria was found in 34% of survivors of acute lymphoblastic leukemia and this study also revealed that exposure to cranial radiation increased the risk of having metabolic syndrome by nearly two times (45).

The presence of these cardiovascular risk factors increases the likelihood of morbidity and mortality from CVD in the cancer survivor population. However, the earlier age of onset and the silent and insidious nature of metabolic syndrome, and the fact that many patients, particularly those who have had bone marrow transplantation, may have a relatively normal body mass index (BMI), make the increase in cardiovascular risk unrecognized by patients and their physicians. The utility of cardiovascular risk calculators for primary prevention in this population is limited as they underestimate the risk due to their relatively young age. Cardiovascular risk factor screening is vital and there are a number of guidelines recommending monitoring (46–49). Despite these recommendations recent surveys have indicated a lack of monitoring CVD risk factors for cancer survivors (50,51).

Weight management is a priority among cancer survivors, especially preventing central fat accumulation, and studies have indicated lifestyle changes can reduce the risk of metabolic syndrome and its components (52,53). When risk factors are identified, primary prevention has been advocated for cancer survivors (54).

Recommendations

Routine cardiovascular risk screening is recommended in patients who have a diagnosis of a brain tumor or who have undergone a stem cell transplant. Endocrine replacement should be optimized and cardiovascular risk factors should be managed.

Other Non-Endocrine Consequences

In the care of cancer survivors, it is also important to be aware of other consequences of cancer therapy that may result in an acute presentation, in particular, the risk of second primary neoplasms and CVD.

- Patients who have had cranial irradiation are at risk of meningiomas or gliomas; cerebrovascular accidents; and SMART ("stroke-like migraine attacks after radiation therapy") syndrome.
- Patients who have had anthracycline chemotherapy are at risk of cardiomyopathy.
- Patients who have had radiation affecting their spleen have a non-functioning spleen and are at risk of overwhelming infection.
- Patients with a diagnosis of Hodgkin's disease or who receive purine analogue chemotherapy agent, such as fludarabine, should receive irradiated blood products unless in an emergency.

Conclusions

Endocrine and metabolic consequences are frequent in cancer survivors. Patients may present acutely and therefore clinicians need to be aware of the impact of cancer therapy on short- and long-term health. To reduce the morbidity and mortality associated with undiagnosed endocrinopathies and metabolic syndrome, patients should be offered routine screening. Further research is required to understand the impact of improving cardiovascular risk in this cohort on the increased risk of CVD. As cancer therapy evolves, ongoing surveillance is required to define consequences of new therapies and follow up required.

References

1 Maddams J, Brewster D, Gavin A, et al. Cancer prevalence in the United Kingdom: estimates for 2008. *Br J Cancer*. 2009;101: 541–547.

2 Maddams J, Utley M, Møller H. Projections of cancer prevalence in the United Kingdom, 2010–2040. *Br J Cancer*. 2012;107:1195–1202.

3 Quaresma M, Coleman MP, Rachet B. 40-year trends in an index of survival for all cancers combined and survival adjusted for age and sex for each cancer in England and Wales, 1971–2011: a population-based study. *Lancet*. 2015;385:1206–1218.

4 Darby SC, McGale P, Taylor CW, Peto R. Long-term mortality from heart disease

and lung cancer after radiotherapy for early breast cancer: prospective cohort study of about 300,000 women in US SEER cancer registries. *Lancet Oncol*. 2005;6:557–565.

5 Haugnes HS, Wethal T, Aass N, et al. Cardiovascular risk factors and morbidity in long-term survivors of testicular cancer: a 20-year follow-up study. *J Clin Oncol*. 2010;28:4649–4657.

6 Hudson MM, Ness KK, Gurney JG, et al. Clinical ascertainment of health outcomes among adults treated for childhood cancer. *JAMA*. 2013;309:2371–2381.

7 Bhatia S, Landier W. Evaluating survivors of pediatric cancer. *Cancer J*. 2005;11: 340–354.

8 Mostoufi-Moab S, Seidel K, Leisenring WM, et al. Endocrine abnormalities in aging survivors of childhood cancer: a report from the Childhood Cancer Survivor Study. *J Clin Oncol*. 2016;34(27): 3240–3247.

9 Joshi MN, Whitelaw BC, Palomar MT, et al. Immune checkpoint inhibitor-related hypophysitis and endocrine dysfunction: clinical review. *Clin Endocrinol (Oxf)*. 2016;85:331–339.

10 Fidler MM, Reulen RC, Winter DL, et al., British Childhood Cancer Survivor Study Steering Group. Long term cause specific mortality among 34 489 five year survivors of childhood cancer in Great Britain: population based cohort study. *BMJ*. 2016;354:i4351.

11 Wallace WH, Blacklay A, Eiser C, Davies H, et al., Late Effects Committee of the United Kingdom Children's Cancer Study Group (UKCCSG). Developing strategies for long term follow up of survivors of childhood cancer. *BMJ*. 2001;323(7307):271–274.

12 Edgar AB, Duffin K, Borthwick S, Marciniak-Stepak P, Wallace WH. Can intensity of long-term follow-up for survivors of childhood and teenage cancer be determined by therapy-based risk stratification? *BMJ Open*. 2013;3(8).

13 Pazderska A, Pearce SH. Adrenal insufficiency: recognition and management. *Clin Med (Lond)*. 2017;17(3): 258–262.

14 Crowne E, Gleeson H, Benghiat H, et al. Effect of cancer treatment on hypothalamic-pituitary function. *Lancet Diabetes Endocrinol*. 2015;3:568–576.

15 Bayman E, Drake AJ. Adrenal suppression with glucocorticoid therapy: still a problem after all these years? *Arch Dis Child*. 2017;102(4):338–339.

16 Zhou J, Ye D, Wu M, Zheng F, et al. Bilateral adrenal tumor: causes and clinical features in eighteen cases. *Int Urol Nephrol*. 2009;41(3):547–551.

17 Ogilvy-Stuart AL, Clark DJ, Wallace WH, et al. Endocrine deficit after fractionated total body irradiation. *Arch Dis Child*. 1992;67(9):1107–1110.

18 Littley MD, Shalet SM, Morgenstern GR, Deakin DP. Endocrine and reproductive dysfunction following fractionated total body irradiation in adults. *Q J Med*. 1991; 78(287):265–274.

19 Clayton PE, Shalet SM. Dose dependency of time of onset of radiation-induced growth hormone deficiency. *J Pediatr*. 1991;118(2):226–228.

20 Appelman-Dijkstra NM, Kokshoorn NE, Dekkers OM, et al. Pituitary dysfunction in adult patients after cranial radiotherapy: systematic review and meta-analysis. *J Clin Endocrinol Metab* 2011;96:2330–2340.

21 Uday S, Murray RD, Picton S, et al. Endocrine sequelae beyond 10 years in survivors of medulloblastoma. *Clin Endocrinol (Oxf)*. 2015;83(5):663–670.

22 Gleeson HK, Stoeter R, Ogilvy-Stuart AL, Gattamaneni HR, Brennan BM, Shalet SM. Improvements in final height over 25 years in growth hormone (GH)-deficient childhood survivors of brain tumors receiving GH replacement. *J Clin Endocrinol Metab*. 2003;88(8):3682–3689.

23 Murray RD, Darzy KH, Gleeson HK, Shalet SM. GH-deficient survivors of childhood cancer: GH replacement during adult life. *J Clin Endocrinol Metab*. 2002;87(1): 129–135.

24 Rose SR, Danish RK, Kearney NS, et al. ACTH deficiency in childhood cancer survivors. *Pediatr Blood Cancer*. 2005; 45(6):808-13.

25 Samaan NA, Schultz PN, Yang KP, et al. Endocrine complications after radiotherapy for tumors of the head and neck. *J Lab Clin Med*. 1987;109(3): 364–372.

26 Kyriakakis N, Lynch J, Orme SM, et al. Pituitary dysfunction following cranial radiotherapy for adult-onset nonpituitary brain tumours. *Clin Endocrinol (Oxf)*. 2016;84(3):372–379.

27 Pui CH, Campana D, Pei D, et al. Treating childhood acute lymphoblastic leukemia without cranial irradiation. *N Engl J Med*. 2009;360(26):2730–2741.

28 Eaton BR, Esiashvili N, Kim S, et al. Endocrine outcomes with proton and photon radiotherapy for standard risk medulloblastoma. *Neuro Oncol*. 2016;18:88–887.

29 Gordijn MS, Rensen N, Gemke RJ, van Dalen EC, Rotteveel J, Kaspers GJ. Hypothalamic-pituitary-adrenal (HPA) axis suppression after treatment with glucocorticoid therapy for childhood acute lymphoblastic leukaemia. *Cochrane Database Syst Rev*. 2015;(8):CD008727.

30 Petersen KB, Müller J, Rasmussen M, Schmiegelow K. Impaired adrenal function after glucocorticoid therapy in children with acute lymphoblastic leukemia. *Med Pediatr Oncol*. 2003;41(2):110–114.

31 Han HS, Park JC, Park SY, et al. A prospective multicenter study evaluating secondary adrenal suppression after antiemetic dexamethasone therapy in cancer patients receiving chemotherapy: A Korean South West Oncology Group Study. *Oncologist*. 2015;20(12):1432–1439.

32 Han HS, Shim YK, Kim JE, et al. A pilot study of adrenal suppression after dexamethasone therapy as an antiemetic in cancer patients. *Support Care Cancer*. 2012;20(7):1565–1572.

33 Armstrong GT, Stovall M, Robison LL. Long-term effects of radiation exposure among adult survivors of childhood cancer: results from the childhood cancer survivor study. *Radiat Res*. 2010;174(6):840–850.

34 Weetman AP. Graves' disease following immune reconstitution or immunomodulatory treatment: should we manage it any differently? *Clin Endocrinol (Oxf)*. 2014;80(5):629–632.

35 Torino F, Barnabei A, Paragliola R, Baldelli R, Appetecchia M, Corsello SM. Thyroid dysfunction as an unintended side effect of anticancer drugs. *Thyroid*. 2013;23(11): 1345–1366.

36 Faje AT, Nachtigall L, Wexler D, Miller KK, Klibanski A, Makimura H. Central diabetes insipidus: a previously unreported side effect of temozolomide. *J Clin Endocrinol Metab*. 2013;98(10):3926–3931.

37 Varan A, Atas E, Aydın B, et al. Evaluation of patients with intracranial tumors and central diabetes insipidus. *Pediatr Hematol Oncol*. 2013;30(7):668–673.

38 Afzal S, Wherrett D, Bartels U, et al. Challenges in management of patients with intracranial germ cell tumor and diabetes insipidus treated with cisplatin and/or ifosfamide based chemotherapy. *J Neurooncol*. 2010;97(3):393–399.

39 Di Iorgi N, Morana G, Napoli F, Allegri AE, Rossi A, Maghnie M. Management of diabetes insipidus and adipsia in the child. *Best Pract Res Clin Endocrinol Metab*. 2015;29(3):415–436.

40 Armenian SH, Hudson MM, Mulder RL, et al., International Late Effects of Childhood Cancer Guideline Harmonization Group. Recommendations for cardiomyopathy surveillance for survivors of childhood cancer: a report from the International Late Effects of Childhood Cancer Guideline Harmonization Group. *Lancet Oncol*. 2015;16(3):e123–e136.

41 Han TS, Lean ME. A clinical perspective of obesity, metabolic syndrome and cardiovascular disease. *JRSM Cardiovasc Dis*. 2016; 5:2048004016633371.

42 Talvensaari KK, Lanning M, Tapanainen P, Knip M. Long-term survivors of childhood cancer have an increased risk of manifesting the metabolic syndrome. *J Clin Endocrinol Metab*. 1996;81:3051–3055.

43 Taskinen M, Saarinen-Pihkala UM, Hovi L, Lipsanen-Nyman M. Impaired glucose tolerance and dyslipidaemia as late effects

after bone-marrow transplantation in childhood. *Lancet.* 2000;356:993–997.

44 Greenfield D, Snowden J, Schoemans H, et al. Metabolic syndrome is common following haematopoietic cell transplantation (HCT) and is associated with increased cardiovascular disease: an EBMT cross-sectional non-interventional study. *Bone Marrow Transplantation.* 2015;50:S89–S90.

45 Nottage KA, Ness KK, Li C, et al. Metabolic syndrome and cardiovascular risk among long-term survivors of acute lymphoblastic leukaemia—from the St. Jude Lifetime Cohort. *Br J Haematol.* 2014;165: 364–374.

46 DeFilipp Z, Duarte RF, Snowden JA, et al., CIBMTR Late Effects and Quality of Life Working Committee; EBMT Complications and Quality of Life Working Party. Metabolic syndrome and cardiovascular disease after hematopoietic cell transplantation: screening and preventive practice recommendations from the CIBMTR and EBMT. *Biol Blood Marrow Transplant.* 2016;22:1493–1503.

47 Scottish Intercollegiate Guidelines Network. Long term follow up of survivors of childhood cancer: a national clinical guideline. www.sign.ac.uk/pdf/sign76.pdf.

48 Shankar SM, Marina N, Hudson MM et al., Cardiovascular Disease Task Force of the Children's Oncology Group. Monitoring for cardiovascular disease in survivors of childhood cancer: report from the Cardiovascular Disease Task Force of the Children's Oncology Group. *Pediatrics.* 2008;121:e387–e396.

49 Bovelli D, Plataniotis G, Roila F, ESMO Guidelines Working Group. Cardiotoxicity of chemotherapeutic agents and radiotherapy-related heart disease: ESMO Clinical Practice Guidelines. *Ann Oncol.* 2010;21 Suppl 5:v277–v282.

50 Sekhar M, Eggenberger C, Coghlan G. How well are patients with myeloproliferative neoplasms assessed for cardiovascular risk: an audit report. *The Online J Clin Audits.* 2015;7:No 3.

51 Kapoor A, P Vineet, Sekhar M, et al. Monitoring cardiovascular disease risk factors in cancer survivors. *Clinical Medicine.* 2017 (in press).

52 Lipshultz SE, Adams MJ, Colan SD, et al. Long-term cardiovascular toxicity in children, adolescents, and young adults who receive cancer therapy: pathophysiology, course, monitoring, management, prevention, and research directions: a scientific statement from the American Heart Association. *Circulation.* 2013;128:1927–1995.

53 Tonorezos ES, Robien K, Eshelman-Kent D, et al. Contribution of diet and physical activity to metabolic parameters among survivors of childhood leukemia. *Cancer Causes Control.* 2013;24:313–321.

54 Slater ME, Ross JA, Kelly AS, et al. Physical activity and cardiovascular risk factors in childhood cancer survivors. *Pediatr Blood Cancer.* 2014;62:305–310.

55 Lam KSL, Tse VKC, Wang C, et al. Effects of cranial irradiation on hypothalamic-pituitary function – a five year longitudinal study in patients with nasopharyngeal carcinoma. *Q J Med.* 1991;78:165–176.

10

Endocrine and Metabolic Emergencies in Transplantation

Robert A. Wermers and Pankaj Shah

Key Points

- Stem cell transplants (SCT) and solid organ transplants (kidney, liver, heart, lung, intestine, and pancreas) are being increasingly performed, but a large number of patients remain on waiting lists for a solid organ transplant.
- There are unique aspects of clinical care to understand when endocrinologists see transplant patients with underlying endocrine disorders, which can include endocrine emergencies. First, one must consider the stage of the transplant (pre-transplant, early post-transplant, and chronic post-transplant). In addition, it is important to be familiar with immunosuppression drugs, including their common side effects (including endocrine dysfunction) and their drug interactions. Finally, since the transplant population often has underlying severe organ dysfunction, one

must appreciate how the disease influences the diagnostic presentation as well as the management of the endocrine emergency.
- There are important specific considerations when diagnosing and managing endocrine emergencies in transplant patients. For example, hypoglycemic emergencies can be encountered with both end-stage liver and kidney disease, especially in the context of predisposing diabetes medications as well as non-antihyperglycemic medications, such as the trimethoprim-sulfamethoxazole combination and fluoroquinolone antibiotics; secondary adrenal insufficiency is a frequent problem in SCT recipients related to corticosteroid therapy discontinuation; and pre-transplant liver and kidney patients can develop significant hypercalcemia that is often multifactorial in nature.

Introduction

Encountering transplant patients in an endocrine practice is becoming an increasingly common challenge, given the expanding number of annual transplants performed. Consider that from 1988–2016 a total of 686,706 solid organ transplants were performed in the USA, and in 2016 alone, there were 33,593 solid organ transplants

performed and another 119,053 patients currently on the waiting list for a solid organ transplant (1). The most common solid organ transplants in the USA are, in descending order, kidney, liver, heart, lung, combined kidney/pancreas, pancreas, intestine, and combined heart/lung. However, the most common transplants done in the USA are stem cell transplants (SCT) with nearly 20,000 completed in 2014 (2). Importantly,

Endocrine and Metabolic Medical Emergencies: A Clinician's Guide, Second Edition. Edited by Glenn Matfin.
© 2018 John Wiley & Sons Ltd. Published 2018 by John Wiley & Sons Ltd.

in the context of other ongoing significant illnesses, as is often the case in the transplant population, abnormalities in endocrine function can lead to emergencies requiring endocrinology assistance.

There are several clinical considerations when endocrinologists see transplant patients that are different from a general practice (3). First, it is critical to understand the type of transplant, the reason for the transplant, and the patient's current clinical status in regard to the specific type of transplant. The transplant process can be broken down into the following clinical phases: pre-transplant, early post-transplant (within the first year), and chronic post-transplant. Each stage of the transplant is associated with unique challenges and expectations in regard to patient management and associated comorbidities (Table 10-1). Second, it is important to be familiar with immuno-suppression drugs (ISDs), including their common side effects and drug interactions, even if you are not managing the immuno-suppressant levels (Table 10-2). The classes of ISDs include glucocorticoids, calcineurin inhibitors: cyclosporine and tacrolimus (nephrotoxic, adverse skeletal effects, neurotoxic, and diabeteogenic), mammalian target of rapamycin (mTOR) inhibitors: sirolimus and everolimus (adverse lipid effects), and anti-proliferative agents: mycophenolate sodium, mycophenolate mofetil, and azathioprine (4). Often these agents are used in combination. Finally, endocrine disease and treatments are influenced by chronic kidney disease which is prevalent in solid organ patients both pre- and post-transplant (5).

Patients undergoing SCT have several unique considerations when compared to solid organ transplant candidates and recipients. This patient population is generally younger, has a shorter interval between diagnosis and transplant, and has received chemotherapy often in conjunction with total body irradiation (TBI) for treatment of their bone marrow disorder and as part of the conditioning regimen for the SCT (6). Additionally, these patients do not receive long-term immunosuppressive therapy. However,

patients with allogeneic SCT, as opposed to autologous SCT, commonly develop graft versus host disease (GvHD) due to the immunocompetent donor cells infused into the host and may require a high dose of immunosuppressive therapy (6).

Hyperglycemia

Acute hyperglycemic complications (both diabetic ketoacidosis and hyperosmolar hyperglycemic state) are described in transplant recipients. Most of the time, the cause of the severe hyperglycemic crisis is apparent. These include the anti-rejection agent tacrolimus (therapeutic and supratherapeutic concentrations), supra-physiologic doses of glucocorticoids, prior hepatitis C infection, and intercurrent infections (7,8). If a person develops acute hyperglycemic complications precipitated by toxic concentrations of tacrolimus, reducing the dose of tacrolimus to achieve therapeutic concentrations or stopping it may improve glycemic control to an extent that the patient may not need anti-hyperglycemic agents (9). Treatment of a hyperglycemic crisis is no different from the treatment in people who have not had organ transplantation. However, renal and cardiac dysfunctions often limit the flexibility of fluid replacement.

Hypoglycemia

After liver transplantation, spontaneous hypoglycemia is an ominous sign of compromised liver recovery and implies primary graft failure with severe graft dysfunction (10). Often intravenous continuous glucose (e.g., 10% dextrose) is required to prevent ongoing hypoglycemia. Sulfonylurea agents as well as insulin are more likely to cause hypoglycemia in people with renal dysfunction (11). Many non-anti-hyperglycemic medications used after transplantation (trimethoprim-sulfamethoxazole combination and fluoroquinolone antibiotics) can

Table 10-1 Endocrine emergencies in relationship to stage of solid organ or stem cell transplant process

	Pre-transplant	Early post-transplant (within the first year)	Chronic post-transplant
Thyrotoxicosis	• Amiodarone • TBI • Reduced metabolism of levothyroxine in liver failure • Iodine through contrast	• Amiodarone • TBI • Stem cell transplantation associated • Reduced renal loss of TBG after kidney transplant • Iodine through contrast	• Iodine through contrast
Hypothyroidism	• Amiodarone • Renal loss of TBG in nephrotic syndrome	• Stem cell transplantation associated • Amiodarone • Accelerated metabolism of levothyroxine after liver transplant	
Hypercalcemia	• CKD associated • Liver failure associated • Diuretic use • Hepatocellular carcinoma producing PTHrP or PTH • Calcitriol use in CKD • Calcium supplements and calcium containing medicines		• Persistent hyperparathyroidism after renal transplant
Hypocalcemia	• Antiresorptive therapies (denosumab, bisphosphonates) • Calcium and vitamin D deficiency • Blood transfusion	• Antiresorptive therapies (denosumab, bisphosphonates) • Early after renal transplant • Blood transfusion • Magnesium deficiency (esp. with cyclosporine use)	• Antiresorptive therapies (denosumab, bisphosphonates) • Post-parathyroidectomy for "tertiary hyperparathyroidism" • Magnesium deficiency (esp. with cyclosporine)
Hyperphosphatemia	• CKD		
Hypophosphatemia	• Antiresorptive therapies (denosumab, bisphosphonates)	• Early after renal transplant	• Antiresorptive therapies (denosumab, bisphosphonates)

(continued)

Table 10-1 *(Continued)*

	Pre-transplant	Early post-transplant (within the first year)	Chronic post-transplant
Hypopituitarism			• Lymphoproliferative disorders • Infections
Secondary adrenal insufficiency			• Prolonged systemic glucocorticoid use (including nonabsorbable intestinal glucocorticoids)
Primary adrenal insufficiency			• CMV adrenalitis
Hyperglycemia	• Hepatitis C infection	• Large dose glucocorticoids	• Tacrolimus and cyclosporine • Chronic glucocorticoid use • Infections
Hypoglycemia	• CKD and liver failure • Spontaneous • Non-diabetes medications (TMP/SMX, Fluoroquinolones) • Antidiabetic medications • Primary liver tumors making IGF-2	• Compromised liver recovery after liver transplant	
Hypertriglyceridemia			• Sirolimus, everolimus
Statin-induced myopathy			• Cyclosporine

TBI = total body irradiation; TBG = thyroid binding globulin; CK = chronic kidney disease; TMP/SMX = trimethoprim/sulfamethoxazole; CMV = cytomegalovirus; PTHrP = parathyroid hormone-related peptide; PTH = parathyroid hormone; IGF-2 = insulin-like growth factor 2.

Table 10-2 Endocrine adverse effects of anti-rejection medications

Drug	Class	Endocrine adverse effects
Basiliximab[2,3]	Interleukin-2 receptor modulator	
Daclizumab[2,3]	Interleukin-2 receptor modulator	
OKT3 (Muromonab-CD3)[2,3]	Anti-CD3 receptor antibody	
Thymoglobulin[2,3]	Antithymocyte globulin	
Methylprednisolone[2,3]	Glucocorticoid	Hyperglycemia
		Secondary adrenal insufficiency
Prednisone[1]	Glucocorticoid	Hyperglycemia
		Secondary adrenal insufficiency
Sirolimus[1]	mTOR inhibitor	Hypertriglyceridemia
		Hypercholesterolemia
Cyclosporine[1]	Calcineurin inhibitor	Diabetes mellitus
		Hypocalcemia
		Hypomagnesemia
		Dyslipidemia
Tacrolimus[1]	Calcineurin inhibitor	Hyperglycemia
Azathioprine[1]	Anti-proliferative agent	
Mycophenolate Mofetil[1]	Anti-proliferative agent	

[1] Maintenance; [2] Induction; [3] Anti-rejection.

cause hypoglycemia (12), especially in the presence of renal and/or liver dysfunction. Spontaneous hypoglycemia, though rare, can occur with stage 5 chronic kidney disease (13) and terminal hepatic failure (14). Patients awaiting liver transplant due to the presence of hepatocellular carcinoma can develop hypoglycemia by production of IGF-2 from the tumor (15). Hypoglycemia has been reported with the liver dysfunction associated with heart failure (16).

Renal and hepatic failure may be associated with prolonged action of the drug causing hypoglycemia. Therefore, correction of hypoglycemia with 15–30 grams of carbohydrates should be followed by a meal or ongoing supply of glucose. Hypoglycemia associated with terminal liver failure may not respond to injections of glucagon, as the main action of glucagon is to release stored glycogen from the liver (17).

Dyslipidemia

Use of mTOR inhibitors (sirolimus and everolimus) as anti-rejection medication is associated with significant dyslipidemia (18), occasionally with a very high concentrations of triglycerides leading to pancreatitis (19). High cholesterol or LDL cholesterol concentrations have no acute health implications. Treatment of severe hypertriglyceridemia induced by sirolimus usually involves putting the patient in NPO status, use of intravenous insulin, and rarely plasmapheresis. Long-term therapy of mTOR inhibitor associated dyslipidemia often involves use of fish oil, fibrates, 3-hydroxy-3-methylglutaryl-coenzyme A (HMG CoA) reductase inhibitors, and occasionally niacin preparations.

Some HMG CoA reductase inhibitors like simvastatin, atorvastatin and lovastatin are metabolized through the cytochrome P450

3A4 pathway. Because cyclosporine is also metabolized by the same pathway, concomitant use of these agents with cyclosporine can dramatically increase the risks of myopathy (20).

Pituitary Disease

Hypopituitarism after transplantation is exceedingly rare. This has been reported to occur with pituitary involvement by post-transplant lymphoproliferative disorder (21), and fungal (22) or bacterial infection (23). Functional corticotropin deficiency after prolonged use of glucocorticoids around the time of transplant is discussed under the section on adrenal disease.

Adrenal Disease

Secondary adrenal insufficiency is a frequent problem in SCT recipients related to corticosteroid therapy discontinuation, and can often be a concern in GvHD where high dose glucocorticoids are utilized. This is further complicated by systemic absorption of "nonabsorbable glucocorticoids" commonly used in the treatment of gastrointestinal GvHD such as budesonide, although the systemic exposure is significantly less than traditional oral glucocorticoids (24). TBI-based conditioning regimens have also been associated with adrenal insufficiency, especially in children (25). Primary adrenal insufficiency caused by adrenalitis associated with cytomegalovirus infections has been reported in patients with immunodeficiency, including after transplantation (26).

Thyroid Disease

Thyroid hormones have a central role in the cardiovascular system, and as such, both hypo- and hyperthyroidism can have significant adverse effects for heart transplant patients (27). A common thyroid emergency in heart transplant patients is amiodarone-induced thyrotoxicosis (AIT) used for management of supraventricular arrhythmias, although any cause of hyperthyroidism can also be seen. Amiodarone contains 2 iodine atoms and a 200 mg daily dose is associated with 6 mg of inorganic iodine release from the liver metabolism which is 20 times above the average daily iodine intake from a diet of 0.3 mg per day (28). When amiodarone is stopped, because it is very lipophilic with a half-life of approximately 100 days, hyperthyroidism or hyperthyroidism can still occur after its discontinuation (29). In general, prior to heart transplant, treatment of hyperthyroidism is advised, and as such, in addition to considering risks and benefits of discontinuing amiodarone, anti-thyroid drugs for patients with iodine-induced hyperthyroidism (Type 1 AIT), prednisone for drug-induced destructive thyroiditis (Type 2 AIT), or both agents ("mixed" AIT), or a total thyroidectomy may also be a consideration (30). However, in patients undergoing surgery, hyperthyroidism can be associated with arrhythmias and thyroid storm (28). Generally, radioiodine is not a treatment option in Type 1 AIT due to the high levels of iodine and low radioiodine uptake. In transplant patients with hyperthyroidism, it is also important to consider the possibility of iodine-induced hyperthyroidism from exposure to excessive iodine through contrast agents for radiographic studies (31).

Endocrinopathies, including thyroid disease, are also a complication of SCT, and TBI in particular predisposes individuals to thyroid dysfunction, with allogenic SCT patients being at higher risk than autologous SCT. Periodic monitoring of thyroid function is recommended in these individuals, but rarely would these individuals present with a thyroid emergency. Although hypothyroidism has been seen in nearly 40% of SCT patients, autoimmune hyperthyroidism can also be encountered, possibly due to the transfer of donor immune cells or immune dysregulation and reconstitution secondary to GvHD (32).

Other unique considerations in the transplant setting are the effects of end-stage renal disease and liver disease on thyroid disease. Thyroid hormone has an important influence on renal hemodynamics, glomerular filtration, and the water and sodium balance, and in addition, with renal protein loss such as would be encountered in nephrotic syndromes, thyroid hormone requirements are often higher due to increased renal protein loss, including thyroid binding globulin (33). After a kidney transplant in patients with nephrotic syndrome, thyroid hormone requirements should lessen and thereby require a preemptive decrease in the thyroid hormone dose.

End-stage liver disease and liver transplants can also be impacted by thyroid dysfunction, given the inherent role of thyroid hormone on regulating the metabolic rate of hepatocytes and normal liver function (34). In addition, the liver is an important site of thyroid hormone metabolism. Indeed, thyroid dysfunction is common in several diseases associated with end-stage liver disease, including primary biliary cirrhosis, primary sclerosing cholangitis, and non-alcoholic fatty liver disease (34). Although there is no data on the treatment of a hyperthyroid crisis in end-stage liver disease or kidney disease, one may consider short-term treatment with anti-thyroid drugs (ATD), preferably methimazole. However, since these medications are metabolized by the liver and excreted by the kidney, a lower dose than is typically used in a thyroid storm could be considered. Also, given the concern with liver toxicity, long-term use of ATD in patients with underlying liver disease would be discouraged. Plasmapheresis to remove thyroid hormone may be another consideration in this population, if there are contraindications to ATD or emergent thyroidectomy is considered, but the benefit is limited to 1–2 days only (35).

Calcium and Phosphate Disorders

When evaluating transplant patients with calcium disorders, either pre- or post-transplantation, it is critical to consider the nuances of calcium measurement. Total serum calcium measurement is influenced by pH and albumin concentrations. Calcium in serum is 40% protein bound, with albumin accounting for 90% of protein binding. Since transplant patients are at risk for changes in albumin levels, correcting for this by adding or subtracting 0.8 mg/dL from total serum calcium for each 1 g/dL decrease or increase respectively in serum albumin from 4 g/dL becomes important. Calcium binding to albumin is pH dependent and acute increases or decreases from a pH of 7.4 will respectively increase or decrease the protein-bound fraction of calcium because carboxy group binding is highly pH dependent. Hence, alkalosis will increase total serum calcium and decrease ionized calcium, while acidosis will do the opposite. Ionized calcium can be useful to measure in critically ill patients were serum protein levels are decreased and pH is abnormal. In addition to these factors, hypovitaminosis D is highly prevalent in transplant patients (36).

Hypercalcemia

There are several specific causes of hypercalcemia that may be encountered in the transplant patient population. In pre-transplant liver patients, non-PTH mediated hypercalcemia can be encountered in individuals who typically have ascites, diuretic use, and impaired renal function (37,38). With liver transplant or improvement of the liver disease, the hypercalcemia generally abates. Another cause of hypercalcemia seen in patients with liver disease is tumor secretion of parathyroid hormone-related peptide (PTHrP) or intact PTH from hepatocellular carcinomas (39–41). Chronic renal failure is also associated with hypercalcemia and can be multifactorial in nature with contributing factures such as vitamin D analogs, calcium containing phosphate binders, reduced renal calcium excretion, and tertiary hyperparathyroidism. Post-transplantation hypercalcemia has been reported in up to 66% of kidney transplant recipients and is most likely mediated by persistent hyperparathyroidism resulting in increased skeletal calcium efflux (42). Treatment of hypercalcemic emergencies in renal failure with bisphosphonates, which are excreted from the kidneys and can be associated with renal toxicity, has been performed and appears to be safe, but there is limited data (43). Denosumab may be another treatment option, especially if the hypercalcemia is refractory to bisphosphonates. However, hypocalcemia can be a consequence of treatment with denosumab (44,45).

Hypocalcemia

Transient hypocalcemia is observed in 41% of kidney transplant recipients within the first postoperative day, possibly due to increased urinary calcium excretion (46), and patients with low PTH and high serum calcium pre-transplantation levels are at higher risk (42). However, the serum calcium levels steadily increase by the second week and stabilize thereafter. Another cause of hypocalcemia in renal transplantation is subtotal parathy-roidectomy or total parathyroidectomy with or with auto-transplantation for tertiary hyperparathyroidism, which can be transient or persistent (47). Recombinant PTH therapy has been reported to potentially benefit patients with severe hypocalcemia both before and after kidney transplantation in such patients (48,49). Antiresorptive osteoporosis therapies which may be utilized in the transplant setting, such as denosumab and potent bisphosphonates, can also be associated with hypocalcemia and patients with CKD are especially at risk (50,51). Other causes of hypocalcemia that may be seen in pre- and post-transplant patients include vitamin D deficiency especially in chronic liver disease or with malabsorption in conditions, such as biliary cirrhosis,

infiltrative hypoparathyroidism associated with hemochromatosis and Wilson's disease, rapid transfusion with large amounts of citrate-containing blood, and renal failure due to reduced calcitriol production or hyperphosphatemia (52). Magnesium deficiency can result in hypocalcemia and may be seen in the context of cyclosporine use, hyperphosphatemia, and ill pre- or post-transplant patients with predisposing medications or conditions (52,53).

Hypophosphatemia

Hypophosphatemia is common shortly after kidney transplant due to increased renal phosphate loss and suppressed calcitriol levels from fibroblast growth factor-23 (FGF-23) (54). Phosphate replacement, however, is generally reserved for when serum phosphate is below 1–1.5 mg/dL (0.32–0.48 mmol/L) unless patients are symptomatic since FGF-23 and phosphorus levels generally return to normal by 1 year after kidney transplant (55).

Conclusions

Solid organ transplant and SCT patients commonly have underlying endocrine conditions, which can be related to both ISDs as well as the severe underlying organ dysfunction. When endocrine emergencies arise in this often critically ill and complex population, there are unique clinical factors that must be considered. The patient's stage in the course of the transplant; pre-transplant, early post-transplant, and chronic post-transplant, also influences the endocrine emergency and management. An understanding of the most common factors associated with endocrine emergencies in transplant patients is important in their management. Also, the effect of end organ dysfunction in the precipitation and management of the specific endocrine crisis should be recognized.

References

1 United Network for Organ Sharing. Data. https://www.unos.org/data/?gclid=Cj0KEQ iAhs3DBRDmu-rVkuif0N8BEiQAWuUJr4 IzabF8_zCKbsgaRpbincBIroX5HfmexrWQC FCZvHMaAljY8P8HAQ (accessed January 16, 2017).

2 Health Resources and Services Administration, U.S. Department of Health and Human Services. Transplant frequently asked questions. https://bloodcell. transplant.hrsa.gov/about/general_faqs/ (accessed January 16, 2017).

3 Wong CJ, Pagalilauan G. Primary care of the solid organ transplant recipient. *Med Clin North Am*. 2015;99:1075–1103.

4 Taylor AL, Watson CJ, Bradley JA. Immunosuppressive agents in solid organ transplantation: Mechanisms of action and therapeutic efficacy. *Crit Rev Oncol Hematol*. 2005;56:23–46.

5 Shaffi K, Uhlig K, Perrone RD, et al. Performance of creatinine-based GFR estimating equations in solid-organ transplant recipients. *Am J Kidney Dis*. 2014;63:1007–1018.

6 Tauchmanova L, Colao A, Lombardi G, Rotoli B, Selleri C. Bone loss and its management in long-term survivors from allogeneic stem cell transplantation. *J Clin Endocrinol Metab*. 2007;92:4536–4545.

7 Sharif A, Cohney S. Post-transplantation diabetes – state of the art. *Lancet Diabetes Endocrinol*. 2016;4:337–349.

8 Montori VM, Basu A, Erwin PJ, Velosa JA, Gabriel SE, Kudva YC. Posttransplantation diabetes: a systematic review of the literature. *Diabetes Care*. 2002;25:583–592.

9 Cho YM, Park KS, Jung HS, Kim YS, Kim SY, Lee HK. A case showing complete insulin independence after severe diabetic ketoacidosis associated with tacrolimus treatment. *Diabetes Care*. 2002;25:1664.

10 Feltracco P, Barbieri S, Galligioni H, Michieletto E, Carollo C, Ori C. Intensive care management of liver transplanted patients. *World J Hepatol*. 2011;3:61–71.

11 Bruderer SG, Bodmer M, Jick SS, Bader G, Schlienger RG, Meier CR. Incidence of and risk factors for severe hypoglycaemia in treated type 2 diabetes mellitus patients in the UK:a nested case-control analysis. *Diabetes Obes Metab*. 2014;16:801–811.

12 Murad MH, Coto-Yglesias F, Wang AT, Sheidaee N, Mullan RJ, Elamin MB, et al. Clinical review: drug-induced hypoglycemia: a systematic review. *J Clin Endocrinol Metab*. 2009;94: 741–745.

13 Rutsky EA, McDaniel HG, Tharpe DL, Alred G, Pek S. Spontaneous hypoglycemia in chronic renal failure. *Arch Intern Med*. 1978;138:1364–1368.

14 Fenves AZ, Schaefer PW, Luther J, Pierce VM. Case records of the Massachusetts General Hospital. Case 21-2016. A 32-year-old man in an unresponsive state. *N Engl J Med*. 2016;375:163–171.

15 Hunter SJ, Daughaday WH, Callender ME, et al. A case of hepatoma associated with hypoglycaemia and overproduction of IGF-II (E-21): beneficial effects of treatment with growth hormone and intrahepatic adriamycin. *Clin Endocrinol (Oxf)*. 1994;41:397–401; discussion 402.

16 Mellinkoff SM, Tumulty PA. Hepatic hypoglycemia; its occurrence in congestive heart failure. *N Engl J Med*. 1952;247: 745–750.

17 Cryer PE. Minireview: glucagon in the pathogenesis of hypoglycemia and hyperglycemia in diabetes. *Endocrinology*. 2012;153:1039–1048.

18 Groth CG, Backman L, Morales JM, et al. Sirolimus (rapamycin)-based therapy in human renal transplantation: similar efficacy and different toxicity compared with cyclosporine. Sirolimus European Renal Transplant Study Group. *Transplantation*. 1999;67:1036–1042.

19 Kella DK, Shoukat S, Sperling L. Plasma exchange for severe hypertriglyceridemia-induced pancreatitis in an orthotopic heart

transplant recipient. *J Clin Lipidol*. 2012;6:474–476.

20 Rodriguez JA, Crespo-Leiro MG, Paniagua MJ, et al. Rhabdomyolysis in heart transplant patients on HMG-CoA reductase inhibitors and cyclosporine. *Transplant Proc*. 1999;31:2522–2523.

21 Meriden Z, Bullock GC, Bagg A, et al. Posttransplantation lymphoproliferative disease involving the pituitary gland. *Hum Pathol*. 2010;41:1641–1645.

22 Vijayvargiya P, Javed I, Moreno J, et al. Pituitary aspergillosis in a kidney transplant recipient and review of the literature. *Transpl Infect Dis*. 2013;15:E196–E200.

23 Leff RS, Martino RL, Pollock WJ, Knight WA, 3rd. Pituitary abscess after autologous bone marrow transplantation. *Am J Hematol*. 1989;31:62–64.

24 Edsbacker S, Andersson T. Pharmacokinetics of budesonide (Entocort EC) capsules for Crohn's disease. *Clin Pharmacokinet*. 2004;43:803–821.

25 Orio F, Muscogiuri G, Palomba S, et al. Endocrinopathies after allogeneic and autologous transplantation of hematopoietic stem cells. *Scientific World Journal*. 2014;282147.

26 Ardalan M, Shoja MM. Cytomegalovirus-induced adrenal insufficiency in a renal transplant recipient. *Transplant Proc*. 2009;41:2915–2916.

27 Kowalczuk-Wieteska A, Baranska-Kosakowska A, Zakliczynski M, Lindon S, Zembala M. Do thyroid disorders affect the postoperative course of patients in the early post-heart transplant period? *Ann Transplant*. 2011;16:77–81.

28 Basaria S, Cooper DS. Amiodarone and the thyroid. *Am J Med*. 2005;118:706–714.

29 Siccama R, Balk AH, de Herder WW, van Domburg R, Vantrimpont P, van Gelder T. Amiodarone therapy before heart transplantation as a predictor of thyroid dysfunction after transplantation. *J Heart Lung Transplant*. 2003;22:857–861.

30 Gough J, Gough IR. Total thyroidectomy for amiodarone-associated thyrotoxicosis

in patients with severe cardiac disease. *World J Surg*. 2006;30:1957–1961.

31 De Leo S, Lee SY, Braverman LE. Hyperthyroidism. *Lancet*. 388:906–918.

32 Sag E, Gonc N, Alikasifoglu A, et al. Hyperthyroidism after allogeneic hematopoietic stem cell transplantation: a report of four cases. *J Clin Res Pediatr Endocrinol*. 7:349–354.

33 Mariani LH, Berns JS. The renal manifestations of thyroid disease. *J Am Soc Nephrol*, 2012; 23:22–26.

34 Burra P. Liver abnormalities and endocrine diseases. *Best Pract Res Clin Gastroentero*. 2013; 27:553–563.

35 Vyas AA, Vyas P, Fillipon NL, Vijayakrishnan R, Trivedi N. Successful treatment of thyroid storm with plasmapheresis in a patient with methimazole-induced agranulocytosis. *Endocr Pract*. 2010; 16:673–676.

36 Stein EM, Shane E. Vitamin D in organ transplantation. *Osteoporos Int*. 2011;22:2107–2118.

37 Kuchay MS, Mishra SK, Farooqui KJ, Bansal B, Wasir JS, Mithal A. Hypercalcemia of advanced chronic liver disease: a forgotten clinical entity! *Clin Cases Miner Bone Metab* 13:15–18

38 Gerhardt A, Greenberg A, Reilly JJ, Jr., Van Thiel DH. Hypercalcemia. A complication of advanced chronic liver disease. *Arch Intern Med*. 1987;147:274–277.

39 Abe Y, Makiyama H, Fujita Y, Tachibana Y, Kamada G, Uebayashi M. Severe hypercalcemia associated with hepatocellular carcinoma secreting intact parathyroid hormone: a case report. *Intern Med*. 2011;50:329–333.

40 Tamura K, Kubota K, Take H, Kurabayashi H, Shirakura T. Parathyroid hormone-related peptide as a possible cause of hypercalcemia in a hepatocellular carcinoma patient. *Am J Gastroenterol*. 1994;89:644–645.

41 Sultan ER, Sharif S, Shah AA. Parathyroid hormone related peptide causing hypercalcaemia in a patient with hepatocellular carcinoma. *J Pak Med Assoc* 63:263–264.

42 Evenepoel P, Van Den Bergh B, Naesens M, et al. Calcium metabolism in the early posttransplantation period. *Clin J Am Soc Nephrol.* 2009;4:665–672.

43 Machado CE, Flombaum CD. Safety of pamidronate in patients with renal failure and hypercalcemia. *Clin Nephrol.* 1996;45:175–179.

44 Hu MI, Glezerman IG, Leboulleux S, et al. Denosumab for treatment of hypercalcemia of malignancy. *J Clin Endocrinol Metab.* 2014;99:3144–3152.

45 de Beus E, Boer WH. Denosumab for treatment of immobilization-related hypercalcaemia in a patient with advanced renal failure. *Clin Kidney J.* 2012;566–571.

46 Nobata H, Tominaga Y, Imai H, Uchida K. Hypocalcemia immediately after renal transplantation. *Clin Transplant.* 2013;27:E644–E648.

47 Triponez F, Clark OH, Vanrenthergem Y, Evenepoel P. Surgical treatment of persistent hyperparathyroidism after renal transplantation. *Ann Surg* 2008;248:18–30.

48 Hod T, Riella LV, Chandraker A. Recombinant PTH therapy for severe hypoparathyroidism after kidney transplantation in pre-transplant parathyroidectomized patients: review of the literature and a case report. *Clin Transplant.* 2015;29:951–957.

49 Nogueira EL, Costa AC, Santana A, et al. Teriparatide efficacy in the treatment of severe hypocalcemia after kidney transplantation in parathyroidectomized patients: a series of five case reports. *Transplantation.* 2011;92:316–320.

50 Wada Y, Iyoda M, Iseri K, et al. Combination therapy of denosumab and calcitriol for a renal transplant recipient with severe bone loss due to therapy-resistant hyperparathyroidism. *Tohoku J Exp Med.* 2016;238:205–212.

51 Torregrosa JV. Dramatic increase in parathyroid hormone and hypocalcaemia after denosumab in a kidney transplanted patient. *Clin Kidney J.* 2013;6:122.

52 Shaffer AL, Shoback D. Hypocalcemia: definition, etiology, pathogenesis, diagnosis, and management. In: Rosen C, ed. *Primer on the Metabolic Bone Diseases and Disorders of Mineral Metabolism. Eigth ed.* Ames, Iowa: John Wiley & Sons, Inc.; 2013: 572–578.

53 Ebeling PR, Thomas DM, Erbas B, Hopper JL, Szer J, Grigg AP. Mechanisms of bone loss following allogeneic and autologous hemopoietic stem cell transplantation. *J Bone Miner Res.* 1999;14:342–350.

54 Evenepoel P, Naesens M, Claes K, Kuypers D, Vanrenterghem Y. Tertiary "hyperphosphatoninism" accentuates hypophosphatemia and suppresses calcitriol levels in renal transplant recipients. *Am J Transplant.* 2007;7:1193–1200.

55 Taweesedt PT, Disthabanchong S. Mineral and bone disorder after kidney transplantation. *World J Transplant.* 2015;5:231–242.

11

Endocrine and Metabolic Changes with Aging

Endocrin-Aging: Recognizing and Managing Care in Older Frail Persons

Angela M. Abbatecola and John E. Morley

Key Points

- Global demographics have consistently underlined a substantial growing trend in the number of elderly persons worldwide. The presence of persons over the age of 65 is projected to increase from 8% in 2012 to 16% by 2050.
- A number of physiological changes in circulating hormones occur with aging. Some of these changes, e.g., low testosterone and 25(OH) vitamin D, insulin-like growth factor-1 and elevated cortisol, play a role in the development of sarcopenia (loss of muscle mass) and frailty.
- The presentation of endocrine disorders in older persons is often subtle and the diagnosis is easily missed.
- Diabetes mellitus is the most common endocrine disorder. New consensus guidelines have suggested that hypoglycemia needs to be avoided, and for healthy older persons glycosylated hemoglobin (HgbA$_{1C}$) targets should be between 7.0–7.5% (53–59 mmol/mol); for the frail, 7.0–8.0% (53–64 mmol/mol); and in persons with dementia, 7.5–8.5% (59–69 mmol/mol). However, all glycemic targets should be individualized.

- Cognitive dysfunction is very common in older people and formal testing needs to be carried out in all persons with diabetes and other conditions to be certain they can follow the clinician's instructions.
- End-of-life care generally focuses on the care of a person in the last two years of their life. Patients with diabetes who are at the end-of-life have a unique set of care needs which includes tailoring glucose-lowering therapy to minimize diabetes-related adverse treatment effects; avoiding metabolic decompensation and diabetes-related emergencies; avoidance of acute foot complications in frail, bed-bound patients with diabetes; avoidance of symptomatic clinical dehydration; and supporting and maintaining the empowerment of the individual patient (in their diabetes self-management) and carers to the last possible stage.
- Common endocrine emergencies in older persons include hyponatremia, hypoglycemia, hyperglycemia, adrenal insufficiency, hypercalcemia, myxedema coma, and rarely thyroid storm.

Introduction

Over the last century, global demographics have consistently underlined a substantial growing trend in the number of elderly persons worldwide. The presence of persons over the age of 65 is projected to increase from 8% in 2012 to 16% by 2050

Endocrine and Metabolic Medical Emergencies: A Clinician's Guide, Second Edition. Edited by Glenn Matfin.
© 2018 John Wiley & Sons Ltd. Published 2018 by John Wiley & Sons Ltd.

Table 11-1   Changes in hormones with aging

Endocrine gland	Increased	Decreased
Pituitary	Follicle stimulating hormone Luteinizing hormone (Females) Corticotropin Oxytocin Thyrotropin (in some long-lived populations)	Growth hormone Luteinizing hormone (Males) Arginine vasopressin (at night)
Thyroid	–	Triiodothyronine (T_3) Calcitonin
Parathyroid	Parathyroid hormone	–
Adrenal	Cortisol Aldosterone	Dehydroepiandrosterone Pregnenolone
Pancreas	Insulin (early) Amylin Glucagon	Insulin (late)
Gonads	–	Estrogen (female) Testosterone (male)
Autonomic nervous system	Norepinephrine	–
Liver and muscle	–	Insulin growth factor-1
Gastrointestinal tract	Cholecystokinin	–

(https://www.census.gov/content/dam/Census/library/publications/2016/demo/p95-16-1.pdf) and those over the age of 80 (the "oldest-old") are projected to grow more rapidly than the older population itself. This growth is predicted to have a large increase of oldest-old within the world's older population, from 16% in 2000 to 24% in 2040, especially in developed countries.

A number of physiological changes in circulating hormones occur with aging (Table 11-1) (1). Some of these changes, e.g., low testosterone and 25(OH) vitamin D, insulin-like growth factor-1 (IGF-1), and elevated cortisol, play a role in the development of sarcopenia (loss of muscle mass) and frailty. Insulin resistance with aging leads to an increase in metabolic syndrome and type 2 diabetes mellitus in older persons. Increases in aldosterone and vasopressin can lead to hypertension and hyponatremia, respectively. Hip fractures are associated not only with the decline in bone and muscle mass, but also due to delirium, which can be due to hypothyroidism, hypoandrenalism, vitamin B_{12} deficiency, hyponatremia, and

hypercalcemia. Finally, diseases such as sleep apnea, which are very common in older persons can lead to hypertension, hyperglycemia, and osteoporosis, due to an increase in cortisol, aldosterone, and catecholamines.

This chapter will focus on endocrine emergencies that are common in older persons. In particular, different presentations that often occur in older persons will be stressed as will the difficulty in diagnosing *hypo*-endocrine disorders whose symptoms can be similar to some of the common changes in normal aging.

Pituitary Dysfunction in the Elderly

The anterior and the posterior lobes of the pituitary gland undergo subtle changes during advanced aging. In particular, the anterior lobe undergoes changes mainly due to fibrosis and vascular alterations. Depending on the degree of clinical consequences of such alterations, treatment may be necessary. Even though fibrosis and vascular alterations may lead to hypopituitarism, most of the causes of hypopituitarism in the elderly are similar to those in younger populations. In older persons, pituitary cell destruction causes more than 95% of hypopituitarism. There is an increase in the percentage of pituitary adenomas found in the elderly (2). Clinical presentation is often insidious, being characterized by non-specific manifestations, such as weight loss, fatigue, reduced appetite, low muscle strength, or hypotension. Considering that many of these signs overlap with those of normal aging, hypopituitarism can be easily underdiagnosed in the elderly.

Usually, hypopituitarism is rarely life-threatening, but evolution may be more dramatic due to pituitary apoplexy. Large adenomas can also compress anterior pituitary cells, thus leading to an insufficient secretion of hormones (3). Pituitary tumors can compress the optic chiasm leading to bitemporal hemianopia. With aging, bitemporal hemianopia is the most common visual field defect with pituitary tumors (which are often large non-functioning adenomas), however, this often goes undiagnosed because visual disturbances related to compression are often attributed to other common causes of visual disturbance in this population (e.g., cataracts, amblyopia, and retinal detachment). This can lead to delayed clinical diagnosis of a pituitary tumor. Other causes of hypopituitarism include infection, traumatic brain injury, cerebral ischemia, which in turn leads to decreased blood supply to pituitary vascularization. Older persons can be afflicted with diverse comorbidities with polypharmacy, which may in turn impact hormonal metabolism (2). The clinical features related to hypopituitarism are related to deficiencies in corticotropin (ACTH), thyrotropin (TSH), follicle stimulating hormone (FSH), luteinizing hormone (LH), growth hormone (GH), sex hormones (estrogen or testosterone) and antidiuretic hormone (ADH, also termed vasopressin).

With aging, there are changes in the circadian rhythm of the release of hypothalamic releasing hormones. This can lead to a reduction in LH and secondary hypogonadism in males. The circadian rhythm changes also lead to an increase in ACTH at night, resulting in a mild increase in cortisol and aldosterone (4). Stressors can also alter the release of hypothalamic hormones with the classical example of hypoxia associated with sleep apnea leading to an increase in cortisol and aldosterone with associated hypertension and hyperglycemia.

Hypothyroidism

Hypothyroidism is more common in older women than in men. Primary hypothyroidism is a more common finding among older adults related to decline in thyroid function and autoimmune disease. Numerous factors have been shown to have diverse degrees of implications on pituitary-thyroid function in old age. There is a generally a fall in free triiodothyronine (FT_3) and TSH, while free thyroxine (FT_4) levels remain preserved. It is important to recall that chronic fatigue, obesity, type 2 diabetes mellitus, and diverse drugs can increase TSH secretion (5), while other common conditions including decreased exercise, use of glucocorticoids (6), iodine, L-DOPA, and depression can inhibit TSH secretion. There is very little clinical evidence that the thyroid hormone effects associated with physiological changes of aging significantly play a role in the development of frailty (7). A subgroup of older persons have mildly elevated TSH levels due to an abnormal TSH. These persons tend to live longer than others and their TSH should not be suppressed.

Symptoms of hypothyroidism are more subtle in older persons and often mimic normal aging complaints. Common symptoms are weight gain, fatigue, hair loss, non-pitting edema, macroglossia, hoarse voice, constipation, memory loss, depression, hypertension, and bradycardia (8). The presence of a goiter or a surgical scar in the neck increases the possibility of hypothyroidism.

Treatment is required to prevent potential dangerous clinical outcomes (myxedema coma, heart failure, hyponatremia, hypothermia). In primary hypothyroidism, levothyroxine dosage should be sufficient to bring TSH into the normal range. In patients with central hypothyroidism, levothyroxine replacement treatment is required and titrated to bring FT_4 levels into the 3rd–4th quartile of target range (9). Levothyroxine should not be used in patients with untreated/undiagnosed adrenal insufficiency, because thyroid hormones may induce acute adrenal crisis by increasing the metabolic clearance of glucocorticoids. In order to prevent adrenal crisis, patients should receive glucocorticoid therapy as indicated before starting thyroid hormonal therapy (10). Alternatively, consideration for excluding adrenal insufficiency by appropriate testing should occur prior to starting thyroxine therapy in both patients with primary or secondary hypothyroidism.

Myxedema coma is a severe form of hypothyroidism with delirium or coma, pericardial effusion, seizures, toxic megacolon, hypothermia, hypoventilation, and bradycardia (11). It is often precipitated by diseases such as infection, myocardial infarction, stroke, trauma, or drugs. Mortality rates range between 25–50%. Treatment involves careful fluid replacement. Hypertonic saline may be needed for severe hyponatremia, but care needs to be taken not to elevate sodium too rapidly (risk of osmotic demyelination syndrome). Hypothermia is treated with external warming. In persons with hypotension, intravenous hydrocortisone (e.g., 50 mg every 6 hours) can be given until it is confirmed that they do not have adrenal insufficiency. Parenteral levothyroxine (loading dose of 200 µg followed by 100 µg daily) is the treatment of choice. Liothyronine (T_3) can be given to obtain a more rapid response.

Hyperthyroidism

With aging, the thyroid gland reduces its production of thyroxine, but circulating levels remain normal because there is a decreased thyroxine clearance. Older persons, therefore, usually need a lower replacement dose of levothyroxine (75 mcg compared to 125 mcg in young persons). Failure to do this can lead to osteoporosis, muscle loss, tachycardia, atrial fibrillation, and heart failure, and should be monitored by TSH levels.

Older persons have fewer symptoms with hyperthyroidism compared to younger persons but are more likely to have fatigue, weight loss, atrial fibrillation, dyspnea, depression and, in some cases, rather than lid lag, they have blepharitis. In older persons, toxic multinodular goiter is more common than Graves' disease. Thyroiditis can produce short-term hyperthyroidism. Amiodarone, an antiarrythmic drug, can produce hyperthyroidism (and hypothyroidism) and its use is questionable in older persons, but when used needs close monitoring.

A low TSH (<0.5 mU/L) usually is indicative of hyperthyroidism (either clinical with elevated FT_4 and/or FT_3; or subclinical with normal FT_4 and FT_3) but can also occur in persons with non-thyroidal illness syndrome. Diagnosis can be confirmed by obtaining a FT_4 and FT_3 sample.

Thyroid storm (crisis) is associated with tachycardia, tremor, hypertension, sweating, diarrhea, and hyperpyrexia; often with confusion and/or coma in older persons. Treatment requires a beta-blocker and anti-thyroid medications (propylthiouracil or methimizole [carbimazole]). Iodine compounds can be given to block the release from the thyroid gland of thyroid hormones but only after anti-thyroid drugs given. This can be done by giving intravenous radio-contrast dyes, e.g., ipodate and iopanoate (if available) or alternative iodine formulations. Glucocorticoids can be given to reduce the conversion of T_4 (pro hormone) to T_3 (active hormone). Plasmapharesis can be used to treat thyroid storm.

Primary Adrenal Insufficiency (Addison's Disease)

This is a rare condition being present in 1 in 25,000 persons. Symptoms are non-specific with weakness, fatigue, abdominal pain, darkening of skin and weight loss.

Causes include autoimmune, tuberculosis, sepsis, adrenal hemorrhage, metastases into the adrenal glands, adrenal amyloidosis. Diagnosis should be suspected in a person with hypotension, increased potassium, low sodium, hypoglycemia, hypercalcemia, and eosinophilia. Adrenal crisis is a medical emergency which can present with nausea and vomiting, abdominal pain, hypotension, hypoglycemia, delirium, fever, and seizures. Diagnosis is made by injecting 250 µg synthetic ACTH (synacthen or cosyntropin) IV or IM and measuring serum cortisol at 30 or 60 minutes. Stimulated cortisol should be >500 nmol/L (18 µg/dL). Acute treatment requires large volumes of a glucose saline solution and intravenous glucocorticoids. Maintenance therapy requires oral glucocorticoids (hydrocortisone or prednisone) and in some cases fludrocortisone for aldosterone deficiency. When patients become ill, they need to increase their dosage and if vomiting, intravenous hydrocortisone should be given.

Type 2 Diabetes Mellitus

The prevalence of type 2 diabetes mellitus is increasing on a worldwide scale due to the substantial increase in number of older persons. It has been reported that over 25% of the US population aged ≥65 years has diabetes (12). Diabetes in older adults is associated with higher mortality, reduced functional status, and increased risk of institutionalization (13). Clinical recognition may pose unique challenges because many age-related physiological changes can disguise the presentation of diabetes and make its diagnosis tricky. The onset of type 2 diabetes is often slow and insidious, and symptoms typical of hyperglycemia, such as polyuria, polydipsia and polyphagia may not be present (14). More common symptoms in older persons include dry mouth, confusion, urinary incontinence, weight loss, and fatigue.

Once diabetes is diagnosed, it remains fundamental to assess the patient's overall health status in order to adapt an anti-diabetic

Table 11-2 Conditions common in older persons with diabetes

- Frailty
- Sarcopenia
- Cognitive decline
- Dehydration
- Pain associated with hyperglycemia
- Functional disability
- Urinary incontinence
- Falls
- Hip fractures
- Infections
- Cataracts
- Pressure sores
- Orthostatic hypotension
- Syncope

treatment strategy. Older persons have numerous and overlapping conditions that complicate managing diabetes. Not only micro- and macrovascular complications of type 2 diabetes have been related to frailty syndrome, but combined metabolic alterations (hypo- and hyperglycemic excursions) are associated with an increased risk for cognitive decline, dementia, falls, bone fractures, and deterioration in muscle function and mass (Table 11-2) (15).

There is growing literature on the difficulties faced when treating frailty mechanisms in older persons with diabetes. Clinicians need to quickly recognize not only type 2 diabetes mellitus, but also need to establish glycemic goals to avoid the irreversible downward spiral of the frailty syndrome. Due to little evidence for specific glycemic and glycosylated hemoglobin levels (HgbA$_{1C}$), data are based on expert opinion and data extrapolation. Various guidelines directly aimed at treating older patients include recommendations from the International Association of Gerontology and Geriatrics (IAGG) (16, 17). Other guidelines such as the American Diabetes Association (ADA) (18), or the ADA/European Association for the Study of Diabetes (EASD)(19), suggest adjustments to their algorithms when treating older patients and was supported in a recent editorial (20) (Table 11-3).

Table 11-3 Modern targets for glycosylated hemoglobin (HbA$_{1C}$) in older persons with diabetes (Targets should be individualized) (18–20)

Status	HbA$_1$C
Healthy elderly	7.0–7.5% (53–59 mmol/mol)
Frail elderly	7.0–8% (53–64 mmol/mol)
Dementia	7.5–8.5% (59–69 mmol/mol)
Nursing home	7.5–8.5% (59–69 mmol/mol)

At the moment, the most validated approach toward obtaining specific glycemic control in older persons is to use an individualized one (21). Intensive glycemic control has been shown to be more harmful than beneficial mainly due to severe hypoglycemic outcomes especially in older persons with frailty syndrome. The complexity of managing diabetes in older frail patients should not only be aimed at correcting chronic hyperglycemia, but also at avoiding severe hypoglycemia. Physical exercise, especially resistance exercise, is a key to treatment of diabetes mellitus. Therapeutic diets in older persons have been shown to be inefficacious and increase mortality rate (22). Available anti-diabetic agents according to potential use in frail older persons are reported in Table 11-4. Clinicians must consider associated comorbidities, drug interactions, geriatric syndromes, as well as functional and cognitive abilities when planning anti-diabetic treatment options. The underlying goal for older frail elders is to maintain the best quality of life.

It is important to recognize that poor cognition is very common in persons with diabetes mellitus (23). Numerous studies, both experimental and clinical, have clearly shown that alterations of the insulin-signaling pathway in neurons are associated with cognitive decline and dementia over aging. Persons with cognitive dysfunction need to have instructions clearly written down and they need to make their caregiver aware of these instructions. The Rapid Cognitive Screen can be used in the emergency department to recognize these diabetic patients requiring extra time when establishing a discharge plan (Figure 11-1).

Hyperglycemic Crisis

Older persons most commonly present with hyperglycemic hyperosmolar state (HHS) but a subset will have diabetic ketoacidosis (DKA). Ketones are present in the urine with both presentations (but <2+ in HHS). The diagnosis of DKA requires an arterial or venous pH <7.3, bicarbonate of <15 mmol/L and an elevated serum beta-hydroxybutyrate (24). HHS is diagnosed with a glucose >600 mg/dL (33 mmol/L), serum osmolality >320 mOm/kg and serum ketones <3.0 mmol/L. Common causes of hyperglycemic crisis include infection, myocardial infarction, and inadequate insulin treatment often due to non-adherence.

Treatment includes fluid resuscitation with 0.9% saline. Persons with elevated serum sodium should receive 0.45% saline. In older persons, care needs to be taken not to produce fluid overload and pulmonary edema. Insulin is given intravenously and dose is adjusted hourly dependent on glucose levels (as per local guidelines). In DKA, 5% dextrose should be added to saline when blood glucose is below 200 mg/dL (11 mmol/L). Levels of serum potassium should be closely monitored and replaced when appropriate.

Lactic acidosis can occur in persons with diabetes receiving metformin or who have severe hypoxia. It is defined as a high calculated anion gap (>12 mmol/L) with a lactate level >5.0 mmol/L. The treatment is supportive care, bicarbonate therapy (even though the literature has conflicting results about its benefit), and hemodialysis to remove metformin.

Hypoglycemia

Hypoglycemia causes tremors, sweating, palpitations, anxiety, hunger, irritability, delirium, and coma. The common causes are overtreatment with insulin or sulfonylureas (deintensification or simplification

Table 11-4 Advantages and disadvantages of different anti-diabetic agents in frailty

Anti-diabetic agent	Advantages	Disadvantages	Use in frailty
Biguanide (metformin)	Low risk of hypoglycemia	Risk of lactic acidosis; GI disturbances; B12 deficiency	++++
Metiglinides (repaglinide, nateglinide)	Rapid action; Short half-life; Weight gain	Hypoglycemia; Contraindicated in hepatic failure	+++ ++(low appetite)
Sulfonylureas 1st generation (chlorpropamide)	None	Very high risk of severe hypoglycemia	No indications
Sulfonylureas 2nd generation (glimepiride, glipizide, glyburide, gliclazide)	Rapid action; Weight gain	High risk of severe hypoglycemia (especially prolonged with glyburide); Contraindicated in hepatic failure	++
α-glucosidase inhibitors(acarbose, miglitol)	Low risk of hypoglycemia	GI disturbances; Contraindicated in renal failure	++
DPP-4 inhibitors (sitagliptin, vildagliptin, saxagliptin, linagliptin, alogliptin)	Low risk of hypoglycemia	Limited data on long-term use; cost	+++
Thiazolidinediones (pioglitazone)	Low risk of hypoglycemia; Improve dyslipidemia (HDL and TG); Weight gain	Fluid retention; Risk of bone fracture; Heart failure	+
SGLT2 inhibitors (canagliflozin#, empagliflozin#, Dapagliflozin*)	Low risk of hypoglycemia	Urinary tract infections; No use in chronic kidney disease Stages 3–5* or 3B–5#; Weight loss; Dehydration; Orthostatic hypotension	Unknown; Lack of data in elderly; Weight loss not indicated in frailty
GLP-1 agonists	Low risk of hypoglycemia	Weight loss	No indications
Insulin	Rapidly effective; Easy dose adjustments; Potential weight gain	Daily glucose monitoring; Multiple daily injections; Problems for cognitively impaired; Self-administration	+++

of complex regimens is recommended), missing meals, infection, Addison's disease, insulinoma, or tumors producing insulin-like factors, carcinomas, and renal and liver failure. Medications that precipitate hypoglycemia include pentamidine, sulfamethoxazole, and trimethoprim. Beta-blockers can mask the symptoms of hypoglycemia.

Recall: Five objects Apple, Pen, Tie, House, Car. [Recall objects after clock drawing: 5 points]

Clock Drawing: Draw with time at ten minutes to eleven o'clock. [4 points]

Insight: Jill was a very successful stockbroker. She made a lot of money on the stock market. She then met Jack, a devastatingly handsome man. She married him and had three children. They lived in Rome. She then stopped work and stayed at home to bring up her children. When they were teenagers, she went back to work. She and Jack lived happily ever after.

What country did they live in? [1 point]

Figure 11-1 The Rapid Cognitive Screen (RCS) – International Version (0–5 = dementia; 6–7 = Mild Cognitive Impairment (MCI); 8–10 = normal). From (39).

Hypercalcemia

The classical signs of hypercalcemia are "painful bones, renal stones, abdominal groans and psychic moans." However, the vast majority of older persons with hypercalcemia suffer a much more subtle effect. These include cognitive impairment (delirium), anorexia, weight loss, polyuria, indigestion (high calcium releases gastrin), constipation, fatigue, muscle weakness, dehydration, cardiac arrhythmias, depression, and hypertension. The highest incidence of hyperparathyroidism in the United States occurs between 65–74 years (63.2 per 100,000 person-years) (25). Hypercalcemia is more common in women than men. Because calcium is bound to albumin, it is essential that the calcium level is corrected for the circulating albumin level.

The most common cause of hypercalcemia in the in-hospital setting is malignancy, especially multiple myeloma, breast or lung cancer. This can be due to hormonal factors (such as parathyroid hormone-related peptide) or direct destruction of bone by metastases. Primary hyperparathyroidism due to an adenoma or hyperplasia of the parathyroid gland is the most common cause of hypercalcemia in the outpatient setting. Other causes of hypercalcemia include hyperthyroidism, hypervitaminosis D, milk-alkali syndrome, Addison's disease, granulomatosis diseases (sarcoid, tuberculosis, lepromatous leprosy, berylliosis, histoplasmosis, and coccidiomycosis), and drug-induced (lithium, vitamin A, thiazide diuretic) (26).

The treatment of symptomatic hypercalcemia in the emergency department is fluid resuscitation with 0.9% saline. Furosemide may be considered to increase urinary calcium excretion, but only after adequate fluid replacement. Bisphosphonates (pamidronate, zolendronic acid) are the drugs of choice for hypercalcemia. They bind to hydroxyapatite and prevent osteoclast attachment to the bone matrix. Denosumab prevents RANK-ligand activation of osteoclasts. It can be used to treat hypercalcemia of malignancy that is refractory to zolendronic acid therapy. Cinacalcet activates the parathyroid calcium-sensing receptor and can be used in parathyroid carcinoma or primary or tertiary hyperparathyroidism to decrease serum calcium. Any drugs that may be increasing serum calcium (e.g., thiazides, vitamin D and calcium supplements) should be held and stopped if possible.

Sarcopenia and Hormones

Sarcopenia is a major predictor of frailty, hip fracture, disability, and mortality in older persons. Hormones play an integral role in maintaining muscle integrity and volume. Anabolic hormones shift the anabolic/catabolic equilibrium of protein metabolism toward the synthesis of new proteins in order to replace the proteins that are continuously catabolized. Hypertrophy requires the proliferation of muscle nuclei (hyperplasia) in order to maintain the nuclear/cytoplasmic ratio. Hormonal factors that have been associated with muscle hypertrophy include: IGF-1, GH, testosterone and dehydroepiandrosterone (DHEA). High IGF-1 concentrations are associated with characteristics that are opposite to those typical of aging, including decreased body fat content, increased muscle mass, and improved metabolic homeostasis of glucose and lipids. At the muscular level, IGF-1 stimulates protein synthesis and satellite cell differentiation in order to maintain muscle mass and function. Circulating IGF-1 concentrations decrease with advancing age. The age-associated decline in IGF-1 plasma concentrations is influenced by reduced GH levels, and also by nutritional status, insulin, and inflammatory cytokines. Specifically, the biological activity of IGF-1 on muscle strength is inhibited by increased Interleukin-6 (IL-6) activity (27). In skeletal muscle, IGF-1 stimulates the rate of protein synthesis via two ways: IGF-1 increases the rate of mRNA transcription of myofilaments such as α-skeletal actin, a major constituent of the muscle contractile apparatus (28); and IGF-1 stimulates the phosphatidylinositol 3 kinase (PI3-K)/Akt (also known as protein kinase B) pathway which activates the mammalian target of rapamycin (mTOR). Furthermore, higher concentrations of pro-inflammatory cytokines found in older persons directly interfere with the IGF-1 gene protein expression and receptor sensibility in muscles (29). High IL-6 and low IGF-1 plasma concentrations are considered risk factors for poor muscle strength, poor lower extremity performance and disability.

The aging process is not only associated with the loss of many anabolic signals to muscle function, but also with an increase in catabolic signals. In fact, impairment of the anabolic IGF-1 signaling pathway has negative effects:

1. Reduced physical activity that is often observed in advanced age causes decreased stretch-activation stimulation of different muscle isoforms of IGF-1.
2. Loss of motor neurons that are essential for skeletal muscle functioning leads to atrophy and increased proteolysis.
3. The progressive loss of appetite with reduced food intake can result in malnutrition and eventually "wasting."
4. An age-related decline of GH influences IGF-1 muscle response.

Other than the age-related decline in GH and IGF-1 levels, there is strong evidence that the dysregulation of GH and IGF-1 on post-receptor signaling strongly contributes

to muscle mass loss (30). Their reduced intracellular signaling efficiency leads to lower muscle mass and strength, decreased protein synthesis, increased proteolytic genes, and increased cell apoptosis leading to reduced exercise capacity, as well as an increased risk for falls and fractures.

Unfortunately, treatment with GH has demonstrated many adverse effects such as, peripheral edema, arthralgias, glucose intolerance, and type 2 diabetes (31). A recent study showed that GH replacement therapy resulted in an increase in the skeletal muscle protein synthesis and mitochondrial biogenesis pathways (32). However, more studies are needed to verify the use of GH in older frail adults.

Testosterone affects muscle mass and muscle strength. Due to evidence that testosterone levels decline with advancing age, a negative impact on muscle function is not surprising. Older men with low circulating levels of testosterone tend to have lower muscle strength than men of the same age with normal testosterone, and a study utilizing supplemental therapy with testosterone showed improved muscle mass and strength in elderly hypogonadal males (33). However, the widespread use of testosterone replacement remains controversial due to safety concerns and inconsistent reports regarding clinically important outcome measures.

The production and the circulating levels of adrenal sex hormone precursors, DHEA and DHEA sulphate (DHEAS), significantly decline with aging. The mechanism by which DHEA acts on muscle function is probably related to the peripheral conversion to testosterone and dihydrotestosterone, but a direct effect of DHEAS cannot be excluded since specific receptors have been identified in muscle tissue. A recent nutrition and exercise intervention study showed significantly greater increases in DHEAS compared to IGF-1 (34)

Estrogen levels also decline with aging. Although estrogen has a direct anabolic effect on muscle cells *in vitro*, several authors believe that the effect of estrogen on muscle is mediated by their conversion to testosterone

(35). Interestingly, both estrogen and testosterone are capable of inhibiting IL-6 production, suggesting that an age-related decline of such hormones would play a pivotal role on catabolic signaling on muscle tissue. However, the available information regarding the effects of supplemental therapy of estrogen on muscle function is limited due to the facts that outcomes have not shown any significant impact on muscle mass or strength in postmenopausal women (36). At the moment, the identification of specific "hormonal" drugs to successfully treat muscle deterioration in older frail individuals is eagerly awaited.

Conclusions

The presentation of endocrine disorders in older persons is often subtle and the diagnosis is easily missed. Diabetes mellitus is the most common endocrine disorder. New consensus guidelines have suggested that hypoglycemia needs to be avoided and glycemic targets should be individualized. Cognitive dysfunction is very common in older persons and formal testing needs to be carried out in all persons with diabetes and other conditions to be certain they can follow the clinician's instructions. Patients with diabetes who are at the end-of-life have a unique set of care needs (37). These include tailoring glucose-lowering therapy to minimize diabetes-related adverse treatment effects; avoiding metabolic decompensation and diabetes-related emergencies; avoidance of acute foot complications in frail, bed-bound patients with diabetes; avoidance of symptomatic clinical dehydration; and supporting and maintaining the empowerment of the individual patient (in their diabetes self-management) and carers to the last possible stage (18, 37). For example, in a recent VA study of 20,329 hospice patients (83% 100-day mortality) with type 2 diabetes, 12% overall experienced hypoglycemia; and approximately 5% overall severe hypoglycemia (BG <50 mg/dL; 2.8 mmol/L). For those patients treated with insulin, the figures were 38% and 18% respectively. Only 12% of patients overall had HbA1c >8%. These results reflect the need to relax and/or discontinue diabetes medication(s) to reduce suffering due to hypoglycemia among hospice patients with type 2 diabetes (38).

Common endocrine emergencies in older persons include hyponatremia, hypoglycemia, hyperglycemia, adrenal insufficiency, hypercalcemia, myxedema coma, and rarely thyroid storm.

References

1 Mooradian AD, Morley JE, Korenman SG. Endocrinology in aging. *Dis Mon.* 1988;34:393-461.

2 Turner HE, Adams CBT, Wass JAH. Pituitary tumours in the elderly: a 20-year experience. *Eur J Endocrinol.* 1999;140: 383–389.

3 Minniti G, Esposito V, Piccirilli M, et al. Diagnosis and management of pituitary tumours in the elderly: a review based on personal experience and evidence of literature. *Eur J Endocrinol.* 2005;153(6): 723–735.

4 Gupta D, Morley JE. Hypothalamic-pituitary-adrenal (HPA) axis and aging. *Compr Physiol.* 2014;4:1495–1510.

5 Pinchera A, Mariotti S, Barbesino G, et al. Thyroid autoimmunity and ageing. *Horm Res.* 1995;43:64–68.

6 Alkemade A, Unmehopa UA, Wiersinga WM, et al. Flucocorticoids decrease thyrotropin-releasing hormone messenger ribonucleic acid expression in the paraventricular nucleus of the human hypothalamus. *J Clin Endocrinol Metab.* 2005;90:323–327.

7 Morley JE. Hormones and the aging process. *J Am Geriatr Soc.* 2003;51(7 Suppl):S333–S337.

8 Dominguez LJ, Bevilacqua M, Dibella G, Barbagallo M. Diagnosing and managing thyroid disease in the nursing home.

J Am Med Dir Assoc. 2008;9(1): 9–17.

9 Persani L, Ferretti E, Borgato S, et al. Circulating thyrotropin bioactivity in sporadic central hypothyroidism. *J Clin Endocrinol Metab.* 2000;85(10):3631–3635.

10 Kim SY. Diagnosis and treatment of hypopituitarism. *Endocrinol Metab.* 2015;30:443–455.

11 Faggiano A, Del Prete M, Marciello F, et al. Thyroid disease in elderly. *Minerva Endocrinol* 2011;38(3):211–231.

12 Centers for Disease Control and Prevention. *National Diabetes Fact Sheet: General Information and National Estimates on Diabetes in the United States, 2011.* Atlanta, Georgia, U.S. Department of Health and Human Services, Centers for Disease Control and Prevention, 2011.

13 Brown AF, Mangione CM, Saliba D, Sarkisian CA; California Healthcare Foundation/American Geriatrics Society Panel on Improving Care for Elders with Diabetes. Guidelines for improving the care of the older person with diabetes mellitus. *J Am Geriatr Soc.* 2003;51(Suppl. Guidelines):S265–S280.

14 Meneilly GS, Tessier D. Diabetes in older adults. *J Gerontol A Biol Sci Med Sci.* 2001;56(1):M5–M13.

15 Morley JE. The complexities of diabetes in older persons. *J Am Med Dir Assoc.* 2016;17:872–874.

16 Sinclair A, Morley JE, Rodriguez-Mañas L, et al. Diabetes mellitus in older people: position statement on behalf of the International Association of Gerontology and Geriatrics (IAGG), the European Diabetes Working Party for Older People (EDWPOP), and the International Task Force of Experts in Diabetes. *J Am Med Dir Assoc.* 2012; 13(6): 497–502.

17 Brown AF, Mangione CM, Saliba D, Sarkisian CA; California Healthcare Foundation/American Geriatrics Society Panel on Improving Care for Elders with Diabetes. Guidelines for improving the care of the older person with diabetes mellitus. *J Am Geriatr Soc.* 2003;51(5 Suppl Guidelines): S265–S280.

18 American Diabetes Association. Standards of medical care in diabetes: 2018. *Diabetes Care.* 2018;41(Suppl 1):S1–S159.

19 Inzucchi SE, Bergenstal RM, Buse JB, et al. (2015) Management of hyperglycaemia in type 2 diabetes, 2015: a patient-centred approach. Update to a position statement of the American Diabetes Association and the European Association for the Study of Diabetes. *Diabetologia.* 58, 429–442.

20 Kalyani RR, Golden SH, Cefalu WT. Diabetes and aging: unique considerations and goals of care. *Diabetes Care.* 2017;40:440–443.

21 Abbatecola AM, Paolisso G, Sinclair AJ. Treating diabetes mellitus in older and oldest old patients. *Curr Pharm Des.* 2015;21(13):1665–1671.

22 Tariq SH, Karcic E, Thomas DR, et al. The use of a non-concentrated-sweets diet in the management of type 2 diabetes in nursing homes. *J Am Diet Assoc.* 2001;101:1463–1466.

23 Liccini A, Malmstrom TK, Morley JE. Metform use and cognitive dysfunction among patients with diabetes mellitus. *J Am Med Dir Assoc.* 2016;17:1063–1065.

24 Trachtenbarg DE. Diabetic ketoacidosis. *Am Fam Physician.* 2005;71:1705–1714.

25 Briebeler ML, Kearns AE, Ryu E, et al. Secular trends in the incidence of primary hyperparathyroidism over five decades (1965–2010). *Bone.* 2015;73:1–7.

26 Dalemo S, Hjerpe P, Bostrom Bengtsson K. Diagnosis of patients with raised serum calcium level in primary care, Sweden. *Scand J Prim Health Care.* 2006;24: 160–165.

27 Bakker AD, Jaspers RT. IL-6 and IGF-1 signaling within and between muscle and bone: How important is the mTOR pathway for bone metabolism? *Curr Osteoporos Rep.* 2015;13(3):131–139.

28 Spangenburg EE, Bowles DK, Booth FW. Insulin-like growth factor-induced transcriptional activity of the skeletal alpha-actin gene is regulated by signaling mechanisms linked to voltage-gated calcium channels during myoblast

differentiation. *Endocrinology*. 2004;145(4):2054–2063.

29 Barbieri M, Ferrucci L, Ragno E, et al. Chronic inflammation and the effect of IGF-I on muscle strength and power in older persons. *Am J Physiol Endocrinol Metab*. 2003;284(3):E481–E487.

30 Perrini S, Laviola L, Carreira MC, et al. The GH-IGF-1 axis and signaling pathways in the muscle and bone: mechanisms underlying age-related skeletal muscle wasting and osteoporosis. *Endocrinology*. 2010;205:201–210.

31 Blackman MR, Sorkin JD, Munzer T, et al. Growth hormone and sex steroid administration in healthy aged women and men: a randomized controlled trial. *JAMA*. 2002;288(18):2282–2292.

32 Brioche T, Kireev RA, Cuesta S, et al. Growth hormone replacement therapy prevents sarcopenia by a dual mechanism: improvement of protein balance and of antioxidant defenses. *J Gerontol A Biol Sci Med Sci*. 2014;69(10):1186–1198.

33 Wittert GA, Chapman IM, Haren MT, et al. Oral testosterone supplementation increases muscle and decreases fat mass in healthy elderly males with low-normal gonadal status. *J Gerontol A Biol Sci Med Sci*. 2003;58:618–625.

34 Yamada M, Nishiguchi S, Fukutani N, Aoyama T, Arai H. Mail-based intervention for sarcopenia prevention increased

anabolic hormone and skeletal muscle mass in community-dwelling Japanese older adults: the INE (Intervention by Nutrition and Exercise) study. *J Am Med Dir Assoc*. 2015;16(8):654–660.

35 Grinspoon S, Corcoran C, Miller K, et al. Body composition and endocrine function in women with acquired immunodeficiency syndrome. *J Clin Endocrinol Metab*. 1997;82:1332–1337.

36 Bea JW, Zhao Q, Cauley JA, et al. Effect of hormone therapy on lean body mass, falls, and fractures: 6-year results from the Women's Health Initiative hormone trials. *Menopause*. 2011;18(1):44–52.

37 Diabetes UK, Association of British Clinical Diabetologists, Training Research and Education for Nurses on Diabetes-UK, Institute of Diabetes for Older People. End of Life Diabetes Care. https://www.diabetes.org.uk/end-of-life-care (accessed June 2017).

38 Petrillo LA, Gan S, Jing B, et al. Hypoglycemia in hospice patients with type 2 diabetes in a national sample of nursing homes. *JAMA Intern Med* (published online December 26, 2017). doi:10.1001/jamaintern-med.2017.7744

39 Malmstrom TK, Voss VB, Cruz-Oliver DM, et al. The Rapid Cognitive Screen (RCS): A point-of-care screening for dementia and mild cognitive impairment. *J Nutr Health Aging*. 2015;19:741–744.

Part IV

Pituitary Disorders

Introduction

Emergency Management of Pituitary Disorders

Edward R. Laws and Ursula B. Kaiser

Key Points

- Endocrine emergencies related to the pituitary are important clinical problems, and they are regularly encountered.
- The pituitary gland can be affected by tumors (primary and metastatic); trauma to the head; hemorrhage, vasospasm and vascular insufficiency; infection; inflammatory and autoimmune processes; by the influence of drugs, and by the reaction to radiation therapy.
- Hypopituitarism can lead to profound fatigue and loss of vital endocrine and metabolic functions. This includes secondary (central) adrenal insufficiency: a true endocrine emergency. If hypopituitarism is suspected, stress doses of intravenous (IV) hydrocortisone should be administered empirically even before hormonal test results are available, together with IV fluids.
- Central hypothyroidism also needs to be considered, and patients may present in myxedema coma, with bradycardia, shock, hypothermia, hypoventilation, and altered mental status.
- Patients with acute pituitary insults can be affected by fluid and electrolyte disturbances manifest as either central diabetes insipidus (DI) or, occasionally, syndrome of inappropriate antidiuretic hormone production (SIADH). Cerebral salt-wasting can also occur.
- Enlargement of the pituitary, acute or chronic, can lead to visual loss from compression or distortion of the optic nerves and chiasm. Sudden visual loss from pituitary apoplexy can be a true endocrine emergency, prompting immediate surgical management.
- The thoughtful clinician should keep in mind the many functions of the pituitary, and the effects on the patient when the "master gland" malfunctions or is injured. A thorough differential diagnosis, and the appropriate gathering of information from laboratory testing and imaging can be lifesaving, and remain a challenge in effective patient care.

Because of its complex control mechanisms over vital hormonal functions, and its strategic location at the base of the brain, endocrine emergencies related to the pituitary are important clinical problems, and they are regularly encountered. Both the blood supply of the pituitary and the hypothalamic stimulatory and inhibitory factors that control its physiology are related to the pituitary stalk (infundibulum) that connects the pituitary gland to the hypothalamus (Figure IV-1). Lodged within the confines of the bony sella turcica, the pituitary is directly related to the optic chiasm superiorly, and to

Endocrine and Metabolic Medical Emergencies: A Clinician's Guide, Second Edition. Edited by Glenn Matfin.
© 2018 John Wiley & Sons Ltd. Published 2018 by John Wiley & Sons Ltd.

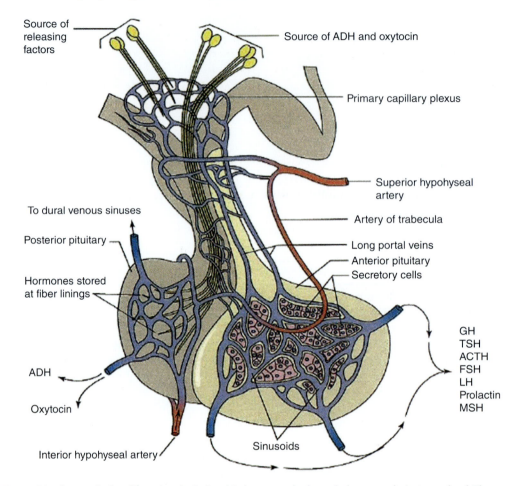

Figure IV-1 Anatomical and functional relationship between the hypothalamus and pituitary gland. The hypothalamic releasing or inhibitory hormones are transported to the anterior pituitary through the portal vessels. Antidiuretic hormone (ADH) and oxytocin are produced by nerve cells in the hypothalamus and then transported through the nerve axons in the infundibulum to the posterior pituitary, where they are released into the circulation.

the cranial nerves of the cavernous sinus laterally. These nerves control pupillary action, extraocular muscle function, and trigeminal nerve sensation.

The pituitary gland can be affected by tumors, primary and metastatic, by trauma to the head, by hemorrhage, vasospasm and vascular insufficiency, by infection, by inflammatory and autoimmune processes, by the influence of drugs, and by the reaction to radiation therapy.

Pituitary insufficiency can lead to profound fatigue and loss of vital endocrine and metabolic functions (1). This can occur as a result of enlarging pituitary tumors and pituitary tumor apoplexy (hemorrhage and/or infarction of a pre-existing pituitary adenoma). Acute and subacute hypopituitarism can also occur following head trauma as a result of damage to the pituitary stalk and the blood supply of the pituitary, during or after pregnancy from Sheehan's syndrome (infarction of the normal pituitary), and as a result of metastatic cancers involving the pituitary gland, its infundibulum, or the hypothalamus. Other primary inflammatory and infectious processes can also result in the abrupt onset of hypopituitarism. These include lymphocytic and other forms of hypophysitis, granulomatous disease, sarcoidosis, tuberculosis, and sellar abscesses.

Afflictions of the pituitary, either sudden or chronic, can cause secondary (central) adrenal insufficiency: a true endocrine emergency. Considering this possibility is of crucial importance in critically ill patients. Patients with acute adrenal insufficiency, or adrenal crisis, often present with shock but may also present with anorexia, weight loss, headache, nausea, vomiting, abdominal pain, weakness, and fatigue, as well as with lethargy, confusion, and coma, frequently accompanied by fever. An adrenal crisis may be precipitated in a patient with chronic adrenal insufficiency by a concurrent infection. If hypopituitarism is suspected, stress doses of intravenous (IV) hydrocortisone should be administered empirically even before hormonal test results are available, together with IV fluids. Central hypothyroidism also needs to be considered, and patients may present in myxedema coma, with bradycardia, shock, hypothermia, hypoventilation, and altered mental status.

Patients with acute pituitary insults can be affected by fluid and electrolyte disturbances manifest as either central diabetes insipidus (DI) or, occasionally, syndrome of inappropriate antidiuretic hormone production (SIADH). Diabetes insipidus occurs rarely in patients with pituitary adenomas, but can manifest in patients with inflammatory or infiltrative pituitary lesions, or after surgery or radiation, typically as a result of hypothalamic or infundibular involvement. Tumors metastatic to the pituitary area may often present clinically with fluid and electrolyte disturbances from DI, the theory being that the network of portal vessels feeding the neurohypophysis may trap circulating tumor cells which then proliferate into a mass lesion. Careful management of the fluid and electrolyte balance is essential, together with desmopressin administration as needed (1,2). Management of these afflictions can be particularly challenging if thirst regulation is also disordered.

Enlargement of the pituitary, acute or chronic, can lead to visual loss from compression or distortion of the optic nerves and chiasm (Figure IV-2). Sudden visual loss from pituitary tumor apoplexy can be a true endocrine emergency, prompting immediate surgical management (3). Progressive failure of visual acuity and visual field deficits can occur with a variety of sellar and parasellar lesions, including not only pituitary adenomas, but also Rathke cleft cysts, craniopharyngiomas, arachnoid cysts, meningiomas, and other problems in this area, making the differential diagnosis broad and often difficult.

Occasionally, cystic pituitary lesions such as Rathke cleft cysts and craniopharyngiomas can rupture, leaking caustic fluid contents into the subarachnoid space. This can produce an acute meningitis-like clinical picture, and the inflammatory response to the cyst contents can contribute to visual loss and hypopituitarism.

Head injury, intracranial hemorrhage and aneurysmal rupture may be accompanied by vasospasm, which may compromise the blood supply to the pituitary and damage the infundibulum and the hypothalamus. These phenomena can lead to DI or SIADH with severe acute electrolyte disturbances (4). Cerebral salt wasting can also occur in these circumstances. The differential diagnosis and correct management can be challenging. In addition to DI and SIADH, head trauma may produce differing degrees of deficiency of anterior pituitary hormones, subsequent to the injury.

A variety of medications can alter or interfere with normal pituitary function. These include psychoactive drugs, therapeutic medications to correct pituitary disorders, some forms of cancer chemotherapy, and a number of hormones that can be toxic or poorly tolerated. One uncommon emergency is the development of cerebrospinal rhinorrhea (CSF leak) from dramatic shrinkage of an invasive prolactin-secreting macroadenoma treated successfully by dopamine agonists (5).

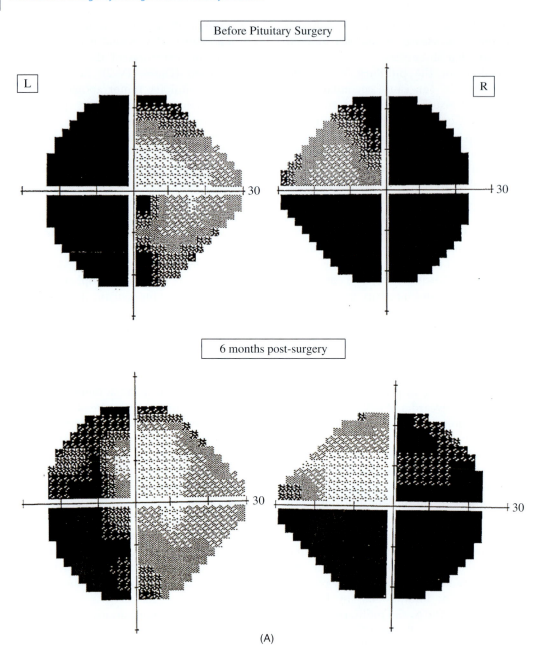

(A)

Figure IV-2 (A) Humphrey visual fields before and 6 months after transsphenoidal surgery. Her eyesight was much improved following surgery with some improvement on formal visual field testing; (B) MRI pituitary coronal and (C) sagittal views of the same patient at baseline showing large macroadenoma (gonadotropin staining non-functioning pituitary tumor). Elevated and compressed optic chiasm not seen on sagittal view but likely in vicinity of arrow.

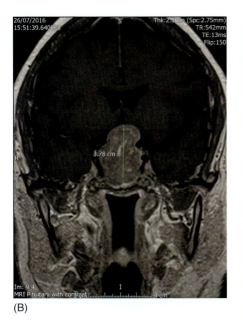

(B)

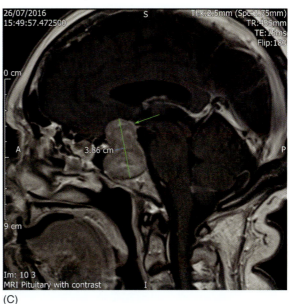

(C)

Figure IV-2 *(Continued)*

Conclusions

The thoughtful clinician, in the office, the Emergency Department, the hospital, or in the operating room, should keep in mind the many functions of the pituitary, and the effects on the patient when the "master gland" malfunctions or is injured. A thorough differential diagnosis, and the appropriate gathering of information from laboratory testing and imaging can be life-saving, and remain a challenge in effective patient care.

References

1 Fleseriu M, Hashim IA, Karavitaki N, et al. Hormonal replacement in hypopituitarism in adults: An Endocrine Society Clinical Practice Guideline. *J Clin Endocrinol Metab*. 2016;101,3888–3921.

2 Prete A, Corsello SM, Salvatori R. Current best practice in the management of patients after pituitary surgery. *Ther Adv Endocrinol Metab*. 2017;8:33–48.

3 Briet C, Salenave S, Bonneville J-F, Laws ER, Chanson P. Pituitary apoplexy. *Endocrine Revs*. 2015;36:622–645.

4 Hannon MJ, Finucane FM, Sherlock M, Agha A, Thompson CJ. Clinical review: disorders of water homeostasis in neurosurgical patients. *J Clin Endocrinol Metab*. 2012;97,1423–1433.

5 Molitch ME. Diagnosis and treatment of pituitary adenomas. *JAMA*. 2017;317:516–524.

12

Hypopituitarism

Nicholas A. Tritos and Anne Klibanski

Key Points

- Hypopituitarism results from complete or partial deficiency in pituitary hormones and includes central hypoadrenalism, central hypothyroidism, central hypogonadism, growth hormone deficiency, and (more rarely) diabetes insipidus.
- Hypopituitarism may be caused by a variety of conditions that either reduce or destroy secretory function or interfere with the hypothalamic secretion of pituitary-releasing hormones.
- Causes of hypopituitarism include pituitary adenomas and other sellar masses, pituitary surgery or radiation therapy, traumatic brain injury, medications, hemorrhage (pituitary apoplexy or subarachnoid hemorrhage), postpartum pituitary infarction (Sheehan's syndrome), inflammation, infection, iron overload, and deleterious mutations of genes involved in pituitary development and function. Hypopituitarism can also be idiopathic in a few cases.
- When considering the diagnosis of hypopituitarism, it is essential to measure both pituitary (e.g., thyrotropin [thyroid stimulating hormone, TSH]) and target organ hormone levels (e.g., free thyroxine) for investigation of central hypoadrenalism, central hypothyroidism and central hypogonadism.
- Pituitary imaging is recommended in patients with biochemical evidence of hypopituitarism in order to identify the underlying cause (such as pituitary adenoma, craniopharyngioma, hypophysitis and others). Magnetic resonance imaging (MRI) of the sella (using a dedicated pituitary protocol) is the imaging modality of choice for sellar imaging. Computed tomography (CT) also has a diagnostic role in pituitary imaging in patients who cannot undergo MRI because of the presence of metal shrapnel or hardware (such as implanted pacemakers). In addition, CT examinations can be particularly helpful in order to demonstrate bony erosions, sellar calcifications, or acute intrasellar hemorrhage.
- Potentially life-threatening manifestations of hypopituitarism include central hypoadrenalism, diabetes insipidus, or, rarely, central hypothyroidism. In contrast, although gonadotropin deficiency and growth hormone deficiency are not life-threatening, they are nevertheless associated with significant morbidity, impaired quality of life and possibly increased mortality.

Endocrine and Metabolic Medical Emergencies: A Clinician's Guide, Second Edition. Edited by Glenn Matfin.
© 2018 John Wiley & Sons Ltd. Published 2018 by John Wiley & Sons Ltd.

- In acutely ill patients at risk for hypopituitarism, glucocorticoid replacement should be administered without awaiting the results of confirmatory diagnostic testing; this can be subsequently performed. Judicious administration of desmopressin, monitoring of fluid balance and serum sodium are essential in the management of diabetes insipidus. Levothyroxine replacement should only be administered after glucocorticoid replacement in order to avoid precipitating adrenal crisis.
- Further studies are needed to optimize the long-term management of hypopituitary patients and minimize associated morbidity and excess mortality.

Introduction

Hypopituitarism may occur as a result of diverse etiologies and lead to substantial morbidity and mortality. Acute manifestations of hypopituitarism may include central hypoadrenalism, due to deficiency of corticotropin (adrenocorticotropic hormone, ACTH), diabetes insipidus or, rarely, central hypothyroidism, due to deficiency of thyrotropin (thyroid stimulating hormone, TSH). In contrast, deficiencies of other pituitary hormones, including gonadotropins, growth hormone (GH) and prolactin, are not immediately life-threatening. Despite advances in the diagnosis and management of pituitary disorders, hypopituitarism is still associated with increased long-term cardiovascular mortality (26,27).

The aims of the present chapter include a review of the causes, pathophysiology, clinical features, diagnosis, and management of hypopituitarism in adults, with emphasis placed on the evaluation and management of acutely ill patients.

Etiology

Pituitary adenomas are the most common cause of hypopituitarism in adult patients seen at pituitary centers. Patients with macroadenomas (defined as lesions 10 mm or larger in greatest diameter) are clearly at risk for anterior hypopituitarism. However, it has been suggested that some patients with microadenomas (<10 mm) may also be at risk (29), especially when ≥6 mm (20). It should be noted that central (neurogenic) diabetes insipidus (CDI) is extremely unlikely to occur in patients with pituitary adenomas before pituitary surgery. As a corollary, the presence of CDI in patients with a sellar mass, who have not had pituitary surgery, strongly suggests that the underlying lesion is not a pituitary adenoma.

In addition, patients with larger (>10 mm) sellar masses other than adenomas (Table 12-1) are at risk of anterior hypopituitarism and in some cases, including those with craniopharyngiomas and metastases, CDI (5). In particular, infiltrating or inflammatory lesions and/or those involving the pituitary stalk may lead to hypopituitarism regardless of size. A minority of patients with primary empty sella may also have anterior hypopituitarism.

Pituitary surgery leads to CDI in ~15% of patients early postoperatively (12). However, persistent CDI only occurs in ~5% of postoperative patients. In addition, new deficits of anterior pituitary hormone secretion may occur in ~10% of patients postoperatively. It is unknown whether some of these patients had marginal anterior pituitary function prior to surgery. Conversely, improvement in pre-existing pituitary function deficits occurs in ~40% of patients undergoing pituitary surgery, presumably due to decompression of the normal anterior pituitary gland.

Radiation therapy to the sella is associated with a lifelong risk of anterior hypopituitarism that becomes more prevalent over time, affecting ~40% of patients at 5 yr and ~60% at 10 yr after therapy (6). In these patients, GH and gonadotropin deficits tend to occur before the development of thyrotropin or corticotropin deficiency. In

Table 12-1 Differential diagnosis of sellar masses. The list includes most pituitary pathologies but is not exhaustive.

Pituitary adenomas (~91%)	Prolactinoma; clinically non-functioning pituitary adenoma; growth hormone secreting adenoma (acromegaly and gigantism); corticotropinoma (Cushing's disease); thyrotropinoma; gonadotroph cell adenoma
Non-adenomatous lesions (~9%)	
Neoplastic	Craniopharyngioma; pituicytoma; meningioma; germ cell tumor; glioma; chordoma; chondrosarcoma; metastases; lymphoma
Cystic	Rathke's cleft cyst; arachnoid cyst; epidermoid cyst; dermoid cyst
Vascular	Aneurysm; cavernous malformation
Inflammatory	Primary hypophysitis (lymphocytic, granulomatous, xanthomatous, necrotizing); secondary hypophysitis (associated with sarcoidosis; Langerhans cell histiocytosis; granulomatosis with polyangiitis [GPA, formerly known as Wegener's granulomatosis]) and drug-induced (e.g., ipilimumab, nivolumab, interferon alpha)
Infectious	Pituitary abscess; Whipple's disease; fungal infection; cysticercosis
Pituitary hyperplasia	Associated with pregnancy, target gland hypofunction (including severe primary hypothyroidism) or ectopic-releasing hormone secretion

addition to gonadotroph failure, radiation-induced hyperprolactinemia may lead to hypogonadism in some cases (22). It may be noted that conventional radiation therapy of brain tumors distant from the sella is also associated with a substantial risk of hypopituitarism. Whether stereotactic radiosurgery, used to treat brain lesions remote from the hypothalamus and pituitary, is safer with regards to pituitary function has not been established.

Traumatic brain injury (TBI) has recently emerged as an important, yet likely underappreciated, cause of hypopituitarism (11,13). It has been estimated that ~25% of patients with TBI severe enough to require hospitalization develop one or more pituitary hormone deficiencies. Of note, at least partial recovery of pituitary function may occur in some of these patients.

A variety of non-traumatic vascular insults have been associated with hypopituitarism, including aneurysmal subarachnoid hemorrhage, pituitary apoplexy (hemorrhage and/or infarction of a pituitary adenoma) and postpartum pituitary infarction in women with severe obstetric hemorrhage resulting in hypovolemic shock (Sheehan's syndrome) (21). It may be noted that

Sheehan's syndrome has become rare in western countries as a result of global improvements in obstetric care.

Medications associated with hypopituitarism include agents that may result in hypophysitis, namely, alpha interferon and immune checkpoint inhibitors, including ipilimumab (in routine clinical use in patients with metastatic melanoma) and, less frequently, nivolumab. Patients with immune checkpoint inhibitor-related hypophysitis usually present with multiple anterior pituitary hormone deficiencies, including central hypoadrenalism and/or central hypothyroidism (8). Hyponatremia is frequent at presentation. In contrast, CDI is very uncommon in this setting.

In addition, some medications may selectively suppress aspects of pituitary function, including pharmacologic doses of glucocorticoids, which inhibit corticotropin, thyrotropin, GH and gonadotropins. Opioids suppress corticotropin and gonadotropins, and bexarotene (retinoic acid receptor agonist) inhibits thyrotropin secretion.

In addition to drug-related hypophysitis, pituitary inflammation may occur as a primary pituitary pathology (classified as lymphocytic, granulomatous, xanthomatous, plasmacytic, or necrotizing) or can be associated with systemic inflammatory/autoimmune conditions (e.g., sarcoidosis, Langerhans cell histiocytosis, granulomatosis with polyangiitis [GPA, formerly known as Wegener's granulomatosis], and immunoglobulin G4-related disease [IgG4-RD]). Infiltrative conditions, including hemochromatosis, may also result in hypopituitarism with a predilection for central hypogonadism. Infectious conditions associated with hypopituitarism include meningitis, pituitary abscess, Whipple's disease, tuberculosis, fungal infection, and cysticercosis.

Genetic causes of hypopituitarism have been identified in some patients with congenital or childhood onset and/or familial hypopituitarism, and may involve inactivating mutations of genes encoding transcription factors having a role in pituitary development (such as *POU1F1 (Pit1), PROP1, LHX3, LHX4, HESX1, OTX2, PITX2, SOX2, SOX3, TPIT*) or inactivating mutations of genes encoding hypothalamic or pituitary hormones or their respective receptors (23).

Pathophysiology

In patients with non-functioning sellar masses, hypopituitarism may occur as a result of mass effect upon the normal secretory cells in the pars distalis or interference with the hypothalamo-hypophyseal portal system. At diagnosis, central hypogonadism and GH deficiency are the most frequent deficits in patients with clinically non-functioning pituitary macroadenomas, followed in prevalence by central hypoadrenalism and hypothyroidism. Stalk transection is associated with multiple pituitary hormone deficits (15). Suprasellar lesions may additionally impinge upon hypothalamic nuclei involved in the secretion of releasing hormones with a critical role in the regulation of pituitary function. Hemorrhage, ischemia, trauma, the chronic effects of radiation therapy, inflammation and infection may all disrupt pituitary function by means of incompletely characterized mechanisms (28). Immune checkpoint inhibitors, including cytotoxic T lymphocyte antigen 4 (CTLA 4)-directed antibodies (such as ipilimumab), may cause hypophyseal inflammation and hypopituitarism by initiating the complement cascade and inducing recruitment of activated macrophages, T and B lymphocytes to the pituitary (3). Secretory pituitary adenomas may selectively inhibit the function of specific anterior pituitary cell populations (including inhibition of gonadotropin secretion by hyperprolactinemia and suppression of GH, gonadotropin and thyrotropin secretion by cortisol excess).

Hypopituitary patients may become acutely ill as a result of severe pituitary hormone deficits (including lack of corticotropin, thyrotropin or vasopressin) or as a consequence of partial pituitary deficiencies when faced with intercurrent homeostatic stressors, such as injury, surgery or infection. Central hypoadrenalism may lead to dehydration, hyponatremia and shock unresponsive to fluid resuscitation and vasopressor therapy before glucocorticoid replacement is administered. Central hypothyroidism may rarely lead to myxedema coma. Vasopressin deficiency causes CDI, which may become clinically apparent only after the initiation of glucocorticoid and thyroid hormone replacement therapies as a result of improvements in renal hemodynamics, glomerular filtration rate and free water clearance.

Clinical Features and Findings

Patients with central hypoadrenalism may present with prostration, headache, nausea, vomiting, orthostatic dizziness, joint aches, dehydration, confusion, shock, or hyponatremia (10,27). Patients with disease of long duration may additionally report fatigue and unexplained weight loss. Notably absent are skin and mucosal hyperpigmentation as well as hyperkalemia (in contrast to patients with Addison's disease).

Patients with central hypothyroidism may rarely present in myxedema coma, characterized by bradycardia, shock, bradypnea, hypoventilation, hypothermia, abnormal mental status, jaundice, hyponatremia, and abnormal liver function tests. If history can be obtained, information elicited may include chronic fatigue, weight gain, constipation, muscle cramps, irregular menses, dry skin, edema, hair loss, and cold intolerance.

In patients with acute pituitary insults affecting the posterior pituitary, including TBI and pituitary surgery, CDI typically presents within 24–48 h and is characterized by polyuria (urine output exceeding 200 ml/h for >2 h) and hyposthenuria (in general, urine specific gravity <1.005 or osmolality <300 mOsm/kg) (7). Serum sodium levels are generally high normal or mildly elevated. However, severe hypernatremic dehydration may occur if patients are unable to compensate for aquaresis by increasing their water intake. Such a scenario is possible in patients with impaired sensorium, deficient thirst, or restricted access to water. Transient CDI may be followed by hyponatremia as a result of the syndrome of inappropriate antidiuretic hormone secretion (SIADH), which generally resolves within two weeks and can be succeeded by recurrent CDI (a sequence of events termed the "triple phase response").

Deficiencies of gonadotropins, prolactin or GH are not likely to be immediately relevant in an acute setting. However, the presence of symptoms and findings suggestive of deficiencies in these hormones should raise the suspicion of the presence of hypopituitarism in patients at risk. Women with gonadotropin deficiency generally note oligomenorrhea or secondary amenorrhea, whereas men may note low libido, erectile dysfunction, fatigue, or increased central adiposity. Patients of both genders may also experience hot flashes, involution of secondary sex characteristics, infertility, and are at risk for bone loss. Women with prolactin deficiency may report failure to lactate in the postpartum state, as is frequently the case in women with Sheehan's syndrome. There are no established consequences of prolactin deficiency in men. In children and adolescents, GH deficiency leads to delays in growth and may also impair the normal accrual of bone mineral and muscle mass. In adults of both genders, GH deficiency is associated with abnormal body composition (increased visceral adiposity, decreased muscle mass, and bone mineral density), decreased exercise capacity, dyslipidemia, insulin resistance and impaired quality of life. The physiologic role of oxytocin has not been completely elucidated. However, emerging data suggest that, in addition to progression of labor and milk letdown, oxytocin may have a role in social bonding and regulation of food intake (14,18).

In addition to symptoms and signs of pituitary hormone deficiencies, patients may note evidence of local mass effect, including headache, vision loss (as a result of compression of the optic apparatus by a sellar mass, most commonly bitemporal hemianopsia) or, less commonly, other cranial neuropathies (involving the III, IV, V, VI cranial nerves). Pituitary apoplexy presents with acute, very severe headache, vision loss and ophthalmoplegia, and constitutes an endocrine and neurosurgical emergency.

Diagnosis

Evaluation of the hypothalamic pituitary adrenal (HPA) axis is the highest diagnostic (as well as therapeutic) priority in patients at risk of hypopituitarism (Table 12-2) (10,27). Morning (or random) serum cortisol levels exceeding 18 µg/dL (~500 nmol/L) assure sufficient adrenocortical function with high specificity but low sensitivity. Conversely, morning serum cortisol levels below 3 µg/dL (~80 nmol/L) are diagnostic of adrenal insufficiency. Intermediate morning cortisol levels are considered non-diagnostic and require additional testing. Measuring plasma corticotropin levels in a concurrent specimen helps to distinguish between central hypoadrenalism (characterized by low or "normal" plasma corticotropin) and primary adrenal insufficiency (characterized by elevated plasma corticotropin). It should be emphasized that acutely ill patients at risk for central hypoadrenalism should be presumed to be adrenally insufficient and treated with stress doses of glucocorticoids (preferably after drawing a blood specimen to assay cortisol and corticotropin) without awaiting the results of diagnostic testing.

Table 12-2 Diagnostic evaluation of adult patients with suspected hypopituitarism (note: use local laboratory reference ranges)

Pituitary function	Test name	Procedure	Test interpretation	Comments
Pituitary adrenal axis	Morning serum cortisol and plasma corticotropin (ACTH)	Draw specimens at 8 a.m.	Serum cortisol >18 µg/dL (~500 nmol/L) assures sufficiency; cortisol <3 µg/dL (~80 nmol/L) is diagnostic of hypoadrenalism Plasma corticotropin levels that are not elevated in patients with untreated hypoadrenalism are diagnostic of a central etiology	Serum cortisol between 3–18 µg/dL (~80–500 nmol/L) are indeterminate and require stimulation testing
	Insulin tolerance test	Short-acting insulin 0.1–0.15 units/kg IV Serum cortisol at 0, 30, 60, 90, 120 min	Peak serum cortisol >18 µg/dL (~500 nmol/L) assures sufficiency	Diagnostic gold standard; nadir plasma glucose <45 mg/dL (~2.2 mmol/L) is needed to assure sufficient corticotroph stimulation Requires physician in attendance; avoid test in the elderly, patients with cardiovascular disease or seizures
	Metyrapone test	Metyrapone (30 mg/kg) po × 1 at 11 p.m. Serum cortisol, ACTH, 11-DOC at 8 a.m. (next morning)	Serum 11-DOC >7 µg/dL (~200 nmol/L) assures sufficiency (ACTH >50 pg/ml [11 pmol/L] is normal; however, ACTH response is less reliable than 11-DOC response) Serum cortisol <5 µg/dL (~140 nmol/L) needed to assure sufficient enzymatic blockade	Avoid test in patients with abnormal cosyntropin stimulation test Risk of precipitating acute adrenal insufficiency
	Short-ACTH stimulation test	Cosyntropin (Cortrosyn or Synacthen) 250 mcg IV or IM × 1* Serum cortisol at 0, 30, 60 min	Peak serum cortisol >18 µg/dL (~500 nmol/L) assures sufficient adrenal function	The test is often falsely normal in patients with corticotroph failure of recent onset (within several weeks)
Pituitary thyroid axis	Serum thyrotropin (TSH) and free T₄	Random serum specimens are drawn to measure thyrotropin and free T₄	Serum free T₄ is low in patients with central hypothyroidism "Normal" serum thyrotropin levels are common in central hypothyroidism	Similar biochemical findings may occur in patients with euthyroid sick syndrome

Posterior pituitary (vasopressin)	Serum sodium and osmolality; urine osmolality (or specific gravity)	Specimens are obtained in patients with polyuria; early morning specimens preferred	Urine osmolality >700 mOsm/kg excludes DI	Exclude hypokalemia, hypercalcemia and hyperglycemia Consider performing a water deprivation test in stable patients with normal serum sodium/osmolality and insufficiently concentrated urine
	Water deprivation test	All fluid intake is withheld with careful monitoring of blood pressure, pulse, urine output, and weight Specimens for serum sodium and osmolality, and urine osmolality are obtained every 2 h until urine osmolality plateaus or evidence of significant dehydration is noted Desmopressin (1–2 mcg SC) is given at the end of the test and urine specimens are obtained in 1 h and 2 h	Urine osmolality >700 mOsm/kg assures sufficient vasopressin secretion and action Patients with severe DI have peak urine osmolality <300 mOsm/kg Serum sodium >145 mmol/L (or serum osmolality >300 mOsm/kg) needed to assure sufficient stimulus for vasopressin stimulation Normalization of urine osmolality (>700 mOsm/kg) after desmopressin administration is consistent with central DI; absence of an increase in urine osmolality after desmopressin is consistent with nephrogenic DI	This test is to performed under close supervision in stable patients; serum potassium, calcium and glucose should be normal; thyroid and adrenal function known to be normal or replaced before test Terminate test if loss of weight >3% over baseline occurs; if clinical evidence of dehydration or hyperosmolality (>300 mOsm/kg) occurs
Gonadotropin gonadal axis	Serum gonadotropins (FSH and LH) Estradiol and menstrual history in women; testosterone and SHBG (or free testosterone) in men	In menstruating women, specimens are preferably drawn on day 3 after onset of menses Morning serum specimens are drawn in men	Regular spontaneous menses suggest that hypogonadism is unlikely; amenorrhea in women and low gonadal steroid levels (in both genders) are consistent with hypogonadism Serum gonadotropin levels that are not elevated in patients with hypogonadism are diagnostic of a central etiology	Avoid testing in hospitalized patients; abnormal results should be confirmed with repeat testing

(continued)

Table 12-2 (*Continued*)

Pituitary function	Test name	Procedure	Test interpretation	Comments
GH	Insulin tolerance test[†]	Short-acting insulin 0.1-0.15 units/kg IV Serum GH at 0, 30, 60, 90, 120 min	Peak GH >3 ng/ml (3 μg/L) is considered a normal response	Diagnostic gold standard; nadir plasma glucose <45 mg/dl (~2.2 mmol/L) is needed to assure sufficient somatotroph stimulation Requires physician in attendance; avoid in the elderly, patients with cardiovascular disease or seizures
	Glucagon stimulation test[†]	Glucagon 1 mg IM × 1 (1.5 mg in patients >90 kg) Serum GH at 0, 30, 60, 90, 120, 150, 180 min	Peak GH >3 ng/ml (3 μg/L) is considered a normal response; a peak GH cut point of 1 ng/ml is likely more accurate in overweight or obese adults	Good diagnostic accuracy in adults
	GHRH arginine stimulation test[†]	GHRH: 1 mcg/kg IV bolus plus arginine 0.5 g/kg (up to 30 g) IV infused over 30 min Serum GH at 0, 30, 60, 90, 120 min	BMI-dependent diagnostic cut points recommended as follows: If BMI <25 kg/m², then peak GH >11.5 ng/ml (11.5 μg/L) is a normal response If BMI: 25-30 kg/m², then peak GH >8 ng/ml (8 μg/L) is a normal response If BMI >30 kg/m², then peak GH >4.2 ng/ml (4.2 μg/L) is a normal response	Good diagnostic accuracy (except in patients with recent brain irradiation)

Test	Procedure	Interpretation	Comments
Arginine stimulation test†	Arginine 0.5 g/kg (up to 30 g) IV infused over 30 min; Serum GH at 0, 30, 60, 90, 120 min	Peak GH >0.4 ng/ml (0.4 µg/L) is considered a normal response	Lower diagnostic accuracy than other tests in adults
IGF-1	Randomly obtained serum specimens are assayed for IGF-1	Normal serum IGF-1 levels occur in ~50% of adults with GH deficiency (low sensitivity); Low serum IGF-1 levels in the presence of 3 or more additional pituitary deficiencies and known pituitary pathology are highly specific for GH deficiency	Low serum IGF-1 levels may also occur in patients on oral estrogen, severe liver disease, uncontrolled diabetes mellitus
Prolactin — Serum prolactin	Specimen for serum prolactin drawn (after overnight fast); Domperidone administration can be used to stimulate prolactin secretion (used in research)	Undetectable serum prolactin levels are diagnostic	Prolactin deficiency generally occurs in patients with multiple additional pituitary hormone deficiencies

* A low dose (1 mcg) short-ACTH stimulation test has been suggested in some studies to be more sensitive than the 250 mcg short-ACTH in the diagnosis of central hypoadrenalism.
† GH stimulation testing is performed after other pituitary hormone deficits are replaced. An overnight fast is required.
ACTH = corticotropin; DI = diabetes insipidus; 11-DOC = 11 deoxycortisol; FSH = follicle-stimulating hormone; GH = growth hormone; GHRH = growth hormone releasing hormone; IGF-1 = insulin-like growth factor 1; IM = intramuscularly; IV = intravenously; LH = luteinizing hormone; PO = by mouth; T_4 = thyroxine.

Stimulation testing is helpful in assessing the integrity of the HPA axis in stable patients, but is not informative or practical in the acute setting. The insulin tolerance test (ITT) is considered the gold standard test in the evaluation of pituitary adrenal function and additionally helps to evaluate GH secretion. However, the test requires the induction of severe hypoglycemia (<45 mg/dL [~2.2 mmol/L]) in order to achieve adequate diagnostic accuracy. As a result, it is often perceived as unpleasant by patients, carries some risk associated with severe hypoglycemia and is contraindicated in the elderly, patients with seizures, or those with cardiovascular disease. The metyrapone test is also reliable in the assessment of the HPA axis. However, the currently limited availability of metyrapone and the potential of precipitating acute adrenal insufficiency, particularly in an unmonitored out-patient setting, have limited use of this test in the USA. The short-ACTH (cosyntropin [Cortrosyn or Synacthen]) stimulation test directly evaluates adrenocortical responsiveness and is quite accurate in the diagnosis of primary adrenal insufficiency. However, the diagnostic accuracy of this test in patients with central hypoadrenalism of recent onset is lower, as it takes several weeks (4–6 weeks) or longer after endogenous corticotropin secretion is blunted for the adrenals to become atrophic and lose responsiveness to exogenous ACTH administration.

Evaluation of the pituitary thyroid axis requires assays for both thyrotropin and free thyroxine (T_4) levels (as serum thyrotropin is often inappropriately "normal" in the presence of low free T_4 levels in patients with central hypothyroidism) (27). Similar biochemical findings may be present in acutely patients with the "euthyroid sick" syndrome. The latter condition may not be reliably distinguished from central hypothyroidism in the critically ill. Unless myxedema coma is suspected, cautious observation with serial laboratory assessments of the pituitary thyroid axis may be appropriate and can help to distinguish between the two diagnostic possibilities, as the biochemical abnormalities in euthyroid sick syndrome improve and eventually resolve in parallel with overall improvement in patients' clinical status.

Evaluation of posterior pituitary function includes careful assessment of urine output, fluid balance, serum sodium and osmolality, and urine specific gravity or osmolality (16). Patients with DI have polyuria with inappropriately dilute urine despite the presence of hypernatremia/hyperosmolality. If needed, a water deprivation test can be performed in stable patients under monitored conditions in order to exclude the presence of primary polydipsia, establish the diagnosis of DI and identify the cause. However, a water deprivation test is not appropriate in acutely ill patients. In patients with DI, a substantial increase in urine osmolality in response to desmopressin administration is consistent with CDI. In contrast, lack of such a response is most consistent with nephrogenic DI. In these patients, the history may also provide important clues, including use of medications, such as lithium, associated with resistance to vasopressin.

Patients with SIADH are euvolemic and have hypotonic hyponatremia with inappropriately concentrated urine (urine osmolality >100–150 mOsm/kg). Hypoadrenalism and hypothyroidism should be excluded before the diagnosis of SIADH can be established as both decrease free water clearance. Review of the medical record helps to exclude medications (such as carbamazepine, opioids or selective serotonin reuptake inhibitors) as potential contributing factors resulting in SIADH.

Assays for vasopressin often lack sufficient accuracy to be clinically useful in the diagnosis of DI and SIADH. An assay for copeptin, which is the C-terminal portion of the vasopressin precursor and is secreted in an equimolar ratio to vasopressin, is being evaluated and appears to hold promise in the differential diagnosis of DI and SIADH (9).

Evaluation of the rest of the anterior pituitary hormones (i.e., gonadotropins, GH, prolactin) may often be confounded by acute illness and is best deferred until patients are medically stable and assessed in the outpatient setting. Obtaining a menstrual history is critical in women, in addition to tests for serum gonadotropins and estradiol. In men, measuring serum testosterone (including total testosterone and sex hormone binding globulin, or free testosterone) and gonadotropins in the morning is advised.

Fasting serum prolactin levels (either at baseline or after stimulation by thyrotropin releasing hormone or domperidone; both stimulation tests being used primarily in research settings) are very low or undetectable in patients with prolactin deficiency. Evaluation of GH secretion generally requires stimulation testing in adults, as serum insulin-like growth factor levels are below normal in only 50% of adults with GH deficiency (19). Several GH stimulation tests are of diagnostic utility in adults, using insulin, glucagon, growth hormone-releasing hormone (GHRH) and arginine, or arginine alone as provocative stimuli (1,27). The role of the recently FDA approved oral ghrelin agonist (macimorelin) for adult GH deficiency testing, remains to be clarified.

Although the diagnosis of hypopituitarism does not rest on imaging, it is nevertheless advisable to obtain pituitary imaging in patients with biochemical evidence of hypopituitarism in order to identify the underlying cause (such as pituitary adenoma, craniopharyngioma, hypophysitis, and others). Magnetic resonance imaging (MRI) of the sella (using a dedicated pituitary protocol) is the imaging modality of choice for sellar imaging. Of note, computed tomography (CT) also has a diagnostic role in pituitary imaging in patients who cannot undergo MRI because of the presence of metal shrapnel or hardware (such as implanted pacemakers). In addition, CT examinations can be particularly helpful in order to demonstrate bony erosions, sellar calcifications or acute intrasellar hemorrhage.

Management

Glucocorticoid replacement is a high priority in patients with known or suspected central hypoadrenalism (Table 12-3) (10,27). Acutely ill, hospitalized patients with central hypoadrenalism should be given stress dose glucocorticoid coverage, including hydrocortisone 50–100 mg intravenously (IV) every 8 hr (or equivalent). Patients with pituitary apoplexy should receive stress dose glucocorticoid replacement, as they are at high risk for hypopituitarism, including central hypoadrenalism (4,21). Of note, neurosurgeons generally recommend pharmacologic doses of glucocorticoids (including dexamethasone 4 mg IV every 6 h) in patients with pituitary apoplexy and cranial neuropathies before surgical decompression is undertaken.

In the outpatient setting, patients with central hypoadrenalism and acute intercurrent illness should be taught to increase their glucocorticoid replacement to 2–3 times their usual maintenance dose until recovery, and then resume taking their usual glucocorticoid replacement (prednisone 2.5–5 mg by mouth daily in a single morning dose or hydrocortisone 15–25 mg by mouth daily in divided doses). Use of a modified release hydrocortisone tablet has been associated with improvements in metabolic profile, including lower body weight, blood pressure and glycemia (17). This medication has been approved for use in Europe but is not currently FDA-approved. Patients with central hypoadrenalism are also advised to wear a medical identification tag.

Levothyroxine replacement should always be deferred until after glucocorticoid replacement has been administered (or hypoadrenalism excluded); failure to do so may precipitate acute adrenal crisis. In acutely ill patients with suspected myxedema coma, 300–500 mcg of levothyroxine is administered IV (after stress dose glucocorticoid replacement is given), followed by 50–100 mcg of IV levothyroxine daily. In the outpatient setting, levothyroxine replacement is given as a single daily dose. Usual levothyroxine replacement doses are ~1.6 mcg/kg. However, patients with mild central hypothyroidism, the elderly, and those with cardiovascular disease are generally advised to begin therapy with a lower levothyroxine dose (25–50 mcg/daily). Careful monitoring of free thyroxine levels is recommended in 6 weeks after dose adjustment. In these patients, serum thyrotropin levels must not

Table 12-3 Management of patients with hypopituitarism in adults

Pituitary function	Acute management	Maintenance therapy	Comments
Pituitary adrenal axis	Hydrocortisone 50–100 mg IV every 8 h (acutely ill hospitalized patients) In outpatients with minor illness: hydrocortisone or prednisone at 2–3 times maintenance can be advised	Hydrocortisone 15–25 mg PO daily (in 2–3 divided doses with the largest dose in the morning) or Prednisone 2.5–5 mg PO daily in a single morning dose	Dose adjustment based on clinical criteria (well-being, weight, blood pressure, glycemia, etc) Patients are advised to wear a medical identification tag
Pituitary thyroid axis*	Suspected myxedema coma: levothyroxine 300–500 mcg IV × 1 followed by levothyroxine 50–100 mcg IV daily	Levothyroxine 1.6 mcg/kg PO daily	Lower starting doses are advised in the elderly, patients with cardiovascular disease or those with mild hypothyroidism Monitor free T_4 levels
Posterior pituitary (vasopressin)	Desmopressin 1–2 mcg SC or IV every 8–24 h as needed	Desmopressin 10–20 mcg intranasally daily–twice daily or Desmopressin 100–400 mcg PO daily–twice daily	Allowing the effect of the medication to wear off between doses may avoid hyponatremia Patients with intact thirst should drink water to thirst only; patients with impaired thirst need to drink water on schedule Monitor fluid balance and serum sodium levels
Gonadotropin gonadal axis	Not recommended	In women: combination oral contraceptive or oral/topical estrogen (with progesterone in women with intact uterus) In men: testosterone in transdermal, intramuscular or subcutaneous implant form	Gonadotropin therapy (rFSH and hCG) is advised to restore fertility in women; hCG alone may be sufficient in men Monitor serum testosterone levels, prostate health and hematocrit in men
GH	Not recommended	Recombinant human GH: 0.2–0.3 mg SC daily (starting dose)	Higher starting doses are appropriate in younger patients or women on oral contraceptives; lower starting doses are appropriate in the elderly Monitor serum IGF-1 levels, body composition and mineral density, serum lipids, quality of life
Prolactin	Not applicable	Not routinely available (used in clinical research)	
Oxytocin	Not applicable	Not routinely available (used in clinical research)	

*Thyroid hormone should only be administered after glucocorticoid replacement is given (or sufficient cortisol secretion assured).

GH = growth hormone; hCG = human chorionic gonadotropin; IGF-1 = insulin-like growth factor 1; IV = intravenously; PO = by mouth; rFSH = recombinant follicle-stimulating hormone; SC = subcutaneously; T_4 = thyroxine.

be relied upon as an index of the adequacy of thyroid hormone replacement.

In hospitalized patients, CDI requires careful monitoring of fluid balance, sodium levels and judicious administration of desmopressin as needed. Patients with intact thirst are advised to drink to thirst. In contrast, patients with impaired thirst sensation need to drink on schedule, guided by changes in fluid balance, body weight, and serum sodium levels. Desmopressin administration is given only on demand in the hospital (desmopressin dose: 1–2 mcg subcutaneously or intravenously every 8–24 h as needed), with careful monitoring of sodium levels as CDI can be transient or can be followed by SIADH. Stable outpatients with persistent CDI generally experience good symptomatic relief from polyuria and excessive thirst on once or twice daily desmopressin therapy, administered either nasally or orally. Patients are advised to drink to thirst and allow for the medication effect to wear off before taking the next desmopressin dose in order to minimize the possibility of hyponatremia. Frequent monitoring of serum sodium levels is important to do, particularly at the start of therapy.

Replacement therapies for other hormone deficiencies (gonadotropins, GH) are not administered in the acute setting because of unclear efficacy and safety in severely ill patients. An overview of sex steroid and GH replacement is outlined in Table 12-3 (10,30). However, a detailed review of these therapies is beyond the scope of this manuscript. Prolactin replacement is not available. However, a recombinant human prolactin preparation has been successfully administered (within the scope of a clinical trial) in women who failed to lactate postpartum and have very low prolactin levels. Oxytocin replacement is strictly investigational at present. Indeed, the therapeutic role of this hormone, administered as nasal spray, is currently under study (18).

Supportive care, including ventilation, correction of volume and electrolyte or temperature abnormalities and treatment of the underlying cause of hypopituitarism are obviously important. Pituitary adenomectomy may improve pituitary function in 30–40% of patients. However, pituitary function rarely, if ever, improves in patients with craniopharyngioma after tumor resection. Similarly, hypopituitarism persists in the majority of patients with immune checkpoint inhibitor-related hypophysitis (8).

Case study

A 35-year-old man, who was previously in good health, was admitted to the intensive care unit after a motor vehicle accident, during which he suffered severe head injury with loss of consciousness, necessitating intubation. He has remained poorly responsive, exhibiting intermittent extensor posturing. He has required vasopressor support in order to maintain adequate circulation. Subarachnoid hemorrhage and frontal contusions, but no obvious sellar mass, were evident on MRI examination. On the third hospital day, the patient was found to be hyponatremic (serum sodium: 129 mmol/L [normal, 135–145], urine sodium: 60 mmol/L and urine osmolality: 450 mOsm/kg). The attending physician noted that hyponatremia was likely caused by SIADH and recommended fluid restriction.

Do you agree with this assessment and recommendation?

The diagnosis of SIADH is always one of exclusion. Hypoadrenalism and hypothyroidism must be excluded as possible explanations before SIADH can be accepted as the cause of hyponatremia.

In this patient, additional laboratory test results were as follows: morning serum cortisol: 2 µg/dL (55 nmol/L); ACTH; 5 pg/ml (normal, 5–70) 1.1 pmol/L (normal, 1.1–15.4); TSH: 1.2 mcu/ml (normal, 0.5–5.0); free T_4: 1.0 ng/dL (normal, 0.9–1.8). These findings are diagnostic of central hypoadrenalism. Hyponatremia resolved within two days after the institution of glucocorticoid replacement in stress doses, confirming the central role of glucocorticoid deficiency in the pathogenesis of hyponatremia in this patient.

Conclusions

Hypopituitarism is caused by a wide variety of pathologies affecting the hypothalamic pituitary unit. Prompt institution of glucocorticoid replacement and careful attention to fluid and electrolyte balance can be lifesaving in acutely ill patients.

Despite substantial advances in the diagnosis and management of pituitary disorders, hypopituitarism remains a serious condition and has been associated with excess mortality, as a result of inadequately treated hypoadrenalism, long-term excess risk of cardiovascular and cerebrovascular disease, and possibly increased risk of malignancy in irradiated patients (2.26). Possible factors contributing to increased cardiovascular risk may include excessive glucocorticoid replacement, lack of appropriate sex steroid and/or GH replacement therapies, and radiation therapy (24,25). Further improvements in the accuracy of diagnostic testing and replacement therapies are needed in order to improve the long-term outlook of these patients.

References

1 Biller BM, Samuels MH, Zagar A, et al. Sensitivity and specificity of six tests for the diagnosis of adult GH deficiency. *J Clin Endocrinol Metab*. 2002;87:2067–2079.

2 Burman P, Mattsson AF, Johannsson G, et al. Deaths among adult patients with hypopituitarism: hypocortisolism during acute stress, and de novo malignant brain tumors contribute to an increased mortality. *J Clin Endocrinol Metab*. 2013;98:1466–1475.

3 Caturegli P, Di Dalmazi G, Lombardi M, et al. Hypophysitis secondary to cytotoxic T-lymphocyte-associated protein 4 blockade: insights into pathogenesis from an autopsy series. *Am J Pathol*. 2016; 186:3225–3235.

4 Chanson P, Lepeintre JF, Ducreux D. Management of pituitary apoplexy. *Expert Opin Pharmacother*. 2004;5:1287–1298.

5 Crowley RK, Hamnvik OP, O'Sullivan EP, et al. Morbidity and mortality in patients with craniopharyngioma after surgery. *Clin Endocrinol (Oxf)*. 2010;73:516–521.

6 Darzy KH. Radiation-induced hypopituitarism. *Curr Opin Endocrinol Diabetes Obes*. 2013;20:342–353.

7 Devin JK. Hypopituitarism and central diabetes insipidus: perioperative diagnosis and Management. *Neurosurg Clin N Am*. 2012;23:679–689.

8 Faje AT, Sullivan R, Lawrence D, et al. Ipilimumab-induced hypophysitis: a detailed longitudinal analysis in a large cohort of patients with metastatic melanoma. *J Clin Endocrinol Metab*. 2014;99:4078–4085.

9 Fenske W, Allolio B. Clinical review: current state and future perspectives in the diagnosis of diabetes insipidus. *J Clin Endocrinol Metab*. 2012;97:3426–3437.

10 Fleseriu M, Hashim IA, Karavitaki N, et al. Hormonal replacement in hypopituitarism in adults: an Endocrine Society Clinical Practice Guideline. *J Clin Endocrinol Metab*. 2016;101:3888–3921.

11 Hannon MJ, Crowley RK, Behan LA, et al. Acute glucocorticoid deficiency and diabetes insipidus are common after acute traumatic brain injury and predict mortality. *J Clin Endocrinol Metab*. 2013;98:3229–3237.

12 Hannon MJ, Finucane FM, Sherlock M, Agha A, Thompson CJ. Clinical review: disorders of water homeostasis in neurosurgical patients. *J Clin Endocrinol Metab*. 2012;97:1423–1433.

13 Hannon MJ, Sherlock M, Thompson CJ. Pituitary dysfunction following traumatic brain injury or subarachnoid haemorrhage: endocrine management in the intensive care unit. *Best Pract Res Clin Endocrinol Metab*. 2011;25:783–798.

14 Hoge EA, Anderson E, Lawson EA. Gender moderates the effect of oxytocin on social

judgments. *Hum Psychopharmacol.* 2014;29:299–304.

15 Ioachimescu AG, Hamrahian AH, Stevens M, Zimmerman RS. The pituitary stalk transection syndrome: multifaceted presentation in adulthood. *Pituitary.* 2012;15:405–411.

16 Jahangiri A, Wagner J, Tran MT. Factors predicting postoperative hyponatremia and efficacy of hyponatremia management strategies after more than 1000 pituitary operations. *J Neurosurg.* 2013;119(6): 1478–1483.

17 Johannsson G, Nilsson AG, Bergthorsdottir R, et al. Improved cortisol exposure-time profile and outcome in patients with adrenal insufficiency: a prospective randomized trial of a novel hydrocortisone dual-release formulation. *J Clin Endocrinol Metab.* 2012;97:473–481.

18 Lawson EA, Marengi DA, Desanti RL, Holmes TM, Schoenfeld DA, Tolley CJ. Oxytocin reduces caloric intake in men. *Obesity (Silver Spring).* 2015;23:950–956.

19 Molitch ME, Clemmons DR, Malozowski S, Merriam GR, Vance ML, Endocrine Society. Evaluation and treatment of adult growth hormone deficiency: an Endocrine Society Clinical Practice Guideline. *J Clin Endocrinol Metab.* 2011;96:1587–1609.

20 Molitch ME. Diagnosis and treatment of pituitary adenomas. *JAMA.* 2017;317: 516–524.

21 Nawar RN, Abdelmannan D, Selman WR, Arafah B. Pituitary tumor apoplexy: a review. *J Intensive Care Med.* 2008; 23:75–90.

22 Pai H0H, Thornton A, Katznelson L, Finkelstein DM, et al. Hypothalamic/pituitary function following high-dose conformal radiotherapy to the base of skull: demonstration of a dose-effect relationship using dose-volume histogram analysis. *Int J Radiat Oncol Biol Phys.* 2001;49:1079–1092.

23 Romero CJ, Nesi-Franca S, Radovic S. The molecular basis of hypopituitarism. *Trends Endocrinol Metab.* 2009;20:506–516.

24 Sherlock M, Reulen RC, Alonso AA, et al. ACTH deficiency, higher doses of hydrocortisone replacement, and radiotherapy are independent predictors of mortality in patients with acromegaly. *J Clin Endocrinol Metab.* 2009;94: 4216–4223.

25 Sherlock M, Stewart PM. Updates in growth hormone treatment and mortality. *Curr Opin Endocrinol Diabetes Obes.* 2013;20:314–320.

26 Stewart, PM, Sherlock M. Mortality and pituitary disease. *Ann Endocrinol (Paris).* 2012;73:81–82.

27 Toogood AA, Stewart PM. Hypopituitarism: clinical features, diagnosis, and management. *Endocrinol Metab Clin North Am.* 2008;37:235–261, x.

28 Tritos, NA, Yuen, KC, Kelly, DF. American Association of Clinical Endocrinologists and American College of Endocrinology. Disease state clinical review: a neuroendocrine approach to patients with traumatic brain injury. *Endocr Pract.* 2015;21:823–831.

29 Yuen, KC, Cook, DM, Sahasranam, P, et al. Prevalence of GH and other anterior pituitary hormone deficiencies in adults with nonsecreting pituitary microadenomas and normal serum IGF-1 levels. *Clin Endocrinol (Oxf).* 2008;69: 292–298.

30 Yuen KC, Tritos NA, Samson Sl, Hoffman AR, Katznelson L. American Association of Clinical Endocrinologists and American College of Endocrinology. Disease state clinical review: update on growth hormone stimulation testing and proposed revised cut-point for the glucagon stimulation test in the diagnosis of adult growth hormone deficiency. *Endocr Pract.* 2016;22: 1235–1244.

13

Pituitary Apoplexy

Claire Briet and Philippe Chanson

Key Points

- Pituitary apoplexy (PA) is a rare clinical syndrome secondary to abrupt hemorrhage or infarction, and is an endocrine emergency.
- It complicates 2–12% of pituitary adenomas, especially nonfunctioning tumors.
- Headache of sudden and severe onset is the main symptom, sometimes associated with visual disturbances or ocular palsy. Signs of meningeal irritation or altered consciousness may complicate the diagnosis.
- In most cases, PA occurs in an undiagnosed, pre-existing pituitary adenoma and the initial diagnosis is often either subarachnoid hemorrhage or bacterial meningitis, until imaging shows the presence of a pituitary adenoma. Diagnosis thus relies on a combination of clinical manifestations (e.g., sudden headache and visual disturbances) and the detection of a pituitary adenoma, whether before or after PA onset.
- Precipitating factors (e.g., increase in intracranial pressure, arterial hypertension,

- major surgery, anticoagulant therapy or dynamic pituitary function testing) may be identified.
- Computed tomography (CT) or magnetic resonance imaging (MRI) confirms the diagnosis by revealing a pituitary tumor with hemorrhagic and/or necrotic components.
- Corticotropic deficiency with adrenal insufficiency may be life threatening if left untreated.
- Formerly considered a neurosurgical emergency, PA always used to be treated surgically. Nowadays, conservative management is increasingly used in selected patients (those without important visual acuity or field defects and with normal consciousness), as successive publications provide converging evidence that a "wait-and-see" approach provides similar outcomes in terms of oculomotor palsy, pituitary function, and subsequent tumor growth.

Introduction

Pituitary apoplexy (PA) is a clinical syndrome due to abrupt hemorrhaging and/or infarction of the pituitary gland, generally within a pituitary adenoma. Headache of sudden and severe onset is the main symptom, sometimes associated with visual disturbances or ocular palsy. PA can reveal an adenoma or can occur in the adenoma's follow-up.

PA is a rare event: according to recent epidemiological studies its prevalence is about 6.2 cases per 100 000 inhabitants (1) and its incidence 0.17 episodes per 100 000 per year (2). Between 2% and 12% of patients with all types of pituitary adenoma experience apoplexy, and the diagnosis of pituitary adenoma was unknown at time of apoplexy. PA can occur at all ages but is most frequent in the fifth or sixth decade, with a

Endocrine and Metabolic Medical Emergencies: A Clinician's Guide, Second Edition. Edited by Glenn Matfin.
© 2018 John Wiley & Sons Ltd. Published 2018 by John Wiley & Sons Ltd.

slight male preponderance ranging from 1.1–2.3/1 (3).

Predisposing and Precipitating Factors

Precipitating factors are identified in 10–40% of cases of PA (3). The temporal relationship between angiographic procedures, such as cerebral angiography, surgical procedure (cardiac surgery and orthopedic surgery), or head trauma and the onset of symptom of PA seems convincing for the link between the two pathologies. PA might be related in these cases to blood pressure fluctuation, anticoagulation, vasospasm, and/or microemboli leading to infarction. PA can also occur after pituitary function dynamic testing (TRH, GnRH, GHRH, and much more rarely CRH). Thus, dynamic testing is not recommended in patients with macroadenoma with extrasellar extension except for CRH or insulin tolerance test when useful for corticotropic axis, the other tests do not add crucial information. Treatment with GnRH agonist for prostate cancer has also been associated with PA (4). PA may be observed in patients under conventional and new classes of anticoagulation therapy very soon after initiation or after a prolonged period of treatment (5,6). Contrary to previous studies, a recent publication suggests that diabetes and arterial hypertension do not predispose patients to pituitary apoplexy (7).

The role of dopamine agonist (DA) is more controversial because PA occurs rarely early after the initiation of treatment, but more often after a long period of treatment (8, 9). Moreover, the rate of PA in macroprolactinomas is not higher than in untreated macroadenoma (10).

The adenoma subtype is a predisposing factor to apoplexy. PA seems more frequent in non-functioning pituitary adenomas (NFPAs) but this may be due to a selection bias: indeed, NFPA are generally discovered late and are usually larger (PA tends to complicate larger macroadenomas) than functioning adenomas (11). Silent ACTH adenomas are more prone to PA (30–64 % of cases), compared with prolactinomas (6.8–20%) (12–15).

Pathophysiology

The pathophysiology of PA is not fully understood, but it is noteworthy that most cases involve patients with macroadenomas (7,16,17).

The vascularization of adenoma is predominantly supported by the direct arterial blood supply rather than portal system for the normal pituitary gland. Pituitary tumors have reduced angiogenesis as shown by reduced density of microvasculature and low contrast-enhanced imaging in MRI.

Pituitary adenomas are five times more prone than other intracranial tumors to bleed and undergo infarction and necrosis, possibly because the pituitary gland has an unique rich vascular structure or because pituitary tumors may outgrow their blood supply or because ischemia (and thus infarction) occur following compression of infundibular or superior hypophyseal vessels against the sellar diaphragm by the expanding tumor mass with intrinsically poor vascularity. In this setting, all clinical situations that acutely decrease systemic BP (see predisposing factors) may decrease the blood supply to the pituitary adenoma and precipitate apoplexy.

Clinical Presentation

Headache is the most prominent symptom of acute apoplexy and is present in more than 80% of patients (18,19). Headache is also generally the initial symptom, with sudden and severe onset described "like a thunderclap in a clear sky" (20). Headache is usually retroorbital but can be bifrontal or diffuse. It is often associated with vomiting and nausea and can mimic migraine or meningitis (21).

Visual disturbances are present in more than half of PA patients due to a compression

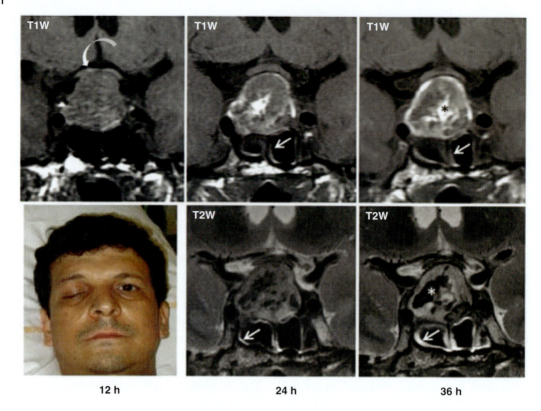

Figure 13-1 Serial MRI studies of a patient with pituitary apoplexy (mainly hemorrhagic). Left row: 12 hours after onset of symptoms (sudden headache, fatigue and right third oculomotor nerve palsy; bottom), T1-weighted (T1W) MRI shows a pituitary mass abutting the optic chiasm (curved arrow) and yielding a heterogeneous signal (top). Middle row: At 24 hours: T1W sequences show peripheral and central areas of spontaneous signal hyperintensity (top), while T2W sequences show mainly central hypointense areas (bottom); note also the typical thickening of the sphenoid sinus mucosa on both T1W and T2W sequences (arrows). Right row: At 36 hours: T1W (top) and T2W (bottom) sequences show an increase in the hyperintense and hypointense areas (asterisk) and further thickening of the sphenoid sinus mucosa (arrows).

of the optic chiasm or optic nerves, from upward expansion of the tumor (22). Variable degrees of visual-field impairment may be observed, bitemporal hemianopsia being most common. Loss of visual acuity and blindness can occur, but are rare (23).

Oculomotor palsies are also frequent, affecting 52% of patients in a compilation of studies and are due to functional impairment of cranial nerves III, IV and VI (24). The third cranial nerve is the most frequently affected (half of cranial nerve palsies) and is characterized by ptosis, limited eye movements in adduction, and mydriasis (24) (Figure 13-1).

Signs or symptoms of meningeal irritation, fever, and reduction of the level of consciousness rarely occur (25).

Scoring System

The UK Pituitary Apoplexy Guidelines Development Group proposed a "Pituitary Apoplexy Score" (PAS) based on the level of consciousness, visual acuity and field defects, and ocular palsies (Table 13-1) in order to enable more uniform clinical description of PA and, thus, better comparison of different management options (26).

Endocrine Dysfunction

Acute endocrine dysfunction may also be present, further complicating the clinical picture. One or more anterior pituitary deficiencies are always present at PA onset.

Table 13-1 Pituitary Apoplexy Score (26). Higher score indicates extensive neuro-opthalmic impairment.

Variable	Points
Level of consciousness	
• Glasgow Coma Scale 15	0
• Glasgow Coma Scale 8–14	2
• Glasgow Coma Scale < 8	4
Visual acuity	
• Normal 10/10 or 6/6 (or no change from pre-PA visual acuity)	0
• Reduced – unilateral	1
• Reduced – bilateral	2
Visual field defects	
• Normal	0
• Unilateral defect	1
• Bilateral defect	2
Ocular paresis	
• Absent	0
• Present unilateral	1
• Present bilateral	2

Corticotropic deficiency is the most common deficit observed in patients with PA, occurring in 50–80% of cases (3). It is also the most life-threatening hormonal complication, potentially causing severe hemodynamic problems and hyponatremia (27,28). Thus, empiric parenteral corticosteroid supplementation should be given to all patients with signs of PA, without waiting for diagnostic confirmation.

Almost all patients with PA have GH deficiency, but it is not often tested at diagnosis. According to reviews of the literature, 30–70% and 40–75% of patients with PA have thyrotropic deficiency and gonadotropic deficiency, respectively, at presentation (3). Finally, PA is one of the rare circumstances in which a pituitary adenoma may be associated with low PRL levels, found in 10–40 % of patient with PA (26,29). Diabetes insipidus is rare at PA onset, being present in fewer than 5% of patients, but may be masked by corticotropic deficiency and can thus emerge after steroid hormone replacement (3).

Pituitary Hypersecretion

PA can occur in a secreting adenoma: prolactinoma, acromegaly or Cushing's disease (3–10% of patients). In some cases, PA leads to resolution of pituitary hypersecretion (3).

Diagnostic Evaluation

Differential Diagnosis

The clinical presentation of PA may raise two major differential diagnoses, namely, subarachnoid hemorrhage and bacterial meningitis. Lumbar puncture is of little help in differentiating SAH and bacterial meningitis from PA, because the latter may be accompanied by a high red cell count, xanthochromia, or pleocytosis, and by an increased cerebrospinal fluid (CSF) protein level, particularly when signs of meningeal irritation are present (3). CSF culture will rule out bacterial meningitis, and a lumbar puncture is thus mandatory if this diagnosis is suspected. The best tools for diagnosing PA are computed tomography (CT) and MRI. By revealing a pituitary tumor, even if no necrosis or hemorrhage is found, these imaging methods offer confident diagnostic confirmation.

Diagnosis thus relies on a combination of clinical manifestations (e.g., sudden headache and visual disturbances) and the detection of a pituitary adenoma, whether before or after PA onset.

Imaging

Before discussing imaging features, it is important to understand that the underlying pathophysiological process in PA can be simple infarction (i.e., with little or no hemorrhagic component), hemorrhagic infarction, mixed hemorrhagic infarction and clot, or pure clot. This explains why imaging rarely shows pure hemorrhage or infarction but rather mixed features.

Computed Tomography (CT)
Given its wide availability, CT is usually the initial emergency examination for patients with severe headache of sudden onset. It has

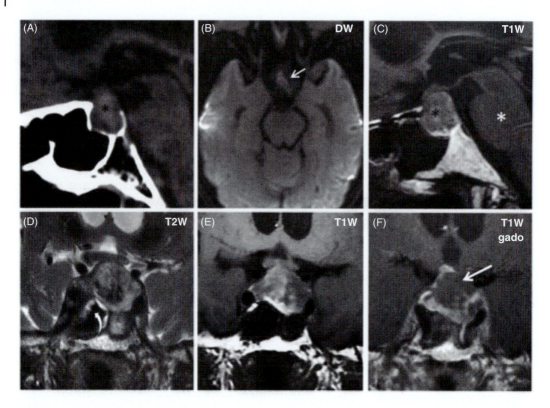

Figure 13-2 Imaging features 24 h after symptom onset in a patient with pituitary apoplexy. (A) Reformatted sagittal CT scan showing a spontaneously hyperdense sellar mass, suggesting hemorrhage within a pituitary adenoma; (B) Diffusion-weighted MRI (DW) at 24 h demonstrates a sellar tumor with a hyperintense central area (straight arrow); (C) T1-weighted MRI: sagittal section showing that the mass (black asterisk) is slightly hyperintense relative to the brain stem (white asterisk); (D) T2-weighted MRI: coronal section showing the mass with central areas of signal hypointensity and thickening of the sphenoid sinus mucosa (curved arrow); T1-weighted MRI: coronal views; (E) before gadolinium injection, the mass shows both hyper- and hypointense areas; (F) after gadolinium injection, only the bottom part of the tumor is enhanced, the central part remaining hypointense, without enhancement (thick arrow).

two advantages: (a) it rules out subarachnoid hemorrhage; and (b) it shows an intrasellar mass in 80% of cases, with hemorrhagic components in 20–30% of cases. After a few days, blood density decreases and may be more difficult to detect. After administration of contrast medium, the pituitary tumor shows inhomogeneous enhancement, occasionally with ring enhancement (3).

Magnetic Resonance Imaging (MRI)

MRI is now the imaging procedure of choice, even in the first days after symptom onset, as it can detect fresh bleeding (Figure 13-2). On T1-weighted (T1W) images, the water (CSF) is black, the gray matter is darker than

the white matter; on T2W images, the water (CSF) is hyperintense, the white matter is darker than gray matter. MRI can identify hemorrhagic and necrotic areas and show the relationship between the tumor and neighboring structures such as the optic chiasm, cavernous sinuses, and hypothalamus. As conventional (T1/T2) MRI sequences may not demonstrate an infarct for 6 hours, and small infarcts may be hard to appreciate on CT for days (Figure 13-3), diffusion weighted imaging (DWI), which provides information about consistency of macroadenomas, is very useful early in the PA process. Indeed, increased DWI signal in ischemic tissue is observed within a few minutes after arterial

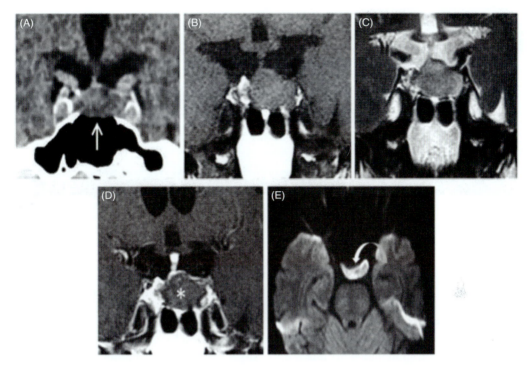

Figure 13-3 CT scan and MRI images of an ischemic form of pituitary apoplexy during the very first hours after the beginning of symptoms. (A) Coronal CT scan. Discrete hypodensity of a pituitary mass and thinning of the sellar floor (white arrow). (B, C, D) T1, T2 and contrast enhanced T1W images. The mass is T1 isointense and T2 hyperintense; a rim enhancement is visible after contrast administration, but the central part of the mass (asterisk) does not enhance. These images give no indication about the pathologic process. (E) Axial DWI shows marked hyperintensity of the lesion (curved arrow) thus confirming the ischemic origin of the apoplexy. Courtesy of Dr C. Magnin.

occlusion. In case of ischemic apoplexy, DWI can show increased signal intensity (Figures 13-2 and 13-3) relative to normal gray and white matter (30).

In the very first hours after onset, frank hyperintensity on T1W may be absent, either because of infarction or because the hemorrhage is still in the form of deoxyhemoglobin (31). A specific pattern of alternating subtly T1W hyperintense and hypointense areas within the sellar mass may suggest apoplexy (Figures 13-2 and 13-4) before the T1W hyperintense signal more characteristic of blood becomes visible (Figure 13-5).

Sequential MRI procedures are able to demonstrate the gradual increase in the T1W hyperintense signal, from the periphery toward the center of the mass, corresponding to the transformation from deoxyhemoglobin to methemoglobin (in methemoglobin, the iron is in the ferric state and, as such, is paramagnetic explaining why it appears hyperintense on T1W) (32); in parallel, T2W sequences demonstrate irregular hypointense areas toward the center of the tumor. Sometimes, the entire lesion can exhibit high signal intensity or a fluid-filled space, possibly associated with a fluid level inside the lesion; in this case, the upper compartment appears hyperintense while the lower compartment appears isointense (Figure 13-6).

T2-star weighted (T2*W) MRI, which is a gradient-echo sequence, is even more sensitive. The signal is dependent on T2 and on heterogeneity of magnetic field. It is generally used to detect deposits of hemosiderin even later after a hemorrhagic event. Thus T2*W MRI can detect intratumoral hemorrhage in pituitary adenomas: it yields a dark "rim,"

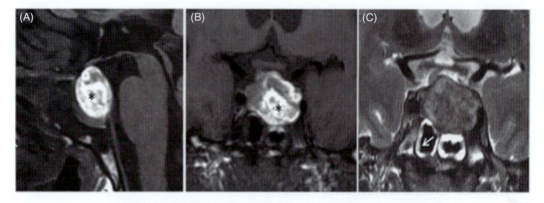

Figure 13-4 Typical aspect of hemorrhagic pituitary apoplexy on MRI, four days after symptom onset. (A) sagittal, and (B) coronal T1W sequences showing a frankly hyperintense pituitary mass (asterisk); (C) on coronal T2W sequences, the lesion is hypointense and the sphenoid sinus mucosa appears hyperintense and thickened (arrow).

"mass," "spot," or "diffuse" aspect or combinations thereof, which can be useful for assessing both recent and old intratumoral hemorrhage (33).

Thickening of the sphenoid sinus mucosa, predominantly in the compartment just beneath the sella turcica (Figures 13-2 and 13-4), was first described by Arita et al. on MRI performed during the acute phase of PA (34). A histological study showed that the subepithelial layer of the sphenoid sinus mucosa was markedly swollen. This thickening of the sphenoid mucosa, confirmed in another study in up to 80% of patients with

PA of variable severity, was shown to correlate with higher grades of PA and with worse neurological and endocrinological outcomes (35). This thickening does not indicate infectious sinusitis nor rule out transsphenoidal surgery, but is likely vascular in nature, from an increase in pressure in the venous system draining the sinus area – an indirect result of the tumor and the increased intrasellar pressure.

If conservative treatment is chosen, spontaneous shrinkage of the sellar mass may be observed within a few weeks (36,37) (Figure 13-6).

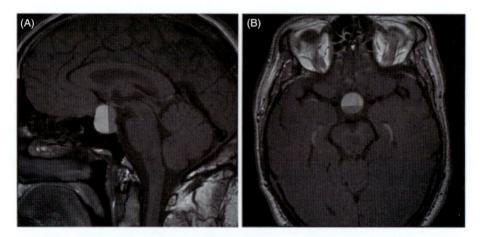

Figure 13-5 MRI in a patient with pituitary apoplexy, showing a fluid level inside the pituitary lesion; the upper compartment is hyperintense while the lower compartment is isointense (T1-weighted sequences, sagittal (A) and axial (B) views).

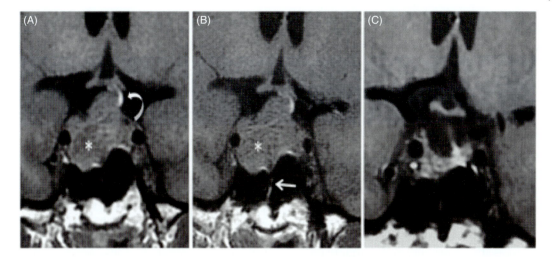

Figure 13-6 Serial imaging studies in a patient with ischemic pituitary apoplexy. (A) Two days after symptom onset, T1W image shows an heterogeneous pituitary mass (asterisk). Note the ectopic position of the posterior pituitary represented by a T1 hyperintense nodule below the optic chiasm (curved arrow); (B) 48 h later, T1W image does not show any hyperintense area within in the pituitary mass, suggesting purely necrotic apoplexy. Note the slight thickening of the sphenoid sinus mucosa (straight arrow). (C). Four months later, after conservative management, T1WI demonstrates a spontaneous shrinkage of the tumor.

Management of Pituitary Apoplexy

A Matter of Debate

The course of PA is highly variable. Histological features may be important for prognostication: simple tumor infarction alone tends to produce less severe clinical features at presentation and have a better outcome than hemorrhagic infarction or frank hemorrhage (38).

Recovery of neurological, ophthalmological, and endocrine function is highly variable. If altered consciousness improves after decompression, altered visual fields and acuity also tend to improve, but permanent visual sequelae may occur, particularly in case of optical nerve atrophy.

The treatment aims are to improve symptoms and relieve compression of local structures, particularly the optic pathways. Surgical decompression is probably the most rapid means of achieving these goals. The dramatic picture presented by many patients explains why PA is considered a neurosurgical emergency and has almost always been treated surgically in the past. However, surgery may also be harmful, with a risk of postoperative CSF rhinorrhea, posterior pituitary damage (risk of permanent diabetes insipidus), and an increased likelihood of hypopituitarism due to removal of or damage to normal pituitary tissue. Fortunately, in experienced pituitary centers these complication are rare and this does not prevent surgery being proposed when symptoms are severe and rapidly installed and/or tumor is large.

As some patients recover normal visual and endocrine function following conservative steroid-based management, the optimal management of acute PA is controversial. At all events, PA must be managed by an expert multidisciplinary team including an ophthalmologist, neuroradiologist, endocrinologist, and neurosurgeon (26).

Steroid Therapy Is Mandatory

As corticotropic deficiency is present in the vast majority of patients at PA onset and may be life-threatening, whether treated surgically or conservatively, corticosteroids should be administered intravenously as soon as the diagnosis is confirmed: it will consist of hydrocortisone 50 mg every 6 h (39,40), or a bolus of 100–200 mg followed by 50–100 mg every 6 h intravenously (or intramuscularly) (41), or 2–4 mg/h by continuous intravenous administration (26).

Surgical Approach

If surgical management is chosen, the transsphenoidal approach is almost always recommended because it allows good decompression of the optic pathways and neuroanatomic structures in contact with the tumor, and because it is associated with low postoperative morbidity and mortality (26).

Even if surgical complications are rare, particularly in experienced hands, CSF leakage and diabetes insipidus (sometimes permanent) may occur (7,22,42,43). It seems that endocrine outcome after elective pituitary surgery is poorer in patients with PA than in patients without PA (7). Much of this, however, is secondary to damage to the normal gland from the initial apoplectic event.

Another important point is that, in this acute setting, the operation may be performed by an on-call neurosurgeon rather than by a skilled pituitary neurosurgeon, as underlined in UK guidelines (26), and this may increase the risk of adverse events.

Conservative Approach

Reports of spontaneous clinical improvement and shrinkage (or disappearance) of apoplectic pituitary adenomas suggest that a conservative approach may be appropriate in selected cases. Pelkonen et al. (1978) were among the first to propose a conservative approach, followed by others, after observing not only spontaneous recoveries but also cases in which the apoplexy appeared to cure hormonal hypersecretion (GH, ACTH, etc.) (44–46).

In 1995, Maccagnan et al. reported the results of a prospective study in which they treated pituitary apoplexy with high-dose steroids (47). Only patients whose visual impairment or altered consciousness failed to improve underwent surgery. Conservative steroid treatment was possible in 7 out of 12 patients, leaving only 5 patients who needed surgery.

Surgical or Conservative Management?

Studies Comparing Outcomes

Five large retrospective studies have compared the outcomes of conservatively and surgically treated patients with pituitary apoplexy (21,48–51). As their authors acknowledged, these studies suffered from a selection bias due to their retrospective design: indeed, the patients in the conservative group generally had less severe ocular defects than those in the surgical group (3). Nevertheless, whatever the outcome (e.g., oculomotor palsy, pituitary function, subsequent tumor growth and even visual defect), immediate surgical treatment has not shown clear superiority over conservative approach (3).

Can Imaging Help to Choose Between Conservative and Surgical Treatment?

Compared to CT, MRI allows more precise evaluation of adjacent anatomical structures (optic apparatus, cavernous sinus, etc.). A single large hypodense area within the tumor on CT might be associated with better subsequent tumor shrinkage than are several small hypodense areas (47). In another study, MRI findings were found to be associated with clinical status and outcome: patients with simple infarction had less severe clinical features and better outcomes than those with hemorrhagic infarction or hemorrhage (52).

UK Guidelines for the Management of Pituitary Apoplexy

In the UK, guidelines were recently proposed for the management of patients with pituitary apoplexy (26). They recommend surgical decompression in case of "significant neuro-ophthalmic signs or reduced level of consciousness." This seems a very reasonable option. A management algorithm is proposed in these guidelines (Figure 13-7). If surgery is chosen, then its timing is important. Visual

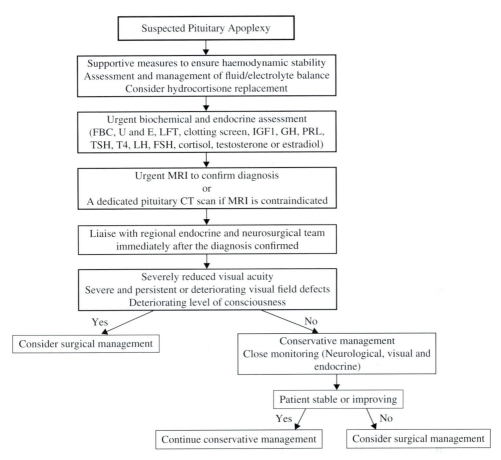

Figure 13-7 Algorithm for the management of pituitary apoplexy (26)
FBC = full (complete) blood count; U and E = urea and electrolytes; LFT = liver function tests;
IGF-1 = insulin-like growth factor 1; GH = growth hormone; TSH = thyroid-stimulating hormone; T4 = thyroxine;
LH = luteinizing hormone; FSH = follicle-stimulating hormone; MRI = magnetic resonance imaging;
CT = computed tomography.

defects used to be considered a neurosurgical emergency, but there seems to be no difference in outcome when surgery is performed in the first three days or during the first week after symptom onset (18,23,53). In contrast, the prognosis of visual defects is less favorable when surgery takes place more than a week after onset (54).

The higher number of patients treated conservatively by the same team nowadays (29.9%) (55) compared as in the past (2.7%) (56) may be related to the lower rates of opthalmoparesis and visual field defects in the current series, which may be explained by earlier diagnosis enabled by MRI.

Conclusions

Pituitary apoplexy, due to sudden hemorrhaging and/or infarction of the pituitary gland, generally within a pituitary adenoma, can be difficult to diagnose. A CT or MRI scan confirms the diagnosis by revealing a pituitary tumor with hemorrhagic and/or necrotic components. Corticotropic deficiency may be life-threatening if left untreated, and glucocorticoids must therefore always be introduced immediately.

Owing to the highly variable course of this syndrome and the lack of randomized prospective studies, optimal management of acute pituitary apoplexy remains controversial. Some authors advocate early transsphenoidal surgical decompression for all patients, whereas others adopt a conservative approach for selected patients, namely, those without visual acuity or field defects and with normal consciousness. The size of the tumor on MRI is also an important part of the clinical decision-making process. If conservative treatment is chosen, then careful monitoring of visual signs and symptoms is necessary, and surgical decompression

is recommended if visual disorders do not improve or if they deteriorate. However, clinical deterioration can be rapid and patients may not be able to be hospitalized for observation, which may limit this approach.

Re-evaluation of pituitary function and the tumor mass in the months following the acute apoplectic episode is mandatory to determine whether or not the pituitary defect is permanent, to determine the possible hypersecretory nature of the adenoma, and to initiate follow-up of a possible tumor remnant.

References

1 Fernandez A, Karavitaki N, Wass JA. Prevalence of pituitary adenomas: a community-based, cross-sectional study in Banbury (Oxfordshire, UK). *Clin Endocrinol (Oxf)*. 2010;72:377–382.

2 Raappana A, Koivukangas J, Ebeling T, Pirila T. Incidence of pituitary adenomas in Northern Finland in 1992-2007. *J Clin Endocrinol Metab*. 2010;95:4268–4275.

3 Briet C, Salenave S, Bonneville JF, Laws ER, Chanson P. Pituitary apoplexy. *Endocrine Reviews*. 2015;36:622–645.

4 Chanson P, Schaison G. Pituitary apoplexy caused by GnRH-agonist treatment revealing gonadotroph adenoma. *J Clin Endocrinol Metab*. 1995;80:2267–2268.

5 Doglietto F, Costi E, Villaret AB, Mardighian D, Fontanella MM, Giustina A. New oral anticoagulants and pituitary apoplexy. *Pituitary*. 2014;19(2):232–234.

6 Uemura M MF, Shimomura R, Fujinami J, Toyoda K. Pituitary apoplexy during treatment with dabigatran. *Neurol Clin Neurosci*. 2013;1:82–83.

7 Moller-Goede DL, Brandle M, Landau K, Bernays RL, Schmid C. Pituitary apoplexy: re-evaluation of risk factors for bleeding into pituitary adenomas and impact on outcome. *Eur J Endocrinol*. 2011;164: 37–43.

8 Chng E, Dalan R. Pituitary apoplexy associated with cabergoline therapy. *J Clin Neurosci*. 2013;20:1637–1643.

9 Balarini Lima GA, Machado Ede O, Dos Santos Silva CM, Filho PN, Gadelha MR. Pituitary apoplexy during treatment of cystic macroprolactinomas with cabergoline. *Pituitary*. 2008;11:287–292.

10 Carija R, Vucina D. Frequency of pituitary tumor apoplexy during treatment of prolactinomas with dopamine agonists: a systematic review. *CNS Neurol Disord Drug Targets*. 2012;11:1012–1014.

11 Semple PL, Jane JA, Jr., Laws ER, Jr. Clinical relevance of precipitating factors in pituitary apoplexy. *Neurosurgery*. 2007;61:956–961; discussion 961–952.

12 Sarwar KN, Huda MS, Van de Velde V, et al. The prevalence and natural history of pituitary hemorrhage in prolactinoma. *J Clin Endocrinol Metab*. 2013;98: 2362–2367.

13 Scheithauer BW, Jaap AJ, Horvath E, et al. Clinically silent corticotroph tumors of the pituitary gland. *Neurosurgery*. 2000; 47:723–729; discussion 729–730.

14 Sahli R, Christ ER, Seiler R, Kappeler A, Vajtai I. Clinicopathologic correlations of silent corticotroph adenomas of the pituitary: report of four cases and literature review. *Pathol Res Pract*. 2006;202: 457–464.

15 Webb KM, Laurent JJ, Okonkwo DO, Lopes MB, Vance ML, Laws ER, Jr. Clinical characteristics of silent corticotrophic

adenomas and creation of an internet-accessible database to facilitate their multi-institutional study. *Neurosurgery*. 2003;53:1076–1084; discussion 1084–1075.

16 Verrees M, Arafah BM, Selman WR. Pituitary tumor apoplexy: characteristics, treatment, and outcomes. *Neurosurg Focus*. 2004;16:E6.

17 Turgut M, Seyithanoglu MH, Tüzgen S. Definition, history, frequency, histopathology and pathophysiology of pituitary apoplexy. In: Turgut M, Mahapatra AK, Powell M, Muthukumar N, eds. *Pituitary Apoplexy*. Berlin: Springer-Verlag; 2014: 3–10.

18 Bi WL, Dunn IF, Laws ER, Jr. Pituitary apoplexy. *Endocrine*. 2014; 48:69–75.

19 Shimon I. Clinical features of pituitary apoplexy. In: Turgut M, Mahapatra AK, Powell M, Muthukumar N, eds. *Pituitary Apoplexy*. Berlin: Springer-Verlag; 2014: 49–54.

20 Garza I, Kirsch J. Pituitary apoplexy and thunderclap headache. *Headache*. 2007; 47:431–432.

21 Sibal L, Ball SG, Connolly V, et al. Pituitary apoplexy: a review of clinical presentation, management and outcome in 45 cases. *Pituitary*. 2004;7:157–163.

22 Dubuisson AS, Beckers A, Stevenaert A. Classical pituitary tumour apoplexy: clinical features, management and outcomes in a series of 24 patients. *Clin Neurol Neurosurg*. 2007;109:63–70.

23 Turgut M, Ozsunar Y, Basak S, Guney E, Kir E, Meteoglu I. Pituitary apoplexy: an overview of 186 cases published during the last century. *Acta Neurochir (Wien)*. 2010;152:749–761.

24 Jenkins TM, Toosy AT. Visual acuity, eye movements and visual fields. In: Turgut M, Mahapatra AK, Powell M, Muthukumar N, eds. *Pituitary Apoplexy*. Berlin: Springer-Verlag; 2014: 75–88.

25 Smidt MH, van der Vliet A, Wesseling P, de Vries J, Twickler TB, Vos PE. Pituitary apoplexy after mild head injury misinterpreted as bacterial meningitis. *Eur J Neurol*. 2007;14:e7–e8.

26 Rajasekaran S, Vanderpump M, Baldeweg S, et al. UK guidelines for the management of pituitary apoplexy. *Clin Endocrinol (Oxf)*. 2011;74:9–20.

27 Grossman AB. Clinical Review#: The diagnosis and management of central hypoadrenalism. *J Clin Endocrinol Metab*. 2010;95:4855–4863.

28 Hahner S, Spinnler C, Fassnacht M, et al. High incidence of adrenal crisis in educated patients with chronic adrenal insufficiency: a prospective study. *J Clin Endocrinol Metab*. 2015;100:407–416.

29 Semple PL, Ross IL. Endocrinopathies and other biochemical abnormalities in pituitary apoplexy. In: Turgut M, Mahapatra AK, Powell M, Muthukumar N, eds. *Pituitary Apoplexy*. Berlin: Springer-Verlag; 2014: 107–115.

30 Rogg JM, Tung GA, Anderson G, Cortez S. Pituitary apoplexy: early detection with diffusion-weighted MR imaging. *AJNR Am J Neuroradiol*. 2002;23:1240–1245.

31 Flanagan EP, Hunderfund AL, Giannini C, Meissner I. Addition of magnetic resonance imaging to computed tomography and sensitivity to blood in pituitary apoplexy. *Arch Neurol*. 2011;68:1336–1337.

32 Glick RP, Tiesi JA. Subacute pituitary apoplexy: clinical and magnetic resonance imaging characteristics. *Neurosurgery*. 1990;27:214–218; discussion 218–219.

33 Tosaka M, Sato N, Hirato J, et al. Assessment of hemorrhage in pituitary macroadenoma by T2*-weighted gradient-echo MR imaging. *AJNR Am J Neuroradiol*. 2007;28:2023–2029.

34 Arita K, Kurisu K, Tominaga A, et al. Thickening of sphenoid sinus mucosa during the acute stage of pituitary apoplexy. *J Neurosurg*. 2001;95:897–901.

35 Liu JK, Couldwell WT. Pituitary apoplexy in the magnetic resonance imaging era: clinical significance of sphenoid sinus mucosal thickening. *J Neurosurg*. 2006;104:892–898.

36 Armstrong MR, Douek M, Schellinger D, Patronas NJ. Regression of pituitary macroadenoma after pituitary apoplexy:

CT and MR studies. *J Comput Assist Tomogr.* 1991;15:832–834.

37 Oldfield EH, Merrill MJ. Apoplexy of pituitary adenomas: the perfect storm. *J Neurosurg.* 2015;122:1444–1449.

38 Semple PL, De Villiers JC, Bowen RM, Lopes MB, Laws ER, Jr. Pituitary apoplexy: do histological features influence the clinical presentation and outcome? *J Neurosurg.* 2006;104:931–937.

39 Chanson P, Lepeintre JF, Ducreux D. Management of pituitary apoplexy. *Expert Opin Pharmacother.* 2004;5:1287–1298.

40 Nawar RN, Abdel-Mannan D, Selman WR, Arafah BM. Pituitary tumor apoplexy: a review. *J Intensive Care Med.* 2008;23:75–90.

41 Vanderpump M, Higgens C, Wass JA. UK guidelines for the management of pituitary apoplexy a rare but potentially fatal medical emergency. *Emerg Med J.* 2011;28:550–551.

42 Gondim JA, Almeida JP, Albuquerque LA, et al. Endoscopic endonasal approach for pituitary adenoma: surgical complications in 301 patients. *Pituitary.* 2011;14:174–183.

43 Berker M, Hazer DB, Yucel T, et al. Complications of endoscopic surgery of the pituitary adenomas: analysis of 570 patients and review of the literature. *Pituitary.* 2012;15:288–300.

44 Pelkonen R, Kuusisto A, Salmi J, et al. Pituitary function after pituitary apoplexy. *Am J Med.* 1978;65:773–778.

45 Jeffcoate WJ, Birch CR. Apoplexy in small pituitary tumours. *J Neurol Neurosurg Psychiatry.* 1986;49:1077–1078.

46 McFadzean RM, Doyle D, Rampling R, Teasdale E, Teasdale G. Pituitary apoplexy and its effect on vision. *Neurosurgery.* 1991;29:669–675.

47 Maccagnan P, Macedo CL, Kayath MJ, Nogueira RG, Abucham J. Conservative management of pituitary apoplexy: a prospective study. *J Clin Endocrinol Metab.* 1995;80:2190–2197.

48 Ayuk J, McGregor EJ, Mitchell RD, Gittoes NJ. Acute management of pituitary apoplexy–surgery or conservative management? *Clin Endocrinol (Oxf).* 2004;61:747–752.

49 Gruber A, Clayton J, Kumar S, Robertson I, Howlett TA, Mansell P. Pituitary apoplexy: retrospective review of 30 patients–is surgical intervention always necessary? *Br J Neurosurg.* 2006;20:379–385.

50 Leyer C, Castinetti F, Morange I, et al. A conservative management is preferable in milder forms of pituitary tumor apoplexy. *J Endocrinol Invest.* 2011;34:502–509.

51 Bujawansa S, Thondam SK, Steele C, et al. Presentation, management and outcomes in acute pituitary apoplexy: a large single-centre experience from the United Kingdom. *Clin Endocrinol (Oxf).* 2014;80:419–424.

52 Ahmed SK, Semple PL. Cerebral ischaemia in pituitary apoplexy. *Acta Neurochir (Wien).* 2008;150:1193–1196; discussion 1196.

53 Agrawal D, Mahapatra AK. Visual outcome of blind eyes in pituitary apoplexy after transsphenoidal surgery: a series of 14 eyes. *Surg Neurol.* 2005;63:42–46; discussion 46.

54 Randeva HS, Schoebel J, Byrne J, Esiri M, Adams CB, Wass JA. Classical pituitary apoplexy: clinical features, management and outcome. *Clin Endocrinol (Oxf).* 1999;51:181–188.

55 Singh TD, Valizadeh N, Meyer FB, Atkinson JL, Erickson D, Rabinstein AA. Management and outcomes of pituitary apoplexy. *J Neurosurg.* 2015;122:1450–1457.

56 Bills DC, Meyer FB, Laws ER, Jr., et al. A retrospective analysis of pituitary apoplexy. *Neurosurgery.* 1993;33:602–608; discussion 608–609.

14

Macroprolactinomas

Mark E. Molitch

Key Points

- Pituitary tumors account for approximately 10–15% of all intracranial tumors.
- The pathogenesis of most pituitary adenomas remains unknown.
- Pituitary adenomas may hypersecrete hormones or cause mass effects (i.e., headache, hypopituitarism, and visual field [VF] defects).
- Pituitary adenomas are divided into microadenomas (<10 mm), macroadenomas (≥10 mm), and giant adenomas (≥40 mm) as demonstrated on magnetic resonance imaging (MRI) or computed tomography (CT) scan. Pituitary carcinomas with distant metastases are rare, occurring in 0.1–0.2% of cases.
- If an MRI shows the tumor impinging on the optic chiasm, then formal VF testing is indicated. An evaluation for hypopituitarism should be carried out in all patients with macroadenomas and even large (6–9 mm) microadenomas. Diabetes insipidus is rarely seen with pituitary adenomas. About two-thirds of pituitary adenomas may secrete excess hormones.
- Treatments include transsphenoidal surgery, medical therapies, and radiotherapy.
- Prolactin-secreting adenomas (prolactinomas), account for approximately 40% of pituitary tumors.
- Several aspects of management of patients with macroprolactinomas may be difficult and, in some cases, can be considered emergencies.
- Visual field defects can be expected in about 40% of patients with macroprolactinomas. Improvement in such defects with dopamine agonist treatment appears to be at least as good as can be achieved by transsphenoidal surgery and can be accomplished with less morbidity. With both treatments, improvements can be delayed and there is no emergency in decompressing the chiasm.
- Cerebrospinal fluid (CSF) rhinorrhea can occur when there is a large, invasive, skull-based prolactinoma that serves as a "cork" in the base of the skull. When the tumor size is reduced substantially through dopamine agonist use, CSF can leak around the tumor into the sphenoid sinus and nasal passages, with a resultant risk of meningitis. Measurement of beta-2 transferrin in the nasal fluid is diagnostic. Surgical repair is usually required.
- Pituitary apoplexy is very rare, although asymptomatic hemorrhage into a pituitary adenoma is common. In patients with apoplexy, rapid assessment for hypopituitarism and treatment of deficits in corticotropin (adrenocorticotropic hormone, ACTH) with stress steroids are important. Although surgical decompression is often required, many patients may be treated conservatively.

Endocrine and Metabolic Medical Emergencies: A Clinician's Guide, Second Edition. Edited by Glenn Matfin.
© 2018 John Wiley & Sons Ltd. Published 2018 by John Wiley & Sons Ltd.

- Macroprolactinoma enlargement during pregnancy occurs in about 22% of women, resulting in headaches or visual symptoms. Visual field monitoring each trimester for women with macroprolactinomas is warranted. Treatment consists of reinstitution of dopamine agonists, surgery if that is not effective, or delivery if the pregnancy is sufficiently advanced.

Introduction

Pituitary tumors account for approximately 10–15% of all intracranial tumors (1,2). The pathogenesis of most pituitary adenomas remains unknown. Pituitary adenomas may hypersecrete hormones or cause mass effects (i.e., headache, hypopituitarism, and visual field [VF] defects). Pituitary adenomas are divided into microadenomas (<10 mm), macroadenomas (≥10 mm), and giant adenomas (≥40 mm) as demonstrated on magnetic resonance imaging (MRI) or a computed tomography (CT) scan (1–3). Pituitary carcinomas with distant metastases are rare, occurring in 0.1–0.2% of cases (3).

If an MRI shows the tumor impinging on the optic chiasm, then formal VF testing is indicated. An evaluation for hypopituitarism should be carried out in all patients with macroadenomas and even large (6–9 mm) microadenomas (3). Diabetes insipidus is rarely seen with pituitary adenomas. About two-thirds of pituitary adenomas may secrete excess hormones. Treatments include transsphenoidal surgery, medical therapies, and radiotherapy.

Prolactin (PRL)-secreting adenomas (prolactinomas) account for approximately 40% of pituitary tumors (1–3). The reported population prevalence of clinically apparent prolactinomas ranges from 6–10 per 100,000 to approximately 50 per 100,000 (1–3). Generally, prolactinomas are diagnosed when patients present with typical findings of hyperprolactinemia, such as galactorrhea, amenorrhea and infertility in women, erectile dysfunction and infertility in men, and lack of libido in both sexes (1). Once hyperprolactinemia is documented and other causes excluded, MRI is performed to characterize a possible tumor (1,3). Prolactinomas are also frequently discovered as a pituitary incidentaloma (previously unsuspected pituitary lesion that is discovered on an imaging study for an unrelated reason), which are present in approximately 10% of the general population and are frequently discovered in acute clinical settings (2). The management of pituitary incidentalomas is discussed in detail in an Endocrine Society Clinical Practice Guideline on pituitary incidentalomas and is summarized in Figure 14-1 (2). However, it should be remembered that PRL levels should be run at 1:100 dilution in patients with large (>3 cm) macro-incidentalomas, to avoid missing a prolactinoma because of the "hook effect" (very high levels of PRL saturating the antibodies in some assays, giving falsely normal or mildly elevated levels) (1–3).

The treatment of patients with microprolactinomas and macroprolactinomas is generally very satisfying for clinicians, primarily due to the excellent efficacy of dopamine agonist therapy in reducing PRL levels (Table 14-1), reducing adenoma size, and restoring gonadal function, and improving other clinical features (1,4). The Endocrine Society guideline on treatment of hyperprolactinemia generally recommends cabergoline as the dopamine agonist of choice, due to higher efficacy in normalizing prolactin levels and pituitary tumor shrinkage (1). Transsphenoidal surgery is a therapeutic option and can achieve a normalization of PRL in 65–85% of patients with microprolactinoma and 30–40% with macroprolactinomas. Radiotherapy is generally reserved for the uncommon patients (<5%) whose hyperprolactinemia and tumor cannot be controlled with dopamine agonists or surgery. The alkylating

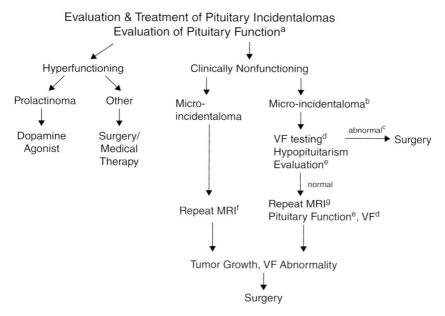

Figure 14-1 Flow diagram for the evaluation and treatment of pituitary incidentalomas. (a) Baseline evaluation in all patients should include a history and physical exam evaluating for signs and symptoms of hyperfunction and hypopituitarism and a laboratory evaluation for hypersecretion. (b) This group may also include large microlesions. (c) The recommendation for surgery includes the presence of abnormalities of visual field (VF) or vision and signs of tumor compression; surgery is also suggested for other findings. (d) VF testing is recommended for patients with lesions abutting or compressing the optic nerves or chiasm at the initial evaluation and during follow-up. (e) Evaluation for hypopituitarism is recommended for the baseline evaluation and during follow-up evaluations. This is most strongly recommended for macrolesions and larger microlesions. (f) Repeat MRI in one year, yearly for three years, and then less frequently thereafter if no change in lesion size. (g) Repeat the MRI in 6 months, yearly for three years, and then less frequently if no change in lesion size.

Table 14-1 Medications used for the treatment of prolactinomas (3). Quinagolide (non-ergot-derived dopamine agonist) is infrequently used in some countries (where approved) when intolerance or lack of efficacy to cabergoline or bromocriptine has occurred. Usual dose is 25 mcg nocte for three days, and then titrated up by 25 mcg every three days to usual maintenance dose of 75–150 mcg nocte.

Medications	Dose	Drug class	Patients achieving hormonal control (%)*	Adverse effects
Bromocriptine	2.5–7.5 mg/d	Dopamine agonist	60–80	Nausea, vomiting, constipation, dizziness, headache, compulsive behavior[#]
Cabergoline	0.5–2.0 mg/wk	Dopamine agonist	80–90	Nausea, vomiting, constipation, dizziness, headache, compulsive behavior[#]
				Cardiac valve disorders (high doses, >2 mg/wk)

*Achieving hormonal control was defined as normal prolactin levels.
[#]Compulsive behavior, such as excessive gambling and hypersexuality, can occur in about 5% of patients on dopamine agonists.

agent, temozolomide, has been used for very aggressive prolactinomas and pituitary carcinomas with limited success (3).

However, there are some aspects of treatment that are more troubling than others and some can even be considered emergencies; most of these aspects occur in patients with macroprolactinomas. Several particular aspects of management fall into these categories of conditions: (a) a VF defect at presentation; (b) the development of cerebrospinal fluid (CSF) rhinorrhea; (c) the development of pituitary apoplexy; and (d) tumor enlargement during pregnancy.

Visual Field Defect at Presentation

Visual field defects can be expected in about 40% of patients with macroprolactinomas (5–8). Visual field testing is only necessary, of course, in patients whose tumors are found to abut the optic chiasm on MRI. While it is recognized that overall, dopamine agonist treatment is more efficacious than transsphenoidal surgery for patients with prolactinomas (1,4), it is worth reviewing some of the data that would allow comparison of the efficacy of dopamine agonist treatment vs. transsphenoidal surgery with respect to improving VF defects.

In a US multicenter study, bromocriptine was found to cause VF defect improvement in 9 of 10 patients who had defects (5). Maximal improvement was found by two weeks in one patient, by three months in five patients and by six months in the remaining three patients (4). In general, the improvement in VF defects parallels the change in tumor size. In their review on bromocriptine-treated macroadenomas, Bevan et al. (6) found that 79% of 271 macroadenomas showed more than 25% shrinkage, and of the 102 patients with chiasmal compression, 85% showed tumor shrinkage of more than 25%. Shrinkage with VF improvement may occur as early as a few days with maximal shrinkage generally occurring by 3–6 months (5–7). A 75–90% tumor shrinkage with VF improvement similarly occurs with cabergoline (1,8–10).

Complete normalization of VF occurred in 9 out of 10 patients in one series, with such normalization occurring by 3 months in 4 patients and by 6–12 months in 5 patients (9).

Because the primary treatment of most patients with prolactinomas is medical rather than surgical currently, the most appropriate comparison is with patients with clinically nonfunctioning pituitary adenomas (CNFA), who have undergone transsphenoidal surgery. In a meta-analysis that analyzed 59 series, 795 patients with CNFAs had visual field defects and transsphenoidal surgery resulted in an improvement in VF defects in 78%, at the expense, however, of a 1% mortality and 3% worsening of VF (11). It is important to note that following surgery, the improvement in VF is not necessarily rapid. There is a rapid recovery of some function within minutes to a few days, a more delayed recovery over weeks to months, and late recovery over months to years (12).

Overall, therefore, the improvement in VF with dopamine agonist treatment appears to be at least as good as can be achieved by transsphenoidal surgery. Furthermore, medical treatment can be accomplished with less morbidity and better achievement of normal PRL levels (4). With both treatments, the improvements in VF can be quite delayed. Dekkers et al. (13) performed repeat VF at a mean of four weeks (range 1–45 weeks) following surgery in 34 patients with CNFAs, finding no change in VFs or visual acuity within that time period. Although some studies show that a longer preoperative duration of symptoms results in worse outcomes after surgery (14), others do not (15). Thus, there is no urgency to rush into surgery for the patient with a VF defect and a trial of a dopamine agonist is indicated unless the VF defect is sudden (see section on Pituitary Apoplexy below). Consultation with an experienced pituitary surgeon can be very helpful in this setting. Given the time periods discussed above, a 3-month trial would appear to be warranted. Monitoring of PRL levels and VF every 4–6 weeks seems reasonable. A full reevaluation with PRL levels, VF and MRI should be carried out at 3 months in such patients. If there is no change in tumor size with continued abutment of the chiasm and no improvement at all in VF and the defect is clinically significant, then surgical decompression is reasonable. If the VF defect is minimal, then perhaps surgery would not be indicated, especially if PRL levels have come down to normal or near normal. If there is substantial tumor shrinkage with relief of pressure on the chiasm, then surgery would not be expected to result in VF improvement despite persistent defects and therefore would not be indicated. Certainly, if there is evidence of tumor growth or a worsening of VF over the initial 3 months or later, surgical decompression of the chiasm would be indicated.

One additional rare complication should be mentioned, and that is a secondary worsening of VF after successful treatment with dopamine agonists due to marked tumor shrinkage with herniation of the optic apparatus into the partially empty sella (16,17). Of course, the same worsening can occur after surgery as well.

Cerebrospinal Fluid (CSF) Rhinorrhea

CSF rhinorrhea can occur when there is a large, invasive, skull-based prolactinoma that serves as a "cork" in the base of the skull. When the tumor size is reduced substantially through dopamine agonist use, CSF can leak around the tumor into the sphenoid sinus and nasal passages (18,29). Because tumor shrinkage may occur rapidly, such CSF rhinorrhea may occur within a week of starting the dopamine agonist (18,19). Although CSF rhinorrhea is relatively rare, such an occurrence has been reported in the literature in 42 patients with prolactinomas through 2012, with the CSF leak occurring following dopamine agonist therapy in 36 (86%) (19). Spontaneous CSF leaks can also occur without medical therapy, but they are much less common (18,19).

Typically, patients will develop excessive rhinorrhea and then the differential diagnosis is between CSF rhinorrhea and a simple upper respiratory infection. With CSF rhinorrhea, the amount of fluid typically is increased if the patient leans forward and down. The fluid should be sent to the laboratory for measurement of beta-2 transferrin, which is an asialo transferrin isoform found only in CSF, ocular fluids, and perilymph and is an accepted marker of CSF leakage (20). The major concern with such leaks is the risk of meningitis, although pneumocephaly may also occur (14–16). The use of prophylactic antibiotics while awaiting surgery is controversial (21). Urgent consultation with an experienced pituitary neurosurgeon is important when CSF rhinorrhea is suspected, as endonasal, endoscopic surgical repair of the leak to prevent meningitis is generally recommended (21). Although such a repair is not emergent, it should be done expeditiously. Conservative approaches of reduction in dopamine agonist dose and reduction of CSF pressure through insertion of a lumbar drain are usually not successful (19).

Case Study

A 38-year-old woman had had previous transsphenoidal surgery and conventional radiotherapy for a large macroadenoma five years previously with resultant hypopituitarism. She required cabergoline for continued management of her residual tumor and hyperprolactinemia. She presented with the new onset of two weeks of persistent, unilateral rhinorrhea.

How Would You Confirm the Diagnosis of CSF Rhinorrhea?

A beta-2 transferrin level was measured in the nasal fluid and was positive, consistent with a diagnosis of CSF rhinorrhea. She subsequently underwent neurosurgical repair with cessation of the CSF rhinorrhea. This patient illustrates a situation of CSF rhinorrhea developing several years after transsphenoidal surgery during cabergoline treatment.

Pituitary Apoplexy

Pituitary apoplexy is a clinical syndrome consisting of severe headache, stiff neck, nausea, vomiting, and often neurologic symptoms such as ophthalmoplegias, cranial nerve palsies, VF defects, ptosis, or altered mental status (22,23). These symptoms are related to a rapid expansion of the contents of the sella into the parasellar and suprasellar spaces due to hemorrhage into or hemorrhagic infarction of an adenoma (22,23). Hemorrhage can be found in 25–36% of pituitary adenomas removed at surgery (22,23) and was found on MRI in 16/79 (20.3%) macroprolactinomas and 9/289 (3.1%) microprolactinomas in a recent series (24). Of these surgical cases, about half of the hemorrhages were entirely asymptomatic, about one third were associated with mild-to-moderate headaches, and only 10–15% had symptoms compatible with pituitary apoplexy. In the prolactinoma series, of the 25/368 patients who had hemorrhage, only 3 were considered to have classic apoplexy (24). This hemorrhagic infarction is to be distinguished from the bland infarction of the normal pituitary that may be seen with hypotension which is most commonly seen following postpartum bleeding (Sheehan's syndrome) (22). Virtually all cases of true pituitary apoplexy are due to hemorrhagic infarction of a preexisting adenoma and not to hemorrhage into normal pituitary tissue and most occur in macroadenomas rather than microadenomas (22,23). In general, the amount of hemorrhage correlates with the severity of symptoms (23). Although bland infarction may cause apoplexy, it usually causes less severe symptoms and a more prolonged course (22). It has been hypothesized that dopamine agonist use may precipitate apoplexy in patients with prolactinomas, but this has not been proven (23). Anticoagulation, especially in the setting of cardiopulmonary bypass, has also been thought to be a precipitating factor (23).

There are several factors to consider in a patient with a prolactinoma who presents with signs and symptoms compatible with pituitary apoplexy. The first issue is to distinguish apoplexy from meningitis and subarachnoid hemorrhage. The CSF may be abnormal, showing increased protein and a pleiocytosis in all three conditions but the finding of bacteria is certainly diagnostic of meningitis (22,23). The finding of hemorrhage into the tumor on a noncontrast CT (hyperdensity within the tumor) is very helpful (22). With MRI (Figure 14-2), within the first 2 hours there are no specific findings, but after 3 hours an acute hemorrhage is usually isointense on T1-weighted images and very hypointense on T2-weighted images (22). Later images may show hyperintense areas on T1-weighted images and variable hypotense and hyperintense areas on T2-weighted images. The intensity changes in these images is due to the progressive breakdown of hemoglobin (22).

A second early issue is that of hypopituitarism. Varying degrees of hypopituitarism are found in up to three-quarters of such patients (22,23,25). A complete hormonal profile should be obtained in all patients and hydrocortisone administered intravenously in stress doses pending return of these levels. If the cortisol level was appropriately elevated for the stress, then hydrocortisone may be discontinued. However, pituitary function may get worse over time following the apoplexy (26), so that repeated cortisol measurements are in order to detect possible later deficiencies. Thyroid hormone can be replaced as necessary after adrenal insufficiency has been either excluded or treated.

Once the patient has been stabilized with appropriate intravenous fluids and hydrocortisone and diagnostic studies have been completed, the decision regarding operative decompression with at least removal of the hemorrhagic adenoma needs to be made. Much depends upon the nature of any neurologic deficits and whether or not they are progressing. A full discussion of the pros and cons of surgery vs. conservative management is discussed elsewhere, but suffice it to say that not all patients need surgery (22,23,26–28). Brisman et al. (29) reported an interesting patient with an untreated macroprolactinoma who presented with pituitary

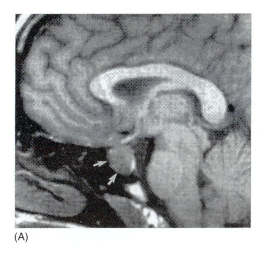

(A)

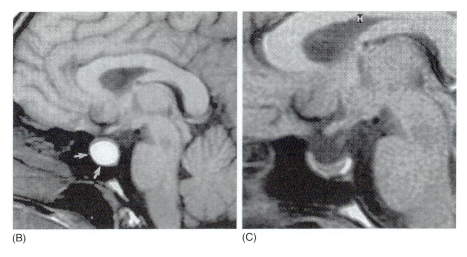

(B)   (C)

Figure 14-2 Macroadenoma with subsequent pituitary hemorrhage. A. The macroadenoma (arrow) appears as an enlarged mass within the sella on the noncontrast T1-weighted sagittal MR image. B. Repeat imaging obtained two years later shows that there is a new high signal (arrow) within the macroadenoma secondary to subacute hemorrhage. The patient had been receiving bromocriptine and was asymptomatic. C. On the examination performed in the same patient one year later, the macroadenoma is no longer present and there is a partially empty sella. Presumably, there has been necrosis of the tumor following the episode of hemorrhage (37). Reproduced with permission from Elsevier.

apoplexy whose tumor mass and clinical findings improved quickly and dramatically following the initiation of bromocriptine along with high dose steroids. Starting a dopamine agonist immediately once PRL levels are found to be elevated in a patient not previously known to have a prolactinoma certainly seems like a reasonable treatment option. Following any surgery or conservative therapy, the decrease in size of the enlarged tumor mass may permit some resolution of

hormonal deficits (22,23) and so a repeat evaluation of pituitary function should be carried out several weeks later.

Tumor Enlargement during Pregnancy

The stimulatory effect of the hormonal milieu of pregnancy and the withdrawal of the dopamine agonist may result in significant

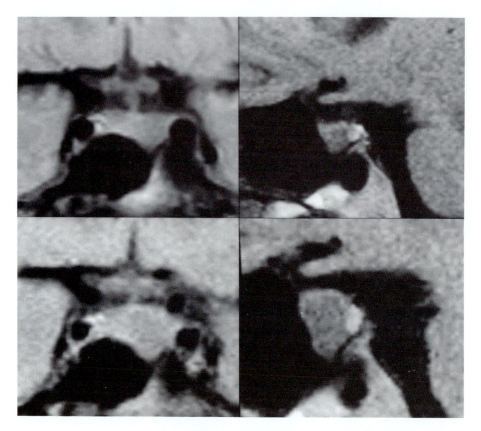

Figure 14-3 Coronal (left) and sagittal (right) MRI scans of an intrasellar prolactin secreting macroadenoma in a woman prior to conception (above) and at 7 months of gestation (below). Note the marked tumor enlargement at the latter point, at which time the patient was complaining of headaches (38). Reproduced with permission from Elsevier.

prolactinoma enlargement (Figure 14-3). Severe headaches or visual disturbances due to tumor enlargement during pregnancy has been reported in 18 of 764 (2.4%) women with microadenomas, 50 of 238 (21.0%) with macroadenomas that had not undergone prior surgery or radiotherapy, and 7/148 (4.7%) with macroadenomas who had undergone prior surgery or radiotherapy (30).

A patient with a microadenoma treated only with a dopamine agonist should be carefully followed throughout gestation. PRL levels do not always rise during pregnancy in women with prolactinomas, as they do in normal women. PRL levels may also not rise with tumor enlargement (31). Therefore, periodic checking of PRL levels is not recommended, as it is of no diagnostic benefit, and may be both misleading and the cause of unnecessary worry. Because of the low incidence of tumor enlargement, routine, periodic VF testing is not cost-effective. Visual field testing and MRI scanning are performed only in patients who become symptomatic when intervention is being considered. There are no data to show that either MRI scans or the use of gadolinium are harmful to the developing fetus (30); nonetheless, many neuroradiology departments are reluctant to do any MRI scan and even more reluctant to give gadolinium to a pregnant patient. In the patient with tumor enlargement who does not respond to reinstitution of a dopamine agonist, surgery or early delivery may be required (30).

For the patient with a small intrasellar or inferiorly extending macroadenoma, dopamine agonists are also favored as the primary therapy. The likelihood that such a tumor will enlarge sufficiently to cause clinically serious complications is probably only marginally higher than the likelihood in patients with microadenomas (30).

In a woman with a larger macroadenoma that may have suprasellar extension, there is a 21% risk of clinically significant tumor enlargement during pregnancy when only dopamine agonists are used. There is no definitive answer as to the best therapeutic approach in such a patient and this has to be a highly individualized decision that the patient has to make after a clear, documented discussion of the various therapeutic alternatives. One approach is to perform a prepregnancy transsphenoidal surgical debulking of the tumor. This greatly reduces the risk of serious tumor enlargement to 4.7%, but cases with massive tumor expansion during pregnancy after such surgery have been reported (30). After surgical debulking, a dopamine agonist is required to restore normal PRL levels and allow ovulation. Although radiotherapy before pregnancy, followed by a dopamine agonist, also reduces the risk of tumor enlargement, it is rarely curative. Furthermore, radiotherapy commonly results in long-term hypopituitarism, so that this approach seems less acceptable than transsphenoidal surgery plus a dopamine agonist. A third approach, that of giving bromocriptine continuously throughout gestation, has been used but data of effects on the fetus are quite meager (3). Data on the effects of continuous cabergoline on the fetus are even fewer (30,32,33); therefore, such treatment cannot be recommended without reservation. Should pregnancy at an advanced stage be discovered in a woman taking bromocriptine or cabergoline, however, the data that exist are reassuring and would not justify therapeutic abortion. A fourth approach, and the one most commonly employed, is to stop the dopamine agonist after pregnancy is diagnosed, as in the patient with a microadenoma.

For patients with macroadenomas treated with a dopamine agonist alone or after surgery or irradiation, careful follow-up with 1–3 monthly formal VF testing is warranted. Repeat MRI scanning is reserved for patients with symptoms of tumor enlargement and/or evidence of a developing VF defect or both. Should symptomatic tumor enlargement occur with any of these approaches, reinstitution of the dopamine agonist is probably less harmful to the mother and child than surgery. There have been a number of cases reported where such reinstitution of the dopamine agonist has worked quite satisfactorily, causing rapid tumor size reduction with no adverse effects on the infant (see above). Any type of surgery during pregnancy results in a 1.5–fold increase in fetal loss in the first trimester and a five-fold increase in fetal loss in the second trimester, although there is no risk of congenital malformations from such surgery (34). Thus, dopamine agonist reinstitution would appear to be preferable to surgical decompression. However, such medical therapy must be very closely monitored, and transsphenoidal surgery or delivery (if the pregnancy is far enough advanced) should be performed if there is no response to the dopamine agonist and vision is progressively worsening.

Rarely, women with pituitary tumors have developed pituitary apoplexy when pregnant and most of these tumors were prolactinomas (35,36). The usual supportive care and hormone replacement are required acutely for such patients (35,36). In their review of their cases and others from the literature, Grand'Maison et al. found that 15/36 (42%) were treated surgically, 11/36 (31%) were treated with dopamine agonists and 12/36 (33%) had at least two forms of treatment (36).

Case Study

A 27-year-old woman presented with galactorrhea and amenorrhea and was found to have an elevated PRL level of 227 ng/mL (4830 mIU/L) and had a 1.3 cm pituitary macroadenoma on MRI scan. She responded well to bromocriptine at the time with normalization of her PRL levels and resumption of ovulatory menstrual cycles and a decrease in the size of her macroadenoma to a maximum diameter of 1.0 cm. She stopped her bromocriptine after she missed a menstrual period and had a positive pregnancy test. At 7 months gestation she called, complaining of progressively severe headaches and an MRI (Figure 14-3) showing tumor enlargement.

How Would You Manage This?

Bromocriptine was resumed and resulted in resolution of her headaches over the next 2–3 weeks. She then continued the medication to term. She delivered a healthy infant at term with no malformations.

Conclusions

Patients with pituitary adenomas should be identified at an early stage so that effective treatment can be implemented. For prolactinomas, therapy is generally very satisfying for clinicians, primarily due to the excellent efficacy of dopamine agonist therapy. However, some aspects of treatment are more troubling than others and some can even be considered emergencies; most of these aspects occur in patients with macroprolactinomas. Several particular aspects of management fall into these categories of conditions: (a) a VF defect at presentation; (b) the development of CSF rhinorrhea; (c) the development of pituitary apoplexy; and (d) tumor enlargement during pregnancy.

References

1 Melmed S, Casaneuva FF, Hoffman AR, et al. Diagnosis and treatment of hyperprolactinemia. an Endocrine Society Clinical Practice Guideline. *J Clin Endocrinol Metab*. 2011;96:273–288.

2 Freda PU, Beckers AM, Katznelson L, et al. Pituitary incidentaloma: an Endocrine Society Clinical Practice Guideline. *J Clin Endocrinol Metab*. 2011;96:894–904.

3 Molitch ME. Diagnosis and treatment of pituitary adenomas. *JAMA*. 2017;317: 516–524.

4 Gillam MP, Molitch MP, Lombardi G, Colao A. Advances in the treatment of prolactinomas. *Endocrine Revs*. 2006; 27:485–534.

5 Molitch ME, Elton RL, Blackwell RE, et al., the Bromocriptine Study Group. Bromocriptine as primary therapy for prolactin-secreting macroadenomas: results of a prospective multicenter study. *J Clin Endocrinol Metab*. 1985;60:698–705.

6 Bevan M, Webster J, Burke CW, Scanlon MF. Dopamine agonists and pituitary tumor shrinkage. *Endocrine Revs*. 1992; 13:220–240.

7 Lesser RL, Zheutlin JD, Boghen D, Odel JG, Robbins RJ. Visual function improvement in patients with macroprolactinomas treated with bromocriptine. *Am J Ophthalmol*. 1990;109:535–543.

8 Colao A, Vitale G, Cappabianca P, et al. Outcome of cabergoline treatment in men with prolactinoma: effects of a 24-month treatment on prolactin levels, tumor mass, recovery of pituitary function, and semen analysis. *J Clin Endocrinol Metab*. 2004;89: 1704–1711.

9 Colao A, Di Sarno A, Landi ML, et al. Long-term and low-dose treatment with cabergoline induces macroprolactinoma shrinkage. *J Clin Endocrinol Metab*. 1997;82:3574–3579.

10 Corsello SM, Libertini G, Altomara M, et al. Giant prolactinomas in men: efficacy of cabergoline treatment. *Clin Endocrinol*. 2003;58:662–670.

11 Murad MH, Fernández-Balsells MM, Barwise A, et al. Outcomes of surgical treatment for nonfunctioning pituitary adenomas: a systematic review and meta-analysis. *Clin Endocrinol*. 2010;73: 777–791.

12 Kerrison JB, Lynn MJ, Baer C, Newman SA, Biousse V, Newman NJ Stages of improvement in visual fields after pituitary

tumor resection. *Am J Ophthalmol.* 2000; 130:813–820.

13 Dekkers OM, de Keizer RJW, Roelfsema F, et al. Progressive improvement of impaired visual acuity during the first year after transsphenoidal surgery for non-functioning pituitary macroadenoma. *Pituitary.* 2007;21:61–65.

14 Yu F-F, Chen L-L, Su Y-H, Huo L-H, Lin X-X, Liao R-D. Factors influencing improvement of visual field after transsphenoidal resection of pituitary macroadenomas: a retrospective cohort study. *J Ophthalmol.* 2015;8:1224–1228.

15 Barzaghi LR, Medone M, Losa M, Bianchi S, Giovanelli M, Mortini P. Prognostic factors of visual field improvement after trans-sphenoidal approach for pituitary macroadenomas: review of the literature and analysis by quantitative method. *Neurosurg Rev.* 2012;35:369–379.

16 Raverot G, Jacob M, Jouanneau E, et al. Secondary deterioration of visual field during cabergoline treatment for macroprolactinoma. *Clin Endocrinol.* 2009;70:588–592.

17 Papanastasiou L, Fountoulakis S, Papa T, et al. Brain and optic chiasmal herniation following cabergoline treatment for a giant prolactinoma: wait or intervene. *Hormones.* 2014;13:290–295.

18 Suliman SGI, Gurlek A, Byrne JV, et al. Nonsurgical cerebrospinal fluid rhinorrhea in invasive macroprolactinoma: incidence, radiological, and clinicopathological features. *J Clin Endocrinol Metab.* 2007; 92:3829–3835.

19 Lam G, Mehta V, Zada G. Spontaneous and medically induced cerebrospinal fluid leakage in the setting of pituitary adenomas: review of the literature. *Neurosurg Focus.* 2012;32:E2. DOI: 10.3171/2012.4.FOCUS1268.

20 Warnecke A, Averbeck T, Wurster U, Harmening M, Lenarz T, Stover T. Diagnostic relevance of beta2-transferrin for the detection of cerebrospinal fluid fistulas. *Arch Otolaryngol Head Neck Surg.* 2004;130:1178–1184.

21 Sherif C, Di Leva A, Gibson D, et al. A management algorithm for cerebrospinal fluid leak associated with anterior skull base fractures: detailed clinical and radiological follow-up. *Neurosurg Rev.* 2012;35:227–37.

22 Nawar RN, AbdelMannan D, Selman WR, Arafah M. Pituitary tumor apoplexy: a review. *J intensive Care Med.* 2008;23: 75–90.

23 Briet C, Salenave S, Bonneville J-F, Laws ER, Chanson P. Pituitary apoplexy. *Endocrine Revs.* 2015;36: 622–645.

24 Sarwar KN, Huda MSB, van de Velde V, et al. The prevalence and natural history of pituitary hemorrhage in prolactinomas. *J Clin Endocrinol Metab.* 2013;98: 2362–2367.

25 Randeva HS, Schoebel J, Byrne J, Esiri M, Adams CT, Wass JAH. Classical pituitary apoplexy: clinical features management and outcome. *Clin Endocrinol.* 1999;51:181–188.

26 Ayuk J, McGregor EJ, Mitchell RD, Gittoes NJL. Acute management of pituitary apoplexy – surgery or conservative management. *Clin Endocrinol.* 2004;61: 747–752.

27 Maccagnan P, Macedo CL, Kayath MJ, Nogueira RG, Abucham J. Conservative management of pituitary apoplexy: a prospective study. *J Clin Endocrinol Metab.* 1995;80:2190–2197.

28 Singh TD, Valizadeh N, Meyer FB, Atkinson JLD, Erickson D, Rabinstein AA. Management and outcomes of pituitary apoplexy. *J Neurosurg.* 2015;122: 1450–1457.

29 Brisman MH, Katz G, Post KD. Symptoms of pituitary apoplexy rapidly reversed with bromocriptine. *J Neurosurg.* 1996;85: 1153–1155.

30 Molitch ME. Endocrinology in pregnancy: management of the pregnant patient with prolactinoma. *Eur J Endocrinol.* 2015; 172:R205–R213.

31 Divers WA Jr, Yen SS. Prolactin-producing microadenomas in pregnancy. *Obstet Gynecol.* 1983;2:425–429.

32 Bajwa SK, Bajwa SJS, Mohan P, Singh A. Management of prolactinoma with cabergoline treatment in a pregnant woman during her entire pregnancy. *Indian J Endocrinol Metab.* 2011;15(Suppl 3):S267–S270.

33 Shahzad H, Sheikh A, Sheikh L. Cabergoline therapy for macroprolactinoma during pregnancy: a case report. *BMC Res Notes.* 2012;5: 606–609.

34 Cohen-Kerem R, Railton C, Oren D, Lishner M, Koren G. Pregnancy outcome following non-obstetric surgical intervention. *Am J Surg.* 2005;190:467–473.

35 Piantanida E, Gallo D, Lombardi V, et al. Pituitary apoplexy during pregnancy: a rare, but dangerous headache. *J Endocrinol Invest.* 2014;37:789–797.

36 Grand'Maison S, Weber F, Bédard M-J, Mahone M, Godbout A. Pituitary apoplexy in pregnancy: a case series and literature review. *Obstet Med.* 2015;8:177–183.

37 Naidich MJ, Russell EF. Current approaches to imaging of the sellar region and pituitary. *Endocrinol Metab Clin N Amer.* 1999;28:45–70.

38 Molitch ME. Medical treatment of prolactinomas. *Endocrinol Metab Clin North Am.* 1999;28:143–170.

Part V

Thyroid Disorders

Introduction

Emergency Management of Thyroid Disorders

Hossein Gharib

Key Points

- Thyroid disorders are very common, affecting approximately 750 million people worldwide.
- Hashimoto thyroiditis, which occurs mostly in women, is the most common cause of diffuse goiter and hypothyroidism in the USA.
- Graves' Disease (GD) is the most common cause of hyperthyroidism in iodine-sufficient parts of the world.
- Immunotherapy including new immune checkpoint inhibitors can cause thyroid dysfunction as well as other endocrine abnormalities (e.g., hypophysitis, primary adrenal insufficiency, and type 1 diabetes mellitus).
- Thyroid emergencies are complex and rare and associated with significant morbidity and excess mortality.

- General axioms related to thyroid emergencies include having a high index of clinical suspicion; general supportive care is critical (e.g., oxygen, vasopressors); initiate treatment before diagnosis is confirmed (treatment is rarely harmful and can be modified or discontinued as more clinical information is acquired); and search for precipitating cause or accompanying illness.
- Thyroid storm is a critical presentation of severe thyrotoxicosis, requiring urgent antithyroid and supportive therapy.
- Myxedema coma is the result of severe hypothyroidism, associated with high mortality, and warrants intravenous use of thyroxine and supportive therapy.

Introduction

Thyroid disorders are very common, affecting 750 million people worldwide according to World Health Organization (WHO) estimates, being possibly even more prevalent than diabetes. Many groups, including primary care physicians and specialists, nurses, physician assistants, health educators, medical clinics, professional medical societies, and public health personnel provide care and assistance to those with thyroid diseases.

Therefore, a discussion of some of the more common, controversial, or challenging issues in thyroid practice should be of great use to those of us who provide regular thyroid care.

Iodine deficiency is arguably the most common global thyroid problem. Consequences of iodine deficiency include endemic goiter, physical and mental retardation, cretinism, hypothyroidism, and poor outcomes in pregnancy, generally referred to as Iodine Deficiency Disorders (IDD). Dietary iodine

Endocrine and Metabolic Medical Emergencies: A Clinician's Guide, Second Edition. Edited by Glenn Matfin.
© 2018 John Wiley & Sons Ltd. Published 2018 by John Wiley & Sons Ltd.

is essential for the production of thyroid hormones, and in 1952 the WHO recommended iodization of all food salts in iodine-deficient regions. Sadly, by 1980, the WHO estimated that anywhere from 20–60% of the world population was still iodine-deficient (1). The USA has been considered iodine-sufficient in the past 100 years, although recent data suggest that pregnant women may be mildly iodine-deficient. A recent review concluded that "Iodine-deficiency remains a significant health problem worldwide and affects both industrialized and developing countries" (2).

Autoimmune thyroiditis is another common thyroid problem with an approximate global prevalence of around 1%. It is estimated that 10% of most populations have anti-thyroid antibodies, and 40–50% of women, and 20% of men, have focal thyroiditis. Hashimoto thyroiditis, which occurs mostly in women, is the most common cause of diffuse goiter and hypothyroidism in the USA. Typically, goiter is diffuse, nontender, and firm. Diagnosis is confirmed by positive anti-thyroid antibodies, characteristic appearance on ultrasound, and occasionally, by cytologic analysis. For patients with elevated thyroid-stimulating hormone (TSH) and/or goiter, thyroxine (T_4) therapy is prescribed.

In recent years, special attention has been paid to thyroid problems in pregnancy (3,4). Adequate iodine intake is critical in pregnancy, because it influences normal fetal development. New trimester-specific ranges are recommended for serum TSH levels in pregnancy. Subclinical hypothyroidism is common in pregnancy, and diagnosed in approximately 2.5% of women. The issue of screening for thyroid function in pregnancy, however, remains a subject of debate. Current guidelines suggest "aggressive case-finding," rather than universal screening, for women planning pregnancy. Postpartum thyroiditis, another form of autoimmune thyroid disease, has a worldwide prevalence of 7.5%. It represents thyroid dysfunction within one year following delivery. The typical course is one of transient hyperthyroidism, followed by hypothyroidism, with the majority of women reverting to a euthyroid state by the end of the postpartum year.

A common and controversial clinical problem is subclinical thyroid disease, which is essentially a biochemical diagnosis. Subclinical hyperthyroidism is defined by a low serum TSH with normal free thyroxine (FT_4) and free triiodothyronine (FT_3) levels; in subclinical hypothyroidism TSH is mildly elevated with normal FT_4. Both subclinical hypo- and hyperthyroidism can be associated with morbidity, and some studies show increased mortality as well. Screening is the only effective way to diagnose these conditions early but, in the absence of controlled, randomized trials, debate continues on the need for screening as well as the benefits of treatment in some patients (5).

Graves' Disease (GD) is the most common cause of hyperthyroidism in iodine-sufficient parts of the world; management options include anti-thyroid drug therapy, radioiodine, or surgical thyroidectomy (6). Treatment should be individualized, based on patient and physician preferences, as well as the availability of resources. Graves' ophthalmopathy is an uncommon but difficult-to-manage complication of GD. Recent reports have looked at risk-benefit ratio for different treatment modalities, including selenium, glucocorticoids, rituximab, and surgical intervention (7). Emerging treatments such as teprotumumab, which is a human monoclonal antibody inhibitor of the insulin growth factor (IGF)-1 receptor, show promise in early proof of concept studies (8).

Another common thyroid problem is nodular disease with an estimated prevalence of around 5% by palpation and 50% by ultrasound examination (9,10). Nodular goiter is more common in women, in the elderly, with iodine deficiency, and in populations exposed to external radiation. According to a WHO report, goiter prevalence between 1993 and 2004 increased by 81% in Africa, 80% in Europe, and by 63% in the Eastern Mediterranean countries. While nodules are common, they are commonly benign. Recent data show that worldwide, the incidence of thyroid cancer has increased in the past 50 years. In the USA for example, the incidence of thyroid cancer has increased three-fold, from 3.6 cases in 1973 to 15.3/100,000 in 2013 (11,12). It seems that this increase is mostly due to widespread use of sensitive imaging and thyroid fine-needle aspiration biopsy (FNA) in clinical practice. Despite this significant increase in prevalence, mortality remains stable. The US Preventive Services Task Force (USPSTF) recently recommended against screening for thyroid cancer in asymptomatic adults (12).

Attention has recently focused on reports describing thyroid-related adverse events in patients treated with new immune checkpoint inhibitors (13). Immunotherapy causes tumor regression in melanoma, lymphoma, and some other malignancies, but can also cause thyroid dysfunction as well as other endocrine abnormalities (e.g., hypophysitis, primary adrenal insufficiency, and type 1 diabetes mellitus). For example, hyper- or hypothyroidism has been reported in almost 15% of melanoma patients treated with pembrolizumab. With more patients receiving immune therapy for cancer and other conditions, it is likely that we will witness more insight into the pathogenesis of this type of inflammatory thyroiditis (which usually just needs supportive care and appropriate monitoring) and the potential implications for harnessing this anti-thyroid immune response in various challenging conditions (e.g., patients with advanced, radioiodine refractory thyroid cancer).

Thyroid Emergencies

Thyroid emergencies are complex and rare and associated with significant morbidity and excess mortality. General axioms related to thyroid emergencies include having a high index of clinical suspicion; general supportive care is critical (e.g., oxygen, vasopressors); initiate treatment before diagnosis is confirmed (treatment is rarely harmful and can be modified or discontinued as more clinical information is acquired); and search for precipitating cause or accompanying illness.

Thyroid Storm

Thyroid storm (also known as thyroid crisis) is a critical presentation of severe thyrotoxicosis, requiring urgent anti-thyroid and supportive therapy (Table V-1).

Table V-1 Thyroid storm (also known as thyroid crisis)

Definition
- A rare, life-threatening condition characterized by severe uncontrolled thyrotoxicosis
- Usually an exacerbation of previously existent thyrotoxicosis with a dramatic clinical picture and fatal outcome in absence of aggressive management

Clinical features
- General features consistent with thyrotoxicosis
- Those typical of storm but worse than usual thyrotoxicosis includes:
  - Fever; tachyarrhythmias including atrial fibrillation; congestive heart failure; abdominal pain, nausea, vomiting, diarrhea, jaundice, dehydration, cachexia; delirium, coma

Precipitating events
- Sepsis; non-thyroid and thyroid surgery; radioiodine therapy; iodine loading (e.g., contrast, amiodarone); labor/delivery; psychosis; acute medical problems such as acute coronary syndromes, diabetic ketoacidosis; poor adherence with anti-thyroid drug (ATD) therapy or patient ATD discontinuation due to perceived ATD (i.e. related or unrelated) adverse effect

Diagnosis
- Thyroid storm is mostly a clinical diagnosis
- Biochemical thyrotoxicosis – degree is not more profound than in typical thyrotoxicosis
- Radioactive iodine uptake test (RAIU) and scan are not necessary to confirm diagnosis
- Scoring systems are helpful (i.e. Burch-Wartofsky [14]; Japanese Thyroid Association [15])

(continued)

Table V-1 (*Continued*)

Treatment
- When treating thyroid storm, one should consider the 5 'Bs':
  - **B**lock synthesis (i.e. ATD)
    - Propylthiouracil (PTU) 200–250 mg q 4 h PO (1200 mg/d)
    - Methimazole or Carbimazole 20–25 mg q 4 h PO (120 mg/d)
  - **B**lock hormonal release
    - Iodine (NB – Give Iodine one hour after ATD)
      - ☐ Lugol's solution or SSKI 5–10 drops q 8 h PO
      - ☐ Sodium Iodide 0.5–1.0 g q 12 h IV
    - Lithium carbonate 300 mg q 6 h PO
  - **B**lock T_4 to T_3 conversion (i.e. high dose PTU, propranolol, corticosteroid)
    - Hydrocortisone 100 mg q 8 h IV
  - **B**eta-blocker (e.g., propranolol or esmolol)
    - Propranolol 60–80 mg q4–6 h PO
    - Esmolol IV (short acting)
  - **B**lock enterohepatic circulation (i.e. cholestyramine) or remove excess thyroid hormone (e.g., plasmapheresis or dialysis)
- General supportive care
  - Manage in intensive care or high dependency unit
  - Treat sepsis and seek and treat precipitants and comorbidities
  - Treat anxiety and agitation (e.g., chlorpromazine)
  - Treat hyperthermia (i.e., cooling, acetaminophen [paracetamol])
  - Correct dehydration (e.g., fluids, electrolytes), glucose, vitamins
  - Oxygen; vasopressors

Prognosis
- Mortality 15–30%

Case Study

A 36-year-old woman presented to the Emergency Department with complaints of severe shortness of breath, nausea, diarrhea, and a feeling of "impending doom." She had been diagnosed with Graves' disease and treated for 6 months with anti-thyroid drugs (ATD). However, she had discontinued them herself several weeks prior because of rash and pruritus.

On exam, she was hyperkinetic and delirious. Pulse 144 (irregularly irregular), BP 106/48, T 103.4 °F (39.7 °C). She was diaphoretic and markedly dyspneic. A goiter estimated at 120 grams (normal 10–25) was noted with a loud bruit. Investigations confirmed severe biochemical thyrotoxicosis; normal bilirubin; pulmonary edema, and atrial fibrillation. Because of the fever, blood cultures are drawn and she is admitted to intensive care unit.

Is This Thyroid Storm?

A clinical diagnosis of thyroid storm is relatively straightforward in this case. This can be confirmed using the Burch-Wartofsky Point Scale for Diagnosis of Thyroid Storm (14). An overall score is obtained by adding the scores from each of seven criteria (range 0–140). The patient's scores are marked in red in the scoring points column. The total score of 115 for this patient is consistent with a diagnosis of thyroid storm (≥45 highly likely thyroid storm). This diagnosis was also confirmed using the Japanese Thyroid Association Diagnostic Criteria for Thyroid Storm scoring system (15).

Burch-Wartofsky Point Scale for Diagnosis of Thyroid Storm (14)

Clinical feature	Scoring points
Thermoregularory dysfunction	
Temperature °F (°C)	
<99 (37.2)	0
99–99.9 (37.2–37.7)	5
100–100.9 (37.8–38.2)	10
101–101.9 (38.3–38.8)	15
102–102.9 (38.9–39.4)	20
103–103.9 (39.5–39.9)	25
≥104 (40)	30
Cardiovascular dysfunction	
Tachycardia (Beats per minute)	
<90	0
90– 109	5
110–119	10
120–129	15
130–139	20
≥140	25
Congestive heart failure	
Absent	0
Mild (Pedal edema)	5
Moderate (Bibasilar rales)	10
Severe (Pulmonary edema)	15
Atrial fibrillation	
Absent	0
Present	10
Central nervous system dysfunction	
Absent	0
Mild (Agitation)	10
Moderate (Delirium, psychosis, extreme lethargy)	20
Severe (Seizures, coma)	30
Gastrointestinal-hepatic dysfunction	
Absent	0
Moderate (Diarrhea, nausea/vomiting, abdominal pain)	10
Severe (Jaundice)	20
Precipitant History	
Absent	0
Present	10
Patient Total	115
≥45	**Highly likely thyroid storm**
25–44	Suggestive of impending storm
<25	Unlikely to represent storm

Table V-2 Myxedema Coma

Definition
- The most extreme, critical, life-threatening presentation of severe hypothyroidism
- Common pathway often is respiratory decompensation with CO_2 narcosis leading to coma and fatal outcome in absence of aggressive management
- Does not require a comatose state for diagnosis

Clinical features
- General features consistent with hypothyroidism
- Those typical of myxedema coma but worse than usual hypothyroidism includes:
  - Hypothermia; edema, dry/coarse skin, hair loss; abdominal/bladder distention; impaired pulmonary ventilation with respiratory acidosis; hyponatremia, hypochloremia; hypoglycemia; bradycardia, congestive heart failure (CHF) and pericardial effusion; shock
- Cause(s) of coma includes:
  - Reduced cardiac output and cerebral blood flow; hypoxia; hypercarbia; hyponatremia; hypoglycemia; hypothermia; traumatic brain injury (e.g., falls); effects of drugs, infection, etc.
- Direct effects of hypothyroidism on pulmonary function includes:
  - Altered Pulmonary Function Tests (PFTs) including increased A-a O_2 gradient, decreased DLCO, and reduced exercise capacity; depressed ventilatory drive; pleural effusion(s); upper airway obstruction (e.g., goiter, tongue); sleep apnea syndrome

Precipitating events
- Infection; drug overdose or exaggerated drug effects (e.g., diuretics, digitalis, sedatives, tranquilizers, narcotics); surgery; cardiovascular (acute coronary syndromes, CHF, cerebrovascular accident); hypothermia; hypoglycemia; loss of blood volume; CO_2 narcosis; poor adherence with thyroid replacement therapy; Addison's disease

Diagnosis
- Myxedema coma is mostly a clinical diagnosis (more common in women)
- Biochemical hypothyroidism
- Scoring system may be helpful but needs more validation (e.g., Popoveniuc-Wartofsky [16]) (see Table 15–2)

Treatment
- General principles:
  - Goals
    - Reversal of coma; normalization of thyroid stimulating hormone (TSH) levels
    - Restoration of normal cardiorespiratory function
  - Treatment
    - Start with parenteral therapy
    - Once conscious, switch to oral once daily dose thyroxine (T_4) (e.g., 1.6 μg/kg/day)
  - Follow-up
    - Monitor TSH levels at 6–8 weeks, after initiation of therapy or dosage change
- Hormone replacement therapy:
  - T_4 7 mcg/kg (350–500 mcg) IV push then 100 mcg IV daily
  - Liothyronine (T_3) 20–40 mcg q 8 h × 3 doses PO or nasogastric tube, then 25 mcg bid
  - Alternatively combination of T_4 + T_3
  - Hydrocortisone 100 mg q 8 h IV × 24 h then taper
- General supportive care:
  - Manage in intensive care or high dependency unit
  - Treat sepsis and seek and treat precipitants and comorbidities
  - Treat hypothermia (i.e. gentle warming)
  - Correct fluids (volume expansion), electrolytes, glucose, and vitamins
  - Oxygen (including non-invasive ventilation [NIV] and mechanical ventilation); vasopressors

Prognosis
- Mortality 30–40%

Myxedema Coma

Myxedema coma is the result of severe hypothyroidism, associated with high mortality, and warrants intravenous use of thyroxine and supportive therapy (Table V-2).

Conclusions

In order to help our patients with thyroid disease, we should continue to improve iodine nutritional status; design studies to determine if screening for thyroid disease, or treatment of subclinical disease, improve outcomes; develop cost-effective screening programs to detect early disease; recognize inflammatory thyroiditis caused by new immune therapies and leverage new insights into other thyroid conditions; encourage healthcare delivery teams to provide appropriate treatment for hypo- and hyperthyroidism (including thyroid emergencies); and promote public education through awareness campaigns and educational materials.

This section, devoted to complex and common thyroid emergencies, discusses pathogenesis, contributing events, diagnosis, treatment and outcomes. Each chapter is written by authors with significant expertise and contribution to the topic area. The chapters are well-written, up-to-date, and concise and should be of great value to clinicians dealing with patients with thyroid disorders.

References

1 Zimmerman MB. Iodine deficiency and excess in children: worldwide status in 2013. *Endocr Pract*. 2013;19:839–846.

2 Pearce EN, Andersson M, Zimmerman MB. Global iodine nutrition: where do we stand in 2013? *Thyroid*. 2013;23:523–528.

3 Alexander EK, Pearce EN, Brent GA, et al. Guidelines of the American Thyroid Association for the diagnosis and management of thyroid disease during pregnancy and the postpartum. *Thyroid*. 2017 Jan 6. DOI: 10.1089/thy.2016.0457. [Epub ahead of print]

4 De Groot L, Abalovich M, Alexander EK, et al. Management of thyroid dysfunction during pregnancy and postpartum: An Endocrine Society Clinical Practice Guideline. *JCEM*. 2012;97:2543–2565.

5 Cooper DS, Biondi B. Subclinical thyroid disease. *Lancet*. 2012;379:1142–1154.

6 Smith TJ, Hegedus L. Graves' disease. *N Eng J Med*. 2016;375:1552–1565.

7 Wiersinga WM. Advances in treatment of active, moderate-to-severe Graves' ophthalmopathy. *The Lancet Diabetes & Endocrinology*. 2017;5:134–142.

8 Smith TJ, Kahaly GJ, Ezra DG, et al. Teprotumumab for thyroid-associated opthalmopathy. *N Eng J Med*. 376:1748–1761.

9 Gharib H, Papini E. Thyroid nodules: clinical importance, assessment, and treatment. *Endocrinol Metabol Clin North Am*. 2007;36:707–735.

10 Gharib H, Papini E, Garber JR et al. American Association of Clinical Endocrinologists, American College of Endocrinology, and Associazione Medici Endocrinologi Medical Guidelines for Clinical Practice for the Diagnosis and Management of Thyroid Nodules–2016 Update. *Endocr Pract*. 2016;22:622–639.

11 Brito JP, Morris JM, Montori VM. Thyroid cancer: zealous imaging has increased detection and treatment of low risk tumours. *BMJ*. 2013;347:14706.

12 US Preventive Services Task Force (USPSTF). Screening for thyroid cancer. *JAMA*. 2017;317:1882–1887.

13 de Fillette J, et al. Incidence of thyroid-related adverse events in melanoma patients treated with pembrozilumab. *JCEM*. 2016;101:4431–4439.

14 Burch HB, Wartofsky L. Life-threatening thyrotoxicosis: thyroid storm. *Endocrinol Metab Clin North Am*. 1993;22:263–277.

15 Akamizu T, Satoh T, Isozaki O, et al. Diagnostic criteria, clinical features, and incidence of thyroid storm based on nationwide surveys. *Thyroid*. 2012;22:661–679.

16 Popveniuc G, Chandra T, Sud A, et al. Diagnostic scoring system for myxedema coma. *Endocrine Pract*. 2014;20:808–817.

15

Myxedema Coma

Natasha Kasid and James V. Hennessey

Key Points

- Myxedema coma is a decompensated state of hypothyroidism resulting from severe and prolonged depletion of thyroid hormones leading to altered mental status and other clinical features related to widespread multiorgan dysfunction.
- While this is a rare condition on the spectrum of thyroid disorders, myxedema coma is considered an endocrine emergency due to the danger of increased mortality with recent rates of 20–29% reported.

- It is often seen in the elderly population and precipitated by several factors in the setting of preexisting hypothyroidism.
- Treatment involves administration of hydrocortisone, levothyroxine, and consideration of liothyronine use, as well as general medical and cardiopulmonary support as needed. It is important to "seek and treat" precipitants.

Introduction

Myxedema coma is a decompensated state of hypothyroidism resulting from severe and prolonged depletion of thyroid hormones leading to altered mental status and other clinical features related to widespread multiorgan dysfunction. In 1877, the term myxedema was first used by William Miller Ord after Sir William Withey Gull correlated this presentation with atrophy of the thyroid gland (1). The term myxedema coma is misleading as most patients are merely obtunded, but not as frequently in a true state of coma. In 1953, the term myxedema coma was used in conjunction with fatal outcomes of four cases where coma was noted in patients in the setting of typical manifestations of myxedema (2).

While this is a rare condition on the spectrum of thyroid disorders, with a reported incidence rate of 0.22/million/year and an estimated 300 or more reported cases in the medical literature (3,4), myxedema coma is considered an endocrine emergency due to the danger of mortality, with 60–80% rates reported in the older literature and 20–25% more recently (3,5,6). In a study assessing an inpatient database in Japan of 149 patients, the in-hospital mortality rate was 29.5% (7). Therefore, it is important to promptly recognize and treat myxedema coma in an attempt to improve outcomes.

Pathophysiology

In the setting of untreated hypothyroidism (both primary and central), after

---

Endocrine and Metabolic Medical Emergencies: A Clinician's Guide, Second Edition. Edited by Glenn Matfin.
© 2018 John Wiley & Sons Ltd. Published 2018 by John Wiley & Sons Ltd.

discontinuation of L-thyroxine (LT4) therapy, or eventually following a total thyroidectomy, there will be an obligatory reduction in intracellular triiodothyronine (T_3) that will interfere with the maintenance of metabolic homeostasis (8). In this situation, myxedema coma can be induced by the additional presence of common inciting factors such as infections like urosepsis or pneumonia or conditions such as heart failure, exposure to a cold environments, trauma, surgery, cerebrovascular accidents, or gastrointestinal bleeding (8–10). Medications that often have been implicated in precipitating myxedema coma are anesthetics, sedatives, narcotics, lithium, amiodarone, sunitinib, and phenytoin (8,11).

Neurological dysfunction may present as severe hypothermia described as core temperatures <90°F (32.2°C) or can be afebrile in the setting of an underlying infectious process (10). Altered mental status in myxedema coma is caused by underlying cerebral tissue hypothyroidism as well as multiple mechanisms such as decreased cerebral blood flow, hyponatremia, and hypoxemia. These can also lower the threshold for precipitation of seizures in the setting of myxedema coma (8, 9). Beside memory impairment, dysarthria, seizures, sensory and motor peripheral neuropathy have also been noted in this severe state of hypothyroidism (12).

Due to innate cardiovascular-related compensatory mechanisms in the setting of reduced availability of thyroid hormone, one can develop diastolic dysfunction and peripheral vasoconstriction which together may result in a reduction of circulating blood volume (13). Further, primary cardiac pump function is directly compromised due to decreased cardiac inotropy which may result in cardiomegaly and negative chronotropy resulting in bradycardia. Nonspecific electrocardiograph (ECG) findings are often seen, and further disruption of cardiac rhythm may result in sustained ventricular tachycardia and torsades de pointes in a severely hypothyroid state (14). Therefore, low cardiac output and hypotension can precipitate cardiogenic shock (8,9). In addition, accumulation of mucopolysaccharides and water can result in pericardial effusions reducing the amplitude of electrical activity, resulting in electrical alternans on the ECG ultimately obscuring ischemic findings but may also result in cardiac tamponade physiology (15). Other ECG findings includes the presence of a J wave if hypothermia is present.

Hypoventilation occurs in the setting of altered respiratory sensitivity to hypoxia and hypercapnia as well as a reduction in respiratory drive. In addition, respiratory muscle dysfunction may occur which further impairs ventilation (8,10). It has been noted in patients with even milder forms of hypothyroidism, compared to controls, that a higher prevalence of cough, sputum production, and airway inflammation may be observed (16). In addition, an underlying anatomic process in the setting of infection or a manifestation of hypothyroidism, such as pleural effusions or macroglossia, can further interfere with the lung volume or airway size (10,15). There is a report of neuropathic oropharyngeal dysphagia that can contribute to aspiration and further respiratory impairment (12).

In myxedema coma, the glomerular filtration rate (GFR) and renal blood flow are reduced as would be expected in the hypothyroid patient (17). The occurrence of hyponatremia is based upon a diminished capacity to clear a free water load which is a consequence of the combined effects of lower renal perfusion and the presence of elevated antidiuretic hormone levels (9,10,18,19). Due to the potential of simultaneous adrenal insufficiency and impaired gluconeogenesis, hypoglycemia can occur (8). It has been observed that reduced intestinal motility may result in symptoms of upper and lower gastrointestinal distress and reduced absorptive efficiency contributing to paralytic ileus with abdominal distention (9,20,21).

Clinical Manifestations

We can document the typical features of hypothyroidism preceding the presentation of myxedema coma, including fatigue, weight gain, cold intolerance, constipation, cool and dry skin. In addition, brittle nails, macroglossia, hoarse voice, muscle cramps, menstrual disturbances, periorbital and non-pitting edema, or delayed deep tendon reflexes may be observed. The clinician should be especially alert to the presence of a goiter, thyroidectomy scar, or history of I^{131} treatment (8,9,22). Myxedema coma is 8-fold more common in women compared to men, and is a frequent cause of hospitalization among women over 60 years of age for a diagnosis of hypothyroidism (4,19). As a consequence of this gender difference, most cases of myxedema coma occur during the winter months in women (13).

The changes in mental status observed are along the spectrum of psychomotor slowing, deficits in memory, confusion, depression, visuo-perceptual skills, paranoia, hallucinations ("myxedema madness"), or dementia (9,19). One may also identify large and small fiber polyneuropathy (9). Hypothermia can be as extreme as temperatures <80°F (26.6°C) (10) or patients with obvious infections will be afebrile (13). In the setting of pericardial and pleural effusions, patients may report progressive dyspnea. With regard to signs of hemodynamic impairment, one may note bradycardia and hypotension when cardiac function is compromised. In the setting of pericardial effusion leading to cardiac tamponade, it is important to evaluate for physical signs such as jugular venous distention, muffled heart sounds, pulsus paradoxus, low voltage QRS complexes, electrical alternans, and tachycardia (10). Respiratory dysfunction may be frequently encountered with up to 80% demonstrating hypoxia and over half having documented hypercapnia (23). In addition to abdominal pain, nausea, and constipation, patients with myxedema coma can develop paralytic ileus and toxic megacolon (8).

Diagnosis

The diagnosis of myxedema coma is made by recognizing the clinical presentation consistent with a change in mental status, hypothermia, hypotension, and clinical signs and symptoms of hypothyroidism (8,22). In addition, the history from family members can reveal a diagnosis of hypothyroidism or past radioiodine therapy in patients with marked mental status changes. When this pattern of findings is identified, it is important to document the potential thyroid etiology biochemically and search for a non-thyroidal precipitating cause. However, treatment should not be withheld pending the results of further evaluation if this endocrine emergency is suspected.

The following laboratory studies (Table 15-1) should be obtained prior to the initiation of pharmacologic treatment: thyroid-stimulating hormone (TSH), free thyroxine (fT_4), a free thyroxine index using

Table 15-1 Aspects of initial evaluation

	Underlying mechanisms	Initial evaluation
Etiology	Primary vs. secondary vs. tertiary hypothyroidism	TSH, fT_4, total T_4, T_3 resin uptake
Precipitating causes	Infectious origin, gastrointestinal bleeding, metabolic derangements	Complete (full) blood count, blood and urine cultures, chest X-Ray, cortisol, cardiac enzymes, and complete history of medications patient is taking
Downstream manifestations	Hyponatremia, hypoglycemia, elevated AST, elevated LDL, elevated creatine kinase, multiorgan failure, and neurologic manifestations	Chemistry panel, liver function tests, and cardiac echo

total T_4 (TT$_4$) and T_3 resin uptake, a complete (full) blood count, and chemistry panel. Evaluation of potential sources of infection with chest X-ray, urine studies, and also blood cultures is also recommended. In the setting of potential myocardial infarction precipitating the crisis, cardiac enzymes should be obtained (8). An elevated TSH will distinguish primary from secondary or tertiary hypothyroidism in which TSH is normal or low (22). Moreover, TSH may not be as elevated in the setting of nonthyroidal illness (NTI) or when the patient is exposed to glucocorticoids or dopamine. However, it is important to recognize that reduced TT$_3$ and increased reverse T_3 levels (if obtained) may be observed in the setting of NTI without thyroid dysfunction, but both would be low in a hypothyroid patient with myxedema coma limiting the clinical utility of these T_3 determinations. Given the risk for co-existent adrenal insufficiency in either polyendocrine failure syndrome or a central hypothyroidism, the collection of a serum cortisol level is essential with the baseline laboratory assessment (19). A short ACTH stimulation test should also be performed under these circumstances.

As mentioned above, laboratory analysis (Table 15-1) can reveal hyponatremia, normocytic anemia, elevated lactate dehydrogenase, elevated aspartate transaminase (AST), elevated low-density lipoprotein (LDL) cholesterol, elevated creatine kinase, and hypoglycemia, which, if observed, should alert the clinician to potential pituitary-adrenal dysfunction (8,9,13,19). An ECG could identify bradycardia, non-specific ST-T wave changes, and/or a prolonged QT interval (8). A baseline ECG prior to initiation of treatment is important as thyroid replacement can precipitate an acute coronary syndrome. A urinalysis and a chest X-ray would be important to evaluate for a potential source of underlying infection as well as the presence of an enlarged cardiac silhouette. A cardiac echo should be obtained to differentiate a dilated cardiomyopathy from the presence of a pericardial effusion (10).

A lumbar puncture, if performed to evaluate the etiology of altered mental status, would note an increase in intracranial pressure and protein. Electroencephalography (EEG) may note low amplitude or a decrease of alpha wave activity with seizure activity that often is related to presence of accompanying hyponatremia, hypoglycemia, or hypoxemia (19).

In the setting of mental status change, change in temperature, and a precipitating event, the diagnosis of myxedema coma if often highly suspected. The most common signs noted in patients with myxedema coma are hypotension and hypothermia (24). Popoveniuc et al. have proposed a diagnostic scoring system for myxedema coma based on the following components of thermoregulatory dysfunction, CNS effects/mental status, gastrointestinal symptoms, presence of precipitating event, cardiovascular dysfunction, and metabolic disturbance (see case study Table 15-2). A maximum of 20 points are accumulated for body temperature <32°C (89.6°F) with no points attributed if the temperature is greater than 35°C (95°F). Central nervous system abnormalities score points from 10 for somnolence/lethargy to 30 for true coma or seizures. Gastroenterological findings contribute only 5 points for anorexia, abdominal pain or constipation up to 20 points in the presence of paralytic ileus. An identifiable precipitating event contributes 10 potential points to this score and cardiovascular abnormalities may account for varying numbers of points in the presence of bradycardia (30 points) if less than 40 beats per minute and 10–20 additional points each for the presence of ECG abnormalities, effusions, congestive heart failure (CHF), cardiomegaly and hypotension. Finally, this system awards risk in the case of metabolic abnormalities ranging from hyponatremia to decreased GFR. They have determined a score ≥60 is "highly suggestive," 25–59 is "suggestive," and ≤25 is "not likely" to indicate myxedema coma. Furthermore, a score of 45–59 would identify patients at risk for myxedema coma (24).

Case Study

A 56-year-old woman was brought to the Emergency Department with progressive fatigue, dyspnea, and confusion. She had constipation but no other abdominal symptoms. No thyroid history was available. On exam, she was disoriented but conversant. Temp 34°C (93°F), BP 120/80, pulse 50/min, respiratory rate 12/min. She had facial edema, course skin and pitting edema.

Investigations confirmed severe hypothyroidism (TSH 258 mIU/L [0.5–4.5]; free thyroxine [FT_4] 0.1 ng/dL [0.7–1.9 ng/dL]); hyponatremia; CHF; hypoxemia but no hypercarbia. She was admitted to the High dependency unit for further management.

Is This Myxedema Coma?

A clinical diagnosis of myxedema coma is made. The Popoveniuc-Wartofsky Diagnostic Scoring System for Myxedema Coma can be potentially diagnostic for myxedema coma (24). An overall score is obtained by adding the scores from each of six criteria. The total score of 70 (case study patient scores marked in red) is consistent with a diagnosis of myxedema coma (≥60 highly likely myxedema coma) (Table 15-2).

Table 15-2 Popoveniuc-Wartofsky Diagnostic Scoring System (24). Case study patients' scores marked in red.

Popoveniuc-Wartofsky Diagnostic Scoring System for Myxedema Coma

Clinical feature	Scoring points
Thermoregularory dysfunction	
Temperature F (C)	
>95 (35)	0
89.6–94.9 (32–35)	**10**
<89.6 (32)	20
Cardiovascular dysfunction	
Bradycardia (Beats per minute)	
Absent (>60)	0
50–59	**10**
40–49	20
<40	30
Other ECG changes (i.e. QT prolongation; or BBB; or low voltage; or non-specific ST changes; or heart block)	10
Pericardial/pleural effusion	10
Pulmonary edema	**15**
Cardiomegaly	15
Hypotension (<90/60)	20
Central nervous system dysfunction	
Absent	0
Somnolent/lethargic	**10**
Obtunded	15
Stupor	20
Coma/seizures	30

Table 15-2 *(Continued)*

Popoveniuc-Wartofsky Diagnostic Scoring System for Myxedema Coma

Clinical feature	Scoring points
Gastrointestinal-hepatic dysfunction	
Absent	0
Anorexia/abdominal pain/constipation	5
Decreased intestinal motility	15
Paralytic ileus	20
Metabolic disturbances	
Hyponatremia	10
Hypoglycemia	10
Hypoxemia	10
Hypercarbia	10
Decreased eGFR	10
Precipitant History	
Absent	0
Present	10
Patient Total	70
≥60	**Highly likely myxedema coma**
25–59	Suggestive of impending myxedema coma
≤25	Unlikely myxedema coma

Another objective tool to screen for the likelihood of myxedema coma by hospitalists and emergency department physicians has been developed by (25) assessing the following criterion of altered mental status (Glasgow Coma Scale [GCS] score 3–10 warranting 4 points); increases in TSH receiving 1 point in the 15–29 mIU/L range; and 2 points if TSH ≥30 mIU/L. Similarly, 1 point is garnered if a low fT_4 is identified and additional single points are accumulated for the presence of hypothermia, bradycardia, and an identifiable precipitating event. A score of 8–10 is considered "most likely" diagnosis of myxedema coma; a score of 5–7 "likely" myxedema coma if no other reason was present; and a score of <5, then the clinical situation is "unlikely" to represent myxedema coma (25).

Management

In a critical care setting, hypoventilation, hypercapnia, as well as airway protection in the setting of a reduced GCS are indications for immediate ventilator support (8,9, 19). As hypotension and hemodynamic strain may be present, careful volume resuscitation with normal saline is recommended while balancing considerations for the management of concomitant hyponatremia (8, 9). Dopamine should be considered if fluid resuscitation does not restore circulatory stability (26). Additionally, the presence of refractory hypotension may also be due to adrenal insufficiency which was discussed above. Consequently, hyponatremia management may not respond until the initiation of glucocorticoids as outlined below (26). For hypothermia, it is recommended to provide gentle warming with blankets, but to avoid excessive rapid external warming as this may lead to peripheral vasodilatation and potentially cardiovascular collapse. Alternatively careful central warming may be attempted (10,19,26).

Given the uncommon risk for co-existent adrenal insufficiency (occurs in 5–10%) in either the setting of polyendocrine failure syndrome or a secondary hypothyroidism, it is important to obtain a baseline assessment of cortisol prior to providing stress dose steroids which should always be given before the administration of thyroid replacement. An adrenal crisis may be precipitated by the initiation of LT_4 as cortisol clearance is accelerated by the thyroid hormone (8,19). Therefore, based on the 2014 American Thyroid Association guidelines (27), empiric glucocorticoids should be administered for initial treatment of myxedema coma. Hydrocortisone 50–100 mg intravenously (IV) every 6–8 hours should be administered for up to 7–10 days or until hemodynamically stable, followed by a taper if adrenal insufficiency is not present (8,19). Due to the frequency with which infections have been reported to result in death in the setting of myxedema coma, it has been recommended that a vigorous search for infectious precipitation of the crisis be pursued with specific antimicrobial intervention being initiated when evidence of infection is present (10).

It is reported that the equivalent of 90 mcg of LT_4 is produced daily in healthy subjects (5). In the setting of primary hypothyroidism and myxedema coma a larger dose of LT_4 is required to make up for the deficit and saturate the excessive binding capacity which is present (5). Differences of opinion persist as to the best approach in replacing the circulating thyroid hormone levels. Some have advocated utilizing LT_4 only, emphasizing the safety of administrating the pro-hormone which would be activated gradually by peripheral metabolism of LT_4. According to the 2014 ATA guidance (27), an initial loading dose of 200–400 mcg IV of LT_4 can be given. Of note, a smaller loading dose should be administered to smaller patients,

elderly patients, or patients with history of coronary artery disease or arrhythmias. Subsequently, a daily LT_4 dose of 1.6 mcg/kg of body weight should be given orally or 75% dose of this if administered via IV route (27). Intravenous and oral routes appeared to have similar survival outcomes in a reported retrospective series (6).

Due to the observed decrease in circulating T_3 and a potential delay in T_4 to T_3 conversion secondary to underlying NTI, a small amount of liothyronine (LT_3) can be given simultaneously. However, there is limited data demonstrating efficacy and necessity of this intervention. Suggested doses have ranged from 2.5 mcg given orally (or via nasogastric tube) at the same time that LT_4 is initiated to doses as high as 25 mcg IV every 12 hours until stabilization of the cardiovascular system or 48 hours have passed (26). Again, from the 2014 ATA guidelines, a suggested liothyronine loading dose of 5–20 mcg can be administered initially with subsequent daily maintenance dose of 2.5–10 mcg every 8 hours. Similar to levothyroxine dose recommendations, lower doses of liothyronine should be administered in elderly patients, smaller patients, or patients with history of coronary artery disease or arrhythmia. Liothyronine therapy can be continued until there are signs of clinical improvement (27). It has been suggested that the use of LT_3 would not be favored in patients with a history of coronary artery disease as it may cause increased oxygen consumption and could lead to an acute coronary syndrome (23). More recently, a middle ground has been suggested to administer 10 mcg IV of LT_3 every 8–12 hours until the patient recovers enough to adequately continue receiving monotherapy with oral LT4 (10). Another approach is to consider LT_3 therapy if clinical status is not improved after 24–48 hours of LT_4 therapy alone (10,13). There are no prospective studies comparing outcomes with these different replacement regimens. Jonklaas et al. suggest monitoring thyroid hormone every 1–2 days in addition to monitoring improvement in clinical parameters such as mental status and cardiac function (27).

Table 15-3 Approach to the management of myxedema coma

	Evaluation	Intervention
Respiratory	Ability to maintain airway protection in setting of altered mental status in setting of reduced Glasgow Coma Scale (GCS) Hypoxemia and hypercapnia	Arterial blood gas Intubation
Cardiovascular	Hypotension Bradycardia Cardiomegaly Pericardial effusions	Volume resuscitation with normal saline Dopamine or other vasopressor ECG: bradycardia, prolonged QT interval Cardiac echo Glucocorticoids in setting of refractory hypotension
Hypothermia	Temperature <90°F (32.2°C) Evaluate for underlying infection	External warming with blankets Empiric antibiotics in setting of suspected infection
Thyroid hormone replacement	Primary: Elevated TSH with low fT_4 Secondary: Low or normal TSH with low fT_4 Teritary: Low TSH and low fT4	Obtain baseline cortisol levels (consider short ACTH stimulation test) Hydrocortisone 50–100 mg IV q6–8h followed by LT_4 bolus 300-600 mcg IV Then, LT_4 50–100 mcg PO or IV daily Consider LT_3 2.5–25 mcg IV or PO daily with concomittent LT_4 initiation
Hyponatremia	Monitor sodium closely	If <120 mmol/L, consider adminstering 3% sodium chloride, avoid increasing sodium more than 10–12 mmol/L in 24 hours

In the setting of severe hyponatremia (105–120 mmol/L), one can administer 3% sodium chloride to achieve a modest increase in sodium level. However, it is very important not to correct sodium more than 10–12 mmol/L in 24 h and 18 mmol/L in 48 h to avoid precipitating osmotic demyelination syndrome (ODS); or more than 8 mmol/L in first 24 h if risk factors for ODS (8,19) (Table 15-3).

Prognosis

As previously noted, mortality rates as high as 25% have been reported in the contemporary literature (18,23). Smaller series have highlighted several factors associated with mortality in those diagnosed with myxedema coma (Table 15-4). Historically, coma has been cited as a poor prognostic factor, while survivors have been noted to be younger, have higher GCS score, and lower APACHE II (Acute Physiology and Chronic Health Evaluation II) scores (3). Others have had associated higher mortality rates in myxedema coma among those with infections especially of the pulmonary system due to aspiration and resulting in respiratory failure (10). In the study of Dutta et al., 23 patients observed over

Table 15-4 Prognostic factors. Compiled from (3,6,10).

Favorable prognosis	Unfavorable prognosis
Higher GCS score	Elderly
Lower APACHE II score	Associated respiratory infections
	Sepsis
	Upper gastrointestinal bleed
	Hypotension
	Bradycardia
	Use of mechanical ventilation
	Unresolved hypothermia
	History of sedative drug use
	Higher SOFA score

a seven-year period had a 52.2% mortality rate with causes of death noted to be sepsis, respiratory failure, and upper gastrointestinal bleed. It was noted that less favorable outcomes occurred with the presence of hypotension, bradycardia, sepsis, use of mechanical ventilation, unresolved hypothermia despite intervention, and history of sedative drug use (6). With respect to the comparison of APACHE II score, GCS score, and the Sequential Organ Failure Assessment (SOFA) score in the accuracy of predicting outcome, Dutta and colleagues concluded a high SOFA score more accurately predicted a higher mortality rate (Table 15-4) (6). In a retrospective observational study using a national database in Japan during a three-year period, there was noted to be a 29.5% in-hospital mortality rate (7).

Conclusions

As summarized in Table 15-3, myxedema coma is a rare but life-threatening condition. It is often seen in the elderly population and precipitated by several factors in the setting of preexisting hypothyroidism. Over time, the mortality rate has improved from 60–70% to 20–29%, which has been attributed to better awareness and more aggressive interventions. Prognosis is less favorable in the elderly, and in the settings of prolonged hypothermia, bradycardia, or lower level of consciousness (19). More specifically, hypotension, bradycardia, sepsis, use of mechanical ventilation, unresolved hypothermia despite intervention, and a history of sedative drug use are factors associated with poor prognosis, and a high SOFA score have correlated with a higher mortality rate (6). Treatment involves administration of hydrocortisone, LT_4 and consideration of LT_3 use, as well as general medical and cardiopulmonary support as needed.

References

1 Hennessey JV. The emergence of levothyroxine as a treatment for hypothyroidism. *Endocrine.* 2017;55(1):6–18.

2 Summers VK. Myxoedema coma. *BMJ.* 1953;366–368.

3 Rodriguez I, Fluiters E, Perez-Mendez LF, Luna R, Paramo I, and Garcia-Mayor RV. Factors associated with mortality of patients with myxedema coma: prospective study in 11 cases treated in a single institution. *J Endocrinol.* 2004;180: 347–350.

4 Wartofsky L. Myxedema coma. *Endocrinol Metab Clin N Am.* 2006;35:687–698.

5 Arlot S, Debussche X, Lalau J-D, et al. Myxoedema coma: response of thyroid hormones with oral and intravenous high-dose L-thyroxine treatment. *Intensive Care Med.* 1991;17:16–18.

6 Dutta P, Bhanasali, Masoodi SR, Bhadada S, Sharma N, Rajput R. Predictors of

outcome in myxedema coma: a study from a tertiary care centre. *Critical Care*. 2008;12(1):R1.

7 Ono Y, Ono S, Yasunaga H, Matsui H, Fushimi K, Tanaka Y. Clinical characteristics and outcomes of myxedema coma: analysis of a national inpatient database in Japan. *J Epidem*. 2017;27:117–122.

8 Mathew V, Misgar RA, Ghosh S, et al. Myxedema coma: a new look into an old crisis. *J Thyroid Res*. 2011:1–7.

9 Yu CHY, Stoval R, Fox S. Chorea: an unusual manifestation in a woman recovering from myxedema coma. *Endocr Pract*. 2012;18:e43–e48.

10 Wartofsky L. Myxedema coma. In: Braverman LE, Cooper CS, eds. *Werner and Ingbar's The Thyroid: A Fundamental and Clinical Text*. 10th ed. Philadelphia, PA: Wolters Kluwer Health; 2013: 600–605.

11 Chakraborty S, Fedderson J, Gums JJ, Toole A. Amiodarone-induced myxedema coma: a case and review of the literature. *Arch Med Sci*. 2014;10 (6):1263–1267.

12 Urquhart AD, Rea IM, Lawson LT, Skipper M. A new complication of hypothyroid coma: neurogenic dysphagia: presentation, diagnosis, and treatment. *Thyroid*. 2001;11:595–598.

13 Wiersinga WM. Myxedma coma. In: Jameson JL, DeGroot LJ, eds. *Endocrinology: Adult and Pediatric*. 6th ed. Philadelphia, PA: Saunders Elsevier; 2010:1618–1619.

14 Schenck JB, Rizvi AA, Lin T. Severe primary hypothyroidism manifesting with torsades de pointes. *Am J Med Sci*. 2006;331(3):154–156.

15 Parving H, Hansen JM, Nielsen SL, Rossing N, Munck O, Lassen NA. Mechanisms of edema formation in myxedema-increased protein extravasation and relatively slow lymphatic drainage. *N Engl J Med*. 1979;301(9):460–465.

16 Birring SS, Patel RB, Parker D, et al. Airway function and markers of airway inflammation in patients with treated hypothyroidism. *Thorax*. 2005;60: 249–253.

17 Kreisman SH, Hennessey JV. Consistent reversible elevations of serum creatinine levels in severe hypothyroidism. *Arch Intern Med*. 1999;159:79–82.

18 Fliers E, Wiersinga WM. Myxedema coma. *Rev Endocrin Metab Dis*. 2003;4:137–141.

19 Klubo-Gwiezdzinska J, Wartofsky L. Thyroid emergencies. *Med Clin N Am*. 2012;96:385–403.

20 Ji JS, Chae HS, Cho YS, et al. Myxedema ascites: case report and literature review. *J Korean Med Sci*. 2006;21:761–764.

21 Chadha JS, Ashby DW, Cowan WK. Fatal intestinal atony in myxoedema. *British Medical Journal*. 1969;3:398.

22 Hamburger S, Collier RE. Myxedema coma. *Ann Emerg Med*. 1982;11:156–159.

23 Reinhardt W, Mann K. Incidence, clinical picture and treatment of hypothyroid coma: results of a survey. *Med Klin (Munich)*. 1997;92:521–524.

24 Popoveniuc G, Chandra T, Sud A, et al. A diagnostic scoring system for myxedema coma. *Endocrine Practice*. 2014;20(8): 808–817.

25 Chiong YV, Bammerlin E, Mariash CN. Development of an objective tool for the diagnosis of myxedema coma. *Translational Res*. 2015;166 (3):233–243.

26 Wiersinga WM. 2013 Myxedema coma. In: DeGroot LJ, ed. *Thyroid Manager*. www.thyroidmanager.org. Last updated December 12, 2013. (accessed December 14, 2013).

27 Jonklaas J, Bianco AC, Bauer AJ, et al. Guidelines to treatment of hypothyroidism. *Thyroid*. 2014;24(12):1670–1751.

16

Life-Threatening Thyrotoxicosis

Thyroid Storm and Adverse Effects of Antithyroid Drugs

Alicia L. Warnock, David S. Cooper, and Henry B. Burch

Key Points

- The spectrum of thyrotoxicosis ranges from asymptomatic subclinical disease to a life-threatening metabolic crisis characterized by multisystem dysfunction and high mortality.
- A number of factors determine where in this continuum a thyrotoxic individual presents, including patient age, the presence of comorbidities, the rapidity of onset of thyroid hormone excess, and the presence or absence of a precipitating event.
- Thyroid storm (or crisis) is triggered when the cumulative effect of these factors surpasses an individual patient's ability to maintain adequate metabolic, thermoregulatory, and cardiovascular compensatory mechanisms.
- The most important determinants of survival in life-threatening thyrotoxicosis are early recognition and institution of appropriate therapy.
- Diagnostic efforts are often frustrated on multiple levels. Laboratory parameters have little value in distinguishing uncomplicated thyrotoxicosis from thyroid storm owing to extensive overlap in circulating thyroid

- hormone levels between these two categories. In addition, diagnostic criteria for thyroid storm have historically been far from uniform.
- Based on these difficulties, the Burch-Wartofsky Point Scale (BWPS) was introduced in 1993 to help distinguish uncomplicated thyrotoxicosis from impending or established thyroid storm. An additional empirically defined diagnostic system was proposed by the Japanese Thyroid Association in 2012. It is important to note that inappropriate application of either system can lead to misdiagnosis, and highlights the importance of clinical judgment in assessing each individual patient.
- An unwavering commitment to an aggressive multifaceted therapeutic intervention is critical to obtaining a satisfactory outcome.
- For the patient successfully treated during the acute stages of thyroid storm, a key objective should be the prevention of a recurrent crisis by planning for definitive therapy with either radioactive iodine ablation or surgery.

Introduction

The spectrum of thyrotoxicosis ranges from asymptomatic subclinical disease to a life-threatening metabolic crisis characterized by multisystem dysfunction and high mortality. A number of factors determine where in this continuum a thyrotoxic

Endocrine and Metabolic Medical Emergencies: A Clinician's Guide, Second Edition. Edited by Glenn Matfin.

individual presents, including patient age, the presence of comorbidities, the rapidity of onset of thyroid hormone excess, and the presence or absence of a precipitating event (1). Thyroid storm (or crisis) is triggered when the cumulative effect of these factors surpasses an individual patient's ability to maintain adequate metabolic, thermoregulatory, and cardiovascular compensatory mechanisms (1). The high morbidity and mortality associated with thyroid storm requires both early recognition and a steadfast commitment to an aggressive multifaceted therapeutic intervention. Since abrupt discontinuation of antithyroid drugs is a common precipitant of thyroid storm, and since the highest doses of antithyroid drugs are used to treat this disorder, a summary of adverse effects associated with thionamide therapy is also included in this chapter.

Clinical Presentation

General Features

The clinical features seen in uncomplicated thyrotoxicosis are generally present and accentuated in thyroid storm (Table 16-1). The heat intolerance and diaphoresis common in simple thyrotoxicosis are often manifested in thyroid storm as moderate-severe hyperpyrexia with large insensible fluid losses as temperatures frequently exceed 104–106°F (40–41°C) (2–4). Cardiovascular findings of sinus tachycardia in uncomplicated thyrotoxicosis become accelerated tachycardia in thyroid storm, with a high propensity for atrial dysrhythmia (3) and varying degrees of ventricular dysfunction and congestive heart failure (1). Anxiety and restlessness are extended in thyroid storm to severe agitation, delirium, or frank psychosis, progressing in some patients to stupor and coma (2,5–7). Gastrointestinal and hepatic involvement, limited to enhanced intestinal transport and mild transaminase elevation in simple thyrotoxicosis, may dominate the presentation in thyroid storm, with nausea, vomiting, frank diarrhea, and marked hepatocellular dysfunction with jaundice (1).

Although not universally present or recognized, a key clinical feature in thyroid storm is the presence of a precipitating event or intercurrent illness. Thyroid surgery, once the most common precipitant of thyroid storm, has become a relatively rare cause of this disorder (4). This is largely attributable to the current practice of rendering the thyrotoxic patient euthyroid before surgery as well as a decrease in the number of patients undergoing surgery for Graves' disease (8), owing to the popularity of radioiodine ablation therapy for hyperthyroidism (8). However, nonthyroidal surgery in patients with unrecognized thyrotoxicosis continues to act as a surgical precipitant of thyroid storm (9,10).

Table 16-1 Comparison of clinical features of uncomplicated thyrotoxicosis to thyroid storm

Clinical feature	Uncomplicated thyrotoxicosis	Thyroid storm
Thermoregulatory	Heat intolerance, diaphoresis	Hyperpyrexia, large insensible fluid losses
Nervous system	Hyperkinesis, nervousness	Confusion, seizure, coma
Cardiovascular	Tachycardia (90–120 bpm)	Accelerated tachycardia (>130 bpm), atrial dysrhythmia, heart failure
Gastrointestinal	Hyperdefecation	Nausea, vomiting, diarrhea
Hepatic	Mild transaminase elevation	Hepatic dysfunction, jaundice
Psychiatric	Agitation, emotional lability	Psychosis
Precipitant history	Absent	Present
Death	Rare	Frequent (10–20%)

Table 16-2 Precipitants or triggers of thyroid storm

Conditions associated with a rapid rise in thyroid hormone levels

- Withdrawal of antithyroid drugs
- Radioiodine therapy
- External beam radiation therapy
- Thyroid "poisoning" (overdose of thyroid hormone)
- Vigorous thyroid palpation
- Iodinated contrast dyes
- Thyroid bed trauma
- Thyroid surgery

Conditions associated with an acute or subacute nonthyroidal illness

- Non-thyroidal surgery
- Infection
- Cerebrovascular accident
- Pulmonary thromboembolism
- Parturition
- Diabetic ketoacidosis
- Emotional stress

A recent survey of Japanese physicians requesting data on thyroid storm cases they had actually managed, found that abrupt withdrawal of antithyroid drugs is the single most commonly recognized precipitant (4). Poor access to medical care has also been implicated as a cause of thyroid storm (11). A list of known triggers or precipitants of thyroid storm is shown in Table 16-2. These can be grouped into those conditions characterized by a rapid rise in circulating thyroid hormone levels, and those associated with an underlying acute or subacute nonthyroidal illness.

Recognition of Thyroid Storm: Diagnostic Criteria

A common theme in early reported series of thyroid storm patients was a rapid downward spiral culminating in death within hours to days of onset (1,12). The most important determinants of survival in life-threatening thyrotoxicosis are early recognition and the institution of appropriate therapy. Yet, diagnostic efforts are often frustrated on

multiple levels. Laboratory parameters have little value in distinguishing uncomplicated thyrotoxicosis from thyroid storm owing to extensive overlap in circulating thyroid hormone levels between these two categories (4,13,14). In addition, diagnostic criteria for thyroid storm have historically been far from uniform (12,15). Based on these difficulties, a diagnostic point scale was proposed by Burch and Wartofsky in 1993 to distinguish uncomplicated thyrotoxicosis from impending or established thyroid storm (Table 16-3). The Burch-Wartofsky Point Scale (BWPS) is an empirically-derived system taking into account three principal observations in patients with thyroid storm, including: (a) the continuum of end organ dysfunction; (b) the high variability of individual patient presentation; and (c) the high mortality associated with a missed diagnosis. An additional empirically defined diagnostic system was proposed by the Japanese Thyroid Association (JTA) in 2012 (4). The JTA system uses combinations of clinical features to assign patients to the diagnostic categories thyroid storm 1 (TS1) or thyroid storm 2 (TS2) (Table 16-4). Data comparing these two diagnostic systems suggest an overall agreement, but a tendency toward under-diagnosis using the JTA categories of TS1 and TS2, compared to a BWPS ≥45. For example, in a recent study including 25 patients with a clinical diagnosis of thyroid storm, the BWPS was ≥45 in 20 patients and 25–44 in the remaining five, but these latter five patients (20%) were not identified using the JTA system (16). In the same series, among 125 patients hospitalized with a clinical diagnosis of compensated thyrotoxicosis but not in thyroid storm, 27 (21.6%) had a BWPS ≥45, and 21 (16.8%) were either TS1 or TS2, suggesting similar rates of over-diagnosis with these two systems. However, an additional 50 patients (40%) hospitalized with a clinical diagnosis of thyrotoxicosis without thyroid storm would have been diagnosed as having impending thyroid storm by the BWPS, which reinforces that a BWPS in the 25–44 range does not replace clinical

Table 16-3 Burch-Wartofsky Point Scale for Diagnosis of Thyroid Storm (1)

Clinical feature	Scoring points
Thermoregularory dysfunction	
Temperature °F (C)	
<99 (37.2)	0
99–99.9 (37.2–37.7)	5
100–100.9 (37.8–38.2)	10
101–101.9 (38.3–38.8)	15
102–102.9 (38.9–39.4)	20
103–103.9 (39.5–39.9)	25
≥104 (40)	30
Cardiovascular dysfunction	
Tachycardia (Beats per minute)	
<90	0
90–109	5
110–119	10
120–129	15
130–139	20
≥140	25
Congestive heart failure	
Absent	0
Mild (Pedal edema)	5
Moderate (Bibasilar rales)	10
Severe (Pulmonary edema)	15
Atrial fibrillation	
Absent	0
Present	10
Central nervous system dysfunction	
Absent	0
Mild (Agitation)	10
Moderate (Delirium, psychosis, extreme lethargy)	20
Severe (Seizures, coma)	30
Gastrointestinal-hepatic dysfunction	
Absent	0
Moderate (Diarrhea, nausea/ vomiting, abdominal pain)	10
Severe (Jaundice)	20

Table 16-3   (*Continued*)

Clinical feature	Scoring points
Precipitant History	
Absent	0
Present	10
Total	
≥45	Highly likely thyroid storm
25–44	Suggestive of impending storm
<25	Unlikely to represent storm

judgment in the selection of patients for aggressive therapy. In another study including 28 patients diagnosed with thyroid storm on the basis of clinical presentation and the BWPS, one patient had a BWPS of 45 but did not meet JTA criteria for thyroid storm (17).

It is important to note that inappropriate application of either system can lead to misdiagnosis. For example, using the JTA system, a thyrotoxic patient with hyperkinesis and a temperature of 100.4°F (38°C) would meet diagnostic criteria for thyroid storm on the basis of "restlessness" and fever alone. This same patient would have a BWPS score of 20, making thyroid storm unlikely. Likewise, using the BWPS, a thyrotoxic patient with tachycardia of 120 and a temperature of 100.0°F (37.8°C) would qualify as impending thyroid* storm, while using the JTA system this same patient would not meet either possible or definite thyroid storm criteria. These cases illustrate the importance of clinical judgment in assessing each individual patient.

Atypical Presentations of Thyroid Storm

Thyrotoxic storm has occasionally been described in patients with masked or "apathetic" hyperthyroidism (18). Although most classically described in the elderly,

Table 16-4 Japanese Thyroid Association diagnostic criteria for thyroid storm. Adapted from (4).

Thyroid storm		Possible thyroid storm	
Combination-1	**Combination-2**	**Combination-1**	**Combination-2**
□ Thyrotoxicosis	□ Thyrotoxicosis	□ Thyrotoxicosis	No T4 or T3 levels
and	*and*	*and*	*and*
□ CNS disturbance	No CNS disturbance	No CNS disturbance	Meeting other criteria for thyroid storm
○ Restlessness			
or			
○ Delirium			
or			
○ Mental aberration/psychosis			
or			
○ Somnolence/lethargy			
and **one** *other:*	*and* **three** *others:*	*and* **two** *others:*	
□ Fever ≥100.4°F (38°C)	□ Fever ≥100.4°F (38°C)	□ Fever ≥100.4°F (38°C)	
or	*and/or*	*and/or*	
□ Tachycardia ≥130 beats per minute	□ Tachycardia ≥130 beats per minute	□ Tachycardia ≥130 beats per minute	
or	*and/or*	*and/or*	
□ Congestive heart failure	□ Congestive heart failure	□ Congestive heart failure	
or	*and/or*	*and/or*	
□ Gastrointestinal/hepatic	□ Gastrointestinal/hepatic	□ Gastrointestinal/hepatic	
○ Nausea	○ Nausea	○ Nausea	
or	*or*	*or*	
○ Vomiting	○ Vomiting	○ Vomiting	
or	*or*	*or*	
○ Diarrhea	○ Diarrhea	○ Diarrhea	
or	*or*	*or*	
○ Bilirubin ≥3 mg/dL	○ Bilirubin ≥3 mg/dL	○ Bilirubin ≥3 mg/dL	

Exclusions and Provisos:
Cases are excluded if other underlying diseases are clearly causing any of the following symptoms: fever (e.g., pneumonia and malignant hyperthermia), impaired consciousness (e.g., psychiatric disorders and cerebrovascular disorders), heart failure (e.g., acute myocardial infarction), and liver disorders (e.g., viral hepatitis and acute liver failure). However, some of these disorders trigger thyroid storm. Therefore, it is difficult to determine whether the symptom is caused by thyroid storm or is simply a symptom of an underlying disease that is possibly triggered by thyroid storm; the symptom should be regarded as being due to a thyroid storm that is caused by these precipitating factors. Clinical judgment in this matter is required (4).

apathetic hyperthyroidism presenting with thyroid storm has been described in all age groups, including pediatric patients. A literature review reported 14 case reports of apathetic thyroid storm with patients most often being in their fourth to sixth decade (19). Additional reports have described thyroid crisis presenting initially as psychosis, coma (2,5,20), status epilepticus (6), and non-embolic cerebral infarction (21). Even less common presentations have included abdominal pain and fever in young women (22,23), small bowel obstruction (24), hypercalcemia (25), and acute renal failure resulting from rhabdomyolysis (26).

Pathophysiology

The pathogenetic mechanisms underlying thyroid storm remain poorly understood. The rarity of this disorder and need for immediate therapeutic intervention, as well as the diversity of precipitants and presenting features, all contribute to this knowledge gap.

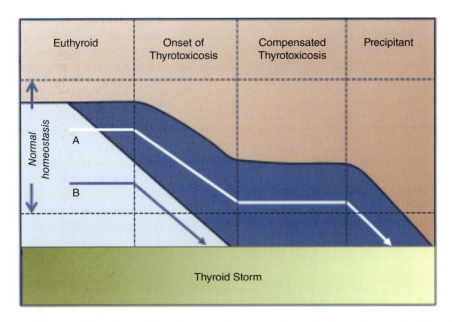

Figure 16-1 Pathways to thyroid storm. Two distinct pathways are shown for the pathogenesis of thyroid storm, as suggested by common precipitants of this disorder. Precipitants associated with an intercurrent illness, such as diabetic ketoacidosis or infection, lead to decompensation from a previously compensated and often unrecognized state of thyrotoxicosis (Pathway A); conversely, precipitants associated with an overwhelming rapid increase in thyroid hormone levels (such as after the abrupt discontinuation of antithyroid medications) lead to rapid systemic decompensation (Pathway B).

Modern hypotheses regarding the pathogenesis of thyroid storm should incorporate advances in our understanding of thyroid hormone action at the cellular level. Further, clues to the pathogenesis of thyroid storm lie in the known precipitants of this disorder. Specifically, precipitants associated with a rapid increase in thyroid hormone levels suggest a sudden and overwhelming intracellular availability of free thyroid hormone, while those triggers related to intercurrent illness suggest that a diminished physiological reserve plays a central role. Both mechanisms cause a failure of normal homeostatic mechanisms, and ultimately lead to life-threatening systemic decompensation (Figure 16-1).

In patients with a rapid increase in circulating thyroid hormone, a transient saturation of plasma binding capacity sufficient to increase concentrations of unbound hormone could lead to increased transporter-mediated intracellular entry of free thyroid hormone. Support for this mechanism comes from observations of a prompt clinical response in patients with refractory life-threatening thyrotoxicosis after rapid normalization of circulating hormone levels through plasmapheresis or charcoal plasmaperfusion (27–29). In addition, the development of thyroid crisis following the acute ingestion of thyroid hormone has been well documented in case reports, although this is not a typical outcome of accidental thyroid hormone overdose (1). While an enhanced availability of free thyroid hormone for cellular entry would intuitively seem central in the development of thyroid storm, no clear distinction from uncomplicated thyrotoxicosis can be made based on absolute levels of circulating thyroid hormones, as has been recently confirmed (4). Conversely, a 1980 report revealed a significant elevation in free T_4 concentrations in five thyroid storm patients compared to a larger group with simple thyrotoxicosis, despite similar levels of total T_4 (30). In some instances of thyroid storm, disproportionate elevation of free thyroid hormone levels have occurred in the setting of only modest elevations in total T_4 and normal levels of total T_3 (1).

Additional mechanisms are likely operative in patients who develop thyroid storm during an underlying acute or subacute non-thyroidal illness. A decoupling of oxidative phosphorylation, leading to an enhanced rate of lipolysis contributes to the heightened oxygen consumption and calorigenesis characteristic of these patients. Preferential production of thermal energy over adenosine triphosphate through this mechanism could also contribute to the hyperthermia seen in thyroid storm (31). A decreased hepatic and renal clearance of thyroid hormone during systemic illness (32) as well as enhanced generation of the metabolically active T_3 congener, triiodoacetic acid (TRIAC), have each been considered to be of possible pathophysiologic significance in patients whose thyroid storm is precipitated by a non-thyroidal illness (1). Lastly, an augmented tissue response to circulating thyroid hormone during non-thyroidal illness has been proposed as a potentiator of thyroid storm. Potential mechanisms for such activity could entail enhanced intracellular transport or nuclear entry of thyroid hormone, an alteration in binding to the nuclear receptor, or altered binding of the thyroid hormone-receptor complex to thyroid hormone response elements in target genes, though experimental evidence in support of this hypothesis is lacking.

Adrenergic system activation plays an important contributory role in the pathogenesis of both uncomplicated thyrotoxicosis and thyroid storm. Many of the clinical features of severe thyrotoxicosis, including agitation, tachycardia, dysrhythmia, and hyperthermia, are related to either direct catecholamine action or an interaction between the adrenergic system and excessive circulating thyroid hormone (33). Probably the best evidence for a significant role of the adrenergic system in this disorder is the dramatic clinical improvement afforded thyroid crisis patients following the addition of specific adrenergic blockade to the therapeutic regimen (1,34). However, a supporting rather than primary role of the adrenergic system is suggested by the observation that circulating levels of catecholamines are normal or low in thyroid storm (35). Furthermore, propranolol, even at high doses, does not prevent or ameliorate thyroid storm (36,37) and propranolol has no effect on thyroid hormone synthesis or release (38). The hyperadrenergic state seen both in thyrotoxicosis and thyroid storm may result from a thyroid hormone-mediated increase in β-adrenergic receptor density on target cells, and post-receptor mechanisms (39), although this remains speculative.

Although the mechanisms underlying thyroid storm remain incompletely understood, important inferences can be derived from the available data. A dramatic increase in free hormone levels is likely a common denominator in the precipitation of thyroid storm. Additional factors, including poor nutrition and the complicating influences of medical, surgical, and emotional stresses on thyroid hormone binding, cellular uptake, metabolic clearance, and an individual patient's physiological reserve are other likely components.

Treatment

General Treatment Strategy

The treatment of impending or established thyroid storm is directed at each therapeutically accessible point in the thyroid hormone synthetic, secretory, and peripheral action pathways. Concurrently, aggressive intervention is directed at the reversal of ongoing or incipient decompensation of normal homeostatic mechanisms. The rigorous level of care, including continuous monitoring and minute-to-minute titration of therapy mandate an intensive care setting for the early management of established thyroid storm. The therapeutic approach to thyroid storm may be grouped as: (a) therapy directed against the thyroid; (b) antagonism of the peripheral actions of the thyroid hormone; (c) reversal or prevention of systemic decompensation; (d) therapy directed at the precipitating event or intercurrent illness; and (e) definitive therapy. These will each be considered separately and are outlined in Table 16-5.

Therapy Directed against the Thyroid Gland

A nearly complete blockade of new hormone synthesis must be established early in the treatment course through the use of the antithyroid drugs propylthiouracil (PTU) or methimazole (MMI). PTU and MMI are thionamides which are thought to inhibit iodine organification, which is the binding of oxidized iodine to tyrosine residues in thyroglobulin, as well as the coupling of iodotyrosine residues to form the iodothyronine thyroid hormones T_4 and T_3.(20). Carbimazole (CBM) is rapidly metabolized to MMI, and can therefore be considered a prodrug for MMI, and is subject to the same dosing regimen and adverse effect profile as MMI. Blockade of iodine organification is established within an hour of administration of any of the ATDs. PTU has the advantage over MMI of decreasing the conversion of T_4 to T_3 (see Section "Treatment directed against peripheral effects of thyroid hormone"). Because of this unique property, thyroid storm continues to be one of a few conditions in which PTU is used preferentially over the more potent MMI (40).

Neither PTU or MMI are commercially available as parenteral formulations and are therefore generally given orally or per nasogastric tube in the stuporous, comatose, or otherwise uncooperative patient. Intravenous (IV), rectal, and even transdermal routes of administration have been utilized (see Section "Non-oral administration of antithyroid drugs"). PTU should be loaded with a dose of 600–1000 mg and then given at doses of 1200–1500 mg daily as 200–250 mg every four hours. MMI is given at a total daily dose of 120 mg in divided doses of 20 mg every 4 h. While a history of antithyroid drug-related agranulocytosis or moderate hepatocellular dysfunction should generally prompt the use of alternate modes of

Table 16-5 Management of thyroid storm

Treatment directed against the thyroid gland

Inhibition of new hormone synthesis

Thionamide drugs (propylthiouracil, methimazole [carbimazole])

Inhibition of thyroid hormone release

Iodine

Potassium iodide (SSKI), Lugol's solution, ipodate

Lithium carbonate

Treatment directed against the peripheral effects of thyroid hormone

Inhibition of T_4-to-T_3 conversion

Propylthiouracil

Corticosteroids

Propranolol

Ipodate, iopanoic acid

B-adrenergic blockade

Propranolol, esmolol (cardioselective β-blocking agents)

Removal of excess thyroid hormone

Plasmapheresis

Charcoal plasmaperfusion

Cholestyramine

Treatment directed against systemic decompensation

Treatment of hyperthermia

Acetaminophen (paracetamol)

Cooling

Correction of dehydration and nutritional deficit

Fluids and electrolytes

Glucose

Vitamins

Supportive therapy

Corticosteroids

Vasopressors

Congestive heart failure management

Treatment directed against the precipitating event

Etiology-dependent

---

therapy, a history of minor adverse reactions such as urticaria or rash is not sufficient cause to abandon these medications in the treatment of thyroid storm. Further, in a patient in whom the addition of an antithyroid drug is felt to be life-saving in nature, a patient with a history of agranulocytosis on one antithyroid drug may be cautiously treated briefly (1–2 weeks) on the alternate antithyroid drug with close monitoring of granulocyte counts. It is important to be aware that antithyroid drug therapy, although highly effective at inhibiting new hormone synthesis, has little effect on release of preformed thyroid hormone, a role which is therefore relegated to inorganic iodine therapy.

Inorganic iodine directly inhibits colloid proteolysis, release of T_4 and T_3 from the thyroid gland, and has transient inhibitory effects on thyroid hormone synthesis, through the Wolff-Chaikoff effect. Recommended oral doses are either Lugol's solution (8 mg/drop [0.05 ml]) 8 drops every 6 h, or saturated solution of potassium iodide (SSKI) (~35–50 mg/drop) 5 drops every 6 h (1). Parenteral administration by slow IV infusion as sodium iodide (NaI), 0.5–1 g every 12 h, has been employed, but sterile NaI for IV usage is not currently commercially available in the USA. Rectal administration of inorganic iodide has been described and recently summarized (41). Sublingual iodine has been used effectively as well, with 0.4 mL of a SSKI sublingually three times daily in a patient with bowel obstruction. By measuring urinary iodine, the authors calculated that 70% of the administered sublingual dose was absorbed (24).

It is generally believed that iodine therapy not be initiated until a blockade of new thyroid hormone synthesis has been established with thionamide antithyroid drugs (approximately 1 hour), as iodine alone will eventually lead to further increases of thyroid hormone stores (particularly in nodular hyperthyroidism), thereby increasing the risk of exacerbating the thyrotoxic state. Further, such "unprotected" use of iodine may complicate any planned management by delaying the effectiveness of antithyroid

drug therapy, increasing surgical risk due to an enrichment of glandular hormone stores, or postponing radioiodine ablation pending clearance of the iodine load. It should be noted that oral iodine therapy has been associated with acute gastrointestinal injury (42). Lithium also reduces the release of hormone from the thyroid, and could be considered in patients unable to be treated with iodide, provided adequate patient monitoring for lithium toxicity is performed (43).

Oral cholecystographic contrast agents such as ipodate and iopanoate (no longer available in the USA) have been used to treat severe thyrotoxicosis (44). These drugs, by virtue of a large content of stable iodine (308 mg/500 mg capsule for ipodate) have beneficial effects on thyroid hormone release similar to inorganic iodide. In addition, these agents are the most potent inhibitors of peripheral conversion of T_4-to-T_3, and may antagonize thyroid hormone binding to nuclear receptors. Ipodate is given at a daily dose of 1–3 g and, as with iodide, should not be used without prior blockade of new thyroid hormone synthesis with PTU or MMI. Although the utility of ipodate in thyroid storm has not been extensively examined, dramatic reductions in circulating T_4 and T_3 levels (by as much as 30–54% within 48 h of initiating therapy) have been reported in uncomplicated thyrotoxicosis (45).

Non-Oral Administration of Antithyroid Drugs
Oral administration of antithyroid drugs can be problematic in a patient with a poorly functioning gastrointestinal tract or who is combative or comatose. Case reports have documented the effective use of IV MMI (46,47). The report by Hodak and colleagues is most informative. These authors prepared IV MMI by reconstituting 500 mg of MMI powder in 0.9% sodium chloride solution to a final volume of 50 mL. The resulting solution of 10 mg/mL was then filtered through a 0.22-mm filter and administered as a slow IV push over 2 minutes, followed by a saline flush (46). Standard sterile pharmacological techniques are obviously required in the preparation process for these alternate medical vehicles.

Rectal administration of antithyroid drugs has also been used successfully (48–51) both as enemas and suppositories, as has been recently reviewed (41). Preparation of a suppository consisting of 1200 mg of MMI dissolved in 12 mL of water with two drops of Span 80 (a non-ionic surfactant), which was then mixed with 52 mL of cocoa butter has been described (48). A retention enema has been tested as well, prepared by dissolving 600 mg of PTU tablets in 90 mL of sterile water, delivered to the rectum by foley catheter with the balloon inflated to prevent leakage (52). Other authors have described the dissolution of 400 mg of PTU in 60 mL of Fleet's mineral oil or in 60 mL of Fleet's phospho soda (49), for use as a retention enema. In this report the enema preparation consisted of 400 mg of PTU dissolved in 90 mL of sterile water, and for the suppository formulation, 200 mg of PTU was dissolved in a polyethylene glycol base and put into suppository tablets. Finally, Zweig and colleagues (51) describe the use of a PTU-based suppository, prepared as follows. A total of 14.4 g of PTU tablets were solubilized in 40 mL of light mineral oil and mixed in 36 g of cocoa butter solid suppository base, melted in a hot water bath, and maintained at less than 60°C. The mixture was then distributed into 36 1-g suppository molds and frozen until solid. Each suppository contained 400 mg of PTU, which was administered every 6 hours, with documentation of therapeutic drug levels (51). Suppository formulations have the benefit of ease of administration compared to retention enema preparations, and appear to have similar clinical effectiveness (50).

Emergent Thyroidectomy

Numerous case reports and small series have described the use of thyroidectomy in thyroid storm patients who continued to deteriorate despite the use of standard medical therapy (53). Scholz and colleagues reviewed 39 cases from the literature and 10 additional cases from their own center, in which thyroidectomy was ultimately used to treat thyroid storm. Early or late postoperative mortality was reported in 5 of 49 (10.2%) of patients

(53). The authors advocated early thyroidectomy to treat thyroid storm, particularly in chronically ill elderly patients with concurrent cardiopulmonary and renal failure, who fail to respond to the standard intensive multifaceted therapy for thyroid storm.

Treatment Directed against Peripheral Effects of Thyroid Hormone

This category includes treatment given to diminish the adrenergic manifestations of severe hyperthyroidism, inhibition of the peripheral conversion of T_4 to T_3, and procedures designed to physically remove thyroid hormone from the circulation. The dramatic clinical response to β-blockers makes them one of the most valuable forms of therapy available for both uncomplicated thyrotoxicosis and thyroid storm. In addition to antiadrenergic effects, these agents have the added benefit of a modest inhibition of the peripheral conversion of T_4 to T_3, although studies have shown minimal changes in the serum levels, certainly not enough to fully account for the clinical response (54). The oral dose of propranolol in thyroid crisis is 60–80 mg every 4 hours, an amount notably higher than that customarily used in uncomplicated thyrotoxicosis. Plasma propranolol levels in excess of 50 ng/mL may be necessary to maintain adequate blockade in thyrotoxicosis (55,56), and it should be noted that the dose required to maintain this level may vary considerably in different thyrotoxic individuals due to the increased rate of plasma clearance (57,58). For a more rapid effect, IV propranolol may be given, using an initial dose of 0.5–1.0 mg with continuous monitoring of the patient's cardiac rhythm. Subsequent IV doses as high as 2–3 mg may be given over 15 minutes, to be repeated every several hours while awaiting the effects of the oral formulation (34).

Inhibition of peripheral conversion of T_4 to T_3, an important aspect of care in thyroid storm, is accomplished as an ancillary effect of other therapeutic agents used for another primary purpose in treating this disorder. These include PTU (but not MMI), propranolol, ipodate (not available in the USA), and glucocorticoids. In regards to PTU, this is achieved through inhibition of the type I deiodinase (D1) located primarily in the liver and thyroid gland. PTU is theoretically most effective in hyperthyroid states such as Graves' disease or toxic nodules where the T1D is upregulated (59,60).

Physical Removal of Thyroid Hormone from the Circulation or Gastrointestinal Tract

Both plasmapheresis and charcoal plasmaperfusion techniques have been used for the physical removal of circulating hormone in thyroid storm with generally positive results (27–29,61–69). Plasmapheresis should be considered in those patients who fail to respond rapidly to conventional therapy, those with a history of antithyroid drug-associated agranulocytosis or moderate hepatocellular dysfunction, and those who are being prepared for emergent thyroidectomy (63,68). It should be recognized, however, that the beneficial effect of plasmapheresis is transient, generally lasting only 24–48 hours (68). Cholestyramine therapy at doses of 4 grams four times daily (70) is another adjunctive measure used to physically remove thyroid hormone, in this setting from the enterohepatic circulation.

Measures Directed against Systemic Decompensation

Combatting systemic decompensation occurring in thyroid storm requires reversal of hyperthermia, dehydration, congestive heart failure, and dysrhythmia, as well as prevention of concomitant adrenal crisis. Hyperthermia should be aggressively treated with measures aimed at both thermoregulatory set point modification and peripheral cooling. Hence, acetaminophen (paracetamol) is given as antipyretic therapy, and cooling techniques such as alcohol washes, ice packs, and cooling blankets are used to enhance the dissipation of thermal energy. Salicylates are specifically avoided owing to their ability to displace thyroid hormone from serum binding sites, which could theoretically aggravate the state of thyrotoxicosis. Gastrointestinal and insensible fluid losses are potentially immense during thyroid crisis and should be aggressively replaced to prevent cardiovascular collapse and shock. Fluid requirements of 3–5 liters/day are not uncommon in thyroid storm. Elderly patients and individuals with evidence of congestive heart failure should be carefully monitored. Depletion of hepatic glycogen stores occurs readily during thyroid storm and has been cited as a characteristic histological finding at autopsy in patients dying from this disorder (9,71). As such, IV fluids containing 5–10% dextrose in addition to required electrolytes should be used in patients with thyroid storm. Vitamin supplementation, particularly thiamine, should be given intravenously to replace any possible coexisting deficiency.

Cardiovascular complications including atrial dysrhythmia and congestive heart failure are treated with conventional means including antiarrhythmic agents, vasodilators, and diuretics. Congestive heart failure occurs largely as a result of impaired myocardial contractility and is aggravated by atrial dysrhythmia, particularly fibrillation. Strong consideration should be given to Swan-Ganz monitoring of central hemodynamics in these patients, since despite modern critical care advances, management of heart failure in thyroid storm continues to prove difficult. With each medication used, careful examination of its effects on thyroid hormones is required to avoid exacerbation of thyrotoxicosis. Beta-blockers are a mainstay of therapy, but there are several special considerations. Propranolol is contraindicated in patients with a history of asthma or chronic obstructive pulmonary disease, who should be considered for other agents such as calcium channel blockers, β1-selective beta-blockers, or reserpine. Propranolol has also been associated with cases of cardiorespiratory arrest in thyroid storm patients (72) further justifying the use of an intensive care setting.

While propranolol has been the beta-blocker of choice for many decades (because of its additional benefit of peripheral inhibition of T_4 to T_3 conversion), more recently the drug esmolol, an ultra-short acting β-blocking agent, has been used successfully in management of severe thyrotoxicosis as well as in thyroid storm (73–77). Esmolol has definite utility over propranolol depending on the clinical circumstance. Because it is β1-selective, it can be used in patients at risk for bronchospasm. Additionally, the half-life of esmolol's β1-selective -blockade property is 9 minutes (versus 2.5 hours with propranolol) allowing minute-to-minute titration of the medication (76). Esmolol should be loaded with a dose of 250–500 µg/kg followed by continuous infusion rates of 50–200 µg/kg per minute, facilitating a rapid titration of drug level to the desired effect (73–75,77).

Other pharmacologic considerations include the following. Furosemide at high doses inhibits T_4 and T_3 binding to TBG, leading to increases in free thyroid hormones. Calcium-channel blockers used for atrial fibrillation can potentially lead to dramatic falls in systemic vascular resistance and consequent severe hypotension (78). In regards to digoxin, somewhat larger loading and maintenance doses may be required in thyrotoxic patients, owing, presumably, to an increased distribution space and/or rapid metabolism of this drug (78). Serum digoxin levels should be closely monitored, particularly as thyrotoxicosis improves, to prevent digitalis toxicity.

The empiric use of glucocorticoids in the treatment of thyroid storm was begun in the 1950s in an attempt to address the accelerated release and turnover of corticosteroids in thyroid storm (1). Indeed, inappropriately normal (rather than elevated) levels of serum cortisol have been observed in thyroid storm compared to other periods of significant stress (14). In addition to these effects, glucocorticoids such as dexamethasone and hydrocortisone have inhibitory effects on the peripheral conversion of T_4 to T_3. Further, the use of these agents appears to have led to improved survival in thyroid storm (7,14). Hydrocortisone is given IV at an initial dose of 300 mg, followed by 100 mg every 8 h during the initial stages of thyroid storm.

The dose may be subsequently reduced and discontinued as allowed by the clinical response of the individual patient.

Measures Directed against Precipitating Events in Thyroid Storm

Although the event precipitating thyroid storm may be quite obvious, such as surgery, labor (79), withdrawal of thionamides (12), or recent use of radioiodine (80), this is frequently not the case. This is particularly true in the instance of an underlying infection. The fever and leukocytosis found in thyroid storm even in the absence of an infection may be difficult to distinguish from an occult infectious process (81). A careful culturing of blood, sputum, and urine is therefore indicated in the febrile thyrotoxic patient. The routine use of broad spectrum antibiotics is, however, not recommended in the absence of other evidence suggestive of infection. In cases of thyroid storm precipitated by hypoglycemia, diabetic ketoacidosis, stroke, or pulmonary embolism, standard therapeutic approaches apply and should be instituted simultaneously with the treatment of thyroid storm. In the stuporous or comatose patient who is unable to provide a history suggestive of a particular precipitating event, a high index of suspicion for these varied etiologies must be maintained. It should be remembered that in some individuals no precipitant will be identified, even in retrospect. In fact, in older clinical series, as many as 25–43% of cases of thyroid storm occurred without an identified precipitating event (1,9,14,15).

After the Storm: Definitive Treatment

For the patient successfully treated during the acute stages of thyroid storm, a key objective should be the prevention of a recurrent crisis by planning for definitive therapy with either radioactive iodine ablation or surgery. As the severely thyrotoxic patient improves clinically, a gradual withdrawal of treatment modalities is often possible. Corticosteroids should be gradually tapered and discontinued, while β-blockade, unless contraindicated, should generally be continued during this period.

Owing to the large load of iodine used in the management of the acute stages of thyroid storm, early subsequent use of radioiodine as ablative therapy is frequently not possible until the excessive iodine has been cleared, as indicated by a return to normal levels of urinary iodine excretion. In the interim, the patient should be continued on antithyroid drug therapy. A surgical ablation with subtotal thyroidectomy is a therapeutic option with the advantage of expediency. Care must be taken, however, to ensure that the patient has adequate control of thyrotoxicosis in order to reduce the risk of another episode of thyroid crisis following anesthesia induction or the surgery itself.

Prevention of Thyroid Storm

In that the vast majority of cases of thyroid crisis today may be considered "medical" rather than a perioperative storm, greater awareness of predisposing factors is warranted. Hence, the clinician and patient alike should be aware that the development of an intercurrent illness during the medical management of thyrotoxicosis warrants scrutiny for signs of metabolic decompensation. Likewise, elective surgical procedures should be deferred until euthyroidism has been established. Likewise, patients requiring thyroidectomy due to a poor response or inability to take antithyroid drugs require rapid preparation using all available pharmacological means to improve thyrotoxicosis preoperatively.

Selective Pre-treatment with Antithyroid Drugs before Radioiodine Therapy

The use of radioiodine ablation for thyrotoxicosis simultaneously exposes patients to two known precipitants of thyroid storm, namely, thionamide withdrawal (in pretreated patients) and the ablation therapy itself.

Treatment of severely thyrotoxic patients with radioiodine can occasionally lead to rapid increases in thyroid hormone levels in the weeks immediately following radioiodine administration. Thyroid storm has even been described following the use of radioiodine in patients with metastatic differentiated thyroid cancer (1). Hence, patients at increased risk for developing thyroid storm such as the elderly, patients with severe thyrotoxicosis and those with extensive comorbidity should receive pre-treatment with antithyroid drugs before radioiodine ablation therapy (40,82). In these patients, an attempt should be made to minimize the duration off antithyroid drugs to 3–5 days before radioiodine is given, as antithyroid drug discontinuation leads to rapid increases in thyroid hormone levels (82). The use of β-adrenergic blockade in the period preceding and immediately following radioiodine provides additional protection in this circumstance. Consideration can also be given to restart antithyroid drugs 3–7 days after radioiodine and then slowly taper this therapy over the ensuing 4–6 weeks (40).

Rapid Preparation for Surgery in the Thyrotoxic Patient

Rapid preoperative preparation is occasionally needed for patients requiring urgent or emergent surgery (Table 16-6) (70). These patients either have insufficient time to be rendered euthyroid by thionamides before surgery or have contraindications to their use. Safe and effective oral therapy with a combination of β-blockers (propranolol 40 mg every 8 h), high dose glucocorticoids (betamethasone 0.5 mg every 6 h) and sodium iopanoate (500 mg every 6 h) has been reported in a small number of patients requiring urgent surgery (83). This regimen was given for 5 days with surgery performed on the 6th day. Dexamethasone and hydrocortisone decrease T_4-to-T_3 conversion and have an important role in this setting. As noted previously, Ipodate and iopanoic acid are no longer available in the USA. Emergent preparation for thyroid surgery at our center in thyrotoxic patients unable to use or

Table 16-6 Rapid preparation of the thyrotoxic patient for surgery. Adapted from (70).

Drug class	Recommended drug	Dose	Mechanism of action	Continue postoperatively?
Beta adrenergic blockade	Propranolol	40–80 mg po tid-qid	Beta adrenergic blockade; decreased T_4-to-T_3 conversion (high dose)	Yes
	Esmolol	50–200 µg/kg/min IV		Change to oral propranolol
Thionamide	Propylthiouracil	200 mg po q 4 h	Inhibition of new thyroid hormone synthesis; decreased T_4-to-T_3 conversion	Stop immediately after near total thyroidectomy; continue after nonthyroidal surgery
	Methimazole (carbimazole)	20 mg po q 4 h	Inhibition of new thyroid hormone synthesis	Stop immediately after near total thyroidectomy; continue after nonthyroidal surgery
Iodine*	SSKI	2 drops q 8 h	Inhibition of new thyroid hormone synthesis; Decreased release of thyroid hormone,	No
	Lugol's	3-5 drops q 8 h		No
Corticosteroid	Dexamethasone	2 mg po or IV q 6 h	Vasomotor stability; decreased T_4-to-T_3	Taper over first 72 h
	Hydrocortisone	100 mg po or IV q 8 h		Taper over first 72 h
Resin agents	Cholestyramine	4 g po q 6 h	Interference with enterohepatic circulation	Stop immediately postoperatively

* In countries where available, cholecystographic agents such as iopanoic acid (500 mg po bid) can be used in place of iodine, with the added benefit of inhibition of T_4-to-T_3 conversion.

responding poorly to antithyroid drugs (70) has successfully involved the following inpatient regimen with rapid correction of thyrotoxicosis when given for 5–10 days before thyroidectomy:

- Propranolol 60 mg orally, twice daily;
- Dexamethasone 2 mg intravenously, four times daily;
- Cholestyramine 4 g orally, four times daily;
- SSKI 2 drops orally, three times daily.

A recent case series has been published using a combination of iodine, dexamethasone, and propranolol to rapidly restore euthyroidism prior to thyroidectomy in 10 patients with Graves' disease (84).

Adverse Effects of Antithyroid Drugs

Antithyroid drugs are generally well tolerated. However, as with any drug, there are side effects that may require cessation of therapy, and the need for alternate treatment. Traditionally, the adverse reactions associated with antithyroid drugs are divided into "minor" and "major" side effects (85). The major side effects, agranulocytosis, hepatotoxicity, and vasculitis are potentially life-threatening. One study suggested that patients with Graves' disease may be more susceptible to allergic reactions to antithyroid drugs, compared to patients with nonautoimmune etiologies of thyrotoxicosis such as toxic multinodular goiter (86).

Minor Drug Reactions

The minor side effects include skin rash, which is typically papular and pruritic, GI distress, nausea, and arthralgias (85). In general, the minor side effects occur in about 2–5% of patients, with skin rash being by far the most common. The development of pruritic skin rash often requires discontinuation of the drug, but some patients may be able to continue therapy along with an antihistamine with eventual resolution of the skin rash. Typically, minor reactions develop within the first few weeks of starting the medication, and while switching to the alternate drug might be possible, there is at least a 50% cross-reactivity between the two antithyroid drugs (85).

Major Drug Reactions

The three major antithyroid drug reactions are: agranulocytosis, hepatotoxicity, and antineutrophil cytoplasmic antibody positive vasculitis. Each of these will be discussed individually.

Agranulocytosis

Agranulocytosis is defined as an absolute granulocyte count $<0.5 \times 10^9$/L, but most patients have granulocyte counts that are close to zero (85). Some patients also have anemia and mild thrombocytopenia. The frequency of antithyroid drug-induced agranulocytosis is in the range of 0.2–0.6% (87), and 99% + cases occur within the first 100 days of therapy (87). The elderly may be more susceptible to agranulocytosis than younger patients (88). Also, agranulocytosis can occur after a prior innocuous first exposure to the

drug many years earlier. The risk of agranulocytosis is dose-related with MMI (89), and is extremely unusual at doses less than 5–10 mg per day. In contrast, there is no dose response relationship with PTU and the risk of agranulocytosis. Patients may have agranulocytosis and be asymptomatic, only developing typical symptoms when they become infected. The classic presentation is that of a fulminant oropharyngeal infection with severe odynophagia, lymphadenopathy, malaise, chills, and high fever (90). Pneumonia, skin, and anorectal infections have also been described. Bone marrow examination typically shows normal or slightly decreased cellularity but absent or markedly decreased myeloid precursors. Bone marrow examination maybe helpful in predicting recovery, since the lack of myeloid precursors makes it unlikely that there will be a normal granulocyte count before 7–14 days (91). On the other hand, if there is preservation of the immature cells, recovery time will be shorter.

Treatment of agranulocytosis induced by antithyroid drugs includes:

- Immediate cessation of the offending drug.
- Hospitalization if there is a fever, with coverage with broad-spectrum antibiotics.
- Avoidance of the other antithyroid drug because of the possibility of cross-reactivity. However, in life-threatening situations (i.e., thyroid storm), where therapeutic options may be limited, the alternate drug might be used for a relatively brief (~1–2 weeks) period of time with monitoring of the leukocyte count, until the patient's clinical status is stable.

Most patients are treated with hematopoietic growth factors (e.g., G-CSF or GM-CSF). In most large cohort studies using retrospective controls and in one meta-analysis, use of these drugs reduced the fatality rate and shortened the time to hematological recovery (92). Mortality rates are in the 5–10% range with worse outcomes in patients over age 65, patients with a neutrophil count that is $<0.1 \times 10^9$/L, and in patients who have severe underlying comorbidities such as renal failure, cardiac disease, or respiratory disease.

Hepatic Involvement

Classically, liver involvement is different for the two antithyroid drugs (85). In the case of PTU, hepatotoxicity is typically "hepatocellular," whereas the pattern of involvement with MMI is "cholestatic." For PTU, the frequency of mild hepatocellular dysfunction is in the 1% range, but the frequency of fulminant, life-threatening hepatic failure is more likely to be in the 1/10,000 range (93). For MMI, there are no reliable data on the prevalence of cholestatic reactions, but it is decidedly rare. There are case reports of liver involvement developing within the first few days of treatment, but in a recent review of case reports involving PTU, the median was 120 days (94). For MMI, the mean duration of therapy before the onset of hepatotoxicity was 36 days (95). In the case of PTU, symptoms and signs of severe hepatic involvement include lethargy, malaise, nausea and vomiting, jaundice, dark urine, and light colored stools. Recognition of the syndrome and immediate discontinuation of PTU is essential. There then should be expectant management of hepatic involvement (coma, prolonged prothrombin time, hepatorenal syndrome, etc.), and consideration of referral to a center that can provide specialized care, including possible liver transplantation. For MMI-induced cholestasis, liver involvement typically resolves over the course of 1–2 months once the drug is stopped. In a recent review of cases reported to the FDA using the MedWatch system, no deaths had been reported from MMI-related hepatotoxicity (94). Two recent surprising studies from Asia suggest that either drug can cause either type of hepatotoxic side effect, although severe hepatocellular disease was still more common with PTU (96,97). In patients with antithyroid drug-induced hepatotoxicity, treatment of the continuing hyperthyroidism may involve switching to the other antithyroid drug, since the two drugs have different hepatotoxicity profiles.

Vasculitis

Antithyroid drug-induced vasculitis may take two forms clinically: (a) drug-induced lupus with fever, palpable purpura, splenomegaly, lymphadenopathy, and serositis involving the pleura and pericardium, or (b) drug-induced vasculitis with malaise, arthritis, myalgias, severe skin involvement, glomerulonephritis, and pulmonary hemorrhage. However, both of these forms likely represent part of a spectrum of antithyroid drug-induced vasculitis with associated anti-neutrophil cytoplasmic antibody (ANCA) positivity (98). In the case of antithyroid drug-related vasculitis, the antibodies are called "pANCA" which stands for "peri-nuclear" ANCA, with the antibody directed against granulocytic myeloperoxidase (MPO). However, antibodies against other neutrophil proteins besides MPO can also be seen. Vasculitis from antithyroid drugs is far more common with PTU than with methimazole, and occurs preferentially in individuals of Asian ethnicity (99). Cross-sectional studies showed the prevalence of circulating pANCA to be in the 10–50% range in asymptomatic individuals taking PTU, and 0–3% in patients taking methimazole (100). Antithyroid drug-related vasculitis typically occurs 1–3 months after starting treatment, but may occur after years of treatment (99). The usual presentation includes fever, arthritis, and palpable purpura involving the extremities and often the earlobes, dermal ulceration, and, more rarely, evidence of organ dysfunction, including glomerulonephritis or pulmonary involvement (99). The syndrome generally resolves after drug cessation, but immunosuppressive therapy, including high-dose glucocorticoids and/or cyclophosphamide have been used in more severe cases.

Birth Defects

Although not classically included in the category of adverse effects, the use of MMI in the first trimester of pregnancy has been associated with rare birth defects, including aplasia cutis, choanal atresia, esophageal atresia and omphalocele (85). Recently, a study from Denmark noted a similar prevalence of birth defects in infants born to mothers exposed to PTU during early pregnancy (101). However, the spectrum of defects differed between those seen with MMI and PTU, the latter being less severe (101). These and other recent similar findings have prompted consideration of definitive therapy in women planning pregnancy who have active Graves' disease, in order to avoid exposure to antithyroid drugs during early pregnancy (102).

Conclusions

While important strides in recognition and therapy have reduced the mortality in thyroid storm from nearly 100% fatality rate noted by Lahey in 1928 (3), survival is by no means guaranteed (103). It is likely that these improvements are a result of early recognition of thyroid storm and the demonstration of beneficial effects of corticosteroid, antithyroid drugs, and antiadrenergic therapies for the treatment of this disorder (14,15) in the decades since Lahey's first description. Relatively recent series have shown fatality rates between 10% and 50% (4,14,104).

Thyroid storm is a dreaded, fortunately rare complication of a very common disorder. Many cases of thyroid storm occur after a precipitating event, such as the abrupt discontinuation of antithyroid drug therapy (frequently due to an adverse effect) or an intercurrent illness. Effective management is predicated on the prompt recognition of impending thyroid storm, which is, in turn, dependent on knowledge of both the typical and atypical presentations of this disorder. An unwavering commitment to an aggressive multifaceted therapeutic intervention is critical to obtaining a satisfactory outcome.

Acknowledgments

The views expressed in this chapter are those of the authors and do not reflect the official policy of the Department of the Army, Navy, the Department of Defense or the United States Government. One or more of the authors are military service members (or employee of the U.S. Government). This work was prepared as part of our official duties. Title 17 U.S.C. 105 provides the "Copyright protection under this title is not available for any work of the United States Government." Title 17 U.S.C. 101 defines a U.S. Government work as a work prepared by a military service member or employee of the U.S. Government as part of that person's official duties. We certify that all individuals who qualify as authors have been listed; each has participated in the conception and design of this work, the analysis of data (when applicable), the writing of the document, and/or the approval of the submission of this version; that the document represents valid work; that if we used information derived from another source, we obtained all necessary approvals to use it and made appropriate acknowledgments in the document; and that each takes public responsibility for it.

References

1 Burch HB, Wartofsky L. Life-threatening thyrotoxicosis: thyroid storm. *Endocrinol Metab Clin North Am*. 1993;22:263–277.

2 Howton JC. Thyroid storm presenting as coma. *Ann Emerg Med*. 1988;17:343–345.

3 Lahey FH. The crisis of exophthalmic goiter. *N Engl J Med*. 1928;199:255–257.

4 Akamizu T, Satoh T, Isozaki O, et al. Diagnostic criteria, clinical features, and incidence of thyroid storm based on nationwide surveys. *Thyroid*. 2012;22:661–679.

5 Laman DM, Berghout A, Endtz LJ, van der Vijver JC, Wattendorff AR. Thyroid crisis presenting as coma. *Clin Neurol Neurosurg*. 1984;86:295–298.

6 Safe AF, Griffiths KD, Maxwell RT. Thyrotoxic crisis presenting as status epilepticus. *Postgrad Med J*. 1990;66:150–152.

7 Waldenstrom J. Acute thyrotoxic encephalo- or myopathy, its cause and treatment. *Acta Medica Scandinavica*. 1945;121:251–294.

8   Burch HB, Burman KD, Cooper DS. A 2011 survey of clinical practice patterns in the management of Graves' disease. *J Clin Endocrinol Metab*. 2012;97:4549–4558.

9   Nelson NC, Becker WF. Thyroid crisis: diagnosis and treatment. *Ann Surg*. 1969;170:263–273.

10 Bish LT, Bavaria JE, Augoustides J. Thyroid storm after coronary artery bypass grafting. *J Thorac Cardiovasc Surg*. 2010;140:6.

11 Sherman SI, Simonson L, Ladenson PW. Clinical and socioeconomic predispositions to complicated thyrotoxicosis: a predictable and preventable syndrome? *Am J Med*. 1996;101:192–198.

12 Rives JD, Shepard RM. Thyroid crisis. *Am Surg*. 1951;17:406–418.

13 Brooks MH, Waldstein SS, Bronsky D, Sterling K. Serum triiodothyronine concentration in thyroid storm. *J Clin Endocrinol Metab*. 1975;40:339–341.

14 Mazzaferri EL, Skillman TG. Thyroid storm: a review of 22 episodes with special emphasis on the use of guanethidine. *Arch Intern Med*. 1969;124:684–690.

15 Waldstein SS, Slodki SJ, Kaganiec GI, Bronsky D. A clinical study of thyroid storm. *Ann Intern Med*. 1960;52:626–642.

16 Angell TE, Lechner MG, Nguyen CT, Salvato VL, Nicoloff JT, LoPresti JS. Clinical features and hospital outcomes in thyroid storm: a retrospective cohort study. *J Clin Endocrinol Metab*. 2015;100:451–459.

17 Swee DS, Chng CL, Lim A. Clinical characteristics and outcome of thyroid storm: a case series and review of neuropsychiatric derangements in thyrotoxicosis. *Endocr Pract*. 2014:1–21.

18 Lahey FH. Apathetic thyroidism. *Ann Surg*. 1931;93:1026–1030.

19 Grossman A, Waldstein SS. Apathetic thyroid storm in a 10-year-old child. *Pediatrics*. 1961;28:447–451.

20 Ghobrial MW, Ruby EB. Coma and thyroid storm in apathetic thyrotoxicosis. *South Med J*. 2002;95:552–554.

21 Jarrett DR, Hansell DM, Zeegen R. Thyroid crisis complicated by cerebral infarction. *Brit J Clin Pract*. 1987;41:671–673.

22 Harwood-Nuss AL, Martel TJ. An unusual cause of abdominal pain in a young woman. *Ann Emerg Med*. 1991;20:574–582.

23 Karanikolas M, Velissaris D, Karamouzos V, Filos KS. Thyroid storm presenting as intra-abdominal sepsis with multi-organ failure requiring intensive care. *Anaesthesia Intensive Care*. 2009; 37:1005–1007.

24 Cansler CL, Latham JA, Brown PM, Jr., Chapman WH, Magner JA. Duodenal obstruction in thyroid storm. *South Med J*. 1997;90:1143–1146.

25 Parker KI, Loftley A, Charles C, Hermayer K. A case of apathetic thyroid storm with resultant hyperthyroidism-induced hypercalcemia. *Am J Med Sci*. 2013;19: 19.

26 Bennett WR, Huston DP. Rhabdomyolysis in thyroid storm. *Am J Med*. 1984;77:733–735.

27 Ashkar FS, Katims RB, Smoak WM, 3rd, Gilson AJ. Thyroid storm treatment with blood exchange and plasmapheresis. *JAMA*. 1970;214:1275–1279.

28 Candrina R, Di Stefano O, Spandrio S, Giustina G. Treatment of thyrotoxic storm by charcoal plasmaperfusion. *J Endocrinol Invest*. 1989;12:133–134.

29 Tajiri J, Katsuya H, Kiyokawa T, Urata K, Okamoto K, Shimada T. Successful treatment of thyrotoxic crisis with plasma exchange. *Crit Care Med*. 1984;12:536–537.

30 Brooks MH, Waldstein SS. Free thyroxine concentrations in thyroid storm. *Ann Intern Med*. 1980;93:694–697.

31 Mackin JF, Canary JJ, Pittman CS. Thyroid storm and its management. *N Engl J Med*. 1974;291:1396–1398.

32 Wartofsky L, Burman KD. Alterations in thyroid function in patients with systemic illness: the "euthyroid sick syndrome." *Endocrine Reviews*. 1982;3:164–217.

33 Landsberg L. Catecholamines and hyperthyroidism. *Clin Endocrinol Metab.* 1977;6:697–718.

34 Das G, Krieger M. Treatment of thyrotoxic storm with intravenous administration of propranolol. *Ann Intern Med.* 1969;70:985–988.

35 Coulombe P, Dussault JH, Walker P. Catecholamine metabolism in thyroid disease. II. Norepinephrine secretion rate in hyperthyroidism and hypothyroidism. *J Clin Endocrinol Metab.* 1977;44: 1185–1189.

36 Anaissie E, Tohme JF. Reserpine in propranolol-resistant thyroid storm. *Arch Intern Med.* 1985;145:2248–2249.

37 Jamison MH, Done HJ. Post-operative thyrotoxic crisis in a patient prepared for thyroidectomy with propranolol. *Brit J Clin Pract.* 1979;33:82–83.

38 Wartofsky L, Dimond RC, Noel GL, Frantz AG, Earll JM. Failure of propranolol to alter thyroid iodine release, thyroxine turnover, or the TSH and PRL responses to thyrotropin-releasing hormone in patients with thyrotoxicosis. *J Clin Endocrinol Metab.* 1975;41: 485–490.

39 Bilezikian JP, Loeb JN. The influence of hyperthyroidism and hypothyroidism on alpha- and beta-adrenergic receptor systems and adrenergic responsiveness. *Endocrine Revs.* 1983;4:378–388.

40 Ross DS, Burch HB, Cooper DS, et al. 2016 American Thyroid Association guidelines for diagnosis and management of hyperthyroidism and other causes of thyrotoxicosis. *Thyroid.* 2016;26:1343–1421.

41 Alfadhli E, Gianoukakis AG. Management of severe thyrotoxicosis when the gastrointestinal tract is compromised. *Thyroid.* 2011;21:215–220.

42 Myung Park J, Seok Lee I, Young Kang J, et al. Acute esophageal and gastric injury: complication of Lugol's solution. *Scand J Gastroenterology.* 2007;42:135–137.

43 Nayak B, Burman K. Thyrotoxicosis and thyroid storm. *Endocrinol Metab Clin North Am.* 2006;35:663–686, vii.

44 Robuschi G, Manfredi A, Salvi M, et al. Effect of sodium ipodate and iodide on free T4 and free T3 concentrations in patients with Graves' disease. *J Endocrinol Invest.* 1986;9:287–291.

45 Wu SY, Chopra IJ, Solomon DH, Johnson DE. The effect of repeated administration of ipodate (Oragrafin) in hyperthyroidism. *J Clin Endocrinol Metab.* 1978;47:1358–1362.

46 Hodak SP, Huang C, Clarke D, Burman KD, Jonklaas J, Janicic-Kharic N. Intravenous methimazole in the treatment of refractory hyperthyroidism. *Thyroid.* 2006;16:691–695.

47 Thomas DJ, Hardy J, Sarwar R, et al. Thyroid storm treated with intravenous methimazole in patients with gastrointestinal dysfunction. *Br J Hosp Med.* 2006;67:492–493.

48 Nabil N, Miner DJ, Amatruda JM. Methimazole: an alternative route of administration. *J Clin Endocrinol Metab.* 1982;54:180–181.

49 Walter RM, Jr., Bartle WR. Rectal administration of propylthiouracil in the treatment of Graves' disease. *Am J Med.* 1990;88:69–70.

50 Jongjaroenprasert W, Akarawut W, Chantasart D, Chailurkit L, Rajatanavin R. Rectal administration of propylthiouracil in hyperthyroid patients: comparison of suspension enema and suppository form. *Thyroid.* 2002;12:627–631.

51 Zweig SB, Schlosser JR, Thomas SA, Levy CJ, Fleckman AM. Rectal administration of propylthiouracil in suppository form in patients with thyrotoxicosis and critical illness: case report and review of literature. *Endocr Pract.* 2006;12: 43–47.

52 Yeung SC, Go R, Balasubramanyam A. Rectal administration of iodide and propylthiouracil in the treatment of thyroid storm. *Thyroid.* 1995;5:403–405.

53 Scholz GH, Hagemann E, Arkenau C, et al. Is there a place for thyroidectomy in older patients with thyrotoxic storm and cardiorespiratory failure? *Thyroid.* 2003;13:933–940.

54 Mintz G, Pizzarello R, Klein I. Enhanced left ventricular diastolic function in hyperthyroidism: noninvasive assessment and response to treatment. *J Clin Endocrinol Metab*. 1991;73:146–150.

55 Feely J, Forrest A, Gunn A, Hamilton W, Stevenson I, Crooks J. Propranolol dosage in thyrotoxicosis. *J Clin Endocrinol Metab*. 1980;51:658–661.

56 Hellman R, Kelly KL, Mason WD. Propranolol for thyroid storm. *N Engl J Med*. 1977;297:671–672.

57 Rubenfeld S, Silverman VE, Welch KM, Mallette LE, Kohler PO. Variable plasma propranolol levels in thyrotoxicosis. *N Engl J Med*. 1979;300:353–354.

58 Shenfield GM. Influence of thyroid dysfunction on drug pharmacokinetics. *Clinical Pharmacokinetics*. 1981;6:275–297.

59 Bianco AC, Salvatore D, Gereben B, Berry MJ, Larsen PR. Biochemistry, cellular and molecular biology, and physiological roles of the iodothyronine selenodeiodinases. *Endocrine Revs*. 2002;23:38–89.

60 Laurberg P, Vestergaard H, Nielsen S, et al. Sources of circulating 3,5,3′-triiodothyronine in hyperthyroidism estimated after blocking of type 1 and type 2 iodothyronine deiodinases. *J Clin Endocrinol Metab*. 2007;92:2149–2156.

61 Horn K, Brehm G, Habermann J, Pickardt CR, Scriba PC. [Successful treatment of thyroid storm by continuous plasmapheresis with a blood-cell separator (author's trans.)]. *Klin Wochenschr*. 1976;54:983–986.

62 Tshirch LS, Drews J, Liedtke R, Schemmel K. [Treatment of thyroid storm with plasmapheresis (author's trans.)]. *Medizinische Klinik*. 1975;70:807–811.

63 Ezer A, Caliskan K, Parlakgumus A, Belli S, Kozanoglu I, Yildirim S. Preoperative therapeutic plasma exchange in patients with thyrotoxicosis. *J Clin Apheresis*. 2009;24:111–114.

64 Herrmann J, Hilger P, Kruskemper HL. Plasmapheresis in the treatment of thyrotoxic crisis (measurement of half-concentration times for free and total T3 and T4). *Acta Endocrinol Suppl*. 1973;173:22–25.

65 Jha S, Waghdhare S, Reddi R, Bhattacharya P. Thyroid storm due to inappropriate administration of a compounded thyroid hormone preparation successfully treated with plasmapheresis. *Thyroid*. 2012;22:1283–1286.

66 Koball S, Hickstein H, Gloger M, et al. Treatment of thyrotoxic crisis with plasmapheresis and single pass albumin dialysis: a case report. *Artif Organs*. 2010;34:1525–1594.

67 Petry J, Van Schil PE, Abrams P, Jorens PG. Plasmapheresis as effective treatment for thyrotoxic storm after sleeve pneumonectomy. *Ann Thorac Surg*. 2004;77:1839–1841.

68 Vyas AA, Vyas P, Fillipon NL, Vijayakrishnan R, Trivedi N. Successful treatment of thyroid storm with plasmapheresis in a patient with methimazole-induced agranulocytosis. *Endocr Pract*. 2010;16:673–676.

69 Pasimeni G, Caroli F, Spriano G, Antonini M, Baldelli R, Appetecchia M. Refractory thyrotoxicosis induced by iodinated contrast agents treated with therapeutic plasma exchange. A case report. *J Clin Apheresis*. 2008;23:92–95.

70 Langley RW, Burch HB. Perioperative management of the thyrotoxic patient. *Endocrinol Metab Clin North Am*. 2003;32:519–534.

71 Ficarra BJ. Thyroid crisis: pathogenesis of hepatic origin. *Am J Surg*. 1945;69.

72 Dalan R, Leow MK. Cardiovascular collapse associated with beta blockade in thyroid storm. *Exp Clin Endocrinol Diabetes*. 2007;115:392–396.

73 Brunette DD, Rothong C. Emergency department management of thyrotoxic crisis with esmolol. *Am J Emerg Med*. 1991;9:232–234.

74 Isley WL, Dahl S, Gibbs H. Use of esmolol in managing a thyrotoxic patient needing emergency surgery. *Am J Med*. 1990;89:122–123.

75 Thorne AC, Bedford RF. Esmolol for perioperative management of thyrotoxic goiter. *Anesthesiology.* 1989;71:291–294.

76 Duggal J, Singh S, Kuchinic P, Butler P, Arora R. Utility of esmolol in thyroid crisis. *Can J Clin Pharmacol.* 2006;13:26.

77 Samra T, Kaur R, Sharma N, Chaudhary L. Peri-operative concerns in a patient with thyroid storm secondary to molar pregnancy. *Indian J Anaesthesia.* 2015;59:739–742.

78 Fadel BM, Ellahham S, Ringel MD, Lindsay J, Jr., Wartofsky L, Burman KD. Hyperthyroid heart disease. *Clin Cardiology.* 2000;23:402–408.

79 Kamm ML, Weaver JC, Page EP, Chappell CC. Acute thyroid storm precipitated by labor. Report of a case. *Obstetrics Gynecology.* 1963;21:460–463.

80 McDermott MT, Kidd GS, Dodson LE, Jr., Hofeldt FD. Radioiodine-induced thyroid storm. case report and literature review. *Am J Med.* 1983;75:353–359.

81 Urbanic RC, Mazzaferri EL. Thyrotoxic crisis and myxedema coma. *Heart Lung.* 1978;7:435–447.

82 Burch HB, Solomon BL, Cooper DS, Ferguson P, Walpert N, Howard R. The effect of antithyroid drug pretreatment on acute changes in thyroid hormone levels after (131)I ablation for Graves' disease. *J Clin Endocrinol Metab.* 2001;86:3016–3021.

83 Baeza A, Aguayo J, Barria M, Pineda G. Rapid preoperative preparation in hyperthyroidism. *Clin Endocrinol.* 1991;35:439–442.

84 Fischli S, Lucchini B, Muller W, Slahor L, Henzen C. Rapid preoperative blockage of thyroid hormone production / secretion in patients with Graves' disease. *Swiss Medical Weekly.* 2016;146:w14243.

85 Cooper DS. Antithyroid drugs. *N Eng J Med.* 2005;352:905–917.

86 Chivu RD, Chivu LI, Ion DA, Barbu C, Fica S. Allergic reactions to antithyroid drugs are associated with autoimmunity a retrospective case-control study. *Revista Medico-Chirurgicala a Societatii de Medici si Naturalisti din Iasi.* 2006;110:830–832.

87 Watanabe N, Narimatsu H, Noh JY, et al. Antithyroid drug-induced hematopoietic damage: a retrospective cohort study of agranulocytosis and pancytopenia involving 50,385 patients with Graves' disease. *J Clin Endocrinol Metab.* 2012;97:E49–E53.

88 Cooper DS, Goldminz D, Levin AA, et al. Agranulocytosis associated with antithyroid drugs: effects of patient age and drug dose. *Ann Int Med.* 1983;98:26–29.

89 Takata K, Kubota S, Fukata S, et al. Methimazole-induced agranulocytosis in patients with Graves' disease is more frequent with an initial dose of 30 mg daily than with 15 mg daily. *Thyroid* 2009;19:559–563.

90 Sheng WH, Hung CC, Chen YC, et al. Antithyroid-drug-induced agranulocytosis complicated by life-threatening infections. *QJM: Monthly Journal of the Association of Physicians.* 1999;92:455–461.

91 Yang J, Zhong J, Xiao XH, et al. The relationship between bone marrow characteristics and the clinical prognosis of antithyroid drug-induced agranulocytosis. *Endocrine J.* 2013;60:185–189.

92 Andres E, Kurtz JE, Perrin AE, Dufour P, Schlienger JL, Maloisel F. Haematopoietic growth factor in antithyroid-drug-induced agranulocytosis. *QJM.* 2001;94:423–428.

93 Cooper DS. Treatment of thyrotoxicosis. In: Braverman LE, Cooper DS, eds. *The Thyroid. 10th ed.* Philadelphia: Lippincott Williams and Wilkins; 2012.

94 Cooper DS, Rivkees SA. Putting propylthiouracil in perspective. *J Clin Endocrinol Metab.* 2009;94:1881–1882.

95 Woeber KA. Methimazole-induced hepatotoxicity. *Endocr Pract.* 2002;8:222–224.

96 Wang MT, Lee WJ, Huang TY, Chu CL, Hsieh CH. Antithyroid drug-related hepatotoxicity in hyperthyroidism

patients: a population-based cohort study. *Brit J Clin Pharmacology.* 2014;78:619–629.

97 Yang J, Li LF, Xu Q, et al. Analysis of 90 cases of antithyroid drug-induced severe hepatotoxicity over 13 years in China. *Thyroid.* 2015;25:278–283.

98 Balavoine AS, Glinoer D, Dubucquoi S, Wemeau JL. Antineutrophil cytoplasmic antibody-positive small-vessel vasculitis associated with antithyroid drug therapy: how significant is the clinical problem? *Thyroid.* 2015;25:1273–1281.

99 Noh JY, Yasuda S, Sato S, et al. Clinical characteristics of myeloperoxidase antineutrophil cytoplasmic antibody-associated vasculitis caused by antithyroid drugs. *J Clin Endocrinol Metab.* 2009;94:2806–2811.

100 Wada N, Mukai M, Kohno M, Notoya A, Ito T, Yoshioka N. Prevalence of serum anti-myeloperoxidase antineutrophil cytoplasmic antibodies (MPO-ANCA) in patients with Graves' disease treated with propylthiouracil and thiamazole. *Endocrine J.* 2002;49:329–334.

101 Andersen SL, Olsen J, Wu CS, Laurberg P. Birth defects after early pregnancy use of antithyroid drugs: a Danish nationwide study. *The Journal of Clinical Endocrinology and Metabolism.* 2013;98:4373–4381.

102 Rivkees SA. Propylthiouracil versus methimazole during pregnancy: an evolving tale of difficult choices. *J Clin Endocrinol Metab.* 2013;98:4332–4335.

103 Parker JL, Lawson DH. Death from thyrotoxicosis. *Lancet.* 1973;2:894–895.

104 Ashkar FS, Miller R, Gilson AJ. Thyroid function and serum thyroxine in thyroid storm. *South Med J.* 1972;65:372–374.

17

Amiodarone-Induced Thyrotoxicosis

Fausto Bogazzi, Luca Tomisti, Luigi Bartalena, and Enio Martino

---

Key Points

- Amiodarone has multiple antiarrhythmic effects that justify its use in supraventricular and ventricular tachyarrhythmias, atrial fibrillation (when other therapies are poorly effective) and in preventing sudden cardiac death in selected patients.
- Amiodarone is a benzofuranic iodine-rich drug structurally similar to thyroid hormones. Using a standard dose of amiodarone (200 mg per day), patients are exposed to a 75-mg daily iodine load, which greatly exceeds the recommended daily iodine intake (150–200 μg).
- This excess iodine load can result in thyroid dysfunction in 15–20% of patients, with either thyroid hormone excess (amiodarone-induced thyrotoxicosis, AIT) or deficiency (amiodarone-induced hypothyroidism, AIH).
- AIT is divided clinically and pathophysiologically into two types (although both can coexist in the same patient).
- Excessive iodine is the cause of type 1 AIT, a form of iodine-induced true hyperthyroidism, in which iodine load reveals

  the underlying thyroid autonomy or latent Graves' disease, and triggers the occurrence of hyperthyroidism (Jod-Basedow).
- Direct drug- (and/or iodine-)induced cytotoxic damage of thyroid follicular cells is considered to be the cause of type 2 AIT (destructive thyroiditis).
- Differentiation of the two main forms of AIT is crucial, although challenging, because treatment and outcome differ.
- AIT occurs in patients with pre-existing cardiac disease and may represent an emergency condition because of the detrimental effects of excess thyroid hormone on underlying heart abnormalities.
- When AIT represents an imminent risk for cardiac function, it should be managed without delay, because the late resolution of thyrotoxicosis is associated with a high mortality rate.
- Under these circumstances, emergent thyroidectomy may represent the most effective and rapid way of resolving thyrotoxicosis.

Introduction

Amiodarone is a benzofuranic iodine-rich drug structurally similar to thyroid hormones (1,2). It is a class III antiarrhythmic drug, which mainly inhibits myocardial Na-K ATPase activity and eventually increases the refractory period. However, amiodarone also has class I (decrease in conduction velocity through blockade of Na channel), class II (antiadrenergic effect reducing β-adrenergic receptor) and class IV (suppression of Ca-mediated action potentials) actions. These multiple antiarrhythmic effects of

Endocrine and Metabolic Medical Emergencies: A Clinician's Guide, Second Edition. Edited by Glenn Matfin.
© 2018 John Wiley & Sons Ltd. Published 2018 by John Wiley & Sons Ltd.

amiodarone justify its use in supraventricular and ventricular tachyarrhythmias, atrial fibrillation (when other therapies are poorly effective) and in preventing sudden cardiac death in selected patients (3–5).

Amiodarone administration is complicated in 15–20% of patients by thyroid dysfunction, with either thyroid hormone excess (amiodarone-induced thyrotoxicosis, AIT) or deficiency (amiodarone-induced hypothyroidism, AIH). Owing to the detrimental effects of thyroid hormone excess on the heart, AIT may represent an endocrine emergency.

Pathophysiology

Abnormal thyroid function tests, not indicative of thyroid dysfunction, are found in all patients who have been given amiodarone. A few weeks after institution of therapy, the serum TSH concentration transiently increases, but usually normalizes thereafter. Serum free thyroxine (FT_4) and reverse triiodothyronine (rT_3) concentrations increase, while serum free T_3 (FT_3) levels decrease because of amiodarone-induced inhibition of hepatic type 1 5'-deiodinase, the enzyme converting T_4 to T_3. In addition, amiodarone and its main metabolite, desethylamiodarone (DEA), due to structural homology with thyroid hormones, may bind to thyroid hormone receptor and act as a weak antagonist. Thus, in addition to changes in serum thyroid hormones concentrations, a "hypothyroid-like effect" in peripheral tissue may also occur.

Amiodarone-induced thyroid dysfunction may result from excessive iodine load and/or the intrinsic properties of the drug (1,6).

Effects of Iodine Load

Using a standard dose of amiodarone (200 mg per day), patients are exposed to a 75-mg daily iodine load, which greatly exceeds the recommended daily iodine intake (150–200 µg). This iodine load may cause either AIH or AIT. After iodine load, the thyroid gland normally blocks thyroid hormone synthesis (the Wolff-Chaikoff effect). This is associated with increased serum TSH concentrations, but is then followed by an "escape" phenomenon driven by a decrease in iodine transport and intrathyroidal concentrations to levels inadequate to maintain the block related to the Wolff-Chaikoff effect. Amiodarone inhibits iodide transport into the thyroid by either an iodine-independent mechanism or a decrease in sodium-iodide symporter mRNA expression.

Failure to escape from the Wolff-Chaikoff effect likely is believed the mechanism responsible for AIH both in patients with normal thyroid glands and those with pre-existing chronic autoimmune thyroiditis. Excessive iodine is the cause of type 1 AIT, a form of iodine-induced true hyperthyroidism, in which iodine load reveals the underlying thyroid autonomy or latent Graves' disease, and triggers the occurrence of hyperthyroidism (Jod-Basedow) (1,2,6).

Effects Intrinsic to the Molecular Structure

Amiodarone and DEA have pro-apoptotic and cytotoxic effects on thyroid follicular cells. Excess iodine may directly contribute to these changes. Histopathological changes look like those seen in other thyroid-destructive processes, such as subacute thyroiditis. A direct drug- (and/or iodine-)induced cytotoxic damage of thyroid follicular cells is considered to be the cause of type 2 AIT (destructive thyroiditis) (1,2,4,6).

The two pathogenetic mechanisms may, however, coexist. Damage of the thyroid follicular cells is expected in any thyroid gland exposed to amiodarone, even though it likely plays a minor role in the pathogenesis of AIT in patients with an underlying thyroid disease.

Amiodarone-Induced Thyroid Disease

The overall prevalence of amiodarone-induced thyroid dysfunction, though widely variable in different series, is between 15% and 20%, but may increase to 36% or 49% in patients with congenital heart disease, β-thalassemia major or under phenytoin therapy (1).

Amiodarone-Induced Thyrotoxicosis

AIT occurs more frequently in iodine-deficient areas and in men. Amiodarone therapy is not associated with *de novo* development of thyroid autoimmunity.

Type 1 AIT is a form of iodine-induced hyperthyroidism with the iodine load revealing pre-existing, latent thyroid autonomy due to Graves' disease or nodular goiter. This explains the relative preponderance of AIT in iodine-deficient regions, where the prevalence of nodular goiter is high, and in men, since iodine-induced thyrotoxicosis is more common in males (4,6). In iodine-replete areas the higher sensitivity of the thyroid gland to generate an iodine-induced turn-off signal for hormone biosynthesis makes it relatively resistant to the iodine load. Iodine load may rapidly trigger thyroidal hyperfunction in type 1 AIT, with a median of 3.5 months from institution of amiodarone therapy to the occurrence of thyrotoxicosis (7).

Type 2 AIT is a thyroid-destructive process, causing the release of preformed thyroid hormones from the damaged thyroid follicular epithelium. This may imply that a high intrathyroidal drug concentration needs to be reached before the damage of thyroid follicular cell becomes evident at a clinical level. In fact, the median time needed between the beginning of amiodarone therapy and the occurrence of thyrotoxicosis is 30 months, much longer than in type 1 AIT (7). Type 2 AIT has been historically considered arising in a normal thyroid gland without signs of autoimmunity. However, a recent study demonstrated that patients with features of a destructive form should be considered as having a type 2 AIT, and consequently treated, irrespective of the presence of anti-thyroglobulin antibodies (TgAb) and/or anti-thyroperoxidase antibodies (TPOAb), if they fulfill other criteria for a thyroid-destructive process (8).

Differentiation of the two main forms of AIT is crucial, although challenging, because treatment and outcome differ. Several diagnostic procedures may be required for an accurate differentiation between type 1 and type 2 AIT, as reported in Table 17-1. Although an increased serum T_4/T_3 ratio (>4) is typical in destructive thyroiditis, it is not useful in individual amiodarone-treated patients, because serum FT_4 is relatively higher than FT_3 due to the peripheral inhibition of type 1 deiodinase (9,10).

Both pathogenic mechanisms, increased synthesis and destructive phenomena, may contribute to the pathogenesis of the challenging, indefinite forms of AIT. These

Table 17-1 Clinical and pathogenic features of the two main forms of AIT

	Type 1 AIT	Type 2 AIT
Pre-existing thyroid disease	YES (Latent Graves' disease, single- or multi-nodular goiter)	NO
FT_4/FT_3 ratio	Often >4	<4
Spontaneous remission	NO	Possible
Thyroid ultrasound CFDS	Increased vascularity	Absent Hypervascularity
Thyroidal RAIU	Low-normal uptake	Absent uptake
TgAb and TPOAb	Not useful in the differential diagnosis	

CFDS = Color-flow Doppler sonography; RAIU = Radioactive iodine uptake.

"mixed" forms might be found in a subset of patients with an underlying multinodular goiter. In fact, a toxic follicular damage it is unlikely to play a relevant role in the pathogenesis of AIT in patients with an underlying Graves' disease or with a toxic adenoma. Likewise, iodine-induced hyperthyroidism is unlikely to play a pathogenic role in patients with a normal thyroid gland.

Mean radioactive iodine uptake (RAIU) values are usually very low to undetectable (<3%) in AIT 2 patients, due to prevalent destructive phenomena, whereas they may be low to inappropriately (for the high iodine load) normal in type 1 AIT, owing to the underlying autonomous function (11,12). Additional radioisotopic techniques using a different tracer still need to be validated (13).

Thyroid ultrasonography may reveal underlying nodules or goiter. However, conventional echography does not provide functional information, and the presence of goiter or nodules does not necessarily imply that an increased thyroid hormone synthesis is the underlying pathogenic mechanism. Color-flow Doppler echography shows an increase in thyroid vascularization in most type 1 AIT patients, whereas an absent hypervascularity, in spite of high serum thyroid hormone concentrations, is almost invariably associated with type 2 AIT (9,14).

In principle, clinical features of AIT are indistinguishable from those of the other forms of thyrotoxicosis. However, some symptoms/signs may herald the occurrence of AIT in a patient under amiodarone therapy:

- Reduced appetite, absence of distal tremors, depression may be frequent features of AIT in the elderly (apathetic hyperthyroidism).
- AIT may worsen the underlying cardiac disease; thus, difficulties in arrhythmias control in patients under chronic amiodarone therapy or occurrence of heart failure may reflect development of AIT.
- Thyrotoxicosis may increase the degradation rate of vitamin K-dependent coagulation factors; thus, unexplained increased

sensitivity to warfarin, in patients under anticoagulant and amiodarone therapy might be related to undiagnosed AIT (15).

Initial Management of AIT

The initial therapeutic choice for AIT patients is the result of a strict interaction between cardiologists and endocrinologists. At this stage the role of the endocrinologist is:

- to differentiate the two main forms of AIT;
- to predict whether the medical therapy could restore euthyroidism (only in type 2 AIT) in a short period of time (ideally <30 days).

On the other hand, the role of the cardiologist is:

- to evaluate the underlying cardiac disease;
- to evaluate the equilibrium of cardiac function;
- to estimate the risk of an impending worsening of cardiologic conditions.

The information resulting from this collaboration leads to the selection of one of the two main therapeutic choices: medical or surgical therapy.

Type 1 AIT

Type 1 AIT is best treated by antithyroid drugs (carbimazole, methimazole, or propylthiouracil). However, the iodine-replete thyroid gland of AIT patients is less responsive to thionamides. Thus, very high daily doses of the drug (40–60 mg/d methimazole or equivalent doses of propylthiouracil) for longer than usual periods of time are needed before euthyroidism is restored (Table 17-2) (16). This is obviously not an ideal situation in patients with underlying cardiac problems, whose hyperthyroidism should be promptly controlled. To increase the sensitivity of the thyroid gland and the response to thionamides, sodium perchlorate, which decreases thyroid iodine uptake, has been used. To minimize the adverse effects of the drug (particularly on the kidney and blood marrow), doses not exceeding 1 g/d should be used

Table 17-2 Medical therapies of AIT

Drugs	Starting dose	Duration
Methimazole	40–60 mg/day	To be tapered gradually until a maintenance dose
Propylthiouracil	400–600 mg/day	To be tapered gradually until a maintenance dose
Carbimazole	40–60 mg/day	To be tapered gradually until a maintenance dose
Sodium perchlorate	≤1 g/day	≤4–6 weeks
Prednisone	0.5–0.7 mg/kg/day	To be tapered gradually based on thyroid hormone levels
Methylprednisolone	0.4–0.6 mg/kg/day	To be tapered gradually based on thyroid hormone levels
Iopanoic acid*	1 g/day	Usually 7–21 days before surgery

*No longer available.

(Table 17-2). In addition, it is recommended not to use the drug for more than 4–6 weeks. Thionamide therapy can be continued until euthyroidism is restored, if this is permitted by the underlying heart disease and cardiocirculatory compensation. After restoration of euthyroidism, definitive therapy of the hyperfunctioning thyroid gland should be considered. If amiodarone can be discontinued, radioiodine therapy can be performed after iodine contamination is over, as suggested by normalized iodine urinary excretion. Otherwise, total thyroidectomy should be considered. In fact, definitive therapy of a type 1 AIT patient with an underlying hyperfunctioning thyroid gland does not differ from those with a spontaneous hyperthyroidism. In type 1 AIT patients not treated with a definitive therapy, the reintroduction of amiodarone therapy leads a high risk of thyrotoxicosis recurrence (73%). The risk may be reduced if patients are treated preventively with a course of thionamides (17).

Type 2 AIT

Type 2 AIT currently is the predominant form of AIT (89%). It is best treated by glucocorticoids. This is usually required, although mild forms may be transient and self-limiting, requiring only watchful waiting, if this is compatible with the underlying cardiac conditions. Initial prednisone dose is about 0.5–0.7 mg/kg body weight per day (or equivalent dose of other steroids) (18), gradually tapering down the drug in keeping with serum thyroid hormone reduction

(Table 17-2). Although response to treatment is often dramatic, with 50% of patients being euthyroid within 4 weeks, response is sometimes delayed (Figure 17-1). Factors possibly delaying the response to glucocorticoids are thyroid volume (>25 ml) and serum FT_4 (>50 pg/ml [ULN 15.5 pg/ml]) at diagnosis (19). Thionamides are not effective in type 2 AIT and should be avoided (Figure 17-2). If amiodarone can be discontinued, restoration of euthyroidism is achieved with a median time of about 30 days. If amiodarone therapy must be continued, glucocorticoids may be started, and euthyroidism can be induced even continuing amiodarone (20), although there may be a higher risk of thyrotoxicosis recurrence during treatment (21).

Discontinuation of amiodarone therapy is advisable, if feasible, to reduce the recurrence rate of thyrotoxicosis, to allow a prompt and stable restoration of euthyroidism, and to shorten the exposure of the heart to thyroid hormone excess (21). After restoration of euthyroidism, periodical assessment of thyroid status is required, because >15% of patients will develop permanent hypothyroidism over time, requiring levothyroxine replacement therapy (22). Radioiodine therapy with 131-I after stimulation with recombinant human TSH (rhTSH) alone or associated with rhTSH and lithium therapy has been proposed for the treatment of AIT patients to overcome the problem of low RAIU values (23). However, owing to very limited experience in this subset of patients and to the risk of exacerbation of

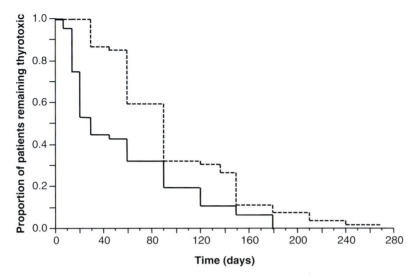

Figure 17-1 Proportion of type 2 AIT patients remaining thyrotoxic during glucocorticoid therapy, considering either the normalization of both T_4 and T_3 (continuous line) or that of TSH (dotted line) (19). Reproduced with permission from the Endocrine Society/OUP.

hyperthyroidism with consequent deleterious cardiac effects, this option should be considered with caution and is not currently recommended (24).

Indefinite AIT Forms
The most difficult challenge is represented by mixed/indefinite forms of AIT because

both pathogenic mechanisms described for type 1 and type 2 AIT are likely operating. From a theoretical point of view, the best medical treatment is a combination of thionamides (with or without potassium perchlorate) and oral glucocorticoids. However, mixed/indefinite forms of AIT, although proposed as a separate entity, have not been

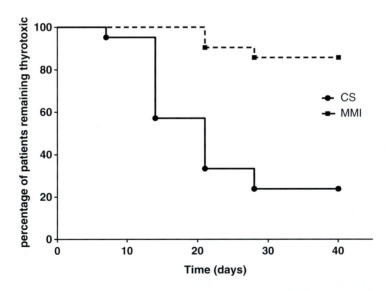

Figure 17-2 Proportion of type 2 AIT patients remaining thyrotoxic during the first 40 days of therapy. Glucocorticoid treated group (corticosteroids [CS] – continuous line) were treated with prednisone and dotted line treated group with methimazole (MMI). Cure of thyrotoxicosis was defined as normalization of serum FT4 and FT3 concentrations at 40 days (18). Reproduced with permission from the Endocrine Society/OUP.

fully characterized so far. If the presence of underlying Graves' disease or toxic adenoma is strongly suggestive of type 1 AIT, while a normal thyroid gland of type 2 AIT patients with multinodular goiter may potentially develop both main forms of AIT type, making it difficult to differentiate the precise etiology.

AIT and Warfarin

Particular attention should be paid to AIT patients who need to start warfarin therapy. In these subjects therapy should be instituted using a very low dose, because amiodarone *per se* and thyrotoxicosis increase the effect of warfarin therapy. In addition, polymorphisms in the genes involved in warfarin metabolism (CYP2C9 and VKORC1), if present, can strongly increase warfarin sensitivity exposing AIT patients to a high risk of bleeding (25).

Reassessing Management of AIT Patients

AIT is a dangerous condition for the patient because of the additional risk posed by thyrotoxicosis to the underlying cardiac abnormalities. Indeed, AIT has been associated with increased morbidity and mortality (Figure 17-3), especially in older patients with impaired left ventricular function (26,27). Thus, a prompt restoration and stable maintenance of euthyroidism should be achieved as quickly as possible, particularly in some patients. Hence, in selected categories of patients, detailed below, emergency management of AIT should be considered in order to obtain a rapid resolution of thyrotoxicosis.

If total thyroidectomy is considered, a multidisciplinary evaluation of the AIT patient involving cardiologists, endocrinologists, surgeons and anesthesiologists is warranted. Two main clinical scenarios should be considered:

1. emergency thyroidectomy
2. urgent thyroidectomy

Emergency Thyroidectomy

- *Patients with deterioration of the cardiac function.* AIT patients with stable cardiac conditions may continue medical therapy and cope with a longer exposure to thyroid hormone excess. At variance, patients with left ventricular systolic dysfunction, as assessed by the left ventricular ejection fraction (LVEF), have an increased mortality risk (Figure 17-4). AIT and left ventricular systolic dysfunction are independent factors associated with high

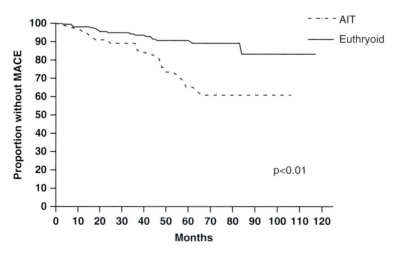

Figure 17-3 Development of major adverse cardiovascular events (MACE) in patients with AIT (dotted line) compared to euthyroid patients under amiodarone therapy (continuous line). MACE was defined as the occurrence of heart failure requiring hospitalization, cardiovascular mortality, myocardial infarction, stroke including transient ischemic attack, and ventricular arrhythmias requiring hospital admission (26). Reproduced with permission from the Endocrine Society/OUP.

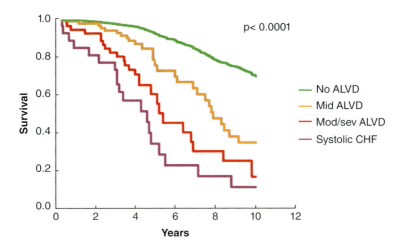

Figure 17-4 Mortality of patients with asymptomatic left ventricular systolic dysfunction (ALVD) according to ejection fraction (EF). Referent group consists of subjects with normal left ventricular systolic function (EF >50%) and no history of congestive heart failure (NO ALVD). Mild ALVD: mild asymptomatic left ventricular systolic dysfunction (EF 40% to 50%). Mod/Sev ALVD: moderate-to-severe asymptomatic left ventricular systolic dysfunction (EF <40%). Systolic CHF: congestive heart failure with EF ≤50%. Modified from (28). Reproduced with permission from Wolters Kluwer Health.

cardiovascular morbidity and mortality. In AIT patients with low LVEF, mortality may be as high as 30–50%. These findings suggest that in patients with severe underlying cardiac disease, prolonged exposure to high thyroid hormone levels may further deteriorate cardiac function and be responsible for the increased mortality rate (28).

- *Patients with a severe underlying cardiac disease* (e.g., arrhythmogenic right ventricular dysplasia) *or patients with malignant arrhythmia* should be considered for thyroidectomy.

Urgent Thyroidectomy

- *Patients unresponsive to medical therapy.* Patients with type 1 AIT often need large doses and a prolonged course of thionamides before achieving euthyroidism because the iodine-replete thyroid gland is less responsive to antithyroid drugs. On the other hand, approximately 20% of glucocorticoid-treated patients with type 2 AIT still are thyrotoxic after 2 months of therapy (more frequently if they have larger thyroid volume and severe thyrotoxicosis) (19).

- *Patients needing to continue amiodarone therapy.* In type 2 AIT patients treated with glucocorticoids, continuation of amiodarone does not significantly affect the first normalization of thyroid hormone. However, patients requiring continuation of amiodarone therapy show a high risk of recurrence of thyrotoxicosis during glucocorticoids therapy (about 70%), causing a delay in achieving stable restoration of euthyroidism (21).

- *Patients with type 2 AIT showing adverse effect to glucocorticoids therapy.* These include severe hyperglycemia, hepatotoxicity, glucocorticoid-induced osteoporosis, and opportunistic infections.

In this subset of patients, total thyroidectomy can represent the only therapeutic approach to guarantee a quick resolution of thyrotoxicosis. In addition, surgery, by rapidly restoring euthyroidism, can improve cardiac function within 2 months, mainly in patients with severe left ventricular systolic dysfunction, thereby reducing the risk of death (29). Therefore, in patients with deteriorated left ventricular function, surgery should be considered without delay. If a total thyroidectomy is considered, a multidisciplinary counseling involving endocrinologists, cardiologists, endocrine surgeons, and anesthesiologists is recommended in order to assess the risk-benefit balance in the individual patient. Older studies have reported frequent postoperative complications, including rehospitalization and deaths (30). Conversely, recent studies have shown that total thyroidectomy can be performed in AIT patients, including those with moderate-to-severe left ventricular dysfunction, without serious complications (31–33). Even though controlled studies are not available, our large personal experience suggests that an optimal preparation to surgery, including glucocorticoids and β-blockers, may reduce the surgical risk. Thus, in AIT patients, who are candidates for total thyroidectomy, a short course with glucocorticoids is mandatory, irrespective of the AIT type. More important, the multidisciplinary interaction of an experienced team is fundamental.

We have extensively used iopanoic acid (for 7–21 days before surgery) to reduce serum FT3 in patients unresponsive to medical therapy (Table 17-2) (34). However, in the absence of controlled studies, the real advantage of preparation with iopanoic acid to thyroidectomy in preventing surgical adverse events remains to be established. In addition, iopanoic acid is no longer available on the market. Whether other iodinated contrast agents may replace iopanoic acid is uncertain.

Plasmapheresis, aimed at removing the excess thyroid hormones from the circulation, has been reported to be efficacious, but this is usually transient and followed by exacerbation of thyrotoxicosis. Thus, its real advantage is unsettled. However, plasmapheresis may be an adjunctive tool to prepare thyrotoxic patients for surgery.

Case Study

A 66-year-old man was referred because of thyrotoxicosis. He had a two-year history of paroxysmal atrial fibrillation treated by electroconversion. In the last 6 months, the sinus rhythm had been maintained by oral amiodarone (200 mg/d) given in association with antiplatelet therapy. There was no information as to his thyroid function and morphology before the initiation of amiodarone therapy, but he had no history of previous thyroid diseases. In the last 4 weeks, he complained of nervousness, palpitations, weight loss (3 kg) not associated with changes in appetite, insomnia, and a modest increase in bowel movements. On physical examination, this patient, whose family history was negative for thyroid disorders, had tachycardic atrial fibrillation (120 beats/min). BP was 145/55 mmHg. The thyroid gland was neither increased in volume nor tender, no nodules were palpable, and no bruit was appreciated over the gland. There were no symptoms or signs of Graves' orbitopathy. There was no distal tremor.

Investigations were as follows: FT_4 65 pg/ml (normal values, 7.5–15.5 pg/ml); FT_3 9.8 pg/ml (3.5–5.7 pg/ml); and TSH <0.01 mU/liter (0.4–3.5 mU/liter). Anti-TPO and anti-TSH receptor antibodies were undetectable. C-reactive protein and complete blood count were normal. Urinary iodine excretion was markedly increased (9100 µg/24 h; normal values, 100–300 µg/24 h). No iodine-containing contrast agents had recently been administered to this patient.

Thyroid ultrasonography evidenced a slightly hypoechogenic gland with an estimated volume of 18 ml and with no nodules; color flow Doppler sonography (CFDS) showed absent hypervascularity; RAIU was 0.7% after 3 h and 0.9% at 24 h.

What Do You Think Is the Cause of His Thyrotoxic State?

The patient had a typical type 2 AIT. His thyroid gland was normal, with absent hypervascularity at CFDS, and thyroid RAIU values were very low. There was no evidence of thyroid autoimmunity. Amiodarone was withdrawn and replaced by β-blocking agents. He was treated with oral prednisone. The initial dose was 30 mg/d and maintained for 2 weeks; the steroid was then gradually tapered and withdrawn after 3 months. Serum free thyroid hormone concentrations normalized after 6 weeks and remained normal afterward. His late follow-up visit confirmed a euthyroid state after 2 years. He had no recurrent paroxysmal atrial fibrillation.

Conclusions

All patients with AIT should be considered potentially at risk of requiring emergency treatment (Figure 17-5). Thyrotoxicosis may precipitate cardiac conditions even in asymptomatic patients. This is unlikely to occur in patients with subtle cardiac abnormalities and more frequent in those with severe heart disease (e.g., congenital or post-infarction heart disease or ventricular arrhythmias).

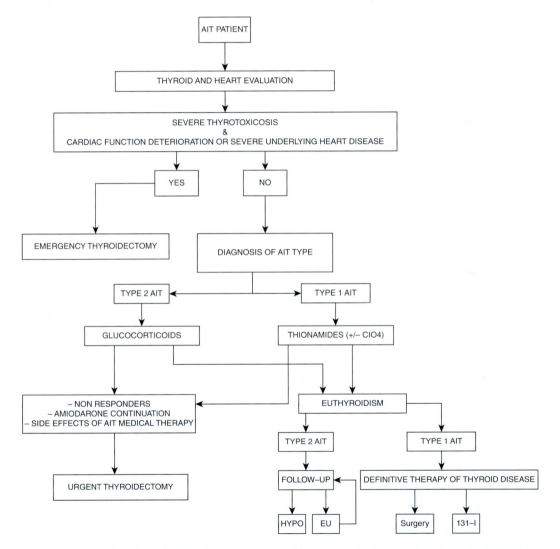

Figure 17-5 A proposed flow-chart for the management of AIT patients. Patients with amiodarone-induced thyrotoxicosis should be considered at high risk at any time; a prompt restoration of euthyroidism is advisable and, in selected patients, may be reached with total thyroidectomy; thyroid surgery may be considered, but should not be considered mandatory, also in patients in whom continuation of amiodarone is necessary. ClO4 = perchlorate.

References

1 Martino E, Bartalena L, Bogazzi F, Braverman LE. The effects of amiodarone on the thyroid. *Endocr Rev.* 2001;22:240–254.

2 Bogazzi F, Bartalena L, Gasperi M, Braverman LE, Martino E. The various effects of amiodarone on thyroid function. *Thyroid.* 2001;11:511–519.

3 Reiffel JA, Estes NA, 3rd, Waldo AL, Prystowsky EN, DiBianco RA. Consensus report on antiarrhythmic drug use. *Clin Cardiol.* 1994;17:103–116.

4 Bogazzi F, Tomisti L, Bartalena L, Aghini-Lombardi F, Martino E. Amiodarone and the thyroid: a 2012 update. *J Endocrinol Invest.* 2012;35:340–348.

5 Doval HC, Nul DR, Grancelli HO, Perrone SV, Bortman GR, Curiel R. Randomised trial of low-dose amiodarone in severe congestive heart failure. Grupo de Estudio de la Sobrevida en la Insuficiencia Cardiaca en Argentina (GESICA). *Lancet.* 1994;344:493–498.

6 Eskes SA, Wiersinga WM. Amiodarone and thyroid. *Best Pract Res Clin Endocrinol Metab.* 2009;23:735–751.

7 Tomisti L, Rossi G, Bartalena L, Martino E, Bogazzi F. The onset time of amiodarone-induced thyrotoxicosis (AIT) depends on AIT type. *Eur J Endocrinol.* 2014;171:363–368.

8 Tomisti L, Urbani C, Rossi G, et al. The presence of anti-thyroglobulin (TgAb) and/or anti-thyroperoxidase antibodies (TPOAb) does not exclude the diagnosis of type 2 amiodarone-induced thyrotoxicosis. *J Endocrinol Invest.* 2016;

9 Eaton SE, Euinton HA, Newman CM, Weetman AP, Bennet WM. Clinical experience of amiodarone-induced thyrotoxicosis over a 3-year period: role of colour-flow Doppler sonography. *Clin Endocrinol (Oxf).* 2002;56:33–38.

10 Bogazzi F, Bartalena L, Dell'Unto E, et al. Proportion of type 1 and type 2 amiodarone-induced thyrotoxicosis has changed over a 27-year period in Italy. *Clin Endocrinol (Oxf).* 2007;67:533–537.

11 Daniels GH. Amiodarone-induced thyrotoxicosis. *J Clin Endocrinol Metab.* 2001;86:3–8.

12 Martino E, Aghini-Lombardi F, Lippi F, et al. Twenty-four hour radioactive iodine uptake in 35 patients with amiodarone associated thyrotoxicosis. *J Nucl Med.* 1985;26:1402–1407.

13 Pattison DA, Westcott J, Lichtenstein M, et al. Quantitative assessment of thyroid-to-background ratio improves the interobserver reliability of technetium-99 m sestamibi thyroid scintigraphy for investigation of amiodarone-induced thyrotoxicosis. *Nucl Med Commun.* 2015;36:356–362.

14 Bogazzi F, Bartalena L, Brogioni S, et al. Color flow Doppler sonography rapidly differentiates type I and type II amiodarone-induced thyrotoxicosis. *Thyroid.* 1997;7:541–545.

15 Kurnik D, Loebstein R, Farfel Z, Ezra D, Halkin H, Olchovsky D. Complex drug-drug-disease interactions between amiodarone, warfarin, and the thyroid gland. *Medicine (Baltimore).* 2004;83:107–113.

16 Bogazzi F, Bartalena L, Martino E. Approach to the patient with amiodarone-induced thyrotoxicosis. *J Clin Endocrinol Metab.* 2010;95:2529–2535.

17 Maqdasy S, Batisse-Lignier M, Auclair C, et al. Amiodarone-induced thyrotoxicosis recurrence after amiodarone reintroduction. *Am J Cardiol.* 2016;117:1112–1116.

18 Bogazzi F, Tomisti L, Rossi G, Dell'Unto E, Pepe P, Bartalena L, Martino E. Glucocorticoids are preferable to thionamides as first-line treatment for amiodarone-induced thyrotoxicosis due to destructive thyroiditis: a matched retrospective cohort study. *J Clin Endocrinol Metab.* 2009;94:3757–3762.

19 Bogazzi F, Bartalena L, Tomisti L, et al. Glucocorticoid response in amiodarone-induced thyrotoxicosis resulting from destructive thyroiditis is predicted by thyroid volume and serum free thyroid hormone concentrations. *J Clin Endocrinol Metab*. 2007;92: 556–562.

20 Eskes SA, Endert E, Fliers E, Geskus RB,et al. Treatment of amiodarone-induced thyrotoxicosis type 2: a randomized clinical trial. *J Clin Endocrinol Metab*. 2012;97:499–506.

21 Bogazzi F, Bartalena L, Tomisti L, Rossi G, Brogioni S, Martino E. Continuation of amiodarone delays restoration of euthyroidism in patients with type 2 amiodarone-induced thyrotoxicosis treated with prednisone: a pilot study. *J Clin Endocrinol Metab*. 2011;96: 3374–3380.

22 Bogazzi F, Dell'Unto E, Tanda ML, et al. Long-term outcome of thyroid function after amiodarone-induced thyrotoxicosis, as compared to subacute thyroiditis. *J Endocrinol Invest*. 2006;29:694–699.

23 Albino CC, Paz-Filho G, Graf H. Recombinant human TSH as an adjuvant to radioiodine for the treatment of type 1 amiodarone-induced thyrotoxicosis (AIT). *Clin Endocrinol (Oxf)*. 2009;70:810–811.

24 Bogazzi F, Tomisti L, Ceccarelli C, Martino E. Recombinant human TSH as an adjuvant to radioiodine for the treatment of type 1 amiodarone-induced thyrotoxicosis: a cautionary note. *Clin Endocrinol (Oxf)*. 2010;72:133–134.

25 Tomisti L, Del Re M, Bartalena L,et al. Effects of amiodarone, thyroid hormones and CYP2C9 and VKORC1 polymorphisms on warfarin metabolism: a review of the literature. *Endocr Pract*. 2013:1–27.

26 Yiu KH, Jim MH, Siu CW, et al. Amiodarone-induced thyrotoxicosis is a predictor of adverse cardiovascular outcome. *J Clin Endocrinol Metab*. 2009;94:109–114.

27 O'Sullivan AJ, Lewis M, Diamond T. Amiodarone-induced thyrotoxicosis: left ventricular dysfunction is associated with increased mortality. *Eur J Endocrinol*. 2006;154:533–536.

28 Wang TJ, Evans JC, Benjamin EJ, Levy D, LeRoy EC, Vasan RS. Natural history of asymptomatic left ventricular systolic dysfunction in the community. *Circulation*. 2003;108:977–982.

29 Tomisti L, Materazzi G, Bartalena L, et al. Total thyroidectomy in patients with amiodarone-induced thyrotoxicosis and severe left ventricular systolic dysfunction. *J Clin Endocrinol Metab*. 2012;97: 3515–3521.

30 Houghton SG, Farley DR, Brennan MD, van Heerden JA, Thompson GB, Grant CS. Surgical management of amiodarone-associated thyrotoxicosis: Mayo Clinic experience. *World J Surg*. 2004;28:1083–1087.

31 Gough J, Gough IR. Total thyroidectomy for amiodarone-associated thyrotoxicosis in patients with severe cardiac disease. *World J Surg*. 2006;30:1957–1961.

32 Pierret C, Tourtier JP, Pons Y, Merat S, Duverger V, Perrier E. Total thyroidectomy for amiodarone-associated thyrotoxicosis: should surgery always be delayed for pre-operative medical preparation? *J Laryngol Otol*. 2012;126:701–705.

33 Kaderli RM, Fahrner R, Christ ER, et al. Total thyroidectomy for amiodarone-induced thyrotoxicosis in the hyperthyroid state. *Exp Clin Endocrinol Diabetes*. 2016;124:45–48.

34 Bogazzi F, Miccoli P, Berti P, et al. Preparation with iopanoic acid rapidly controls thyrotoxicosis in patients with amiodarone-induced thyrotoxicosis before thyroidectomy. *Surgery*. 2002;132: 1114–1117; discussion 1118.

18

Thyrotoxic Periodic Paralysis

Mark Vanderpump

Key Points

- Thyrotoxic periodic paralysis (TPP) is a rare complication of thyrotoxicosis characterized by acute, reversible episodes of muscle weakness and hypokalemia.
- TPP is often precipitated by heavy exercise or high-carbohydrate meals and is most commonly described in Asian men.
- Although the pathogenesis remains unclear, the recurrent paralytic muscle weakness is caused by hypokalemia resulting from a shift of potassium (K^+) into the intracellular space without a total K^+ deficit.
- The clinical features of TPP and the factors precipitating the acute paralysis episodes are similar to those of familial periodic paralysis (FPP) associated with hypokalemia, which is an autosomal dominant channelopathy more common in Caucasians.

- Although rare, early treatment of TPP is necessary to avoid reversible but potentially life-threatening complications, such as cardiac arrhythmias and respiratory failure.
- Symptoms and signs of thyrotoxicosis may be subtle in TPP so the diagnosis requires an awareness of precipitants and clinical features with recognition of biochemical and electrocardiography abnormalities.
- Treatment doses of potassium chloride required to recover from paralysis need to be minimized to avoid rebound hyperkalemia.
- Non-selective β-blockers can prevent paradoxical hypokalemia associated with hyperadrenergic activity.
- Treatment of the underlying cause of thyrotoxicosis (usually Graves' disease) should completely abolish further attacks of TPP.

Introduction

Periodic paralyses (PPs) are rare autosomal dominantly inherited channelopathies that manifest as abnormal, often K-sensitive, muscle membrane excitability leading to episodic flaccid paralysis. PPs are classified as hypokalemic (HypoPP) when episodes occur in association with low K^+ blood levels or hyperkalemic when episodes can be induced by elevated K^+ (1,2). HypoPP is the most common of the PPs, but is rare with an estimated prevalence of 1 in 100,000. Acquired sporadic cases of HypoPP have been described in association with all causes of thyrotoxicosis (3–6). Episodes of painless muscle weakness may be precipitated by heavy exercise or high-carbohydrate meals. Although the association of thyrotoxicosis and PP was first described in 1902 in a White person, TPP is most common among Asian populations with an incidence among

Endocrine and Metabolic Medical Emergencies: A Clinician's Guide, Second Edition. Edited by Glenn Matfin.
© 2018 John Wiley & Sons Ltd. Published 2018 by John Wiley & Sons Ltd.

patients with hyperthyroidism of 2% compared to 0.1–0.2% in non-Asian populations. In contrast to other thyroid disorders, over 95% of cases occur in men and the reported incidence in Asian men is 9–13% (7,8). Symptoms and signs of thyrotoxicosis may be subtle so the diagnosis requires an awareness of precipitants, clinical features, biochemical and ECG abnormalities associated with TPP. Prompt diagnosis and effective treatment avoid the life-threatening complications such as cardiac arrhythmias and respiratory failure (3–6).

Pathophysiology

The mechanisms by which thyrotoxicosis can produce HypoPP are not well understood. Thyroid hormone increases tissue responsiveness to beta-adrenergic stimulation, which increases Na^+-K^+ ATPase activity on the skeletal muscle membrane and drives K^+ into cells. TPP is thought to be due to over-activity of Na^+-K^+ ATPase by stimulation from excessive thyroid hormone, which leads to greater intracellular shifts of potassium, hypokalemia and hyperpolarization of skeletal muscle membranes (5). Activation of Na^+-K^+ ATPase cannot be the only mechanism for TPP, because only a minority of patients develop HypoPP. Excess thyroid hormone may predispose to paralytic episodes by increasing the susceptibility to the hypokalemic action of adrenaline. The increased Na^+-K^+ ATPase activity in muscle may be compensated by increased potassium efflux preventing development of hypokalemia. Insulin also activates the Na^+-K^+ ATPase pump and may act synergistically with the thyroid hormone to drive K^+ into cells. This is consistent with the observation that a heavy meal can be a precipitant for attacks of TPP (9). However, less than one-third of TPP patients receiving an oral glucose load develop glucose-induced acute hypokalemia with paralysis and those with provocable attacks have similar insulin responses to those without induced paralysis so insulin-independent factors must be involved in the pathogenesis.

The increased incidence of TPP among Asian people suggests a genetic predisposition and many clinical features, other than thyrotoxicosis, are similar to those found in familial PP (FPP). HypoPP and hyperkalemic PP are genetically heterogeneous with mutations in genes encoding three skeletal muscle ion channels (i.e., calcium [CACN1AS]; sodium [SCN4A]; and potassium [KCNE3]) accounting for at least 70% of the identified cases (1,10)). The resting membrane potential should hyperpolarize when extracellular K^+ decreases but muscle fibers in HypoPP depolarize under low extracellular K^+ concentrations (3 mmol/L). This hypokalemia-induced paradoxical depolarization of the resting membrane potential leads to inactivation of Na^+ channels, rendering them unexcitable. The most common mutation is in the gene that codes for the alpha-1 subunit of the dihydropyridine-sensitive calcium channel in skeletal muscle (CACNA1S) found in about 60% of patients (10). It is not known how the calcium channel defect leads to episodic potassium movement into cells and causes weakness. A mutation in the skeletal muscle sodium channel, SCN4A, is responsible for the majority of the remainder where an anomalous gating pore current may cause aberrant depolarization during attacks of weakness (10).

Patients with TPP do not have the genetic mutations associated with HypoPP but susceptible individuals are suspected to have an ion channel defect that is not sufficient to produce symptoms when euthyroid (3). Defects of the skeletal muscle-specific K^+ channel (Kir2.6) encoded by the KCNJ18 gene, are associated with a proportion of TPP patients, mainly from the United States, Brazil, France, and Singapore but less commonly in Thailand (11). Loss-of-function mutations in Kir2.6 channels cause an imbalance between inward leak current and outward K^+ current resulting in paradoxical depolarization (12,13).

Clinical Features

TPP is known to occur predominately in men despite a higher incidence of thyrotoxicosis in women (14). In 80% of patients the first episode of TPP occurs between the ages of 20–40 years in contrast to the younger onset (less than 20 years) of familial HypoPP (2). Although attacks of weakness may occur at any time of the day, a higher frequency is seen at night or early in the morning. There is a seasonal incidence with attacks more frequent in warmer summer months. Patients may experience recurrent episodes of weakness that last from a few hours up to 72 hours, with complete recovery between attacks (14,15). Intervals between attacks can vary from weeks to months, and some patients can experience several per week.

Events which are associated with release of adrenaline or insulin, both of which result in movement of K^+ into cells and hypokalemia, are associated with approximately one-third of episodes of TPP (14). Reported precipitating factors which precede the acute attack of TPP within 24 hours include high carbohydrate ingestion (12%), strenuous exercise (7%), trauma, acute upper respiratory tract infection, high-salt diet, emotional stress, cold exposure, alcohol ingestion, menstruation, and use of drugs such as corticosteroids, epinephrine, acetazolamide, and non-steroidal anti-inflammatory drugs (14).

The clinical features of TPP are virtually indistinguishable from those of HypoPP, except for the presence of thyrotoxicosis. The differential diagnosis includes Guillain-Barré syndrome, acute spinal cord compression, metabolic myopathies, myelitis, myesthenic crisis, botulism, and tic paralysis. The attacks in TPP are characterized by recurrent, transient episodes of muscle weakness that range from mild weakness to complete flaccid paralysis associated with preserved consciousness (14–16). Prodromal symptoms can include myalgia (<50%), cramps and muscle stiffness. Weakness usually begins in the proximal muscles of the legs which can progress to flaccid quadriplegia. Hypotonia with hypo- or areflexia is typical. Sensory function, bladder, and bowel function are not affected. The paralysis is usually symmetrical and bulbar and ocular muscles are usually spared. Tachycardia at presentation may distinguish TPP from familial HypoPP (17). In exceptional cases, respiratory weakness requiring ventilator support and fatal arrhythmias including ventricular tachycardia and ventricular fibrillation have been reported.

By definition, biochemical evidence of thyrotoxicosis is required for the diagnosis of TPP and paralysis only occurs when thyrotoxic and not when euthyroid. Classic symptoms such as weight loss, heat intolerance, palpitations, increased appetite, agitation, and diaphoresis may be subtle and precede the onset of TPP by months or even years, occur at the same time (50%) or follow the development of PP (15%) (14,15,17,18). Using the Wayne's index (a validated quantitative score of hyperthyroid severity), only 17% of a large series of TPP patients had a score >19 at the time of presentation (i.e., <11 euthyroid; 11–19 equivocal; and >19 toxic), confirming that most TPP patients have mild to equivocal hyperthyroid symptoms (14). Only a third have a known personal or family history of hyperthyroidism (14). The underlying cause of thyrotoxicosis in the majority is Graves' disease but TPP has rarely been associated with thyroiditis (autoimmune or viral), toxic nodular goitre, toxic adenoma, thyroid-stimulating hormone (TSH) secreting pituitary adenoma, thyroid hormone excess or iodine excess (5). For those who have no known personal or family history of overt clinical thyrotoxicosis, the rapid and correct diagnosis of TPP relies on the characteristic clinical and laboratory findings (Table 18-1).

Diagnosis

Patients presenting with hypokalemic paralysis and thyrotoxicosis are generally considered to have TPP as the initial diagnosis. However, this may be erroneous in

Table 18-1 Diagnostic features of thyrotoxic periodic paralysis (TPP)

Clinical
- Adult Asian men first onset aged 20-40 years
- Periodic symmetrical paralysis of proximal muscles, legs > arms
- Precipitating factors (e.g. high carbohydrate meals and extreme exercise)
- Subtle clinical features of thyrotoxicosis (e.g. tachycardia)
- Familial history of thyrotoxicosis

ECG findings
- Sinus tachycardia or sinus arrhythmia
- Prominent U wave and prolonged PR interval
- First degree AV block
- Atrial and ventricular arrhythmias

Biochemistry
- Hypokalemia with low spot urine [K^+]
- Normal blood acid-base balance
- Hypophosphatemia with hypophosphaturia
- Normal or increased serum calcium with hypercalciuria
- Hypomagnesemia
- Hypocreatininemia (increased glomerular filtration rate [GFR])
- Elevated creatine kinase (CK)
- Suppressed serum TSH, elevated free T_4 ± free T_3 (i.e. consistent with thyrotoxicosis)

---

rare circumstances owing to other conditions that cause renal or non-renal K^+ loss including diuretic therapy, gastrointestinal loss and chronic alcohol abuse (19) (Figure 18-1 and Table 18-2). Incorrect diagnosis may result in inappropriate K^+ repletion and recurrent hypokalemia. The use of simple, fast, and inexpensive tests of blood and urine electrolytes, and acid-base status may aid in differentiating such disorders as supporting thyroid function tests may not always be immediately available.

During an attack of paralysis or weakness the serum K^+ level is usually <3 mmol/L and can be less than 1.5 mmol/L. If the patient is at the recovery stage of the paralysis, serum K^+ may be normal. Usually the severity of weakness corresponds to the degree of hypokalemia (20). Renal K^+ excretion assessment allows for determination as to whether hypokalemia is due to renal or extra-renal causes. Low renal K^+ excretion in response to acute hypokalemia and relatively normal acid-base status are characteristic findings in TPP, in contrast to non-HypoPP disorders which usually have metabolic acidosis or alkalosis associated with large total K^+ deficits (21). A spot urine K^+ less than 15–20 mmol/L suggests an extra-renal cause of hypokalemia. Polyuria is common in patients with hypokalemia due to thirst or defective renal concentration in chronic hypokalemia (i.e., nephrogenic diabetes insipidus) so a low urine K^+ concentration can be seen even if significant renal K^+ wasting is present. The urine K^+-creatinine ratio can be used to differentiate between TPP and non-HypoPP with a diagnostic cutoff value of <2.5 mmol/mmol (i.e., hypokalemia consistent with trancellular potassium shift) (21).

Other characteristic biochemical abnormalities include hypomagnesemia and mild to moderate hypophosphatemia with low urine phosphate excretion (22). A low/normal serum creatinine concentration due to hyperdynamic renal changes is common. Increased urine calcium excretion rate due to the direct or indirect effect of thyroid hormone on bone and kidney is also found in TPP. Hypercalciuria and hypophosphaturia are unique and an early index of acute TPP. Serum creatine kinase (CK) is raised in two-thirds of patients, particularly if those attacks precipitated by exercise (23,24) (Table 18-1).

Electrocardiographic (ECG) changes associated with hypokalemia including ST depression, sinus tachycardia, U waves, abnormal PR interval, high QRS voltage and various AV and right bundle branch blocks, VT, ventricular fibrillation, and cardiac arrest have been reported (25,26).

Once TPP is established, the underlying etiology for thyrotoxicosis must be identified and effectively treated to avoid missing a potentially curable cause of TPP. In addition to history and physical examination, the assessment of serum TSH, free thyroxine (T_4) and free triiodothyronine (T_3), TSH-receptor

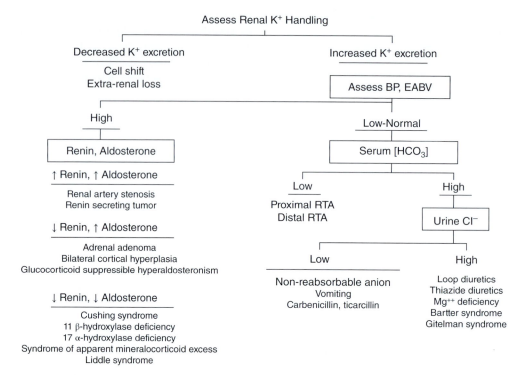

Figure 18-1 Approach to the patient with hypokalemia. A primary increase in mineralocorticoid levels gives rise to disorders characterized by hypokalemia, metabolic alkalosis, and hypertension. Disorders characterized by a primary increase in distal Na^+ delivery are differentiated by acid base status and urinary chloride [Cl^-] concentration. Both result in increased K^+ urinary loss. Hypokalemia due to cell shift and non-renal losses which are associated with low urinary [K^+] are listed in Table 18.2 (28). BP = Blood pressure; EABV = effective arterial blood volume; RTA = renal tubular acidosis.

antibodies, and, rarely, a thyroid diagnostic uptake scan can determine the underlying cause.

Acute Emergency Management

In view of acute hypokalemia, close cardiac monitoring is warranted in acute TPP (27). Unlike in non-HypoPP disorders, patients with TPP do not have a large K^+ deficit so the aim of K^+ supplementation is to raise serum K^+ concentration rather than to replace a large K^+ deficit. Required doses of potassium supplementation are variable and range from 10–200 mmol (5). Correction of hypomagnesemia is recommended but serum phosphate level spontaneously returns to normal without supplementation on recovery from paralysis.

The use of oral potassium supplements during the early phase of weakness can sometimes help to prevent the further progression of paralysis. Intravenous (IV) KCl therapy (10 mmol/hr) usually results in a rapid reversal of paralysis (28) although a delayed response can be seen (21). Intravenous K^+ should be administered in saline without glucose to avoid rapid shifts into the intracellular compartment (28). KCl administration carries a risk of rebound hyperkalemia because K^+ is released from cells rapidly when the paralysis subsides (2,4,5). Rebound hyperkalemia (>5.0 mmol/L) on recovery occurs in approximately 50% of patients with TPP receiving KCl but the risk is markedly reduced if the total KCl dose given is <50 mmol (29).

"Paradoxical hypokalemia" defined as a further fall in plasma K^+ concentration

Table 18-2 Etiology of hypokalemia associated with decreased renal K$^+$ excretion (28)

Cell shift

Insulin administration and overdose

β2 adrenergic stimulation
- Stress or exercise-induced adrenaline release

Drugs
- Theophylline intoxication, ritodrine, terbutaline, albuterol, clenbuterol

Anabolism
- Treatment of pernicious anemia
- Rapidly proliferating leukemias and lymphomas

Hypokalemic periodic paralysis
- TPP
- Familial
- Sporadic

Toxins/herbs
- Barium intoxication
- Chloroquine intoxication
- Cesium salts (in herbal preparations marketed as anti-tumor agent)

Extra-renal loss

Celiac disease

Tropical sprue

Infectious diarrhea
(e.g., Salmonella enteritis, Strongyloides enteritis, Yersinia enterocolitis)

Short bowel syndrome

(>0.1 mmol/L) occurs in approximately 25% of patients with TPP during KCl therapy (30) and is associated with more severe hyperthyroidism and hyperadrenergic activity. Higher KCl doses are required to restore muscle strength and consequently more severe rebound hyperkalemia is likely after recovery. Those who do not develop paradoxical hypokalemia usually need a smaller KCl dose to achieve recovery and have a much lower risk of rebound hyperkalemia. A higher dose of K$^+$ is rarely still urgently warranted in patients who develop the life-threatening ventricular arrhythmias and impending respiratory failure. A more rapid KCl 3–6 mmol can be administered IV in one minute or more to transiently raise K$^+$ concentration by 1–2 mmol/L with 20–40 mmol/hr as the recommended maximum infusion dose (30, 31).

High-dose non-selective β-blockers via the suppression of β$_2$ adrenergic activity and inhibition of insulin secretion have been reported to be used as an alternate therapy based on the implication of hyperadrenergic activity and hyperinsulinemia in the pathogenesis of TPP (32). Non-selective β-blockers like propranolol (oral 3–4 mg/kg or IV 1–2 mg/Kg every 10 minutes up to a maximum of 3 mg) but not the selective β$_1$ receptor blockers (e.g., metoprolol) shorten the duration of the attack and promote recovery. Those with paradoxical hypokalemia may be more suitable for non-selective β blockers to block K$^+$ uptake via Na$^+$-K$^+$ ATPase. Whether the combination of low dose KCl and non-selective β-blockers is more effective in reversal of paralysis and prevention of rebound hyperkalemia is not known. A treatment algorithm for TPP is shown in Figure 18-2.

Preventive Management

Once the cause of thyrotoxicosis has been identified, achieving euthyroidism as quickly as possible is the definitive way to completely abolish TPP attacks. Thionamides are recommended initially with early consideration of definitive treatment options (i.e., radioiodine therapy or elective thyroidectomy) depending on the etiology and patient choice to avoid the potential risk of relapse (33). Propranolol but not regular KCl supplementation is also effective in preventing recurrent attacks of TPP until euthyroid (5). Patients should be advised to avoid any identifiable precipitating factors such as high carbohydrate diet, high-salt diet, extreme exercise, and alcohol excess, which are also known to precipitate acute paralysis in HypoPP. Acetazolamide (which is commonly used in patients with familial HypoPP) can precipitate recurrent attacks of TPP and should not be used (34).

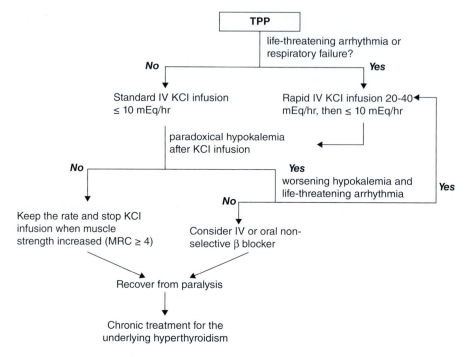

Figure 18-2 Therapeutic algorithm for thyrotoxic periodic paralysis (TPP).
Note: Medical Research Council (MRC) scale for assessment of muscle power (MRC ≥ 4, can move against gravity and some resistance exerted by examiner.

Case Study

A 34-year-old Filipino-American physician was seen in the Emergency Department because of a sudden onset marked by unknown quadriplegia, tachycardia and sweating. Symptoms appeared at a Super Bowl party where he had consumed excessive beer, popcorn, cake, sweets, and other snacks. He had no prior health issues.

On exam, he had flaccid paralysis, depressed distal tendon reflexes, and a normal sensory exam. A goiter estimated at 35 grams (normal 10–25) was noted. BP was 130/80; P 140; R 20.

Labs showed serum K^+ 2.1 mmol/L, Na^+ 133 mmol/L, TSH 0.01 (0.5–5.0), FT4 3.9 ng/dL (0.7–1.9 ng/dL), T3 222 ng/dL (80–180 ng/dL), TSH-receptor antibody positive, glucose was 108 mg/dL (5.5 mmol/L), creatinine 1.0 mg/dL (0.6–1.2).

Is the Diagnosis Consistent with TPP?

The clinical and biochemical features are consistent with TPP. The thyrotoxic state was due to hyperthyroidism secondary to Graves' disease. The likely precipitant was the excessive carbohydrate intake during the sporting celebration. He was admitted to the hospital and treated with IV fluids (normal saline not dextrose), IV K^+ (being careful not to overtreat and cause rebound hyperkalemia), anti-thyroid drugs (methimazole 20 mg/day) and propranolol were initiated. He was well in 48 hrs and discharged. He was treated with radioiodine 4 weeks later. Although this classical TPP case was an Asian male, it is important to appreciate that females and other ethnicities (e.g., Hispanics) can also be affected by TPP and therefore a high index of clinical suspicion is needed in order to make the correct diagnosis and prevent serious morbidity and potential mortality (i.e., cardiac arrhythmias) (35).

Conclusions

TPP is a rare endocrine emergency with diagnostic and therapeutic challenges. Most patients with TPP do not manifest typical symptoms and signs of thyrotoxicosis. The diagnosis requires an awareness of the clinical features, laboratory findings of blood and urine electrolytes, and ECG changes. The KCl dose required to correct hypokalemia should be minimal to avoid rebound hyperkalemia except in case of ventricular arrhythmia and impending respiratory insufficiency. High-dose non-selective β-blockers can help terminate muscle paralysis, especially for those patients who develop paradoxical hypokalemia associated with evidence of hyperadrenergic activity. Long-term management relies on definitive treatment of the etiology of the thyrotoxicosis, non-selective β-blockers and avoidance of the known precipitating factors.

Acknowledgments

The author wishes to acknowledge the contributions to the previous edition by Chih-Jen Cheng and Shih-Hua Lin, upon which portions of this chapter are based.

References

1 Venance SL, Cannon SC, Fialho D, et al. CINCH investigators. The primary periodic paralyses: diagnosis, pathogenesis and treatment. *Brain*. 2006;129:8–17.

2 Alkaabi JM, Mushtaq A, Al-Maskari FN, Moussa NA, Gariballa S. Hypokalemic periodic paralysis: a case series, review of the literature and update of management. *Eur J Emerg Med*. 2010;17:45–47.

3 Kung AW. Clinical review: Thyrotoxic periodic paralysis: a diagnostic challenge. *J Clin Endocrinol Metab*. 2006;91:2490–2495.

4 Pothiwala P, Levine SN. Analytic review: thyrotoxic periodic paralysis: a review. *J Intensive Care Med*. 2010; 25:71–77.

5 Vijayakumar A, Ashwath G, Thimmappa D. Thyrotoxic periodic paralysis: clinical challenges. *J Thyroid Res*. 2014;2014: 649502.

6 Chaudhry MA, Wayangankar S. Thyrotoxic periodic paralysis: A concise review of the literature. *Curr Rheumatol Rev*. 2016;12:190–194.

7 McFadzean AJ, Yeung R. Periodic paralysis complicating thyrotoxicosis in Chinese. *Br Med J*. 1967;1(5538):451–455.

8 Patel H, Wilches LV, Guerrero J. Thyrotoxic periodic paralysis: diversity in America. *J Emerg Med*. 2014;46:760–762.

9 Soonthornpun S, Setasuban W, Thamprasit A. Insulin resistance in subjects with a history of thyrotoxic periodic paralysis (TPP). *Clin Endocrinol (Oxf)*. 2009;70:794–797.

10 Vicart S, Sternberg D, Arzel-Hézode M, et al. Hypokalemic periodic paralysis. In: Pagon RA, Adam MP, Ardinger HH, et al., eds. *GeneReviews*®. Seattle (WA): University of Washington, Seattle; 1993–2017. http://www.genereviews.org/ (accessed March 9, 2017).

11 Ryan DP, da Silva MR, Soong TW, et al. Mutations in potassium channel Kir2.6 cause susceptibility to thyrotoxic hypokalemic periodic paralysis. *Cell*. 2010;140:88–98.

12 Cheung CL, Lau KS, Ho AY, et al. Genome-wide association study identifies a susceptibility locus for thyrotoxic periodic paralysis at 17q24.3. *Nat Genet*. 2012;44: 1026–1029.

13 Park S, Kim TY, Sim S, et al. Association of KCNJ2 Genetic variants with susceptibility to thyrotoxic periodic paralysis in patients with Graves' disease. *Exp Clin Endocrinol Diabetes*. 2017;125:75–78.

14 Chang CC, Cheng CJ, Sung CC, et al. A 10-year analysis of thyrotoxic periodic paralysis in 135 patients: focus on

symptomatology and precipitants. *Eur J Endocrinol.* 2013;169:529–536.

15 Hsieh MJ, Lyu RK, Chang WN, et al. Hypokalemic thyrotoxic periodic paralysis: clinical characteristics and predictors of recurrent paralytic attacks. *Eur J Neurol.* 2008;15:559–564.

16 Lin SH, Davis MR, Halperin ML. Hypokalemia and paralysis. *QJM.* 2003;96: 161–169.

17 Rhee EP, Scott JA, Dighe AS. Case records of the Massachusetts General Hospital. Case 4-2012. A 37-year-old man with muscle pain, weakness, and weight loss. *N Engl J Med.* 2012;366:553–560.

18 Wong P. Hypokalemic thyrotoxic periodic paralysis: a case series. *CJEM.* 2003;5: 353–355.

19 Tsai MH, Lin SH, Leu JG, Fang YW. Hypokalemic paralysis complicated by concurrent hyperthyroidism and chronic alcoholism: a case report. *Medicine (Baltimore).* 2015; 94:e1689.

20 Li J, Yang XB, Zhao Y. Thyrotoxic periodic paralysis in the Chinese population: clinical features in 45 cases. *Exp Clin Endocrinol Diabetes.* 2010;118:22–26.

21 Lin SH, Lin YF, Chen DT, Chu P, Hsu CW, Halperin ML. Laboratory tests to determine the causes for hypokalemia and paralysis. *Arch Intern Med.* 2004;164: 1561–1566.

22 Manoukian MA, Foote JA, Crapo LM. Clinical and metabolic features of thyrotoxic periodic paralysis in 24 episodes. *Arch Intern Med.* 1999;159:601–606.

23 Lin YF, Wu CC, Pei D, Chu SJ, Lin SH. Diagnosing thyrotoxic periodic paralysis in the ED. *Am J Emerg Med.* 2003;21:339–342.

24 Lin SH, Chu P, Cheng CC, Chu SJ, Hung YJ, Lin YF. Early diagnosis of thyrotoxic periodic paralysis: urine calcium to phosphate ratio. *Crit Care Med.* 2006; 34:2984–2989.

25 Hsu YJ, Lin YF, Chau T, Liou JT, Kuo SW, Lin SH. Electrocardiographic manifestations in patients with thyrotoxic periodic paralysis. *Am J Med Sci.* 2003; 326:128–132.

26 Lopez S, Henderson SO. Electrocardiogram changes in thyrotoxic periodic paralysis. *West J Emerg Med.* 2012;13:512–513.

27 Ashurst J, Sergent SR, Sergent BR. Evidence-based management of potassium disorders in the Emergency Department. *Emerg Med Pract.* 2016;18:1–24.

28 Palmer BF, Clegg DH. Physiology and pathophysiology of potassium homeostasis. *Adv Physiol Educ.* 2016;40:480–490.

29 Tassone H, Moulin A, Henderson SO. The pitfalls of potassium replacement in thyrotoxic periodic paralysis: a case report and review of the literature. *J Emerg Med.* 2004;26:157–161.

30 Lu KC, Hsu YJ, Chiu JS, Hsu YD, Lin SH. Effects of potassium supplementation on the recovery of thyrotoxic periodic paralysis. *Am J Emerg Med.* 2004;22: 544–547.

31 Shiang JC, Cheng CJ, Tsai MK, et al. Therapeutic analysis in Chinese patients with thyrotoxic periodic paralysis over six years. *Eur J Endocrinol.* 2009;161:911–916.

32 Lin SH, Lin YF. Propranolol rapidly terminates the hypokalemia, hypophosphatemia and paralysis in thyrotoxic periodic paralysis. *Am J Kidney Dis.* 2001;37:620–623.

33 Chang RY, Lang BH, Chan AC, Wong KP. Evaluating the efficacy of primary treatment for Graves' disease complicated by thyrotoxic periodic paralysis. *Int J Endocrinol.* 2014;2014:949068.

34 Cheng CJ, Kuo E, Huang CL. Extracellular potassium homeostasis: insights from hypokalemic periodic paralysis. *Semin Nephrol.* 2013;33:237–247.

35 Matfin G, Durand D, D'Agostino A, et al. Thyrotoxic hypokalemic periodic paralysis in an Hispanic female. *Hospital Practice* 1998;1:23–26.

19

Sight-Threatening Graves' Orbitopathy

Rebecca S. Bahn and James A. Garrity

Key Points

- Graves' orbitopathy is an autoimmune condition with heterogeneous expression ranging from mild ocular discomfort to severe and potentially sight-threatening disease.
- Almost half of all patients with hyperthyroidism due to Graves' disease can be identified as having some degree of orbital involvement. Patients may report a sensation of ocular "grittiness," diplopia, or eye redness and periorbital edema that can fluctuate in degree during the course of a single day or from day to day.
- The disease progresses in approximately 20% of patients who may experience eye

pain, frequent diplopia, severe periorbital erythema and swelling or excessive proptosis. In 3–5%, sight-threatening corneal breakdown or compressive optic neuropathy, a condition termed dysthyroid optic neuropathy (DON), may develop. The rare patient experiences anterior displacement or subluxation of the globe.
- Prompt recognition of the signs and symptoms of these sight-threatening conditions allows the clinician to arrange appropriate urgent or emergency referral to a specialist ophthalmologist.

Introduction

Graves' orbitopathy (GO), also known as Graves' ophthalmopathy or thyroid eye disease, is an autoimmune disorder with heterogeneous expression ranging from mild ocular discomfort to sight-threatening disease (1). Almost half of all patients with hyperthyroidism due to Graves' disease can be identified as having some degree of orbital involvement. Patients may report a sensation of ocular "grittiness," diplopia, or eye redness and periorbital edema that can fluctuate in degree during the course of a single day or from day to day (2). The disease progresses

in approximately 20% of patients who may experience eye pain, frequent diplopia, severe periorbital erythema and swelling or excessive proptosis. In 3–5%, sight-threatening corneal breakdown or compressive optic neuropathy, a condition termed dysthyroid optic neuropathy (DON), may develop (3). While the management of patients with mild GO is generally supportive, disease that is moderate to severe may require immunosuppressive therapy or surgical intervention (4). Sight-threatening disease requires urgent or emergency evaluation. Early intervention is especially important for patients with corneal breakdown as this can lead to corneal ulcers

Endocrine and Metabolic Medical Emergencies: A Clinician's Guide, Second Edition. Edited by Glenn Matfin.
© 2018 John Wiley & Sons Ltd. Published 2018 by John Wiley & Sons Ltd.

with loss of vision, possible globe perforation, and potential loss of the eye itself. While treatment of DON is less urgent, case series suggest that about 20% of untreated eyes may be left with visual acuity of 20/100 or less, with most having vision ranging from finger counting to no light perception (5). In our experience, orbital decompression improved or stabilized visual acuity by at least 3 lines of Snellen visual acuity in 110/205 eyes having visual acuity of 20/40 or less, and improved or resolved field defects in 246/291 eyes (6).

Patients with GO, except those with the mildest of manifestations, are optimally evaluated and cared for jointly by an endocrinologist and an ophthalmologist with special expertise in the treatment of patients with GO. However, most endocrinologists have not managed a large number of patients with this disorder and few practice in the setting of a thyroid-eye clinic where ophthalmologic expertise is readily available. This chapter focuses on the key features of impending or established sight-threatening GO that clinicians should recognize in order that appropriate urgent or emergency referral to a specialist ophthalmologist can be made.

Pathophysiology

The observation that Graves' hyperthyroidism and GO are often diagnosed in the same individual within a span of only a few months long suggested to clinicians that these two conditions might be initiated by a common stimulus. It is known that the thyrotropin receptor (TSHR) is the target antigen on thyroid follicular cells against which stimulatory TSHR autoantibodies (TRAb) are directed, resulting in uncontrolled and excessive release of thyroid hormone. The more recent finding that TSHR is also expressed on orbital fibroblasts, the target cells in GO, supported the notion of a common autoantigen and shared pathophysiology (7). Immune cells and TRAb, both directed against TSHR on these cells, work in tandem to trigger the disease process within the orbit. Some orbital fibroblasts are stimulated to overproduce hyaluronic acid (HA) while others, termed preadipocyte fibroblasts, undergo differentiation into mature fat cells. It has been further shown that orbital fibroblasts from GO patients express high levels of insulin-like growth factor-1 receptor (IGF-1R). Recent studies suggest that TSHR and IGF-1R on orbital fibroblasts engage in cross-talk induced by TSHR ligation to synergistically enhance HA production, adipogenesis and the secretion of inflammatory mediators within the GO orbit (7).

Excessive HA synthesis by interstitial fibroblasts within the extraocular muscles leads to their characteristic enlargement. Likewise, *de novo* adipogenesis as well as HA production within the orbital connective tissue compartment leads to expansion of these tissues. This combined increase in tissue volume within the confines of the bony orbit results in elevated intraorbital pressure. As a result, proptosis may ensue as the globe is anteriorly displaced. If quite pronounced, proptosis may contribute to incomplete eyelid closure with resulting corneal damage and, in rare cases, subluxation of the globe. If the extraocular muscles are especially enlarged at the orbital apex, they may compress the optic nerve, leading to the development of DON. Extraocular muscle dysfunction is caused, early in the disease, by swelling of the muscle bodies. The production of cytokines and chemokines by infiltrating immune cells and activated orbital fibroblasts underlies the inflammatory component of the disease. Periorbital and conjunctival edema may develop, owing to decreased venous and lymphatic drainage from the orbit, secondary to compression of these channels.

Environmental and genetic factors combine with the autoimmune process to produce the myriad clinical manifestations of the disease with their variable severity. Among the environmental contributions, smoking is the risk factor most consistently linked to the development of the disease and appears to be a major contributor to the occurrence of sight-threatening manifestations.

In addition, the presence of uncontrolled hyperthyroidism or hypothyroidism, a history of radioactive iodine therapy, or very high TRAb levels predispose to more severe disease in patients with GO (1).

Dysthyroid Optic Neuropathy (DON)

DON is multifactorial in etiology and occurs secondary to the orbital tissue remodeling that characterizes the disease. The neuropathy typically results from direct apical compression of the optic nerve or less likely impingement of its vascular supply by enlarged extraocular muscles at the orbital apex (8). A contributing factor in some patients is a tight orbital septum preventing the auto-decompression of orbital pressures by forward protrusion of the globe. Rarely, DON develops in the setting of extreme proptosis or corneal subluxation as the optic nerve is stretched between the orbital apex and the globe. Men, older patients, smokers, and patients with diabetes mellitus are at particular risk for the development of DON (9).

Clinical characteristics were studied in 47 patients considered to have features suspicious of DON who were evaluated at seven European centers over a one-year period (10). While most patients had moderate to severe inflammatory signs and symptoms with excessive proptosis at presentation, 25% had only modest inflammation and a third had proptosis of <21 mm on exophthalmometry (>21 mm usually considered abnormal). Visual acuity was reduced in 75% (6/9 Snellen or worse) and formal color vision assessment showed abnormalities in essentially all patients. Double vision was present in most patients and was frequently inconstant (present with side gaze) or constant in primary gaze. Keratopathy was evident in 20 and corneal ulceration was found in three patients. DON was unilateral in about half of the patients.

Because changes in visual acuity and color vision may be insidious, some patients with DON may not notice any visual changes.

Subtle color vision issues in association with a unilateral optic neuropathy can be identified with a red-desaturation test where a red colored object is shown to each eye independently. The eye with optic neuropathy will appear washed-out and less intense. The report of new onset blurred or dimmed vision that is not corrected by blinking (which regenerates the tear film) or by closing one eye (which distinguishes the visual changes from incipient diplopia) should alert the physician to the possibility of DON (11). Similarly, the presence of optic nerve involvement should be suspected in patients who show "frozen eyes" or significant restriction of eye movement, particularly to upward gaze, or who suffer from constant diplopia (10).

The finding of a relative afferent pupillary defect (RAPD; asymmetric pupillary response in association with GO to a light stimulus, often tested using a "swinging flashlight") is very suggestive, if not diagnostic, of DON. However, the RAPD may be absent if DON is bilateral and symmetrical. While the presence of disc edema can be one of the cardinal features of DON, about 50–75% of patients with this diagnosis show normal optic disc morphology or only minimal retinal venous congestion (Figure 19-1). The signs with the greatest specificity for DON are impairment of color perception and optic

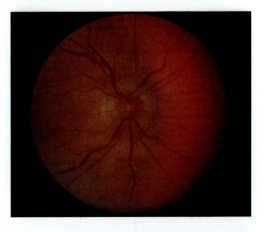

Figure 19-1 Optic disc edema (right eye) in a patient with DON showing elevation of the optic disc with indistinct margins. Retinal veins are congested.

disc swelling (10). Ballottement of the globe revealing a tense, rather than soft, consistency is not a sensitive test but may occasionally be useful.

Once DON is suspected, the patient should be referred urgently to a specialist ophthalmologist who can obtain and interpret additional testing. Because no single test confirms or refutes the diagnosis, the decision either to immediately treat or closely observe a patient is based on a constellation of findings. Further assessment generally includes formal visual acuity assessment, determination of pupillary responses and color vision testing, although this latter test will not be helpful in

the 10% of males who are congenitally color blind. Automated perimetry is performed to identify visual field defects which are generally central, paracentral and/or inferior when DON is present (2). However, these tests may be difficult to interpret in the setting of visual impairment caused by confounding ocular pathology, such as glaucoma, cataracts or macular degeneration. Imaging with computed tomography (CT) scanning or magnetic resonance imaging (MRI) is commonly used to support the diagnosis of DON in patients with impairment in any of these parameters (Figure 19-2). The combination of apical crowding (effacement of perineural

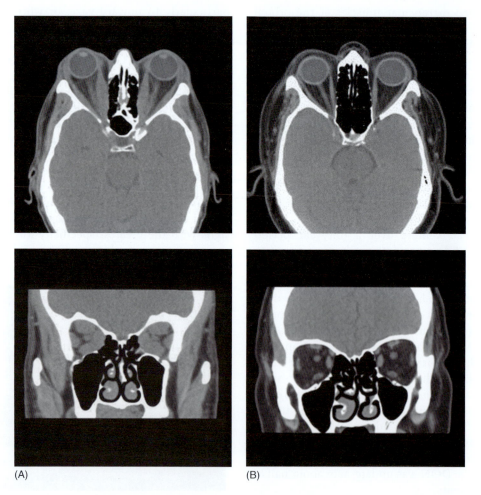

(A)   (B)

Figure 19-2 Axial (A top) and coronal (A bottom) CT scans of a patient (also shown in Figure 19.1) with DON showing compression of the optic nerve at the apex of the orbit by enlarged extraocular muscles with apical crowding (effacement of perineural fat at the apex). Axial (B top) and coronal (B bottom) CT scans of a normal orbit are shown for comparison.

fat at the apex) and evidence of fat herniation through the superior orbital fissure seen on axial images has a specificity of 91% and a sensitivity of 94% for DON (12).

Therapy for DON involves intravenous (IV) pulse therapy with methylprednisolone, orbital decompression surgery or both modalities. Orbital radiotherapy is not recommended in this setting except as an adjunct to these two proven therapies (4). Perhaps because of the rarity of the condition and the lack of well-defined diagnostic criteria, only one randomized controlled trial (15 patients) comparing the two modalities has been performed (13). In this study, 5/6 patients who initially underwent orbital decompression surgery subsequently deteriorated or failed to improve visual acuity and subsequently required treatment with IV methylprednisolone (1.0 g daily for 3 consecutive days, repeated once after 1 week) followed by a 4-month course of oral prednisone (2 weeks of 40 mg daily, 4 weeks of 30 mg, 4 weeks of 20 mg, tapering off by 2.5 mg per week until finished). Conversely, 4/9 IV methylprednisolone-treated patients subsequently required orbital decompression. While neither approach was uniformly successful as an initial therapy, DON ultimately resolved in all cases as patients failing one approach responded to the other. Case studies report some visual function improvement in 76–90% of patients within a few days of orbital decompression surgery (13).

The recent management guidelines from the European Group on Graves' Orbitopathy (EUGOGO) advises as first-line therapy for DON very high doses of IV glucocorticoids (e.g., 0.5 g–1.0 g of methylprednisolone) for 3 consecutive days or on alternate days during the first week (4). This course can be repeated after a week and is effective in approximately 40% of patients with recovery of normal or near-normal vision (14). If DON has resolved or improved after 2 weeks of therapy, pulses of weekly IV methylprednisolone should be continued using a regimen similar to that recommended in the EUGOGO guidelines for the treatment of moderate-to-severe and active GO, with the total cumulative dose not exceeding 8.0 g (4). If the initial response to glucocorticoids is absent or poor, or when there is rapid deterioration in visual function (acuity/visual field), urgent decompression surgery should be performed. Surgery may be indicated as first line therapy if visual acuity is <20/200, the corneal exposure from proptosis is significant, if congestive features are prominent or steroid side-effects are to be avoided (6).

Corneal Breakdown

Severe eye pain in a patient with GO, especially if new in onset, sharp in quality and associated with blurred vision, is a worrisome feature that is suggestive of severe corneal exposure, breakdown, or corneal ulcer. While much less common than DON, suspicion of corneal breakdown requires emergency, rather than urgent, referral to an ophthalmologist (4). Corneal ulceration can develop when corneal protection is limited (Figure 19-3). This can result from extreme proptosis, excessive eyelid retraction, ineffective blinking with poor tear production or incomplete eyelid closure. In some patients with GO, the cornea remains exposed when the eyelids are approximated because the reflex upwards motion of the globe is prevented by a tight inferior rectus muscle (absent Bell's phenomenon). Such patients, especially those unable to completely close their eyes (lagophthalmos) owing to excessive lid

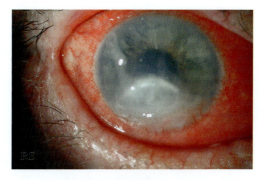

Figure 19-3 Slit-lamp photograph showing a corneal ulcer in a patient with lid retraction and lagophthalmos

retraction, are particularly at risk for corneal breakdown (2).

Initial treatment for corneal exposure includes the frequent use of topical lubricants and intensive topical antibiotics where appropriate. Eyelids may be taped closed or a moisture chamber may be used for protection of the healing cornea. When corneal exposure is more severe (large epithelial and/or stromal defects), temporary globe coverage may be achieved by injecting botulinum toxin into the levator (although there is typically a 3–4 day delay in therapeutic effect), or surgically by tarsorrhaphy. Pulse therapy with IV methylprednisolone or orbital decompression surgery may be considered in refractory cases. In the setting of corneal decompensation, amniotic membrane grafts, conjunctival flaps or even corneal transplant may be required (4). The recent EUGOGO management guidelines recommend that severe corneal exposure be treated medically or by means of progressively more invasive surgeries as soon as possible in order to avoid progression to corneal breakdown. The latter should be immediately addressed surgically (4).

Subluxation of the Globe

Axial globe subluxation is defined as anterior displacement of the globe equator beyond the orbital rim, lid retraction behind the equator, and tethering of the optic nerve. A retrospective study of 4000 patients with GO found the incidence of globe subluxation to be 0.01% (15). Examination of the CT scans of four of these patients uniformly revealed increased orbital fat without significant extraocular muscle enlargement. The authors concluded that the increased orbital

Table 19-1 Features of sight-threatening Graves' orbitopathy

Sight-threatening condition	Risk factors	Suggestive signs/symptoms	Referral to ophthalmologist; treatment options
Dysthyroid optic neuropathy (DON)	Diabetes mellitus Smoking Older patients Severe inflammation (but may occur in patients with little inflammation)	Complaint of blurry vision not corrected by blinking or closing an eye Dulling of color vision Constant diplopia Optic disc edema Relative afferent pupillary defect	Urgent referral Therapy may include pulse therapy with IV methylprednisolone, orbital decompression surgery, or both modalities
Corneal exposure	Extreme proptosis Lagophthalmos/ excessive lid retraction Absent Bell's phenomenon	Severe eye pain, especially if new in onset, sharp in quality, and associated with blurry vision	Emergency referral Depending on severity, treatment may include medical measures to protect the globe, tarsorrhaphy, IV methylprednisolone pulses, or emergency orbital decompression surgery
Subluxation of the globe	Extreme proptosis with lid retraction Excessive orbital fat enlargement with relatively normal extraocular muscle volume	Patient may describe an episode compatible with subluxation	Urgent referral Generally urgent orbital decompression surgery or a tarsorraphy is indicated

fat content results in increased compliance of the soft tissues and the normal caliber of the muscles allows them to be more extensible, permitting acute contraction of the eyelids posterior to the equator of the globe. With subluxation, vision may be acutely threatened by either corneal exposure or DON. Tarsorrhaphy may be performed at presentation as a temporary measure prior to urgent orbital decompression surgery. Patients with significant proptosis and lid retraction, particularly those with excessive orbital fat enlargement, should be made aware of this condition and instructed regarding manual repositioning of the globe with axial pressure should it occur.

Conclusions

Optimum care for the patient with GO is achieved through team work between endocrinologist and ophthalmologist. Because sight-threatening GO may require prompt intervention by an ophthalmologist, at each clinic visit the endocrinologist should assess key signs, symptoms, and risk factors that might suggest the need for urgent or emergency ophthalmologic consultation (Table 19-1). In particular, a patient who describes severe eye pain, especially if new in onset, sharp in nature, and associated with visual blurring, should be emergently referred to an ophthalmologist for possible corneal breakdown. Reported deterioration in vision that does not clear with blinking, especially if disc edema is detected, suggests impending or established DON and requires urgent referral to an ophthalmologist. A history compatible with subluxation of the globe warrants urgent ophthalmologic referral to prevent recurrent episodes with possible corneal or optic nerve damage.

References

1 Bahn RS. Graves' ophthalmopathy. *N Engl J Med.* 2010;362:726–738.

2 Dickinson AJ, Perros P. Controversies in the clinical evaluation of active thyroid associated orbitopathy: use of a detailed protocol with comparative photographs for objective assessment. *Clin Endocrinol (Oxf).* 2001;55:283–303.

3 Ben Simon GJ, Syed HM, Douglas R, Schwartz R, Goldberg RA, McCann JD. Clinical manifestations and treatment outcome of optic neuropathy in thyroid-related orbitopathy. *Ophthalmic Surg Lasers Imaging.* 2006;37:284–290.

4 Bartalena L, Baldeschi L, Borboridis K, et al. on behalf of the European Group on Graves' Orbitopathy (EUGOGO) The 2016 European Thyroid Association/European Group on Graves' orbitopathy. Guidelines for the management of Graves' orbitopathy *Eur Thyroid J.* 2016;5:9–26.

5 Trobe JD, Glaser JS, Laflamme P. Dysthyroid optic neuropathy: clinical profile and rationale for management. *Arch Ophthalmol.* 1978;96:1199–1209.

6 Soares-Welch CV, Fatourechi V, Bartley GB, et al. Optic neuropathy of Graves' disease: results of transantral orbital decompression and long-term follow-up in 215 patients. *Am J Ophthalmol.* 2003;136:433–441.

7 Krieger CC, Place RF, Bevilacqua C, et al. TSH/IGF-1 receptor cross talk in Graves' ophthalmopathy pathogenesis. *J Clin Endocrinol Metab.* 2016;101:2340–2347.

8 Dosso A, Safran AB, Sunaric G, Burger A. Anterior ischemic optic neuropathy in Graves' disease. *J Neuroophthalmol.* 1994;14:170–174.

9 Kalmann R, Mourits MP. Diabetes mellitus: a risk factor in patients with Graves' orbitopathy. *Br J Ophthalmol.* 1999;83:463–465.

10 McKeag D, Lane C, Lazarus JH, Baldeschi L, et al. Clinical features of dysthyroid optic neuropathy: a European Group on Graves'

Orbitopathy (EUGOGO) survey. *Br J Ophthalmol*. 2007;91:455–458.

11 Bahn RS, Bartley GB, Gorman CA. treatment of Graves' ophthalmopathy. *Baillieres Clin Endocrinol Metab*. 1992;6:95–105.

12 Birchall D, Goodall KL, Noble JL, Jackson A. Graves' ophthalmopathy: intracranial fat prolapse on CT images as an indicator of optic nerve compression. *Radiology*. 1996;200:123–127.

13 Wakelkamp IM, Baldeschi L, Saeed P, Mourits MP, Prummel MF, Wiersinga WM. Surgical or medical decompression as a first-line treatment of optic neuropathy in Graves' ophthalmopathy? A randomized controlled trial. *Clin Endocrinol (Oxf)*. 2005;63:323–328.

14 Currò N, Covelli D, Vannucchi G, et al. Therapeutic outcomes of high-dose intravenous steroids in the treatment of dysthyroid optic neuropathy. *Thyroid*. 2014;24:897–905.

15 Rubin PA, Watkins LM, Rumelt S, Sutula FC, Dallow RL. Orbital computed tomographic characteristics of globe subluxation in thyroid orbitopathy. *Ophthalmology*. 1998;105:2061–2064.

Part VI

Adrenal Disorders

Introduction

Emergency Management of Adrenal Disorders

Anand Vaidya

Key points

- Genomics has transformed our understanding and approach to adrenal diseases.
- Today, we recognize that at least a dozen genes may predispose to an inheritable pheochromocytoma-paraganglioma syndrome (PPS) and that 35–40% of all pheochromocytomas and paragangliomas may be attributable to germline mutations in one of these genes, while several other somatic mutations have also been found.
- It is now recommended that all patients with pheochromocytomas and paragangliomas be counseled on the value of genetic testing, and that those who are discovered to have a genetic susceptibility be enrolled in a prospective surveillance program.

- Primary hyperaldosteronism (PA) is traditionally considered to manifest with severe hypertension. However, an accruing number of studies have demonstrated that when employing a more permissive, or indiscriminate, strategy for PA screening, the prevalence of overt PA and milder autonomous aldosterone secretion is high, ranging from 8–20% in the hypertensive population and 3–14% in the normotensive population.
- Despite the remarkable insights gained from genetic, molecular, and metabolomic studies, we still await the translation of many of these findings into robust clinical and randomized interventional trials to develop high-grade evidence that will confidently impact patient (including emergency) care.

Introduction

The twenty-first century has witnessed remarkable progress in our understanding of the pathogenesis of adrenal disorders. Much of this enlightenment can be attributed to the renaissance in genomics that has transformed, and is still transforming, our understanding and approach to adrenal diseases. The ongoing lessons learned from genomic and molecular studies have transferred to clinical practice; we now employ genetic testing to explain the pathogenesis, inform diagnosis, and dictate management of adrenal disorders.

Pheochromocytoma and Paraganglioma

In 1886, Felix Fränkel described an 18-year-old woman (Minna Roll) in Germany who died after episodic paroxysms of anxiety, palpitations, dizziness, and headaches (1,2).

Endocrine and Metabolic Medical Emergencies: A Clinician's Guide, Second Edition. Edited by Glenn Matfin.
© 2018 John Wiley & Sons Ltd. Published 2018 by John Wiley & Sons Ltd.

Post-mortem examination revealed bilateral adrenal tumors that were described at the time as sarcoma and angiosarcoma (1,2). The recognition of chromaffin tumors and the term pheochromocytoma were not coined until many years later, but by the mid-1960s it was generally recognized that neurofibromatosis type 1, the syndrome of multiple endocrine neoplasia, and the von Hippel-Lindau syndrome were three inheritable conditions that were associated with the risk for developing pheochromocytomas. Interestingly, in 2007, Neumann et al. traced the family lineage of Minna Roll in Germany and found that multiple family members carried *RET* mutations and features of multiple endocrine neoplasia type 2; therefore, Minna Roll is considered to be the first patient with an inheritable pheochromocytoma-paraganglioma syndrome (PPS). A seismic change in our understanding of pheochromocytomas occurred in 2000, when Baysal et al. discovered that germline mutations in a new gene (*SDHD*) were a source of inheritable PPS (3). In the subsequent years, mutations in other succinate dehydrogenase genes were implicated as causes of inheritable PPS and it became clearer that a substantial proportion of what were previously considered to be "sporadic" pheochromocytomas and paragangliomas were in fact attributable to an inheritable germline susceptibility (4). Today, we recognize that at least a dozen genes may predispose to an inheritable PPS and that 35–40% of all pheochromocytomas and paragangliomas may be attributable to germline mutations in one of these genes (5,6), while several other somatic mutations have also been found.

This new paradigm of pheochromocytomas and paragangliomas as syndromic tumors that are a part of an inheritable genetic syndrome has changed our approach to management. It is now recommended that all patients be counseled on the value of genetic testing, and that those who are discovered to have a genetic susceptibility be enrolled in a prospective surveillance program (5,6). Further, family members can be counseled based on the results of the genetic testing of the proband, thereby identifying other at-risk individuals. Although more longitudinal studies to determine the most effective and precise surveillance strategy are still needed, imaging is widely used to survey for new tumors. Since most of the PPS increase the lifetime risk for developing not only pheochromocytoma and paraganglioma, but also other tumors (such as renal cell carcinoma, gastrointestinal stromal tumors, and others), unbiased imaging may be the optimal approach to detect tumors in their infancy, before metastases and other complications occur. It is anticipated that future studies will increase our understanding of genotype-phenotype correlations and the most efficacious manner by which to survey patients with PPS. Multi-disciplinary *tour de force* efforts such as the Cancer Genome Atlas have already provided new data that may be used to reorganize the pathogenic framework and nomenclature of PPS based on genotype-phenotype correlations (7).

Primary Aldosteronism

Jerome Conn first described the condition of primary aldosteronism (PA) in the setting of hypertension, sodium retention, volume expansion, and a unilateral adrenal adenoma (8). The condition is characterized by autonomous secretion of aldosterone, independent of its dominant regulators (angiotensin II, potassium, and corticotropin) and in the face of a high sodium balance. Since Conn first described it, PA has been diagnosed by demonstrating "renin-independent aldosteronism," as manifested by a suppression of renin and a high aldosterone-to-renin ratio, along with the failure to suppress aldosterone with sodium loading (9). Given the lack of a true gold standard for PA diagnosis, it can be argued that most current clinical definitions of PA are designed to detect fairly overt and severe autonomous aldosteronism. However, this paradigm is slowly changing as it is becoming clearer that autonomous aldosteronism is more common than previously perceived and the molecular and genetic underpinnings of autonomous aldosterone secretion are increasingly understood.

PA is traditionally considered to manifest with severe hypertension; therefore, clinical guidelines have usually recommended screening for PA when patients have multi-drug or resistant hypertension (9,10). However, an accruing number of studies have demonstrated that when employing a more permissive, or indiscriminate, strategy for PA screening, the prevalence of overt PA and milder autonomous aldosterone secretion is high, ranging from 8–20% in the hypertensive population (11–13) and 3–14% in the normotensive population (14,15). These studies, and others, suggest that the spectrum of primary (or autonomous) aldosteronism is much more expansive than we had previously realized: PA likely begins in normotension as a mild form of autonomous aldosteronism, and may progress to hypertension where it is overtly detected in early and late stages (11–13). These insights then raise the question how we should change our screening practices to detect autonomous aldosteronism earlier in its pathogenesis, and when and how we should implement interventions (such as mineralocorticoid receptor antagonists) to mitigate the cardiovascular risks associated with inappropriate aldosterone secretion. Since large cohort studies have shown that inappropriate aldosterone secretion increases the risk for developing incident hypertension in normotensives (16,17), we await future studies that focus on early interventions to mitigate mineralocorticoid receptor activation in these susceptible individuals.

Why is autonomous aldosteronism so common? For decades only one established genetic mechanism for PA was recognized: familial hyperaldosteronism type 1, whereby a fusion of the promoter for CYP11B1 to CYP11B2 resulted in ACTH-dependent aldosterone secretion. However, the last five years have witnessed an explosion in genetic mechanisms that contribute to autonomous aldosterone secretion, almost all of which involve alterations in cell membrane channels that increase intra-cellular calcium flux. We now recognize that mutations in zona glomerulosa cell *KCNJ5* (outward rectifying potassium channel), voltage gated calcium channels (*CACNA1D, CACNA1H*), and ATPases (*ATP1A1, ATP2B3*) can all result in autonomous aldosterone secretion and PA. These are overwhelmingly somatic mutations found in resected aldosterone producing adenomas; however, rarely some of them are inheritable. In parallel, it has been observed that normal adrenal glands obtained from post-mortem studies exhibit abnormal CYP11B2 expression. The use of specific CYP11B2 antibodies in the last 5 years has dramatically expanded our ability to investigate foci of aldosterone synthase activity. Nishimoto et al. showed that even normal adrenal glands harbor abnormal islands of CYP11B2 activity (termed aldosterone-producing cell clusters or APCCs) that exhibit autonomous and non-suppressible expression and harbor somatic gene mutations known to induce aldosterone secretion (18,19). Further, APCCs have been observed to increase in quantity with age; therefore, a prevailing hypothesis that has emerged is that APCCs may underlie the pathogenesis of age-related incident hypertension and the increased prevalence of autonomous aldosterone secretion that is observed in both normotensive and hypertensive populations.

Incidentally Discovered Adrenal Tumors

The rising use of cross-sectional abdominal imaging worldwide has increased the detection of incidental adrenal neoplasia. Hundreds of millions of abdominal CT and MRI scans are performed annually (20). Although the exact prevalence and incidence of adrenal tumor detection are not known, even if it represented only 1% of all scans, the absolute number observed per year would be expected to be huge. The vast majority of these incidentally discovered adrenal masses are benign and non-functional; however, a notable proportion of these benign tumors may still hypersecrete adrenal cortical hormones, such as cortisol. Elegant studies using steroid metabolomics have shown that even "nonfunctional" adrenal tumors hypersecrete glucocorticoids, thereby implicating a spectrum of glucocorticoid excess that extends well beyond our traditional ability to detect circulating cortisol (21). Much focus has been placed on defining and detecting this subclinical hypercortisolism in the clinical setting (also defined as autonomous cortisol secretion). Currently, the minimal definition is a cortisol concentration >50 nmol/L (1.8 µg/dL) following an overnight 1 mg dexamethasone suppression test, whereas values >138 nmol/L (5.0 µg/dL) are universally accepted as abnormal. When these results of autonomous cortisol secretion are accompanied by overt Cushing's syndrome, the decision to localize and treat the source of cortisol excess is appropriate and recommended. However, when this excess cortisol is not accompanied by any clear evidence of Cushing's syndrome (hence the term subclinical), evidence-based recommendations remain more nebulous and reliant on expert opinion.

Numerous cross-sectional studies have suggested that subclinical hypercortisolism is associated with higher blood pressure, impaired glycemia, and low bone density (22), and meta-analyses of anecdotal reports have suggested that surgical resection of the source of hypercortisolism may correct these abnormalities (23). Longitudinal studies have shown that subclinical hypercortisolism in patients with adrenal tumors is associated with higher risk for developing cardiovascular disease and diabetes (24,25). Although these observational studies strongly suggest that even low-grades of subclinical hypercortisolism may increase the risk for cardiometabolic disease, robust intervention studies (specifically randomized controlled studies) to investigate whether directed treatment significantly improves incident cardiometabolic risk have not been reported. Therefore, current recommendations advise the screening and surveillance of cortisol autonomy in patients with adrenal incidentalomas, but do not provide specific indications for surgery when the excess is subclinical (22). These situations continue to require physicians to practice the "art of medicine" and assess each patient on a case-by-case basis to determine the risk-to-benefit ratio of treatment versus on-going monitoring.

Conclusions

In summary, the last 5–10 years in adrenal medicine and science have been transformative. Despite the remarkable insights gained from genetic, molecular, and metabolomic studies, we still await the translation of many of these findings into robust clinical and randomized interventional trials to develop high-grade evidence that will confidently impact patient (including emergency) care. Thus, as we celebrate and revel in these recent accomplishments, we must remain vigilant and determined to continue to expand and cultivate new evidence to best serve our patients.

References

1 Frankel F. Ein Fall von doppelseitigem, völlig latent verlaufenen Nebennierentumor und gleichzeitiger Nephritis mit Veränderungen am Circulationsapparat und Retinitis. *Arch Pathol Anat Physiol Klin Med.* 1886;103:244–263.

2 Neumann HP, Vortmeyer A, Schmidt D, et al. Evidence of MEN-2 in the original description of classic pheochromocytoma. *N Engl J Med.* 2007;357:1311–1315.

3 Baysal BE, Ferrell RE, Willett-Brozick JE, et al. Mutations in SDHD, a mitochondrial complex II gene, in hereditary

paraganglioma. *Science*. 2000;287:848–851.

4 Neumann HP, Bausch B, McWhinney SR, et al. Germ-line mutations in nonsyndromic pheochromocytoma. *N Engl J Med*. 2002;346:1459–1466.

5 Lenders JW, Duh QY, Eisenhofer G, et al. Pheochromocytoma and paraganglioma: an endocrine society clinical practice guideline. *J Clin Endocrinol Metab*. 2014;99:1915–1942.

6 Rana HQ, Rainville IR, Vaidya A. Genetic testing in the clinical care of patients with pheochromocytoma and paraganglioma. *Curr Opin Endocrinol Diabetes Obes*. 2014;21:166–176.

7 Fishbein L, Leshchiner I, Walter V, et al. Comprehensive molecular characterization of pheochromocytoma and paraganglioma. *Cancer Cell*. 2017;31:181–193.

8 Conn JW. Primary aldosteronism. *J Lab Clin Med*. 1955;45:661–664.

9 Funder JW, Carey RM, Mantero F, et al. The management of primary aldosteronism: case detection, diagnosis, and treatment: an Endocrine Society Clinical Practice Guideline. *J Clin Endocrinol Metab*. 2016;101:1889–1916.

10 Funder JW, Carey RM, Fardella C, et al. Case detection, diagnosis, and treatment of patients with primary aldosteronism: an endocrine society clinical practice guideline. *J Clin Endocrinol Metab*. 2008;93:3266–3281.

11 Baudrand R, Guarda FJ, Torrey J, Williams G, Vaidya A. Dietary sodium restriction increases the risk of misinterpreting mild cases of primary aldosteronism. *J Clin Endocrinol Metab*. 2016:jc20161963.

12 Mosso L, Carvajal C, Gonzalez A, et al. Primary aldosteronism and hypertensive disease. *Hypertension*. 2003;42:161–165.

13 Monticone S, Burrello J, Tizzani D, et al. Prevalence and clinical manifestations of primary aldosteronism encountered in primary care practice. *J Am Coll Cardiol*. 2017;69:1811–1820.

14 Markou A, Pappa T, Kaltsas G, et al. Evidence of primary aldosteronism in a predominantly female cohort of normotensive individuals: a very high odds ratio for progression into arterial hypertension. *J Clin Endocrinol Metab*. 2013;98:1409–1416.

15 Baudrand R, Brown JM, Hundemer G, Williams GH, Vaidya A. The continuum of renin-independent aldosteronism in normotension. *Hypertension*. 2017;in press.

16 Newton-Cheh C, Guo CY, Gona P, et al. Clinical and genetic correlates of aldosterone-to-renin ratio and relations to blood pressure in a community sample. *Hypertension*. 2007;49:846–856.

17 Vasan RS, Evans JC, Larson MG, et al. Serum aldosterone and the incidence of hypertension in nonhypertensive persons. *N Engl J Med*. 2004;351:33–41.

18 Nishimoto K, Nakagawa K, Li D, et al. Adrenocortical zonation in humans under normal and pathological conditions. *J Clin Endocrinol Metab*. 2010;95: 2296–2305.

19 Nishimoto K, Tomlins SA, Kuick R, et al. Aldosterone-stimulating somatic gene mutations are common in normal adrenal glands. *Proc Natl Acad Sci U S A*. 2015;112:E4591–E4599.

20 OECD. OfEC-oaD. *Health at a Glance 2013*: OECD Indicators, Paris: OECD Publishing; 2013.

21 Arlt W, Biehl M, Taylor AE, et al. Urine steroid metabolomics as a biomarker tool for detecting malignancy in adrenal tumors. *J Clin Endocrinol Metab*. 2011;96:3775–3784.

22 Fassnacht M, Arlt W, Bancos I, et al. Management of adrenal incidentalomas: European Society of Endocrinology Clinical Practice Guideline in collaboration with the European Network for the Study of Adrenal Tumors. *Eur J Endocrinol*. 2016;175:G1–G34.

23 Bancos I, Alahdab F, Crowley RK, et al. Therapy of endocrine disease: improvement of cardiovascular risk factors after adrenalectomy in patients with adrenal tumors and subclinical Cushing's syndrome: a systematic review and

meta-analysis. *Eur J Endocrinol.* 2016;175:R283–R295.

24 Di Dalmazi G, Vicennati V, Garelli S, et al. Cardiovascular events and mortality in patients with adrenal incidentalomas that are either non-secreting or associated with intermediate phenotype or subclinical Cushing's syndrome: a 15-year

retrospective study. *The Lancet Diabetes Endocrinol.* 2014;2:396–405.

25 Lopez D, Luque-Fernandez MA, Steele A, Adler GK, Turchin A, Vaidya A. "Nonfunctional" adrenal tumors and the risk for incident diabetes and cardiovascular outcomes: a cohort study. *Ann Intern Med.* 2016;165:533–542.

20

Acute Adrenal Insufficiency

Glenn Matfin

Key Points

- Symptomatic acute adrenal insufficiency (adrenal crisis) is associated with significant morbidity and mortality and should be managed as a medical emergency requiring immediate treatment with parenteral hydrocortisone and intravenous saline.
- Adrenal crisis is brought about by lack of production of the adrenal hormone cortisol and/or mineralocorticoids and requires immediate treatment.
- The severity of this condition is related to the central role of these hormones in energy, salt, and fluid homeostasis.
- There are two forms of adrenal insufficiency: primary and secondary.
- Primary adrenal insufficiency (also termed Addison's disease), is caused by the inability of the adrenal cortex to produce sufficient amounts of glucocorticoids and/or mineralocorticoids (e.g., due to autoimmune-mediated destruction of adrenocortical tissue).

- Secondary adrenal insufficiency (also termed central hypoadrenalism) results from deficient adrenal glucocorticoid production only, because of corticotropin (adrenocorticotropic hormone [ACTH]) deficiency due to impairment of hypothalamic-pituitary axis. The most common cause of secondary adrenal insufficiency is chronic exogenous glucocorticoid treatment.
- Symptoms of adrenal insufficiency are non-specific and a high level of clinical suspicion is required to make the correct diagnosis.
- Effective chronic care of primary and secondary adrenal insufficiency is critical, as this is an important opportunity to reduce future admissions by reiterating sick-day rules and other crisis preventative measures, improve quality of life, and decrease morbidity and mortality.

Introduction

The adrenal glands are small, bilateral structures that weigh approximately 5 g each and lie retroperitoneally at the apex of each kidney. The medulla or inner portion of the gland (which constitutes approximately 10% of each adrenal) secretes epinephrine (adrenaline) and norepinephrine (noradrenaline) and is part of the sympathetic nervous system. The cortex forms the bulk of the adrenal gland (approximately 90%) and is responsible for secreting three types of hormones: glucocorticoids, mineralocorticoids, and adrenal androgens (1). Because epinephrine and norepinephrine can also be derived from non-adrenal sources (e.g., norepinephrine from the sympathetic

Endocrine and Metabolic Medical Emergencies: A Clinician's Guide, Second Edition. Edited by Glenn Matfin.
© 2018 John Wiley & Sons Ltd. Published 2018 by John Wiley & Sons Ltd.

Table 20-1 Clinical features of primary adrenal insufficiency and adrenal crisis. Adapted from (5).

Symptoms	Signs	Routine laboratory tests
Adrenal insufficiency		
Darkened complexion/increased pigmentation/easier suntanning	Hyperpigmentation (primary only), particularly of sun-exposed areas, skin creases, mucosal membranes, scars, areola of breast	Hyponatremia Hyperkalemia Uncommon: hypoglycemia, hypercalcemia
Postural dizziness	Low blood pressure with increased postural drop	
Anorexia, abdominal discomfort, weight loss		
Fatigue		
Adrenal crisis		
Syncope	Hypotension	Hyponatremia
Abdominal pain, nausea, vomiting; may mimic acute abdomen	Abdominal tenderness/guarding	Hyperkalemia Hypoglycemia Hypercalcemia
Confusion	Reduced consciousness, delirium	
Back pain		
Severe weakness		

Most symptoms are non-specific and present chronically, often leading to delayed diagnosis. Hyponatremia and, later, hyperkalemia are often triggers to diagnosis, requiring biochemical confirmation of adrenal insufficiency. Hyperpigmentation is a specific sign, but it is variably present in individuals and must be compared with the patient's background pigmentation, such as that in siblings. Adrenal crisis is a medical emergency with hypotension, marked acute abdominal symptoms, and marked laboratory abnormalities, requiring immediate treatment. Additional symptoms and signs may arise from the underlying cause of adrenal insufficiency, e.g., associated autoimmune disorders, neurological features of adrenoleukodystrophy, or disorders that may lead to adrenal infiltration.

nervous system and mesentery), adrenal medullary function is not essential for life, but adrenal cortical function is. If untreated, the total loss of adrenal cortical function is fatal in 4–14 days.

Cortisol is the principal glucocorticoid; aldosterone is the principal mineralocorticoid; and together with adrenal androgens constitutes the major hormones of the more than 30 produced by the adrenal cortex. All of the adrenal cortical hormones have a similar structure in that all are steroids, and each of the steps involved in the synthesis of the various hormones requires a specific enzyme. The secretion of both glucocorticoids and adrenal androgens is controlled by corticotropin (adrenocorticotropic hormone [ACTH]) secreted by corticotrophs in the anterior pituitary gland, as part of the hypothalamic-pituitary-adrenal (HPA) axis. The mineralocorticoids are controlled predominantly by the renin-angiotensin system.

Acute adrenal insufficiency, also termed adrenal crisis, is a life-threatening endocrine emergency (2–4). Adrenal crisis is brought about by lack of production of the adrenal hormone cortisol and/or mineralocorticoids. It presents with marked symptoms and signs, characteristic laboratory abnormalities, and requires immediate treatment (Table 20-1). The severity of this condition is related to the

Table 20-2 Clinical findings of adrenal insufficiency

Finding	Primary (%)	Secondary/Tertiary (%)
Anorexia and weight loss	Yes (100)	Yes (100)
Fatigue and weakness	Yes (100)	Yes (100)
Gastrointestinal symptoms, nausea, vomiting	Yes (50)	Yes (50)
Myalgia, arthralgia	Yes (10)	Yes (10)
Orthostatic hypotension	Yes	Yes
Hyponatremia	Yes (85–90)	Yes (60)
Hyperkalemia	Yes (60–65)	No
Hyperpigmentation	Yes (>90)	No
Secondary deficiencies of gonadal, growth hormone, thyroxine, and antidiuretic hormone may occur	No	Yes
Associated autoimmune conditions	Yes	No

The numbers are representative, some symptoms and signs can be subtle. In acute adrenal crisis, these symptoms and signs can be more common and pronounced (e.g., abdominal pain ~90%, with abdominal rigidity or rebound tenderness in ~20%).

central role of these hormones in energy, salt, and fluid homeostasis.

There are two forms of adrenal insufficiency: primary and secondary (Table 20-2). Recent Endocrine Society Clinical Practice Guidelines have reviewed both primary adrenal insufficiency (5), and secondary adrenal insufficiency (6). Primary adrenal insufficiency (also termed Addison's disease), is caused by the inability of the adrenal cortex to produce sufficient amounts of glucocorticoids and/or mineralocorticoids (e.g., due to autoimmune-mediated destruction of adrenocortical tissue). Secondary adrenal insufficiency (also termed central hypoadrenalism) results from deficient adrenal glucocorticoid production only, because of ACTH deficiency due to impairment of hypothalamic-pituitary axis (i.e., hypopituitarism). The most common cause of secondary adrenal insufficiency is chronic exogenous glucocorticoid treatment. Central hypoadrenalism due to impaired hypothalamic corticotropin-releasing hormone (CRH) release is sometimes termed "tertiary" adrenal insufficiency, but will be grouped with secondary for discussion in this chapter.

Since the last decade, reference has also been made to "relative adrenal insufficiency" in the context of critical illness (7–9). It refers to the condition in which, despite a maximally ACTH-activated adrenal cortex in response to critical illness, cortisol production is still insufficient to generate enough glucocorticoid and mineralocorticoid receptor activation to maintain hemodynamic stability (10). Recently, the Adrenal Scientific Committee of the American Association of Clinical Endocrinologists (AACE) have proposed a diagnostic algorithm to diagnose adrenal insufficiency in critically ill patients, with different cut-offs depending on the blood albumin concentration and the presence or absence of septic shock (11). Hopefully, ongoing studies will provide more clarity regarding diagnosis and optimal management of relative adrenal insufficiency/failure.

In primary adrenal insufficiency, cortisol deficiency results in a decrease in feedback to the HPA axis and subsequent enhanced stimulation of the adrenal cortex by elevated levels of plasma ACTH. In addition, consequent to disruption of adrenal

Table 20-3 Glucocorticoids commonly used in hospitalized patients

Name	IV Dosing	PO Dosing	Relative potency (Ratio*)	Duration of metabolic effect	Typical dosing
Hydrocortisone	yes	yes	20 mg (1)	8 hours	20–300 mg/day
Prednisone (Prednisolone)	no	yes	5 mg (4)	16 hours	5–100 mg/day
Methylprednisolone	yes	yes	4 mg (5)	16 hours	50–1000 mg/day
Dexamethasone	yes	yes	0.8 mg (25)	24 hours	2–24 mg/day

Cortisone dose equivalence to hydrocortisone 20 mg is 25 mg, however, this is not commonly used in hospital setting. IV = Intravenous; PO = Oral. *Potency is based on anti-inflammatory properties with hydrocortisone arbitrarily denoted as 1.

mineralocorticoid synthesis, renin release by the juxtaglomerular cells of the kidneys increases. This is of clinical, diagnostic, and therapeutic relevance because primary adrenal insufficiency needs to be distinguished from secondary adrenocortical insufficiency due to insufficient production of ACTH and without an impact on the renin-angiotensin-aldosterone system.

Cortisone was first identified by the American chemist Edward Kendall, and he was awarded the 1950 Nobel Prize for Physiology or Medicine with Philip Hench and Tadeus Reichstein for the discovery of adrenal cortex hormones, their structures, and their functions. Cortisone was an instant success in a wide range of diseases, including adrenal insufficiency. However, while management of adrenal insufficiency using hydrocortisone (and other glucocorticoid formulations) is life-saving, fine-tuning of therapy has always been a challenge with periods of glucocorticoid over- and under-replacement the norm for most patients. Despite much effort it has been impossible (at least in clinical studies) to dissect out the transrepressive, anti-inflammatory effects of glucocorticoids from the transactivating "Cushingoid" effects. Glucocorticoid-induced side-effects with so-called "tertiary adrenal suppression" now contribute to morbidity and premature mortality in the 1–3% or so of Western populations taking exogenous steroids (including those commonly used in the in-hospital setting, Table 20-3); its diagnosis and management remain challenging. This balance is probably best illustrated by the late US President John F. Kennedy, who was diagnosed with Addison's disease in the 1940s. Gravely ill, Kennedy was admitted to a London hospital in 1947, his doctor's verdict: "He hasn't got a year to live" (12). Despite this rather stark prognosis, Kennedy survived until his untimely death in 1963 using various formulations of glucocorticoids, mineralocorticoids, and androgens. During this period he appeared occasionally Cushingoid (reflective of over-replacement), while at other times was deeply pigmented (suggesting under-replacement).

More recently, several advances in our understanding of adrenal replacement therapy have occurred (e.g., using smaller daily doses). Irrespective, replacement therapy in adrenal insufficiency remains sub-optimal. It certainly fails to mimic normal circadian secretion patterns and undoubtedly earlier regimens did result in over-replacement with all the added risks of long-term, albeit usually mild, Cushing's syndrome (although with associated increased risks of metabolic and cardiovascular disease) (13). This, together with the ongoing and unacceptable management of patients with adrenal crises, even in Centers of Excellence, is likely to explain the increased mortality (standardized mortality ratio ~2:1) in patients with primary and secondary adrenal insufficiency. It remains to be seen whether emerging developments in glucocorticoid therapies (e.g., plenadren, which is modified-release hydrocortisone available in several countries) or different routes of administration such as continuous subcutaneous hydrocortisone infusion (CSHI) (14) that deliver closer "physiological" replacement impact upon failure of care (15).

Adrenal insufficiency, like type 1 diabetes mellitus, is a chronic metabolic disorder that requires lifetime hormone replacement therapy. In both conditions, increased morbidity can occur as a result of the primary life-saving therapy (i.e., insulin vs glucocorticoid); poor adherence to treatment is common; and failure to observe "sick day rules" is an important precipitant of crises; substantial healthcare burden exists (16), including increasing costs of the hormone replacement therapy itself (i.e., glucocorticoid and insulin costs are spiraling upwards); psychological distress and psychiatric disorders are prevalent; and health-related quality of life is often reduced. In addition, based on prospective data, about one in 12 patients with primary adrenal insufficiency will experience a life-threatening adrenal crisis in the coming year (similar to the common occurrence of glucose-related crises – severe hypoglycemia and diabetic ketoacidosis – in type 1 diabetes).

It is therefore important that all clinicians understand the normal physiology of the HPA axis, its derangements in pathological states, the different modes of diagnostic test procedures used to demonstrate a deficiency, the optimal type of replacement therapy, and the information needed by the patient to sustain a normal life with minimal morbidity. When acute adrenal insufficiency or crisis occurs, it is imperative that it is quickly diagnosed with appropriate emergency management and follow-up, and this will be discussed in this chapter.

Pathophysiology

Glucocorticoids

The glucocorticoid hormones, mainly cortisol, are synthesized in the zona fasciculata and the zona reticularis of the adrenal cortex. ACTH controls the release of cortisol mainly through G-coupled melanocortin receptor-2 in the adrenal cortex, increasing cholesterol delivery and expression of steroidogenic enzymes. ACTH is released in a pulsatile fashion from the pituitary corticotrophs, which are regulated by a multitude of neuroendocrine signals, but mostly by CRH from the hypothalamic paraventricular nucleus. Cortisol is also released in pulses, and this pulsatile nature of production for both ACTH and cortisol is maintained in stress and illness. Both ACTH and cortisol displays a circadian variation, with peaks before awakening in the morning, and troughs late at night. Cortisol suppresses both CRH and ACTH through a negative feedback mechanism operating at various levels of the HPA axis.

In the circulation, about 80% of cortisol is bound to cortisol-binding globulin (CBG), nearly 15% to albumin, with only around 5% being free and bioavailable. CBG is more than a reservoir for cortisol, and serves an important role in the targeted delivery of cortisol to tissues and its bioavailability (17). Tissue-specific cleavage of CBG can enable release of bound cortisol for targeted, local activity. CBG is also nearly fully saturated, and an increase in cortisol or a decrease in CBG concentrations can increase the free, bioavailable cortisol fraction significantly.

Cortisol acts by binding to both glucocorticoid and mineralocorticoid receptors (GR and MR, respectively). Cortisol has a several-fold higher affinity for MR than for GR. A complex control of glucocorticoid bioactivity in different tissues is made possible by different ratios of MR to GR in various organs and cell types, different receptor capacities and affinities resulting in different receptor occupancies, as well as fluctuations in cortisol that can differentially change the occupancy of the non-genomic and the two genomic receptors. Furthermore, in tissues such as the kidneys upon which mineralocorticoids act, 11β-hydroxysteroid dehydrogenase type 2 deactivates cortisol and allows aldosterone to bind to the MR (inhibition of this enzyme by licorice or genetic mutations can lead to apparent mineralocorticoid excess due to overstimulation of the MR by cortisol).

Glucocorticoids influence a vast array of cellular activities in different cell types (1). They orchestrate responses to stress, and are key mediators of physiological and behavioral adaptations against injury and illness. They mobilize stored fuel to meet demand, regulate the inflammatory response, and have direct and indirect effects on various tissues. By far the best-known metabolic effect of cortisol and other glucocorticoids is their ability to stimulate gluconeogenesis (glucose production) by the liver. Cortisol also influences multiple aspects of immunologic function and inflammatory responsiveness. Large quantities of cortisol are required for an effective anti-inflammatory action. This is achieved by the administration of pharmacologic rather than physiologic doses of cortisol. The increased cortisol blocks inflammation at an early stage by decreasing capillary permeability and stabilizing the lysosomal membranes so that inflammatory mediators are not released. Cortisol suppresses the immune response by reducing humoral and cell-mediated immunity. During the healing phase, cortisol suppresses fibroblast activity and thereby lessens scar formation. Cortisol also inhibits prostaglandin synthesis, which may account in large part for its anti-inflammatory actions.

Mineralocorticoids

The mineralocorticoids play an essential role in regulating potassium and sodium levels and water balance. They are produced in the zona glomerulosa or the outer layer of cells of the adrenal cortex. Aldosterone secretion is regulated by the renin-angiotensin system and by blood levels of potassium. Increased levels of aldosterone promote sodium retention by the distal tubules of the kidney while increasing urinary losses of potassium.

Adrenal Androgens

The adrenal androgens are synthesized primarily by the zona reticularis and zona fasciculata of the adrenal cortex. These sex hormones probably exert little effect on normal sexual function in women (the effects in men is minimized by coexisting testicular-derived androgen). There is evidence, however, that adrenal androgens (the most important of which is dehydroepiandrosterone [DHEA] and its sulfate conjugate [DHEAS]) contribute to the pubertal growth of body hair, particularly pubic and axillary hair in women. Lack of adrenal androgens has no relevance during acute adrenal insufficiency/crisis.

The adrenal cortex has a large reserve capacity, and the manifestations of adrenal insufficiency usually do not become apparent until approximately 90% of the cortex has been destroyed in primary or inactive in secondary adrenal insufficiency. These clinical manifestations are related primarily to glucocorticoid deficiency, mineralocorticoid deficiency (in primary), and hyperpigmentation (in primary).

Etiology of Adrenal Insufficiency

Primary Adrenal Insufficiency

In 1855, Thomas Addison, an English physician, provided the first detailed clinical description of primary adrenal insufficiency, also called Addison's disease (18). The use of this term is reserved for primary adrenal insufficiency in which adrenal cortical hormones are deficient and ACTH levels are elevated because of lack of feedback inhibition.

Addison's disease is a relatively rare disorder in which all layers of the adrenal cortex are destroyed (19). Autoimmune destruction with specific autoantibodies against 21-hydroxylase (CYP21A2) is the most common cause of Addison's disease (up to 90%) in Western countries, and can be an isolated finding or associated with other autoimmune conditions as part autoimmune polyendocrinopathy syndrome (APS) types 1 and 2 (20). Before 1950, tuberculosis was the major cause of Addison's disease in Western countries, and continues to be a common etiology where active infection is prevalent.

Other causes of primary adrenal insufficiency include fungal infections (particularly histoplasmosis), and infiltrative disorders such amyloid disease and hemochromatosis affecting the adrenals. Bilateral adrenal hemorrhage can be caused by meningococcal septicemia (i.e., Waterhouse-Friderichsen syndrome), major trauma, anticoagulant therapy, anti-cardiolipin syndrome, adrenal vein thrombosis, or adrenal metastases. Bilateral adrenalectomy for conditions such as intractable Cushing's syndrome or bilateral pheochromocytoma requires life-long adrenal replacement therapy.

Drugs (e.g., ketoconazole, etomidate, and metyropone) that inhibit synthesis or cause excessive breakdown of glucocorticoids can also result in adrenal insufficiency. Attention has recently focused on reports describing primary and secondary adrenal insufficiency adverse events in patients treated with new immune checkpoint inhibitors (21). Immunotherapy causes tumor regression in melanoma, lymphoma, and some other malignancies, but can also cause thyroid dysfunction as well as other endocrine abnormalities (e.g., hypophysitis with secondary adrenal insufficiency, primary adrenal insufficiency, and type 1 diabetes mellitus).

Due to the growing number of chronically and severely ill patients requiring chronic intensive care, which includes multiple concomitant pharmacological therapies and additional iatrogenic factors (such as adrenal hemorrhage related to anticoagulants, inhibition of cortisol synthesis by aminoglutethimide or etomidate, activation of glucocorticoid metabolism by anticonvulsants like phenytoin or phenobarbital, or antibiotics like rifampicin) that increasingly contributes to the ultimate manifestation of primary and secondary adrenal insufficiency in this complex setting.

Adrenal insufficiency can be caused by human immunodeficiency virus (HIV)-1 infection and acquired immune deficiency syndrome (AIDS). Adrenal dysfunction is common in both treated and untreated HIV infection, due to multiple etiologies. Unrecognized, hypoadrenalism is associated with significant morbidity and mortality risk. Prior to the introduction of combined anti-retroviral therapy (cART), infection and infiltration were the most common causes of adrenal abnormalities. Cytomegalovirus infection is the most common infective cause of adrenal failure and is known to affect both the adrenal medulla and cortex. There is often bilateral adrenal gland involvement and the spectrum of severity can range widely, from mild adrenalitis to necrosis with severe, generalized systemic infection. In addition, the HIV virus itself may cause adrenalitis. HIV-specific infiltrative processes that can result in primary adrenal insufficiency include lymphoma, malignancy, and Kaposi sarcoma, all reported in advanced HIV infection or AIDS. Since the advent of cART, the most common form of adrenal failure appears to be medication-induced (iatrogenic) adrenal suppression, including cART-corticosteroid interactions For example, the azole antifungal agents, such as ketaconazole and itraconazole, impair and inhibit adrenal steroidogenesis. Furthermore, protease inhibitors, a frequent component of cART, inhibit hepatic cytochrome P450 CYP3A4 drug metabolic pathways. This will potentiate the half-life of medications that can affect adrenal steroidogenesis, particularly synthetic glucocorticoids. This can result in iatrogenic Cushing's syndrome and HPA suppression. Iatrogenic Cushing's syndrome in HIV-infected patients receiving ritonavir and inhaled fluticasone has been reported (22). The degree of HPA suppression in these cases can be substantial, leading to adrenal insufficiency and crisis if the inhaled (or other modes of administration) steroids are ceased without corticosteroid support (22).

Genetic causes of primary adrenal insufficiency include congenital adrenal hyperplasia (CAH), an autosomal recessive trait in which there is a deficiency of any of the enzymes necessary for the synthesis of cortisol (23). A common characteristic of all types of CAH is a defect in the synthesis of cortisol results in increased levels of ACTH and adrenal hyperplasia. The increased levels of ACTH overstimulate the pathways for production of adrenal androgens. Mineralocorticoids may be produced in excessive or insufficient amounts, depending on the precise enzyme deficiency. The two enzymes most commonly deficient are 21-hydroxylase (accounting for >90% of cases) and 11-β-hydroxylase. A spectrum of 21-hydroxylase deficiency states exists, ranging from simple virilizing CAH to a complete salt-losing enzyme deficiency. The salt-losing form is accompanied by deficient production of aldosterone and its intermediates. This results in fluid and electrolyte disorders including hyponatremia, hyperkalemia, vomiting, dehydration, and shock.

Other genetic causes include adrenal congenita hypoplasia which is associated with primary adrenal insufficiency and hypogonadotropic hypogonadism (24).

Young males and males without 21-hydroxylase autoantibodies should be screened for adrenoleukodystrophy by measuring very-long chain fatty acids (25). Adrenal insufficiency may be the only presenting sign of adrenoleukodystrophy, which is an inherited disorder of long chain fatty acid metabolism, and most often occurs in boys between 2 and 10 years of age. It may progress to severe neurological problems and dementia.

Secondary Adrenal Insufficiency

Secondary adrenal insufficiency can occur as the result of hypopituitarism and/or hypothalamic dysfunction. Hypopituitarism may occur as a result of diverse etiologies and lead to substantial morbidity and mortality (6). Hypopituitarism is characterized by a decreased secretion of pituitary hormones that causes hypofunction of the secondary organs that depend on trophic stimuli from the pituitary. It may selectively involve one subset of pituitary cells (e.g., corticotrophs) or all of the pituitary cells, in which case it is referred to as panhypopituitarism. The cause may be congenital or result from a variety of acquired abnormalities that cause destruction of the anterior pituitary or a secondary

phenomenon resulting from deficiency of hypothalamic hormones normally acting on the pituitary (i.e., CRH in central hypoadrenalism). Space-occupying lesions cause hypopituitarism by destroying the pituitary gland or hypothalamic nuclei or by disrupting the hypothalamic-hypophyseal portal system.

Anterior pituitary hormone loss is usually gradual, especially with progressive loss of pituitary reserve due to tumors (26) or previous pituitary radiation therapy (which may take 10–20 years or more to produce hypopituitarism). When the pituitary begins to fail non-acutely, there is generally a specific sequential failure of pituitary hormones, starting with growth hormone (**G**H), continuing through luteinizing hormone (**L**H) and follicle-stimulating hormone (**F**SH) deficiency, and culminating in loss of thyroid-stimulating hormone (**T**SH) and ACTH (easily remembered by the acronym 'Go Look For The Adenoma'). Generally, ACTH is the last to be lost, and teleologically this may reflect that it is vital to survival (27). However, it should be recalled that with certain pituitary lesions, such as lymphocytic hypophysitis, ACTH deficiency may occur first or alone. "Isolated pituitary deficiency" should also raise the possibility of HPA suppression due to exogenous glucocorticoids.

Glucocorticoid Suppression of Adrenal Function

A highly significant aspect of long-term therapy with exogenous pharmacologic preparations of the glucocorticoids (i.e. doses ≥5 mg prednisolone equivalent for more than 4 weeks) is adrenal insufficiency upon withdrawal of the drugs. Similarly, patients with Cushing's syndrome due to endogenous glucocorticoid production, when treated, can result in transient or life-long adrenal insufficiency. The deficiency results from suppression of the HPA system. Chronic suppression causes atrophy of the adrenal gland, and the abrupt withdrawal of glucocorticoids in exogenous or endogenous causes can result in acute adrenal insufficiency especially during periods of stress or when surgery is performed. Recovery to a state of normal adrenal function may be prolonged, requiring up to 12 months or more (28).

Clinical Assessment

It is crucial to recognize clinical features suggestive of adrenal insufficiency, because if present, they identify symptomatic patients who may require urgent corrective measures. The severity of signs and symptoms depends both on the absolute degree of glucocorticoid and mineralocorticoid deficiency and the rapidity of its onset. The rapid onset of adrenal insufficiency in the postsurgical setting, adrenal hemorrhages, or in children with salt-losing forms of CAH, can present dramatically and in a manner that demands immediate and aggressive intervention. In comparison, patients with chronic adrenal insufficiency can have more insidious presentation.

It is important to ask patients, relatives or health care providers about any relevant history, including any exposure to steroid therapy in any formulation, including over-the-counter agents. Any previous HPA disorders and treatment should also be explored. Family history may also be useful (e.g., autoimmune conditions and rarer disorders). It is also imperative to elicit any signs of previous steroid exposure resulting in Cushingoid phenotype that may result in HPA suppression. Checking for medic alert jewellery (or tattoos!), steroid cards, and medication reconciliation are all valuable. Manifestations of the primary pathological disorder can also be present (e.g., vitiligo in autoimmune disorders).

Primary Adrenal Insufficiency

The clinical findings of primary adrenal insufficiency (Figure 20-1) are mainly based on the deficiency of glucocorticoids and mineralocorticoids and the resultant weight loss, abdominal tenderness and guarding; fever; orthostatic hypotension with dizziness due to dehydration (≥20 mmHg drop in BP from supine to standing position) and in severe case hypovolemic shock; confusion, somnolence, delirium and coma; electrolyte changes; and hypoglycemia (Tables 20-1 and 20-2). Enhanced secretion of ACTH and other pro-opiomelanocortin derived peptides (e.g., melanocyte-stimulating hormone [MSH]) often leads to the characteristic hyperpigmentation of the skin and mucous membranes. The skin looks bronzed or suntanned in exposed and unexposed areas, and the normal creases and pressure points tend to become especially dark (Figure 20-2). The gums and oral mucous membranes may become bluish-black (Figure 20-3). Hyperpigmentation occurs in more than 90% of persons with Addison disease, and is helpful in distinguishing the primary and secondary forms of adrenal insufficiency (Tables 20-1 and 20-2). In women, loss of adrenal androgens results in loss of axillary (Figure 20-2) and pubic hair. Except for salt craving, the symptoms of primary adrenal insufficiency are rather nonspecific and include weakness, fatigue; musculoskeletal pain and cramps; weight loss, abdominal pain, nausea and vomiting; depression, and anxiety. As a result, the diagnosis is frequently delayed, resulting in a clinical presentation with an acute life-threatening adrenal crisis (which is the presentation in more than half of patients with adrenal insufficiency).

In individuals with HIV/AIDS, the HPA axis requires evaluation when symptomatic of fatigue, weight loss, nausea, postural hypotension, or with hypoglycemia or hyponatremia.

Secondary Adrenal Insufficiency

Central hypoadrenalism may lead to dehydration, hyponatremia (due to dilution and not mineralocorticoid deficiency) and shock, unresponsive to fluid resuscitation and vasopressor therapy before glucocorticoid replacement is administered. Vasopressin deficiency causes cranial diabetes insipidus (CDI), which may become clinically apparent only after the initiation of glucocorticoid

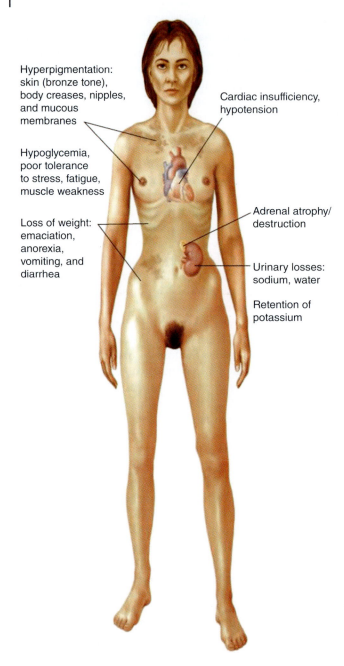

Figure 20-1 Clinical manifestations of primary adrenal insufficiency

Hyperpigmentation: skin (bronze tone), body creases, nipples, and mucous membranes

Cardiac insufficiency, hypotension

Hypoglycemia, poor tolerance to stress, fatigue, muscle weakness

Loss of weight: emaciation, anorexia, vomiting, and diarrhea

Adrenal atrophy/ destruction

Urinary losses: sodium, water

Retention of potassium

and/or thyroid hormone replacement therapies as a result of improvements in renal hemodynamics, glomerular filtration rate, and free water clearance.

Patients with central hypoadrenalism may present with prostration, headache, nausea, vomiting, orthostatic dizziness, joint and muscle aches, dehydration, confusion, shock, and hyponatremia (6). Patients with disease of long duration may additionally report fatigue and unexplained weight loss. Notably absent are skin and mucosal hyperpigmentation as well as hyperkalemia (in contrast to patients with Addison's disease) (Table 20-2).

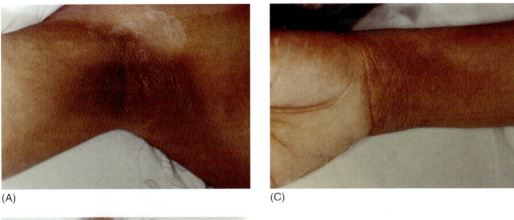

(A)

(C)

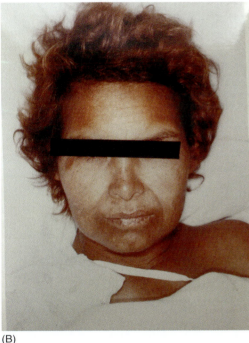

(B)

Figure 20-2 Clinical features in primary adrenal insufficiency: (A) Hyperpigmented axilla with no axillary hair; (B) Hyperpigmented facies; and (C) Hyperpigmented wrist

Acute secondary adrenal insufficiency is seen in two-thirds of patients with pituitary tumor apoplexy and is a major source of morbidity and rarely mortality associated with the condition (29,30). Indications of empirical glucocorticoid treatment are hemodynamic instability, altered consciousness level, reduced visual acuity or severe visual field defects. Steroid replacement is potentially life-saving in these patients.

Diagnostic Testing of Adrenal Insufficiency

The increased requirements for cortisol during physiological stress make it crucially important not to miss a diagnosis of adrenal insufficiency in acute and critically ill patients. However, *diagnostic measures should never delay prompt treatment of suspected adrenal crisis.*

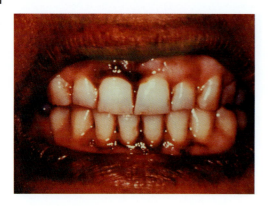

Figure 20-3 Mouth hyperpigmentation in primary adrenal insufficiency

The initial laboratory evaluation of patients should include a determination of plasma glucose, blood urea nitrogen (BUN, or urea), creatinine, electrolytes, urinalysis, complete (full) blood count with differential, and ESR or CRP (if indicated). Thyroid function tests should be performed as thyrotoxicosis can precipitate an adrenal crisis (acute adrenal insufficiency can also increase TSH, so do not replace with thyroxine if TSH ≤ 10 mU/L – and only then after glucocorticoid is started). An electrocardiogram (ECG), chest X-ray, and urine, and blood cultures should also be considered where comorbidity is possible (sepsis is the most common precipitant (13), although poor adherence to chronic glucocorticoid therapy and failure to observe "sick day rules" are also common). Other investigations are performed as warranted by the clinical situation (e.g., cardiac troponins, serum lactate, and appropriate imaging).

Specific investigations targeting the HPA axis for suspected adrenal insufficiency or adrenal crisis are only needed in patients without a prior diagnosis of adrenal insufficiency, those with pre-existing diagnosis should have general investigations as needed and be treated promptly.

The acute laboratory assessment of the HPA axis is generally limited to measuring cortisol and ACTH. A CBG assay, which would be very useful for assessing free cortisol index, is not routinely available in clinical settings. A random cortisol is usually unhelpful although >400 nmol/L (14.5 µg/dL) makes adrenal insufficiency unlikely in an unstressed person. A morning (8–9 a.m.) cortisol of >500 nmol/L (18 µg/dL) in an unstressed person excludes HPA pathology, and one of >400 nmol/L (14.5 µg/dL) is usually associated with adequate reserve. Preferably, a stimulated cortisol is evaluated for investigation of adrenal hypofunction. For this, an insulin stress (tolerance) test (IST [ITT]), a CRH test, or a short corticotopin (IV or IM 250 µg synthetic ACTH, e.g., cosyntropin or synacthen) stimulation test is used to assess the HPA axis, the PA axis or only the adrenal response, respectively. The short ACTH stimulation test is the most commonly used test, and shows good correlation with IST (ITT), since chronic ACTH deficiency leads to adrenal atrophy and an abnormal cortisol response to short ACTH stimulation testing (31). A cortisol of >500 nmol/L (18 µg/dL) 30 min. or 60 min. after short ACTH stimulation testing excludes adrenal insufficiency, and <500 nmol/L (18 µg/dL) may suggest a need for steroid replacement during acute illness. However, assays cross-react differently with cortisol, and the target and threshold values are assay-dependent and local normal ranges should be used (e.g., in the UK using the Abbott Architect platform, the normal cortisol value cut-off 30 minutes post short ACTH testing varies from 420–450 nmol/L [15.2–16.3 µg/dL]).

Another variation of the cosyntropin or synacthen test uses a low-dose 1 µg for adrenal stimulation. However, based on the currently available data, the 1 µg test dose does not provide better diagnostic accuracy than the 250 µg corticotropin test and is not recommended in routine clinical practice to exclude adrenal insufficiency or 'relative adrenal insufficiency' (9,32).

There are, however, caveats regarding the interpretation of post-ACTH stimulation cortisol results. A low plasma CBG concentration results in a smaller increment in total cortisol concentrations, thereby increasing the risk of false positive results (17). For example, reduced CBG levels can occur in certain situations including nephrotic syndrome, liver disease, and postoperative and critical care patients. In contrast, elevated

CBG levels occur in pregnancy (which should be excluded in the acute presentation) or when using estrogens (oral contraceptive or estrogen replacement therapy which should be stopped if possible for 6 weeks prior to stimulation testing) and may alter the interpretation of cortisol levels. Furthermore, assays cross-react differently with cortisol, and laboratories should use established, assay-specific increments in cortisol to interpret the short ACTH test results. An assessment of the recent medications is also necessary, as exogenous cortisol assays have 30–40% cross-reactivity with prednisolone, which is also generated from prednisone.

In patients with severe adrenal insufficiency symptoms or adrenal crisis, immediate therapy with IV hydrocortisone at an appropriate stress dose prior to the availability of the results of diagnostic tests should be administered.

Primary Adrenal Insufficiency

The 2016 Endocrine Society Clinical Practice Guideline (5) recommended diagnostic testing for the exclusion of primary adrenal insufficiency in acutely ill patients with otherwise unexplained indicative clinical symptoms or signs (e.g., volume depletion, hypotension, hyponatremia, hyperkalemia, fever, abdominal pain, hyperpigmentation or, especially in children, hypoglycemia), as well as in patients with predisposing factors. This is also recommended for pregnant women with unexplained persistent nausea, fatigue, and hypotension.

The short corticotropin test (250 µg given IV or IM) is considered the "gold standard" confirmatory tool to establish the diagnosis of primary adrenal insufficiency in patients with suggestive symptoms and signs (31). This test should be performed when the patient's condition and circumstances allow. Peak cortisol levels below 500 nmol/L (18 µg/dL) (assay dependent) at 30 or 60 minutes indicate adrenal insufficiency. Plasma ACTH should also be measured with the baseline sample, and a plasma ACTH >2-fold the upper limit of normal is consistent with primary adrenal insufficiency. The

simultaneous measurement of plasma renin and aldosterone in primary adrenal insufficiency is also indicated to determine the presence of mineralocorticoid deficiency.

If a short corticotropin test is not possible in the first instance, an initial screening procedure comprising the measurement of morning plasma ACTH and cortisol levels is recommended until confirmatory testing with short corticotropin test is possible. Morning cortisol <140 nmol/L (5 µg/dL) is suggestive of adrenal insufficiency (and needs confirmatory testing).

Measuring plasma corticotropin levels in a concurrent specimen may help to distinguish between central hypoadrenalism (characterized by low or "normal" plasma corticotropin) and primary adrenal insufficiency (characterized by elevated plasma corticotropin).

Diagnosing the underlying cause in all patients with confirmed disease should include a validated assay of autoantibodies against 21-hydroxylase (Figure 20-4). In autoantibody-negative individuals, other causes should be sought. Young males and males without autoantibodies should be screened for adrenoleukodystrophy by measuring very-long chain fatty acids (25). Adrenal insufficiency may be the only presenting sign of adrenoleukodystrophy. In 21-hydroxylase (CYP21A2) autoantibody-negative individuals with primary adrenal insufficiency of unknown etiology, computer tomography (CT) scan of the adrenals to identify infectious diseases such as tuberculosis and tumors should be performed. CT scanning for these conditions is generally not specific for the infiltrative disorder, and not all patients with infiltrative adrenal conditions such as tuberculosis causing primary adrenal insufficiency have enlarged adrenals. Genetic diseases should also be investigated (after appropriate genetic counselling) as indicated.

Secondary Adrenal Insufficiency

Evaluation of the HPA axis is the highest diagnostic (as well as therapeutic) priority in patients at risk of hypopituitarism

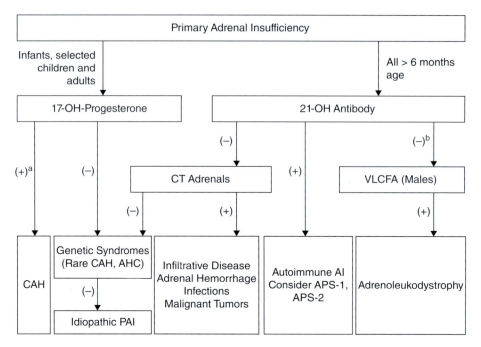

Figure 20-4 Algorithm for the diagnostic approach to the patient with Primary adrenal insufficiency (PAI) (5). The most common causes of PAI are autoimmune destruction of the adrenal cortex in adults and CAH in children. These etiologies can be screened for using 21-hydroxylase antibodies and a baseline serum 17-hydroxyprogesterone level. Males with negative 21-hydroxylase antibodies should be tested for adrenoleukodystrophy with plasma VLCFAs. If these diagnoses are excluded, a CT scan of the adrenals may reveal evidence of adrenal infiltrative processes or metastases. The individual's clinical picture and family history may render some steps in the algorithm redundant or suggest specific genetic syndromes. The latter includes subtypes of autoimmune polyglandular syndromes or specific rare genetic disorders where adrenal failure is part of a broader phenotype. VLCFA should be measured in the initial evaluation of preadolescent boys. 17-OH-progesterone >1000 ng/dL is diagnostic for 21-OH deficiency (23).
AHC = adrenal hypoplasia congenita; AI = adrenal insufficiency; VLCFA = very long chain fatty acid.

(6). It should be emphasized that acutely ill patients at risk for central hypoadrenalism should be presumed to be adrenally insufficient and treated with stress doses of glucocorticoids (preferably after drawing a blood specimen to assay cortisol and corticotropin) without awaiting the results of diagnostic testing.

Morning (or random) serum cortisol levels exceeding 18 μg/dL (~500 nmol/L) assure sufficient adrenocortical function with high specificity but low sensitivity. Morning serum cortisol levels below 3 μg/dL (~80 nmol/L) are diagnostic of adrenal insufficiency. Intermediate morning cortisol levels are considered non-diagnostic and require additional testing. Measuring plasma corticotropin levels in a concurrent specimen may help to distinguish between primary and secondary adrenal insufficiency.

Stimulation testing is helpful in assessing the integrity of the HPA axis in stable patients, but is not informative or practical in the acute setting. The insulin stress (tolerance) test (IST or ITT) is considered the gold standard test in the evaluation of pituitary adrenal function and additionally helps to evaluate GH secretion. However, the test requires the induction of severe hypoglycemia (<45 mg/dL [~2.2 mmol/L]) in order to achieve adequate diagnostic accuracy. As a result, it is often perceived as unpleasant by patients, carries some risk associated with severe hypoglycemia and is contraindicated in the elderly, patients with seizures or those with cardiovascular disease.

The metyrapone test is also reliable in the assessment of the HPA axis. However, the currently limited availability of metyrapone and the potential of precipitating acute adrenal insufficiency, particularly in an unmonitored out-patient setting, have limited use of this test in the USA. The short-ACTH stimulation test directly evaluates adrenocortical responsiveness and is quite accurate in the diagnosis of primary adrenal insufficiency. However, the diagnostic accuracy of this test in patients with central hypoadrenalism of recent onset is lower, as it takes several (4–6) weeks or longer after endogenous corticotropin secretion is blunted for the adrenals to become atrophic and lose responsiveness to exogenous ACTH administration.

Relative Adrenal Insufficiency

From large association studies, relative adrenal insufficiency in critically ill patients is thought to be identifiable by an insufficient rise (<9 µg/dL [250 nmol/L]) in plasma cortisol in response to a 250 µg ACTH bolus, and carries a poor chance of survival, irrespective of the baseline plasma cortisol concentration which is usually much higher than in healthy humans (10). In such a condition of insufficiently increased cortisol production, a very high plasma ACTH concentration would be expected. However, the recent robust findings that ACTH plasma concentrations are suppressed, that cortisol production is not much elevated, if at all, and that instead reduced cortisol breakdown plays a major role during critical illness, further complicate the issue of diagnostic criteria for adrenal failure in that setting. The concept of relative adrenal insufficiency based on delta cortisol response to corticotropin stimulation test is flawed and can lead to adrenal insufficiency over-diagnosis and inappropriate treatment (11).

Alternatively, a random total cortisol of <10 µg/dL (275 nmol/L) with low serum albumin levels, or 10–15 µg/dL (275–414 nmol/L) in those patients with normal albumin levels during critical illness has been suggested for the diagnosis of 'relative adrenal insufficiency' (7, 11). However, total plasma cortisol concentration is the net effect of adrenal production and secretion, distribution, binding, and elimination of cortisol. Judging the adequacy of the adrenal cortisol production in response to critical illness based on a single measurement of total plasma cortisol is merely indicative. Furthermore, circulating total cortisol concentrations do not reveal the glucocorticoid effect. Since only free cortisol can pass the cell membrane to bind to GR, and suppressed circulating levels of the binding proteins, CBG and albumin, as well as decreased CBG binding affinity via increased cleavage from CBG at inflammatory loci or by increased temperature, were established (17), plasma free cortisol may be more appropriate to assess HPA-axis function (9, 11). However, more research is needed as plasma free cortisol assays are not readily available and normal ranges for plasma free cortisol during critical illness have not been defined. Finally, assays to quantify plasma cortisol concentrations are often inaccurate and vary substantially, making it impossible to identify one cut-off value for clinical practice (10).

Treatment

Acute Intervention

This could be in the outpatient setting (e.g., rapid access clinic) for selected cases of mild adrenal insufficiency/crisis. However, the majority of patients will be hospitalized and managed in an emergency care setting such as emergency department, acute medical unit (AMU) or equivalent, as well as more advanced step-up facilities such as high dependency unit (HDU), or intensive care unit (ICU). As with all acute medical patients, prompt assessment and management of the ABCDEs should occur (i.e. Airway; Breathing; Circulation; Disability [i.e., conscious level]; and Exposure [i.e., examination]).

General Supportive Care

Supportive care includes inserting large bore intravenous (IV) cannulae and starting appropriate IV fluid resuscitation, electrolyte replacement, nutritional support including monitoring and maintaining blood glucose levels, continuous cardiac monitoring, and pulse oximetry. Co-incident comorbidities should be treated appropriately. It is also imperative to exclude unknown pregnancy by performing pregnancy test in appropriate patient. All patients with adrenal crisis should receive low molecular weight heparin (LMWH) for the full duration of admission unless contraindicated.

Acute Adrenal Crisis

For acute adrenal insufficiency or crisis, the five **Ss** of management should be followed: (a) **S**alt replacement (i.e., normal 0.9% saline); (b) **S**ugar replacement (i.e., 5% or 10% Dextrose); (c) **S**teroid replacement (i.e., glucocorticoid ± mineralocorticoid);(d) **S**upportive care; and(e) **S**eek and treat precipitants (e.g., infection is the most common precipitant (13). Where available, the endocrine inpatient team should be involved as early as is practical after admission.

Acute adrenal crisis is treated with extracellular fluid restoration and glucocorticoid replacement therapy (2,3,5). Extracellular fluid volume should be restored with several liters of 0.9% saline and 5% dextrose. Rapid infusion of 1000 mL isotonic saline within the first hour or 5% glucose in isotonic saline, followed by continuous IV isotonic saline guided by individual patient needs (usually 4–6L in 24 h; monitor for fluid overload). If hyponatremia is present, the rate of sodium correction should be limited maximum of 12 mmol/L within 24 h; or 18 mmol/L within 48 hours to avoid precipitating osmotic demyelination syndrome (ODS); or 8 mmol/L over any 24-h period in patients at high risk of ODS (33,34).

Treatment of adrenal crisis (Table 20-4) requires an immediate bolus injection of 100 mg hydrocortisone IV or IM followed by continuous IV infusion of 200 mg hydrocortisone per 24 h (alternatively 50 mg hydrocortisone IM injection every 6 h). Reduce hydrocortisone dose to 100 mg/d the following day.

Glucose monitoring is also required as hypoglycemia is common. Check for any medic alert jewellery (or tattoos!) or steroid cards.

Oral hydrocortisone replacement therapy can be resumed once the saline infusion has been discontinued and the patient is taking food and fluids by mouth. Mineralocorticoid therapy is not required when large amounts of hydrocortisone are being given, but as the dose is reduced, it usually is necessary to add fludrocortisone (primary adrenal insufficiency only). Glucocorticoid and mineralocorticoid replacement therapy is monitored using heart rate and blood pressure measurements, serum electrolyte values, and titration of plasma renin activity into the upper-normal range. Since bacterial infection frequently precipitates acute adrenal crisis, broad-spectrum antibiotic therapy may be needed.

Although dexamethasone can be given acutely (e.g., 4 mg IV stat) if short ACTH testing is performed, as it will not be measured by the cortisol assay (both hydrocortisone and a portion of prednisone can be detected in standard cortisol assays). However, it should be noted that dexamethasone does not have any mineralocorticoid activity and this should not be standard practice as biochemical confirmation is not required in the acute emergency setting.

Treatment of Precipitating Illness

For patients with adrenal crisis, consider any precipitating causes and treat appropriately.

Chronic Treatment of Primary Adrenal Insufficiency

The 2016 Endocrine Society Clinical Practice Guideline recommends glucocorticoid therapy in patients with confirmed primary adrenal insufficiency (5)) (Table 20-4). Hydrocortisone (15–25 mg/d) or cortisone acetate replacement (20–35 mg/d) divided into two to three daily doses in adults, with the highest dose being given in the morning on wakening, the next either in the early afternoon (2 h after lunch; two-dose regimen)

Table 20-4 Recommended therapeutic approach to adrenal insufficiency. Adapted from (5,15).

Diagnosis	Recommendations
Acute adrenal insufficiency	
Glucocorticoid replacement	Start on physiological saline infusions, initial rate 1 liter/h under continuous cardiac monitoring conditions
	Administer 100 mg hydrocortisone as an IV injection, followed by 100–200 mg hydrocortisone in glucose 5% per continuous IV infusion (alternatively, administer hydrocortisone IM at a dose of 50 mg four times daily)
Mineralocorticoid replacement	Only in primary adrenal insufficiency
	Not required as long as hydrocortisone dose >50 mg per 24 h
Adrenal androgen replacement	Not required
Chronic adrenal insufficiency	
Glucocorticoid replacement	Primary adrenal insufficiency: start on 20–25 mg hydrocortisone per 24 h
	Secondary adrenal insufficiency: 15–20 mg hydrocortisone per 24 h; if borderline fail in short-ACTH (cosyntropin or synacthen) stimulation test consider 10 mg or stress dose cover only
	Administer in two to three divided doses with two-thirds and half of the dose, respectively, administer first dose immediately after waking up
	Alternatively use prednisolone 3–5 mg/day
	Consider modified-release hydrocortisone formulation where approved
Monitoring	Check body weight, calculate body mass index (BMI)
	Check for signs of under-replacement (weight loss, fatigue, nausea, myalgia, lack of energy)
	Check for signs of over-replacement (weight gain, central obesity, stretch marks, osteopenia/osteoporosis, pre-diabetes/diabetes, hypertension)
	Take a detailed account of stress-related glucocorticoid dose self-adjustments since last visit, potential adverse events including emergency treatment and/or hospitalization
Mineralocorticoid replacement	Only required in primary adrenal insufficiency
	Not required as long as hydrocortisone dose >50 mg per 24 h
	Start on 100 µg fludrocortisone (doses vary between 50–250 µg per 24 h) administered as a single dose in the morning immediately after waking up
Monitoring	Blood pressure sitting and erect (postural drop ≥20 mmHg indicative of under-replacement, high blood pressure may indicate over-replacement)
	Check for peripheral edema (indicative of over-replacement)
	Check serum sodium and potassium
	Check plasma renin activity (at least every 2–3 yr, upon clinical suspicion of over- and under-replacement and after significant changes in the hydrocortisone dose (40 mg hydrocortisone = 100 µg fludrocortisone)

(continued)

Table 20-4 *(Continued)*

Diagnosis	Recommendations
Adrenal androgen replacement	Consider in patients with impaired well-being and mood despite apparently optimized glucocorticoid and mineralocorticoid replacement and in women with symptoms and signs of androgen deficiency (e.g., dry, itchy skin; reduced libido)
	DHEA 25–50 mg as a single morning dose; in women also consider using transdermal testosterone (300 μg/d, i.e., two patches per week)
Monitoring	In women, serum testosterone and SHBG (to calculate free androgen index)
	In men and women on DHEA replacement, serum DHEAS and androstenedione levels
	Blood should be sampled at steady state (i.e., 12–24 h after the last preceding DHEA dose)
Additional management:	Regular follow-up in specialist center every 6–12 months
	In primary adrenal insufficiency of autoimmune origin (isolated Addison's or APS) • Serum TSH every 12 months • In female patients: check regularity of menstrual cycle, consider measurement of ovarian autoantibodies if family planning not finalized
	Check emergency bracelet/steroid card, update as required
	Check knowledge of "sick day rules 1 and 2" and reinforce emergency guidelines involving partner/family members/lay-persons
	Prescribe hydrocortisone emergency self-injection kit, in particular if delayed access to acute medical care is likely (rural areas, travel)
	Give emergency contact numbers
	Check if other medication includes drugs known to induce (e.g., rifampicin, mitotane, anticonvulsants such as phenytoin, carbamazepine, oxcarbazepine, phenobarbital, topiramate) or inhibit (e.g., antiretroviral gents) hepatic cortisol inactivation by CYP3A4, which may require glucocorticoid dose adjustment

ACTH = adrenocorticotropic hormone; APS = autoimmune polyglandular syndromes; CYP3A4 = cytochrome P450 3A4; DHEA(S) = dihydroepiandrosterone (sulfate); IM = intramuscular; IV = intravenous; SHBG = sex-hormone binding globulin; TSH = thyroid stimulating hormone.

or at lunch and afternoon (three-dose regimen). As an alternative to hydrocortisone, prednisolone (3–5 mg/d) administered orally once or twice daily, especially in patients with reduced compliance can be used (15). Appropriate monitoring glucocorticoid replacement using clinical assessment including body weight, postural blood pressure, energy levels, and signs of frank glucocorticoid excess (Table 20-4).

All patients with confirmed aldosterone deficiency should receive mineralocorticoid replacement with fludrocortisone (starting dose, 50–100 μg in adults) and not restrict their salt intake (4). Appropriate monitoring mineralocorticoid replacement is primarily based on clinical assessment (salt craving, postural hypotension, or edema), and blood electrolyte measurements (Table 20-4). In patients who develop hypertension while receiving fludrocortisone, reducing the dose of fludrocortisone would be a reasonable initial step. If blood pressure remains elevated, initiating antihypertensive treatment and continuing fludrocortisone are recommended.

Patients should be educated about stress dosing and equipped with a steroid card and glucocorticoid preparation for parenteral emergency administration. Follow-up should aim at monitoring appropriate dosing of glucocorticoids and reviewing underlying primary pathology. For example, associated autoimmune diseases, particularly autoimmune thyroid disease are common. In one recent observational study of autoimmune Addison's disease (n = 660), 62% had ≥1 associated autoimmune disease with hypothyroidism the most common (15).

Secondary Adrenal Insufficiency

Glucocorticoid replacement is a high priority in patients with known or suspected central hypoadrenalism (6,27). Acutely ill, hospitalized patients with central hypoadrenalism should be given stress-dose glucocorticoid coverage, including stat dose of IV Hydrocortisone 100–200 mg followed by a hydrocortisone IV infusion at a rate of 2–4 mg/hour; or 50–100 mg intramuscular hydrocortisone every 6 hours. If the patient is hypotensive, resuscitation with IV hydration is indicated.

Patients with pituitary apoplexy should receive stress-dose glucocorticoid replacement, as they are at high risk for hypopituitarism, including central hypoadrenalism (29,30). Of note, neurosurgeons generally recommend pharmacologic doses of glucocorticoids (including dexamethasone 4 mg IV every 6 h) in patients with pituitary apoplexy and cranial neuropathies before surgical decompression is undertaken.

In the outpatient setting, patients with central hypoadrenalism and acute intercurrent illness should be taught to increase their glucocorticoid replacement to 2–3 times their usual maintenance dose until recovery, and then resume taking their usual glucocorticoid replacement (prednisone 2.5–5 mg by mouth daily in a single morning dose or hydrocortisone 15–20 mg by mouth daily in divided doses).

Levothyroxine replacement for primary or secondary hypothyroidism should always be deferred until after glucocorticoid replacement has been administered (or hypoadrenalism excluded); failure to do so may precipitate acute adrenal crisis (thyroxine enhances clearance of cortisol). Starting GH may also unmask HPA deficiency resulting in adrenal crisis (GH blocks conversion of cortisone to cortisol), or change dosing requirements for existing adrenal insufficiency therapy.

Relative Adrenal Insufficiency

It is generally accepted that patients with an established diagnosis of primary or secondary adrenal insufficiency or patients on chronic treatment with systemic glucocorticoids prior to critical illness, should receive additional coverage to cope with the acute stress (10). Patients with septic shock who are pressor-dependent or refractory to fluid resuscitation can be given a short course of hydrocortisone regardless of their serum cortisol levels. Also, patients who are diagnosed with an acute adrenal crisis in the ICU are typically treated with high doses of glucocorticoids. This therapeutic strategy is based on the assumption that cortisol production is several-fold increased in critical illness. The conventional treatment proposes the administration of a bolus of 100 mg of hydrocortisone followed by 50–100 mg every 6 h on the first day, 50 mg every 6 h on the second day, and 25 mg every 6 h on the third day, tapering to maintenance dose by the fourth to fifth day. Currently, the Endocrine Society Clinical Practice Guideline still recommends a high loading dose on the first day, but more rapid tapering. Initially, a bolus of 100 mg of hydrocortisone is recommended, followed by 200 mg/d for the first 24 h and reduced to 100 mg/d on the following day (5).

The doses of hydrocortisone advised for treatment of "relative adrenal insufficiency" are another controversial issue. The proposed dose of 200–300 mg of hydrocortisone per day, referred to as "low dose" in the literature, is approximately 6–10 times higher than the normal amount of daily cortisol production in healthy humans (10) and between 2- to 6-fold higher than the production which has been quantified in critically ill patients. In view of the substantially reduced cortisol breakdown during critical illness, the currently proposed doses for adrenal insufficiency during critical illness may be too high. This may further explain why the multi-center randomized controlled trials which assessed the effect of hydrocortisone treatment during severe sepsis/septic shock (who are pressor-dependent) could not confirm the benefit that was originally observed in the pilot study (35–37).

Also the duration of treatment is under debate. Treating critically ill patients with glucocorticoids in too high a dose for too long a time could inferentially aggravate the loss of lean tissue, increase the risk of myopathy and prolong the ICU dependence, which could increase the susceptibility to potentially lethal complications (7, 38).

Based on the results of stable isotope studies, a dose of approximately 60–75 mg/day (10,11) of hydrocortisone, equivalent to about a doubling of the normal daily cortisol production, may be warranted. A fast tapering down to the lowest effective dose should limit the adverse effects of excessive amounts of glucocorticoids during critical illness.

Special Populations

HIV/AIDS Patients

In patients with HIV/AIDS, protease inhibitor-recipients also treated with inhaled or other formulation glucocorticoids, care should be taken in abruptly ceasing any steroid-containing medications, due to the risk of precipitating an adrenal crisis, as has been described (22). Patients with evidence of hypocortisolism, regardless of the etiology, should be treated with physiological replacement doses of corticosteroids (with fludrocortisone if there is evidence of mineralocorticoid deficiency) and have regular clinical and biochemical monitoring to avoid over-replacement.

Pregnancy

The diagnosis of primary adrenal insufficiency in pregnant women is particularly challenging due to its extreme rarity, overlapping symptoms like nausea and hypotension as well as physiological changes (e.g., increased cortisol production and CBG levels during pregnancy), making the diagnosis difficult. Because untreated adrenal insufficiency in pregnant women is associated with a high mortality, whereas sufficiently treated patients can expect a normal pregnancy course and outcome, early recognition and diagnosis are critical.

In addition to a paired sample of cortisol and ACTH, the adrenal reserve is appropriately and safely assessed in pregnancy by corticotropin stimulation, if indicated (39). Interpretation of the diagnostic results requires thorough consideration of pregnancy-associated physiological changes of adrenocortical function (40). A strong recommendation for immediate treatment before the availability of test results (but after the relevant samples have been procured) is driven by placing high value on preventing major harm. The corticotropin stimulation test is the test of choice in pregnant women if adrenal insufficiency is suspected. In a small cohort of healthy pregnant women, the peak total cortisol response after ACTH injection was significantly higher in comparison to the nonpregnant state (median, 1000 nmol/L [37 µg/dL]) in the second and third trimesters, whereas their responses returned to pre-pregnancy levels during the postpartum period (median, 700 nmol/L [26 µg/dL]) (40). Thus, it has been suggested to use higher diagnostic cortisol cut-offs of 700 nmol/L (25 µg/dL), 800 nmol/L (29 µg/dL), and 900 nmol/L (32 µg/dL) for the first, second, and third trimesters, respectively (39,40).

Hydrocortisone dose should be increased by 20–40% from the 24th week onward to reflect the physiological increase in free cortisol. A hydrocortisone dose equivalent to that used for major surgical stress should be initiated at the onset of active labor (cervix dilation >4 cm and/or contractions every 5 min. for the last hour) with a bolus injection of 100 mg hydrocortisone IV followed by continuous infusion of 200 mg hydrocortisone/24 h. After delivery, hydrocortisone can be quickly tapered back to pre-pregnancy doses.

Management of adrenal insufficiency in pregnancy requires a multidisciplinary approach and should involve endocrinologist, obstetrician, and paediatrician and/or neonatologist.

Case Study

A 30-year-old female with well-controlled type 1 diabetes mellitus with no obvious complications complains of intermittent chronic abdominal pain for 6 months. Her celiac screening laboratory evaluation was normal. She becomes pregnant. Her average HbA1c during pregnancy was 5.9% (41 mmol/mol) and intermittent hypoglycemia was a complication with significant reduction in insulin dosing during her third trimester. A morning cortisol during her third trimester was 15 µg/dL (415 nmol/L). She had a normal full-term delivery of a 7 lb 4 oz baby. She had difficulty breast feeding and lost all of her weight gain during pregnancy within 6 weeks post-partum.

She returns to the clinic with a continued complaint of abdominal pain and fatigue. Her blood pressure is 100/70 mmHg, HR 99 and BMI is 21 kg/m². She is tachycardic on exam, but otherwise the exam is unremarkable. Her insulin requirements have decreased by 20% compared to her pre-pregnancy dosing. An AM cortisol is 5 µg/dL (138 nmol/L) with ACTH 120 pg/mL (10–50 pg/mL); ACTH stimulated cortisol was 8 µg/dL (220 nmol/L); TFTs normal.

What Is the Diagnosis and Likely Etiology? What Urgent Treatment Is Indicated?

This case illustrates the increased incidence of primary adrenal insufficiency in individuals with type 1 diabetes. Non-specific symptoms such as abdominal pain can be easily missed, but more classic symptoms such as weight loss, frequent and unexplained hypoglycemia and fatigue should warrant an evaluation for adrenal insufficiency in this population.

Diagnosis of adrenal insufficiency in pregnancy can be complicated by the increase in CBG related to increased estrogen, giving a falsely elevated total cortisol level, as was the case in this patient. Trimester-specific cortisol levels should be used to interpret these results. A morning cortisol level of less than 11 µg/dL (300 nmol/L); 16.3 µg/dL (450 nmol/L); and 21.7 µg/dL (600 nmol/L) in the 1st, 2nd, and 3rd trimester respectively raises the suspicion of hypocortisolism (39,40). Our patient's third trimester morning cortisol level was 15 µg/dL (415 nmol/L), which is below the optimum level 21.7 µg/dL (600 nmol/L) and should have been followed promptly by treatment and confirmatory short ACTH stimulation test. Similarly, the optimal cut-off for the 60-minute cortisol level as part of the short ACTH stimulation test during pregnancy should be greater than 25.3 µg/dL (700 nmol/L), 29 µg/dL (800 nmol/L) and 32.6 µg/dL (900 nmol/L) in the 1st, 2nd, and 3rd trimester respectively (39, 40). Our patient's post-pregnancy short ACTH stimulation test was abnormal (normal > 18 µg/dL [500 nmol/L]) confirming adrenal insufficiency, which was primary in nature (i.e., raised ACTH > 2 ULN).

Additionally, this is an opportunity to consider screening for other potential autoimmune diseases such as pernicious anemia or hypothyroidism. Many of these patients will satisfy criteria for polyglandular autoimmune syndrome, type 2 (41).

She is started on hydrocortisone PO 10 mg in the AM and 5 mg in the early afternoon. Within a few days she feels generally much better. She will need appropriate monitoring and consideration of the need for mineralocorticoid replacement (5). She also needs education regarding "sick-day" rules; and the need for a medic alert bracelet or similar. She will likely need higher insulin doses now she is eating better with glucocorticoid replacement.

Prevention of Adrenal Crisis

For the prevention of adrenal crisis, adjusting the glucocorticoid dose according to severity of illness or magnitude of the stressor is critical (Table 20-4). Patient education concerning glucocorticoid adjustments in stressful events, and adrenal crisis prevention strategies, including parenteral self- or lay-administration of emergency glucocorticoids, are of value. All patients should be equipped with a steroid emergency card and medical alert identification to inform health personnel of the need for increased glucocorticoid doses to avert or treat adrenal crisis and the need for immediate parenteral steroid treatment in the event of an emergency. Every patient (including family members or key lay-persons) should be equipped with a glucocorticoid injection kit for emergency use and be educated on how to use it.

All adults with adrenal insufficiency should be evaluated by an endocrinologist or a healthcare provider with endocrine expertise at least annually for symptoms and signs of over- and under-replacement. For those patients with autoimmune primary adrenal insufficiency, screening for other autoimmune diseases known to be more prevalent in this population should also occur.

Conclusions

Symptomatic acute adrenal insufficiency (adrenal crisis) is associated with significant morbidity and mortality and should be managed as a medical emergency. Adrenal crisis is brought about by lack of production of the adrenal hormone cortisol and/or mineralocorticoids. It presents with marked signs and symptoms, characteristic laboratory abnormalities, and requires immediate treatment. The severity of this condition is related to the central role of these hormones in energy, salt, and fluid homeostasis. There are two forms of adrenal insufficiency: primary and secondary. Primary adrenal insufficiency (also termed Addison's disease) is caused by the inability of the adrenal cortex to produce sufficient amounts of glucocorticoids and/or mineralocorticoids (e.g., due to autoimmune-mediated destruction of adrenocortical tissue). Secondary adrenal insufficiency (also termed central hypoadrenalism) results from deficient adrenal glucocorticoid production only, because of ACTH deficiency due to impairment of hypothalamic-pituitary axis. The most common cause of secondary adrenal insufficiency is chronic exogenous glucocorticoid treatment. Effective chronic care of primary and secondary adrenal insufficiency is critical; as this is an important opportunity to reduce further admissions by reiterating sick-day rules and other crisis preventative measures, improve quality of life, and decrease morbidity and mortality.

References

1 Matfin G. Disorders of endocrine function. In: Matfin G, Porth CM. eds. *Pathophysiology: Concepts of Altered Health States*. 8th edn. New York: Lippincott; 2008: 1021–1046.

2 Allolio B. Extensive expertise in endocrinology: adrenal crisis. *Eur J Endocrinol*. 2015;172:R115–R124.

3 Arlt W, and the Society for Endocrinology Clinical Committee. Emergency

management of acute adrenal insufficiency (adrenal crisis) in adult (2016). DOI: 10.1530/EC-16-0054.

4 Pazderska A, Pearce SH. Adrenal insufficiency: recognition and management. *Clin Med (Lond).* 2017;17(3):258–262.

5 Bornstein SR, Allolio B, Arlt W, et al. Diagnosis and treatment of primary adrenal insufficiency: an Endocrine Society Clinical Practice Guideline. *J Clin Endocrinol Metab.* 2016;101: 364–389.

6 Fleseriu M, Hashim IA, Karavitaki N, et al. Hormonal replacement in hypopituitarism in adults: an Endocrine Society Clinical Practice Guideline. *J Clin Endocrinol Metab.* 2016;101,3888–3921.

7 Annane D, Pastores SM, Rochwerg B, et al. Guidelines for the diagnosis and management of critical illness-related corticosteroid insufficiency (CIRCI) in critically ill patients (Part I): Society of Critical Care Medicine (SCCM) and European Society of Intensive Care Medicine (ESICM) 2017. *Intensive Care Med.* 2017;43:1751–1763.

8 Cooper MS, Stewart PM. Corticosteroid insufficiency in acutely ill patients. *N Engl J Med.* 2003;348:727–734.

9 Hamrahian AH, Oseni TS, Arafah BM. Measurements of serum free cortisol in critically ill patients. *N Engl J Med.* 2004;350:1629–1638.

10 Boonen E, Bornstein SR, Van den Berghe G. New insights into the controversy of adrenal function during critical illness. *Lancet Diabetes Endocrinol.* 2015;10: 805–815.

11 Hamrahian AH, Fleseriu M, Committee AAS. Evaluation and management of adrenal insufficiency in critically ill patients: disease state review. *Endocr Pract.* 2017 DOI:10.4158/EP161720.RA.

12 Matfin G. Something old, something new…*Ther Adv Endocrinolo Metab.* 2010;1:99–100.

13 Stewart PM, Biller BM, Marelli C, et al. Exploring inpatient hospitalizations and morbidity inpatients with adrenal insufficiency. *J Clin Endocrinol Metab.* 2016;101:4843–4850.

14 Gagliardi L, Nenke MA, Thynne TR, et al. Continuous subcutaneous hydrocortisone infusion therapy in Addison's disease: a randomized, placebo-controlled clinical trial. *J Clin Endocrinol Metab.* 2014;99: 4149–4157.

15 Arlt W. The approach to the adult with newly diagnosed adrenal insufficiency. *J Clin Endocrinol Metab.* 2009;94(4): 1059–1067.

16 Gunnarsson C, Ryan MP, Marelli C, et al. Health care burden in patients with adrenal insufficiency. *J Endocr Soc.* 2017;1:512–523.

17 Meyer EJ, Nenke MA, Rankin W, Lewis JG, Torpy DJ. Corticosteroid-binding globulin: a review of basic and clinical advances. *Horm Metab Res.* 2016;48:359–371

18 Addison T. *On the Constitutional and Local Effects of Disease of the Supra-renal Capsules.* London: Samuel Highley; 1855.

19 Bornstein SR. Predisposing factors for adrenal insufficiency. *N Engl J Med.* 2009;360:2328–2339.

20 Winqvist O, Karlsson FA, Kämpe O. 21-Hydroxylase, a major autoantigen in idiopathic Addison's disease. *Lancet.* 1992;339:1559–1562.

21 Corsello SM, Barnabei A, Marchetti P, et al. Endocrine side effects induced by immune checkpoint inhibitors. *J Clin Endocrinol Metab.* 2013;98:1361–1375.

22 Samaras, K., et al., Iatrogenic Cushing's syndrome with osteoporosis and secondary adrenal failure in human immunodeficiency virus-infected patients receiving inhaled corticosteroids and ritonavir-boosted protease inhibitors: six cases. *J Clin Endocrinol Metab.* 2005;90(7):4394–4398.

23 Speiser PW, Azziz R, Baskin LS, et al. Congenital adrenal hyperplasia due to steroid 21-hydroxylase deficiency: an Endocrine Society Clinical Practice Guideline. *J Clin Endocrinol Metab.* 2010;95:4133–4160.

24 Matfin G, Sheaves R, Muscatelli F, et al. Gene deletion causing adrenal hypoplasia congenita and hypogonadotrophic

hypogonadism. *Clinical Endocrinology*. 1994;40:807–808.

25 Horn MA, Erichsen MM, Wolff AS, et al. Screening for X-linked adrenoleukodystrophy among adult men with Addison's disease. *Clin Endocrinol (Oxf)*. 2013;79:316–320.

26 Molitch ME. Diagnosis and treatment of pituitary adenomas. *JAMA*. 2017;317: 516–524.

27 Grossman AB. The diagnosis and management of central hypoadrenalism. *J Clin Endocrinol Metab*. 2010:95(11): 4855–4863.

28 Prete A, Corsello SM, Salvatori R. Current best practice in the management of patients after pituitary surgery. *Ther Adv Endocrinol Metab*. 2017;8:33–48.

29 Briet C, Salenave S, Bonneville J-F, Laws ER, Chanson P. Pituitary apoplexy. *Endocrine Revs*. 2015;36:622–645.

30 Baldeweg SE, Vanderpump M, Drake W, the Society for Endocrinology Clinical Committee. Emergency management of pituitary apoplexy in adult patients. 2016. DOI: 10.1530/EC-16-0057.

31 Kazlauskaite R, Evans AT, Villabona CV, et al. Corticotropin tests for hypothalamic-pituitary-adrenal insufficiency: a meta-analysis. *J Clin Endocrinol Metab*. 2008;93:4245–4253.

32 Dekkers OM, Timmermans JM, Smit JW, Romijn JA, Pereira AM. Comparison of the cortisol responses to testing with two doses of ACTH in patients with suspected adrenal insufficiency. *Eur J Endocrinol*. 2011;164:83–87.

33 Verbalis JG, Goldsmith SR, Greenberg A, et al. Diagnosis, evaluation, and treatment of hyponatremia: expert panel recommendations. *Am J Med*. 2013;126(10 Suppl 1):S1–S42.

34 Ball S, Barth J, Levy M, the Society for Endocrinology Clinical Committee. Emergency management of severe symptomatic hyponatraemia in adult patients. 2016. DOI: 10.1530/EC-16-0058.

35 Dalin F, Eriksson GN, Dahlqvist P, et al. Clinical and immunological characteristics of autoimmune Addison disease: a nationwide Swedish multicenter study. *J Clin Endocrinol Metab*. 2017;102:379–389.

36 Annane D, Sébille V, Charpentier C, et al. Effect of treatment with low doses of hydrocortisone and fludrocortisone on mortality in patients with septic shock. *JAMA*. 2002;288(7):862–871.

37 Sprung CL, Annane D, Keh D, et al. Hydrocortisone therapy for patients with septic shock. *N Engl J Med*. 2008;358(2):111–124.

38 Keh D, Trips E, Marx G, et al. Effect of hydrocortisone on development of shock among patients with severe sepsis: The HYPRESS randomized clinical trial. *JAMA*. 2016;316(17):1775–1785.

39 Hermans G, De Jonghe B, Bruyninckx F, Van den Berghe G. Clinical review: critical illness polyneuropathy and myopathy. *Crit Care*. 2008;12(6):238.

40 Lebbe M, Arlt W. What is the best diagnostic and therapeutic management strategy for an Addison patient during pregnancy? *Clin Endocrinol (Oxf)*. 2013;78:497–502.

41 Langlois F, Lima D, Fleseriua M. Update on adrenal insufficiency: diagnosis and management in pregnancy. *Curr Opin Endocrinol Diabetes Obes*. 2017. DOI: 10.1097/MED.0000000000000331

42 Betterle C, Lazzarotto F, Presotto F. Autoimmune polyglandular syndrome type 2: the tip of an iceberg? *Clin Exp Immunol*. 2004;137(2):225–233.

43 Husebye ES, et al. Consensus statement on the diagnosis, treatment and follow-up of patients with primary adrenal insufficiency. *J Intern Med*. 2014;275:104–115.

44 Arlt W. *J Clin Endocrinol Metab*. April 2009;94(4):1059–1067.

45 Amin A, Sam AH, Meeran K. Glucocorticoid replacement. *BMJ*. 2014;349:g4843.

21

Acute Medical Aspects Related to Florid Cushing's Syndrome

Krystallenia I. Alexandraki and Ashley B. Grossman

Key Points

- Cushing's syndrome (CS) is defined by long-standing exposure to supraphysiologic levels of circulating glucocorticoids.
- Uncontrolled CS (i.e., florid CS), produces high morbidity and mortality rates because of the metabolic and cardiovascular derangement as well as the risk of infection.
- These conditions are intensified when the hypercortisolemia (or synthetic glucocorticoid levels) is severe and thus leads to an urgent situation requiring emergency management.
- In the acute care setting, prompt diagnosis of florid CS (i.e., florid clinical features; and serum cortisol usually >1000 nmol/L [36 μg/dL]) should be followed by urgent therapy to normalize the excess glucocorticoid state, treat the metabolic complications, such as diabetes and hypertension, stabilize any psychotic state, and vigorously treat any suspected sepsis or perforated viscus. This takes precedence over establishing the specific cause.
- Florid clinical features of CS includes: sepsis, opportunistic infection, uncontrolled hypertension, edema, heart failure, gastrointestinal hemorrhage, glucocorticoid-induced acute psychosis, progressive debilitating myopathy, thromboembolism, or uncontrolled hyperglycemia, and diabetic ketoacidosis.
- In suspected cases of florid CS caused by exogenous glucocorticoid exposure, a detailed drug history (including over-the-counter agents) is mandatory and any relevant drug-drug interactions should be addressed.
- In suspected cases of florid CS caused by endogenous glucocorticoid exposure, the cause is likely to be severe hypercortisolemia secondary to a macroadenoma causing Cushing's disease, the ectopic ACTH syndrome, or an adrenal carcinoma.
- Rapid control of endogenous CS is achieved with oral metyrapone and/or ketoconazole, but if parenteral therapy is required, then intravenous etomidate is rapidly effective in almost all cases, but all measures require careful supervision and monitoring.

Introduction

Cushing's syndrome (CS) is defined by long-standing exposure to supraphysiologic levels of circulating glucocorticoids (1). Uncontrolled CS (i.e., florid CS), produces high morbidity and mortality rates because of the metabolic and cardiovascular derangement as well as the risk of infection. These conditions are intensified when the hypercortisolemia (or synthetic glucocorticoid levels) is severe and thus leads to an urgent situation

Endocrine and Metabolic Medical Emergencies: A Clinician's Guide, Second Edition. Edited by Glenn Matfin.
© 2018 John Wiley & Sons Ltd. Published 2018 by John Wiley & Sons Ltd.

and requires acute admission to hospital. In the acute care setting, prompt diagnosis of florid CS should be followed by urgent therapy to normalize the excess glucocorticoid state, which may take precedence over establishing the specific cause. The description of a real clinical case admitted via the emergency department some years back when there were fewer tools to manage florid CS may be used to indicate the important steps that must be followed in these situations.

Case Study

A 65-year-old man was admitted to the emergency department with collapse and coma in July 1997. On clinical examination, he was Cushingoid with abdominal adiposity, a moon face, easy bruising, thin skin, abdominal striae, lower limb edema up to his hips, and an infective exacerbation of venous ulcers. He was treated with antibiotics (ciprofloxacin and erythromycin, flucoxacillin), an intensified insulin regimen, ascorbic acid, vitamin B complex, acetylsalicylic acid, slow potassium, furosemide, enalapril, and warfarin. His clinical status improved and he recovered from the coma. On direct questioning and focused examination, it was noted that over the last three years he had experienced a 7-kg weight gain, no erectile function (last ejaculation three years before admission), proximal weakness, lethargy, tiredness, nocturia, polydipsia, pigmentation (started 11 months before admission), abdominal bloating, blurred vision, anxiety, and low mood. He also had diabetes mellitus type 2, hypertension (with silver wiring on fundoscopy), cardiac decompensation with cardiac failure, an episode of pulmonary embolism the year before admission, osteoporosis diagnosed three years earlier, and resistant fungal infection in his toe nails.

Investigations showed: Midnight total serum cortisol levels were increased (1028 and 1290 nmol/L [37.3–46.8 μg/dL]) and an increased mean (at 5-point) daily cortisol level (1055 nmol/L [38.2 μg/dL]) was seen. ACTH was detectable at levels of 200 ng/L and 160 ng/L (0–40 ng/L normal range) on two consecutive mornings. Pituitary magnetic resonance imaging (MRI) scan showed a large tumor arising from the pituitary with a significant suprasellar extension. A diagnosis of an ACTH-secreting pituitary adenoma (i.e., Cushing's disease [CD]), was made. Adrenal targeted therapy (a combination of metyrapone, ketoconazole, and mitotane) was commenced but the CS could not be controlled and the decision to proceed to bilateral adrenalectomy was taken. However, during the postoperative period persistent venous oozing from the adrenal bed occurred, and he developed a urinary tract infection and pre-renal failure; the patient succumbed to sepsis on the 39th postoperative day.

Etiology

Classically, the most common cause of CS is the exogenous administration of glucocorticoids for medical reasons; a meticulous drug history will shed light on the use of any medication or over-the-counter agents which may be involved. Topical, inhaled, injected preparations or remedies taken over-the-counter may be responsible for the apparent steroid excess, particularly if a drug interaction is involved. This is the case for the severe glucocorticoid status caused by the anti-retroviral drugs used in human immunodeficiency virus (HIV) patients in combination with synthetic glucocorticoids administered even by way of intraocular drops or intra-articular injection. The concomitant use of synthetic glucocorticoids (triamcinolone, budesonide, fluticasone, dexamethasone, and prednisolone) along with agents, such as ritonavir and atazanavir, results in increased serum concentrations of glucocorticoids. This is due to the inhibition of the hepatic enzyme CYP3A4 and P-glycoprotein (PGP) export pump by the protease inhibitors, since both mediators participate in the metabolism of glucocorticoids (2–4).

In terms of endogenous CS, for ACTH-dependent CS, CD is more prevalent (80–85%) compared to ectopic CS (ECS) caused by a neoplasm, usually a neuroendocrine neoplasm (NEN) secreting ACTH. Pituitary microadenomas, defined as adenomas with a size less than 1 cm in diameter, comprise the majority of CD cases, but macroadenomas (5–10%), with or without extrasellar extension or invasion, particularly result in florid CS as the case described here. Pituitary corticotroph carcinomas are defined by extra-pituitary metastases and, if large, may also cause severe disease (5). Generally, CD is more common in women and tends to present between the ages of 25–40 years of age, as opposed to the case described above, suggesting that long-standing CS was undiagnosed and then caused an emergency admission. On the other hand, ECS is more common in men, and usually presents one decade older than CD, after the age of 40 years. The neoplasms associated with ECS are NENs arising from the lung, pancreas, thymus, adrenal medulla (pheochromocytomas) or as medullary thyroid carcinoma, while a neoplasm cannot be identified in some cases (6). These neoplasms usually show an indolent natural history but the neoplastic cells may secrete increased levels of ACTH independent of tumor size. When the primary site of the ECS is identified, *overt* ECS is defined, while when it is identified at a later evaluation or follow-up, *covert* ECS is defined: *occult* ECS is defined when the tumoral source has not been identified over time.

For ACTH-independent hypercortisolemia, unilateral or bilateral cortisol-secreting adenomas have not usually been associated with florid CS, as opposed to a cortisol-secreting adrenocortical carcinoma (ACC), present in 40% of ACTH-independent CS which by size criteria may result rapidly in uncontrolled hypercortisolemia (Figure 21-1). ACC is slightly more common in women, displaying a bimodal age distribution, with peaks in childhood and adolescence and then later in life.

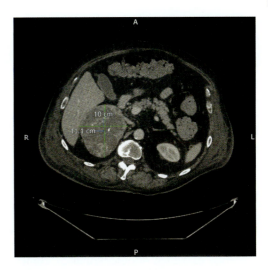

Figure 21-1 CT scan showing 11 × 10 cm cortisol secreting adrenocortical tumor. The patient presented with florid Cushing's syndrome.

Florid Cushing's Syndrome Investigation

The most important step in the natural history of florid CS is clinical suspicion. In an urgent clinical setting, a detailed past medical and drug history may be not available in the first instance but it should be targeted as soon as possible (7).

The most accepted definition for florid CS (i.e., when due to severe hypercortisolemia), includes a massively elevated random serum cortisol (more than 1000 nmol/L [36 µg/dL]), or a 24-hr urinary free cortisol (UFC) more than 4-fold the upper limit of normal and/or severe hypokalemia (<3.0 mmol/L), along with the recent onset of one or more of the following clinical conditions: sepsis, opportunistic infection, uncontrolled hypertension, edema, heart failure, gastrointestinal hemorrhage, glucocorticoid-induced acute psychosis, progressive debilitating myopathy, thromboembolism, or uncontrolled hyperglycemia, and diabetic ketoacidosis (8–10).

However, it should be noted that ACTH and cortisol are stress hormones, and may be elevated during any severe metabolic or systemic stressor such as sepsis, myocardial infarction, and in patients in intensive care

(11). In this situation, clinical stigmata or their absence are crucial.

Finally, the rare occasions of exogenous florid CS must be considered, particularly when patients suffering from chronic diseases are taking drugs with potential unknown drug-to-drug interactions, as is the case of anti-viral medical therapy in HIV patients.

Clinical Signs and Features

Hypercortisolemia has characteristic signs, symptoms, and other comorbidities, the presence of which should enhance clinical suspicion. The most specific signs are skin thinning, limb wasting, and muscle weakness, a plethoric red face, and spontaneous bruising. The major exception to this phenotype is the paraneoplastic wasting syndrome which can mask the hypercortisolism in cases of ECS, but this case is usually characterized by a rapid onset with severe metabolic features, often secondary to small cell lung cancers (SCLCs). The duration of CS has been suggested to be the major determinant of the clinical features rather than the degree. The gradual establishment of signs may be seen with NENs, as opposed to SCLC, which usually have a rapid onset with an absence of overt Cushingoid features but profound weakness, ankle edema, and hyperpigmentation. Moreover, severe hirsutism and virilization in a female strongly suggest an adrenal carcinoma when an adrenal mass is present (1,7). The comorbidities usually seen in CS are metabolic such as hypertension, pre-diabetes or diabetes and hypokalemia; osteoporotic fractures, and psychiatric features, such as severe psychosis, may also be present.

Management

The goals of treatment of florid CS differ compared to the conventional management of CS, which target the normalization of glucocorticoid levels aiming at the reversal of clinical symptoms with the long-term objective of avoiding the consequences of excess glucocorticoid exposure. In florid CS, the priority is the stabilization of the patient, saving them from a life-threatening condition while simultaneously attempting to lower glucocorticoid levels.

Acute Intervention for Hemodynamic Stabilization

The metabolic derangements should be attended to urgently, and then measures taken to lower the cortisol levels.

Diabetes often requires insulin to be controlled with or without oral medications, although insulin is often required; care should be given when hypercortisolemia is controlled and there is then a serious risk of hypoglycemia.

Hypertension therapy follows conventional paradigms, and no specific agents are recommended. However, the combination of fluid retention with ankle edema and hypertension may be associated with cardiac failure, and special care should be addressed in the older population. Hypokalemia is present in almost all patients with severe CS, mostly in patients with ECS. A potassium-sparing anti-hypertensive drug is the most appropriate. Spironolactone at a dose of 50 or 100 mg daily is a good candidate as initial treatment with triamterene or amiloride as alternatives if spironolactone is not well tolerated. Potassium replacement may be needed in the first days of admission, as in our case study patient.

A significant pro-thrombotic tendency has recently been confirmed in CS, and the use of anticoagulant treatment should be considered as prophylaxis in patients admitted with severe hypercortisolemia. The precise form this should take has not been decided; while in milder cases a prophylactic dose of heparin may be appropriate, in more severe cases, especially when there is evidence of pulmonary embolism and/or deep vein thrombosis, low molecular weight heparins should be used at therapeutic doses, particularly since these patients are often bed-ridden or of poor mobility (12,13).

When the mental status is altered as the occasion of acute psychosis, management may be problematic and haloperidol may be useful to calm the patient. Newer agents such as olanzapine have been successfully used in isolated cases.

If osteoporotic fractures cause symptoms, drug therapy to relieve the pain is necessary along with other supportive measures as indicated.

It is important to note that many of these supportive treatments may be needed for the acute deleterious effects of the excess glucocorticoid state, and may rapidly reverse when hypercortisolemia is resolved. Careful continuous monitoring is mandatory to avoid overtreatment or other serious sequelae, and particularly acute adrenal failure on cortisol-lowering regimes.

Sepsis remains the most life-threatening complication of florid CS, especially as the usual indicators and signs of its presence may be masked by hypercortisolemia *per se*. Any infection, bacterial, fungal and viral, must be vigorously treated as soon as possible when recognized, since patients with hypercortisolemia are the classically immune-suppressed patients. Prophylaxis with trimethoprim-sulfamethoxazole (or dapsone in allergic patients) is highly effective for pneumocystis pneumonia (PCP), and has been suggested as routine therapy for patients receiving a glucocorticoid dose equivalent to ≥20 mg of prednisone daily for one month or longer; it is mandatory for patients who have an additional cause for immunodepression, such as patients under treatment with chemotherapy with ECS as paraneoplastic condition (14). However, in one published case, a hypercortisolemic patient developed PCP in spite of the administration of prophylactic treatment, questioning the necessity of prophylactic or curative doses of antibiotics (15). On the other hand, resolution of CS should improve the immune status of these patients. It is also of note that when severe infection is present, serum cortisol should be lowered to a level compatible with that seen with severe metabolic or systemic stressors i.e., 600–1000 nmol/L (22–36 µg/dL). Despite intensive efforts to treat infection, in our case, infection and sepsis were the complications that resulted in death, demonstrating how important this factor is and how vigorously it should be treated.

Finally, perforation of a viscus may occur with minimal evidence of peritonitis, especially in the elderly with underlying diverticular disease; if surgery is performed as essential, vigorous resuscitation should be undertaken.

Drug Interactions Documentation

When a drug interaction is documented as the culprit of severe CS, after acute intervention, special measures should be taken. Regarding synthetic glucocorticoid therapy, alternative therapeutic options should be considered such as substituting an inhaled glucocorticoid with beclomethasone since it is not metabolized by CYP3A4. If there is no alternative medication, such as in the case of the intra-articular administration of triamcinolone, close follow-up of the patient may prevent complications. The shift from ritonavir-containing anti-retroviral therapy to a non-interacting compound, such as an integrase inhibitor, might also be considered (2–4).

Adrenal-Specific Therapy

In the emergency setting, during the attempt to obtain hemodynamic stabilization no diagnostic procedure is necessary to identify the source of hypercortisolemia. However, as soon as the acute intervention has been initiated, medical treatment should aim to reduce glucocorticoid levels. This is similar to the case in a non-emergency setting before surgery; to reverse cardiometabolic consequences and poor healing; or in patients who cannot be submitted to surgical procedures because of comorbidities; in patients who are unwilling to receive other types of treatment; and as chronic therapy when surgical treatment fails. However, in an emergency setting, if adrenal-specific therapy fails to fully control the severe hypercortisolemic state, then bilateral adrenalectomy should also be considered.

Lowering of the elevated serum cortisol levels may be attempted using drugs which are directed at adrenal steroidogenesis (Figure 21-2). Metyrapone is generally the first initial choice since it is rapid in onset and highly effective, but high doses up to 1 g four times a day may be required with a final dose not exceeding 6 g daily in divided doses. The effect is usually seen within hours, with initial dose 500–750 mg 3 times daily and a 4-times regimen at higher doses. Lower doses may be required in cases of ECS or adrenal tumors compared to CD, since in this later situation there is feedback which may overcome the blockade. Metyrapone is an 11β-hydroxylase (CYP11B1) inhibitor and for this reason its adverse effects include acne and hirsutism caused by the accumulation of androgenic precursors as well as hypertension, hypokalemia, and edema, due to an increase in mineralocorticoid precursors, but these are rarely problematic in the acute situation; dizziness and gastrointestinal upset are minimized when metyrapone is taken with food or milk (16,17). It should be noted that cortisol measured with most assays other than LC-MS may measure precursors such as 11-deoxycortisol and thus the "true" cortisol may be at least 20% lower.

Osilodrostat (LCI699) is a newer potent oral 11β-hydroxylase and aldosterone synthase (CYP11B2) inhibitor. It has shown encouraging efficacy and safety in one proof-of-concept study and recently in a long-term phase 3 study (18). Displaying a similar therapeutic profile to metyrapone, it promises to be a useful new treatment.

Ketoconazole is an imidazole-blocking cytochrome P450 enzyme, and can be used

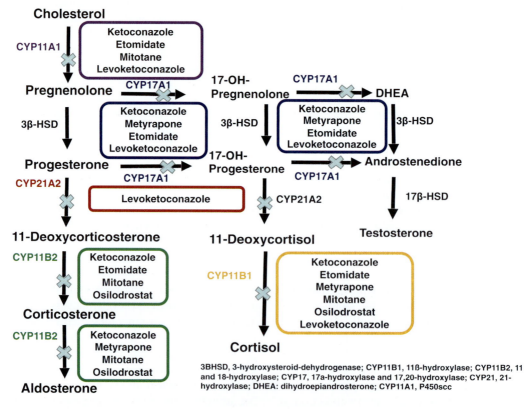

Figure 21-2 Drugs used for the management of florid Cushing's syndrome

either additionally or in place of metyrapone. It has an onset of action more rapid than previously thought and it is usually started at 400 mg/day (divided into two doses) and increased to a maximum of 1.2–1.6 g/day in three or four divided doses. However, it is still unclear as to whether it works within hours, as metyrapone, or over several days. Gastric acidity is necessary to metabolize ketoconazole into the active compound and this should be taken in consideration when an acute intervention includes drugs for gastroprotection. Ketoconazole may cause mild liver enzyme elevation, and very rarely acute liver failure, so this needs to be monitored; mild asymptomatic elevations of serum transaminases when therapy starts or when doses increase may occur, but usually do not require cessation of therapy. Care should be given to consider the extremely low occasion of fatal hepatotoxicity. Other adverse effects such as gastrointestinal symptoms, gynecomastia, decreased libido and impotence, irregular menses, and teratogenicity are not problematic in the acute setting, while drug interactions need to be considered since it displays a potent inhibitory effect on cytochrome P450 enzymes (CYP3A4, CYP2C9, CYP1A2) (19,20). Levoketoconazole is a new investigational agent, the single 2S,4R enantiomer of ketoconazole that has been designed to provide better safety and efficacy than the currently used racemic ketoconazole. Even though it has not been used in the acute setting, it is expected to be a promising therapy for severe hypercortisolemia (21).

When these drugs or their counterparts alone or in combination are not effective or tolerated, then the glucocorticoid antagonist mifepristone, at a starting dose of 300 mg/day, can be slowly titrated up to 400–800 mg daily (Figure 21-2). Mifepristone may rapidly reduce the symptoms and signs of hypercortisolemia, but as serum cortisol cannot be used as a marker of efficacy and safety, the patient can become unwittingly Addisonian. Hence, despite the fact that there are case reports published for its use in a severe CS situation, increased care has to be taken,

since high doses of mifepristone expose patients to adverse effects with hypokalemia and adrenal insufficiency, rendering this generally an unsuitable choice in critically ill patients since it is difficult to determine whether any change in clinical state is due to the treatment or to the underlying disease. Hypokalemia may be severe but respond promptly to spironolactone, but it should not be administered with drugs that are metabolized by CYP3A or CYP2C (15,22).

If all else fails, or the severely ill patient cannot receive *per os* medical therapy, intravenous administration of etomidate, an imidazole potently blocking 11β-hydroxylase and side chain cleavage enzymes but also aldosterone synthase, may be life-saving at sub-anesthetic doses (Figure 21-2). Etomidate may be used as first-line treatment in an acute situation since it acts within hours and is almost always highly effective with a starting loading dose of 3–5 mg to be followed by a continuous infusion of 0.03–0.10 mg/kg/h (2.5–3.0 mg/hr), with dose titration. If complete rather than partial blockade is desired ("block-and-replace"), a hydrocortisone infusion may be added. This drug needs to be very carefully monitored, and the clinicians who are using this should be highly experienced in its use or otherwise, as the recent guidelines suggest, the patient should be admitted to an intensive care unit (ICU) or high-dependency unit (HDU) setting. Sedation could be (but rarely is) problematic if care is not taken, and adjustments should be made with regards to renal failure and stressed situations such as sepsis, i.e., titrating the infusion rate to achieve a stable serum cortisol level between 280–560 nmol/L (10.1–20.3 µg/dL) in physiologically stressed patients or to 150–300 nmol/L (5.4–10.9 µg/dL) in unstressed patients (12,23,24). Again, as noted of metyrapone, serum cortisol levels may be contaminated by precursors in some assays and judicious assessment is vital.

After all such treatments for hemodynamic stabilization and control of hypercortisolemia, when rapid control of hypercortisolemia has not been achieved by other means, bilateral adrenalectomy can induce rapid resolution of the clinical features and may be life-saving. However, it must be considered that patients will need lifelong treatment with glucocorticoids and mineralocorticoids along with careful education to prevent adrenal insufficiency. Since, even with a good laparoscopic technique, surgery in the presence of florid CS is far from ideal, every attempt should be made to lower the cortisol levels preoperatively with medical therapy.

Diagnostic Considerations

Following clinical suspicion of endogenous CS, hypercortisolemia must be established biochemically (i.e., 24-h UFC, low-dose or overnight dexamethasone suppression test, and midnight serum cortisol or late-night salivary cortisol) before any attempt at differential diagnosis. This is not the case for florid CS where no further diagnostic tests are essential, and plasma ACTH levels, together with appropriate imaging, are the most useful non-invasive investigations to determine the etiology. When ACTH is readily detectable, then the patient either has CD or ECS. An obvious pituitary macroadenoma may be seen when the cause of the hypercortsolemia is the pituitary gland, as in our case, or an ectopic source which in most – but not all – occasions is apparent on imaging studies. Axial imaging with thin-cut multi-slice-computed tomography (CT) of the chest and abdomen and a pelvic MRI have the highest detection rate for the identification of an ectopic source. CT of the adrenals on scanning may also support a diagnosis, since adrenals may be enlarged in patients with CD and ECS, but a pheochromocytoma may also be identified as the ECS source. Somatostatin receptor scintigraphy (SRS) may prove helpful as ECS may be caused by a small NET expressing SSTRs, adding supportive functional data to conventional imaging techniques, although it may be not possible to perform this in an acute setting. The same is valid for the other functional imaging studies such as positron emission tomography (PET) with [18]fluorodeoxyglucose (FDG-PET) or whole-body PET with ^{11}C-5-hydroxytryptophan may be performed when the emergency is over. On the contrary, when ACTH is very low or undetectable, imaging of the adrenals with high-resolution CT scanning provides the best resolution of adrenal anatomy for masses over 1 cm, allowing evaluation of the contralateral gland. Florid CS will be caused usually by a mass over 5 cm in diameter which by definition must be considered to be malignant until proven otherwise (Figure 21-1).

Despite all this diagnostic work-up, definitive proof of the source of CS source requires complete resolution of the clinical and biochemical features after tumor resection or partial resolution after tumor debulking, and/or demonstration of ACTH immunohistochemical staining in the tumor tissue or in metastatic deposits in ACTH-dependent cases.

Comments on the Case Study

The case described demonstrates the value of medical treatments to control hypercortisolemia. The combination of mitotane, metyrapone, and ketoconazole concomitantly introduced was recently shown to be an effective alternative to bilateral adrenalectomy in 11 patients with severe ACTH-dependent CS after 24–48 h of combination treatment (25), although this combination was not tolerated in the specific case described here. We would generally recommend metyrapone and/or ketoconazole, with etomidate being reserved for patients requiring parenteral therapy, and we rarely use mitotane or mifepristone.

What Alternatives Have Been Used in Recent Years?

The use of etomidate can be used in unconscious patients and could have controlled the excess cortisol secretion. We may speculate that our patient was not promptly controlled and he had more complications from the hypercortisolemia. Future oral medical management such as levoketoconazole and osilodrostat may also prove to be valuable tools for CS since they may have a better adverse effect profile. Moreover, for ACTH-secreting adenomas, one could consider targeted medical therapy such as pasireotide, a newer multi-ligand SA, which has a high binding affinity to somatostatin receptor (SSTR) 5 and 1, 2 and 3 subtypes (26), recently approved (in the USA and Europe) for the treatment of patients with CD for whom surgery is not possible; this compound was also used in florid CS cases with success (27). However, we would generally not recommend its use for severe cases as it is usually only effective for mild CD.

Conclusions

In an acute situation in a patient with florid CS, this can be confirmed in most instances with a single grossly elevated serum cortisol level taken at any time of the day. In exogenous CS, a detailed drug history is mandatory and any relevant drug-to-drug interactions should be urgently addressed. The most urgent priority is to treat the metabolic complications such as diabetes and hypertension, stabilize any psychotic state, and vigorously treat any suspected sepsis or perforated viscus. Rapid control of endogenous CS is achieved with oral metyrapone and/or ketoconazole (Figure 21-2), but if parenteral therapy is required, then intravenous etomidate is rapidly effective in almost all cases, but all measures require careful supervision and monitoring.

References

1 Newell-Price J, Bertagna X, Grossman AB, Nieman LK. Cushing's syndrome. *Lancet.* 2006;367:1605–1617.

2 Eeftinck Schattenkerk JK, Lager PS. Cushing;s syndrome during HIV treatment: pharmacological interaction during use of ritonavir. *Ned Tijdschr Geneeskd.* 2013;157:A5509 (in Dutch).

3 From HIV i-Base. Case Reports: Cushing's Syndrome with atazanavir/ritonavir. Available at: http://www.thebody.com/content/63748/case-reports-cushings-syndrome-with-atazanavirrito.html (accessed November 25, 2013).

4 Hall JJ, Hughes CA, Foisy MM, Houston S, Shafran S. Iatrogenic Cushing syndrome after intra-articular triamcinolone in a patient receiving ritonavir-boosted darunavir. *Int J STD AIDS.* 2013;24:748–752.

5 Kaltsas GA, Nomikos P, Kontogeorgos G, Buchfelder M, Grossman AB. Clinical review: diagnosis and management of pituitary carcinomas. *J Clin Endocrinol Metab.* 2005;90:3089–3099.

6 Alexandraki KI, Grossman AB. The ectopic ACTH syndrome. *Rev Endocr Metab Disord.* 2010;11:117–126.

7 Alexandraki KI, Grossman AB. Cushing's syndrome. In: Bandeira F, Gharib H, Golbert A, Griz L, Faria M (Eds.) *Endocrinology and Diabetes: A Problem Oriented Approach.* New York: Springer Science+Business Media; 2014: 99–111.

8 Sarlis NJ, Chanock SJ, Nieman LK. Cortisolemic indices predict severe infections in Cushing syndrome due to ectopic production of adrenocorticotropin. *J Clin Endocrinol Metab.* 2000;85:42–47.

9 Corcuff JB, Young J, Masquefa-Giraud P, et al. Rapid control of severe neoplastic hypercortisolism with metyrapone and ketoconazole. *Eur J Endocrinol.* 2015;172:473–478.

10 Reincke M, Ritzel K, Osswald A, et al. A critical re-appraisal of bilateral adrenalectomy for ACTH-dependent Cushing's syndrome. *Eur J Endocrinol.* 2015;173:M23–M32.

11 Boonen E, Bornstein SR, Van den Berghe G. New insights into the controversy of adrenal function during critical illness. *Lancet Diabetes Endocrinol.* 2015;3: 805–815.

12 Nieman LK, Biller BM, Findling JW, et al. Treatment of Cushing's syndrome: an Endocrine Society Clinical Practice Guideline. *J Clin Endocrinol Metab.* 2015;100:2807–2831.

13 Stuijver DJ, van Zaane B, Feelders RA, et al. Incidence of venous thromboembolism in patients with Cushing's syndrome: a multicenter cohort study. *J Clin Endocrinol Metab.* 2011;96:3525–3532.

14 Thomas CF, Limper AH. Treatment and prevention of pneumocystis pneumonia in non-HIV-infected patients. *UpToDate.* Section Editor Marr KA, Deputy Editor Thorner AR http://www.uptodate.com/contents/treatment-and-prevention-of-pneumocystis-pneumonia-in-non-hivinfectedpatients (accessed November 24, 2013).

15 Oosterhuis JK, van den Berg G, Monteban-Kooistra WE, et al. Life-threatening pneumocystis jiroveci pneumonia following treatment of severe Cushing's syndrome. *Neth J Med.* 2007;65:215–217.

16 Verhelst JA, Trainer PJ, Howlett TA, et al. Short- and long-term responses to metyrapone in the medical management of 91 patients with Cushing's syndrome. *Clin Endocrinol.* 1991;35:169–178.

17 Daniel E, Aylwin S, Mustafa O, et al. Effectiveness of metyrapone in the treatment of Cushing's Syndrome: a retrospective multicenter study in 195 patients. *J Clin Endocrinol Metab.* 2015;100:4146–4154.

18 Bertagna X, Pivonello R, Fleseriu M, et al. LCI699, a potent 11β-hydroxylase inhibitor, normalizes urinary cortisol in patients with Cushing's disease: results from a multicenter, proof-of-concept study. *J Clin Endocrinol Metab.* 2014;99:1375–1383.

19 Castinetti F, Morange I, Jaquet P, et al. Ketoconazole revisited: a preoperative or postoperative treatment in Cushing's disease. *Eur J Endocrinol.* 2008;158:91–99.

20 Castinetti F, Guignat L, Giraud P, et al. Ketoconazole in Cushing's disease: is it worth a try? *J Clin Endocrinol Metab.* 2014;99:1623–1630.

21 Salvatori R, DelConte A, Geer EB, et al. An open-label study to assess the safety and efficacy of levoketoconazole (COR-003) in the treatment of endogenous Cushing's Syndrome. In: Program of the 97th annual meeting of The Endocrine Society, March 5–8, 2015; San Diego, CA. *Abstract Endocrine Reviews.* 2015;36:376.

22 Fleseriu M, Findling JW, Koch CA, et al. Changes in plasma ACTH levels and corticotroph tumor size in patients with Cushing's disease during long-term treatment with the glucocorticoid receptor antagonist mifepristone. *J Clin Endocrinol Metab.* 2014;99:3718–3727.

23 Preda VA, Sen J, Karavitaki N, Grossman AB et al. Etomidate in the management or hypercortisolaemia in Cushing's syndrome: a review. *Eur J Endocrinol.* 2012;167: 137–143.

24 Schulte HM, Benker G, Reinwein D, et al. Infusion of low dose etomidate: correction of hypercortislemia in patients with Cushing's syndrome and dose–response relationship in normal subjects. *J Clin Endocrinol Metab.* 1990;70:1426–1430.

25 Kamenický P, Droumaguet C, Salenave S, et al. Mitotane, metyrapone, and ketoconazole combination therapy as an alternative to rescue adrenalectomy for severe ACTH-dependent Cushing's syndrome. *J Clin Endocrinol Metab.* 2011;96:2796–2804.

26 Boscaro M, Ludlam WH, Atkinson B, et al. Treatment of pituitary-dependent Cushing's disease with the multireceptor ligand somatostatin analog pasireotide (SOM230): a multicenter, phase II trial. *J Clin Endocrinol Metab.* 2009;94:115–122.

27 Feelders RA, de Bruin C, Pereira AM, et al. Pasireotide alone or with cabergoline and ketoconazole in Cushing's disease. *N Engl J Med.* 2010;362:1846–1848.

22

Endocrine Hypertensive Emergencies

Graeme Eisenhofer, Andrzej Januszewicz, Christina Pamporaki, and Jacques W.M. Lenders

---

Key Points

- Hypertension may be the initial clinical presentation for at least 15 endocrine disorders.
- Hypertensive emergencies are defined by situations of uncontrolled hypertension resulting in acute or looming end-organ damage.
- Endocrine causes of hypertensive emergencies are easily overlooked when patients present with uncontrolled hypertension in association with evidence of end-organ damage.
- Emergencies arising from hypertensive crises due to pheochromocytoma can be particularly dangerous. To ensure appropriate therapeutic counter-measures and a favorable outcome, the presence of a catecholamine-producing tumor should be distinguished from more common etiologies as well as other uncommon endocrine causes, such as primary hyperaldosteronism, Cushing's syndrome and thyrotoxicosis.
- However, pheochromocytoma diagnosis at the time of the emergency can be made difficult by activation of the sympathoadrenal system resulting from the physiological stress of the clinical condition. Tests of catecholamine excess are therefore rendered problematic to interpret, with reliable diagnosis often only possible once and if the patient recovers.
- Because of this and time delays in obtaining test results, recognition of a possible endocrine cause in the emergency setting requires careful attention to patient history, presentation and precipitating causes that may provide clues to the underlying etiologies for guiding therapeutic interventions.
- Acute hypertensive emergency suspected to be related to an endocrine cause represents one situation where imaging studies to locate a tumor (e.g., pheochromocytoma) may be carried out directly, without adhering to recommendations that imaging should only be carried out once biochemical evidence is clear. Such imaging studies, nevertheless, are only reasonable to consider when there is sufficient evidence to suspect an endocrine cause or when carried out as part of other investigations into associated pathology (e.g., investigation of an aortic dissection).
- Management of the patient presenting with an endocrine cause of hypertensive emergency is not only directed at safely lowering blood pressure, but also must be tailored according to affected end-organs and underlying etiology. The latter can be particularly important in endocrine causes of hypertensive emergencies in which additional therapeutic strategies may be considered (e.g., steroidogenesis inhibitors in Cushing's syndrome) or in which other therapies are contraindicated (e.g., beta-adrenergic blockers in pheochromocytoma).

Endocrine and Metabolic Medical Emergencies: A Clinician's Guide, Second Edition. Edited by Glenn Matfin.

Introduction

Hypertensive emergencies are defined by situations of uncontrolled hypertension resulting in acute or looming end-organ damage (1). Such end-organ involvement includes serious cardiac, vascular, cerebral, and renal complications (Table 22-1). In the severest forms, a hypertensive emergency can present as or progress to multi-organ failure, cardiovascular collapse, and death. Lack of acute life-threatening end-organ damage distinguishes hypertensive emergency, requiring rapid therapeutic intervention, from hypertensive urgency, which may be managed by slower-acting agents and without the necessity for transfer of the patient to an intensive care unit (2,3).

In general, for the patient with a hypertensive emergency, quick-acting antihypertensive drugs are required to bring the blood pressure down and prevent the progression of target organ damage. The nature of end-organ involvement dictates the choice of antihypertensive agent and targeted blood pressure falls. Endocrine causes of hypertensive emergencies require specific drug considerations in view of the underlying pathology. For the patient with pheochromocytoma, certain agents, such as beta-adrenergic receptor blockers, are contraindicated. Thus, management of the patient presenting with a hypertensive emergency is not only directed at safely lowering blood pressure, but also must be tailored according to affected end-organs and underlying etiology (4).

Table 22-1 Spectrum of cardiovascular end organ damage in patients with hypertensive emergencies

- Acute left ventricular failure
- Acute coronary syndrome
- Aortic dissection
- Encephalopathy
- Intracerebral hemorrhage
- Subarachnoidal hemorrhage
- Acute ischemic stroke
- (Sub)acute renal failure
- Eclampsia
- Advanced retinopathy

Hypertensive Emergencies

Hypertensive emergencies presenting as acute coronary syndromes or left ventricular failure are the most common presentation (5). Even in patients without coronary artery disease, myocardial ischemia may result from acute large increases in blood pressure that evoke increases in cardiac oxygen consumption and left ventricular wall stress. Patients presenting with severe hypertension and stroke represent another common emergency situation in which severe elevations of blood pressure may represent the acute precipitating cause overlaying other contributing pathogenic causes. Such emergency conditions are relatively easily identified by standard history, physical, and laboratory evaluations (Table 22-2).

Hypertensive encephalopathy can occur even with mild hypertension (4) and this may be evoked when the mean arterial blood pressure level exceeds the upper blood pressure limit of cerebral blood flow autoregulation. In normotensive individuals this upper limit of mean arterial blood pressure is around 150 mmHg (6). Above this, autoregulation can become overwhelmed, leading to increases in cerebral blood flow proportional to those in blood pressure. This induces cerebral vasodilation, cerebral edema, and subsequent clinical characteristics of acute lethargy, confusion, headache, visual disturbances, and seizures. In patients with established hypertension the window for cerebral blood flow autoregulation is shifted to the right so that a much higher blood pressure may be required to evoke breakthrough of the blood-brain barrier. If untreated, cerebral edema can progress to cerebral hemorrhage, coma, and death.

Among less common hypertensive emergencies, aortic dissection carries the highest risk for rapid fatality (Figure 22-1). Rapid onset severe, sharp or tearing pain in the chest or back is the most common presenting symptom. Patients may have aortic regurgitation, widened pulse pressure, and discrepancies in right and left arm blood pressure

Table 22-2 Tests for patients with hypertensive emergencies

Initial tests for all patients in the emergency situation
- Serum creatinine and estimated glomerular filtration rate (eGFR), plasma sodium and potassium, glucose.
- Urinalysis: protein, cells and cell casts.
- Blood count/smear for microangiopathic hemolysis.
- Electrocardiogram.
- Chest X-ray.
- Fundoscopy to document advanced stage retinopathy.

Optional when indicated in the emergency situation
- Troponin in case of ischemic heart disease.
- Echocardiography in case of suspicion of heart failure.
- CT or MRI of the brain in case of neurological signs/symptoms.
- Transesophageal echocardiography, magnetic resonance angiography or computed tomography angiogram of thorax and abdomen when aortic dissection is suspected.
- CT of abdomen if pheochromocytoma is suspected.

Initital screening tests for endocrine pathologies (for the stabilized patient)
- Plasma free metanephrines or 24-hour urinary fractionated metanephrines.
- Plasma aldosterone and plasma renin concentration or activity.
- 24-hour urinary cortisol or midnight salivary cortisol.

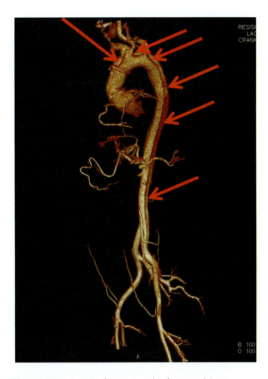

Figure 22-1 Aortic dissection (red arrows) in a 37-year-old male patient with severe hypertension. Computed tomographic volume rendering projection shows aortic dissection type A Stanford after surgical repair of ascending aorta.

readings. In case of a large dissection or rupture, patients can even present with syncope, hypotension or shock. With low cardiac output, patients may present with acute myocardial infarction, stroke, paraplegia, renal failure or limb and visceral ischemia.

In addition to a history of hypertension, evidence of atherosclerotic disease, a vascular inflammatory disorder, cocaine use, pregnancy, or previously diagnosed vascular abnormalities (e.g., aortic aneurysm, bicuspid aortic valve, aortic coarctation) are all risk factors to consider when evaluating the possibility of aortic dissection. Other risk factors include connective tissue diseases, such as due to Marfan or Ehlers-Danlos syndrome. Aortic dissection may also occur as a result of trauma following surgery or an accident. Definitive diagnosis requires transesophageal echocardiography, magnetic resonance angiography or a computed tomography (CT) angiogram.

Pathogenesis

Beyond the originating cause of increased blood pressure, the pathogenesis of end-organ damage in many cases of hypertensive emergencies is suggested to involve disruption of vascular endothelial integrity, increased endothelial permeability with edema and associated inflammatory responses (1). This may be accompanied by arteriolar fibrinoid necrosis and thrombotic microangiopathic hemolysis. Disseminated intravascular coagulation may also follow from loss of endothelial fibrinolytic activity combined with activation of coagulation. It has been postulated that endothelial damage from high blood pressure also triggers release of the prothrombotic von Willebrand factor, which activates intravascular coagulation.

The above pathological processes are considered to follow abrupt vasoconstrictor responses as the initiating step, which may follow the impact of endogenous vasoconstrictors, such as norepinephrine or angiotensin II. Activated sympatho-adrenomedullary, hypothalamo-pituitary-adrenocortical and renin-angiotensin-aldosterone systems underlie endocrine hypertensive emergencies. However, the same systems may also be involved in other situations such as psychogenic stress leading to severe hypertension and Takotsubo cardiomyopathy. Drugs such as cocaine, which alter the disposition of endogenous vasoconstrictors, represent other situations whereby neuronal or endocrine systems may act as mediators of initiating vasoconstrictor responses.

Autocrine/paracrine release of nitric oxide and other vasodilators by the vascular endothelium helps to buffer vasoconstrictor responses. However, these compensatory responses can be overwhelmed when hypertension is severe or sustained. The result can be ischemia with failure of affected end organs; this may involve pro-inflammatory responses with secretion of cytokines and further endothelial damage and vasoconstrictor responses. Breakdown in endothelial integrity may primarily manifest as edema, such as that affecting pulmonary and cerebral organs. Increased platelet aggregation may further promote vasoconstriction and inflammation and lead to thrombosis and ischemic injury to end organs.

Hypertensive Emergencies Associated with Pheochromocytoma

Pheochromocytoma stands out from primary hyperaldosteronism, Cushing's

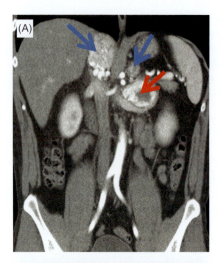

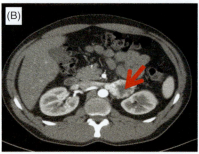

Figure 22-2 Paragangliomas (indicated by arrows) associated with paraganglioma syndome 1 (due to a mutation of the succinate dehydrogenase subunit D gene) in a 39-year-old male patient with severe hypertension. Computed tomographic multiplanar reconstruction of upper abdomen scans show multiple contrast enhanced periaortic masses (panel A). An axial scan at the level of the kidneys and the lower of the three paragangliomas is shown in panel B.

syndrome and thyrotoxicosis as the most prominent endocrine cause of hypertensive emergencies (Figure 22-2). The literature is replete with case reports involving highly diverse situations in which a pheochromocytoma hypertensive crisis involves serious end-organ involvement, in many instances culminating in death (7,8). Acute complications of pheochromocytoma are reported to occur in about 10–20% of all patients (9,10). Although the overall mortality rate of a pheochromocytoma crisis is 15%, patients presenting with acute cardiovascular complications have even a higher mortality rate

(11). Hypertension due to pheochromocytoma results in more severe end-organ damage than that resulting from similarly increased blood pressure in patients with essential hypertension (12), suggesting a blood pressure independent effect due to high catecholamine levels.

As reviewed in detail elsewhere (11), hypertensive emergencies due to pheochromocytoma are wide-ranging. Severe hypertension may be accompanied by myocardial ischemia or infarction (13,14), bradyarrhythmias or tachyarrhythmias (15,16), as well as hypertrophic cardiomyopathy and heart failure (17,18). Strokes and other cerebrovascular accidents have also been reported repeatedly (19–22), including their combination with hypertrophic cardiomyopathy (23, 24). In the above situations, an underlying pheochromocytoma is often difficult to recognize, but should always be considered when acute heart failure is not accompanied by evidence of valvular or coronary artery disease.

Increasingly now described in conjunction with pheochromocytoma are cases of Takotsubo cardiomyopathy (Figure 22-3). Apart from severe hypertension, this form of cardiomyopathy may present with signs and symptoms of an acute coronary syndrome but without significant obstructive coronary artery disease. It has been postulated that pheochromocytoma-related Takotsubo cardiomyopathy is mediated by excessive local myocardial levels of catecholamines, resulting in hyperkinesis of the basal part of the ventricle with apical ballooning. The shape of the left ventricle resembles a Japanese octopus fishing pot, a so-called Takotsubo. In patients diagnosed with symptoms of acute coronary syndrome without coronary artery stenosis or spasm, pheochromocytoma-induced Takotsubo cardiomyopathy should be considered, particularly when accompanied by pronounced blood pressure variability or shock (8,25,26).

Pheochromocytomas occurring in association with acute aortic dissection pose a

Figure 22-3 Echocardiagraphic evidence by apical four chamber (panel A) and two chamber (panel B) views of systolic ballooning of the apical and midportions of the left ventricle associated with significant systolic dysfunction in a 53-year-old patient with Takotsubo cardiomyopathy

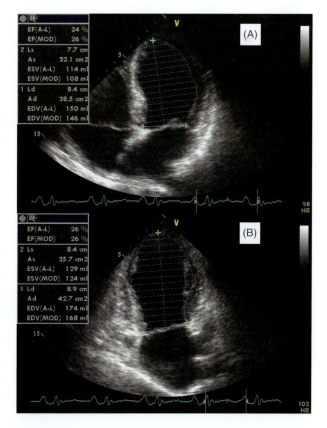

particularly difficult dilemma, with the need for rapid aortic repair balanced against adequate adrenergic blockade in preparing the patient for surgery (27,28). If immediately operated on without blockade, there is a high risk of life-threatening complications secondary to tumoral catecholamine release. Thus, when evaluating imaging studies carried out to diagnose aortic dissection, it is important not to dismiss any adrenal or abdominal mass that could represent the underlying endocrine cause of the condition.

Pulmonary edema, either cardiac or non-cardiac and presenting as severe respiratory distress, is a particularly common emergency condition associated with pheochromocytoma that may present either with other life-threatening conditions or alone as the primary feature of the tumor (29,30). Presumably as a reflection of the vasoconstriction-associated reduced vascular perfusion, pheochromocytomas can also present as acute renal failure or reversible functional renal artery stenosis (31–33). Ischemia combined with actions of catecholamines to reduce intestinal peristalsis and motility is also believed responsible for emergency presentations of intestinal pseudo-obstruction, megacolon, and ischemic colitis in other cases of pheochromocytoma (34–36). In some cases peripheral ischemia may be severe enough to result in gangrene and tissue necrosis (37,38).

Presentation as unexplained shock is one of the most dangerous situations for a patient with an unsuspected pheochromocytoma (39–41). Pheochromocytoma in such situations should be suspected when accompanied by significant abdominal pain, pulmonary edema, intense mydriasis unresponsive to light stimulation, profound weakness, diaphoresis, cyanosis, hyperglycemia, and leukocytosis. Abrupt cessation of catecholamine secretion by the tumor in a patient with a constricted circulatory volume and densensitized adrenoceptors, following prolonged exposure to catecholamines, is thought to represent the main mechanism responsible for shock in this setting. Decreased cardiac output due to catecholamine-induced cardiomyopathy or myocardial infarction may also be contributing factors.

Shock in patients with pheochromocytoma may be accompanied or followed by multiple organ dysfunction syndrome, where early detection of the tumor can be crucial to improve a patient's chances of survival (42–44). Pheochromocytoma multisystem crisis is defined as multiple organ failure, lactic acidosis, temperature often greater than 40°C, encephalopathy and hypertension, and/or hypotension (45). The presentation can easily be mistaken for septicemia, delaying appropriate treatment. Fever and acute inflammatory symptoms may be due to interleukin-6 production by the tumor (46). Therefore, pheochromocytoma should be included in the differential diagnosis of patients with shock.

The hypertensive emergency in a pregnant patient with pheochromocytoma, a situation frequently mistaken for pre-eclampsia, carries a particularly high risk of both maternal and fetal mortality if the tumor remains undiagnosed (47,48). However, if pheochromocytoma is recognized and appropriate countermeasures are made, the prognosis is considerably improved with now close to 85–90% chance of survival for both mother and neonate. Potentially fatal hypertensive crises in unrecognized pregnancies may be precipitated by anesthesia, vaginal delivery, mechanical effects of the gravid uterus, uterine contractions and vigorous fetal movements, and drugs. One of the potentially dangerous drugs frequently used for nausea in pregnancy is the D2-receptor antagonist metoclopramide. This drug may provoke a pheochromocytoma crisis by stimulating tumoral catecholamine release (49,50).

Other Endocrine Causes of Hypertensive Emergencies

A recent Endocrine Society Scientific Statement suggested that hypertension may be the initial clinical presentation for at least 15 endocrine disorders (Figure 22-4) (51).

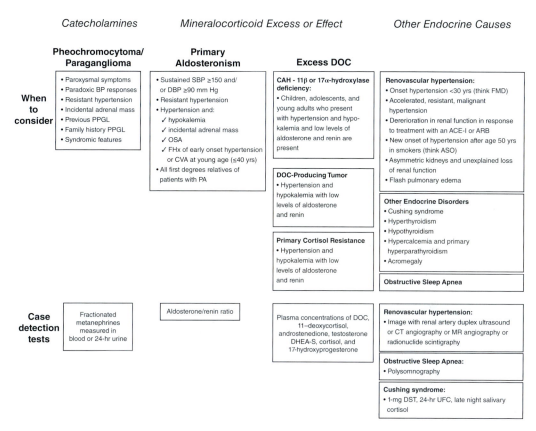

Figure 22-4 When to consider and how to test for endocrine hypertension (51)
ARB = angiotensin II receptor blockers; ASO = arterial switch operation; CT = computerized tomography; CVA = cerebrovascular accident; DBP = diastolic blood pressure; DST = dexamethasone suppression test; FMD = fibromuscular dysplasia; FHx = family history; MR = magnetic resonance; SBP = systolic blood pressure; UFC = urinary free cortisol; PPGL = pheochromocytoma and paraganglioma; DOC = deoxycorticosterone; OSA = obstructive sleep apnea.

Hypertensive emergencies due to Cushing's syndrome can be similarly dangerous as those occurring with pheochromocytoma, but are more rarely described. Patients with hypertension due to hypercortisolism can present with left ventricular failure, pulmonary edema and other end-organ complications (52,53). Cushing's syndrome during pregnancy with uncontrolled hypertension, masquerading as pre-eclampsia, has also been described (54,55). Associated clinical conditions of hypercortisolism, also requiring immediate therapeutic attention, can exacerbate dangers and further increase the high risk of mortality. Such conditions that may contribute to morbidity include electrolyte and metabolic imbalances as well as opportunistic infections or even sepsis related to immune-suppression.

Primary hyperaldosteronism (Figure 22-5) carries a high risk for end-organ damage to the heart, kidney, and arterial walls (56). This is due not only to the high blood pressure, but also the direct deleterious effects of high levels of circulating aldosterone and downstream actions on electrolyte balance (57). Thus, patients with hypertension due to hyperaldosteronism have more severe end-organ damage than those with essential hypertension and similar increases in blood pressure. The mechanism is thought to involve mineralocorticoid receptor activation, which induces oxidative stress, dysfunction, inflammation, and fibrosis of

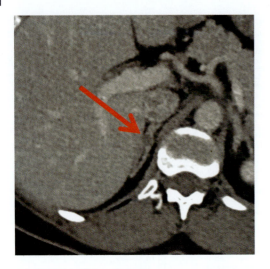

Figure 22-5 Computed tomographic scan of a 43-year-old male patient with primary hyperaldosteronism showing a small hypodense mass in the right adrenal gland.

the vascular wall (58). Current evidence convincingly demonstrates that both surgical and medical treatment strategies have beneficial long-term effects on cardiovascular outcomes and mortality (59). Despite significant end-organ damage in patients with hyperaldosteronism, reports of hypertensive emergencies in the condition are relatively rare (60). This may reflect the typically sustained nature of the associated blood pressure increases and the chronically progressive rather than acute nature of end-organ damage resulting from primary hyperaldosteronism, particularly common in patients with resistant hypertension (61). In a large group of patients with resistant hypertension, the diagnosis of primary aldosteronism was established by confirmatory testing in 11.3% of the population (62). This suggests that the prevalence of PA in patients with resistant hypertension is lower than that reported in the previous smaller studies.

Acute emergencies that do occur in patients with hyperaldosteronism may relate to associated hypokalemia leading to arrhythmias, ventricular fibrillation, and rhabdomyolysis, the latter usually presenting as muscular weakness, limb pain and in severe cases, muscular paralysis. Pulmonary edema has also been reported in isolated cases of severe hypertension in patients with primary hyperaldosteronism (63).

Thyrotoxicosis, presenting in its extreme form as a thyrotoxic crisis (or thyroid storm), can be accompanied by hypertension, though this is not a consistent or a usually primary feature. The more usual key manifestations include fever, often with profuse sweating, tachycardia, arrhythmias and respiratory distress (64). The latter may reflect pulmonary hypertension and right ventricular failure, other manifestations increasingly reported in patients with severe thyrotoxicosis (65–67). The etiology is most commonly Graves' disease, with transition to thyrotoxic crisis usually requiring a secondary contributing cause, such as infection, trauma, or surgery. The condition can involve multi-organ failure with mortality rates reaching 10–20%.

Diagnostic Considerations

In addition to standard laboratory studies (e.g., urinalysis, serum electrolytes, creatinine and derived estimated glomerular filtration rate [eGFR], urea or blood urea nitrogen, blood count) useful to pinpoint end-organ involvement, blood or urine specimens may also be collected for measurements of specific hormones should an endocrine cause of the hypertensive emergency be suspected (Table 22-2). Recommended tests for diagnosis of pheochromocytoma include plasma or urinary fractionated metanephrines (68). For primary hyperaldosteronism, measurements of plasma aldosterone and renin, to yield a ratio of aldosterone to renin, are the recommended first-line test (69). First-line diagnostic tests for Cushing's syndrome include urinary or salivary measurements of cortisol (70).

For patients presenting with hypertensive emergencies, the requirement to immediately institute therapeutic counter-measures supersedes requirements for any useful information that might be provided by endocrine diagnostic testing. Availability of results for these tests invariably involves considerable delay. Some tests, such as those involving

24-hour urine collections for measurements of urinary metanephrines or cortisol, are moreover impractical in the emergency setting for timely delivery of diagnostic test results. Furthermore, since the compounds measured are either stress hormones or metabolites of stress hormones, the very nature of the acute emergency situation renders a high likelihood of false-positive results.

Problems with stress-associated influences on diagnostic test results are particularly problematic for measurements of catecholamines and their O-methylated metabolites, the metanephrines (Figure 22-6).

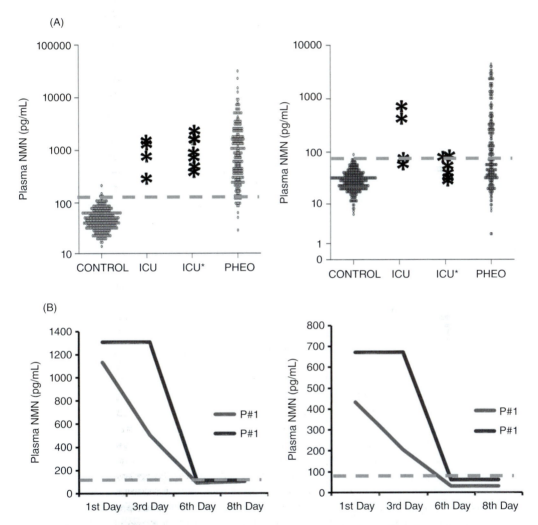

Figure 22-6 (A) Dot-plot logarithmic distributions of plasma concentrations of free normetanephrine (NMN) and metanephrine (MN) in a reference population (CONTROL, n = 262) and a population of patients with pheochromocytoma (PHEO, n = 198) compared to patients without pheochromocytoma sampled in an intensive care unit (ICU) with (ICU*, n = −7) and without (ICU, n = −4) infusions of norepinephrine. Dashed horizontal lines show the upper cut-offs (97.5 percentiles) for the reference population. Note that both groups of ICU patients have concentrations of NMN well above the upper cut-offs of reference intervals that are indistinguishable from concentrations in patients with pheochromocytoma. Additionally, two of the four ICU patients not receiving IV norepinephrine also had plasma concentrations of MN well above the upper cut-offs. (B) Repeated measurements of plasma free NMN and MN in two of the four ICU patients not receiving IV norepinephrine over the 8 days of hospitalization. Note normalization of plasma concentrations of NMN and MN with clinical stabilization.

Although the metanephrines are produced within chromaffin cells and chromaffin cell tumor derivatives by a process that is independent of exocytotic release, the metabolites can also be produced by extra-neuronal metabolism of norepinephrine released by sympathetic nerves and to a minor extent from epinephrine released from the adrenal medulla (71). From this understanding it can be appreciated that there is absolutely no benefit in measurements performed during hypertensive crises. In fact, blood sampling for measurements of plasma metanephrines is most ideally performed under conditions of minimal stress; patients should be lying supine for 30 minutes before blood sampling to minimize sympatho-adrenal activation and reduce likelihood of false-positive results (72).

Precautions to minimize false-positive results are largely impractical in the acute emergency setting. As a result, plasma concentrations of normetanephrine, metanephrine and parent amines in blood samples collected during hypertensive emergencies in patients without pheochromocytoma can run well into the range of concentrations commonly observed in patients with the tumor (Figure 22-6). Plasma levels reaching 10-fold or more above upper cut-offs of reference intervals in such patients without pheochromocytoma can make interpretation of positive test results nearly impossible. Confirming any endocrine cause of a hypertensive emergency by biochemical testing invariably also requires follow-up testing, also impractical in the acute emergency setting. Endocrine diagnostic testing may of course yield negative results that can be used to rule out the tumors. Nevertheless such results are likely to remain unavailable during the critical time of the acute emergency when initial decisions about best management practices must be made.

Taking into account the above considerations, the acute hypertensive emergency represents one situation where imaging studies to locate a tumor may be carried out directly, without adhering to recommendations that imaging should only be carried out once biochemical evidence is clear. Such imaging studies, nevertheless, are only reasonable to consider when there is sufficient evidence to suspect an endocrine cause or when carried out as part of other investigations into associated pathology (e.g., investigation of an aortic dissection). For suspicion of an underlying endocrine cause, awareness of clinical clues is essential (Figure 22-4) (51).

Clues to Endocrine Causes of Hypertensive Emergencies

Apart from sustained or episodic hypertension, patients with pheochromocytoma often present with symptoms of catecholamine excess. While knowledge of the classic symptoms of pheochromocytoma – such as diaphoresis, palpitations, and headaches – may be useful general pointers, such symptoms also commonly occur in patients with hypertensive emergencies. Consideration of familial disease, preceding history, and precipitating factors are more important than symptoms alone for raising the level of suspicion for an underlying pheochromocytoma (Table 22-3).

Among the above considerations, any knowledge gained from the patient or family members on the presence of a mutation in a pheochromocytoma or paraganglioma tumor-susceptibility gene should immediately arouse strong suspicion that the hypertensive emergency results from a catecholamine-producing tumor. Such suspicion need not just require knowledge of a diagnosed mutation in the patient, but can also include a previous history of pheochromocytoma or associated clinical syndrome (e.g., multiple endocrine neoplasia type 2, neurofibromatosis type 1, von Hippel-Lindau syndrome) in family members. If the patient has a history of pheochromocytoma, this should also raise immediate suspicion that the emergency reflects a residual of recurrent

Table 22-3 Clinical clues for considering pheochromocytoma when a patient presents with a hypertensive emergency

- Previous history of pheochromocytoma
- Presence of paroxysmal signs and symptoms known to be associated with pheochromocytoma
- Use of a medication know to elicit a pheochromocytoma crisis
- Pheochromocytoma in first- or second-degree relatives
- Presence of an adrenal incidentaloma
- Family history of hereditary syndromes known to be associated with pheochromocytoma: von Hipple-Lindau syndrome, multiple endocrine neoplasia type 2, neurofibromatosis type 1, familial paraganglioma syndromes
- Diagnosed mutation in a known pheochromocytoma- or paraganglioma-susceptibility gene

disease. A previous history of paroxysmal hypertension or other clinical conditions such as panic attacks can also raise the level of suspicion for a catecholamine-producing tumor.

Among precipitating factors, considerations of medications and drugs known to provoke tumoral catecholamine release can provide particularly useful clues to the possibility of an underlying pheochromocytoma (50). D2-dopamine-receptor antagonists, such as metoclopramide, and beta-adrenergic receptor blockers are better-known classes of drugs established to provoke hypertensive emergencies in patients with pheochromocytoma. Features of hypertensive emergencies due to pheochromocytoma precipitated by beta-adrenergic receptor blockers commonly include severe hypertension, pulmonary edema, in some cases progressing to shock. When such adverse reactions occur in a patient taking beta-adrenergic receptors blockers, pheochromocytoma should be immediately suspected.

Other drugs documented to result in hypertensive emergencies in patients with pheochromocytoma include tricyclic antidepressants, monoamine oxidase inhibitors, and sympathomimetics (50). Corticosteroids, including dexamethasone, prednisone and hydrocortisone, are also agents now increasingly recognized to cause hypertensive crises in patients with an unsuspected pheochromocytoma, in some cases culminating in multi-organ failure and death (73,74). Thus, pheochromocytoma should be strongly suspected in any patient presenting with a hypertensive emergency after administration of steroids.

Other emergencies where pheochromocytoma should be strongly suspected are those occurring during surgical anesthesia or physical procedures, insults or changes in physiology involving compression of an unsuspected catecholamine-producing tumor. Included among the latter are pregnancy, childbirth, and micturition-induced hypertensive emergencies in cases of patients with bladder paraganglioma.

Clues to other endocrine causes of hypertensive emergencies, such as Cushing's syndrome, primary hyperaldosteronism and thyrotoxicosis are in most cases best provided from physical and routine laboratory evaluations. For Cushing's syndrome, features such as the classic moon face, buffalo hump, abdominal striae, ecchymoses, osteoporosis, depression, and hirsutism in women should arouse suspicion. Extremely low potassium should arouse suspicion of primary hyperaldosteronism, but apart from this, there are only few clear physical or laboratory findings that might immediately signal aldosterone excess in such patients. Plasma potassium is, however, only decreased in one out of every three patients with primary hyperaldosteronism. Another factor complicating the use of potassium is the fact that when the patient presents with a hypertensive emergency, potassium is usually low, due to the activation of the renin-aldosterone-angiotensin system. An enlarged thyroid gland, extreme tachycardia, history of weight loss, diarrhea, and exophthalmos can signal thyrotoxicosis, but often there should also be a history of Graves' disease or another recognized contributing condition.

Treatment of Hypertensive Emergencies

In most cases of hypertensive emergencies, the first goal is a partial reduction and not necessarily normalization of blood pressure (75). Guidelines recommend that treatment of hypertensive emergencies should take into consideration the nature of the associated organ damage, with a range in treatment from no or extremely cautious lowering of blood pressure in acute stroke to prompt and aggressive blood pressure reduction in acute pulmonary edema or aortic dissection. Except for acute stroke, these recommendations are not based on randomized controlled trials comparing aggressive with conservative blood pressure lowering but only on long-standing clinical experience.

Rapid lowering of blood pressure is particularly contraindicated in patients with cerebrovascular end-organ involvement, in whom excessive reduction of blood pressure can lead to extension of stroke (76). In contrast, in the patient with aortic dissection, rapid lowering of systolic blood pressure to at least to 120 mmHg within 20 minutes has been advocated.

There are a number of parenteral agents that may be used for first-line acute lowering of blood pressure, with choice tailored according to the presentation, type of emergency, and etiology (Table 22-4). In acute coronary syndrome, the use of intravenous (IV) nitroglycerine as vasodilator can be combined with a beta-adrenergic receptor blocker such as esmolol or metoprolol to reduce heart rate and myocardial oxygen consumption. Among these agents, esmolol is most useful due to its rapid onset and short duration of action allowing titration of dosage. The combined alpha- and beta-adrenergic blocking agent, labetalol, is an alternative.

For control of volume over-load in patients with a hypertensive emergency and left ventricular heart failure, IV nitroglycerine or sodium nitroprusside should be combined with a loop diuretic. In cases of aortic dissection, labetalol or the combination of esmolol and nitroprusside can be used to minimize stress on the aortic wall and prevent spread of the dissection.

Use of antihypertensives in acute stroke can be complicated by impaired autoregulation of cerebral blood flow in ischemic areas such that blood pressure reduction may further reduce flow to affected brain areas and expand the size of the infarct. Because of this it has been suggested to consider antihypertensive therapy in patients with ischemic stroke only when blood pressures exceed 220/120 mmHg (76). Even then, blood pressure should be reduced only gradually. Labetalol is most commonly used for this indication. Lower blood pressure thresholds (systolic >180 mmHg) for initiating antihypertensive therapy are, however, called for in patients with cerebral hemorrhage. Nicardipine or labetalol and sodium nitroprusside can be used for patients with acute hemorrhagic stroke. In the case of hypertensive encephalopathy, either labetalol or nicardipine can be used.

Treatment of Pheochromocytoma-Related Hypertensive Emergencies

Hypertensive emergencies in patients with pheochromocytoma are best treated with IV infusions of rapidly acting alpha-adrenergic receptor antagonists such as phentolamine or urapidil, but sodium nitroprusside, and nicardipine are reasonable alternatives. More recently employed antihypertensive agents include clevidipine, an ultra-short acting IV dihydropyridine calcium-channel blocker approved by the Food and Drug Administration (FDA) for use in treatment of hypertensive emergencies (77). The agent has some unique pharmacodynamic and pharmacokinetic properties that in clinical trials have shown promise in comparison to other agents, including nicardipine, nitroglycerin and sodium nitroprusside. Use of the drug during intra-operative management of patients with pheochromocytoma

Table 22-4 Available drugs for acute treatment of hypertensive emergencies

Drug	Indication	Dose	Adverse effects
Sodium nitroprusside	Most hypertensive emergencies except in ischemic heart disease and eclampsia. Not when renal or liver failure is present	Start: 0.3–10 µg/kg/min; increase by 0.5 µg/kg/min every 5 minutes	Cyanide toxicity, Methemoglobinemia, Increased intracranial pressure
Nitroglycerine	Ischemic heart disease	Start: 5–100 µg/min; increase by 5 µg/min every 5 minutes	Flushing Headache Tolerance
Nicardipine	Most hypertensive emergencies Not for ischemic heart disease and heart failure	Start: 5 mg/hr, increase by 2.5 mg every 15–30 minutes until 15 mg/hr	Reflex tachycardia Increased intracranial pressure
Clevidipine	Most hypertensive emergencies Not for ischemic heart disease and heart failure	Start: 1–2 mg/hr then titrate to maximum of 16 mg/hr	Reflex tachycardia Increased intracranial pressure Soy allergy
Labetalol	Most hypertensive emergencies except pheochromcytoma, acute heart failure 2nd or 3rd degree AV block and bronchoconstrictive disease	Start: 1–2 mg/min. Increase every 10 minutes by 1 mg/min until maximum dose of 20 mg/24 hr	
Esmolol	Most hypertensive emergencies except for pheochromcytoma, acute heart failure 2nd or 3rd degree AV block and bronchoconstrictive disease	Start: 80 mg bolus in 30 seconds, then 150 µg/kg/min	
Phentolamine	Hypertensive emergencies due to catecholamine excess, e.g., pheochromcoytoma	2.5–5 mg bolus and repeat after 5–10 minutes Continuous: 0.5–1.0 mg/hr	Flushing Headache Tachycardia
Fenoldopam	Most hypertensive emergencies, in particular acute renal failure	0.1–0.6 µg/kg/min	Flushing Headache Tachycardia
Urapidil	Hypertensive emergencies due to catecholamine excess, e.g., pheochromcoytoma	12.5–50 mg as bolus. Continuous: 1–10 µg/kg/min	Headache

has been described (78,79). Phentolamine may be given as an IV bolus of 2.5 mg to 5 mg at 1 mg/min, with the dose repeated every 5–10 minutes, or as a continuous infusion (100 mg of phentolamine in 500 mL of 5% dextrose in water) of 0.5–1.0 mg/hour

with doses adjusted to the blood pressure response.

A less used but effective predominantly arterial vasodilator is magnesium sulfate. To achieve a rapid effect, a bolus (4 g in 5 minutes) is administered intravenously, followed by a continuous infusion of 1 g/hr (Table 22-4). The agent inhibits catecholamine release, blocks adrenergic receptors, and improves hemodynamic control and is also effective in treating catecholamine-induced arrhythmias (80,81). Magnesium sulfate has an acceptable safety profile and is well suited for children and pregnant women with a pheochromocytoma. It should not be combined with calcium antagonists because of an increased risk of hypotension. During continuous infusion it is advised to check plasma magnesium levels which should remain between 2–4 mmol/L. Urapidil, a selective alpha$_1$-adrenoceptor blocker, can also be administered in IV bolus doses or by infusion (Table 22-4).

Beta-adrenergic blockers may be used to treat arrhythmias or tachycardia, the latter often arising as a reflex to vasodilators, but only after adequate blockade of alpha-adrenoceptor-mediated vasoconstriction. The danger of using beta-adrenergic receptor blockers without first blocking alpha-adrenergic receptors has been documented in numerous case studies of hypertensive emergencies in patients with unsuspected pheochromocytoma receiving beta-adrenergic receptor blockers (for review, see [50]). The mechanism is believed to involve inhibition of beta$_2$-adrenoceptor-mediated vasodilation, leaving alpha-adrenoceptor-mediated vasoconstrictor response to catecholamines unopposed. Importantly, such adverse reactions have been documented in numerous reports for the mixed adrenoceptor blocker, labetalol (82–88). This is likely due to the fact that the non-selective beta-adrenergic receptor blocking actions of labetalol predominate over the alpha-adrenergic receptor blocking actions at a 7:1 ratio (when used intravenously). Therefore, labetalol should not be used in any patient with a hypertensive emergency when there is real suspicion of pheochromocytoma.

For patients presenting with shock and multiorgan failure, therapeutic options are limited in circumstances when an underlying pheochromocytoma is suspected. In some patients with catecholamine-induced shock, vasoconstriction may be so severe that reliable blood pressure measurements are compromised, obscuring severe central hypertension. In this situation, assessment of volume status and cardiac function is critical. Volume expansion becomes important once hypovolemic shock is clearly identified.

For the patient with multisystem crisis or shock, it is imperative to correct metabolic acidosis and improve peripheral perfusion with judicious use of colloids and/or crystalloids. Renal function should also be assessed and protected as necessary. Identification and correction of hypocalcemia may also be particularly important in patients with pheochromocytoma-associated cardiogenic shock (89). In such situations, replacement of ionized calcium may preserve cardiac function and reduce mortality.

Pulmonary edema is common in cases of pheochromocytoma-associated hypertensive emergencies and may require intubation and lung-protective ventilatory strategies to maintain oxygenation. Hypertensive encephalopathy, hyperthermia, hyperglycemia and hepatic failure may further complicate prognosis and therapeutic options in patients with multisystem organ failure and add to the high mortality of this condition.

If pheochromocytoma is suspected in a patient with a hypertensive emergency, any requirement for biochemical confirmation of catecholamine excess is largely made impractical by the seriousness of the patient's condition and likely delay in obtaining laboratory results. Immediate attempts are better made to localize the lesion, with abdominal CT the most practical imaging option in patients on cardiac and ventilatory support. Carefully considered and planned surgery may present the only chance for a successful outcome in patients with multisystem crisis (40, 44,90,91). However, emergency resection of pheochromocytoma without adequate preoperative preparation is associated with high surgical morbidity and mortality and thus remains controversial (92). If the patient can be stabilized, it is preferable that surgery be carried out after preparation with recommended alpha-adrenergic receptor blockers or other agents to block the hemodynamic effects of catecholamines produced by the tumors (93).

Treatment of a hypertensive emergency in a pregnant patient with a pheochromocytoma remains one of the most difficult therapeutic challenges for a clinician since the life of both the mother and the fetus is at stake. Once the pheochromocytoma is discovered, acute treatment of the hypertensive crisis, with some caveats, is not different from a non-pregnant woman with pheochromocytoma. Nicardipine might be the drug to start with but some prefer phentolamine. In pregnancy the use of IV magnesium sulfate has been advocated, with a mechanism of action thought to involve vasodilation as well reductions in the release and effects of catecholamines (80). Combined adminstration of nicardipine and magnesium sulfate might act synergistically and cause unwanted excessive blood pressure reductions. Some drugs such as sodium nitroprusside are not desirable due to the risk of fetal cyanide intoxication. A multidisciplinary approach by obstetrician, surgeon, endocrinologist and anesthesiologist is essential to achieve optimal outcome.

Treatment of Other Endocrine Hypertensive Emergencies

In severe enough cases of hypertensive emergencies in Cushing's syndrome, IV etomidate or administration of other fast-acting steroidogenesis inhibitors may be initiated to provide immediate relief, but as in pheochromocytoma, surgical intervention provides the only cure (51,52,94). Bilateral adrenalectomy may be employed as an emergency surgical procedure even in the more common cases of ACTH-dependent Cushing's syndrome (95). In such cases steroid replacement therapy must be initiated immediately during surgery to avoid associated dangers of adrenal insufficiency, particularly cardiovascular collapse.

Conclusions

Most of the numerous blood pressure lowering drugs can be used to treat patients with hypertensive emergencies, with treatment practices varying considerably due to paucity of evidence-based randomized trials to support use of one agent over another (96). Nevertheless, lower-level evidence and inferential reasoning strongly suggest that choice of therapeutic agents and mode of therapy should be tailored according to clinical presentation and affected end-organs, with additional considerations of etiology. The latter can be particularly important in endocrine causes of hypertensive emergencies in which additional therapeutic strategies may be considered (e.g., steroidogenesis inhibitors in Cushing's syndrome) or in which other therapies are contraindicated (e.g., beta-adrenergic blockers in pheochromocytoma). Standard blood or urine tests to diagnose endocrine causes of hypertensive emergencies are rendered largely irrelevant due to issues of time and stress-associated false-positive results. Rather, recognition of endocrine causes of hypertensive crises primarily requires appreciation of clinical features and precipitating stimuli.

References

1 Vaughan CJ, Delanty N. Hypertensive emergencies. *Lancet*. 2000;356(9227): 411–417.

2 Moser M, Izzo JL, Jr., Bisognano J. Hypertensive emergencies. *J Clin Hypertens (Greenwich)*. 2006;8(4):275–281.

3 Rosei EA, Salvetti M, Farsang C. European Society of Hypertension Scientific Newsletter: treatment of hypertensive urgencies and emergencies. *J Hypertension*. 2006;24(12): 2482–2485.

4 Kaplan NM. Management of hypertensive emergencies. *Lancet*. 1994;344(8933): 1335–1338.

5 Zampaglione B, Pascale C, Marchisio M, Cavallo-Perin P. Hypertensive urgencies and emergencies: prevalence and clinical presentation. *Hypertension*. 1996;27(1):144–147.

6 Strandgaard S, Jones JV, MacKenzie ET, Harper AM. Upper limit of cerebral blood flow autoregulation in experimental renovascular hypertension in the baboon. *Circulation Res*. 1975;37(2):164–167.

7 Brouwers FM, Eisenhofer G, Lenders JW, Pacak K. Emergencies caused by pheochromocytoma, neuroblastoma, or ganglioneuroma. *Endocrin Metab Clin North Am*. 2006;35(4):699–724.

8 Prejbisz A, Lenders JW, Eisenhofer G, Januszewicz A. Cardiovascular manifestations of phaeochromocytoma. *J Hypertension*. 2011;29(11):2049–2060.

9 Amar L, Eisenhofer G. Clinical question: diagnosing phaeochromocytoma/ paraganglioma in a patient presenting with critical illness: biochemistry versus imaging. *Clin Endocrin*. 2015.

10 Riester A, Weismann D, Quinkler M, et al. Life-threatening events in patients with pheochromocytoma. *European J Endocrin/European Federation of Endocrine Societies*. 2015;173(6):757–764.

11 Whitelaw BC, Prague JK, Mustafa OG, et al. Phaeochromocytoma [corrected] crisis. *Clinic Endocrin*. 2014;80(1):13–22.

12 Stolk RF, Bakx C, Mulder J, Timmers HJ, Lenders JW. Is the excess cardiovascular morbidity in pheochromocytoma related to blood pressure or to catecholamines? *J Clin Endocrin Metab*. 2013;98(3):1100–1106.

13 Garg A, Banitt PF. Pheochromocytoma and myocardial infarction. *South Med J*. 2004;97(10):981–984.

14 Brown H, Goldberg PA, Selter JG, et al. Hemorrhagic pheochromocytoma associated with systemic corticosteroid therapy and presenting as myocardial infarction with severe hypertension. *J Clin Endocrin Metab*. 2005;90(1):563–569.

15 Petit T, de Lagausie P, Maintenant J, Magnier S, Nivoche Y, Aigrain Y. Thoracic pheochromocytoma revealed by ventricular tachycardia: clinical case and review of the literature. *Eur J Pediatr Surg*. 2000;10(2):142–144.

16 Tzemos N, McNeill GP, Jung RT, MacDonald TM. Post exertional broad complex tachycardia in a normotensive patient: a rare presentation of phaeochromocytoma. *Scott Med J*. 2001;46(1):14–15.

17 Wood R, Commerford PJ, Rose AG, Tooke A. Reversible catecholamine-induced cardiomyopathy. *Am Heart J*. 1991;121(2 Pt 1):610–613.

18 Giavarini A, Chedid A, Bobrie G, Plouin PF, Hagege A, Amar L. Acute catecholamine cardiomyopathy in patients with phaeochromocytoma or functional paraganglioma. *Heart*. 2013.

19 Moritani H, Sakamoto M, Yoshida Y, Nasu H, Nemoto R, Nakamura I. Pheochromocytoma of the urinary bladder revealed with cerebral hemorrhage. *Intern Med*. 2001;40(7):638–642.

20 Van YH, Wang HS, Lai CH, Lin JN, Lo FS. Pheochromocytoma presenting as stroke in two Taiwanese children. *J Pediatr Endocrinol Metab*. 2002;15(9): 1563–1567.

21 Chuang HL, Hsu WH, Hsueh C, Lin JN, Scott RM. Spontaneous intracranial hemorrhage caused by pheochromocytoma in a child. *Pediatr Neurosurg*. 2002;36(1):48–51.

22 Petramala L, Cavallaro G, Polistena A, et al. Multiple catecholamine-secreting paragangliomas: diagnosis after hemorrhagic stroke in a young woman. *Endoc Prac*. 2008;14(3):340–346.

23 Cohen JK, Cisco RM, Scholten A, Mitmaker E, Duh QY. Pheochromocytoma crisis resulting in acute heart failure and cardioembolic stroke in a 37-year-old man. *Surgery*. 2013.

24 Vindenes T, Crump N, Casenas R, Wood K. Pheochromocytoma causing cardiomyopathy, ischemic stroke and acute arterial thrombosis: a case report and

review of the literature. *Connecticut Med.* 2013;77(2):95–98.

25 Gianni M, Dentali F, Grandi AM, Sumner G, Hiralal R, Lonn E. Apical ballooning syndrome or takotsubo cardiomyopathy: a systematic review. *Europ Heart J.* 2006;27(13):1523–1529.

26 De Backer TL, De Buyzere ML, Taeymans Y, Kunnen P, Rubens R, Clement DL. Cardiac involvement in pheochromocytoma. *J Hum Hypertension.* 2000;14(7):469–471.

27 Triplett JC, Atuk NO. Dissecting aortic aneurysm associated with pheochromocytoma. *South Med J.* 1975;68(6):748, 53.

28 Bowen FW, Civan J, Orlin A, Gleason T. Management of type A aortic dissection and a large pheochromocytoma: a surgical dilemma. *Ann Thor Surg.* 2006;81(6):2296–2298.

29 de Leeuw PW, Waltman FL, Birkenhager WH. Noncardiogenic pulmonary edema as the sole manifestation of pheochromocytoma. *Hypertension.* 1986;8(9):810–812.

30 Desai AS, Chutkow WA, Edelman E, Economy KE, Dec GW, Jr. Clinical problem-solving: a crisis in late pregnancy. *N Eng J Med.* 2009;361(23):2271–2277.

31 Shemin D, Cohn PS, Zipin SB. Pheochromocytoma presenting as rhabdomyolysis and acute myoglobinuric renal failure. *Arch Int Med.* 1990;150(11):2384–2385.

32 Kuzmanovska D, Sahpazova E, Kocova M, Damjanovski G, Popov Z. Phaeochromocytoma associated with reversible renal artery stenosis. *Nephr, Dial, Transp.* 2001;16(10):2092–2094.

33 Gillett MJ, Arenson RV, Yew MK, Thompson IJ, Irish AB. Diagnostic challenges associated with a complex case of cystic phaeochromocytoma presenting with malignant hypertension, microangiopathic haemolysis and acute renal failure. *Nephr, Dial, Transp.* 2005;20(5):1014.

34 Turner CE. Gastrointestinal pseudo-obstruction due to pheochromocytoma. *The American J Gastroenterology.* 1983;78(4):214–217.

35 Sweeney AT, Malabanan AO, Blake MA, de las Morenas A, Cachecho R, Melby JC. Megacolon as the presenting feature in pheochromocytoma. *J Clin Endocrin Metab.* 2000;85(11):3968–3972.

36 Wu HW, Liou WP, Chou CC, Chen YH, Loh CH, Wang HP. Pheochromocytoma presented as intestinal pseudo-obstruction and hyperamylasemia. *Am J Emerg Med.* 2008;26(8):971 e1–e4.

37 Tack CJ, Lenders JW. Pheochromocytoma as a cause of blue toes. *Arch Int Med.* 1993;153(17):2061.

38 Lutchman D, Buchholz S, Keightley C. Phaeochromocytoma-associated critical peripheral ischaemia. *Int Med J.* 2010;40(2):150–153.

39 Bergland BE. Pheochromocytoma presenting as shock. *Am J Emerg Med.* 1989;7(1):44–48.

40 Mohamed HA, Aldakar MO, Habib N. Cardiogenic shock due to acute hemorrhagic necrosis of a pheochromocytoma: a case report and review of the literature. *Can J Cardiol.* 2003;19(5):573–576.

41 Hanna JS, Spencer PJ, Savopoulou C, Kwasnik E, Askari R. Spontaneous adrenal pheochromocytoma rupture complicated by intraperitoneal hemorrhage and shock. *World J Emerg Surg.* 2011;6(1):27.

42 Kolhe N, Stoves J, Richardson D, Davison AM, Gilbey S. Hypertension due to phaeochromocytoma–an unusual cause of multiorgan failure. *Nephr, Dial, Transp.* 2001;16(10):2100–2104.

43 Herbland A, Bui N, Rullier A, Vargas F, Gruson D, Hilbert G. Multiple organ failure as initial presentation of pheochromytoma. *Am J Emerg Med.* 2005;23(4):565–566.

44 Moran ME, Rosenberg DJ, Zornow DH. Pheochromocytoma multisystem crisis. *Urology.* 2006;67(4):846 e19–e20.

45 Newell KA, Prinz RA, Pickleman J, et al. Pheochromocytoma multisystem crisis: a surgical emergency. *Arch Surg.* 1988;123(8):956–959.

46 Kang JM, Lee WJ, Kim WB, et al. Systemic inflammatory syndrome and hepatic inflammatory cell infiltration caused by an interleukin-6 producing pheochromocytoma. *Endocr J.* 2005;52(2):193–198.

47 Mannelli M, Bemporad D. Diagnosis and management of pheochromocytoma during pregnancy. *J Endocrin Invest.* 2002;25(6):567–571.

48 Lenders JW. Pheochromocytoma and pregnancy: a deceptive connection. *European J Endocrin/European Federation of Endocrine Societies.* 2012;166(2): 143–150.

49 Takai Y, Seki H, Kinoshita K. Pheochromocytoma in pregnancy manifesting hypertensive crisis induced by metoclopramide. *Int J Gynaecol Obstet.* 1997;59(2):133–137.

50 Eisenhofer G, Rivers G, Rosas AL, Quezado Z, Manger WM, Pacak K. Adverse drug reactions in patients with phaeochromocytoma: incidence, prevention and management. *Drug Saf.* 2007;30(11):1031–1062.

51 Young WF, Calhour DA, Lenders JWM, Stowasser M, Textor SC. Screening for endocrine hypertension: an endocrine society scientific statement. *Endocr Rev.* 2017;38(2):103–122. doi: 10.1210/er.2017-00054

52 Kamenicky P, Droumaguet C, Salenave S, et al. Mitotane, metyrapone, ketoconazole combination therapy as an alternative to rescue adrenalectomy for severe ACTH-dependent Cushing's syndrome. *J Clin Endocrinol Metab.* 2011;96(9): 2796–2804.

53 von Stempel C, Perks C, Corcoran J, Grayez J. Cardio-respiratory failure secondary to ectopic Cushing's syndrome as the index presentation of small-cell lung cancer. *BMJ Case Reports.* 2013;2013.

54 Choi WJ, Jung TS, Paik WY. Cushing's syndrome in pregnancy with a severe maternal complication: a case report. *J Obstet Gyn Res.* 2011;37(2):163–167.

55 Lim WH, Torpy DJ, Jeffries WS. The medical management of Cushing's syndrome during pregnancy. *European J Obstet, Gyn, Rep Biol.* 2013;168(1):1–6.

56 Prejbisz A, Warchol-Celinska E, Lenders JW, Januszewicz A. Cardiovascular risk in primary hyperaldosteronism. *Horm. Metab. Res = Hormon- und Stoffwechselforschung = Hormones et metabolisme.* 2015;47(13):973–980.

57 Born-Frontsberg E, Reincke M, Rump LC, et al. Cardiovascular and cerebrovascular comorbidities of hypokalemic and normokalemic primary aldosteronism: results of the German Conn's Registry. *J Clin Endocrinol Metab.* 2009;94(4): 1125–1130.

58 Marney AM, Brown NJ. Aldosterone and end-organ damage. *Clin Sci (Lond).* 2007;113(6):267–278.

59 Reincke M, Fischer E, Gerum S, et al. Observational study mortality in treated primary aldosteronism: the German Conn's registry. *Hypertension.* 2012;60(3):618–624.

60 Labinson PT, White WB, Tendler BE, Mansoor GA. Primary hyperaldosteronism associated with hypertensive emergencies. *Am J Hypertension.* 2006;19(6):623–627.

61 Calhoun DA. Aldosteronism and hypertension. *Clin J Am Soc Nephr: CJASN.* 2006;1(5):1039–1045.

62 Douma S, Petidis K, Doumas M, et al. Prevalence of primary hyperaldosteronism in resistant hypertension: a retrospective observational study. *Lancet.* 2008;371(9628):1921–1926.

63 Prejbisz A, Klisiewicz A, Januszewicz A, et al. 22-year-old patient with malignant hypertension associated with primary aldosteronism. *J Hum Hyper.* 2013;27(2):138–140.

64 Carroll R, Matfin G. Endocrine and metabolic emergencies: thyroid storm. *Ther Advances Endocrin Metab.* 2010;1(3):139–145.

65 Soroush-Yari A, Burstein S, Hoo GW, Santiago SM. Pulmonary hypertension in men with thyrotoxicosis. *Respiration.* 2005;72(1):90–94.

66 Paran Y, Nimrod A, Goldin Y, Justo D. Pulmonary hypertension and predominant

right heart failure in thyrotoxicosis. *Resuscitation*. 2006;69(2):339–341.

67 Suk JH, Cho KI, Lee SH, et al. Prevalence of echocardiographic criteria for the diagnosis of pulmonary hypertension in patients with Graves' disease: before and after antithyroid treatment. *J Endocrin Inves*. 2011;34(8):e229–e234.

68 Pacak K, Eisenhofer G, Ahlman H, et al. Pheochromocytoma: recommendations for clinical practice from the First International Symposium. *Nature Clin Prac Endocrin Metab*. 2007;3(2):92–102.

69 Funder JW, Carey RM, Mantero F, et al. The management of primary aldosteronism: case detection, diagnosis, treatment: an Endocrine Society Clinical Practice Guideline. *J Clin Endocrin Metab*. 2016;101:1889–1916.

70 Nieman LK, Biller BM, Findling JW, et al. The diagnosis of Cushing's syndrome: an Endocrine Society Clinical Practice Guideline. *J Clin Endocrin Metab*. 2008;93(5):1526–1540.

71 Eisenhofer G, Huynh TT, Hiroi M, Pacak K. Understanding catecholamine metabolism as a guide to the biochemical diagnosis of pheochromocytoma. *Rev Endocr Metab Disord*. 2001;2(3):297–311.

72 Grossman A, Pacak K, Sawka A, et al. Biochemical diagnosis and localization of pheochromocytoma: can we reach a consensus? *Ann New York Acad Sci*. 2006;1073:332–347.

73 Rosas AL, Kasperlik-Zaluska AA, Papierska L, Bass BL, Pacak K, Eisenhofer G. Pheochromocytoma crisis induced by glucocorticoids: a report of four cases and review of the literature. *Europ J Endocrin/ European Federation of Endocrine Societies*. 2008;158(3):423–429.

74 Barrett C, van Uum SH, Lenders JW. Risk of catecholaminergic crisis following glucocorticoid administration in patients with an adrenal mass: a literature review. *Clin Endocrinol*. 2015;83(5):622–628.

75 Elliott WJ. Management of hypertension emergencies. *Current Hypertension Rep*. 2003;5(6):486–492.

76 Bath P, Chalmers J, Powers W, et al., International Society of Hypertension (ISH): Statement on the management of blood pressure in acute stroke. *J Hypertension*. 2003;21(4):665–672.

77 Sarafidis PA, Georgianos PI, Malindretos P, Liakopoulos V. Pharmacological management of hypertensive emergencies and urgencies: focus on newer agents. *Exp Opin Inves Drugs*. 2012;21(8):1089–1106.

78 Kline JP. Use of clevidipine for intraoperative hypertension caused by an undiagnosed pheochromocytoma: a case report. *AANA*. 2010;78(4):288–290.

79 Bettesworth JG, Martin DP, Tobias JD. Intraoperative use of clevidipine in a patient with Von Hippel-Lindau disease with associated pheochromocytoma. *J Cardio Vasc Anes*. 2013;27(4):749–751.

80 James MF, Cronje L. Pheochromocytoma crisis: the use of magnesium sulfate. *Anesthes Analg*. 2004;99(3):680–686.

81 Herroeder S, Schonherr ME, De Hert SG, Hollmann MW. Magnesium: essentials for anesthesiologists. *Anesthesiology*. 2011;114(4):971–993.

82 Briggs RS, Birtwell AJ, Pohl JE. Hypertensive response to labetalol in phaeochromocytoma. *Lancet*. 1978;1(8072):1045–1046.

83 FitzGerald GA. Hypertensive response to labetalol in phaeochromocytoma. *Lancet*. 1978;1(8076):1259.

84 Feek CM, Earnshaw PM. Hypertensive response to labetalol in phaeochromocytoma. *BMJ*. 1980;281 (6236):387.

85 Sheaves R, Chew SL, Grossman AB. The dangers of unopposed beta-adrenergic blockade in phaeochromocytoma. *Postgrad Med J*. 1995;71(831):58–59.

86 Chung PC, Li AH, Lin CC, Yang MW. Elevated vascular resistance after labetalol during resection of a pheochromocytoma (brief report). *Can J Anaesth*. 2002;49(2):148–150.

87 Petrie J, Lockie C, Paolineli A, et al. Undiagnosed phaeochromocytoma masquerading as eclampsia. *BMJ Case Reports*. 2012;2012.

88 Kuok CH, Yen CR, Huang CS, Ko YP, Tsai PS. Cardiovascular collapse after labetalol for hypertensive crisis in an undiagnosed pheochromocytoma during cesarean section. *Acta Anaesthesiologica Taiwanica*. 2011;49(2):69–71.

89 Olson SW, Deal LE, Piesman M. Epinephrine-secreting pheochromocytoma presenting with cardiogenic shock and profound hypocalcemia. *Ann Intern Med*. 2004;140(10):849–851.

90 Uchida N, Ishiguro K, Suda T, Nishimura M. Pheochromocytoma multisystem crisis successfully treated by emergency surgery: report of a case. *Surg Today*. 2010;40(10):990–996.

91 Salinas CL, Gomez Beltran OD, Sanchez-Hidalgo JM, Bru RC, Padillo FJ, Rufian S. Emergency adrenalectomy due to acute heart failure secondary to complicated pheochromocytoma: a case report. *World J Surg Oncol*. 2011;9:49.

92 Scholten A, Cisco RM, Vriens MR, et al. Pheochromocytoma crisis is not a surgical emergency. *J Clin Endocrin Metab*. 2013;98(2):581–591.

93 Lenders JWM, Duh QY, Eisenhofer G, et al. Pheochromocytoma and paraganglioma: An Endocrine Society Clinical Practice Guideline. *J Clin Endocrinol Metab*. 2014;99:1915–1942.

94 Lutgers HL, Vergragt J, Dong PV, et al. Severe hypercortisolism: a medical emergency requiring urgent intervention. *Critl Care Med*.2010;38(7):1598–1601.

95 Biller BM, Grossman AB, Stewart PM, et al. Treatment of adrenocorticotropin-dependent Cushing's syndrome: a consensus statement. *J Clin Endocrinol Metab*. 2008;93(7):2454–2462.

96 Perez MI, Musini VM. Pharmacological interventions for hypertensive emergencies: a Cochrane Systematic Review. *J Hum Hyper*. 2008;22(9):596–607.

Part VII

Calcium, Phosphate, and Metabolic Bone Diseases

Introduction

Emergency Management of Calcium, Phosphate, and Metabolic Bone Diseases

John P. Bilezikian

Key points

- Clinical disorders of calcium, phosphate, and metabolic bone diseases are now being defined in biochemical, structural, and molecular terms.
- The most prevalent of these diseases is osteoporosis, a disorder of skeletal microstructure, usually typified by reduced bone mineral density, leading to an increased risk of fracture.
- The therapeutic landscape of osteoporosis continues to move forward with various formulations of bisphosphonates; another antiresorptive class, RANKL inhibition, in the formulation of denosumab; and with availability of two osteoanabolic therapies, teriparatide rhPTH(1-34) and abaloparatide (an analogue of PTHrP). In development is an antisclerostin agent, romosozumab.
- Disorders of the parathyroid glands, as seen in primary and secondary hyperparathyroid states, and, in hypoparathyroidism, have led to new insights into how parathyroid hormone controls mineral metabolism. More recently, hypoparathyroidism is the last of the classical endocrine deficiency diseases for which the replacement hormone, rhPTH(1-84) has become available.

The field of bone and mineral metabolism has become established, over the past 5 decades, as a key endocrinological discipline. With the great Fuller Albright leading the way, even earlier, clinical disorders of calcium metabolism are now being defined in biochemical, structural, and molecular terms. The most prevalent of these diseases is osteoporosis, a disorder of skeletal microstructure, usually typified by reduced bone mineral density, leading to an increased risk of fracture. The diagnosis of osteoporosis can be made by the occurrence of the fragility fracture itself or by a bone density measurement. The advent of the dual energy x-ray absorptiometer (DXA) in the late 1980s ushered in a new era in this field because now the diagnosis of osteoporosis could be made, by this key and powerful risk factor, before the outcome of the disease, namely, a fracture event, occurred. Osteoporosis is defined as a bone density measurement that is 2.5 standard deviations lower than peak bone mass values (e.g. T-score < -2.5). The other seminal moment in this field was a therapeutic one, namely the development of safe and effective drugs that prevent the incidence of fragility fractures. One can point to the approval of the bisphosphonate, alendronate, for the prevention and treatment of osteoporosis in 1995 as a watershed event in our field. Since then, there have been other bisphosphonates

---

Endocrine and Metabolic Medical Emergencies: A Clinician's Guide, Second Edition. Edited by Glenn Matfin.

that have become available in formulations that permit weekly or monthly (oral) or quarterly or yearly (intravenous) administration. The therapeutic landscape of osteoporosis continues to move forward with another antiresorptive class, RANKL inhibition, in the formulation of denosumab, and with the availability of two osteoanabolic therapies, teriparatide rhPTH(1-34) and abaloparatide (an analogue of PTHrP). In development is an antisclerostin agent, romosozumab.

Although osteoporosis dominates the field of bone and mineral metabolism because of its major world-wide prevalence, in the hundreds of millions, and the devastating effects of its most important consequence, the hip fracture, other abnormalities of bone and mineral metabolism are also important. For example, disorders of the parathyroid glands, as seen in primary and secondary hyperparathyroid states, and in hypoparathyroidism, have led to new insights into how parathyroid hormone (PTH) controls mineral metabolism. Primary hyperparathyroidism is a relatively common disorder characterized, classically, by hypercalcemia and elevated levels of PTH. Even if the PTH is not frankly elevated, its measurable presence is abnormal in the setting of hypercalcemia. Primary hyperparathyroidism is seen most often among postmenopausal women, but it occurs in men and in both sexes at any age. We have gained new insights through the study of primary hyperparathyroidism with regard to parathyroid hormone's target effects at bone and the kidney as well as off-target effects on the cardiovascular or neurocognitive systems that conceivably could be related to the disease. The secondary hyperparathyroid states are seen when the parathyroid glands respond appropriately to a lowering of the serum calcium with increased PTH secretion. Most commonly, secondary hyperparathyroidism is associated with kidney or gastrointestinal disorders. Management of secondary hyperparathyroidism associated with gastrointestinal disease (e.g., malabsorption) is handled by treating the gastrointestinal tract disorder.

With regard to chronic kidney disease, guidelines are established as to how to deal with that form of secondary hyperparathyroidism.

Hypoparathyroidism occurs when the parathyroid glands are no longer functional because they have all been removed or they have been irreversibly damaged. This is due most commonly to their removal in the course of parathyroid, thyroid, or other neck surgery. Less commonly, autoimmune destruction of the parathyroid glands is responsible for the disease. Even less commonly, genetic defects in which the calcium sensing receptor binds extracellular calcium with enhanced sensitivity, or in which PTH synthesis is disturbed, can lead to hypoparathyroidism. The co-presence of hypocalcemia and levels of PTH that are undetectable or very low help to establish the diagnosis. The hypocalcemia can present as a medical emergency with life-threatening neuromuscular irritability such as laryngeal spasm, and seizures. Recent advances in the therapeutic use of PTH in hypoparathyroidism have led to the approval of rhPTH(1-84) as a therapy. Hypoparathyoridism is the last of the classical endocrine deficiency diseases for which the replacement hormone has become available.

Paget's disease of bone is a focal or multifocal disorder of excessive osteoclast-mediated bone resorption. It can be treated effectively with amino-substituted bisphosphonates (e.g., zoledronic acid). In some cases, patients achieve a remission that appears to be permanent. While Paget's disease has diminished in incidence and is generally now rather easily treatable, it is important to note that it can also present as an emergency. If the Pagetic bone is in a vulnerable site, such as the femur, or the cervical vertebrae, it may be urgent to treat, thus preventing devastating orthopedic and/or neurological sequellae.

Nutritional issues are becoming more noteworthy in the field of bone and mineral metabolism. Vitamin D sufficiency is a key physiological requirement for normal bone and mineral metabolism. Sufficient Vitamin D helps to optimize calcium and phosphate absorption. When the vitamin D level is insufficient, for whatever reason, the serum calcium will tend to be in the lower range of normal and the parathyroid hormone level will rise. The serum phosphate will also be low. The definition of vitamin D insufficiency continues to be a matter of debate but most experts agree that levels < 20 ng/mL (50 nmol/L) are deficient. Others feel that levels of 25-hydroxyvitamin D should be > 30 ng/mL (>75 nmol/L). Whatever the outcome of this uncertainty turns out to be, no one disagrees that vitamin D insufficiency is detrimental to bone and must be corrected.

In the context of nutrition, it is also important to mention phosphate. Circulating phosphate is in a steady state with the circulating calcium level, with one often affecting the other. The serum phosphate can be very low in the context of vitamin D deficiency, malabsorption syndromes or renal tubular abnormalities. When the serum phosphate is exceedingly low (<1.5 mg/dL [<0.48 mmol/L]), musculoskeletal weakness, platelet and white cell dysfunction, and reduced oxygen delivery to tissues can present. When the serum phosphate is high, as in hypoparathyroidism or in uncontrolled renal failure, the associated elevated calcium-phosphate product can lead to the ectopic deposition of calcium-phosphate complexes in soft tissues.

In Part VII, these various disorders will be discussed with a focus on when they require urgent or emergency attention.

23

Hypocalcemia

Glenn Matfin

Key Points

- Approximately 99% of total body calcium (1 kg) is found in bone. Most of the remainder is located in the intracellular compartment with only a small amount present in extracellular fluid.
- The free (ionized) calcium is the physiologically important ion and is tightly regulated.
- Calcium homeostasis is directly or indirectly regulated by vitamin D metabolites and parathyroid hormone (PTH) via the kidney, intestine, and bone.
- PTH is secreted by the chief cell of the parathyroid glands. A unique calcium receptor on the cell membrane (extracellular calcium-sensing receptor [CaSR]) responds rapidly to changes in serum free (ionized) calcium.
- Low total plasma calcium (hypocalcemia) may be due to a reduction in albumin-bound calcium, the free fraction of calcium, or both.
- Hypocalcemia is a common electrolyte disturbance complicating approximately 15–26% of hospital admissions, and up to 88% of critically ill patients admitted to an intensive care unit.
- There are a large number of recognized causes of hypocalcemia in the inpatient setting, such as anterior neck surgery (including thyroid and parathyroid surgery), acute pancreatitis, blood transfusions, and numerous medications.
- Hypocalcemia with neurological, muscular, or cardiac dysfunction is associated with

significant morbidity and mortality and should be managed as a medical emergency.
- Symptomatic patients (e.g., tetany, seizures, laryngospasm or cardiac arrhythmias or dysfunction) or those with adjusted calcium (i.e., corrected for albumin concentration) <8 mg/dL (2 mmol/L); or free (ionized) calcium <4 mg/dL (1 mmol/L) should prompt emergency intervention with intravenous calcium replacement.
- It is important to evaluate and treat the underlying cause(s). In postoperative parathyroid-related hypocalcemia and other cases of hypoparathyroidism, undetectable or inappropriately low PTH levels in the context of hypocalcemia are consistent with the diagnosis. Treatment consists of calcium and vitamin D and/or vitamin D analogs (alfacalcidol or calcitriol). PTH (1-34) and PTH (1-84) therapies also have an evolving role in this setting.
- Hypomagnesemia should always be corrected as it causes inhibition of PTH secretion as well as resistance to its action; correction of hypocalcemia may be difficult with uncorrected hypomagnesemia. The underlying cause of hypomagnesemia should also be diagnosed and treated.
- Effective chronic care of the hypocalcemic patient is an important opportunity to prevent/reduce further acute presentations related to both hypocalcemia and iatrogenic hypercalcemia.

Endocrine and Metabolic Medical Emergencies: A Clinician's Guide, Second Edition. Edited by Glenn Matfin.
© 2018 John Wiley & Sons Ltd. Published 2018 by John Wiley & Sons Ltd.

Introduction

Calcium is required for the mineralization of bone and is a key regulator of many body processes. Calcium ions play critical roles in intracellular signaling, in the regulation of events at the plasma membrane, and in the function of extracellular proteins such as those involved in blood coagulation. Deviations of the concentration of free (unbound) calcium outside its very narrow reference interval can cause morbidity and mortality. The importance of the tight regulation of free calcium is underscored by the recognition that skeletal health is allowed to suffer markedly to allow physiologic processes in other organs to be maintained.

In blood, virtually all of the calcium is found in the plasma, which has a mean calcium concentration of 9.5 mg/dL (2.38 mmol/L) with a narrow reference range (8.5–10.5 mg/dL; 2.1–2.6 mmol/L). Calcium exists in three physicochemical states in plasma: 50% is free (ionized), 40% is bound to plasma proteins, and 10% is complexed with small diffusible inorganic and organic anions, including bicarbonate, lactate, phosphate, and citrate.

Calcium homeostasis is tightly regulated through multiple interactions between dietary intake of bone minerals and serum levels of homeostatic hormones (principally parathyroid hormone [PTH], vitamin D metabolites, and phosphaturic agents, such as osteocyte-secreted fibroblast growth factor 23 [FGF23]), acting principally on bone, intestine, and kidneys. Hypocalcemia (low total plasma calcium, which may be due to a reduction in albumin-bound calcium, the free fraction of calcium, or both), represents a serious disruption of calcium homeostasis, in which these homeostatic mechanisms have been overwhelmed by specific pathological state(s).

Vitamin D deficiency has the greatest contribution to hypocalcemia in the community (although rarely causes symptomatic hypocalcemia), with surgical hypoparathyroidism being the most significant cause of acute hypocalcemia in the hospital setting.

However, multiple other drugs and etiologies can interact to amplify the impact of any principal pathological process.

Hypocalcemia is a common electrolyte disturbance complicating approximately 15–26% of hospital admissions, and up to 88% of critically ill patients admitted to an intensive care unit (ICU) (1,2). There are a large number of recognized causes (see Table 23-1) and, though much of the acute management is generic, the overall quality of management is greatly enhanced by an appropriate diagnosis (3). Chronic hypocalcemia may be asymptomatic even at very low levels of serum calcium, but severe or acute hypocalcemia is associated with predictable signs. Hypocalcemia with neurological, muscular or cardiac dysfunction is associated with significant morbidity and mortality and should be managed as a medical emergency (4,5).

Pathophysiology

Calcium, phosphate, and magnesium are the major divalent cations in the body (6). They are ingested in the diet, absorbed from the intestine, filtered in the glomerulus of the kidney, reabsorbed in the renal tubules, and eliminated in the urine. Only a small amount of these three ions are present in extracellular fluid (ECF). The calcium is regulated within a narrow range by vitamin D metabolites and PTH through their action on the bowel, the skeleton, and the kidneys.

Vitamin D

Vitamin D is structurally similar to steroid and retinoid hormones and is functionally more of a prohormone than what is classically understood by the term "vitamin" (7–9). It regulates the plasma levels of calcium and phosphate by increasing their absorption from the bowel and plays a crucial role in the normal bone formation by promoting the mineralization of osteoid.

Unless specified otherwise in the text, vitamin D (calciferol) is used to encompass both its D3 (cholecalciferol) and D2

Table 23-1 Etiology of hypocalcemia

Reduced entry of calcium into circulation	Increased movement of calcium out of circulation

Parathyroid dysfunction
• Hypoparathyroidism
  • Autoimmune
  • Autoimmune polyglandular syndrome
  • Postoperative
  • Infiltrative (e.g., hemochromatosis, amyloidosis)
• Hypomagnesemia
• Hypermagnesemia
• Congenital disorders of the parathyroid glands, such as:
  • DiGeorge syndrome
  • Activating mutations in CaSR
• Pseudohypoparathyroidism secondary to G-protein defects
• Drugs (including cinacalcet)
 	
Vitamin D deficiency
• Dietary or malabsorption (especially post bariatric surgery)
• Lack of sunlight exposure
• CKD
 	
Reduced bone resorption
• Drugs (including bisphosphonates and denosumab)
	Movement into bone stores
	• "Hungry bone" syndrome
	• Osteoblastic metastases (e.g., prostate, breast cancer)
	
	Chelation of free (ionized) calcium
	• Acute pancreatitis
	• Hyperphosphatemia
	• CKD
	• Tumor lysis syndrome
	• Rhabdomyolysis
	• Citrate or EDTA in context of transfusions
	• Phlebotomy
	
	Miscellaneous
	• Sepsis
	• Drugs (including chemotherapeutic agents and foscarnet)

CKD = chronic kidney disease; CaSR = calcium sensing receptor.

(ergocalciferol) forms, which undergo a similar metabolism to 25-(OH)D (calcidiol) and 1,25-(OH)D (calcitriol), respectively, but differ in their side-chains. Determination of circulating vitamin D status generally refers to the plasma levels of the 25-hydroxylated forms of both vitamins, 25-(OH)D$_3$ and 25-(OH)D$_2$ (i.e., the chole- and ergo- forms of calcidiol, respectively).

D3 is mainly synthesized by ultraviolet (UV) irradiation (UVB: around 300 nm wavelength) of 7-dehydrocholesterol in the skin (Figure 23-1), though in winter dietary sources may predominate. Circulating D2 (manufactured by UV irradiation of sterol precursors by algae, fungi, or marine plankton), derives exclusively from consumption of oily fish or food supplements. It is less bioactive than cholecalciferol by a factor of around 25%. Some foods are statutorily fortified with vitamin D, but this varies hugely from country to country.

Once it enters the circulation from the skin or intestine, calciferol is concentrated in the liver and hydroxylated to form 25-hydroxyvitamin D3 (25-(OH)D3) (calcidiol). It is then transported to the kidney, where it is transformed into active 1,25-dihydroxyvitamin D3 (1,25-(OH)2D3, or calcitriol). However, some 1-alpha hydroxylation also takes place in macrophages and, in a paracrine manner, in peripheral tissues (10). The normal production rate of calcitriol is 0.5–1 mcg/day. The major action of calcitriol is to increase the absorption of calcium from the intestine, but it also sensitizes bone to the resorptive actions of PTH, limits parathyroid gland growth and suppresses the synthesis and secretion of PTH. Calcitriol formation is regulated in feedback fashion by plasma levels of calcium, phosphate, FGF23 (a potent phosphaturic agent, or phosphatonin) and calcitriol itself. Hyperphosphatemia is sensed by osteocytes,

Figure 23-1 Metabolism of vitamin D

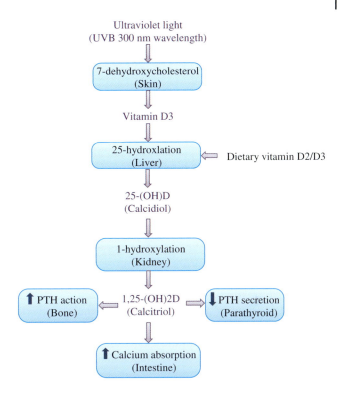

which respond by secreting FGF23. High levels of FGF23, as found in chronic kidney disease (CKD) or rarely tumor-induced osteomalacia, block 1 alpha hydroxylation of vitamin D, thereby contributing to hypocalcemia in these patients (11). Increased FGF23 is also found in hypoparathyroidism. When PTH production is absent or deficient, the expected calcium-conserving effects of PTH on the renal tubule are lost. The phosphaturic effects of PTH are also lost. These two pathophysiological processes are responsible, in part, for the characteristic hypocalcemia and hyperphosphatemia of hypoparathyroidism. PTH deficiency also leads to decreased 1,25-(OH)2D (calcitriol) production. The resultant hyperphosphatemia stimulates FGF23 levels, which in turn further inhibits 1,25-(OH)2D (calcitriol) production, exacerbating the hypocalcemia.

Parathyroid Hormone (PTH)

PTH, a major regulator of plasma calcium and phosphate, is secreted by the four parathyroid glands located on or near the posterior surface of the thyroid gland. The dominant regulator of PTH is the ECF calcium concentration. A unique receptor on the parathyroid cell membrane (the calcium-sensing receptor, or CaSR) responds rapidly to changes in ECF calcium levels (12,13). The main function of PTH is to maintain the calcium concentrations in the ECF. It performs this function by promoting the release of calcium from bone, increasing the activation of vitamin D as a means of enhancing intestinal absorption of calcium, and by stimulating calcium conservation by the kidney while increasing phosphate excretion. Most renal calcium conservation is through reabsorption at proximal tubule level (65%). By promoting phosphate excretion, PTH keeps the calcium-phosphate product low, so as to prevent calcium phosphate salt formation in the ECF. When the plasma calcium level is high, PTH secretion is inhibited and vice versa; the PTH response to a change in plasma calcium is prompt, occurring within seconds. There is also a direct, calcium-independent effect of calcitriol to inhibit PTH secretion (11).

Etiology

Calcium homeostasis is maintained through interactions involving the parathyroid glands, kidneys, bones and vitamin D metabolism (6). Hypocalcemia is defined as a free (ionized) serum calcium concentration that falls below the lower limit of the normal range. Hypocalcemia occurs with either decreased entry of calcium into the blood supply, or through sequestration and effective removal of calcium (see Table 23-1). The most frequent cause of chronic hypocalcemia in the general population and among hospitalized patients is vitamin D deficiency, however, this rarely causes symptomatic hypocalcemia (14,15). The most commonly encountered cause of acute symptomatic hypocalcemia is postoperative hypoparathyroidism in the context of recent head and neck surgery (>75% of all cases of hypoparathyroidism) (16,17). However, the prevalence of post-surgical hypoparathyroidism in patients undergoing thyroidectomy or surgery for primary hyperparathyroidism (PHPT) is generally uncommon but depends on how it is defined (i.e., acute versus chronic hypoparathyroidism), the extent of the neck surgery, and also the skill of the surgeon. It is more common in patients undergoing radical neck surgery for treatment of head and neck malignancies. In general, transient postsurgical hypoparathyroidism-related hypocalcemia lasting <6 months, has been estimated to occur in 25.4–83% of patients worldwide after neck surgery (17). In comparison, permanent hypoparathyroidism after anterior neck surgery occurs in between 0.1–4.6% (16,17). A history of prior neck radiotherapy may also point toward hypoparathyroidism. Even in individuals with well-known hypoparathyroidism, needs for supplemental calcium and active vitamin D can change, or in those who are poorly or non-compliant can result in acute presentation. Other common causes of hypocalcemia are moderate to advanced CKD (i.e., CKD stages 3B-5), and hypomagnesemia. In CKD, hypoproteinemia, hyperphosphatemia, low plasma 1,25(OH)2D (caused by reduced renal synthesis), and skeletal resistance to PTH can all contribute to hypocalcemia.

In practice, many cases of hypocalcemia are multifactorial, comprising two or more different risk factors (e.g., vitamin D deficiency ± drug-induced hypomagnesemia ± thyroid/parathyroid post-surgery effect) (8). Reversible hypoparathyroidism is also seen in severe hypomagnesemia (mild hypomagnesemia tends to promote PTH secretion), which can thereby predispose to hypocalcemia. For example, the magnesium-wasting effects of loop diuretics, proton-pump inhibitors (PPIs), and alcohol abuse (particularly in combination) potentially cause resistant secondary hypocalcemia.

Rare causes of hypocalcemia include genetic/epigenetic, autoimmune and infiltrative conditions (18). The latter include amyloidosis and iron/copper overload from hemochromatosis and Wilson's disease respectively. Tumor metastases can also infiltrate and destroy the parathyroids (19). Other causes of hypocalcemia related to malignancy include osteoblastic bone disease due to metastatic cancer (e.g., breast or prostate cancer) which can cause a "hungry bones" scenario; neck surgery and irradiation; tumor lysis syndrome; magnesium depletion related to chemotherapy (e.g., cisplatin, cetuximab) and other causes; vitamin D deficiency; and adverse effects of potent bone resorption inhibitors including bisphosphonates and denosumab (19).

Genetic disorders cause hypocalcemia through defects in calcium- or PTH-signaling. They are comprised of a number of syndromic (i.e., associated with other glands and systems, including polyglandular autoimmune syndromes, DiGeorge's syndrome, and Bartter's syndrome) and non-syndromic isolated forms. Activating

CaSR mutations cause autosomal dominant hypocalcemia type 1 (ADH1) with hypercalciuria, which is associated with hypocalcemic symptoms in ~50% of cases (12,13). Bartter syndrome type 5, which is characterized by renal salt-wasting, hypokalemia and hyperreninemic hyperaldosteronism, may also have gain-of-function CaSR mutations with hypocalcemic symptoms in 75% of cases (13). Pseudohypoparathyroidism typically arises from epigenetic G-protein defects causing post-receptor inhibition of PTH action. Patients have hypocalcemia and hyperphosphatemia as per true hypoparathyroidism, but a high PTH level. They may also exhibit syndromic features of the most common form, pseudohypoparathyroidism type 1 (Albright's hereditary osteodystrophy [AHO]), such as moon faces and short third, fourth and fifth metacarpals and metatarsals. The molecular basis for this condition is an inactivating mutation in the gene coding for the stimulatory guanine nucleotide-binding protein in the adenylate cyclase complex, resulting in an inability to produce the second-messenger cyclic adenosine monophosphate (cAMP). Hence, decreased urinary cAMP levels in response to exogenous bioactive PTH are found on modified Ellsworth-Howard testing (based on the Chase-Aurbach test) (17). Autoimmune hypoparathyroidism (which is the second commonest cause of hypoparathyroidism after anterior neck surgery (16)) can be an isolated autoimmune process or part of polyglandular autoimmune syndrome type 1 (AIRE1 gene) which is a familial disorder associated with adrenal insufficiency, fulminant liver disease, vitiligo, and mucocutaneous candidiasis.

Hypocalcemia arising from "hungry bone syndrome" (due to excessive movement of ECF calcium into bone) can occur with osteoblastic bone disease, including metastatic cancer (e.g., breast or prostate cancer), following correction of long-standing hypercalcemia due to hyperparathyroidism, and less commonly with treatment of hyperthyroidism and osteomalacia due to rapid remineralization (20). Routine post-thyroidectomy prophylactic vitamin D and calcium supplementation may be helpful in reducing the occurrence of transient symptomatic hypocalcemia (21), and seems to be more cost-effective than calcitriol in this context and also improves quality of life (22). However, at least some postoperative hypocalcemic crises ascribed to hungry bone syndrome may simply reflect undiagnosed severe vitamin D deficiency. Along those lines, a recent study suggested that pre-operative vitamin D deficiency increased risk of transient post-operative hypocalcemia (but not permanent hypoparathyroidism) and increased the length of stay following thyroidectomy (23). It seems sensible to treat these patients pre-surgery with standard vitamin D therapy (24).

Hyperphosphatemia, most commonly seen in renal impairment, but also a feature of tumor lysis syndrome and rhabdomyolysis, causes hypocalcemia through sequestration and complexing of ionized calcium. Acute pancreatitis is associated with the formation of calcium complexes within the abdominal cavity. Calcium chelation can occur with ethylenediaminetetraacetic acid (EDTA), or citrate, but is rare in patients being transfused with normal renal and hepatic function. Sepsis-related hypocalcemia is multifactorial, but significant factors include renal impairment, magnesium abnormalities, release of inflammatory cytokines, and frequent transfusions. It is particularly associated with gram-negative septicemia. Mortality rates are increased compared with matched septic patients without hypocalcemia (25).

Drug history is important, as a number of medications are associated with hypocalcemia (26). These include inhibitors of bone turnover, such as high-dose bisphosphonates and denosumab; the CaSR-agonist cinacalcet; drugs causing renal tubular magnesium loss, either reversibly (diuretics), and potentially irreversibly (e.g., cisplatin, carboplatin, aminoglycosides); PPIs seem to cause a dose-dependent gastrointestinal magnesium leak;

and calcium-chelation by foscarnet and fluoride. Finally, phenytoin, rifampicin, theophylline, and phenobarbital cause vitamin D deficiency through induction of cytochrome P450 enzyme activity which accelerates calcidiol metabolism.

Diagnostic Considerations

ECF calcium is normally maintained within a narrow reference range 8.5–10.5 mg/dL (2.1–2.6 mmol/L). Hypocalcemia is defined as a serum calcium level of less than 8.5 mg/dL (<2.1 mmol/L) or a free (ionized) calcium level of less than ~4.25 mg/dL (<1.1 mmol/L). Some 40% of total serum calcium is protein bound with the majority bound to albumin, while 50% is ionized and active. Hypoalbuminemia is the most common cause of apparent hypocalcemia on a standard biochemical profile, particularly in hospitalized patients, because 1 g/dL (1 g/L) of albumin binds approximately 0.8 mg/dL (0.02 mmol/L) of calcium. For example, for every 1g/dL (1 g/L) reduction in the serum albumin (corrected to normal albumin level of 4 g/dL [40 g/L]), the total calcium is adjusted upward by 0.8 mg/dL (0.02 mmol/L). Albumin levels should therefore be considered when assessing possible hypocalcemia, although most laboratories now provide corrected or adjusted calcium (ACa) level. However, in states of acute albumin fluctuations, such as sepsis, measurement of ionized calcium may be a more reliable assessment of calcium status if an accurate, direct ionized serum calcium can be obtained. Alkalosis tends to decrease free (ionized) calcium levels due to increased binding to albumin. Apparent hypocalcemia after gadolinium-based magnetic resonance imaging (MRI) contrasts is due to assay interference and, as contrast is rapidly excreted in urine, the effect is transient with normal renal function (27).

While not delaying the emergency treatment outlined below, the finding of acute hypocalcemia should always prompt biochemical testing to elicit a cause, comprising renal function, PTH, phosphate, alkaline phosphatase (ALP), magnesium, bicarbonate and vitamin D levels (Table 23-2 and Figure 23-2). Measurement of PTH level is crucial in identifying the underlying cause, as undetectable or inappropriately low levels suggests hypoparathyroidism (diagnosis of hypoparathyroidism is outlined in Table 23-3), whereas high levels confirm physiological PTH response to hypocalcemia arising from other etiology. Exceptions to this rule include severe magnesium deficiency or excess, both of which can impair PTH release. In addition, pseudohypoparathyroidism

Table 23-2 Investigation of hypocalcemia

Routine investigations	Specific investigations
• Free (ionized) and/or corrected calcium (ACa); phosphate • Parathyroid hormone (PTH) – second- or third-generation assay • Alkaline phosphatase (ALP) • Magnesium • Vitamin D level • Blood urea nitrogen (BUN); creatinine/eGFR • Liver function tests • Bicarbonate level; arterial or venous blood gas • ECG – looking for prolonged QTc interval or arrhythmia	• Amylase/lipase – pancreatitis • Fecal elastase/bowel investigation/breath testing – malabsorption/bacterial overgrowth • Urinary magnesium – urinary magnesium loss • X-rays – osteomalacia (due to vitamin D deficiency) • Bone scan and other imaging – malignancy • Genetic tests – genetic/epigenetic causes • Urinary cAMP – pseudohypoparathyroidism

QTc = corrected QT interval duration; cAMP = cyclic AMP; eGFR = estimated glomerular filtration rate

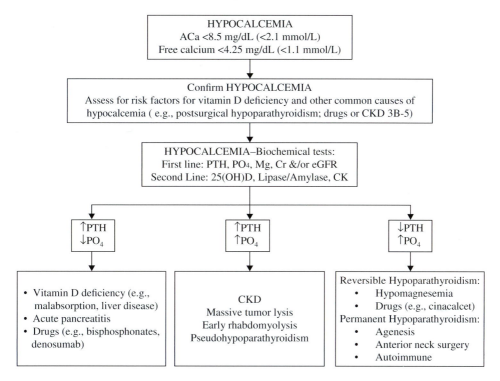

Figure 23-2 Clinical approach to investigation of causes of hypocalcemia. Adapted from (17). Reproduced with permission from OUP.
ACa = Adjusted or corrected calcium; CKD = chronic kidney disease; CK = creatine kinase; eGFR = estimated glomerular filtration rate; Cr = creatinine; 25(OH)D = 25 Hydroxyvitamin D

Table 23-3 Diagnosis and evaluation of hypoparathyroidism (17)

- Hypocalcemia (ACa) confirmed on at least two occasions separated by at least 2 weeks
- PTH concentration, by second- or third-generation immunoassay, that is undetectable or inappropriately low in the presence of hypocalcemia on at least two occasions
- Phosphate levels in the upper normal or frankly elevated range (helpful but not mandatory)
- After neck surgery, chronic hypoparathyroidism is established only after 6 months

is associated with high PTH levels due to end-organ PTH resistance.

Measurement of calcidiol (25-(0H)D) level is crucial, as deficiency thereof is one of

the commonest causes of hypocalcemia. Why some patients with hypovitaminosis D develop hypocalcemia and others do not is unclear, but likely reflects the interplay of dietary calcium intake, concomitant medication(s) and individual factors, including robustness of PTH response. Measurement of serum calcitriol is surprisingly unhelpful in this context, due to compensatory hyperparathyroidism leading to "normal" levels. In vitamin D deficiency, both hypocalcemia and hypophosphatemia may be present, whereas patients with hypoparathyroidism, tumor lysis syndrome and renal failure tend to hypocalcemia with hyperphosphatemia.

Both hypo- and hypermagnesemia can be associated with hypocalcemia due to inhibition of PTH release from the parathyroid. High urinary magnesium excretion levels point toward renal magnesium-wasting.

Acid base assessment is also important as alkalosis can cause reduction in free (ionized) calcium due to increased protein binding. Amylase/lipase should be measured in suspected pancreatitis.

Finally, detailed physical examination and diagnostic imaging are crucial to the assessment of patients with osteoblastic metastases. High bone turnover may be associated with elevated levels of ALP and other serum or urine bone turnover markers.

Clinical Assessment

Clinical Manifestations of Hypocalcemia

It is crucial to identify the clinical manifestations, because if present, they identify symptomatic patients who may require urgent corrective measures. The severity of signs and symptoms depends both on the absolute degree of hypocalcemia (especially free calcium decrease) and the rapidity of its onset, with the majority of features relating to neuromuscular dysfunction. The rapid onset of hypocalcemia in the postsurgical setting can present dramatically and in a manner that demands immediate and aggressive intervention. In comparison, patients with hypocalcemia due to chronic hypoparathyroidism can be nearly asymptomatic despite profound biochemical disturbances (24).

Perioral tingling and acral paraesthesia (regions of relative ischemia/hypoxia) are the earliest symptoms and almost always present in symptomatic cases, while other frequently reported features include muscle stiffness, myalgia, and confusion (Tables 23-2 and 23-3). In more severe cases, intense, painful spasm of the fingers and toes develops (tetany) and may be sustained for several minutes. In the most severe cases, life-threatening laryngospasm may occur.

Chvostek's sign describes ipsilateral twitching of the facial muscle groups including the perioral, nasal, and ocular regions, when the facial nerve is tapped 2 cm anterior to the earlobe beneath the zygomatic bone. However, perioral twitching is also seen in up to 25% of normal individuals and, conversely, this sign is negative in approximately 30% of those with hypocalcemia (28). However, Trousseau's sign is more sensitive (94%) and specific for hypocalcemia and describes flexion of the wrist and metacarpophalangeal joints, hyperextension of the fingers and flexion of the thumb producing a characteristic deformity known as *main d'accoucheur*. It is elicited by occluding the brachial artery 20 mmHg above systolic pressure for 3 minutes and is positive in only 1% of normocalcemic patients (29).

Neurological manifestations of acute hypocalcemia include irritability, confusion, and seizures. In known epilepsy, hypocalcemia lowers the threshold for seizure activity. Features of chronic hypocalcemia include depression, dementia, extrapyramidal features, hair and nail changes, cataracts, and papilledema. Patients who present with acute-on-chronic hypocalcemia can exhibit both sets of features.

Cardiac features of hypocalcemia include electrocardiographic (ECG) changes and cardiac failure (30). The ECG hallmark of hypocalcemia is prolongation of the corrected QT interval (QTc), the duration of which is proportional to the degree of hypocalcemia. The more prolonged the QTc interval, the more likely an arrhythmia. The most common arrhythmia associated with prolonged QTc is *torsade de pointes* which, if untreated, can progress to ventricular fibrillation and cardiac arrest. Other recognized abnormalities include reduced voltage or negative T waves, although T waves are normal in more than half of those with hypocalcemia, and include changes that mimic acute anterior myocardial infarction. Low calcium levels may cause resistance to digoxin. Hypocalcemia can lead to cardiac failure, particularly if associated with severe hypovitaminosis D.

Hypocalcemia can affect the function of most organs, but in hypoparathyroidism, the most obvious organ systems that become dysfunctional are neurological, cognitive, muscular, and cardiac. The divalent cationic imbalance renders these systems subject to an irritability that can be subtle (e.g., paresthesia, "brain fog," and prolonged QTc on ECG) or life-threatening as described. Chronic hypocalcemia and hyperphosphatemia, with an increased serum calcium-phosphate product, can lead over the years to soft tissue calcifications. These calcifications are typically seen in the brain (in basal ganglia in particular) and in the kidney (stones and nephrocalcinosis) but can also be seen in joints, eyes, skin, vasculature, and other organ systems (16,31). One of the most frequent complaints in hypoparathyroidism is diminished quality of life.

Medical History

This is central to the initial assessment of hypocalcemia and helps to signpost key priorities in the diagnostic workup. Onset in childhood is obviously consistent with congenital etiology, though environmental factors must also be considered, such as severe hypovitaminosis D in the breast-fed child of a dark-skinned mother living at high latitudes. When the evaluation suggests a genetic cause as, for example, young age, family history, candidiasis, or multiple endocrine gland failure, genetic counseling, and germline mutation testing should be considered (16).

Abdominal pain or jaundice may suggest the possibility of pancreatitis; and a history of massive/multiple transfusions, particularly in trauma patients, points toward transfusion-related hypocalcemia. Risk factors should also be identified (or a defined history established), for malabsorption of calcium, vitamin D and/or magnesium (e.g., Crohn's, celiac disease, chronic pancreatitis, and malabsorptive bariatric surgery). A history of renal disease, liver disease and/or anticonvulsant therapy might indicate a defect of vitamin D hydroxylation/metabolism. Recent neck surgery, particularly thyroidectomy or parathyroidectomy, suggests acute hypoparathyroidism due to removal/devascularization of parathyroid glands, though other risk factors might also coexist (Table 23-3).

Hyperventilation and history of anxiety disorder are compatible with a (reversible) fall in ionized calcium due to induced respiratory alkalosis, and recent contrast-MRI with gadolinium-induced pseudohypocalcemia due to assay interference. Drug history is also important, as noted previously. Hypoalbuminemia associated with malnutrition or chronic illness may lead to apparently low total and ACa levels, hence the need for measurement of free (ionized) calcium. Finally, a history of malignancies with propensity for osteoblastic metastases, such as breast and prostate cancer, should not be missed.

In summary, a full medical history and traditional "head-to-toe" examination may not only elicit signs of hypocalcemia, but also help differentiate acute from chronic; syndromic from non-syndromic hypocalcemia; and will usually signpost other underlying diagnoses.

Acute Intervention

Once severe hypocalcemia is recognized, the patient should be managed in an appropriate emergency setting such as an acute medical unit (AMU), high dependency unit (HDU) or intensive care unit (ICU). Prompt assessment and management of the ABCDEs should occur (i.e., Airway; Breathing; Circulation; Disability [i.e., conscious level]; and Exposure [i.e., examination and evaluation]).

Intravenous Calcium

The symptoms of hypocalcemia do not always strictly follow the extent to which the calcium level is low. The severity of symptoms (paresthesias, carpopedal spasm, broncho- or laryngospasm, tetany, seizures, or mental status changes) and signs (Chvostek's or Trousseau's signs, bradycardia, impaired cardiac contractility, and prolongation of the QTc interval) all depends upon the absolute level of calcium, the rate of decrease, and individual variability.

Symptomatic patients (e.g., tetany, seizures, laryngospasm or cardiac arrhythmias or dysfunction) or those with an ACa below 2 mmol/L (<8 mg/dL) or ionized calcium <1 mmol/L (<4 mg/dL) should prompt emergency intervention with IV calcium replacement (Table 23-4). In addition, although some patients with marked hypocalcemia (i.e., ACa <7.0 mg/dL [<1.75 mmol/L]) may not be symptomatic, IV therapy may be indicated because at those levels, life-threatening features can appear rather suddenly, such as laryngeal spasm and seizures. Patients who become unable to take or absorb oral supplements can quickly become symptomatic, although the serum calcium may not have fallen dramatically at the time they present with symptoms. Finally, there are some women who typically become symptomatic during the luteal phase of their menstrual cycle. In these situations, clinical judgment and prompt decision-making to opt for IV calcium are required (31).

IV calcium should be given in hospital and calcium levels carefully monitored (usually at least 4–6 hourly). Ten to twenty ml (1–2 standard ampoules equals 1–2 g calcium gluconate or 90–180 mg elemental calcium) 10% calcium gluconate should be infused slowly in 50–100 ml 0.9% saline (or 5% dextrose) over 10–20 minutes (with cardiac monitoring) (Figure 23-3). IV calcium should not be given more rapidly because of the serious risk of cardiac dysfunction, including systolic arrest.

Calcium gluconate is the preferred formulation for acute calcium replacement and should be repeated until the patient is symptom-free. Some 10 ml of 10% calcium chloride can also be used (which contains

Table 23-4 Assessment of the hypocalcemic patient

Features of acute hypocalcemia	Features of chronic hypocalcemia	Features of the underlying cause
• Perioral and digital paraesthesia • Muscle weakness, twitching, Tetany and carpopedal spasm • Chvostek's sign – less specific (present in 25% normocalcemic subjects) • Trousseau's sign – more specific (present in 1% normocalcemic subjects) • Laryngospasm and bronchospasm – shortness of breath, stridor • Seizure (partial or generalized) • Altered mental status • Hypotension and cardiac failure • Arrhythmias – check pulse and electrocardiogram (ECG)	• Features of Parkinsonism or other extrapyramidal movement disorders • Dementia • "Brain fog" • Nail dystrophy • Hair loss • Dry skin • Papilledema • Ectopic calcifications (e.g., eyes)	• Evidence of neck surgery – hypoparathyroidism (temporary or permanent) • Abdominal tenderness – e.g., pancreatitis • Previous abdominal surgery (especially bariatric surgery) – malabsorption and refeeding syndrome • Proximal muscle weakness - osteomalacia • Syndromic features (e.g., moon facies, short third, fourth and fifth metacarpals) – suggestive of genetic/epigenetic cause • Evidence of malignancy – e.g., breast, prostate cancer • Features of infiltrative diseases – e.g., bronzed skin discoloration (hemochromatosis); Kayser-Fleischer rings (Wilson's disease) • Features of Addison's disease, mucocutaneous candidiasis, vitiligo – autoimmune polyglandular syndrome type 1

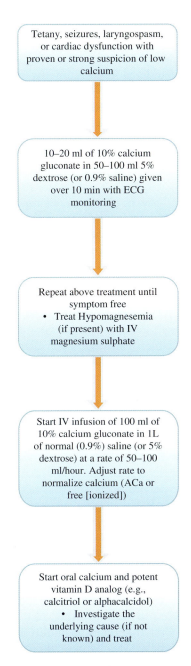

Figure 23-3 Management of acute severe hypocalcemia. Adapted from (5).

273 mg of elemental calcium), but is more irritating to the veins than calcium gluconate and extravasation can lead to tissue necrosis. This will increase the serum calcium levels for 2–3 hours, and should be followed by a slow infusion of 100 ml (10 standard ampoules) 10% calcium gluconate in 1L 0.9% saline (or 5% dextrose). A solution of 10% calcium gluconate contains 10 g of calcium gluconate in 100 ml, and 10 g of calcium gluconate contains about 900 mg of elemental calcium. Therefore, adding 100 ml of 10% calcium to 1 L of fluid gives a preparation close to 1 mg/ml of elemental calcium. The infusion should be commenced at 50–100 ml/hour (equivalent to 50–100 mg/h) and titrated to increase serum calcium to the lower end of the normal range (5,16). Calcium infusion is usually given at 0.5–1.5 mg/kg of elemental calcium per hour. Over 8–10 hours, this infusion protocol will deliver as much as 15 mg/kg body weight of elemental calcium, raising the serum calcium levels by approximately 2 mg/dL (0.5 mmol/L). Infusion of calcium compounds is occasionally associated with the induction of cardiac arrhythmias and myocardial infarction (hence, the need for cardiac monitoring), and may cause chelation with resultant end-organ deposition if hyperphosphatemia is present and not addressed. Care should be taken if the patient has a known history of coronary artery disease or arrhythmias but in most situations correction of severe hypocalcemia would take priority.

Hypomagnesemia should always be corrected as it causes inhibition of PTH secretion as well as resistance to its action; correction of hypocalcemia may be difficult with uncorrected hypomagnesemia. Administer IV Mg^{2+}, 24 mmol/24 hours, made up as 6 g of magnesium sulfate (i.e., 30 ml of 20%, 800 mmol/L, MgSO4) in 500 ml normal (0.9%) saline or 5% dextrose. Monitor serum Mg^{2+} and aim to achieve normal serum magnesium level (5). If magnesium administration is too rapid, excessive urinary losses of both magnesium and calcium can occur. Underlying cause(s) of hypomagnesemia should be diagnosed and treated. Specifically, PPIs should always be stopped unless absolutely necessary and a diuretic replaced with alternative agents wherever feasible. Even if cessation is not possible, any dose reduction will be useful.

There are three situations where extra caution must be observed with parenteral calcium administration (5). First, patients taking digoxin (whose action is blunted by hypocalcemia) might develop clinical digoxin toxicity as calcium levels improve. Second, aggressive calcium replacement in patients with hyperphosphatemia can lead to precipitation of calcium phosphate salts and metastatic calcification, most typically in tumor lysis syndrome. Finally, correction of acidemia in renal failure patients with hypocalcemia can result in tetany, due to increased protein-binding of calcium, so hypocalcemia should always be corrected before correction of acidemia.

The serum calcium level should be measured frequently in the acute setting. The recurrence of symptoms caused by hypocalcemia may indicate the need to increase the infusion rate and should be correlated with a simultaneous serum calcium value to assess the progress of treatment. Intravenous calcium should be continued until the patient is receiving an effective regimen of oral calcium and vitamin D. Intravenous infusions are generally tapered off slowly (over a period of 24–48 h or longer) while oral therapy is adjusted. Oral calcium and parent vitamin D therapy (i.e., calciferol), in addition to calcitriol, should be initiated as soon as is practical.

There are limited data on the use of PTH in human subjects who are acutely hypocalcemic. In addition, there are no systematic data available on the use of PTH (1-34) or PTH (1-84) in the more common setting of acute hypocalcemia against a backdrop of chronic hypoparathyroidism. At the moment, injectable PTH therapy cannot be recommended for the treatment of acute hypocalcemia (16).

Oral Therapies

For patients who need transitioning from parenteral calcium therapy; and also those patients with "mild" hypocalcemia (i.e., asymptomatic or ACa >8 mg/dL [>2 mmol/L]), oral calcium replacement therapy (plus magnesium or phosphate as required) should be initiated as soon as possible. Oral calcium supplements, such as Sandocal 1000 (contains 1000 mg elemental calcium) two tablets twice daily (or equivalent), should be initiated. In the post-bariatric surgery setting, calcium citrate is the preferred form of supplementation, owing to its superior absorption in conditions of reduced stomach acid production, including surgical alteration to the stomach (e.g., gastric sleeve). Calcium should be given 8 hourly and also potentially at increased dose. Chewable or liquid formulations may be required for these patients especially in the initial post-operative phase. Increased requirements for vitamin D may also be required in this setting (sometimes 100,000 IU or more after malabsorptive procedures). Injectable active vitamin D are also available (calcitriol and alfacalcidol) and may be useful following malabsorptive procedures.

Vitamin D deficiency should also be corrected as promptly as possible, because this will facilitate subsequent stabilization of patients on oral replacement. Load with ~300,000 IU chole- or ergocalciferol over ~6–8 weeks (1 mcg = 40 IU). Although there are no protocols specific to the context of acute hypocalcemia, pharmacokinetic studies in patients with severe vitamin D deficiency indicate that a single oral dose of 200,000–300,000 IU normalizes serum calcidiol levels within 48–72 hours, without risk of "overshoot-hypercalcemia," whereas the same dose given intramuscularly can take weeks to achieve this (32). Other "front-loaded" regimens include 60,000 IU daily for 5 days. Meanwhile, calcitriol (1,25-(OH)2D3), which has a more rapid onset of action (hours) than unhydroxylated D3, can be started immediately at an initial dose of 0.25 mcg–0.5 mcg/day (5). Its rapid onset of action and biological half-life of 4–6 hours make it a useful adjunct in the management of acute hypocalcemia. Moreover, the calcemic response to calcitriol can persist for more than 24 hours after a single oral dose. Injectable formulations of active vitamin D are also available (alfacalcidol and calcitriol).

If the patient is post-thyroidectomy and asymptomatic, repeat ACa and PTH levels in 24 hrs (PTH levels can also be assessed at 4 hrs post-op). If ACa <8 mg/dL (2 mmol/L) and the PTH level is low (e.g., <10–15 pg/mL), the patient is at risk of permanent hypoparathyoidism and should be treated with calcium and a vitamin D analog (e.g. calcitriol 0.5 mg twice daily) as well as having overnight observation (24). If ACa is >8.5 mg/dL (2.1 mmol/L), the patient can be discharged with repeat ACa in 1 week. If ACa remains 8–8.5 mg/dL (2–2.1 mmol/L), Sandocal 1000 (or equivalent) can be increased to three tablets twice daily. If the patient remains in the mild hypocalcemic range beyond 72 hrs post-operatively despite calcium supplementation, a vitamin D analog (e.g., calcitriol or alfacalcidol) 0.25–0.5 mcg/day can be started with close monitoring.

Maintenance Therapy

This may not be required for vitamin D-replete patients who merely experienced transient postoperative hypoparathyroidism. Indeed, it may even be possible to gradually wean off therapy patients who have been taking oral replacement for many years after neck surgery. For patients with intact parathyroid function, but prior hypovitaminosis D, avoidance of other precipitating factors or drugs, and maintenance therapy with oral vitamin D so as to achieve optimum serum levels of 25-OHD will suffice. The prolonged effective half-life and large volume of distribution of vitamin D, necessarily arising from its marked lipophilicity (33), mean that repeat assessment of 25-OHD levels should be deferred for around 3 months after commencing therapy (9). Due the impossibility of monitoring any meaningful serum levels, its comparative expense and risk of overtreatment (i.e., hypercalcemia), vitamin D analogs (e.g., calcitriol/alfacalcidol) should not be used for routine vitamin D replacement therapy. However, these short-acting (~6

hours) agents are really useful for patients with permanent hypoparathyroidism, who require a more nuanced approach.

Permanent Hypoparathyroidism

There are six goals of management of the chronic hypocalcemia of hypoparathyroidism (31): (a) to prevent signs and symptoms of hypocalcemia; (b) to maintain the serum calcium concentration slightly below normal (i.e., no more than 0.5 mg/dL [0.13 mmol/L] below normal) or in the low normal range; (c) to maintain the calcium-phosphate product to below 55 mg^2/dL^2 (4.4 $mmol^2/L^2$); (d) to avoid hypercalciuria; (e) to avoid hypercalcemia; and (f) to avoid renal (nephrocalcinosis/nephrolithiasis) and other extraskeletal calcifications.

The standard medical treatment for hypoparathyroid patients includes oral elemental calcium supplementation 0–3000 mg/day. As it has been observed that only ~500 mg calcium is absorbed at any one administration, smaller doses may need to be spread out throughout day (i.e., typically 500–1000 mg two to three times daily). Calcium carbonate is the preferred option, although calcium citrate can be useful when achlorhydia is present; if PPIs are used; in the post-bariatric surgical patient who has abnormal stomach anatomy (e.g., gastric sleeve); or if carbonate causes excessive constipation. Vitamin D analogs (i.e., calcitriol 0.25–2 mcg once or twice daily [doses above 0.75 mcg/day are usually divided into twice daily dosing]; or alfacalcidol 0.25–4 mcg/day) are given (34). Titrating upward the dose of active vitamin D formulations can help reduce the amount of calcium supplementation that patients require. Some experts also advocate adding vitamin D (chole- or ergocalciferol 800–1000 IU/day) as these agents can have beneficial "off-target" effects and provide smoother control (half-life 2–3 weeks) given the short half-life of vitamin D analogs (31,34). Vitamin D analogs may also be too expensive for some patients.

Having achieved consistent target-range 25-OHD levels through supplementation or lifestyle adjustments, the dose of short-acting agents, calcitriol/alfacalcidol ($\pm$ oral calcium $\pm$ vitamin D), should be adjusted so as to maintain appropriate serum ACa levels. Because a deficiency of PTH action at the renal tubule predisposes to unopposed calciuria, repletion of calcium in these patients to levels within the upper half of the normal range reported by most laboratories will lead to excessive urinary calcium excretion; hence favoring nephrolithiasis or nephrocalcinosis. Thus, a serum ACa level at, or just below, the lower end of the normal range that relieves the patient's symptoms should therefore be the therapeutic goal. Urinary calcium excretion and calcium/creatinine ratio should be measured once a satisfactory serum level has been achieved (ACa generally checked 1 week after starting vitamin D analogs, then if satisfactory at 1, 3 and then 6 months), ideally on a 24-hour collection of urine or, failing that, a "spot" urine sample. If excessive excretion is detected, a lower serum calcium target should be set. If use of a lower target is associated with hypocalcemic symptoms, adjunctive treatments such as a low dose of thiazide diuretic could potentially be beneficial due to the reduced tubular calcium excretion (see below). Even in stable patients, serum and urinary calcium levels should be monitored every 6 months to check for hypercalcemia and hypercalciuria (16,31).

Adjunctive Treatment

Thiazide diuretic can be used as an adjunctive treatment to increase distal renal tubular calcium reabsorption, usually in conjunction with a low-salt diet to promote calcium retention (31,34). Effects on calcium excretion can be noted within 3 or 4 days of starting treatment. The dose of hydrochlorothiazide is 25–100 mg daily. Due to the short plasma half-life of hydrochlorothiazide, twice daily dosing is most often needed (i.e., 25–50 mg twice daily). Chlorthalidone is another thiazide diuretic that can be used. Doses at the higher end of the range are usually necessary to significantly lower urinary calcium with thiazide therapy, but these higher doses can be associated with hypokalemia, hypomagnesemia, and hyponatremia. Potassium supplementation or a potassium- and magnesium-sparing diuretic (e.g., amiloride 2.5–5 mg twice a day) may be used in conjunction with hydrochlorothiazide to prevent hypokalemia and hypomagnesemia.

Phosphate binders or low-phosphate diets are generally not used in hypoparathyroidism unless hyperphosphatemia is particularly troublesome.

Pregnancy

Management of hypoparathyroidism in pregnancy and breastfeeding requires more frequent calcium monitoring (ACa or free calcium every 2–3 weeks (34) and dose-adjustment (35). Calcium levels should be kept at the lower end of normal range. Replacement doses may need to be reduced during the third trimester perhaps due to enhanced hydroxylation of vitamin D to its active form by placental 1 alpha hydroxylase activity, although generally doses need to be maintained or even increased (34). A multidisciplinary approach should occur with endocrinologist, obstetrician, and paediatrician, or neonatologist. The latter should be involved in the immediate care and monitoring of the infant for possible consequences of the treatment of the mother and the underlying maternal disorder (which may be genetic or epigenetic in origin) (34).

Emerging Therapies

Hypoparathyroidism was until recently the only life-threatening hormone deficiency for which bioidentical replacement therapy was not routinely available. However, PTH (1-84) was approved in the USA in 2015 (16,31).

PTH (1-34)

Prior to this, teriparatide, a synthetic injectable human PTH (1-34), which is currently licensed only for the treatment of osteoporosis, had been used off-label as part of the treatment of chronic hypoparathyroidism. Several randomized controlled trials have shown that when compared with conventional therapies (i.e., calcium and vitamin D/vitamin D analogs), administration of teriparatide achieves similar restoration of normal calcium levels and prevents bone demineralization in patients with hypoparathyroidism (36). In addition, urinary calcium levels remain "normal" (but are not reduced) in the teriparatide group, in contrast to the frequent hypercalciuria observed in the conventionally treated patients (with consequent increased risk of nephrocalcinosis or renal calculi). Patients were treated with 20 mcg teriparatide SC once a day, but can achieve even better control when administered in twice-daily dosing regimens (i.e., 20 mcg 12 hrly). More recently, a pump delivery system has been adapted by which teriparatide could be administered continuously (37). Under these conditions, urinary calcium excretion fell and markers of bone turnover normalized. A smaller daily dose was required with pump delivery vs multiple daily dosing regimens. An open-label trial of PTH (1-34) 20 mcg twice daily in adult subjects with postsurgical hypoparathyroidism showed improvement in quality of life (38). In addition, PTH (1-34) administration to hypocalcemic hospitalized patients following thyroidectomy was safe and it can rapidly limit symptoms linked to low calcium levels; furthermore, this treatment was associated with reduced hospital length of stay (39). The THYPOS trial evaluated PTH (1-34) in the primary prevention of postthyroidectomy hypocalcemia by administering PTH (1-34) 20 mcg every 12 hours to subjects with low PTH level 4 hours post-surgery, who were at high risk of hypocalcemia. In comparison to the control group who got standard care for postoperative hypocalcemia, the PTH (1-34) may have prevented some cases of hypocalcemia, shortened the length of stay, and reduced the need for calcium and active vitamin D supplementation (40). PTH (1-34)

has also been studied in ADH1 patients but may not always prevent hypercalciuric renal complications (13).

Major issues with PTH (1-34) include the development of tachyphylaxis which can revert when switched to PTH (1-84). Since teriparatide was introduced as a treatment for osteoporosis in 2002, ongoing surveillance has not revealed any information that might suggest that human subjects are at risk for osteosarcoma. However, because of increased risk of osteosarcoma in pre-clinical studies, PTH (1-34) is limited to 2 years duration of therapy. Hypercalcemia can also occur with resultant hypercalciuria.

PTH (1-84)

There is also growing evidence for the efficacy of recombinant human PTH (1-84) in the treatment of primary hypoparathyroidism. Theoretically, PTH (1-84) is more attractive as a replacement hormone in hypoparathyroidism because the full-length peptide is exactly what is missing in this disease. It is longer *in vivo* and its biological half-life makes once-daily dosing more feasible than PTH (1–34). Several investigative groups that have studied rhPTH (1-84) over the past decade have made the following observations: a substantial reduction, often as much as 50%, in the need for calcium and active vitamin D in both short- and long-term studies; only transient reductions in urinary calcium excretion; improvements in quality of life with protocols that minimized hypercalcemia; and it is associated with improvements in histomorphometric and biochemical indices of skeletal dynamics. Structural bone changes are consistent with an increased remodeling rate in both trabecular and cortical compartments. These changes suggest that PTH (1-84) may improve abnormal skeletal properties in hypoparathyroidism by restoring bone metabolism toward normal euparathyroid levels (31,41).

These observations were followed by a pivotal, multinational, randomized, double-blinded, placebo-controlled phase 3 clinical trial of rhPTH (1-84) in hypoparathyroidism. Results from the REPLACE study, which was a large randomized placebo-controlled double blind trial, are encouraging in this regard (42). In this 6-month trial, rhPTH (1-84) added to standard treatment was compared with standard treatment with calcitriol and calcium supplements. Adding rhPTH (1-84) at a dose between 50–100 mcg once daily to the standard regimen resulted in more than 50% reduction in doses of vitamin D analogs and calcium with reduction in phosphate levels, but no significant change in urinary calcium. However, urinary calcium did not rise in spite of improvement in plasma calcium in the rhPTH (1-84) treatment group. In comparison, only 2% of patients in the placebo arm achieved a dose reduction of vitamin D and calcium. More recently, long-term, continuous therapy of hypoparathyroidism for 6 years with rhPTH(1–84) was associated with reductions in supplemental calcium and calcitriol requirements, stable serum calcium concentration, and reduced urinary calcium excretion. The safety profile was reassuring (43).

PTH (1-84) treatment of hypoparathyroidism is indicated for subjects with hypoparathyroidism of any etiology, except ADH, who cannot be well controlled on calcium and active vitamin D. The recommendations from the labeling are as follows (31). The lowest dose of 50 mcg is initiated once daily SC into the thigh. Simultaneously, the dose of active vitamin D is reduced by 50%. The serum calcium concentration is monitored within the first week of initiation and similarly whenever the dose of rhPTH (1-84) is changed or as often as needed. The goals of therapy with rhPTH (1-84) are to minimize or eliminate the use of active vitamin D, to reduce supplemental calcium to 500 mg daily, and to maintain the serum calcium in the lower range of normal. An alternative approach would be to start by reducing oral calcium by 50% instead of active vitamin D. The dose of rhPTH (1-84) can be increased in 25-mcg steps to 100 mcg daily. There are no factors that can predict which ultimate dose will work best for a given patient.

If rhPTH (1-84) is to be discontinued for any reason, due regard for acute manifestations of hypocalcemia are very important because PTH in any form has a short half-life. The 25-(OH)D level in all patients should generally be in the range 20–30 ng/mL(50–80 nmol/L), and particularly so in individuals who are discontinuing rhPTH (1-84). The dosing of calcium and active vitamin D should be increased or started with careful frequent monitoring for signs and symptoms of hypocalcemia. In view of a recent example of abrupt hypocalcemia developing in two subjects who stopped teriparatide therapy (44), a recommendation to double or triple the ambient calcium and active vitamin D regimen should be seriously considered, as well as a regimen to taper the dose of rhPTH (1-84).

The US FDA approved rhPTH (1-84) with a "black box" warning because of the history of rat osteosarcoma using all forms of PTH that have been studied so far but did not limit the duration of use. Hypercalcemia can also occur with resultant hypercalciuria. However, in a 6-year experiential study of 33 subjects with hypoparathyroidism treated with rhPTH (1-84), only 12 episodes of hypercalcemia were detected over 6 y; representing 2.5% of all values (43). Since being approved for primary hypoparathyroidism therapy, routine use of rhPTH (1-84) is still limited due to its cost and need for more clinical/trial evidence. Interestingly, an European Society of Endocrinology Clinical Guideline on treatment of chronic hypoparathyroidism recently recommended against the routine use of replacement therapy with PTH (1-84) or PTH analogs (i.e., PTH [1-34]) (34). An oral PTH formulation is also in advanced clinical development.

Calcilytics

Finally, drugs that antagonize the CaSR by negative allosteric modulation (termed calcilytics), thereby increasing PTH secretion, are being explored and may also have a role in the management of mild/moderate hypoparathyroidism and ADH1 patients (13,45).

Conclusions

Hypocalcemia is a common electrolyte disturbance, especially in the inpatient setting. Acute hypocalcemia is associated with significant morbidity and mortality and should be managed as a medical emergency. Management of chronic hypocalcemia can seem complex due to the varying underlying diagnoses and different calcium and vitamin D formulations available, but there is an underlying logic that is based on physiological first principles. Patients on long-term, potent hydroxylated vitamin D-analog products (e.g., calcitriol/alfacalcidol) should be closely monitored for complications of therapy (i.e., hypercalcemia, hypercalciuria, nephrocalcinosis, or renal calculi). These products should not be used to replace vitamin D deficiency itself, for which cholecalciferol, or ergocalciferol is logical, safer and cheaper (9,33).

Acknowledgments

The current author wishes to acknowledge the contributions to the previous edition by previous co-authors, Richard Quinton and Muhammad Asam, upon which portions of this chapter are based.

References

1 Zivin J, Gooley T, Zager R, Ryan M. Hypocalcemia: A pervasive metabolic abnormality in the critically ill. *Am J Kidney Dis*. 2001;37;689–698.
2 Hannan FM, Thakker RV. Investigating hypocalcemia. *BMJ*. 2013;346:f2213.
3 Schafer AL, Shoback D. Hypocalcemia: definition, etiology, pathogenesis, diagnosis, and management. In: Rosen CJ, ed. *Primer on the Metabolic Bone Diseases and Disorders of Mineral Metabolism, 8 edn*, Washington, DC, American Society for Bone and Mineral Research, 2013; 572–578.
4 Carroll R, Matfin G. Endocrine and metabolic emergencies: hypocalcaemia. *Therap Adv Endocrin Metab*. 2010;1:29–33.
5 Turner J, Gittoes N, Selby P, the Society for Endocrinology Clinical Committee. Emergency management of acute hypocalcaemia in adult patients. 2016. DOI: 10.1530/EC-16-0056.
6 Favus MJ, Goltzman D. Regulation of calcium and magnesium. In: Rosen CJ, ed: *Primer on the Metabolic Bone Diseases and Disorders of Mineral Metabolism, 8 edn*, Washington, DC, American Society for Bone and Mineral Research. 2013; 173–179.
7 Holick MF. Vitamin D deficiency. *N Engl J Med*. 2007;357;266–281.
8 Pearce SHS, Cheetham, TD. Diagnosis and management of vitamin D deficiency. *BMJ*. 2010;340:142–147.
9 National Osteoporosis Society 2013. *Vitamin D and Bone Health: A Practical Clinical Guideline for Patient Management*. http://www.nos.org.uk/document.doc?id=1352 (accessed January 20, 2014).
10 Monkawa T, Yoshida T, Hayashi M, Saruta T. (2000) Identification of 25-hydroxyvitamin D3 1alpha-hydroxylase gene expression in macrophages. *Kindnet Int*. 2000;58(2):559–568.
11 Jüppner H. Phosphate and FGF-23. *Kidney Int*. 2011;79:S24–S27.
12 Egbuna OI, Brown EM. Hypercalcaemic and hypocalcaemic conditions due to calcium-sensing receptor mutations. *Best Pract Res Clin Rheumatol*. 2008;22: 129–148.
13 Hannan FM, Babinsky VN, Thakker RV. Disorders of the calcium-sensing receptor and partner proteins: insights into the

molecular basis of calcium homeostasis. *J Molecular Endocrinology.* 2016;57: R127–R142.

14 Asam M, Pawlak A, Matfin G, Quinton R. Disorders of calcium homeostasis. *Foundation Years Journal.* 2014;5;14–23.

15 Munns CF, Shaw N, Kiely M, et al. Global consensus recommendations on prevention and management of nutritional rickets. *J Clin Endocrinol Metab.* 2016;101: 394–415.

16 Brandi ML, Bilezikian JP, Shoback D, et al. Management of hypoparathyroidism: summary statement and guidelines. *J Clin Endocrinol Metab.* 2016;101:2273–2283.

17 Clarke BL, Brown EM, Collins M, et al. Epidemiology and diagnosis of hypoparathyroidism. *J Clin Endocrinol Metab.* 2016;101:2284–2299.

18 Shoback D. (2008). Hypoparathyroidism. *N Engl J Med* 359; 391–403.

19 Schattner A, Dubin I, Huber R, Gelber M. Hypocalcaemia of malignancy. *Neth J Med.* 2016;74:231–239.

20 Brasier AR, Nussbaum SR. Hungry bone syndrome: clinical and biochemical predictors of its occurrence after parathyroid surgery. *Am J Med.* 1988;84(4): 654–660.

21 Alhefdhi, A, Mazeh H, Chen, H. Role of Postoperative vitamin D and/or calcium routine supplementation in preventing hypocalcemia after thyroidectomy: a systematic review and meta-analysis. *Oncologist.* 2013;18(5):533–542.

22 Wang TS, Roman SA, Sosa JA. Postoperative calcium supplementation in patients undergoing thyroidectomy. *Curr Opin Oncology.* 2012;24:22–28.

23 Alkhalili E, Ehrhart MD, Ayoubieh H, Burge MR. Does preoperative vitamin D deficiency predict postoperative hypocalcemia after thyroidectomy? *Endocrine Pract.* (2016) DOI:10.4158/ EP161411.OR.

24 Shoback D, Bilezikian JP, Costa AG, et al. Presentation of hypoparathyroidism: etiologies and clinical features. *J Clin Endocrinol Metab.* 2016;101:2300–2312.

25 Desai TK, Carlson RW, Geheb MA. Prevalence and clinical implications of hypocalcemia in acutely ill patients in a medical intensive care setting. *Am J Med.* 1988;84(2):209–214.

26 Liamis G, Milionis H, Elisaf M. A review of drug induced hypocalcemia. *J Bone Miner Metab.* 2009;27;635–642.

27 Doorenbos CJ, Ozyilmaz A, van Wijnen M. Severe pseudohypocalcemia after gadolinium-enhanced magnetic resonance angiography. *N Engl J Med.* 2003;349(8): 817–818.

28 Hoffman E. The Chvostek sign: a clinical study. *Am J Surg.* 1958;96;33–37.

29 Jesus JE, Landry A. Chvostek's and Trousseau's signs. *N Engl J Med.* 2012;367:e 15.

30 Hurley K, Baggs D. Hypocalcemic cardiac failure in the emergency department. *J Emerg Med.* 2005;28(2):155–159.

31 Bilezikian JP, Brandi ML, Cusano NE, et al. Management of hypoparathyroidism: present and future. *J Clin Endocrinol Metab.* 2016;101:2313–2324.

32 Romagnoli E, Mascia ML, Ciprianj C, et al. Short- and long-term variations in serum calciotropic hormones after a single very large dose of ergocalciferol (vitamin D2) or cholecalciferol (vitamin D3) in the elderly. *J Clin Endocrinol Metab.* 2008;93(8): 3015–3020.

33 Holick MF, Brinkley NC, Bischoff-Ferrari HA, et al. Evaluation, treatment, and prevention of vitamin D deficiency: an Endocrine Society Clinical Practice Guideline. *J Clin Endocrinol Metab.* 2011;96:1911–1930.

34 Bollerslev J, Rejnmark L, Marcocci C, et al. European Society of Endocrinology Clinical Guideline: Treatment of chronic hypoparathyroidism in adults. *Europ J Endocrinology.* 2015;173:G1–G20.

35 Bilezikian JP, Khan A, Potts JT Jr, et al. Hypoparathyroidism in the adult: epidemiology, diagnosis, pathophysiology, target-organ involvement, treatment, and challenges for future research. *J Bone Miner Res.* 2011;26:2317–2337.

36 Winer KK, Ko CW, Reynolds JC, et al. Long-term treatment of hypoparathyroidism: a randomized controlled study comparing parathyroid hormone-(1-34) versus calcitriol and calcium. *J Clin Endocrinol Metab*. 2003;88; 4214–4220.

37 Winer KK, Fulton KA, Albert PS, Cutler GB Jr. Effects of pump versus twice-daily injection delivery of synthetic parathyroid hormone 1–34 in children with severe congenital hypoparathyroidism. *J Pediatr*. 2014;165:556–563.

38 Santonati A, Palermo A, Maddaloni E, et al. PTH(1–34) for surgical hypoparathyroidism: a prospective, open-label investigation of efficacy and quality of life. *J Clin Endocrinol Metab*. 2015;100:3590–3597.

39 Shah M, Bancos I, Thompson GB, et al. Teriparatide therapy and reduced postoperative hospitalization for postsurgical hypoparathyroidism. *JAMA Otolaryngo Head Neck Surgery*. 2015;141: 822–827.

40 Palermo A, Mangiameli G, Tabacco G, et al. PTH (1-34) for the primary prevention of postthyroidectomy hypocalcemia: The TYPHOS Trial. *J Clin Endocrinol Metab*. 2016;101:4039–4045.

41 Rubin MR, Dempster DW. (2011) PTH(1-84) administration reverses abnormal bone-remodeling dynamics and structure in hypoparathyroidism. *J Bone Miner Res*. 2011;26(11):2727–2736.

42 Mannstadt B, et al. Efficacy and safety of recombinant human parathyroid hormone (1-84) in hypoparathyroidism (REPLACE): a double-blind, placebo-controlled, randomised, phase 3 study. *Lancet Diabetes & Endocrinology*. 2013;1: 275–283.

43 Rubin MR, Cusano NE, Fan WW, et al. Therapy of hypoparathyroidism with PTH(1–84): a prospective six year investigation of efficacy and safety. *J Clin Endocrinol Metab*. 2016;101: 2742–2750.

44 Gafni RI, Guthrie LC, Kelly MH, et al. Transient increased calcium and calcitriol requirements after discontinuation of human synthetic parathyroid hormone 1-34 (hPTH 1–34) replacement therapy in hypoparathyroidism. *J Bone Miner Res*. 2015;30:2112–2118.

45 Saidek Z, Brazier M, Kamel S, Mentaverri R. Agonists and allosteric modulators of the calcium-sensing receptor and their therapeutic applications. *Mol Pharmacol*. 2009;76;1131–1144.

24

Hypercalcemia

Glenn Matfin

Key Points

- The skeleton is the major store of calcium. Approximately 99% of total body calcium (1 kg) is found in bone. Most of the remainder is located in the intracellular compartment with only a small amount present in extracellular fluid.
- The free (ionized) calcium is the physiologically important ion and is tightly regulated.
- Calcium homeostasis is directly or indirectly regulated by vitamin D metabolites and parathyroid hormone (PTH) via the kidney, intestine, and bone.
- PTH is secreted by the chief cells of the parathyroid glands. A unique calcium receptor on the cell membrane (extracellular calcium-sensing receptor [CaSR]) responds rapidly to changes in serum ionized calcium.
- Hypercalcemia (serum calcium >10.5 mg/dL [2.6 mmol/L], measured on at least two occasions) affects about 0.5% of hospitalized patients and is usually well tolerated if adjusted calcium (i.e., corrected for albumin concentration) levels are <12 mg/dL (3.0 mmol/L).
- Adjusted calcium above this threshold is associated with nephrogenic diabetes insipidus, increasingly severe volume contraction, neurological, cardiac, and gastrointestinal dysfunction, and requires urgent treatment to prevent life-threatening consequences.
- Measurement of intact PTH level is pivotal in the differential diagnosis of calcium disorders. The causes of hypercalcemia can be conveniently divided into those associated with an elevated or inappropriately normal PTH level, and those where PTH output is appropriately suppressed.
- In an ambulatory population, primary hyperparathyroidism (PHPT) accounts for the vast majority of detected hypercalcemia (>90%).
- Hypercalcemia of malignancy (HCM) complicates 5–30% of malignancies and is the commonest cause of inpatient hypercalcemic crises (>50%).
- The final common pathway for many types of severe hypercalcemia is increased mobilization of calcium from bone due in part to activation of osteoclasts by RANK/RANKL pathway.
- For treatment of severe hypercalcemia, the underlying cause should be identified and multitargeted therapies should be started as soon as possible.
- The cornerstone of acute management of hypercalcemia is fluid resuscitation with correction of the volume state (rapid-acting). Other treatment options include short-term calcitonin; and for slower onset, longer term control, the most effective antiresorptive agents (e.g., bisphosphonates, denosumab) should be considered. Glucocorticoids can also be used for vitamin D-related hypercalcemia (e.g., vitamin D overdose, and granulomatous disorders) and in certain malignancies (e.g., myeloma).

Endocrine and Metabolic Medical Emergencies: A Clinician's Guide, Second Edition. Edited by Glenn Matfin.
© 2018 John Wiley & Sons Ltd. Published 2018 by John Wiley & Sons Ltd.

- If the diagnosis is PHPT, then surgical removal of parathyroid adenoma(s) should be planned. If surgical intervention is not an option or is delayed, a calcimimetic (cinacalcet) can be used to lower calcium levels.

- For HCM, further therapy will be determined by the diagnosis, extent of the disease, and overall prognosis of the associated malignancy.

Introduction

The skeletal system is one of the largest organs in the body and is one of the hallmarks that distinguishes vertebrates from invertebrates. It is the storehouse for 98–99% of the body's 1 kg of calcium. Bones are mineralized connective tissue in which type I collagen forms a network of flexible fibers with a smaller cellular fraction. Mineralization of this network, or matrix, with calcium salts is required to produce the rigid skeleton.

The skeleton is not only a storehouse for ions but is essential for locomotion, protection of vital organs, and production and maturation of major components of the hematopoietic system. The structural component of bone required for locomotion and protection of organs is the outer cortical shell, which accounts for 80% of skeletal mass. The less robust inner cancellous (trabecular) bone also has a role in the mechanical stability and flexibility of the skeleton, in that disruption of its microarchitecture is the dominant contributor to minimal-trauma fractures (i.e., osteoporosis). In addition, bone is increasingly recognized as having endocrine functions playing an important role in regulating metabolic processes.

Bone is a dynamic tissue that is under continuous turnover or remodeling, which enables bone to repair damage and adjust strength. Osteoclasts and osteoblasts are two main types of bone cells located on bone surfaces and are responsible for bone resorption and formation, respectively. Osteocytes, the most abundant cells in mature bone, are located in lacunae within the bone matrix. Osteoclasts resorb bone, osteoblasts lay down new bone at a site of previous bone resorption, and osteocytes nourish the skeleton and regulate bone cell activity. Bone remodeling does not occur at random, but occurs instead in discrete packets known as "bone remodeling units." Bone resorption and bone formation normally are coupled, with synthesis of new bone following the resorption of old. An estimated 10–30% of the skeleton is remodeled each year, with wide variation among individuals. During the perimenopause and under the influence of various states and medications, the remodeling rate is often increased, but with excess resorption (a negative bone balance) resulting in net loss of bone (i.e., secondary osteoporosis, when resulting osteoporosis is secondary to diseases or medications).

Calcium is required for the mineralization of bone and is a key regulator of many body processes. Calcium ions play critical roles in intracellular signaling, in the regulation of events at the plasma membrane, and in the function of extracellular proteins such as those involved in blood coagulation. The circulating concentration of calcium ions is kept constant under the control of the parathyroid hormone (PTH) and metabolites of vitamin D (1). Deviations of the concentration of free (unbound) calcium outside its very narrow reference interval can cause morbidity and mortality. The importance of the tight regulation of free calcium is underscored by the recognition that skeletal health is allowed to suffer markedly to allow physiologic processes in other organs to be maintained.

In blood, virtually all of the calcium is found in the plasma, which has a mean calcium concentration of 9.5 mg/dL (2.38 mmol/L) with a narrow reference range (8.5–10.5 mg/dL; 2.1–2.6 mmol/L). Calcium exists in three physicochemical states in plasma: 50% is free (ionized), 40% is bound to plasma proteins, and 10% is complexed with small diffusible inorganic and organic anions, including bicarbonate, lactate, phosphate, and citrate.

Hypercalcemia (serum calcium >10.5 mg/dL [2.6 mmol/L], measured on at least two occasions) affects about 0.5% of hospitalized patients and is usually well tolerated if adjusted calcium (ACa) (i.e., corrected for albumin concentration) levels are <12 mg/dL (3.0 mmol/L). Hypercalcemia is commonly seen in the context of parathyroid dysfunction and malignancy, and when severe, can be life-threatening. Measurement of intact PTH level is pivotal in the differential diagnosis of hypercalcemia.

Adjusted calcium >12 mg/dL (3.0 mmol/L) is associated with nephrogenic diabetes insipidus (DI), increasingly severe volume contraction, neurological, cardiac, and gastrointestinal dysfunction, and requires urgent treatment to prevent life-threatening consequences. The term "hypercalcemic crisis" is frequently used to describe the severely compromised patient with profound volume depletion, altered sensorium, which may be manifest as coma, cardiac decompensation (including dysrhythmias), and abdominal pain that may mimic an acute surgical abdomen (2). Hypercalcemic crises usually occur when ACa levels >14 mg/dL (3.5 mmol/L) (3). Hypercalcemia of malignancy is the commonest cause of inpatient hypercalcemic crises (>50%) and complicates 5–30% of malignancies (4).

Severe hypercalcemia requires urgent treatment (5). Although there are multiple, overlapping causes of calcium imbalance, much of the acute management is generic, logical and intuitive. However, making a correct diagnosis remains important for the quality of management and long-term outcomes (6).

Pathophysiology

Calcium is ingested in the diet, absorbed from the intestine, filtered in the glomerulus of the kidney, reabsorbed in the renal tubules, and eliminated in the urine (1,7). Approximately 99% of total body calcium (1 kg) is found in bone. Most of the remainder is located in the intracellular compartment with only a small amount present in extracellular fluid (ECF). Calcium homeostasis is tightly regulated through multiple interactions between the dietary intake of bone minerals and the serum levels of homeostatic hormones (principally PTH, vitamin D metabolites, and phosphaturic agents such as osteocyte-secreted Fibroblast Growth Factor 23 [FGF23]), acting principally on bone, intestine and kidneys (7–9). Hypercalcemia represents a serious disruption of calcium homeostasis, wherein these homeostatic mechanisms have become overwhelmed by a specific pathological process.

PTH is secreted by the chief cells of the parathyroid glands (four glands classically located on or near the posterior surface of the thyroid gland). A unique calcium receptor on the cell membrane (the extracellular calcium-sensing receptor [CaSR]) responds rapidly to changes in serum free (ionized) calcium (10,11). When the free (ionized) calcium is high, appropriate inhibition of PTH synthesis and release occurs, while a decrease in free (ionized) calcium prompts a rapid adaptive increase in PTH release (Figure 24-1). The main function of PTH is to maintain the calcium concentration of the ECF by promoting the release of calcium from bone by osteoclast resorption, increasing the activation of 25-hydroxyvitamin D (25-(OH)D, calcidiol) to 1,25-dihydroxyvitamin D (1,25-(OH)2D, calcitriol), which increases the calcium absorption from the intestine plus sensitizes bone to the resorptive actions of PTH, and stimulates calcium conservation by the kidney while increasing phosphate excretion (which prevents calcium phosphate salt formation in the ECF) (Figure 24-1) (7).

At least one of the following mechanisms is involved in the pathophysiology of hypercalcemia: (a) increased intestinal calcium absorption; (b) increased bone resorption; and (c) increased renal calcium reabsorption or decreased calcium excretion. Hypercalcemia often results when the influx of calcium into the ECF compartment from the skeleton, intestine, or kidney is greater than

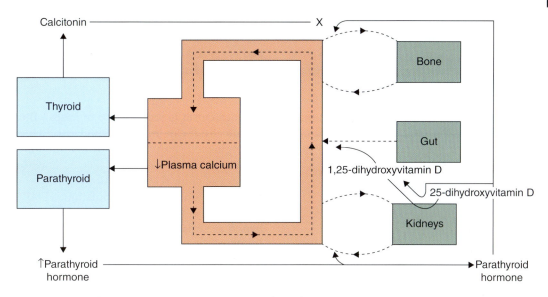

Figure 24-1 Parathyroid hormone (PTH) response to a fall in free (ionized) calcium. A decrease in free (ionized) calcium is detected by the calcium-sensing receptor (CaSR) on the chief cells of the parathyroid gland to stimulate PTH release and synthesis. PTH acts on the osteoblasts and osteoclasts promoting calcium release via bone resorption; on the kidneys promoting calcium reabsorption and 1,25-(OH)2D (calcitriol) production which stimulates calcium absorption via the intestine, thus increasing circulating ionized calcium.

the efflux as, for example, when excessive resorption of bone mineral occurs in malignancy. Hypercalciuria often develops in such situations. When the capacity of the kidney to excrete filtered calcium is exceeded, hypercalcemia develops; where renal failure is present and calcium excretion is decreased, hypocalciuria may paradoxically be present. Hypercalcemia can be caused by increased intestinal absorption (e.g., vitamin D intoxication [rare]); increased renal retention (e.g., thiazide diuretics); increased skeletal resorption (e.g., immobilization); or a combination of mechanisms (e.g., primary hyperparathyroidism [PHPT]). When the 24 h urinary calcium concentration exceeds 400 mg/dL (10 mmol/L) (plasma concentration approximately 12 mg/dL [3.0 mmol/L]), nephrogenic DI results with impaired urine concentrating ability due to effects on vasopressin binding, with aquaporin downregulation, and altered renal interstitial sodium concentration. Volume depletion can also result from associated vomiting. The resultant intravascular volume contraction and subsequent reduction in glomerular

filtration rate (GFR) severely limit the ability of the kidneys to excrete calcium. If continued calcium mobilization from bone occurs, hypercalcemia can rapidly increase. The patient becomes progressively worse until hypercalcemia is treated and the vicious cycle is broken. This chain of events highlights the extreme importance of volume resuscitation in the management of hypercalcemia (12).

Hypercalcemia predominantly results from increased mobilization of calcium from bone. The final common pathway for increased bone resorption is activation of one of the key signaling pathways, known as the RANK/RANKL/OPG system (13). RANK (receptor activator of nuclear factor–κB) is a membrane protein expressed on the surface of osteoclasts. Its ligand (RANK ligand, or RANKL) is found on the surface of osteoblasts (also on stromal and T cells). Binding of RANK to RANKL activates osteoclasts. Osteoprotegerin (OPG, literally means "bone protector") is a cytokine (a member of the tumor necrosis factor [TNF] receptor superfamily) and a RANK homolog that can inhibit the production and maturation of osteoclasts by acting as a decoy receptor blocking the interaction of RANK with its ligand RANKL. Activation of RANK by RANKL is increased in many causes of severe hypercalcemia. Knowledge of this pathway has resulted in the development of a new therapy (i.e., denosumab, which prevents RANKL activating RANK on osteoclasts) for hypercalcemia (14–16) and some metabolic bone diseases.

Etiology

The two most common causes of hypercalcemia are PHPT and malignancy. PHPT tends to be more common in outpatient settings, whereas malignancy is most commonly seen in inpatients (17,18). Vitamin D (cholecalciferol or ergocalciferol) or vitamin D analog therapy has become one of the most common causes of hypercalcemia detected in laboratory practice (vitamin D toxicity is defined as hypercalcemia and serum 25-(OH)D >250 nmol/L [sufficient is >50 nmol/L], with hypercalciuria and suppressed PTH) (19). Together, these causes account for 90–95% of all cases of hypercalcemia.

The causes of hypercalcemia can be conveniently divided into those associated with an elevated or inappropriately normal PTH level (PTH increases hydroxylation of vitamin D to its active form in the kidneys and increases bone resorption resulting in hypercalcemia), and those where PTH output is appropriately suppressed (Table 24-1) (20). Notable exceptions to this paradigm include hypercalcemia due to familial hypocalciuric hypercalcemia (FHH), where PTH output is appropriate to the level of ambient calcium sensed by the abnormal CaSR; or treatment with lithium (10,11). FHH is a rare disorder and comprises three genetically distinct conditions, designated FHH types 1–3 (11). As such, FHH is characterized by life-long mild-moderate hypercalcemia (usually <12 mg/dL [3 mmol/L]) and is usually asymptomatic (FHH3 has symptomatic

hypercalcemia in >20% cases). FHH1 is the most common type (~65% of all FHH cases) and is caused by an inactivating mutation in the CaSR. Reduced sensing of extracellular calcium leads to a rise in PTH levels, resulting in hypercalcemia without hypercalciuria (hypocalciuria is seen in 95% of cases). Biochemically, it can look very similar to PHPT, distinguished only by a lower fractional excretion of urine calcium (FeCA) and the absence of clinical complications.

In an ambulatory population, PHPT accounts for the vast majority of detected hypercalcemia (>90%) (7,21–23). PHPT is often characterized by increased secretion of PTH that results in hypercalcemia. Inappropriate autonomous PTH secretion is found in the context of parathyroid adenomas which may be solitary (80% to 85% of cases) or multiple (7). Parathyroid adenomas are most commonly sporadic but may be part of an endocrine neoplastic syndrome especially if numerous or found in the young, such as multiple endocrine neoplasia (MEN) type 1 (MEN1); MEN2A (MEN2); and MEN4. Hereditary forms of PHPT occur in 5–10% overall, including syndromic (i.e., associated with other glands and systems) and non-syndromic types, but can be even higher in younger patients or with atypical features (e.g., age less than 45 years, multi-gland involvement, parathyroid carcinoma). Parathyroid hyperplasia without an obvious physiological stimulus can also occur, and usually involves all four glands (~15% of PHPT). Rarely, parathyroid carcinoma may occur (<1% of PHPT cases). Secondary hyperparathyroidism (SHPT) is an appropriate physiological adaptation to many situations in which hypocalcemia is seen, including vitamin D deficiency, advanced chronic kidney disease (CKD), and gastrointestinal malabsorption of calcium (7,9). However, parathyroid autonomy often develops if the stimulus persists, and when hypercalcemia results, the condition is redefined as tertiary hyperparathyroidism (THPT). Vitamin D deficiency is typically severe and long-standing before

Table 24-1 Etiology of hypercalcemia

Elevated or inappropriately normal PTH	Suppressed PTH
Primary hyperparathyroidism (PHPT) • Adenoma (solitary or multiple), hyperplasia, carcinoma • Familial (e.g., familial hypocalciuric hypercalcemia [FHH]; multiple endocrine neoplasia [MEN] type 1 [MEN1], MEN2A [MEN2], and MEN4; hyperparathyroidism jaw tumor syndrome; familial isolated PHPT) *Tertiary hyperparathyroidism (THPT)* • Advanced chronic kidney disease (CKD) • Severe vitamin D deficiency • Malabsorption of calcium (e.g. celiac disease) *Miscellaneous* • Lithium • PTH therapy – PTH (1-84) • Ectopic PTH secretion	*Malignancy* • Humoral mediators (e.g., PTHrP) • Vitamin D mediated • Multiple myeloma • Lytic bone metastases *Drug-induced* • Calcium ± vitamin D • Vitamin D intoxication • Vitamin A intoxication • Thiazide diuretics *Endocrinopathies* • Thyrotoxicosis • Acute adrenal insufficiency • Pheochromocytoma • VIPoma • Acromegaly *Granulomatous disorders* • Sarcoidosis; tuberculosis; berylliosis *Miscellaneous* • Immobilization • Milk-alkali syndrome

PTH = Parathyroid hormone; PTHrP = Parathyroid hormone-related peptide; VIP = Vasoactive inhibitory peptide.

THPT develops. Lithium therapy produces biochemistry that mimics FHH as the intracellular calcium concentration threshold at which PTH, that continues to be produced and secreted, is raised, while hypocalciuria is also seen.

Hypercalcemia of malignancy (HCM) is the commonest cause of inpatient hypercalcemic crises (>50%) and complicates 5–30% of malignancies (2,4). Hypercalcemia secondary to malignancy usually presents in the context of advanced clinically obvious disease and portends an ominous prognosis with survival typically on the order of months. It results either from humoral mediated bone resorption (>80%); or direct destruction of bone, either in myeloma or lytic metastatic disease (~20%). Increased calcitriol production due to increased 1α-hydroxylase activity in some lymphomas, and ectopic PTH are rare and account <1% HCM (4). The majority of humoral hypercalcemia of malignancy (HHM) (>80%) is induced by parathyroid hormone-related peptide (PTHrP), a peptide with significant amino terminal homology to PTH. PTHrP induces bone resorption by binding to PTH receptor type 1 and can also induce phosphaturia/hypophosphatemia. Many solid tumors are associated with hypercalcemia and include squamous cell carcinomas of the lung, head and neck, esophagus, renal cell carcinoma, and breast carcinoma. Humoral mediated bone resorption stimulated by PTHrP accounts for the majority of hypercalcemia in these malignancies (24) even when lytic metastatic bone disease is present. Signs and symptoms of hypercalcemia are more evident in patients with HHM because the plasma calcium increases rapidly and often reaches concentrations higher than those usually seen in PHPT. Hematological malignancies such as multiple myeloma can be associated with hypercalcemia via locally produced osteolytic peptides, which can include PTHrP.

Increased expression of 1α-hydroxylase by lymphoproliferative tissues including lymphoma occasionally results in clinically significant hypercalcemia as a result of significantly increased synthesis of 1,25 dihydroxyvitamin D (25). Between 5% and 15% of patients with hypercalcemia and malignancy have coexisting PHPT.

A number of administered drugs can cause hypercalcemia. Thiazide diuretics reduce renal calcium excretion, increase renal calcium reabsorption and, as a result, mild hypercalcemia is frequently seen, and they can unmask PHPT. The effect of lithium is discussed above. Calcium (± vitamin D) supplementation rarely causes hypercalcemia if normal physiological mechanisms of calcium regulation are intact. In milk-alkali syndrome, a high intake of milk or calcium carbonate (used to treat dyspepsia or more commonly now osteoporosis) may lead to hypercalcemia mediated by the high calcium intake plus metabolic alkalosis, which augments calcium reabsorption in the distal tubule. This usually occurs in the presence of renal impairment and reducing GFR, which decreases calcium excretion, thus increasing serum ACa. Hypercalcemia in the context of vitamin D intoxication is recognized but rare (8,19), but treatment with vitamin D analogs (alfacalcidol, calcitriol) especially in CKD and osteoporosis is increasingly recognized as a cause of hypercalcemia (26). Hypercalcemia is of particular concern in individuals treated with large doses of parent vitamin D (ergo- or cholecalciferol), which can accumulate in large amounts in fat stores and, when released, can result in prolonged hypercalcemia. Prolonged immobilization (including the post-acute care setting) may be associated with hypercalcemia due to a marked increase in bone resorption. Patients with underlying high bone turnover states are at particular risk (e.g., active polyostotic Paget's disease). Granuloma-associated macrophages occasionally express 1α-hydroxylase with consequent increased conversion to active 1,25-(OH)2D (calcitriol), and hypercalcemia will complicate over 10% of cases of sarcoidosis (26). A number of endocrinopathies are associated with hypercalcemia. Hypercalcemia in thyrotoxicosis is postulated to be secondary to increased bone resorption (27,28). Volume depletion in Addison's disease is claimed to promote hypercalcemia. PTHrP secretion by pheochromocytomas occasionally results in clinically significant hypercalcemia. The very rare vasoactive intestinal peptide (VIP) secreting tumor, VIPoma, is associated with hypercalcemia possibly through VIP mediated stimulation of the PTH receptor.

Diagnostic Considerations

Calcium status is more accurately determined by measuring free (ionized) calcium, the tightly regulated, biologically active species. Interpretation of the total serum calcium value is complicated by its association with protein and inorganic and organic ions. Interpretation of free calcium concentration is less complicated, provided the specimen has been properly obtained, handled, and analyzed.

Severe hypercalcemia is defined as a total serum calcium >14 mg/dL (3.5 mmol/L) (29). Some 40% of total serum calcium is protein bound with the majority bound to albumin, while 50% is ionized and active. Albumin concentrations should therefore be considered when assessing hypercalcemia, and most laboratories provide a calcium level adjusted for the prevailing albumin (ACa). However, in states of acute albumin fluctuations such as sepsis, infections and in many emergency situations, measurement of ionized calcium may be a more reliable assessment of calcium status (although alkalosis increases binding to albumin and therefore decreases free calcium levels). Overall free (ionized) calcium measurement may be more useful than total calcium determination in hospitalized patients. The reference interval of free calcium (in adults) has been reported as 4.6–5.3 mg/dL (1.15–1.33 mmol/L). Hypercalcemia is defined >5.4 mg/dL (1.34 mmol/L) when measuring free calcium.

Severe hypercalcemia, suspected clinically or detected biochemically, should prompt immediate treatment. The first step in the evaluation of hypercalcemia which must be performed prior to commencing any treatment is to obtain samples for PTH measurement to establish whether the hypercalcemia is PTH dependent (30).

PTH can be unstable in serum and therefore blood samples should be taken in the appropriate preservative and delivered to the laboratory promptly. The "intact" molecule (PTH [1-84]) is now assayed routinely and was thought to have eliminated the problems of measured bio-inactive C-terminal fragments (especially in patients with impaired renal function). It has become clear that the "intact" assays measure some PTH fragments (particularly PTH (7-84)) which are biologically inactive but accumulate with impaired renal function. The percentage of PTH (7-84) fragments increase proportionally with decreasing renal function. New "whole" PTH assays have been developed that do not cross-react with the PTH (7-84) fragment, but these have not been shown to be offer any major clinical usefulness when investigating calcium abnormalities compared to the "intact" assays. It should be remembered that PHPT is a common condition and is therefore occasionally (5–15% of patients with HCM) the cause of hypercalcemia in patients with concurrent cancer (24,29).

Other tests include measurement of creatinine and calculation of estimated GFR (eGFR). Renal function may be abnormal due to dehydration or may indicate THPT. Raised alkaline phosphatase is associated with osteoblastic bone metastases, but also with vitamin D deficiency and acute fracture. Full (complete) blood count may point to hematological disorders such as lymphoma, whereas serum electrophoresis is used to diagnose myeloma. Levels of blood markers such as 1,25-(OH)2D (calcitriol) and angiotensin converting enzyme (ACE) may be raised in sarcoidosis. Assessment of calcitriol level is also required if the patient is receiving vitamin D analogs, or has a confirmed or suspected diagnosis of lymphoproliferative disorders. Thyroid disease and acute adrenal insufficiency should be investigated if clinical manifestations are present (Table 24-2). FeCa (fractional excretion of calcium) is used to differentiate between PHPT and FHH, but the definitive diagnosis of FHH requires genetic testing (11). Next generation genetic sequencing for hereditary forms of PHPT is now cheaper and more widely available. PTHrP can be measured but adds little to the management if malignancy associated hypercalcemia is already obvious. Other investigations should be directed by the clinical situation and include electrocardiogram (ECG) and imaging tests as required (Table 24-2).

Clinical Signs and Features

Most patients with mild hypercalcemia are asymptomatic and hypercalcemia is an incidental finding on blood testing (including 80% of PHPT patients). However, severe hypercalcemia is usually symptomatic and symptoms can vary from malaise to severe dehydration and coma (Table 24-3). In practice, most cases of severe, acute hypercalcemia are due to cancer, though excess intake of calcium-containing products elicits a similar biochemical picture with suppressed PTH and biochemical alkalosis.

A history of smoking, persistent cough, hemoptysis, and weight loss suggests lung cancer as the most likely underlying diagnosis. Back pain can be due to bone metastases, myeloma, osteoporotic fracture, vitamin D deficiency or, rarely, Paget's disease, but can also be unrelated (e.g., due to degenerative disease). Night sweats and lymphadenopathy may be suggestive of lymphoma or tuberculosis. If the patient is known to have cancer, then hypercalcemia is most likely malignancy-related, but other causes, particularly PHPT, should be ruled out. Long-standing, relatively asymptomatic hypercalcemia is usually most likely due to PHPT, but the diagnosis should always

Table 24-2 Investigation of hypercalcemia (22)

Routine investigations	Specific investigations
• Corrected (ACa) or free (ionized) calcium; phosphate – low phosphate suggests PHPT or PTHrP related • Urea (BUN)/creatinine – raised due to dehydration or acute kidney injury (AKI) or suggests THPT; eGFR <60 ml/min – PHPT* • Alkaline phosphatase (ALP) - raised with bone metastases or osteomalacia (which can coexist with PHPT or THPT) • PTH • Vitamin D levels – raised in toxicity or other states (specify if calcidiol or calcitriol levels needed) • Urine calcium excretion (24 h) – hypercalciuria (>400 mg/dL [10 mmol/L] – PHPT*; or hypocalciuria (e.g., FHH) • Spot urine calcium and creatinine to calculate calcium:creatinine clearance ratio – FHH (<0.01 in 80%; 0.01–0.02 "gray area"; majority PHPT >0.015)	• Blood film/markers – lymphoma • Serum and urine electrophoresis – myeloma • CXR/chest CT scan – lung cancer or granulomatous disease • Bone scan/MRI – bone metastases • DEXA scan – low – PHPT* • Vertebral fracture by CT, MRI, or vertebral fracture analysis (VFA) – PHPT* • Imaging/scopes/biopsy/calcitriol/ACE – granulomatous diseases • PTHrP – malignancy • Kidney ultrasound or CT – kidney stones/nephrocalcinosis – PHPT*; renal cancer • Ultrasound parathyroid/sestamibi scan – PHPT or THPT • Thyroid function tests – thyrotoxicosis • Cortisol level/Short ACTH stimulation test – acute adrenal insufficiency • Genetic tests – syndromic and non-syndromic familial causes (e.g., FHH, MEN) • X-ray hands – periosteal calcification due to vitamin A toxicity • Vitamin A /theophylline level – toxicity

* Indications for surgery in PHPT include age >50 and any one of ACa >1 mg/dL (0.25 mmol/L) above ULN; eGFR <60 ml/min; osteoporosis diagnosed by DEXA or fragility fractures; nephrocalcinosis or renal calculi; 24 hr urine calcium >400 mg/day (10 mmol/day); PHPT = primary hyperparathyroidism; THPT = tertiary hyperparathyroidism; PTH = parathyroid hormone; PTHrP = parathyroid hormone-related peptide; ACE = angiotensin converting enzyme; MEN = multiple endocrine neoplasia; FHH = familial hypocalciuric hypercalcemia; ACTH = adrenocorticotropic hormone; BUN = blood urea nitrogen

Table 24-3 Assessment of the hypercalcemic patient

Features of hypercalcemia	Features of the underlying cause
• Malaise, fatigue, lethargy • Anorexia, nausea, vomiting, weight loss • Mental status change: depression, confusion, coma • Bone pain • Polydipsia and polyuria • Abdominal pain suggestive of pancreatitis/peptic ulcer/reflux/renal calculi • Features of bowel distension due to fecal impaction (constipation) • Fracture due to osteoporosis in PHPT or malignancy • Metastatic calcification • ECG changes: short QT interval	• Lymphadenopathy – cancer, lymphoma or tuberculosis • Clubbing, chest dullness, hemoptysis – lung cancer • Abdominal masses, visceromegaly – solid organ malignancy or lymphoma • Neck mass – cancer (including parathyroid) or goitre • Tachycardia, goitre, sweating - thyrotoxicosis • Hyperpigmentation and hypotension – Addison's disease • End-stage CKD/dialysis – THPT • Syndromic features – MEN1; MEN2A (MEN2); MEN4; Hyperparathyroid Jaw tumor syndrome

PHPT = primary hyperparathyroidism; THPT = tertiary hyperparathyroidism; MEN = multiple endocrine neoplasia; CKD = chronic kidney disease.

be confirmed. Family history may indicate genetic causes (which constitute 5–10% PHPT) such as FHH, MEN syndromes or familial hyperparathyroidism-jaw tumor syndrome. Thiazide diuretics, lithium, calcium (including antacids), vitamin D supplements and high-dose vitamin A supplements may promote hypercalcemia that is typically reversible on stopping the medication.

Examination of patients with hypercalcemia should explore the effects of hypercalcemia itself as well as search for the underlying cause. Features of severe hypercalcemia usually affect multiple organ systems (Table 24-3). Patients with chronic hypercalcemia may present with renal failure, renal stones, or osteoporotic fractures. Palpable masses (including breast exam), enlarged lymph nodes, or visceromegaly on abdominal examination, point toward malignancy as a likely cause. Finger clubbing, cough, hemoptysis, and pleural effusions suggest lung cancer. Back pain, leg weakness, and spinal tenderness indicate spinal disease (including possibility of spinal cord compression, which is an oncologic emergency), which may be metastases from a different site. If features of thyrotoxicosis or adrenal insufficiency are present, they should be considered as a possible etiology. Granulomatous diseases usually produce signs in the chest or bowel, but other organ systems may also be affected.

The symptoms and signs of hypercalcemia predominantly relate to the rapidity of onset or chronicity of the abnormality and the effects on volume contraction that accompany increased ACa, and the neuromuscular dysfunction that occurs. Aside from underlying specific features (i.e., bone pain in metastatic neoplastic disease), the symptoms can be the same irrespective of the etiology, and relate more to the level of hypercalcemia. Overt symptoms are unlikely to occur if the ACa is <12 mg/dL (3.0 mmol/L), although a thorough search for symptoms in patients with milder degrees of hypercalcemia will often elicit abdominal or neuropsychiatric features not necessarily initially volunteered by the patient. While the differential diagnosis of hypercalcemia is broad, a finding of ACa increased to the extent that overt symptoms are present nearly always indicates either PHPT or malignancy. Acute onset of hypercalcemia and rapidly increasing calcium strongly favors a diagnosis of neoplastic disease, although sudden volume contraction secondary to diarrhea, vomiting, surgery, or immobilization can dangerously exacerbate pre-existing hypercalcemia.

As a consequence of hypercalcemia-induced nephrogenic DI, the initial symptoms relate to polyuria and the resultant adaptive increased thirst. Neurological dysfunction, secondary to the central neuronal depressant effect of increased calcium, is prominent and may manifest as confusion, drowsiness, agitation, stupor, or coma. Myopathy is occasionally seen. Hypertension as a consequence of calcium-mediated vasoconstriction can occur in chronic disease but is less likely in the acute volume contracted state. Bradyarrhythmias or heart block are frequently seen in severe hypercalcemia, however, and relate to detrimental effects on the cardiac action potential as a consequence of increased extracellular calcium. Gastrointestinal symptoms resulting in part from reduced smooth muscle contraction include constipation, nausea, anorexia, vomiting, and abdominal pain, which are often severe. Renal stones and pancreatitis can occur. The term "hypercalcemic crisis" is frequently used to describe the severely compromised patient with profound volume depletion, and altered sensorium, which may be manifest as coma, cardiac decompensation, and abdominal pain, that may mimic an acute abdomen (2).

The diagnosis of hypercalcemic crisis can sometimes be difficult to make clinically when associated with malignancy. This is because the patient may already be debilitated, anorexic, nauseated, constipated, weak or confused, from the underlying malignancy, concurrent medications, complications of chemo- or radiotherapy, as well as comorbid disorders. Clinical vigilance is crucial in this setting to prevent unnecessary morbidity and mortality.

Management of Severe Hypercalcemia

Acute Intervention

Once severe hypercalcemia is recognized, the patient should be managed in an appropriate emergency setting such as an acute medical unit, high dependency area or intensive care unit. Prompt assessment and management of the ABCDEs should occur (i.e., Airway; Breathing; Circulation; Disability [i.e., conscious level]; and Exposure [i.e., examination and evaluation]).

The acute management of hypercalcemia will depend on a number of factors, including severity of symptoms, comorbidities that may affect treatment options, and the patient's prognosis. In malignancy-related severe hypercalcemia, it may be appropriate to adopt a palliative approach that will emphasize comfort, care, and symptom control.

General Supportive Care

The cornerstone of acute management of hypercalcemia is fluid resuscitation with correction of the volume state (3). As described above, hypercalcemia potently induces a diuresis, and the subsequent volume contraction (i.e., at least 4 L deficit can occur) and reduction in GFR compound renal calcium clearance. Appropriate fluid administration should depend on an assessment of volume depletion, but in most situations of hypercalcemic crises 500–1000 ml of intravenous (IV) 0.9% saline should be given over the first hour, and 3–6 litres (i.e., 125–250 ml/hr) over the first 24 hours (Figure 24-2). This regimen should be continued for 1–3 days with careful monitoring of cardiac status and total body hydration. While historical approaches advocated the use of loop diuretics (e.g., furosemide) to induce further renal calcium losses in the acute

management, more recent treatment strategies have warned of the risk of aggravating volume contraction if these medications are used and also potentially aggravating arrhythmias by decreasing magnesium and potassium levels (31). However, loop diuretics do have a role in those patients where vigorous fluid resuscitation may provoke cardiogenic fluid overload. In these situations, once euvolemia has been attained, aggressive fluid administration (i.e., 3 L 0.9% saline over 24 h), should be balanced with IV furosemide treatment (20–40 mg every 2–4 h) to maintain a neutral fluid balance. In most circumstances this can be achieved by inducing a forced diuresis of 2.5 litres over 24 h (i.e., urine output 100 ml/hr) and allowing for 500 ml of insensible fluid loss. Potassium and magnesium levels should be cautiously monitored whenever furosemide is used, and replaced appropriately if required. Central line insertion with central venous pressure (CVP) measurements should be considered in patients where external features of fluid state are difficult to assess, or in those who poorly tolerate initial attempts at aggressive fluid administration. Overall fluid resuscitation can decrease ACa levels by at least 2 mg/dL (0.5 mmol/L) with immediate onset.

Any possible agents causing hypercalcemia should be discontinued as soon as possible. Immobilization promotes osteoclastic bone resorption, hence early ambulation should be encouraged whenever possible. Dietary calcium restriction is only rarely warranted in patients with vitamin D/vitamin D metabolite/vitamin D analog dependent hypercalcemia (26).

For treatment of severe hypercalcemia, where possible, the cause should be identified, and multitargeted therapies should be started as soon as possible. Rapid-acting (hours) approaches including rehydration, possibly forced diuresis, short-term calcitonin and in the longer term, the most effective anti-resorptive agents (i.e., bisphosphonates, denosumab) should be considered (unless imminent parathyroid surgery is planned when there is an increased risk of postoperative hypocalcemia due to "hungry

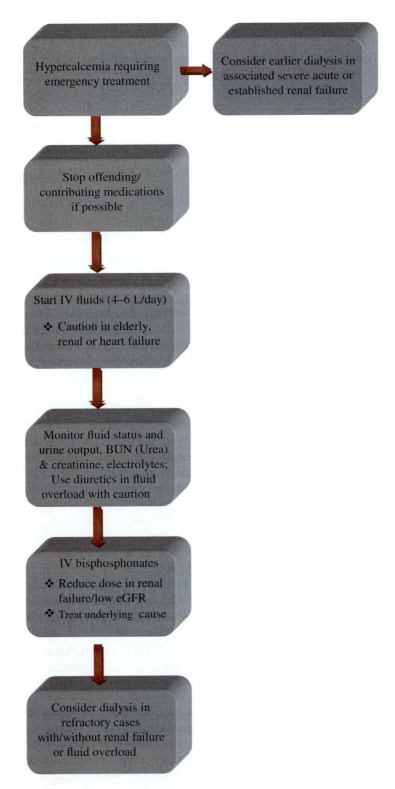

Figure 24-2 Algorithm for treatment of acute hypercalcemia. Adapted from (3).

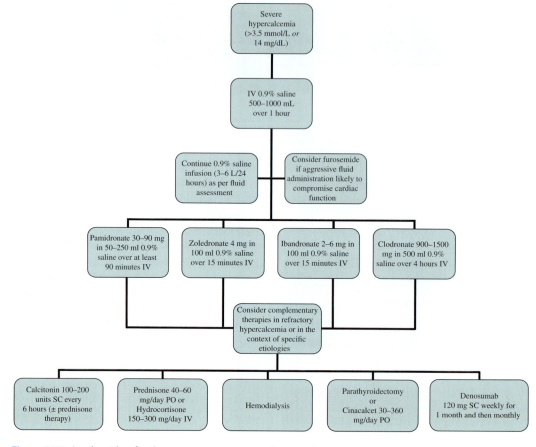

Figure 24-3 An algorithm for the acute management of hypercalcemia.

bone" syndrome). If the diagnosis is PHPT, then surgical removal of parathyroid adenoma(s) should be planned, ideally when the patient is stabilized but occasionally emergency surgery may be required (Figure 24-3).

Calcium-Specific Therapy

Bisphosphonates

Irrespective of the etiology, severe hypercalcemia predominantly results from increased mobilization of calcium from bone. Bisphosphonate therapy directly addresses this feature by inhibiting osteoclast activity (4,32). Several IV bisphosphonate formulations are available; in order of potency, the nitrogen-containing zoledronate, pamidronate and ibandronate, and the non-nitrogen-based

clodronate. Zoledronate and pamidronate are the most potent (zoledronate is 1000x even more potent than pamidronate). Analyses of randomized controlled trials (RCTs) suggest a superior effect of zoledronate over pamidronate in the management of HCM (normalizing ACa levels in 90% vs 70% using zoledronate compared with pamidronate respectively) (33). Intravenous bisphosphonates (Table 24-4) should be administered as soon as possible following rehydration (12 h) for severe hypercalcemia because there is latency until peak effect of 2–4 days. The dose of pamidronate depends on the level of hypercalcemia (i.e., 30 mg over 2 hours with calcium <12 mg/dL [<3 mmol/L] or significant renal impairment [see later]; 60 mg over 4 hours with calcium 12–14 mg/dL

Table 24-4 Medical therapy in severe hypercalcemia

Drug	Dose	Infusion rate	Notes
Bisphosphonates			
Pamidronate	30–90 mg	2 hours in 50–250 ml 0.9% saline (or slower over 6 hours)	Acute phase response, nephrotoxic, ONJ. Calcium lowering effect may last 3–4 weeks
Zoledronate	4 mg	15 minutes in 50–100 ml 0.9% saline	Acute phase response, nephrotoxic, ONJ, hypocalcemia (check vitamin D status), AF. Calcium lowering effect may last 3–4 weeks
Ibandronate	2–6 mg	15 minutes in 100 ml 0.9% saline	Acute phase response, ONJ, nausea/vomiting. Calcium lowering effect may last 2–4 weeks
Clodronate	900–1500 mg	4 hours in 500 ml 0.9% saline	Acute phase response, nausea, diarrhea, skin reactions, bronchospasm, ONJ. Calcium lowering effect may last 2 weeks
Additional options			
Calcitonin	100–200 IU 6 hrly (or 4–8 IU/kg 12 hrly) (Test dose: 10–50 units)	IM/SC	Hypersensitivity reaction (test dose required). flushing, nausea/vomiting
	10 IU/kg	6 hours in 500 ml 0.9% saline	
Glucocorticoids			
Prednisone Hydrocortisone	40–60 mg once daily 150–300 mg/day (given 50-100 mg 8 hrly)	Oral IV	Hyperglycemia, neutrophilia, immunosuppression, adrenal suppression, psychosis
Calcimimetic			
Cinacalcet	30–360 mg/day (given 30 mg/day to 90 mg 6 hrly)	Oral	Nausea/vomiting/diarrhea hypocalcemia, hypotension, myalgia, parasthesia, headache
Denosumab	120 mg/week for 1 month, then monthly	SC	Arthralgias, hypocalcemia (10%, check vitamin D status), ONJ

ONJ = Osteonecrosis of the jaw; AF = Atrial fibrillation.

[3.0–3.4 mmol/L]; and 90 mg over 6 hours with calcium >14 mg/dL [3.5 mmol/L]). Caution should be exercised in renal impairment, and both pamidronate and zoledronate are relatively contraindicated if the GFR is less than 30 mL/min/1.73 m^2. However, the clinician should assess the perceived benefit of treatment in severe hypercalcemia, and must also consider that renal impairment may be a consequence of the hypercalcemia and dehydration. In such cases, renal impairment may be seen to improve as the hypercalcemia abates. Some 60–90% of patients will have a significant decrease in ACa following a bisphosphonate infusion, and ongoing treatment should be considered if the hypercalcemia is likely to recur at a later date (usually in HCM). Due to the long duration of effect of these agents, second doses are usually not required for some time (at least 7–14 days) and should be based on the prescribing information for the agent used. Bisphosphonates may have additional putative benefits in neoplastic disease such as analgesic properties if bone metastases; decreasing the likelihood of pathological fracture; and anti-tumor effects.

Bisphosphonates are not generally necessary in patients with PHPT as these patients often respond to rehydration alone. Bisphosphonates should be particularly avoided if parathyroid surgery is imminent as their use can result in profound postoperative hypocalcemia. Calcimimetics, such as cinacalcet, which activate CaSR, reduce PTH secretion and, subsequently, a decrease in calcium levels may be a better option in these circumstances (21).

Calcitonin

Calcitonin acts by inhibiting osteoclast action and therefore calcium mobilization from bone (34). It can be given as a subcutaneous (SC) or intramuscular (IM) injection (100–200 units every 6 h) or as an IV infusion in emergencies (10 units/kg over 6 h). A test dose (10–50 units) should precede a treatment as hypersensitivity reactions are reported. Flushing, nausea, and vomiting can occur as milder side-effects. Tachyphylaxis is often seen with calcitonin administration

(within 3 days) and can be reduced by the co-administration of glucocorticoid therapy (which can extend activity for at least 5 days). Calcitonin administration can result in more rapid decreases in ACa (rate of onset 2–6 h), and so it can be used early in treatment to get a more rapid decrease in calcium while waiting for the bisphosphonate therapy to take effect, and in patients with refractory hypercalcemia as the absolute effect on lowering ACa is small (typically 2 mg/dL [0.5 mmol/L]) (29).

Glucocorticoid

Glucocorticoid therapy may also be useful in cases of hypercalcemia resulting from increased exogenous (i.e., vitamin D or vitamin D analog toxicity) or endogenous 1,25-dihydroxyvitamin D (i.e granulomatous or lymphoproliferative disorders), due to increased metabolism of vitamin D in the context of glucocorticoid therapy and also decreased conversion of 25 vitamin D to 1,25 vitamin D (8,26). Prednisone can be prescribed at a dose of 40–60 mg once daily or if IV therapy is required, hydrocortisone at a dose of 100–300 mg/day (i.e., 50–100 mg 8 hourly). They are typically effective in 2–4 days and reduce ACa >3 mg/dL (0.75 mmol/L). They are used for at least 3–10 days, but depend on the underlying condition. Glucocorticoids may also be useful in HCM involving cytokine release (e.g., some myelomas). An overall management plan should be established in liaison with a hematologist for lymphoproliferative disorders and myeloma. Glucocorticoids may also be of value in treating other neoplastic problems in addition to HCM (e.g., spinal cord compression, brain metastases). Hydroxychloroquine may also be useful in sarcoid-related hypercalcemia.

Hemodialysis

Hemodialysis against a low or calcium free diasylate is effective and should be considered in any patient already on dialysis therapy or with new onset oliguric renal failure (Figure 24-3 and Figure 24-4) (3). In refractory hypercalcemia, it should be considered

Figure 24-4 The effect of PTHrP on the response to bisphosphonate. Circulating parathyroid hormone-related peptide (PTHrP) higher than 2.6 pmol/L (Nichols Institute Assay) significantly decreases the percentage of patients normalizing adjusted calcium (ACa) and shortens the length of time of response to 60 mg Pamidronate (APD) infusion.

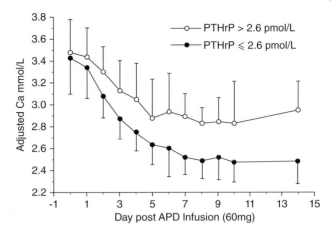

as an additional therapy even in those without underlying renal dysfunction. It is the most potent and rapid means of decreasing ACa levels in severe hypercalcemia (i.e., 3–5 mg/dL [0.75–1.25 mmol/L] decrease within 2–4 h).

Miscellaneous

Medications that interfere with osteoclast action and therefore bone resorption include gallium nitrate and mithramycin. These preparations are associated with significant side-effects and are very rarely used. Gallium nitrate appears to be at least as effective as pamidronate in achieving decreases in ACa, but is limited by the long duration of infusion with typical dosing 200 mg per square meter of body surface administered over 24 hours for 5 consecutive days (35). Significant nephrotoxicity seen with rapid infusions is ameliorated by the longer duration of infusion (36). Onset is usually within 4 days and duration of activity about 2 weeks. Mithramycin (plicamycin) is a tumoricidal antibiotic that has significant renal and hepatic toxicity. It is currently only available for research purposes but has significant hypocalcemic properties.

Phosphate infusion efficiently reduces the serum calcium level within minutes of administration, but the resultant tissue deposition of calcium phosphate makes it inappropriate for use in most hypercalcemia cases. The only indications are for life-threatening cardiac arrhythmias or severe encephalopathy when dialysis is not immediately available.

Treatment of Precipitating Illness

After the acute treatment of severe hypercalcemia (ACa can be decreased by 3–9 mg/dL [0.7–2.2 mmol/L] within 24–48 h in most patients), the underlying cause should be established. Further therapy will be determined by the diagnosis.

Parathyroid Disease

All patients with underlying parathyroid disease (e.g., parathyroid adenoma or carcinoma), who present with hypercalcemic crisis, should be considered for elective parathyroidectomy at the earliest safest opportunity unless there is good reason not to (i.e., comorbidities, poor prognosis, non-localizable disease, or strong patient preference). Urgent parathyroidectomy can be considered in all patients with hypertensive crises as a result of hyperparathyroidism (37) or in cases of severe hypercalcemia due to hyperparathyroidism refractory to medical treatment. However, initial curative success rates differ only marginally between elective and urgent cases, and long-term outcomes appear similar, therefore elective surgery when the patient is stabilized may be preferred in these circumstances (38).

Alternatively, cinacalcet, a calcimimetic which activates the CaSR thereby reducing

PTH secretion, is in current use in treatment of PHPT (including parathyroid carcinoma, and additionally PHPT deemed unsuitable for surgery), SHPT and THPT (7,23). It decreases ACa significantly in most patients with PHPT, and in approximately two-thirds of those with parathyroid carcinoma (39,40). The use of cinacalcet in the management of hypercalcemic crisis has not yet been the subject of a RCT, but many case studies and reports demonstrate safety and effectiveness of its application in the context of refractory hyperparathyroid disease. It is commenced at a dose of 30 mg once- or twice-daily orally and titrated to a maximum dose of 90 mg 6 hrly (180 mg per day in renal dialysis patients). ACa should be checked one week after starting treatment or after dose adjustments. Bisphosphonates may be used in combination with cinacalcet (cinacalcet alone does not improve bone mineral density). Ethanol injection directly into the parathyroid adenoma may be another option if surgery is declined or contraindicated.

Treatment of Underlying Neoplastic Disease

Definitive treatment of a primary solid tumor with expression of PTHrP may prevent further hypercalcemic events. PTHrP secretion by a tumor significantly decreases bisphosphonate efficacy restoring normocalcemia and will result in earlier rebound hypercalcemia (Figure 24-4). Occasionally patients with non-humoral hypercalcemia as a result of lytic bone metastases may find improvement with radiation therapy directed at the lesion.

Miscellaneous

Treatment of granulomatous disorders with standard therapy including glucocorticoids and immunosuppressants may reduce circulating 1,25-(OH)2D (calcitriol) concentrations resulting in decreased ACa (26). Hydroxychloroquine may also be useful in this setting.

On the rare occasions where severe hypercalcemia is felt to be secondary to drug therapy, the offending drug must be stopped and ACa monitored for 3–6 months. This may be particularly difficult in those on lithium therapy. However, newer psychotropic agents effective in bipolar disease can effect this change more safely than in the past. Drug cessation must also occur in the more common scenario where a drug is felt to have contributed to the hypercalcemic state (i.e., thiazide therapy in a patient with HCM), unless significant benefit to risk ratios can be demonstrated.

Emerging Treatments

Osteoclast recruitment with resultant bone resorption is in part mediated by the RANK/RANKL system (13). Activation of the RANK receptor located on immature osteoclasts by osteoblast-derived RANKL promotes maturation and differentiation of the osteoclast. Denosumab, a monoclonal antibody which binds to RANKL, preventing binding to the RANK receptor, has been shown to decrease bone resorption in metastatic bone disease and in osteoporosis with a good safety profile (14). Recent reports have demonstrated the efficacy of denosumab in patients with HCM who have become "resistant" to bisphosphonates (15,16). For example, in one study of bisphosphonate refractory HCM patients (n = 33, baseline ACa 13.5 mg/dL [3.4 mmol/L]), administration of denosumab (120 mg SC weekly for 4 weeks; and then monthly thereafter) resulted in a normalization in ACa in 64% of patients by, on average, day 9 (Day 50 ACa ~10.2 mg/dL [2.4 mmol/L]) (16). This has translated into a proposed regime of 120 mg weekly for one month followed by monthly injections (which can be self-administered). Onset is usually within 7–10 days and duration of activity of 3–4 months. Denosumab may also be of value in parathyroid cancer with refractory hypercalcemia if adjuvant treatments such as chemotherapy and radiotherapy are declined or ineffective (41).

Case Study

A 76-year-old man presents confused, with increased thirst, lower back and hip pain, lower limb weakness, no bowel movement for several days, and decreased urine output for 48 hours prior to admission. He has a past history of prostate cancer and had a previous prostatectomy. Investigations reveal PSA >100 ng/mL (normal <4); ACa 3.5 mmol/L (14 mg/dL), PTH suppressed. Widespread osteoblastic lesions on spine and pelvic X rays (Figure 24-5A).

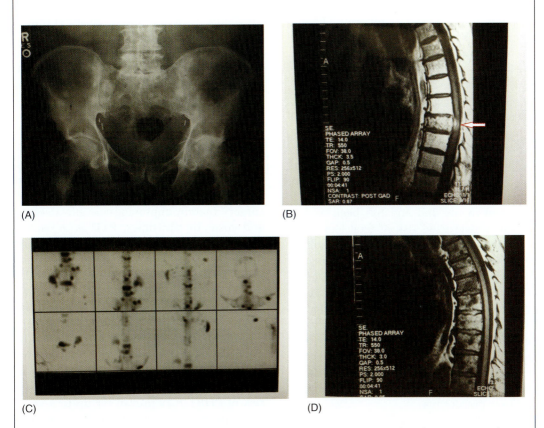

(A)

(B)

(C)

(D)

Figure 24-5 A) Osteoblastic bone metastases in lower spine and pelvis; B) Spinal cord metastases with obstruction (red arrow shows obstruction); C) Widespread metastases on bone scanning; D) Widespread lytic bone metastases but no spinal cord compression.

What Oncological Emergency Needs to Be Excluded?

This patient has spinal cord compression (Figure 24-5B, red arrow) secondary to widespread metastatic prostate cancer (Figure 24-5C). He also has hypercalcemia of malignancy with high calcium and appropriately suppressed PTH. He received rehydration, urinary catheter, pain relief, IV zoledronate, high-dose dexamethasone, emergency neurosurgical review and radiation treatment to the spine. He was reviewed by urology for further management of the prostate cancer. Compare Figure 24-5B showing spinal metastases with spinal cord compression (red arrow), to Figure 24-5D from a patient with widespread metastatic lytic lesions due to lung cancer and hypercalcemia of malignancy but no evidence of spinal cord compression.

Hypercalcemia in Pregnancy

Hypercalcemia in pregnancy is an uncommon event (although may be the third most common endocrinopathy after diabetes and thyroid disorders in pregnancy when screened for) but can be associated with significant maternal morbidity (and rarely mortality) and/or fetal or neonatal morbidity and mortality (23,42). Numerous changes in calcium homeostasis occur during normal pregnancy and lactation. This translates into lower diagnostic thresholds in pregnancy such that serum calcium >9.8 mg/dL (2.4 mmol/L) may be suggestive of hypercalcemia. Subsequently surgery for PHPT (which is the major cause of hypercalcemia in pregnancy) may also be warranted at lower calcium levels than in non-pregnant patients (e.g., >11 mg/dL [2.75 mmol/L]). Surgery can be performed in any trimester but is preferred in the 2nd and has been associated with decreased risk of fetal loss when ACa >11.4 mg/dL (2.85 mmol/L). Maternal issues with significant hypercalcemia include hyperemesis, PHPT-associated hypertension and pre-eclampsia, nephrolithiasis, and pancreatitis. In view of the young population being affected with PHPT, genetic causes such as MEN should be considered. Fetal issues include intrauterine growth defect, in utero fetal demise, and increased miscarriage. Tetany can occur in the neonatal period due to hypocalcemia.

As with all comorbid conditions in pregnancy, multidisciplinary team (MDT) management is critical; it is important to be aware that at least 2 lives are involved; prompt senior review should be available at all times; and many standard of care investigations (e.g., nuclear scans) and drugs (e.g., bisphosphonate) may be contraindicated or need to be modified or have not been tested in the pregnant setting. The majority of cases are asymptomatic (>80%). However, when treatment is warranted, medical management can be a reasonable approach with increased hydration, IV phosphate, IV magnesium sulfate, and calcitonin being well tolerated. Cinacalcet, although not approved in pregnancy, has been used with good effect (it appears that CaSR is not pivotal in placental maternal-to-fetal calcium transport). IV bisphosphonates should not be used as they cross the placenta and can be deposited in fetal bones.

When PHPT surgery is warranted, an experienced parathyroid surgeon should be sought ("the most important localization procedure"). Parathyroid localization procedures rely on ultrasound and other non-nuclear imaging (although lower radioactive doses when using sestamibi scanning have been used in pregnancy). It is critical to measure intraoperative PTH levels to confirm successful removal of abnormal parathyroid gland(s). Because of the short half-life of PTH (≤5 minutes), intraoperative determination of intact PTH can be used to assess the completeness of parathyroidectomy and to facilitate minimally invasive parathyroid surgery, thereby improving cost-effectiveness and cosmetic outcomes. PTH is measured just before the incision and again at 20 minutes after resection of the hyperfunctioning parathyroid tissue. The surgeon should not massage the patient's neck at baseline (this can increase PTH) or following parathyroidectomy (when PTH can be released from injured parathyroid glands). A decline of 50% or more is usually considered indicative of the removal of all hyperfunctioning tissue. It is important to be aware that increased risk of PHPT may prevail for up to 5 years post-operatively in this population, so regular screening is needed.

Conclusions

Severe hypercalcemia is an endocrine emergency that requires prompt action to prevent severe neurological, cardiac, and renal consequences. The diagnosis should be considered in any patient with known parathyroid disease or neoplasm who presents with acute deterioration, especially in the context of neurological dysfunction. The cornerstone of management is to perform appropriate investigations to make an accurate diagnosis;

fluid resuscitation; and the administration of calcium-specific therapies such as bisphosphonates. Additional therapies, including calcimimetics in certain situations and drugs that affect the RANKL system, are likely to become more widely used in the future although further studies are required to define their role.

References

1 Favus MJ, Goltzman D. Regulation of calcium and magnesium. In: Rosen CJ, ed. *Primer on the Metabolic Bone Diseases and Disorders of Mineral Metabolism*, 8 ed, Washington, DC, American Society for Bone and Mineral Research, 2013; 173–179.

2 Ahmad S, Kuraganti G, Steenkamp D. Hypercalcemic crisis: a clinical review. *Am J Med*. 2015;128:239–245.

3 Walsh J, Gittoes N, Selby P, the Society for Endocrinology Clinical Committee. *Emergency Management of Acute Hypercalcaemia in Adult Patients* (2016). DOI: 10.1530/EC-16-0055.

4 Sternlicht H, Glezerman IG. Hypercalcemia of malignancy and new treatment options. *Therapeutics Clin Risk Management*. 2015;11:1779–1788.

5 Carroll R, Matfin G. Endocrine and metabolic emergencies: hypercalcaemia. *Therap Advances Endocrinol Metab*. 2010;1:225–334.

6 Schafer AL, Shoback D. Hypocalcemia: definition, etiology, pathogenesis, diagnosis, and management. In: Rosen CJ. ed., *Primer on the Metabolic Bone Diseases and Disorders of Mineral Metabolism*, 8th ed. Ames, Iowa: John Wiley & Sons, Inc., 2013.

7 Fraser WD. Hyperparathyroidism. *Lancet*. 2009;11;374(9684):145–158.

8 Holick MF. Vitamin D deficiency. *N Engl J Med*. 2007;357; 266–281.

9 Holick MF, Brinkley NC, Bischoff-Ferrari HA, et al. Evaluation, treatment, and prevention of vitamin D deficiency: an Endocrine Society Clinical Practice Guideline. *J Clin Endocrinol Metab*. 2011;96:1911–1930.

10 Egbuna OI, Brown EM. Hypercalcaemic and hypocalcaemic conditions due to calcium-sensing receptor mutations. *Best Pract Res Clin Rheumatol*. 2008;22: 129–148.

11 Hannan FM, Babinsky VN, Thakker RV. Disorders of the calcium-sensing receptor and partner proteins: insights into the molecular basis of calcium homeostasis. *J Mol Endocrinol*. 2016;57: R127–R142.

12 Asam M, Pawlak A, Matfin G, Quinton R. Disorders of calcium homeostasis. *Foundation Years J*. 2014;5;14–23.

13 Tanaka S, Nakamura K, Takahasi N, Suda T. Role of RANKL in physiological and pathological bone resorption and therapeutics targeting the RANKL–RANK signaling system. *Immunol Rev*. 2005;208;30–49.

14 Body JJ, Lipton A, Gralow J, et al. Effects of denosumab in patients with bone metastases with and without previous bisphosphonate exposure. *J Bone Miner Res*. 2010;25;440–446.

15 Hu MI, Glezerman I, Leboulleux S, et al. Denosumab for patients with persistent or relapsed hypercalcemia of malignancy despite recent bisphosphonate treatment. *J Natl Cancer Inst*. 2013;105(18):1417–1420.

16 Hu MI, Glezerman I, Leboulleux S, et al. Denosumab for treatment of hypercalcemia of malignancy. *J Clin Endocrinol Metab*. 2014;99:3144–3152.

17 Fenech, ME, Turner, JJO. Hypercalcaemia and primary hyperparathyroidism. *Medicine (United Kingdom)*. 2013; 41/10(573–576):1357–3039, 1365–4357.

18 Minisola S, Pepe J, Piemonte S, Cipriani C. The diagnosis and management of hypercalcaemia. *BMJ*. 2015;350:h27323. DOI:10.1136/bmj.h2723.

19 Munns CF, Shaw N, Kiely M, et al. Global consensus recommendations on prevention and management of nutritional

rickets. *J Clin Endocrinol Metab*. 2016; 101:394–415.

20 Endres, DB. Investigation of hypercalcemia. *Clinical Biochemistry*. 2012;45/12(954–963): 0009-9120, 1873–2933.

21 Marcocci C, Cetani F. Clinical practice: primary hyperparathyroidism. *N Engl J Med*. 2011;365:2389–2397.

22 Bilezikian JP, Brandi ML, Eastell R, et al. Guidelines for the management of asymptomatic primary hyperparathyroidism: summary statement from the Fourth International Workshop. *J Clin Endocrinol Metab*. 2014;99: 3561–3569.

23 Khan AA, Hanley DA, Rizzoli R, et al. Primary hyperparathyroidism: review and recommendations on evaluation, diagnosis, and management: a Canadian and iInternational consensus. *Osteoporosis Int*. 2017;28:1–19.

24 Fraser WD, Robinson J, Lawton R, et al. Clinical and laboratory studies of new immunoradiometric assay of parathyroid hormone related protein. *Clin Chem*. 1993;39:414–419.

25 Hewison M, Burke F, Evans KN, et al. Extra-renal 25-hydroxyvitamin D3-1-hydroxylase in human health and disease. *J Steroid Biochem*. 2007;103;316–321.

26 Tebben PJ, Singh RJ, Kumar R. Vitamin D-mediated hypercalcemia: mechanisms, diagnosis, and treatment. *Endocrine Rev*. 2016;37: 521–547.

27 Fraser WD, Logue FC, MacRitchie K, et al. Intact parathyroid hormone concentration and cyclic AMP metabolism in thyroid disease. *Acta Endocrinology*. 1991a;124:652–657.

28 Igbal AA, Burgess EH, Gallina DL, Nanes MS, Cook CB. Hypercalcemia in hyperthyroidism: patterns of serum calcium, parathyroid hormone, and 1,25-dihydroxyvitamin D3 levels during management of thyrotoxicosis. *Endocr Pract*. 2003;9:517–521.

29 Stewart A. Hypercalcaemia associated with cancer. *N Engl J Med*. 2005;352:373–379.

30 Fraser WD, Logue FC, Gallacher SJ, et al. Direct and indirect assessment of the parathyroid hormone response to pamidronate therapy in Paget's Disease of bone and hypercalcaemia of malignancy. *Bone & Mineral*. 1991;2:113–121.

31 LeGrand SB, Leskuski D, Zama I. Narrative review: furosemide for hypercalcemia: an unproven yet common practice. *Ann Intern Med*. 2008;149;259–263.

32 Maraka S, Kennel KA. Bisphosphonates for the prevention and treatment of osteoporosis. *BMJ*. 2015;351:h3783.

33 Major P, Lortholary A, Hon J, et al. Zoledronic acid is superior to pamidronate in the treatment of hypercalcemia of malignancy: a pooled analysis of two randomized, controlled clinical trials. *J Clin Oncol*. 2001;19;558–567.

34 Chesnut CH, Azria M, Silverman S, Engelhardt M, Olson M, Mindeholm M. Salmon calcitonin: a review of current and future therapeutic indications. *Osteoporos Int*. 2008;19:479–491.

35 Cvitkovic F, Armand J-P, Tubiana-Hulin M, Rossi J-F, Warrell R. Randomized, double-blind, phase ii trial of gallium nitrate compared with pamidronate for acute control of cancer-related hypercalcemia. *Cancer J*. 2006;12; 47–53.

36 Chitambar CR. Medical applications and toxicities of gallium compounds. *Int J Environ Res Public Health*. 2010;7(5):2337–2361.

37 Young WF, Calhour DA, Lenders JWM, Stowasser M, Textor SC. Screening for endocrine hypertension: an Endocrine Society Scientific Statement. *Endocr Rev*. 2017;38(2):103–122. DOI: 10.1210/er.2017-00054.

38 Cannon J, Lew J, Solorzano J. Parathyroidectomy for hypercalcemic crisis: 40 years' experience and long-term outcomes. *Surgery*. 2010;148;807–813.

39 Marcocci C, Chanson P, Shoback D, et al. Cinacalcet reduces serum calcium concentrations in patients with intractable primary hyperparathyroidism. *J Clin Endocr Metab*. 2009;94;2766–2772.

40 Silverberg SJ, Rubin MR, Faiman C, et al. Cinacalcet hydrochloride reduces the serum calcium concentration in inoperable parathyroid carcinoma. *J Clin Endocr Metab*. 2007;92;3803–3808.

41 Tong CV, Hussein Z, Noor NM, et al. Use of denosumab in parathyroid carcinoma with refractory hypercalcemia. *QJ Med*. 2015;108:49–50.

42 Rey E, Jacob CE, Koolian M, Morin F. Hypercalcemia in pregnancy – a multifaceted challenge: case reports and literature review. *Clinical Case Reports*. 2016;4:1001–1008.

25

Acute Medical Aspects Related to Phosphate Disorders

Anda R. Gonciulea and Suzanne M. Jan de Beur

Key Points

- Plasma contains both inorganic and organic phosphate, but only inorganic phosphate is measured.
- Regulation of phosphate is a complex process involving the kidneys, intestine, and skeleton and is under the regulation of parathyroid hormone (PTH), vitamin D metabolites, and fibroblast growth factor 23 (FGF23). FGF23 is also termed a *phosphatonin* (a class of factors regulating phosphate homeostasis).
- Acute hypophosphatemia with phosphate depletion is common in the hospital setting (observed in up to 5% of hospitalized patients) and results in significant morbidity.
- Acute hypophosphatemia may be mild (2–2.5 mg/dL [0.65–0.81 mmol/L]), moderate (1–1.9 mg/dL [0.32–0.61 mmol/L]) or severe (<1 mg/dL [0.32 mmol/L]) and commonly occurs in clinical settings such as refeeding, alcoholism, diabetic ketoacidosis, malnourishment/starvation, postoperatively and in the intensive care unit.
- Clinical manifestations of hypophosphatemia include dysfunction of the central nervous system, skeletal and smooth muscle, cardiopulmonary system, and hematopoietic system.

- Phosphate replacement can be given either orally, intravenously, in dialysate or in total parenteral nutrition. The rate and amount of replacement are empiric and several algorithms are available. Treatment should be tailored to symptoms, severity, anticipated duration of illness and presence of comorbid conditions, such as renal failure, volume overload, hypo- or hypercalcemia, hypo- or hyperkalemia, and acid-base status.
- Hyperphosphatemia results from acute exogenous phosphate loads, redistribution of intracellular phosphate to the extracellular space, decreased renal excretion, and pseudohyperphosphatemia.
- Severe, acute hyperphosphatemia most commonly results from tumor lysis syndrome and administration of phosphate-based purgatives.
- Complications of the acute hyperphosphatemia include acute kidney injury and profound hypocalcemia with resultant tetany, cardiac arrhythmias, hypotension, and seizures.
- Severe, acute hyperphosphatemia is a medical emergency requiring prompt treatment.

Introduction

Unlike serum calcium, which is tightly regulated and constant throughout the day and throughout the lifespan, serum phosphorus values are greater in infancy and childhood and show considerable diurnal variation (1, 2). The normal range for serum phosphorus in adults is 2.5–4.5 mg/dL (0.8–1.4 mmol/L). Hypophosphatemia is generally divided into acute and chronic. Acute hypophosphatemia with phosphate depletion is common in the hospital setting and, when severe, can result in significant morbidity (3,4). Chronic hypophosphatemia presents as rickets in children with lower extremity deformity and abnormal growth and as osteomalacia in adults, and is generally associated with genetic or acquired renal phosphate-wasting disorders. Acute hypophosphatemia with severe phosphate depletion often is a metabolic emergency and will be the focus of this chapter. While chronic hypophosphatemia requires treatment, it generally is not a metabolic emergency and will not be discussed in this review. Details of its pathophysiology and treatment can be found elsewhere (5–7). While hyperphosphatemia is commonly seen in chronic kidney disease (CKD), hypoparathyroidism, pseudohypoparathyroidism and tumoral calcinosis, hyperphosphatemia is not a metabolic emergency in these disorders and will not be discussed. However, acute hyperphosphatemia which develops after endogenous phosphate release in tumor lysis syndrome or after exogenous use of phosphate bowel preparations is often a metabolic emergency and its management will be reviewed.

Pathophysiology of Phosphate Homeostasis

Phosphate plays a vital role in physiological processes, such as nucleic acid synthesis, cell membrane structure, intracellular signaling, protein synthesis, energy stores via adenosine triphosphate (ATP), oxygen delivery via 2,3-diphosphoglycerate (2,3-DPG), acid excretion and bone mineralization. Approximately 85% of whole body phosphate content resides in bone, with the remainder in the intracellular pool except for less than 1% in the extracellular pool. Phosphate balance is maintained by ingestion/intestinal absorption, release from bone and renal excretion via the apical brush border sodium phosphate cotransporters NaPi2a and NaPi2c (Figure 25-1) (8,10). Important hormonal regulators of phosphate include parathyroid hormone (PTH) and fibroblast growth factor 23 (FGF23), both of which increase renal phosphate excretion. In contrast, they have opposite actions on 1,25-dihydroxyvitamin D (1,25D), which increases intestinal phosphate absorption (Figure 25-1). PTH increases synthesis of 1,25D and FGF23 decreases synthesis and increases degradation 1,25D. While it is clear that both PTH and FGF23 have critical roles in controlling phosphate homeostasis, it is controversial how PTH and FGF23 actions are integrated. Approximately 80% of the ingested dietary phosphate is absorbed in the small intestine via sodium dependent (in part, via the NaPi2b) and independent pathways and under the regulation of vitamin D. The exact mechanisms through which vitamin D controls intestinal phosphate absorption remain largely unknown. Some studies suggest an increase in NaPi2b expression under stimulation of vitamin D, while others found a vitamin D independent upregulation of NaPi2b after a low phosphate diet (9). Moreover, changes in the phosphate status directly affect production of 1,25D. Hypophosphatemia stimulates 1,25D production, increasing intestinal phosphate absorption while hyperphosphatemia suppresses 1,25D production decreasing intestinal phosphate absorption. Whether the effects of vitamin D on serum phosphate are through direct action or indirectly via modulation of PTH and FGF23 levels is the subject of ongoing research (10,11).

Serum phosphate is affected by the serum calcium modulation of PTH. Phosphate

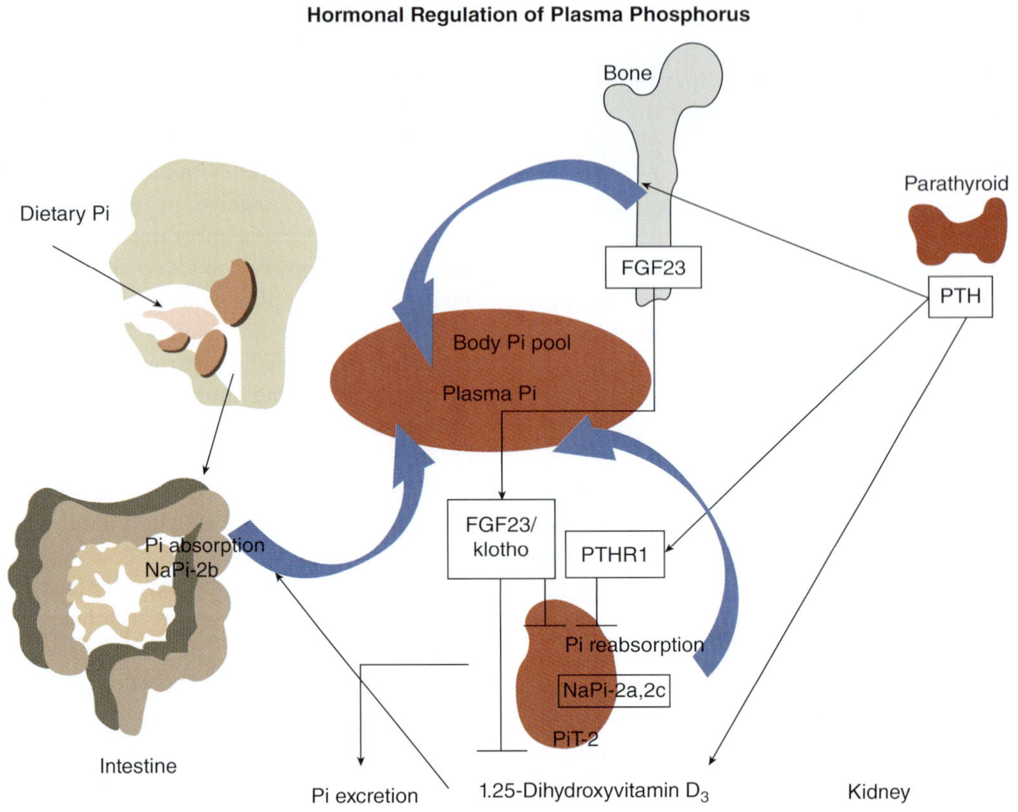

Figure 25-1 Inorganic phosphate homeostasis. The PTH-vitamin D3-FGF23 endocrine system as well as dietary Pi play an important role in regulating renal and intestinal absorption of Pi. FGF23 is an endocrine hormone that is secreted by osteocytes and osteoblasts, and it achieves target cell specificity through binding to the FGFR1 receptor-α-Klotho complex. FGF23 increases renal Pi excretion by the downregulation of NaPi-2a and NaPi-2c, and it decreases circulating 1,25 D concentrations. PTH increases renal Pi excretion by the downregulation of NaPi-2a and NaPi-2c and stimulates 1,25 D production. In turn, PTH is inhibited by increased 1,25 D. In contrast, FGF23 inhibits PTH and 1,25 D production, whereas 1,25 D stimulates FGF23 synthesis. Blue lines signify phosphate entering circulation.

loading decreases serum calcium by reducing the calcium efflux from bone and complexing with calcium. This relative hypocalcemia stimulates PTH secretion to correct serum calcium which also increases renal phosphate excretion and thereby lowers serum phosphorus. Hyperphosphatemia may also directly stimulate PTH secretion (12). In contrast, phosphate depletion increases the calcium efflux from bone, decreasing PTH values, and decreases PTH secretion from the parathyroid gland (6). In addition to PTH, FGF23 has a central role in phosphate homeostasis. By interaction with its coreceptor FGFR1/α-Klotho, FGF23 inhibits transcription, translation, and apical translocation of the NaPi2a and NaPi2c transporters, promoting phosphaturia. It also suppresses 1-α-hydroxylase activity and stimulates 24-α-hydroxylase, therefore decreasing 1,25 D levels (13). Phosphate loading in humans increases serum FGF23, but the response is not immediate and less robust than expected (14). Phosphate loading results in a dose-dependent increase in serum PTH concentration followed by an increase in FGF23 levels and reduction in 1,25 D. Whether phosphate loading or subsequent PTH elevation is responsible for the increased FGF23 production is debatable (15). Moreover, a reciprocal pathway exists between FGF23 and 1,25D with 1,25D stimulating FGF23 secretion (16). More recent data support the role of calcium and iron in regulating FGF23 production with hypercalcemia and iron deficiency being associated with higher circulating FGF23 concentrations (17,18). Controversy exists about the role of PTH in FGF23 regulation (19).

Hypophosphatemia as a Metabolic Emergency

Etiology of Acute Hypophosphatemia

In adults, hypophosphatemia occurs in up to 5% of hospitalized patients and its incidence may be as high as 30–50% in clinical settings such as alcoholism, sepsis or intensive care unit (ICU) admissions (3). Other medical conditions in which acute hypophosphatemia is commonly seen include: refeeding after starvation/malnutrition; or large weight losses, in anorexia nervosa and with kwashiorkor/marasmus (4). Postsurgical conditions associated with hypophosphatemia include hepatic surgery and after parathyroidectomy for severe primary or secondary hyperparathyroidism due to hungry bone syndrome. Finally, hypophosphatemia is commonly seen in the ICU during continuous renal replacement therapy (CRRT).

Phosphate depletion results from decreased absorption/intake, renal/extracorporeal losses and shifts of phosphate into bone (hungry bone syndrome) while transcellular shifts of phosphate are a major cause of hypophosphatemia (Figure 25-2). Although severe hypophosphatemia is often associated with phosphate depletion, the serum phosphorus value especially on presentation may not be representative of total body phosphorus. An example of the failure of serum phosphate to indicate phosphate depletion is the poorly controlled diabetic patient who presents to the Emergency Department with a normal or even elevated serum phosphorus value despite continuous renal phosphate losses and decreased phosphate intake (4).

Hypophosphatemia only develops after treatment with insulin due to a marked shift of phosphate into the intracellular compartment. Another cause of hypophosphatemia is that associated with the infusion of fructose which results in the sequestration of phosphate in extracellular sites or intracellular pathways that do not produce ATP or 2,3-DPG. Finally, awareness of the factors that can cause pseudohypophosphatemia is important because phosphate treatment is not necessary and can be harmful. Mannitol, myeloma protein, and hyperbilirubinemia can interfere with the colorimetric assay for serum phosphorus. In acute leukemia, phosphate uptake by abundant white blood cells in the test tube can cause a hypophosphatemic reading (Figure 25-2).

Transcellular shifts of phosphate are an interesting phenomenon because they can occur with or without phosphate depletion. When free intracellular phosphate is moved into glycolytic or protein synthesis pathways, free intracellular phosphate concentrations decrease and extracellular phosphate shifts into cells (20). Examples include the decrease in serum phosphate from insulin and glucose infusion and from respiratory alkalosis (Figure 25-2). Treatment of hypophosphatemia is not necessary in these situations because ATP and 2,3-DPG concentrations are maintained. Of interest, a precipitous decrease in serum phosphorus after initiating glucose-containing solutions may indicate phosphate depletion (21).

Clinical Manifestations

Acute hypophosphatemia with phosphate depletion is associated with a broad range of clinical manifestations and increases morbidity. The primary mechanism responsible for acute clinical manifestations with hypophosphatemia is depletion of ATP and 2,3-DPG, which results in reduced energy stores and impaired oxygen delivery, respectively (2,10). Central nervous system manifestations of severe hypophosphatemia include parathesias, metabolic encephalopathy, delirium, seizures, and coma. In the ICU

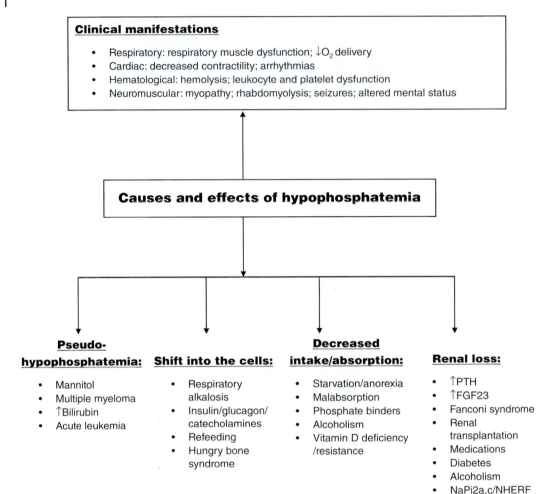

Figure 25-2 Causes and effects of hypophosphatemia/phosphate depletion. Hypophosphatemia may be acute or chronic and results from decreased intake and/or absorption, gastrointestinal and renal/extracorporeal losses, internal redistribution, or a combination of these factors. Pseudohypophosphatemia may occur in acute leukemias due to increased uptake of phosphate by leukemic cells *in vitro*, or may result from interference with the phosphate assay by mannitol, bilirubin or dysproteinemia.

setting, hypophosphatemia is associated with longer duration of mechanical ventilation and hospitalization, decreased left ventricular stroke index and blood pressure, an increased incidence of ventricular tachycardia and postoperative complications (3,4,22). Correction of severe hypophosphatemia improves myocardial and respiratory performance (4,20). Hypophosphatemia-induced manifestations of muscle dysfunction include a proximal myopathy, dysphagia, and ileus. Hypophosphatemia can affect each of the components of the hematopoietic system: hemolysis, reduced granulocyte phagocytosis and chemotaxis, and thrombocytopenia.

Treatment of Hypophosphatemia

In certain situations, hypophosphatemia may be anticipated and prevented by judicious phosphate supplementation. During refeeding in malnutrition, the intake of fluids, electrolytes and energy should be introduced gradually (4). Careful monitoring of serum phosphorus is important. During hyperalimentation, symptomatic hypophosphatemia can be prevented by administering 11–14 mmol of potassium phosphate per 1000 calories in the parenteral feeding. In patients undergoing CRRT, hypophosphatemia can be prevented by adding phosphate to the dialysate or administering phosphate when serum phosphorus falls below normal (4).

Phosphate repletion for acute hypophosphatemia associated with phosphate depletion can be given orally or intravenously (IV) (Table 25-1). The oral route is preferred, if clinically indicated, as it is a safer alternative. Intravenous repletion corrects hypophosphatemia more rapidly, but adverse effects may include hypocalcemia, arrhythmias, ectopic calcification, and acute kidney injury (AKI). The severity of hypophosphatemia is important in determining the urgency and mode of treatment. In most instances, mild (serum phosphorus 2–2.5 mg/dL, 0.65–0.81 mmol/L) or moderate (serum phosphorus 1–1.9 mg/dL, 0.32-0.61 mmol/L) hypophosphatemia can be treated by increasing dietary phosphate or giving oral phosphate supplementation (Table 25-1). In severe acute hypophosphatemia (<1 mg/dL, < 0.32 mmol/L) with phosphate depletion, treatment with IV phosphate is generally necessary, especially in patients in the ICU. Intravenous therapy also is indicated in hypophosphatemic patients unable to tolerate or ingest oral phosphate.

The amount of phosphate needed to restore serum phosphorus and/or replete total-body phosphate is empirical because the volume of distribution is highly variable (23). When giving oral supplementation for mild to moderate hypophosphatemia, 32–65 mmol/day of phosphate for 7–10 days is usually adequate to replenish stores. However, doses as high as 97 mmol/day may be needed initially for severe deficiency. Cow's milk, preferably skim milk to avoid diarrhea, is a good source of phosphate containing 1 mg/ml. Oral sodium- and potassium-based phosphate preparations are also available (Table 25-1).

In the first studies with IV phosphate replacement in severely hypophosphatemic patients (<1 mg/dL [<0.32 mmol/L]), 9 mmol (~0.14 mmol/kg) of IV phosphate was administered every 12 hours. Three additional doses were needed to achieve normal serum phosphorus at 48 hours (4). In a subsequent study, a 0.32 mmol/kg per 12 hours dose was given, which was increased to 0.48 mmol/kg per 12 hours if serum phosphorus did not increase by 0.2 mg/dL (0.065 mmol/L) at 6 hours (4). Seven of 10 patients attained a serum phosphorus ≥ 2 mg/dL (≥0.65 mmol/L) by 24 hours and all 10 by 48 hours. Because the hypophosphatemic patient in the ICU with myocardial or respiratory compromise may need more rapid correction, higher doses of IV phosphate have been used. In severe hypophosphatemia, doses as high as 10–20 mmol/hour given for 1–3 hours have been used without reported adverse effects (4). Perhaps in a better suited approach, doses of 42–67 mmol have been given over 6–9 hours (Table 25-1) (4). In moderate hypophosphatemia, lower doses of IV phosphate have been used. In most studies, either potassium or sodium phosphate was used based on a pre-infusion serum potassium value of 4 meq/L (4 mmol/L). Finally, in the presence of decreased renal function, the dose of phosphate replacement should be reduced, with serum phosphorus carefully monitored during repletion, and use of potassium phosphate replacement minimized. Key considerations for treatment of hypophosphatemia are shown in Table 25-2.

Hyperphosphatemia as a Metabolic Emergency

There are four general mechanisms whereby phosphate entry into the extracellular fluid can outstrip the rate of renal excretion and lead to hyperphosphatemia: (1) acute exogenous phosphate loads; (2) redistribution of intracellular phosphate to the extracellular space; (3) decreased renal excretion;

Table 25-1 Oral and intravenous phosphate preparations and replacement guidelines

Preparation	Phosphate content grams	Sodium Meq (mmol)	Potassium Meq (mmol)
Oral preparations			
Skim milk (1 liter)	1.0	28	38
Phospho-soda (1 ml)	0.150	4.8	0
K-phos original #1 (1 tablet)	0.114	0	3.70
K-phos original #2 (1 tablet)	0.250	5.80	2.80
K-phos neutral (1 tablet)	0.250	13.0	1.10
Commonly used intravenous preparations			
Sodium phosphate (1 ml)	0.011	4.0	0
Potassium phosphate (1 ml)	0.011	0	4.4

	Intravenous replacement guidelines			
	Intensive care unit setting		Ward setting	
Serum phosphorus mg/dL (mmol/L)	Amount[*] (mmol/kg bwt)	Duration (hours)	Amount[*] (mmol/kg bwt)	Duration (hours)
<1 (<0.32)	0.6	6	0.64	24–72
1-1.7 (0.32-0.55)	0.4	6	0.32	24–72
1.8-2.2 (0.58-0.71)	0.2	6	0.16	24–72

Complications may include diarrhea (oral), thrombophlebitis (K phos infusion), hypocalcemia, acute kidney injury, nephrocalcinosis, hyperkalemia, hypernatremia/volume overload, hyperphosphatemia, and metabolic acidosis.
When providing IV phosphate, serum calcium, phosphate, potassium, magnesium, and creatinine should be closely monitored (at least every 6 hours), and telemetry is recommended.
Conversion factor for phosphorus in mg/dL to mmol/L, x0.3229.
[*] In patients who are >130% of their ideal body weight (bwt), an adjusted body weight should be used.

and (4) pseudohyperphosphatemia caused by interference with analytical detection methods. Specific etiologies of these general mechanisms are enumerated in Table 25-3.

Acute hyperphosphatemia is a metabolic emergency and is most commonly caused by release of intracellular phosphate into the extracellular space as in tumor lysis syndrome (TLS) and after exogenous administration of phosphate bowel preparations, especially phosphate-containing enemas. These two disorders are briefly discussed below.

Tumor Lysis Syndrome (TLS)

Several recent comprehensive reviews of TLS are available (24–26). TLS occurs when bulky, rapidly growing tumors with high sensitivity to cytotoxic chemotherapy are treated. Heading the list of these tumors are hematologic malignancies such as acute lymphoblastic/cytic and myeloid leukemias, and Burkitt's lymphoma. However, treatment of other rapidly growing, chemosensitive tumors can also result in TLS. Besides tumor bulk and chemosensitivity, a pre-existing decrease in renal function (serum creatinine >1.4 mg/dL, >123 μmol/L) increases the risk of TLS (15).

Rapid cellular destruction releases uric acid and phosphate, both of which are toxic to renal tubules. Until recently, the decision whether to treat the hyperuricemia or hyperphosphatemia was challenging because a post-treatment observation period was

Table 25-2 Key considerations for treatment of hypophosphatemia and hyperphosphatemia

- Severity: Mild (2–2.5 mg/dL, 0.65–0.81 mmol/L) or moderate (1–1.9 mg/dL, 0.32–0.61 mmol/L) hypophosphatemia can usually be treated with increased dietary phosphate or oral phosphate supplements. Severe acute hypophosphatemia (<1 mg/dL, <0.32 mmol/L) with phosphate depletion, particularly in the ICU setting, is often a metabolic emergency requiring IV phosphate replacement.
- Comorbid conditions: When the contribution of hypophosphatemia to symptoms is unclear, the severity of illness should be a determining factor in deciding whether oral or IV treatment is preferred.
- Hypocalcemia, hypercalcemia: Phosphate therapy can exacerbate hypocalcemia. In hypercalcemic patients, phosphate therapy can lead to calcium-phosphate precipitation, nephrocalcinosis and AKI.
- Renal failure: In renal failure, the dose of phosphate replacement should be reduced by at least 50%.
- Use of potassium or sodium phosphate treatment: With hypokalemia, potassium containing phosphate supplements are preferred, but with hyperkalemia, sodium-containing supplements should be used. With volume overload, avoid sodium-containing phosphate supplements if possible. In CKD, sodium phosphate replacement is generally preferred.
- Pseudohypophosphatemia: Pseudohypophosphatemia is important to recognize because treatment is not needed and can result in hyperphosphatemia (see Figure 25-2 for causes).
- Hyperphosphatemia in TLS: When severe, hyperphosphatemia in TLS is a metabolic emergency because of the risk of AKI. The decision to treat with CRRT depends on the magnitude of hyperphosphatemia, the rate of increase in serum phosphorus, the deterioration in renal function and the adequacy of the urine output.
- Hyperphosphatemia from phosphate bowel preparations: Severe hyperphosphatemia from phosphate enemas and OSPs is associated with AKI and catastrophic effects such as hypotension and severe metabolic acidosis. The risk is greatest in elderly patients and anyone with decreased kidney function. Awareness of potential toxicity is the best preventive.

AKI = acute kidney injury; CKD = chronic kidney disease; CRRT = continuous renal replacement therapy; IV = intravenous; OSP = oral sodium phosphate purgative; TLS = tumor lysis syndrome.

needed to decide whether hyperuricemia or hyperphosphatemia predominated. Hydration with IV crystalloid, at least 3 liters per day as long as urine output is adequate, is the recommended treatment for TLS. For marked hyperuricemia, IV sodium bicarbonate is recommended to alkalinize the urine which greatly increases the solubility of uric acid. However, if hyperphosphatemia predominates, the solubility of calcium-phosphate is greater in acidic urine and IV sodium chloride is recommended.

Currently, there are several agents available to prevent and treat hyperuricemia associated with TLS. Allopurinol is available in oral and IV formulations and may be used for treatment and prevention of hyperuricemia in TLS. It blocks the conversion of hypoxanthine to xanthine and xanthine to uric acid, resulting in rapid clearance. Use is usually restricted to patients at low or intermediate risk for TLS, given that the risk of xanthine nephropathy is substantial with underlying renal impairment (26). Febuxostat is a selective xanthine oxidase inhibitor that effectively reduces uric acid levels. Its biliary elimination makes it an attractive option for patients with pre-existing nephropathy both for preventing and treating TLS. Rasburicase is a recombinant form of urate oxidase which lowers serum uric acid dramatically by converting insoluble uric acid into the more soluble allantoin. Because of the high cost of rasburicase, our approach is not to administer it prophylactically, but rather to observe uric acid values after completion of chemotherapy and to give a single dose if marked hyperuricemia develops. Because rasburicase also generates hydrogen peroxide, patients should be tested for glucose-6-phosphatase deficiency before treatment. Since it is highly effective, rasburicase should be considered in patients with pre-existing hyperuricemia before anti-cancer therapy as well as in patients at high risk for TLS.

Complications of the acute hyperphosphatemia include AKI and profound hypocalcemia with resultant tetany, cardiac

Table 25-3 Causes of hyperphosphatemia

Mechanism	Etiology
Decreased renal excretion	Renal insufficiency/failure
	Hypoparathyroidism
	Pseudohypoparathyroidism
	Tumoral calcinosis
	Acromegaly
	Bisphosphonates
Acute phosphate load	Phosphate containing laxatives
	Fleet's phosphosoda enemas
	Intravenous phosphate
	Parenteral nutrition
Redistribution to the extracellular space	Tumor lysis
	Rhabdomyolysis
	Acidosis
	Hemolytic anemia
	Severe hyperthermia
	Fulminant hepatitis
	Systemic infections
Pseudohyper-phosphatemia	Hyperglobulinemia
	Hyperlipidemia
	Hemolysis
	Hyperbilirubinemia

arrhythmias, hypotension, and seizures. The decision to treat hyperphosphatemia depends on the magnitude of hyperphosphatemia, the rate of rise of serum phosphate, the adequacy of the urine output and the deterioration of the renal function. Because phosphate clearance is time-dependent, phosphate removal is best accomplished with CRRT rather than intermittent hemodialysis.

Nephropathy from Phosphate Bowel Preparations

Acute phosphate nephropathy has been observed after both oral sodium phosphate (OSP) purgatives for colonoscopy and phosphate enemas. The former often results in subacute kidney injury without obvious clinical symptomatology in which the patient presents several months later with decreased kidney function (27). In one study, 28% of patients receiving OSP (11.6 grams of phosphate) for colonoscopy had serum phosphorus values >8 mg/dL (2.58 mmol/L) after taking the OSP (16). Kidney biopsies obtained when serum creatinine was discovered to be increased several months later, showed calcium phosphate deposition in the tubular epithelial cells. Pre-existing risk factors for nephrotoxicity include decreased kidney function, volume depletion, age, female gender, hypertension, diabetes, and use of ACE-inhibitors/angiotensin receptor blockers, diuretics, and non-steroidal anti-inflammatory drugs.

Acute phosphate nephropathy associated with phosphate enemas often presents as a metabolic emergency. In a retrospective study of 11 patients hospitalized after a sodium phosphate (Fleet) enema, 7 patients presented in the first 24 hours (28). Mean age of the patients was 80 years and 10 patients received the Fleet enema for constipation. Presenting findings included hypotension, volume depletion, severe hyperphosphatemia, profound hypocalcemia, metabolic acidosis, hypernatremia, and both hypo- and hyperkalemia. The mean serum phosphorus and calcium on presentation were 18.8 mg/dL (6.06 mmol/L) and 5.9 mg/dL (1.47 mmol/L) respectively. Five patients died and three patients required prolonged hospitalizations. Eight patients received the standard Fleet enema dose of 250 ml, which contains 10.7 grams elemental phosphorus, and 3 patients received doses between 500 and 798 ml. Awareness that phosphate enemas in the elderly population can result in a metabolic emergency is the most important preventive. Pre-existing chronic kidney disease, common in the elderly, magnifies the risk for developing phosphate nephropathy. In a retrospective cohort study of 70,499 VA patients, the use of sodium phosphate enemas versus polyethylene glycol powder was associated with increased risk of long-term estimated glomerular filtration rate (eGFR) decline.

Patients with non-iron deficient anemia were at higher risk for eGFR decline (29). Key considerations for the development and treatment of hyperphosphatemia are presented in Table 25-2.

Conclusions

Treatment of hypophosphatemia has largely been based on empirical administration of different doses of oral and IV phosphate. In the setting of severe hypophosphatemia, especially in the ICU, IV phosphate administration is generally necessary. Hyper-phosphatemia and the severe metabolic toxicities associated with phosphate bowel preparations can be prevented by awareness of the patient population at risk. Hyper-phosphatemia associated with TLS requires prompt treatment to prevent renal toxicity.

Acknowledgments

The current authors wish to acknowledge the contributions to the previous edition by the previous authors, Arnold Felsenfeld and Barton Levine, upon which portions of this chapter are based.

References

1 Bielesz B, Bacic D, Honegger K, et al. Unchanged expression of the sodium-dependent phosphate cotransporter NaPi-IIa despite diurnal changes in renal phosphate excretion. *Pflügers Archiv*. 2006;452(6):683–689. Epub 2006 May 19.

2 Portale AAL, Halloran BP, Morris RC Jr. Dietary intake of phosphorus modulates the circadian rhythm in serum concentration of phosphorus: implications for the renal production of 1,25-dihydroxyvitamin D. *J Clin Invest*. 1987 Oct;80(4):1147–1154.

3 Brunelli SM, Goldfarb S. Hypophosphatemia: clinical consequences and management. *J Am Soc Nephrol*. 2007;18:1999–2003.

4 Felsenfeld AJ, Levine BS. Approach to treatment of hypophosphatemia. *Am J Kidney Dis*. 2012;60:655–661.

5 Gonciulea A, Jan de Beur SM. Bone disorders: FGF-23 mediated bone disease. *Endocr Metab Clin N Amer*. 2017;46:19–39.

6 Imel EA, Econs MJ. Approach to the hypophosphatemic patient. *J Clin Endocrinol Metab*. 2011;97:696–706.

7 Prie D, Friedlander G. Genetic disorders of renal phosphate transport. *N Engl J Med*. 2010;362:2399–2409.

8 Forster IC, Hernando N, Biber J, Murer H. Proximal tubular handling of phosphate: a molecular perspective. *Kidney Int*. 2006;70(9): 1548–1559.

9 Brown AJ, Zhang F, Ritter CS. The vitamin D analog ED-71 is a potent regulator of intestinal phosphate absorption and NaPi-IIb. *Endocrinology*. 2012;153(11): 5150–5156. doi: 10.1210/en.2012-1587.

10 Lederer E. Regulation of serum phosphate. *J Physiol*. 2014;592(18):3985–3995. doi: 10.1113/jphysiol.2014.273979.

11 Bergwitz C, Jüppner H. Regulation of phosphate homeostasis by PTH, vitamin D, and FGF23. *Annu Rev Med*. 2010;61: 91–104.

12 Silver J, Naveh-Many T. Phosphate and the parathyroid. *Kidney Int*. 2009;75:898–905.

13 Shimada T, Hasegawa H, Yamazaki Y, et al. FGF-23 is a potent regulator of vitamin D metabolism and phosphate homeostasis. *J Bone Miner Res*. 2004;19(3):429–435.

14 Nishida Y, Taketani Y, Yamanaka-Okumura H, et al. Acute effect of oral phosphate loading on serum fibroblast growth factor 23 levels in healthy men. *Kidney Int*. 2006;70:2141–2147.

15 Scanni R, von Rotz M, Jehle S, et al. The human response to acute enteral and parenteral phosphate loads. *J Am Soc*

Nephrol. 2014;25(12):2730–2739. doi: 10.1681/ASN.2013101076.

16 Quarles LD. Endocrine functions of bone in mineral metabolism regulation. *J Clin Invest.* 2008;18:3820–3828.

17 Quinn SJ, Thomsen AR, Pang JL, et al. Interactions between calcium and phosphorus in the regulation of the production of fibroblast growth factor 23 in vivo. *Am J Physiol Endocrinol Metab.* 2013;304(3):E310–20. DOI: 10.1152/ajpendo.00460.2012.

18 Braithwaite V, Prentice AM, Doherty C, Prentice A. FGF23 is correlated with iron status but not with inflammation and decreases after iron supplementation: a supplementation study. *Int J Pediatr Endocrinol.* 2012;2012(1):27. DOI: 10.1186/1687-9856-2012-27.

19 Lanske B, Razzaque MS. Molecular interactions of FGF23 and PTH in phosphate regulation. *Kidney Int.* 2014;86(6):1072–1074.

20 Rubin MF, Narins RG. Hypophosphatemia: pathophysiological and practical aspects of its therapy. *Semin Nephrol.* 1990;10: 536–545.

21 Ritz E. Acute hypophosphatemia. *Kidney Int.* 1982;22:84–94.

22 Bacchetta J, Salusky IB. Evaluation of hypophosphatemia: lessons from patients with genetic disorders. *Am J Kidney Dis.* 2012;59:152–159.

23 Lentz RD, Brown DM, Kjellstrand CM. Treatment of severe hypophosphatemia. *Ann Intern Med.* 1978;89:941–944.

24 Coiffier B, Altman A, Pui C-H, Younes A, Cairo MS. Guidelines for the management of pediatric and adult tumor lysis syndrome: an evidence-based review. *J Clin Oncol.* 2008;26:2767–2778.

25 Wilson FP, Berns JS. Onco-nephrology: tumor lysis syndrome. *Clin J Am Soc Nephrol.* 2012;7:1730–1739.

26 Alakel N, Middeke JM, et al. Prevention and treatment of tumor lysis syndrome, and the efficacy and role of rasburicase. *Oncol Targets Ther.* 2017;10:597–605.

27 Markowitz GS, Perazella MA. Acute phosphate nephropathy. *Kidney Int.* 2009;76:1027–1034.

28 Ori Y, Rozen-Zvi B, Chagnac A, et al. Fatalities and severe metabolic disorders associated with the use of sodium phosphate enemas. *Arch Intern Med.* 2012;172:263–265.

29 Schaefer M, Littrell E, et al. Estimated GFR decline following sodium phosphate enemas versus polyethylene glycol for screening colonoscopy: a retrospective cohort study. *Am J Kidney Dis.* 2016;67(4):609–616.

26

Acute Medical Aspects Related to Osteoporosis and Its Therapy

Dima L. Diab and Nelson B. Watts

Key Points

- Osteoporosis is a generalized skeletal disorder characterized by compromised bone strength, predisposing to an increased risk of fractures.
- Osteoporotic fractures (fragility fractures, low-trauma fractures) are those occurring from a fall from a standing height or less, without major trauma.
- Laboratory evaluation to assess for causes of secondary osteoporosis is important.
- There are several safety concerns (some of which can present as emergencies) with the use of non-pharmacologic and pharmacologic agents for the treatment of osteoporosis.
- There is some evidence (suggestive but not conclusive) that excessive use of calcium supplements may lead to an increased risk of kidney stones and possibly cardiovascular disease.
- Excessive vitamin D supplementation, especially combined with calcium supplementation, may cause hypercalcemia, hypercalciuria, and kidney stones.
- Raloxifene (a selective estrogen receptor modulator) is associated with an increased risk of venous thromboembolic events and fatal strokes.
- Safety issues with bisphosphonate therapy include gastrointestinal side effects (when given orally); and acute phase reaction, hypocalcemia, musculoskeletal pain, renal safety, atrial fibrillation, and ocular side effects.

- Safety concerns with denosumab (a fully human monoclonal antibody to the receptor activator of nuclear factor kappa-B ligand [RANKL]) include hypocalcemia, infections, skin reactions, malignancy, and risk of "rebound" multiple vertebral fractures after discontinuation.
- Osteonecrosis of the jaw and atypical femur fractures have been reported with both bisphosphonates and denosumab.
- The main adverse events with teriparatide use (recombinant form of parathyroid hormone [1-34]) are hypercalcemia and hypercalciuria.
- Initial management of osteoporotic vertebral compression fractures should include pain control, with resumption of activity as quickly as possible, and physical therapy. The evaluation includes assessment for neurologic findings.
- Hip fractures are the most devastating osteoporotic fractures and are associated with increased morbidity and mortality. Initial care of the patient with a hip fracture consists primarily of providing adequate analgesia and consulting an orthopedic surgeon. Because the occurrence of fall and fracture often signals underlying ill-health, a comprehensive multidisciplinary approach is required from presentation to subsequent follow-up, including the transition from hospital to community.

Endocrine and Metabolic Medical Emergencies: A Clinician's Guide, Second Edition. Edited by Glenn Matfin.
© 2018 John Wiley & Sons Ltd. Published 2018 by John Wiley & Sons Ltd.

Introduction

Osteoporosis is a generalized skeletal disorder characterized by compromised bone strength, predisposing to an increased risk of fractures (1). Osteoporosis has no clinical manifestations until there is a fracture. The annual incidence of osteoporotic fractures in the USA is higher than two million, which is expected to rise to more than three million by the year 2020 (2). The gold standard for establishing the diagnosis of osteoporosis is the measurement of bone mineral density (BMD) by dual-energy x-ray absorptiometry (DXA) of the lumbar spine, femoral neck, total hip, and/or 33%radius. While osteoporosis has traditionally been diagnosed based on T-scores less than -2.5 at any of these sites, the National Bone Health Alliance (NBHA) and American Association of Clinical Endocrinologists (AACE) propose that osteoporosis may also be diagnosed in patients with osteopenia and increased fracture risk using FRAX® country-specific thresholds (3). A clinical diagnosis of osteoporosis can also be made in individuals who sustain a fragility fracture regardless of the T-score. There are numerous effective pharmacologic treatment options for osteoporosis, with different safety profiles (4). This chapter provides a thorough updated review of the safety of osteoporosis therapy, with a focus on the acute medical aspects related to such therapy. This chapter also discusses the work-up and management of the acute fragility fracture.

Safety Concerns with Osteoporosis Therapy

Calcium

Adequate intake of calcium is an important component in the prevention and treatment of osteoporosis. The recommended calcium intake for postmenopausal women is 1200 mg daily, with the preferred source being diet (5,6). Supplementation is recommended if this cannot be obtained through diet alone. Although there appears to be a wide margin of safety, excessive calcium supplementation may cause hypercalcemia, hypercalciuria, and kidney stones. In general, the concern that high dietary calcium increases the risk of nephrolithiasis is unfounded, as the incidence of stone formation appears to be reduced in both men and women with high dietary calcium intake (7). However, calcium supplements have been associated with an increased risk of kidney stones in randomized clinical trials. The Women's Health Initiative (WHI) trial reported an increased risk of kidney stones in postmenopausal women who were supplemented with calcium and vitamin D when compared with placebo (2.5% versus 2.1%, [hazard ratio] HR 1.17, 95% CI 1.02–1.34), although the total calcium intake in the intervention group exceeded 2000 mg/day (8). Patients with a history of kidney stones should be evaluated for this prior to deciding about calcium supplementation.

The effect of calcium supplementation on the risk of cardiovascular disease remains controversial. In the WHI trial described above, there was no effect of calcium and vitamin D supplementation on cardiovascular disease (9). However, the findings of two meta-analyses evaluating calcium or calcium with or without vitamin D supplementation raised some concern about an increased risk of myocardial infarction in patients randomly assigned to calcium versus placebo (10,11). Some prospective studies also showed an increased cardiovascular risk with calcium supplements, but no relationship between dietary calcium intake and cardiovascular disease (12,13). On the other hand, data from a 5-year randomized, controlled trial and 4.5 years of post-trial follow-up revealed that daily calcium supplementation of 1200 mg did not increase the risk of atherosclerotic vascular disease in elderly women (14). In fact, a meta-analysis of trials comparing vitamin D with or without calcium with no treatment or placebo showed that calcium plus vitamin D were associated with reduced all-cause mortality in older adults (HR 0.91, 95% CI 0.84–0.98) (15). Furthermore, a recent systematic review and meta-analysis showed that calcium intake within tolerable upper intake levels is not associated with cardiovascular risk in generally healthy adults (16). The National Osteoporosis Foundation and American Society for Preventive Cardiology have adopted the position that calcium intake (from food or supplements) has no relationship to the risk for cardiovascular and cerebrovascular disease, mortality, or all-cause mortality in generally healthy adults at this time (17).

Other potential side effects of high calcium intake include bloating and constipation, especially with the intake of calcium carbonate supplement formulations. In addition, calcium supplements may interfere with the absorption of other medications (such as thyroid hormone) and, in such cases, these medications should be taken several hours apart.

In summary, the total intake of calcium (diet plus supplements) should not exceed 1500 mg/day because of the possibility of adverse effects related to excessive calcium intake. Existing studies suggest that dietary calcium may be preferred over supplemental calcium.

Vitamin D

Vitamin D deficiency is common and supplementation is essential for the maintenance of bone and muscle strength. Vitamin D status is assessed by measurement of its major circulating metabolite, 25-hydroxy vitamin D or 25-(OH) D, with the minimum desirable level being 30 ng/mL (75 nmol/L) (18,19). Many people require supplements of vitamin D, 2000 IU daily or more, to achieve this level. The Endocrine Society Task Force, in July 2011, published guidelines for the evaluation, treatment, and prevention of vitamin D deficiency (18). Based on these guidelines, patients with confirmed vitamin D deficiency should be treated with 50,000 IU of vitamin D2 weekly for 8 weeks, followed by maintenance therapy of 50,000 IU every other week or 1500–2000 IU daily to achieve and maintain a blood level of 25-(OH) D above 30 ng/mL (75 nmol/L). It is important to use the available expert

recommendations in conjunction with clinical judgment to determine the proper vitamin D requirement for any given patient. For example, obese patients, patients with malabsorption, and patients on medications affecting vitamin D metabolism may require higher doses of vitamin D to maintain a desirable 25-(OH) D level. A repeat 25-(OH) D level should be obtained approximately 3 months after initiating therapy in patients being treated for vitamin D deficiency to assure obtaining the goal serum 25-(OH) D level. Based on the result, the dose of vitamin D may require further adjustment and additional measurements of 25-(OH) D.

Excessive vitamin D, especially combined with calcium supplementation, may cause hypercalcemia, hypercalciuria, and kidney stones. High-dose vitamin D (300,000–500,000 units) administered once yearly is not recommended due to an increase in the risk of falls and fracture (20,21). Furthermore, chronically high levels of 25-(OH) D (exceeding 50 ng/mL [125 nmol/L]) have been found in some association studies to be linked to a modest increase in the risk of some cancers (such as pancreatic) and all-cause mortality (22–24). Therefore, until further evidence is available, a reasonable upper limit for 25-(OH) D is 50 ng/mL (125 nmol/L), based on levels in sun-exposed healthy young adults.

Raloxifene

Raloxifene, a selective estrogen receptor modulator, has been shown to reduce the risk of vertebral fractures but not to reduce the risk of hip or non-vertebral fractures (25). It is also indicated to reduce the risk of breast cancer. Safety concerns with raloxifene include an increased risk of thromboembolic events and fatal strokes (26). Patients taking raloxifene should be advised to discontinue use, if possible, at least 2 weeks before prolonged travel or expected immobilization (such as recovery time from some surgical procedures). When raloxifene is stopped, the skeletal benefits appear to be lost during the following 1 or 2 years.

Bisphosphonates

Bisphosphonates reduce osteoclastic bone resorption by entering the osteoclast, causing loss of resorptive function and accelerating osteoclast apoptosis. Alendronate was the first bisphosphonate approved by the Food and Drug Administration (FDA) in 1995 for the treatment of osteoporosis, followed by risedronate in 1998, zoledronic acid in 2001 and ibandronate in 2005. Approval of bisphosphonates in the USA was based on studies of 3–4 years' duration, although some of these studies have been extended, with zoledronic acid, risedronate, and alendronate suggesting efficacy for up to 6 years, 7 years, and 10 years, respectively (27–30).

Gastrointestinal side effects have been the primary concern for patients taking oral bisphosphonates, which may irritate the esophagus and cause reflux esophagitis, esophageal ulcers, and, rarely, bleeding. The incidence of these side effects is low with good patient selection when proper instructions for administration are followed. Bisphosphonates should not be given orally to patients who cannot remain upright, who have active upper gastrointestinal symptoms or have delayed esophageal emptying such as in patients with esophageal strictures, achalasia, or severe dysmotility.

Intravenous (IV) bisphosphonates are often associated with an acute-phase reaction within 24–72 hours of the infusion, characterized by fever, myalgias, and arthralgias (31–33). Treatment with antipyretic agents generally improves the symptoms, and these rarely recur with subsequent infusions.

Hypocalcemia may occur with bisphosphonate use but is usually mild and not clinically important except in patients with hypoparathyroidism, calcium or severe vitamin D deficiency (34). Disturbances of mineral metabolism should be corrected before initiating bisphosphonate therapy.

In terms of renal safety, bisphosphonates appear to be safe and effective in individuals with mild or moderate renal impairment and no dosage adjustment is recommended for these patients. Intravenous bisphosphonates should be used with caution, if at all, in patients with glomerular filtration rate (GFR) <35 mL/min. There is a dearth of data on use of bisphosphonates in patients with severe renal impairment and in end-stage renal disease (ESRD) (35).

Cases of severe musculoskeletal pain (bone, joint and/or muscle pain) in adults taking oral and IV bisphosphonates have been reported to the FDA (36). In a series of 117 cases, pain was not isolated to a particular anatomical site and could occur at any time after starting bisphosphonate therapy. Some patients experienced immediate improvement in their symptoms after discontinuation of the drug, although for most patients the improvement was gradual or partial. The frequency and mechanism for this adverse effect are not known. There is no clear evidence supporting a causal relationship between this side effect and bisphosphonate use.

Bisphosphonates in general have not been associated with atrial arrhythmias. However, the Health Outcomes and Reduced Incidence with Zoledronic Acid Once Yearly (HORIZON) Pivotal Fracture Trial (PFT) raised concerns of cardiac safety issues surrounding use of bisphosphonates when it unexpectedly reported that zoledronic acid increased the risk for atrial fibrillation reported as a serious adverse event (1.3% of the zoledronic acid group compared with 0.5% of the placebo group) (37). In the HORIZON Recurrent Fracture Trial (RFT), a smaller and shorter study in which careful evaluation of atrial fibrillation (AF) and its serious adverse events was performed, (38), there was no increase in the rate of AF in the treatment group. Similarly, no increase in the rate of AF was noted in an extension of the HORIZON pivotal trial up to 6 years (27). However, in the extension study up to 9 years, there was a small increase in cardiac arrhythmias (combined serious and non-serious) in the group that received zoledronic acid for 9 years compared to 6 years (39). While the data regarding this issue are discordant, the overall evidence still does not support a causal relationship between bisphosphonate exposure and atrial fibrillation. In the absence of more definitive data, the benefits of fracture prevention must be weighed against the potential risk of atrial fibrillation in patients with serious underlying heart disease or a history of atrial fibrillation when considering intravenous bisphosphonates.

Ocular side effects, including pain, blurred vision, conjunctivitis, iritis, uveitis, and scleritis, have been reported with most bisphosphonates (more with intravenous than oral agents) but these complications are a rare occurrence, approximately 1 per 1000 (40). It would be prudent to avoid bisphosphonates in patients with a history of serious inflammatory eye disease.

Denosumab

Denosumab is a fully human monoclonal antibody to the receptor activator of nuclear factor kappa-B ligand (RANKL), an osteoclast differentiating factor. It inhibits osteoclast formation, resulting in decreased bone resorption (41). Denosumab was first approved by the FDA in 2010. It is administered as a subcutaneous injection every 6 months. Up to eight years of denosumab exposure in postmenopausal women with osteoporosis in the Fracture Reduction Evaluation of Denosumab in Osteoporosis Every 6 Months (FREEDOM) Extension trial was associated with a favorable risk/benefit profile (42,43). Denosumab was also generally safe and well tolerated after 8 years of exposure in an open-label phase 2 clinical trial (44).

The FDA label includes a caution about the possibility of hypocalcemia after denosumab administration, and there have been post-marketing reports of severe, symptomatic hypocalcemia after denosumab injections (45–48). While all antiresorptive agents may induce a small and transient hypocalcemic effect after administration, clinically significant hypocalcemia is not typically observed in patients with adequate calcium and vitamin D intake. Thus, it is important to ensure that patients maintain an adequate amount of calcium and vitamin D supplementation, especially with conditions that predispose to hypocalcemia, such as chronic kidney disease (CKD) or malabsorption syndromes. Denosumab should not be given to patients with pre-existing hypocalcemia until it is corrected. In the FREEDOM trial discussed above, there was no difference in reported hypocalcemia between the treated and the placebo groups either in the registration (first 3 years – 3 cases in the placebo group and none with denosumab) or the extension trial (5 more years).

The major safety concerns with denosumab have been the potential risks for infections and malignancy because of the ubiquitous presence of RANKL throughout many tissues, including cells of the immune system. There was no increase in the overall risk of infection or cancer in the FREEDOM trial; however, serious adverse events of cutaneous infections, namely cellulitis and erysipelas, occurred in 1 (<0.1%) placebo subject and 12 (0.3%) denosumab subjects (P = 0.002). Dermatologic adverse events such as dermatitis, eczema, and rashes also occurred at a significantly higher rate in the treated versus placebo groups (10.8% versus 8.2%, p <0.0001) (49). A detailed post-hoc analysis of this trial examining the incidence and types of infections revealed that serious adverse events of infections (namely, skin, gastrointestinal, ear, urinary, and cardiac valvular infections) were numerically higher in the denosumab group, although the number of events were small and the differences between groups were not statistically significant (50). Comparison of these events during the 3-year blinded trial and the following 3 years in which patients received 3 more years of denosumab or crossed over from placebo to denosumab did not suggest an increase or causal association (51).

Starting in 2015, there have been reports of patients experiencing multiple vertebral fractures after discontinuation of denosumab therapy (52–57).

Osteonecrosis of the Jaw (ONJ) and Atypical Femur Fractures (AFF)

In terms of long-term safety, concerns about two uncommon but possible time-related adverse events have emerged: osteonecrosis of the jaw (ONJ) and atypical femur fractures (AFF) related both to bisphosphonates (58,59) and denosumab.

ONJ is defined as exposed necrotic bone in the maxillo-facial region, not healing after 8 weeks in patients with no history of craniofacial radiation. It appears as areas of exposed yellow-white hard bone with smooth or ragged borders and can be associated with pain, swelling, paresthesias, suppuration, soft tissue ulceration, intra- or extra-oral sinus tracks and loosening of teeth (see Figure 26-1) (60). This can occur spontaneously but is generally associated with invasive dental procedures such as tooth extraction. ONJ has been described in patients receiving chronic bisphosphonate therapy but appears to be much more common in cancer patients receiving bisphosphonates in 10–12 times higher doses than those used to treat osteoporosis (61). The 3-year FREEDOM trial reported no cases of ONJ in either denosumab or placebo group. ONJ was observed in the extension period, approximately 5 cases per 10,000 person-years exposure to denosumab) (43,62).

In patients already receiving antiresorptive therapy, there is concern for patients scheduled for invasive dental procedures that involve the jaw, such as extractions or implants. Guidelines for oral surgeons have also been published by the American Association of Oral and Maxillofacial Surgeons (63,64), who suggest performing dentoalveolar surgery as usual in patients who have been treated with oral bisphosphonates for less than 4 years, and to discontinue the oral bisphosphonate for 2 months prior to performing the dental surgery if a patient has been treated for more than 4 years, aiming to restart it when the bone has healed. However, there is no evidence to support that this would lower ONJ risk, especially since bisphosphonates stay in the bone for years. In fact, the American Dental Association guidelines state that the benefit provided by antiresorptive therapy outweighs the low risk of developing osteonecrosis of the jaw, and that discontinuing bisphosphonate therapy may not lower the risk but may have a negative effect on low-bone-mass-treatment outcomes (65). Useful information for patients is also available on their website (www.ada.org) (65,66) and recent guidelines from an international group (67). Good oral hygiene and regular dental visits should be recommended for everyone.

AFF are thought to be stress fractures which are frequently bilateral. These "chalkstick" fractures have characteristic radiographic findings including cortical hypertrophy, a transverse fracture pattern, and medial cortical spiking (Figure 26-2). They are typically associated with minimal or no trauma and often present with prodromal pain in the region of the fracture (68,69). These fractures had been described in patients who have not received any treatment for osteoporosis. A case-control study found that longer use of bisphosphonates (5–9 years) was associated with a greater risk of atypical fractures (OR 117, 95% CI 34–402) compared with shorter use (<2 years) (OR 35, 95% CI 10–124) (70). A 2013 systematic review and meta-analysis of 11 published studies examining the association of bisphosphonates with AFF showed that bisphosphonate exposure was associated with an increased risk of AFF with

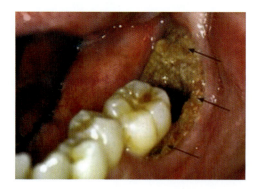

Figure 26-1 Bisphosphonate-related osteonecrosis of the jaw at extraction site of tooth. Necrotic, nonhealing exposed bone extends up the ramus and to the buccal aspect of adjacent tooth (60). Adapted or reprinted with permission from Bisphosphonate-Related Osteonecrosis of the Jaw in Patients with Osteoporosis, June 15, 2012, Vol 85, No 12, American Family Physician. Copyright © 2012 American Academy of Family Physicians. All Rights Reserved.

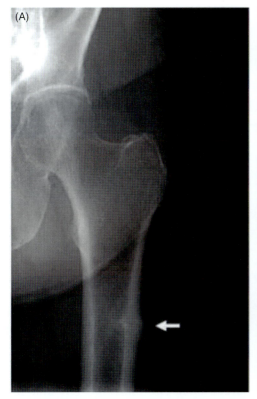 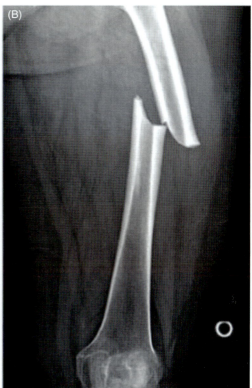

Figure 26-2 X-rays showing an impending femoral shaft fracture (A) and a representative "atypical" diaphyseal femoral fracture (B) with thickened cortices and a "beak" or "spike" (59). Courtesy of Drs. Joseph Lane and Aasis Unnanuntana, Hospital for Special Surgery, New York, N.Y. From Watts NB and Diab DL, Long-Term Use of Bisphosphonates in Osteoporosis, JCEM 2010; 95:1555-1565. Copyright 2010, The Endocrine Society.

an adjusted RR of 1.70 (95% CI 1.22-2.37) (71). Atypical femur fractures were not seen in the FREEDOM trial but occurred at a low rate, approximately 1 per 10,000 person-years exposure, in the FREEDOM extension (43,72).

The FDA currently recommends that patients with new-onset groin or thigh pain be further evaluated (73). Conventional radiography is usually the initial imaging procedure of choice, followed by magnetic resonance imaging (MRI) or bone scintigraphy if clinical suspicion is high and conventional radiography is unrevealing. In patients confirmed to have an atypical fracture, antiresorptive medications should be discontinued and these fractures should be reported. A high index of suspicion for a contralateral fracture should be maintained in patients with such fractures.

No causal relationship has been established between prolonged bisphosphonate exposure and either of these outcomes. Even though the risks of ONJ and AFF may increase after 5 years of bisphosphonate therapy, the likelihood remains low. The FDA suggests re-evaluation of the need for continuing bisphosphonate therapy beyond 3–5 years in individual patients (74). A "drug holiday" is not recommended with denosumab.

Teriparatide and Abaloparatide

In contrast to the previously-discussed therapies for osteoporosis, all of which reduce bone resorption, teriparatide (recombinant form of 1-34 parathyroid hormone, PTH) and abaloparatide (an analog of parathyroid hormone-related peptide, PTHrp) are anabolic agents that stimulate bone remodeling, preferentially increasing bone formation over resorption. Teriparatide (75) was approved by the FDA in 2002 and abaloparatide (76) in 2017. Both are administered as daily subcutaneous injections.

Hypercalcemia and hypercalciuria are the two most common short-term side effects of teriparatide treatment. Following once-daily subcutaneous administration, teriparatide produces a modest but transient increase in serum calcium, consistent with the known effects of endogenous PTH on mineral metabolism. The excursion in serum calcium is brief, due to the short length of time that teriparatide concentrations are elevated (77). Significant hypercalcemia rarely occurs, and persistent hypercalcemia after discontinuation of therapy should lead to an evaluation for other causes. There are small increases from baseline in urinary calcium excretion, which are clinically not significant for the majority of patients, although it may be prudent to consider urinary calcium monitoring for patients with a history of nephrolithiasis (78). When measuring serum calcium in patients taking teriparatide, it is advisable to wait at least 16 hours after the last dose (e.g., patients taking teriparatide in the morning should have labs in the morning, before taking that day's dose and patients taking teriparatide at bedtime should have labs in the late afternoon). Abaloparatide is less likely to cause hypercalcemia than teriparatide (76).

There have been only three cases of osteosarcoma reported in over 1 million subjects who have received teriparatide since 2002, which is lower than epidemiologic expectations (79,80). Furthermore, in a post-marketing study where 549 of 1448 patients diagnosed with osteosarcoma in the USA between 2003 and 2009 were interviewed, none reported a history of teriparatide use (81).

Nevertheless, both drugs carry a "black box warning" and are contraindicated in patients with existing risk factors for osteosarcoma, including Paget's disease of bone, prior skeletal radiation, and children with open epiphyses. The FDA recommends that both be limited to 2 years of treatment. Anabolic therapy should be followed by the use of antiresorptive agents to prevent bone density decline and loss of fracture efficacy.

Work-Up and Management of the Acute Fragility Fracture

Osteoporotic fractures (fragility fractures, low-trauma fractures) are those occurring from a fall from a standing height or less, without major trauma. Risk factors for falling and fracture include neurologic disorders, impaired vision, impaired hearing, frailty and deconditioning, proximal myopathy, sarcopenia, medications, and environmental factors (see Table 26-1). Several measures can be taken to prevent falls, including anchoring rugs, minimizing clutter, installing handrails in bathrooms and halls, and keeping hallways and rooms well lit (see Table 26-2).

Vertebral compression fractures are the most common type of osteoporotic fracture. About two-thirds of vertebral fractures are asymptomatic and are diagnosed as an incidental finding on imaging. In some patients, the presence of vertebral fractures may become apparent because of height loss and/or kyphosis. In patients who have a symptomatic vertebral fracture, there is often no history of preceding trauma. Typically patients present with acute back pain after bending, coughing, or lifting. The pain from a vertebral compression fracture may be sharp or dull and often radiates bilaterally into the anterior abdomen in the distribution of contiguous nerve routes. Sitting and movement aggravate the discomfort. Acute episodes of pain usually resolve after 4–6 weeks, but mild pain may persist for up to 3 months (82). In some patients, the pain may persist beyond 3 months, sometimes due to paraspinal spasm. However, severe back pain that persists longer should raise the question of more fractures or another diagnosis (e.g., osteomalacia, infections, or malignancy). Posterior wedging is uncommon and may indicate an underlying destructive lesion. A solitary vertebral fracture in vertebrae higher than T4 is also unusual with

Table 26-1 Factors that increase risk of falling and fracture (3)

Neurologic disorders

- Parkinson's disease
- Seizure disorder
- Peripheral neuropathy
- Prior stroke
- Dementia
- Impaired gait and/or balance
- Autonomic dysfunction with orthostatic hypotension

Impaired vision

Impaired hearing

Frailty and deconditioning

Proximal myopathy

Sarcopenia

Medications
- Sedatives and hypnotics
- Antihypertensive agents
- Narcotic analgesics

Environmental factors
- Poor lighting
- Stairs
- Slippery floors
- Wet, icy, or uneven pavement
- Uneven roadways
- Electric or telephone cords
- Walking large dogs, being tripped up by small dogs
- Throw rugs
- Positioning in a wet or dry bathtub

osteoporosis and should prompt further evaluation. Patients should be assessed for neurologic findings which may indicate fracture fragments in the spinal canal that demand surgical intervention. A bone density scan should be performed on a non-urgent basis if not already done.

Initial laboratory testing for osteoporosis should include:

- complete (full) blood count;
- complete metabolic panel including creatinine, calcium, phosphorus, alkaline phosphatase, and liver function tests;

Table 26-2 Measures for prevention of falls (3)

- Anchor rugs
- Minimize clutter
- Remove loose wires
- Use nonskid mats
- Install handrails in bathrooms, halls, and long stairways
- Light hallways, stairwells, and entrances
- Encourage patient to wear sturdy, low-heeled shoes
- Recommend hip protectors for patients who are predisposed to falling
- Keep all items within reach and avoid using stepstools

- 25-OH D to evaluate for vitamin D deficiency;
- testosterone in men to test for hypogonadism;
- 24-h urine calcium, sodium, and creatinine to check for calcium malabsorption or hypercalciuria.

This work-up identifies about 90% of occult disorders at a reasonable cost (83). Patients who have abnormalities on the initial laboratory testing or who have suspicious findings on history and physical examination may also require additional laboratory tests (84).

Initial management of osteoporotic vertebral compression fractures should include pain control, with resumption of activity as quickly as possible, and physical therapy. Aquatic therapy may be helpful in the management of back pain in these patients. Acute pain requires non-opioid or opioid analgesics and may require some limitation of activity. Options include acetaminophen (paracetamol), non-steroidal anti-inflammatory medications, or opioids combined with acetaminophen (paracetamol). A short course of nasal calcitonin, 200 units (one spray) once daily in alternating nostrils, can be a useful adjunct to traditional analgesics in the acute setting for patients who do not have adequate pain relief with oral analgesics.

Treatment should be aimed at the underlying disease, and with osteoporosis, medications such as bisphosphonates, denosumab or teriparatide should be initiated. Muscle relaxants, back braces, vertebroplasty and/or kyphoplasty are not recommended for the routine management of acute pain due to osteoporotic compression fractures (85–87). Short-term complications of vertebral augmentation procedures include cement extravasation and rarely pulmonary cement embolism or infectious complications. Both vertebroplasty and kyphoplasty have been suggested to increase the risk of vertebral fractures in adjacent vertebrae but this has not been proven in randomized trials. The American Academy of Orthopedic Surgeons recommends against vertebroplasty and provides only a limited recommendation for kyphoplasty as an option for neurologically intact patients due to the quality of the evidence available (88). These modalities have also not been adequately evaluated for the treatment of chronic pain. Exercise has beneficial effects on BMD and an exercise program can be initiated when pain has diminished.

Hip fractures are the most devastating osteoporotic fractures and are associated with increased morbidity and mortality. Initial care of the patient with a hip fracture consists primarily of providing adequate analgesia and consulting an orthopedic surgeon. Because the occurrence of fall and fracture often signals underlying ill-health, a comprehensive multidisciplinary approach is required from presentation to subsequent follow-up, including the transition from hospital to community.

Conclusions

There are several treatment options for osteoporosis with different side effect profiles and safety concerns. The evaluation of an osteoporotic compression fracture includes assessment for neurologic findings and laboratory evaluation to assess for causes of secondary osteoporosis. Oral analgesics are first-line therapy for the relief of acute pain due to vertebral compression fractures. Calcitonin may be a useful adjunct. Muscle relaxants, back braces, vertebroplasty and/or kyphoplasty are not recommended for the routine management of acute pain due to osteoporotic compression fractures. Osteoporosis therapy should be initiated to decrease the risk of new fractures.

References

1 NIH Consensus Statement. Osteoporosis prevention, diagnosis, and therapy. 2000;17:1–45. www.aafp.org/afp/2002/0701/p161.html

2 Clark WA, Burnes JP, Lyon SM. Vertebroplasty for acute osteoporotic fractures: position statement from the Interventional Radiology Society of Australasia. *J Med Imaging Radiat Oncol.* 2011;55:1–3.

3 Camacho PM, Petak SM, Binkley N, et al. American Association of Clinical Endocrinologists and American College of Endocrinology Clinical Practice Guidelines for the Diagnosis and Treatment of Postmenopausal Osteoporosis – 2016. *Endocr Pract.* 2016;22:1–42.

4 Diab DL, Watts NB. Postmenopausal osteoporosis. *Curr Opin Endocrinol Diabetes Obes.* 2013;20:501–509.

5 Tang BM, Eslick GD, Nowson C, et al. Use of calcium or calcium in combination with vitamin D supplementation to prevent fractures and bone loss in people aged 50 years and older: a meta-analysis. *Lancet.* 2007;370:657–666.

6 Verbrugge FH, Gielen E, Milisen K, Boonen S. Who should receive calcium and vitamin D supplementation? *Age Ageing.* 2012;41:576–580.

7 Curhan GC, Willett WC, Speizer FE, et al. Comparison of dietary calcium with supplemental calcium and other nutrients as factors affecting the risk for kidney

stones in women. *Ann Intern Med.* 1997;126:497–504.

8 Jackson RD, LaCroix AZ, Gass M, et al. Calcium plus vitamin D supplementation and the risk of fractures. *N Engl J Med.* 2006;354:669–683.

9 Hsia J, Heiss G, Ren H, et al. Calcium/ vitamin D supplementation and cardiovascular events. *Circulation.* 2007;115:846–854.

10 Bolland MJ, Avenell A, Baron JA, et al. Effect of calcium supplements on risk of myocardial infarction and cardiovascular events: meta-analysis. *BMJ.* 2010;341:c3691.

11 Bolland MJ, Grey A, Avenell A, et al. Calcium supplements with or without vitamin D and risk of cardiovascular events: reanalysis of the Women's Health Initiative limited access dataset and meta-analysis. *BMJ.* 2011;342:d2040.

12 Xiao Q, Murphy RA, Houston DK, et al. Dietary and supplemental calcium intake and cardiovascular disease mortality: the National Institutes of Health-AARP diet and health study. *JAMA Intern Med.* 2013;173:639–646.

13 Van Hemelrijck M, Michaelsson K, Linseisen J, Rohrmann S. Calcium intake and serum concentration in relation to risk of cardiovascular death in NHANES III. *PLoS One.* 2013;8:e61037.

14 Lewis JR, Calver J, Zhu K, et al. Calcium supplementation and the risks of atherosclerotic vascular disease in older women: results of a 5-year RCT and a 4.5-year follow-up. *J Bone Miner Res.* 2011;26:35–41.

15 Rejnmark L, Avenell A, Masud T, et al. Vitamin D with calcium reduces mortality: patient level pooled analysis of 70,528 patients from eight major vitamin D trials. *J Clin Endocrinol Metab.* 2012;97:2670–2681.

16 Chung M, Tang AM, Fu Z, et al. Calcium intake and cardiovascular disease risk: an updated systematic review and meta-analysis. *Ann Intern Med.* 2016;165:856–866.

17 Kopecky SL, Bauer DC, Gulati M et al. Lack of evidence linking calcium with or without vitamin D supplementation to cardiovascular disease in generally healthy adults: a clinical guideline from the National Osteoporosis Foundation and the American Society for Preventive Cardiology. *Ann Intern Med.* 2016;165:867–868.

18 Holick MF, Binkley NC, Bischoff-Ferrari HA, et al. Evaluation, treatment, and prevention of vitamin D deficiency: an Endocrine Society Clinical Practice Guideline. *J Clin Endocrinol Metab.* 2011;96:1911–1930.

19 Holick MF, Binkley NC, Bischoff-Ferrari HA, et al. Guidelines for preventing and treating vitamin D deficiency and insufficiency revisited. *J Clin Endocrinol Metab.* 2012;97:1153–1158.

20 Sanders KM, Stuart AL, Williamson EJ, et al. Annual high-dose oral vitamin D and falls and fractures in older women: a randomized controlled trial. *JAMA.* 2010;303:1815–1822.

21 Smith H, Anderson F, Raphael H, et al. Effect of annual intramuscular vitamin D on fracture risk in elderly men and women: a population-based, randomized, double-blind, placebo-controlled trial. *Rheumatology (Oxf).* 2007;46:1852–1857.

22 Helzlsouer KJ. Overview of the Cohort Consortium Vitamin D Pooling Project of Rarer Cancers. *Am J Epidemiol.* 2010;172:4–9.

23 Stolzenberg-Solomon RZ, Jacobs EJ, Arslan AA, et al. Circulating 25-hydroxyvitamin D and risk of pancreatic cancer: Cohort Consortium Vitamin D Pooling Project of Rarer Cancers. *Am J Epidemiol.* 2010;172:81–93.

24 Melamed ML, Michos ED, Post W, Astor B. 25-hydroxyvitamin D levels and the risk of mortality in the general population. *Arch Intern Med.* 2008;168:1629–1637.

25 Ettinger B, Black DM, Mitlak BH, et al. Reduction of vertebral fracture risk in postmenopausal women with osteoporosis treated with raloxifene: results from a 3-year randomized clinical trial. Multiple Outcomes of Raloxifene Evaluation (MORE) Investigators. *Jama.* 1999;282:637–645.

26 Barrett-Connor E, Grady D, Sashegyi A, et al. Raloxifene and cardiovascular events in osteoporotic postmenopausal women: four-year results from the MORE (Multiple Outcomes of Raloxifene Evaluation) randomized trial. *JAMA*. 2002;287: 847–857.

27 Black DM, Reid IR, Boonen S, et al. The effect of 3 versus 6 years of zoledronic acid treatment of osteoporosis: a randomized extension to the HORIZON-Pivotal Fracture Trial (PFT). *J Bone Miner Res*. 2012;27:243–254.

28 Mellstrom DD, Sorensen OH, Goemaere S, et al. Seven years of treatment with risedronate in women with postmenopausal osteoporosis. *Calcif Tissue Int*. 2004;75:462–468.

29 Black DM, Schwartz AV, Ensrud KE, et al. Effects of continuing or stopping alendronate after 5 years of treatment: the Fracture Intervention Trial Long-term Extension (FLEX): a randomized trial. *JAMA*. 2006;296:2927–2938.

30 Schwartz AV, Bauer DC, Cummings SR, et al. Efficacy of continued alendronate for fractures in women with and without prevalent vertebral fracture: the FLEX trial. *J Bone Miner Res*. 2010;25:976–982.

31 Knopp JA, Diner BM, Blitz M, et al. Calcitonin for treating acute pain of osteoporotic vertebral compression fractures: a systematic review of randomized, controlled trials. *Osteoporos Int*. 2005;16:1281–1290.

32 Molina V, Court C, Dagher G, et al. Fracture of the posterior margin of the lumbar spine: case report after an acute, unique, and severe trauma. *Spine (Phila Pa 1976)*. 2004;29:E565–E567.

33 McDonough PW, Davis R, Tribus C, Zdeblick TA. The management of acute thoracolumbar burst fractures with anterior corpectomy and Z-plate fixation. *Spine (Phila Pa 1976*. 2004;29:1901–1908; discussion 1909.

34 Heini PF. The current treatment: a survey of osteoporotic fracture treatment. Osteoporotic spine fractures: the spine

surgeon's perspective. *Osteoporos Int*. 2005;16 Suppl 2:S85–S92.

35 Miller PD. Diagnosis and treatment of osteoporosis in chronic renal disease. *Semin Nephrol*. 2009;29:144–155.

36 Wysowski DK, Chang JT. Alendronate and risedronate: reports of severe bone, joint, and muscle pain. *Arch Intern Med*. 2005;165:346–347.

37 Black DM, Delmas PD, Eastell R, et al. Once-yearly zoledronic acid for treatment of postmenopausal osteoporosis. *N Engl J Med*. 2007;356:1809–1822.

38 Lyles KW, Colon-Emeric CS, Magaziner JS, et al. Zoledronic acid and clinical fractures and mortality after hip fracture. *N Engl J Med*. 2007;357:1799–1809.

39 Black DM, Reid IR, Cauley JA, et al. The effect of 6 versus 9 years of zoledronic acid treatment in osteoporosis: a randomized second extension to the HORIZON-Pivotal Fracture Trial (PFT). *J Bone Miner Res*. 2015;30:934–944.

40 Lewiecki EM. Safety of long-term bisphosphonate therapy for the management of osteoporosis. *Drugs*. 2011;71:791–814.

41 Josse R, Khan A, Ngui D, Shapiro M. Denosumab, a new pharmacotherapy option for postmenopausal osteoporosis. *Curr Med Res Opin*. 2013;29:205–216.

42 Bone HG, Chapurlat R, Brandi ML, et al. The effect of three or six years of denosumab exposure in women with postmenopausal osteoporosis: results from the FREEDOM extension. *J Clin Endocrinol Metab*. 2013;98:4483–4492.

43 Papapoulos S, Lippuner K, Roux C, et al. The effect of 8 or 5 years of denosumab treatment in postmenopausal women with osteoporosis: results from the FREEDOM Extension study. *Osteoporos Int*. 2015;26:2773–2783.

44 McClung MR, Lewiecki EM, Geller ML, et al. Effect of denosumab on bone mineral density and biochemical markers of bone turnover: 8-year results of a phase 2 clinical trial. *Osteoporos Int*. 2013;24:227–235.

45 Martin-Baez IM, Blanco-Garcia R, Alonso-Suarez M, et al. Severe

hypocalcaemia post-denosumab. *Nefrologia*. 2013;33:614–615.

46 McLachlan JM, Marx GM, Bridgman M. Severe symptomatic hypocalcaemia following a single dose of denosumab. *Med J Aust*. 2013;199:242–243.

47 Okada N, Kawazoe K, Teraoka K, et al. Identification of the risk factors associated with hypocalcemia induced by denosumab. *Biol Pharm Bull*. 2013.

48 Ungprasert P, Cheungpasitporn W, Srivali N, et al. Life-threatening hypocalcemia associated with denosumab in a patient with moderate renal insufficiency. *Am J Emerg Med*. 2013;31:756 e751–e752.

49 Cummings SR, San Martin J, McClung MR, et al. Denosumab for prevention of fractures in postmenopausal women with osteoporosis. *N Engl J Med*. 2009;361:756–765.

50 Watts NB, Roux C, Modlin JF, et al. Infections in postmenopausal women with osteoporosis treated with denosumab or placebo: coincidence or causal association? *Osteoporos Int*. 2012;23:327–337.

51 Watts NB, Brown JP, Papapoulos S, et al. Safety Observations with 3 years of denosumab exposure: comparison between subjects who received denosumab during the randomized FREEDOM Trial and subjects who crossed over to denosumab during the FREEDOM Extension. *J Bone Miner Res*. 2017.

52 Aubry-Rozier B, Gonzalez-Rodriguez E, Stoll D, Lamy O. Severe spontaneous vertebral fractures after denosumab discontinuation: three case reports. *Osteoporos Int*. 2016;27:1923–1925.

53 Lamy O, Gonzalez-Rodriguez E, Stoll D, et al. Severe rebound-associated vertebral fractures after denosumab discontinuation: 9 clinical cases report. *J Clin Endocrinol Metab*. 2017;102:354–358.

54 Anastasilakis AD, Polyzos SA, Makras P, et al. Clinical features of 24 patients with rebound-associated vertebral fractures after denosumab discontinuation: systematic review and additional cases. *J Bone Miner Res*. 2017.

55 Popp AW, Zysset PK, Lippuner K. Rebound-associated vertebral fractures

after discontinuation of denosumab-from clinic and biomechanics. *Osteoporos Int*. 2016;27:1917–1921.

56 Anastasilakis AD, Makras P. Multiple clinical vertebral fractures following denosumab discontinuation. *Osteoporos Int*. 2016;27:1929–1930.

57 Polyzos SA, Terpos E. Clinical vertebral fractures following denosumab discontinuation. *Endocrine*. 2016;54: 271–272.

58 Diab DL, Watts NB. Bisphosphonates in the treatment of osteoporosis. *Endocrinol Metab Clin North Am*. 2012;41:487–506.

59 Watts NB, Diab DL. Long-term use of bisphosphonates in osteoporosis. *J Clin Endocrinol Metab*. 2010;95:1555–1565.

60 Heng C, Badner VM, Vakkas TG, et al. Bisphosphonate-related osteonecrosis of the jaw in patients with osteoporosis. *Am Fam Physician*. 2012;85:1134–1141.

61 Khosla S, Burr D, Cauley J, et al. Bisphosphonate-associated osteonecrosis of the jaw: report of a task force of the American Society for Bone and Mineral Research. *J Bone Miner Res*. 2007;22:1479–1491.

62 Diab DL, Watts NB. Denosumab in osteoporosis. *Expert Opin Drug Saf*. 2013.

63 American Association of Oral and Maxillofacial Surgeons. Position paper on bisphosphonate-related osteonecrosis of the jaws. *JOral Maxillofacial Surgery*. 2007;65:369–376.

64 http://www.aaoms.org/docs/govt_affairs/ advocacy_white_papers/mronj_position _paper.pdf. 2014.

65 Hellstein JW, Adler RA, Edwards B, et al. Managing the care of patients receiving antiresorptive therapy for prevention and treatment of osteoporosis: executive summary of recommendations from the American Dental Association Council on Scientific Affairs. *J Am Dent Assoc*. 2011;142:1243–1251.

66 Osteoporosis medications and your dental health. *J Am Dent Assoc*. 2011;142:1320.

67 Khan AA, Morrison A, Hanley DA, et al. Diagnosis and management of osteonecrosis of the jaw: a systematic

review and international consensus. *J Bone Miner Res.* 2015;30:3–3.

68 Dell RM, Adams AL, Greene DF, et al. Incidence of atypical nontraumatic diaphyseal fractures of the femur. *J Bone Miner Res.* 2012;27:2544–2550.

69 Shane E, Ebeling PR, Abrahamsen B, et al. Atypical subtrochanteric and diaphyseal femoral fractures: Second report of a task force of the American society for bone and mineral research. *J Bone Miner Res.* 2013.

70 Meier RP, Perneger TV, Stern R, et al. Increasing occurrence of atypical femoral fractures associated with bisphosphonate use. *Arch Intern Med.* 2012;172:930–936.

71 Gedmintas L, Solomon DH, Kim SC. Bisphosphonates and risk of subtrochanteric, femoral shaft, and atypical femur fracture: a systematic review and meta-analysis. *J Bone Miner Res.* 2013;28:1729–1737.

72 http://www.mhra.gov.uk/Safety information/DrugSafetyUpdate/CON 239411. (accesed May 1, 2017).

73 Bach SM, Holten KB. Guideline update: what's the best approach to acute low back pain? *J Fam Pract.* 2009;58:E1.

74 Whitaker M, Guo J, Kehoe T, Benson G. Bisphosphonates for osteoporosis–where do we go from here? *N Engl J Med.* 2012;366:2048–2051.

75 Neer RM, Arnaud CD, Zanchetta JR, et al. Effect of parathyroid hormone (1-34) on fractures and bone mineral density in postmenopausal women with osteoporosis. *N Engl J Med.* 2001;344:1434–1441.

76 Miller PD, Hattersley G, Riis BJ, et al. Effect of abaloparatide vs placebo on new vertebral fractures in postmenopausal women with osteoporosis: a randomized clinical trial. *JAMA.* 2016;316:722–733.

77 Satterwhite J, Heathman M, Miller PD, et al. Pharmacokinetics of teriparatide (rhPTH1-34]) and calcium pharmacodynamics in postmenopausal women with osteoporosis. *Calcif Tissue Int.* 2010;87:485–492.

78 Miller PD, Bilezikian JP, Diaz-Curiel M, et al. Occurrence of hypercalciuria in patients with osteoporosis treated with teriparatide. *J Clin Endocrinol Metab.* 2007;92:3535–3541.

79 Subbiah V, Madsen VS, Raymond AK, et al. Of mice and men: divergent risks of teriparatide-induced osteosarcoma. *Osteoporos Int.* 2010;21:1041–1045.

80 Cipriani C, Irani D, Bilezikian JP. Safety of osteoanabolic therapy: a decade of experience. *J Bone Miner Res.* 2012;27:2419–2428.

81 Andrews EB, Gilsenan AW, Midkiff K, et al. The US postmarketing surveillance study of adult osteosarcoma and teriparatide: study design and findings from the first 7 years. *J Bone Miner Res.* 2012;27: 2429–2437.

82 Venmans A, Klazen CA, Lohle PN, et al. Natural history of pain in patients with conservatively treated osteoporotic vertebral compression fractures: results from VERTOS II. *AJNR Am J Neuroradiol.* 2012;33:519–521.

83 Tannenbaum C, Clark J, Schwartzman K, et al. Yield of laboratory testing to identify secondary contributors to osteoporosis in otherwise healthy women. *J Clin Endocrinol Metab.* 2002;87:4431–4437.

84 Diab D, Watts N. Secondary osteoporosis: differential diagnosis and work-up. *Clinical Obstetrics and Gynecology.* Oct. 2013.

85 Abudou M, Chen X, Kong X, Wu T. Surgical versus non-surgical treatment for thoracolumbar burst fractures without neurological deficit. *Cochrane Database Syst Rev.* 2013; 6:CD005079.

86 Hoshino M, Tsujio T, Terai H et al. Impact of initial conservative treatment interventions on the outcomes of patients with osteoporotic vertebral fractures. *Spine (Phila Pa 1976).* 2013;38:E641–E648.

87 Lee HM, Park SY, Lee SH, et al. Comparative analysis of clinical outcomes in patients with osteoporotic vertebral compression fractures (OVCFs): conservative treatment versus balloon kyphoplasty. *Spine J.* 2012;12:998–1005.

88 http://www.aaos.org/research/guidelines/ SCFguideline.pdf.

27

Acute Medical Aspects Related to Paget's Disease of Bone

Ethel S. Siris and Dorothy A. Fink

Key Points

- Paget's disease is a localized disorder of bone remodeling that typically presents in both men and women after age 40–50.
- It may continue to be an active, progressive process for the rest of an individual's life.
- The structural changes that occur with time result in a poorer quality bone that is prone to bone deformity or fracture.
- Paget's disease may be completely asymptomatic at presentation, or it may be associated over time with a variety of complications, some of which require urgent or emergency management (e.g., severe bone pain that may indicate fracture or neoplastic process; neurological complications; hypercalcemia; and high output cardiac failure).
- Bisphosphonate treatment is warranted in most patients with active Paget's disease who are at risk for future complications; as well as those with complications. Surgery and other treatment modalities (e.g., glucocorticoids, chemotherapy) may also be required depending on the clinical setting.

Introduction

Paget's disease is a localized disorder of bone remodeling that typically presents in both men and women after age 40–50 and may continue to be an active, progressive process for the rest of an individual's life. It is initiated by excessive bone resorption caused by increased numbers of larger than normal osteoclasts. The increased bone resorption is subsequently coupled with secondary increases in new bone formation by apparently normal osteoblasts, but the new bone that is deposited at the previously resorbed sites is disorganized woven bone rather than neatly aligned lamellar bone and is thus less compact, taking up more space, and it has greater vascularity. Paget's disease may be found in a part of a single bone (monostotic disease) or in multiple bones (polyostotic disease). It is believed that once the condition declares itself to be present at specific skeletal sites, it can progress within those bones but is unlikely to appear years later in previously unaffected bones. The structural changes that occur with time result in a poorer quality bone that is prone to bone deformity or fracture.

The localized increase in bone remodeling is reflected in elevations of bone turnover markers, such as the bone resorption marker serum C-telopeptide (CTX) and the bone formation marker total serum alkaline phosphatase (SAP). High turnover and increased blood flow are the basis for the increased uptake of radiotracers at pagetic sites noted

Endocrine and Metabolic Medical Emergencies: A Clinician's Guide, Second Edition. Edited by Glenn Matfin.
© 2018 John Wiley & Sons Ltd. Published 2018 by John Wiley & Sons Ltd.

on bone scans. However, neither the elevations of markers nor the increased uptake on a bone scan are specific to Paget's disease. The diagnosis should be made only when the characteristic changes seen on skeletal radiographs (and in some cases elaborated upon by magnetic resonance imaging [MRI] or computed tomography [CT] scanning) are found. These radiographic and imaging studies not only allow for a diagnosis, but help to characterize the causes of some of the complications of Paget's disease that may occur.

Table 27-1 Symptoms and complications of Paget's disease of bone (1)

	Complication
Musculoskeletal	Bone pain
	Bone deformity
	Osteoarthritis of adjacent joints
	Acetabular protrusion
	Fractures
	Spinal stenosis
Neurological	Hearing loss
	Tinnitus
	Cranial nerve deficits (rare)
	Basilar impression
	Increased cerebrospinal fluid pressure
	Spinal stenosis
	Paraplegia, quadriplegia, vascular steal syndrome
Cardiovascular	Congestive heart failure
	Increased cardiac output
	Aortic stenosis
	Generalized atherosclerosis
	Endocardial calcification
Metabolic	Immobilization hypercalciuria
	Hypercalcemia
	Hyperuricemia
	Nephrolithiasis
Neoplasia	Sarcoma (osteosarcoma, chondrosarcoma, and fibrosarcoma)
	Giant cell tumor

For example, during the osteolytic phase in the femur or tibia, an advancing "blade of grass" or lytic wedge viewed on a radiograph may slowly progress along the length of the bone from one end, and there is the potential for fracture. After the osteoblastic phase fills in previously resorbed regions, the poor structure of the newly made bone subjects it to the potential for cortical thickening and bone enlargement, with subsequent bone deformity. Enlargement of the skull and bowing deformities of extremities are possible outcomes. Based upon the location of pagetic sites and the highly variable magnitude of the increase in bone remodeling as suggested by the levels of SAP and CTX, Paget's disease may be completely without symptoms at presentation, or it may be associated over time with a variety of complications (Table 27-1), some of which require urgent or emergency management. Both a clinical guideline of Paget's disease of bone from the Endocrine Society and a comprehensive review have recently been published (1,2), and both provide greater detail about this disease and its management. The present chapter will focus on those complications that require immediate attention and treatment (Table 27-2).

Severe Bone Pain in Persons with Paget's Disease

Severe Bone Pain that May Indicate Fracture or Impending Fracture

What patients perceive as pagetic bone pain may result from one or more of several causes, some of which pose acute, intermittent or chronic, non-emergency issues, and some of which are much more serious. Examples of non-emergency complaints include non-specific aches and pains that may result from minor micro-fractures along the convex surfaces of bowed extremities, pain from arthritis at a major joint due to pagetic bone enlargement and/or deformity in one or both of the bones at that joint, headache or a band like tightening in the skull in the setting of skull enlargement, or radiculopathy from

Table 27-2 Emergencies in Paget's disease of bone

Type	Symptoms
Orthopedic	New, severe bone pain from new or impending fracture
Oncological	New, severe bone pain from osteosarcoma, fibrosarcoma, or chondrosarcoma; benign giant cell tumor; or bone metastases from a primary cancer (e.g., breast, prostate, lung)
Neurological	Spinal cord compression (or vascular steal syndrome); platybasia of the skull with basilar invagination and hydrocephalus or brain stem compression; cranial nerve compression syndromes
Metabolic	Rare instances of hypercalcemia in very high turnover polyostotic Paget's disease with immobilization
Cardiac	High-output cardiac failure in very high turnover polyostotic Paget's disease

nerve root compression by pagetic vertebrae in the lumbar spine.

However, severe new pain at a previously asymptomatic or minimally uncomfortable site of Paget's disease, with or without bone enlargement or deformity such as bowing, warrants immediate examination and imaging with radiographs to rule out fracture or impending fracture (Figure 27-1). If an x-ray is not conclusive but there is a high level of suspicion of a fracture, a CT scan should be performed, and orthopedic consultation is mandatory. The orthopedic treatment of a fracture through pagetic bone is more complex than that for normal or osteoporotic bone, and a skilled orthopedic surgeon with experience managing Paget's disease fractures – or being able to consult with someone else who has more experience – is desirable (3). In medically untreated Paget's disease where the SAP is 2–3 or more times above the upper limit of normal, there is the potential for greater than normal bleeding at the time of a complete fracture and during an operation to internally fix the fractured bone. Thus, in some cases treatment with an intravenous (IV) infusion of 5 mg of zoledronic acid and a delay of a few days (ideally at least 3) before doing an open repair may be appropriate, if the repair can safely wait without posing other medical risks to the typically older patient. Impending fracture of a pagetic femur or tibia may sometimes require placement of orthopedic hardware to prevent a complete fracture, and the same issues regarding bleeding and bisphosphonate therapy would apply. Alternatively, medical management with an infusion of zoledronic acid

Figure 27-1 Paget's disease of bone involving pelvis and hips. Fracture of left neck of femur is also present.

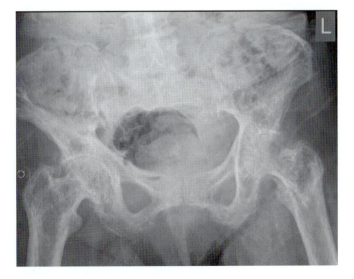

and a period of non-weight bearing on an unoperated extremity, together with careful orthopedic follow-up may be possible and safer.

A painful acute vertebral fracture at a site of Paget's disease is typically managed conservatively, with an MRI as indicated by the patient's presentation to confirm that the fracture is not causing neural entrapment. There is very little experience with kyphoplasty or vertebroplasty of a bone affected by Paget's disease (4,5) and it is difficult to know if the procedure is safe and effective in this setting, especially if adjacent vertebrae also have pagetic features. If such a patient has active Paget's disease with elevated markers of bone turnover, it may be prudent to offer an infusion of zoledronic acid to reduce vascularity. It is not proven that this will reduce pain, but it should reduce the high bone turnover and the associated increased vascularity at the site, restoring these features toward normal.

Severe Bone Pain due to a Neoplastic Process

Bone destruction due to a neoplastic process in pagetic bone also presents with severe new pain typically at a previously quiescent site. In addition to plain radiographs, MRI scanning is critical as it will typically reveal a soft tissue mass adjacent to the affected bone. CT scanning may also be useful in some cases to evaluate the status of the bone that is being eroded.

Neoplastic changes within bone affected by Paget's disease can include any of several types of lesions. Rarely, likely in less than 1% of patients, pagetic bone is the site of an osteosarcoma, a serious malignancy with a very poor prognosis (6). Fibrosarcoma and chondrosarcoma have also been described at pagetic sites. Osteosarcoma is managed by oncologists and orthopedic oncologic surgeons with aggressive surgery and chemotherapy, sometimes adding radiation therapy, even though these lesions are relatively radio-resistant. Early metastasis to

the lungs is a common complication, and the condition is often fatal within a year.

A second type of neoplasm arising at a site of Paget's disease is a benign giant cell tumor, a highly vascular lesion consisting of osteoclast-like giant cells that cause aggressive bone destruction at the localized site. These tumors are relatively rare single lesions that even more uncommonly can present over time at multiple sites within more than one pagetic bone. Often initially thought to be osteosarcoma until a biopsy correctly makes the diagnosis, these benign giant cell tumors usually shrink away dramatically and fairly quickly after treatment with high doses of dexamethasone in the range of 16–24 mg per day in divided doses (7). Prolonged use of dexamethasone if the tumor recurs locally after periods of remission has led to some of the problems associated with iatrogenic Cushing's syndrome, and other approaches to management have been attempted. In our own clinical experience, a course of thalidomide, 100 mg per day for up to several months was effective in stopping the cycle of recurrence after a remission of a large, locally destructive giant cell tumor in a pagetic spine, although the year-long course of treatment led to the development of peripheral neuropathy. A second patient with a periodically recurring giant cell tumor, also in the spine, appears to be in a prolonged remission while receiving denosumab (i.e., RANKL inhibitor), currently 60 mg every 4–5 months. The safety of long-term denosumab in this setting is not known, however. There is no specific protocol for use of glucocorticoids, thalidomide, or denosumab in patients with Paget's disease-associated giant cell tumors and treatment is empirical, provided by an oncologist working closely with the patient's endocrinologist.

Finally, clinical experience has demonstrated that bones affected by Paget's disease may be sites of painful bone metastases from common primary tumors, such as breast or prostate cancer or other solid tumors that metastasize to bone. Whether the heightened vascularity of metabolically active, high turnover Paget's disease makes pagetic bone more susceptible to attracting tumor cells from distant primaries is unknown. In this situation, severe, acute bone pain is the presenting complaint, and it must be addressed with imaging studies such as an MRI and possibly biopsy to determine if a neoplasm is present. A bone scan, normally useful in locating sites of malignancy in cancer patients will not be helpful if the patient's metastatic disease is at a site of Paget's disease, since the scan is going to be positive as a consequence of the pagetic change.

A metastasis from a distant primary may also manifest itself as an "ivory vertebra," a radio-dense vertebral body that could reflect a pagetic vertebra, an osteoblastic bone metastasis from a distant primary cancer, or a hemangioma. Paget's disease is most likely if the posterior elements as well as the vertebral body light up on a bone scan. Positron-emission tomography (PET) scans of sites of active Paget's disease display substantially less activity than what is seen when there is a malignant tumor at a site, and this may be helpful in differential diagnosis (8). A full patient work-up is needed to diagnose the cause of an ivory vertebra, including the patient's history, symptoms and other clinical and radiographic or imaging findings.

Whether the destructive bone lesion found at a severely painful site of Paget's disease is osteosarcoma, benign giant cell tumor, or bone metastasis from a remote primary, help from an oncologist is critical, and an orthopedic surgeon is required in most cases to biopsy the bone for pathological confirmation of the tumor type. Treatment will depend on that diagnosis. In the case of metastatic disease at a pagetic site, cancer doses of zoledronic acid may be used. It has not been demonstrated that bisphosphonates have any benefit in giant cell tumors at pagetic sites, though they will offer benefit in the management of the patient's underlying Paget's disease. There is limited experience with bisphosphonates as a component of the management of osteosarcoma in Paget's disease, and there is not clear evidence that there is benefit. Pamidronate is sometimes used in non-pagetic osteosarcomas, but the use of that therapy for Paget's sarcoma should be made in conjunction with the managing oncologist or oncologic orthopedic surgeon.

Neurological Complications of Paget's Disease

Pagetic bone tends to be larger than normal bone, and with its poorer structure, hypervascularity and potential for deformity, it may give rise to a number of neurological complications (9). Some of these represent medical emergencies which, while relatively uncommon, require timely diagnosis and prompt medical and neurosurgical intervention as required.

Paget's disease of the skull may be associated with headache or hearing loss, but extensive changes in the skull and facial bones after years of progressive abnormal bone remodeling with thickening, enlargement, and deformation of these bones can also lead to a variety of less common problems that may constitute emergencies. Cranial nerve palsies from narrowing of cranial nerve foramina can acutely affect cranial nerves I, II, V, VII and VIII. Flattening of the skull base, termed platybasia, can produce basilar invagination that uncommonly results in acute compression symptoms referable to the brain stem. Hydrocephalus can result when basilar invagination leads to obstruction of cerebrospinal fluid flow, presenting as ataxia, dementia and urinary incontinence, and even more rarely with symptoms of Parkinsonism (10).

Imaging studies of the brain are needed to characterize the process causing the symptoms and urgent neurological and neurosurgical consultations are mandatory. In some cases, direct compression of neural tissue by thickened and deformed pagetic bone is the primary problem, in which case surgical decompression typically after acute use of high dose glucocorticoids, at the discretion of the neurologist/neurosurgeon, will be necessary, if feasible. Hydrocephalus may be relieved through the placement of a ventricular shunt, a relatively less invasive procedure.

Intravenous zoledronic acid should probably be the empirical treatment prior to surgery. Since high turnover pagetic bone is highly vascular, and vascular steal syndromes promote ischemia in neural structures as blood flow increases in the adjacent bone, it is reasonable to use a potent IV bisphosphonate, that is zoledronic acid, possibly calcitonin, if a bisphosphonate cannot be used in these circumstances. By reducing elevated bone resorption fairly quickly with a subsequent reduction in elevated formation, it is possible to reduce the degree of blood flow through the pagetic bone and minimize the vascular steal phenomenon. In some cases vascular steal and not direct bony compression is causal, in which case the primary treatment would be the IV bisphosphonate.

For certain cranial nerve syndromes such as trigeminal neuralgia or hemi-facial spasm, carbamazepine has been described to be useful and surgical decompression has been used successfully to alleviate facial nerve palsy (9).

Paget's disease of the vertebral bodies can be a part of the basis for spinal stenosis or nerve root compression in the lumbar spine, though this is usually a chronic non-emergent problem, managed with zoledronic acid and, if it is needed and likely to help, with surgery. Often concomitant osteoarthritic changes contribute to the problem, and the degree to which the pagetic changes causing enlarged vertebral bodies or pagetic vertebral fracture play a role in lumbar stenosis can be challenging to discern. In cases of lumbar stenosis, bisphosphonate therapy is most likely to be effective when there is high turnover and less likely to help if there is very minimal increased turnover.

Sub-acute or acute spinal cord compression, typically in the thoracic spine, with acute or sub-acute loss of motor function, is a much rarer but very serious complication that constitutes an emergency. How much of the syndrome is a result of direct pagetic bony impingement on neural structures in the thoracic area, where the spinal canal is narrow, and how much results from vascular steal can be difficult to know, even with excellent imaging. While neurosurgical decompression has been recommended by some for acute spinal cord compression (9), experience at our institution has indicated that aggressive use of a short course of high dose dexamethasone and immediate treatment with zoledronic acid, particularly when indices of turnover are high, may obviate the need for surgery.

Whenever acute zoledronic acid is provided in these emergency situations, it is important to assure that patients are both vitamin D- and calcium-sufficient to avoid hypocalcemia. Serum calcium corrected for levels of serum albumin should be monitored in the setting of acute treatment.

Hypercalcemia

When hypercalcemia is discovered in someone with Paget's disease, bone diagnostic testing is needed to determine if the cause is parathyroid-mediated or non-parathyroid-mediated, and management will depend on the underlying cause. Primary hyperparathyroidism can certainly co-exist with Paget's disease – and may make the pagetic process more metabolically active than it would be if parathyroid hormone (PTH) levels were normal. Clinically significant acute hypercalcemia is a very unusual complication of Paget's disease, but if a patient with polyostotic Paget's disease and very high baseline bone turnover is immobilized for some reason, such as bed rest following an illness, it may occur. With immobilization the elevated bone resorption continues and may even increase, while bone formation, previously well coupled to resorption, decreases, and hypercalcemia can develop. As with other forms of acute hypercalcemia, serum PTH should be measured, hydration initiated, and IV zoledronic acid, 4 or 5 mg, can be given as required.

High Output Cardiac Failure

Patients with polyostotic Paget's disease and current levels of high turnover have the potential for an increased vascularity in the bone, as has been described earlier, and in some cases have been shown to have increases in cardiac output as a consequence. An echocardiographic study described lower peripheral vascular resistance and higher cardiac stroke volume in patients with Paget's disease than in controls, especially in those with more extensive bone disease and evidence of higher turnover (11). Since Paget's disease predominantly affects older individuals who may have underlying cardiovascular disease, a high output state may be detrimental. Thus, if a patient with Paget's disease experiences congestive heart failure, an evaluation of the possibility that high bone turnover is contributing to the condition is needed. In addition to standard medical management of the cardiac problem, zole-dronic acid should be administered as needed to manage the Paget's disease process.

Conclusions

Paget's disease may be completely asymptomatic at presentation, or it may be associated over time with a variety of complications, some of which require urgent or emergency management (e.g., severe bone pain that may indicate fracture or neoplastic process; neurological complications; hypercalcemia; and high output cardiac failure). Bisphosphonate treatment is warranted in most patients with active Paget's disease who are at risk for future complications; as well as those with complications. Other therapeutic modalities (e.g., surgery, glucocorticoids, chemotherapy) may also be required.

References

1 Singer F, Bone HG, Hosking DJ, et al. Paget's disease of bone: an Endocrine Society Clinical Practice Guideline, *J Clin Endocrinol Metab*. 2014;99(12):4408–4422.

2 Siris ES, Roodman GD. Paget's disease of bone. In: Rosen CJ, ed. *Primer on the Metabolic Bone Diseases and Disorders of Mineral Metabolism*. 8th edn. Washington, DC: American Society for Bone and Mineral Research, 2013: 659–668.

3 Parvizi J, Klein GR, Sim FH. Surgical management of Paget's disease of bone. *J Bone Mineral Res*. 2006;21 Suppl 2:P75–P82.

4 Pedicelli A, Papacci F, Leone A, et al. Vertebroplasty for symptomatic monostotic Paget's disease. *J Vasc Interventional Rradiology*. 2011;22(3):400–403.

5 Tancioni F, Di Ieva A, Levi D, et al. Spinal decompression and vertebroplasty in Paget's disease of the spine. *Surgical Neurology*. 2006;66(2):189–191.

6 Hansen MF, Seton M, Merchant A. Osteosarcoma in Paget's disease of bone. *J Bone Min Res*. 2006;21 Suppl 2:P58–P63.

7 Jacobs TP, Michelsen J, Polay JS, D'Adamo AC, Canfield RE. Giant cell tumor in Paget's disease of bone: familial and geographic clustering. *Cancer*. 1979;44(2):742–747.

8 Sundaram M. Imaging of Paget's disease and fibrous dysplasia of bone. *J Bone Min Res*. 2006;21 Suppl 2:P28–P30.

9 McCloskey EV, Kanis JA. Neurological complications of Paget's disease. *Clinical Rev Bone Minl Metab*. 2002;1:135–143.

10 Botez MI, Bertrand G, Leveille J, Marchand L. Parkinsonism-dementia complex, hydrocephalus and Paget's disease. *Can J Neurological Sciences/Le journal canadien des sciences neurologiques*. 1977;4(2):139–142.

11 Morales-Piga AA, Moya JL, Bachiller FJ, Munoz-Malo MT, Benavides J, Abraira V. Assessment of cardiac function by echocardiography in Paget's disease of bone. *Clinical and Experimental Rheumatology*. 2000;18(1):31–37.

28

Acute Medical Aspects Related to Kidney Stones

Hasan Fattah and David S. Goldfarb

Key Points

- Kidney stones are a common diagnosis in the USA, affecting approximately 1 in 11 people at least once in their lifetime.
- Epidemiologic studies suggest an increasing prevalence worldwide, the cause is of uncertain etiology but may be attributable to changing dietary practices (including calcium supplementation), migration from cooler rural settings to warmer urban settings, and even global warming. Obesity, hypertension, metabolic syndrome, and diabetes are now recognized as important risk factors.
- The term "renal colic" is widely used to describe the pain resulting from passage of kidney stones through the urinary tract. This "colicky" renal pain is among the most common symptoms leading to emergency care presentation, and often prompts extensive differential diagnosis and work-up.
- The most common crystal composition of kidney stones is calcium oxalate. About 20% of calcium stones are predominantly calcium phosphate. Although calcium stones are occasionally secondary to a systemic disease, on most occasions they are idiopathic. Calcium phosphate stones should

lead to consideration of primary hyperparathyroidism.
- The most common urinary risk factor for calcium stones remains hypercalciuria. In most cases, the etiology of hypercalciuria remains unexplained and is usually termed idiopathic hypercalciuria.
- Uric acid stones are associated with the metabolic syndrome, obesity, and diabetes, all of which lead to impaired ammoniagenesis and acid urine.
- Laboratory evaluation should include a urinalysis, complete (full) blood count, and comprehensive metabolic profile. The most important use of the urinalysis is to rule out urinary tract infection.
- Unenhanced, non-contrast CT KUB (kidney, ureter, bladder) is the gold standard imaging modality for the initial evaluation of kidney stones.
- Acute management of renal colic consists of pain management and medical expulsive therapy (MET).
- Kidney stone prevention is relatively inexpensive, cost-effective, and infrequently practiced.

Endocrine and Metabolic Medical Emergencies: A Clinician's Guide, Second Edition. Edited by Glenn Matfin.
© 2018 John Wiley & Sons Ltd. Published 2018 by John Wiley & Sons Ltd.

Introduction

The term "renal colic" is widely used to describe the pain resulting from the passage of kidney stones through the urinary tract. The severe intermittent flank pain that radiates to the lower abdomen, genitalia, and groin, may be associated with other gastroenterological or urological symptoms. This "colicky" renal pain is one of the most common symptoms leading to emergency care presentation, and often prompts extensive differential diagnosis and work-up.

In this chapter we focus on the pathophysiology of renal colic, the evaluation and acute management of kidney stones, and the measures taken to prevent stone recurrence. We will briefly review appropriate surgical management of ureteral stones.

Epidemiology

Kidney stones are a common diagnosis in the USA, affecting approximately 1 in 11 people at least once in their lifetime (1). Although kidney stones are becoming more frequent in women, there continues to be a gender prevalence difference, with a male:female ratio of about 2:1. Some data suggest women are catching up (2). Stones affect as many as 6–15% of American men, and up to 7% of American women. This ratio appears to be consistent with that observed in other countries as well (3).

Moreover, epidemiologic studies suggest an increasing prevalence worldwide, best demonstrated in the USA by the National Health and Nutrition Examination Survey (NHANES) III cohort (1988–1994 and 2007–2010) (2). This increasing prevalence is of uncertain etiology but may be attributable to changing dietary practices, increasing prevalence of diabetes and obesity, migration from cooler rural settings to warmer urban settings, and even global warming. These increasing prevalence rates are also associated with an increase in the cost of kidney stone management to an estimated $2.1 billion in 2000 in the USA (4).

Renal colic affects approximately 1.2 million people each year in the USA, accounts for about 1% of all ED visits and is the main diagnosis for about 1% of all hospital admissions (5). A related estimate is that urolithiasis leads to approximately 4000 emergency room visits each day in the USA (6).

Pathophysiology

The pain of renal colic may simply be thought to arise from the muscular contraction of the ureter in response to the irritating, descending stone. In fact, the mechanism seems to be more complicated. The ureteral smooth muscle contracts in a peristalsis-like manner, which could expel the stone. However, prolonged isotonic contraction leads eventually to increased production of lactic acid which irritates the sub-mucosal nerve endings located in the upper urinary tract. Pain radiates to, and can be perceived in, any organ with similar innervation such as the gastrointestinal organs and other components of the genitourinary system (7). Denervation due to kidney transplant surgery makes the development of typical renal colic unlikely. More than 50% of kidney transplant patients with *de novo* or donor-gifted stones present with no specific symptoms.

In animal models of acute unilateral upper-tract obstruction, renal pelvic pressure and renal blood flow both increase initially within 1–2 h, likely from the increased level of prostaglandin E2 (8). In turn, there is afferent arteriolar vasodilatation leading to further increases in renal blood flow and diuresis that may worsen the intra-pelvic pressure. Over the next several hours, renal blood flow starts to decline, initially due to efferent arteriolar vasoconstriction. Both renal pelvic pressure and renal blood flow start to decline, and a progressive reduction ensues in glomerular filtration rate, renal plasma flow, and renal oxidative metabolism (8–10). These reductions occur within hours, and reach a nadir by 2 weeks of complete unilateral ureteral occlusion.

Calcium Stones

The most common crystal composition of kidney stones is calcium oxalate (11). About 20% of calcium stones are predominantly calcium phosphate (12). Although calcium stones are occasionally secondary to a systemic disease, on most occasions they are idiopathic. Calcium phosphate stones should lead to consideration of primary hyperparathyroidism, if serum calcium is at the high end of the normal range or high; and renal tubular acidosis, in which case, serum bicarbonate concentration is low.

Uric Acid Stones

Uric acid stones occur as the result of low urine pH; hyperuricosuria is less important as a risk factor (13). Uric acid stones have recently been associated with the metabolic syndrome, obesity, and diabetes, all of which lead to impaired ammoniagenesis and acid urine (14). The growing prevalence of diabetes and metabolic syndrome, leading to increasing prevalence of uric acid stones, likely contributes to increasing kidney stone prevalence. Occasionally the diagnosis of diabetes is first made or suspected when uric acid stones present; measurement of glycosylated hemoglobin may be appropriate.

Struvite stones

Struvite stones are composed of "triple phosphate" crystals composed of calcium ammonium magnesium phosphate. They result exclusively in the presence of very high urine pH (≥ 7.5) as the result of urease-producing organisms, particularly species of *Proteus* (15). Struvite stones are more common in women because women are more often affected by urinary tract infections.

Cystine Stones

Cystinuria is a genetic cause of stones, accounting for 1% of all stones, and up to 7% of stones in children (16). It is due to mutations in two genes responsible for expression of the cystine transporter in the nephron.

Pathology

New ideas about the origins of calcium stones have recently resulted from a series of examinations of renal pathology obtained from renal papillary biopsies during endoscopic stone management (17). Calcium oxalate kidney stones appear to grow over deposits of "Randall's plaque" on the papillary surface exposed to urine.

The most common urinary risk factor for calcium stones remains hypercalciuria. In most cases, the etiology of hypercalciuria remains unexplained and is usually termed idiopathic hypercalciuria. One possible mechanism by which hypercalciuria occurs and causes urinary supersaturation, promoting stone formation, is the reduction of proximal tubular calcium reabsorption (18). The etiology of this reduced reabsorption is unclear but has been linked to effects of insulin.

Differential Diagnosis

Kidney stones are the most frequent cause of flank pain in an emergency room. A variety of other urinary tract and extrarenal causes should also be considered when evaluating a patient with acute flank pain. In one study, only 25–60% of patients with flank pain who had a non-contrast computed tomography (CT) study, proved to have a stone (19). The remainder, 20–35%, had a non-urinary cause of pain, such as appendicitis, diverticulitis, unsuspected bowel obstruction, or twisted ovarian cyst.

Risk Factors

Evaluation of a patient with possible kidney stones should address several important risk factors. Table 28-1 addresses many of the risk factors for stones. Kidney stones in the general population clearly result from genetic influences. About 40% of patients with renal colic in an emergency room have a first degree relative with stones. Twin studies

Table 28-1 Suggested initial evaluation of kidney stone risk factors in emergency care setting

Lifestyle and medical history	Risk factor
Past medical history • Kidney diseases like polycystic kidney disease • Anatomic abnormalities such as medullary sponge kidney, horseshoe kidney • Metabolic disorders such as gout, hyperparathyroidism, renal tubular acidosis, diabetes, obesity • Genetic disorders such as cystinuria • Short bowel syndrome, Inflammatory bowel disease, ileostomy • Sarcoidosis, urinary tract infections	Increased risk of calcium and uric acid stones
Spinal cord injury requiring intermittent catheterization, bladder dysfunction, neurogenic bladder	Increased risk of struvite stones
Dietary habits: • High protein intake • Low fluid intake • High sodium intake • Any vitamin C • Low dietary calcium intake	Increased risk of calcium stones
Positive family history	Increased risk of kidney stones
Medication use	Exclude medications associated increased risk of kidney stones
Occupational history: athletes, hot environments, teachers	Increased risk of kidney stones

support this genetic effect in that monozygotic twin pairs are more than twice as likely to be concordant for the condition compared with dizygotic, or non-identical twins (20). However, the genes accounting for this significant heritability remain obscure. Polymorphisms in candidate genes coding for proteins involved in calcium metabolism such as the vitamin D receptor or the calcium-sensing receptor have been demonstrated to account for only small proportions of calcium stone formers (21,22).

Environmental risk factors include low urine volume due to ambient heat, and occupational factors that cause reduced fluid intake and result in a concentrated urine (23). Dietary factors have been extensively studied as well (24). Increased risk arises from higher amounts of animal protein ingestion, and lower quantities of ingested fruits and vegetables (25,26). Prospective epidemiologic studies have also shown that men and women with the highest dietary calcium ingestion (mostly via dairy products, but non-dairy foods contribute as well) have the lowest associated prevalence of stones (27). This effect is attributed to the ability of ingested calcium to serve as a binder of oxalate in the intestinal lumen, diminishing its absorption into the blood and subsequent excretion by the kidneys. Obesity, hypertension, metabolic syndrome, and diabetes are now recognized as important risk factors as well (28).

Other medical conditions may be associated with higher risk of kidney stone formation as well. For example, nephrolithiasis is strongly associated with prior pregnancy due to pregnancy-related effects like hydronephrosis, urinary stasis, and altered urinary pH. The odds for stones more than double in women who had been pregnant compared with those never pregnant (29). Metabolic and urodynamic abnormalities associated with kidney transplant might contribute to formation of kidney stones in certain conditions.

Medications

A number of medications have been implicated in stone formation. Calcium supplements are consistently associated with small absolute increases in stone incidence, even when the preferred calcium citrate is used (30). Whether administration of vitamin D is associated with an increased risk of stones is uncertain and little evidence suggests that it is. We administered 50,000 units of vitamin D2 to hypercalciuric calcium stone formers with 25-OH-vitamin D levels less than 30 ng/ml (75 nmol/L) and found that the mean urine calcium excretion did not change after 8 weeks (31). However, some patients experienced increases; we recommend repeating 24 h urine collections after supplementing vitamin D. Mutations in CYP24A1, which codes for 24-hydroxylase, an enzyme that deactivates 1,25-dihydroxy vitamin D, will predispose affected patients to vitamin D toxicity, manifesting as hypercalcemia, hypercalciuria, and suppressed parathyroid hormone (32).

Emergency Care Evaluation

Typical presenting symptoms of urolithiasis are intermittent colicky flank pain associated with an inability to find a comfortable position. This presentation is in contrast to the lack of movement of the typical patient with peritonitis. However, we have been fooled when these stereotypical responses are reversed. The pain may radiate to the lower abdomen or groin, and later into the genitalia. Often renal colic is associated with nausea and diaphoresis, and sometimes with vomiting. As the stone descends into the distal ureter, lower genitourinary symptoms such as dysuria, urinary frequency, or urgency occur as well.

Laboratory Studies

Laboratory evaluation should include a urinalysis, complete (full) blood count, and comprehensive metabolic profile. The most important use of the urinalysis is to rule out urinary tract infection. Infection of an obstructed urinary tract is a urologic emergency and requires relief of obstruction before bacteremia supervenes (33). Surprisingly, microhematuria is neither sensitive nor specific for kidney stones (34). High urine pH ($\geq$6.5) is suggestive of renal tubular acidosis and may suggest urinary tract infection as well. Values $\geq$7.5 are most consistent with urease-producing organisms such as the *Proteus* species, which may be causative for destructive struvite stones. Low urine pH suggests uric acid stones but is neither sensitive nor specific. A complete blood count is useful to detect leukocytosis, which is not expected with stones without urinary tract infection, but expected with peritonitis and other abdominal pathology. A comprehensive metabolic profile is most important to assess kidney function. Significant reductions in glomerular filtration rate (GFR) may result from bilateral obstruction, obstruction of a solitary kidney, or obstruction of one kidney in a patient with chronic kidney disease. Hypercalcemia can suggest primary hyperparathyroidism or sarcoidosis or CYP24A1 mutations. Low serum bicarbonate may suggest metabolic acidosis (or respiratory alkalosis due to pain and anxiety), and could be the initial presentation of renal tubular acidosis.

Radiologic Studies

When newly diagnosed renal colic is suspected due to nephrolithiasis, abdominal imaging is often indicated for diagnosis. Imaging may not be necessary in every case, however. It is important to note that many patients seek emergency care knowing full well what the correct diagnosis is, based on their previous history. Our strong recommendation is to trust them! Adequate pain relief for recurrent stones is a goal worth achieving, and while "drug-seeking behavior" is often suspected, our experience is that far more stone formers are treated inadequately and with suspicion, than opiate seekers are granted their inappropriate wishes.

Unenhanced, non-contrast CT is clearly today the gold standard for the initial evaluation of kidney stones. It will also provide a thorough quantitation of total stone burden, and stone characteristics that aid in planning urologic interventions if warranted later. An expectation of clinicians today should be analysis of the density of stones in Hounsfield units, as that value may be useful in determining kidney stone composition (35). Lower values are most consistent with uric acid stones, higher values with calcium stones, but significant overlap reduces the accuracy of this analysis. Dual energy CT scanning is significantly more accurate at suggesting stone composition when available. All kidney stones are visible on CT, except for stones induced by some protease inhibitors used for the treatment of HIV: indinavir, saquinavir, nelfinavir, and, most recently, atazanavir (36). While CT is clearly the best and most accurate study, there is growing concern about the potential detrimental effects of ionizing radiation, especially when used repeatedly in chronic kidney stones formers. This worry will be mitigated as the development of low-dose stone protocols continue to be developed and disseminated (37).

Management

Acute management of renal colic consists of pain management and medical expulsive therapy (MET). We also offer an opinion regarding intravenous (IV) fluids. We briefly review the indications for admission, for urologic consultation, and the choices of urologic intervention.

Pain Control

Both IV narcotics and non-steroidal anti-inflammatory drugs (NSAIDs) lead to pain relief, with NSAIDs leading, in some studies, to better outcomes with fewer adverse effects

(38). Prostaglandin E2 may play an important role in the pathogenesis of pain by increasing the intra-renal pressure from disruption of vascular autoregulation, and by increasing ureteral muscular spasm. Ureteral edema may also delay stone passage and be reduced by anti-inflammatories. Hence NSAIDs may be a perfect initial acute therapy in such patients.

Most recommendations then are to start with NSAIDs if the patient has no history of peptic ulcer disease, or acute or chronic estimated GFR (eGFR) decline to less than 50 ml/min. The usual practice in the emergency room is parenteral administration of ketorolac, for rapid achievement of pain control. If an opioid is used, we often prescribe combinations with acetaminophen (paracetamol), which will soon be unavailable in the USA. Meperidine is associated with more nausea, and sometimes vomiting, than morphine. Combining NSAIDs and opiates is also rational, and may allow adverse effects of both to be minimized.

Medical Explusive Therapy (MET)

No study has demonstrated that IV fluid administration has any benefit in promoting kidney stone passage. In the only well-done randomized controlled trial (RCT) of which we are aware, patients with renal colic were randomly assigned to receive either 1 liter or 20 ml of normal saline per hour for 2 hours (39). The results suggested that both fluid regimens had little impact on stone passage or pain. It is in fact unlikely that any significant proportion of IV fluids will find their way to an obstructed urinary tract. We suggest administration of normal saline or lactated Ringer solution only to patients with vomiting who are unable to take food or liquids by mouth.

The evidence regarding the use of alpha-blockers for MET remains controversial. Stones less than or equal to 5 mm have greater than 75% chance of spontaneous passage in the course of four weeks (2) so that the benefit of MET, if any, is likely to be small. The likelihood drops to less than 25% for stones larger than 9 mm. One meta-analysis suggests the benefit of alpha blockers for 5–10 mm stones (40) but the most recent major studies are negative (41). Current American Urological Association guidelines suggest MET as a reasonable treatment in stable patients with kidney stones of less than 10 mm, but the guidelines remain in flux. The most frequently used medication has been tamsulosin 0.4 mg each evening. Often NSAIDs, such as naproxen, are given to outpatients for both analgesia and MET.

Some studies have shown efficacy of calcium channel blockers, specifically nifedipine. Alpha-blockers are expected to cause less lowering of blood pressure than calcium channel blockers; the effect may be mitigated by taking the drug at bedtime. MET can be used in association with other urologic interventions, such as shock wave lithotripsy for larger stones to aid passage of stone fragments (42).

Hospitalization

The most important indications for admission, and consultation with urology, are evidence of infection and renal failure. In patients with adequate pain control, effective relief of nausea and vomiting, the presence of two kidneys and a normal mental status, prescription of MET, and discharge are considered safe.

Urologic Intervention

The decision to perform a urologic procedure, and whether to perform extracorporeal shockwave lithotripsy, or laser ureteroscopy, is of course left to an urologist. The management of ureteral stones is comprehensively reviewed by the American Urological Associations guidelines (43). Shock wave lithotripsy continues to decline in favor of flexible ureteroscopy. A summary of suggested management of stones is presented in Figure 28-1.

Prevention of Recurrence

Kidney stone prevention is relatively inexpensive, cost-effective, and infrequently practiced (44). Patients with stones should be notified that this is a highly recurrent disorder and when offered therapy, many patients will indicate that episodes of renal colic, though seemingly transient and not life-threatening, are sufficiently painful, time-consuming, and humiliating to motivate them to do whatever is necessary so that "this never happens again." A recent systematic review of medical prevention of nephrolithiasis, emphasizing only RCTs, was recently published (45). Increasing fluid intake is the first line therapy proven to be safe and most effective in most kidney stones formers, regardless of the kidney stones' composition (46). This is true in first and recurrent kidney stone formers. There should be an emphasis on taking in at least 96 ounces, or 3 liters, of fluid, to achieve more than 2.5 liters of urine output each day. All fluids are considered acceptable, including coffee and alcohol, which are often proscribed despite epidemiologic data demonstrating that their ingestion is associated with fewer, not more stones (47).

Calcium stones should not lead to a restriction of dairy products. The only RCT to demonstrate prevention of stones from a dietary manipulation had four components: 3–4 servings of dairy per day, to total 1000–1200 mg of calcium; reduced animal protein, sodium and oxalate ingestion (48). Dietary restriction of high oxalate food, and increasing consumption of calcium-rich food to accompany oxalate containing food are the mainstays of therapy for patients with hyperoxaluria. See https://regepi.bwh. harvard.edu/health/Oxalate/files for a complete and up-to-date listing of high and low oxalate-containing foods. Uric acid stones may be benefited by reductions in animal protein ingestion, which reduces uric acid production and net acid excretion.

Pharmacologic therapy is appropriate when fluid intake and dietary manipulation fail, or when fluid intake is difficult given

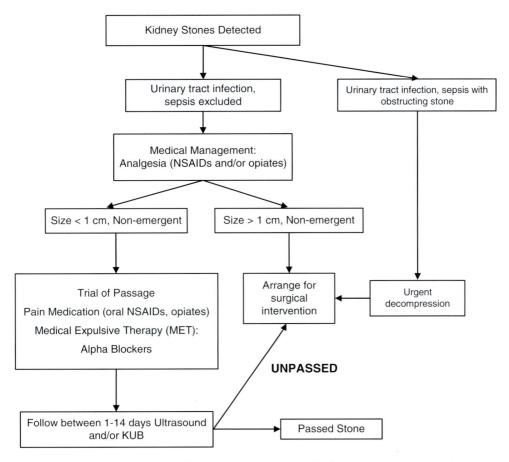

Figure 28-1 Suggested management of kidney stones causing renal colic.

occupational concerns (lack of toilet facilities) or medical considerations (benign prostatic hypertrophy or incontinence). Urinary calcium excretion is reduced by thiazides (indapamide and chlorthalidone are longer-acting than hydrochlorothiazide and therefore preferred). Trials of thiazides which lasted at least two years were almost uniformly associated with benefit (49). Supplementation with potassium citrate can prevent hypokalemia and increase urinary citrate excretion, further contributing to an increase in calcium solubility. Patients with hypocitraturia can also be given potassium citrate at doses of 10–30 meq twice a day (50). Sodium citrate is avoided as sodium excretion will increase calcium excretion. One trial of allopurinol was effective in preventing calcium stones in patients who had hyperuricosuria, and not hypercalciuria (51).

Since uric acid stones are attributable to uric acid's poor solubility at urine pH of less than 5.5, urinary alkalinization to pH greater than 6.0 is desirable (52). Allopurinol is reserved for patients with persistently acidic urine who do not alkalinize easily, such as in the presence of bowel disease.

Surgical treatment is of paramount importance for struvite stones because urinary sterilization is usually ineffective when bacteria remain in the kidneys. Thorough removal of stone material via endourologic intervention may suffice. Several RCTs have shown the efficacy of the urease inhibitor acetohydroxamic acid (53). Its adverse effects lead to it being reserved for patients who are poor surgical candidates.

Increasing urine volume, restricting animal protein and salt intake, alkalinizing the urine, and prescribing cystine-binding thiol drugs (tiopronin and d-penicillamine) are the available therapies for cystinuria (16).

Conclusions

Kidney stones are a disorder of high and increasing prevalence. They are now linked to a wide range and diversity of disease processes making them, if not a risk factor for other, significant disorders such as metabolic syndrome and diabetes, at least a warning sign of other morbidities. They account for a large number of emergency care and clinician visits. Prevention of kidney stones should not be left to the urologists, who most often see the patients, but to the internists whose responsibilities include disease prevention. This responsibility should fall to endocrinologists, as well as general internists and primary care practitioners.

References

1 Stamatelou KK., Francis ME, Jones CA, et al. Time trends in reported prevalence of kidney stones in the United States: 1976–1994. *Kidney Int*. 2003;63: 1817–1823.

2 Scales CD, Smith AC, Hanley JM, et al. Prevalence of kidney stones in the United States. *Eur Urol*. 2012;62:160–165.

3 Romero V, Akpinar H, Assimos DG. Kidney stones: a global picture of prevalence, incidence, and associated risk factors. *Rev Urol*. 2010;12:e86–e96.

4 Saigal CS, Joyce G, Timilsina AR, et al. Direct and indirect costs of nephrolithiasis in an employed population: opportunity for disease management? *Kidney Int*. 2005;68:1808–1814.

5 Brown J. Diagnostic and treatment patterns for renal colic in US emergency departments. *Int Urol Nephrol*. 2006;38:87.

6 Foster G, Stocks C, Borofsky MS. Emergency department visits and hospital admissions for kidney stone disease, 2009: Statistical brief #139. In: *Healthcare Cost and Utilization Project (HCUP) Statistical Briefs*. Rockville, MD: Agency for Healthcare Research and Quality. 2006.

7 Clark AJ, Norman RW. "Mirror pain" as an unusual presentation of renal colic. *Urology*. 1998;51:116–118.

8 Huland H, Leichtweiss HP, Augustin HJ. Changes in renal hemodynamics in experimental hydronephrosis. *Invest Urol*. 1981;18:274–277.

9 Cadnapaphornchai P, Aisenbrey G, McDonald KM, et al. Prostaglandin-mediated hyperemia and renin-mediated hypertension during acute ureteral obstruction. *Prostaglandins*. 1978;16:965–971.

10 Moody TE, Vaughn ED, Jr., Gillenwater JY. Relationship between renal blood flow and ureteral pressure during 18 hours of total unilateral uretheral occlusion. Implications for changing sites of increased renal resistance. *Invest Urol*. 1975;13:246–251.

11 Goldfarb DS. In the clinic: nephrolithiasis. *Ann Int Med*. 2009;151:ITC2.

12 Goldfarb DS. A woman with recurrent calcium phosphate kidney stones. *Clin J Am Soc Nephrol*. 2012;7:1172.

13 Maalouf NM, Cameron MA, Moe OW, et al. Novel insights into the pathogenesis of uric acid nephrolithiasis. *Curr Opin Nephrol Hypertens*. 2004;13:181–189.

14 Cameron MA, Maalouf NM, Adams-Huet B, et al. Urine composition in type 2 diabetes: predisposition to uric acid nephrolithiasis. *J Am Soc Nephrol*. 2006;17:1422–1428.

15 Rodman JS. Struvite stones. *Nephron*. 1999;81(Suppl 1):50.

16 Mattoo A, Goldfarb DS. Cystinuria. *Semin Nephrol*. 2008;28:181–191.

17 Evan AP, Lingeman JE, Coe FL, et al. Randall's plaque of patients with nephrolithiasis begins in basement membranes of thin loops of Henle. *J.Clin.Invest.* 2003;60:111–119.

18 Worcester EM, Coe FL. Evidence for altered renal tubule function in idiopathic calcium stone formers. *Urological Res.* 2010;38:263–269.

19 Talner L, Vaughan M. Nonobstructive renal causes of flank pain: findings on noncontrast helical CT (CT KUB). *Abdom Imaging.* 2003;28:21–216.

20 Goldfarb DS, Fischer ME, Keich Y, et al. A twin study of genetic and dietary influences on nephrolithiasis: a report from the Vietnam Era Twin (VET) Registry. *Kidney Int.* 2005;67:1053.

21 Vezzoli G, Terranegra A, Rainone F, et al. Calcium-sensing receptor and calcium kidney stones. *J Translational Med.* 2011;9: 201.

22 Vezzoli G, Terranegra A, Arcidiacono T, et al. Genetics and calcium nephrolithiasis. *Kidney Int.* 2011;80:587–593.

23 Goldfarb DS. The exposome for kidney stones. *Urolithiasis.* 2016;44(1):3–7.

24 Heilberg IP, Goldfarb DS. Optimum nutrition for kidney stone disease. *Adv Chronic Kidney Dis.* 2013;20: 165–174.

25 Curhan GC, Willett WC, Rimm EB, et al. A prospective study of dietary calcium and other nutrients and the risk of symptomatic kidney stones. *N Engl J Med.* 1993;328:833–838.

26 Taylor EN, Fung TT, Curhan GC. DASH-style diet associates with reduced risk for kidney stones. *J Am Soc Nephrol.* 2009;20:2253–2259.

27 Curhan GC, Willett WC, Speizer FE. et al. Comparison of dietary calcium with supplemental calcium and other nutrients as factors affecting the risk for kidney stones in women. *Ann Intern Med.* 1997;126:497–504.

28 Obligado SH, Goldfarb DS. The association of nephrolithiasis with hypertension and obesity: a review. *Am J Hypertens.* 2008;21:257–264.

29 Reinstatler L, Khaleel S, Pais VM, Jr. Association of pregnancy with stone formation among women in the United States: a NHANES analysis 2007 to 2012. *J Urol.* 2017.

30 Wallace RB, Wactawski-Wende J, O'Sullivan MJ, et al. Urinary tract stone occurrence in the Women's Health Initiative (WHI) randomized clinical trial of calcium and vitamin D supplements. *Am J Clin Nutr.* 2011;94:270–277.

31 Leaf DE, Korets R, Taylor EN, et al. Effect of vitamin D repletion on urinary calcium excretion among kidney stone formers. *Clin J Am Soc Nephrol.* 2012;7:829–834.

32 Tebben PJ, Singh RJ, Kumar R. Vitamin D-mediated hypercalcemia: mechanisms, diagnosis, and treatment. *Endocr Rev.* 2016;37:521–547.

33 Borofsky MS, Walter D, Shah O, et al. Surgical decompression is associated with decreased mortality in patients with sepsis and ureteral calculi. *J Urol.* 2013;189:946.

34 Bove P, Kaplan D, Dalrymple N, et al. Reexamining the value of hematuria testing in patients with acute flank pain. *J Urol.* 1999;162:685.

35 Nakada SY, Hoff DG, Attai S, et al. Determination of stone composition by noncontrast spiral computed tomography in the clinical setting. *Urology.* 2000;55:816–819.

36 Hamada Y, Nishijima T, Watanabe K, et al. High incidence of renal stones among HIV-infected patients on ritonavir-boosted atazanavir than in those receiving other protease inhibitor-containing antiretroviral therapy. *Clin Infect Dis.* 2012;55:1262–1269.

37 Ferrandino MN, Bagrodia A, Pierre SA, et al. Radiation exposure in the acute and short-term management of urolithiasis at 2 academic centers. *J Urol.* 2009;181:668–673.

38 Larkin GL, Peacock WF, Pearl SM, et al. Efficacy of ketorolac tromethamine versus meperidine in the ED treatment of acute renal colic. *Am J Emerg Med.* 1999;17:6–10.

39 Springhart WP, Marguet CG, Sur RL, et al. Forced versus minimal intravenous hydration in the management of acute renal colic: a randomized trial. *J Endourol.* 2006;20: 713–716.

40 Hollingsworth JM, Canales BK, Rogers MA, et al. Alpha blockers for treatment of ureteric stones: systematic review and meta-analysis. *BMJ.* 2016;355:i6112.

41 Pickard R, Starr K, MacLennan G, et al. Use of drug therapy in the management of symptomatic ureteric stones in hospitalised adults: a multicentre, placebo-controlled, randomised controlled trial and cost-effectiveness analysis of a calcium channel blocker (nifedipine) and an alpha-blocker (tamsulosin) (the SUSPEND trial). *Health Technol Assess.* 2015;19:vii.

42 John TT, Razdan S. Adjunctive tamsulosin improves stone free rate after ureteroscopic lithotripsy of large renal and ureteric calculi: a prospective randomized study. *Urology.* 2010;75:1040–1042.

43 Assimos D, Krambeck A, Miller NL, et al. Surgical management of stones: American Urological Association/Endorological Society Guideline, PART I. *J Urol.* 2016;196:1153.

44 Parks JH, Coe FL. The financial effects of kidney stone prevention. *Kidney Int.* 1996;50:1706.

45 Fink HA, Wilt TJ, Eidman KE, et al. *Recurrent Nephrolithiasis in Adults: Comparative Effectiveness of Preventive Medical Strategies.* Rockville, MD: Agency for Healthcare Research and Quality, 2012.

46 Cheungpasitporn W, Rossetti S, Friend K, et al. Treatment effect, adherence, and safety of high fluid intake for the prevention of incident and recurrent kidney stones: a systematic review and meta-analysis. *J Nephrol.* 2016;29: 211–219.

47 Curhan GC, Willett WC, Rimm EB, et al. Prospective study of beverage use and the risk of kidney stones. *Am J Epidemiol.* 1996;143:240.

48 Borghi L, Schianchi T, Meschi T, et al. Comparison of two diets for the prevention of recurrent stones in idiopathic hypercalciuria. *N Engl J Med.* 2002;346:77–84.

49 Pearle MS, Roehrborn CG, Pak CY. Meta-analysis of randomized trials for medical prevention of calcium oxalate nephrolithiasis. *J Endourol.* 1999;13:679–685.

50 Fabris A, Lupo A, Bernich P, et al. Long-term treatment with potassium citrate and renal stones in medullary sponge kidney. *Clin J Amer Soc Nephrology.* 2010;5:1663–1668.

51 Ettinger B, Tang A, Citron JT, et al. Randomized trial of allopurinol in the prevention of calcium oxalate calculi. *N Engl J Med.* 1986;315:1386–1389.

52 Mehta TH, Goldfarb DS. Uric acid stones and hyperuricosuria. *Adv Chronic Kidney Dis.* 2012;19:413–418.

53 Griffith DP, Gleeson MJ, Lee H, et al. Randomized, double-blind trial of Lithostat (acetohydroxamic acid) in the palliative treatment of infection-induced urinary calculi. *Eur Urol.* 1991;20:243–247.

Part VIII

Neuroendocrine Tumors

Introduction

Emergency Management of Neuroendocrine Tumors

Kjell Oberg

Key Points

- Neuroendocrine tumors (NETs, also termed neuroendocrine neoplasms [NENs]) constitute a heterogeneous group of malignant solid tumors that arise in hormone-secreting tissues of the diffuse neuroendocrine system.
- Consequently, they can have various clinical presentations and courses. Some tumors present an indolent course, whereas others are more aggressive with shorter survival. The overall 5-year survival for metastatic NETs is 35%.
- All subtypes of NETs can be divided into functional tumors, which are associated with hormone-related symptoms, whereas nonfunctional tumors do not cause any clinically apparent hormone-related symptoms.
- The so-called functional tumors can result in various endocrine and metabolic emergencies.
- Treatment options include a combination of different treatment modalities to control the clinical manifestations. These may include surgery; radiotherapy; peptide receptor radionuclide therapy (PRRT); and various medical therapies (e.g., somatostatin analogs); chemotherapy; and targeted therapies such as the mTOR (mammalian target of rapamycin) inhibitor everolimus; or the tyrosine kinase inhibitor, sunitinib.

- Supportive care and treatments aimed at the major end-result of the excess hormone secreted are also important (e.g., intravenous glucose to treat hypoglycemia caused by excessive insulin secretion from an insulinoma; proton-pump inhibitors to counteract excessive gastrin secretion from gastrinomas).
- Small intestinal NETs with the production of serotonin, tachykinins, and bradykinin present as the carcinoid syndrome with flushing, diarrhea, and specific carcinoid heart disease (right-sided). A new drug which inhibits the synthesis of serotonin, telotristat ethyl can significantly reduce diarrhea in patients with the carcinoid syndrome.
- Carcinoid syndrome can manifest as a life-threatening medical emergency – carcinoid crisis. Somatostatin analogs are useful to both prevent and treat carcinoid crisis.
- The most common clinical syndrome related to pancreatic NETs (pNETS) are hypoglycemia syndrome caused by insulinoma with the production of excessive insulin/proinsulin by the tumor resulting in hypoglycemia; and Zollinger-Ellison syndrome related to excess gastrin production, resulting in high gastric acid output with repeated gastrointestinal ulcers and significant risk of bleeding.

Endocrine and Metabolic Medical Emergencies: A Clinician's Guide, Second Edition. Edited by Glenn Matfin.
© 2018 John Wiley & Sons Ltd. Published 2018 by John Wiley & Sons Ltd.

- Ongoing challenges for clinicians caring for patients with NETs include earlier disease detection and diagnosis before metastasis. This may result in treatment that prevents progression to more advanced disease, which can lead to the well-defined and debilitating clinical syndromes that can be associated with endocrine and metabolic emergencies.

Introduction

Neuroendocrine tumors (NETs) constitute a heterogeneous group of malignant solid tumors that arise in the hormone-secreting tissues of the diffuse neuroendocrine system. Consequently, they can have various clinical presentations and courses. Some tumors present an indolent course, whereas others are more aggressive with shorter survival. The incidence of these relatively rare tumors is estimated to be about 6.2 cases per 100,000/year, and they have a prevalence of about 35 per 100,000 (USA Surveillance Epidemiology and End Results [SEER] 2012). The overall 5-year survival for metastatic NETs is 35% (1). The major subtypes of neuroendocrine tumors are bronchial NETs (30%), small intestinal NETs (25%), rectal NETs (17%), colonic NETs (10%), pancreatic NETs (7.5%), and thymic NETs (5%).

According to the World Health Organization (WHO) 2017 classification system for NETs (also termed neuroendocrine neoplasms [NENs]), they are divided into three categories. The first category is well-differentiated NETs: NET G1 with a Ki-67 index proliferation <3%; NET G2 with proliferation 3–20%; and NET G3 with >20% dividing cells. The second category is poorly differentiated neuroendocrine carcinomas (NEC): NEC G3 with >20% proliferation. NEC G3 is further subdivided into small cell and large cell types. The final category is mixed neuroendocrine-nonneuroendocrine neoplasm (also termed mixed endocrine-nonendocrine neoplasms [MENEM/MINEN]). The European Neuroendocrine Tumor Society (ENETS) as well as the National Comprehensive Cancer Center (NCCN)/Union for International Cancer Control (UICC) have developed a staging system with clear features for each of the stages (2–4). In addition, all subtypes of NETs can be divided into functional tumors which are associated with hormone-related symptoms, whereas nonfunctional tumors do not cause any clinically apparent hormone-related symptoms. The so-called functional tumors can result in various endocrine and metabolic emergencies.

Small Intestinal NETs

Small intestinal NETs, which produce serotonin, tachykinins, and bradykinin, present as the carcinoid syndrome with flushing, diarrhea, and specific carcinoid heart disease (right-sided). This syndrome can manifest as a life-threatening medical emergency during different interventional procedures, such as surgery, embolization, and biopsies. The so-called carcinoid crisis presents with tachycardia, severe flushing, and low blood pressure and is related to the release of tachykinins and serotonin, in particular (5). With the introduction of somatostatin analogs for the treatment of patients with carcinoid tumors, this emergency is nowadays rather rare but it is important to prepare the patient very carefully for surgery or other therapeutic and investigational interventions (5). A new drug that inhibits the synthesis of serotonin, telotristat ethyl can significantly reduce diarrhea in patients with carcinoid syndrome (6).

Pancreatic NETs

With regard to pancreatic NETs, the most significant clinical syndromes are the Zollinger-Ellison syndrome, insulinoma (hypoglycemic syndrome), as well as Verner-Morrison syndrome (vasoactive intestinal polypeptide [VIP] secreting tumor, termed VIPoma syndrome). The Zollinger-Ellison syndrome is related to excess gastrin production by the tumor, resulting in high gastric acid output with repeated gastrointestinal ulcers, sometimes down to the jejunum with significant risk of bleeding. Today, these patients are treated with high doses of proton-pump inhibitors (PPIs), sometimes in combination with somatostatin analogs, to reduce this risk. For long-term management, it is important to try to find the primary tumor as well as metastases in order to resect as much tumor tissue as possible. Peptide receptor radionuclide therapy (PRRT) is commonly used to reduce hormone levels and clinical symptoms in these patients. More recently, new targeted therapies such as the mTOR (mammalian target of rapamycin) inhibitor everolimus; or the tyrosine kinase inhibitor (TKI), sunitinib have also been effective (7,8).

The most common clinical syndrome related to pancreatic NETs is hypoglycemia syndrome caused by insulinoma with the production of insulin/proinsulin resulting in hypoglycemia. This condition is sometimes missed because the symptoms are initially nonspecific and the patient is often misdiagnosed as having psychiatric problems. The definitive diagnosis is established by the demonstration of low blood glucose in the presence of high levels of insulin or proinsulin. The primary clinical objective in these patients has been to detect the primary tumor and attempt resection. This can be challenging because the tumor is usually small (i.e. less than 2 cm in size in approximately 90% of cases) and is located in the pancreas. For these reasons, traditional localization studies such as anatomic imaging modalities (i.e. computed tomography [CT], and magnetic resonance imaging [MRI]), selective arterial secretagogue injection (SASI), and ultrasound (both standard and intraoperative) may not always identify insulinomas. Newer imaging modalities which target somatostatin receptors such as ^{68}Ga-DOTATATE positron emission tomography (PET)/CT scanning may be considered an adjunct imaging study when all of the standard imaging modalities are negative and especially when a focused or minimally invasive surgical approach is planned (Figure VIII-1) (9). ^{68}Ga-DOTATATE PET/CT may also be of value in detecting other gastroentero-pancreatic NETs (10). For malignant insulinomas, treatment with cytotoxic agents has been the standard care over the years (11). Other therapies are targeted agents such as Everolimus and Sunitinib (7,8).

The Verner-Morrison syndrome is a severe condition with extremely high volumes of liquid stools and loss of potassium, magnesium, and bicarbonate, resulting in the typical features of VIPoma syndrome. Excessive VIP secretion is the cause of this syndrome and tumors may be located either in the pancreas (most commonly) or in the lung. Surgery is important to try to reduce as much tumor bulk as possible and treatment with somatostatin analogs, alpha interferon, and everolimus can result in significant reduction of hormone levels and improvement of the clinical condition (12).

The glucagonoma syndrome (related to a glucagon-producing tumor) rarely results in medical emergencies, but sometimes can cause significant hyperglycemia, anemia, and thromboembolic complications, which need appropriate urgent care (11).

Syndromes Related to Ectopic Hormonal Secretion

Occasionally the substances secreted by gastrointestinal NET are not directly related to the tissue of origin, and the corresponding clinical syndromes are related to these ectopically secreted compounds. Appreciation of the presence of such syndromes is highly relevant, as, if the clinical presentation is not identified, it may delay the diagnosis of the underlying neoplasia and lead to increased morbidity and mortality. Hypersecretion of parathyroid hormone-related peptide (PTHrP) by metastatic pancreatic NET can cause severe hypercalcemia, resulting in "hypercalcemis crisis," which might be life-threatening (13).

Bronchial and thymic NETs can cause Cushing's syndrome, due to ectopic production of the adrenocorticotropic hormone

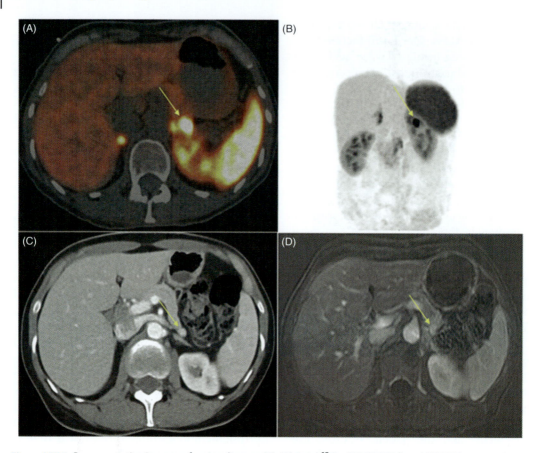

Figure VIII-1 Representative images of an insulinoma (9). (A) Axial ^{68}Ga-DOTATATE fused PET/CT arrow pointing to the uptake in the pancreas. (B) ^{68}Ga-DOTATATE anterior three-dimensional maximum intensity projection; arrow pointing to the uptake in the pancreas. (C) Axial arterial phase CT; arrow pointing to the arterially enhancing lesion in the tail of the pancreas. (D) MRI axial three-dimensional with arterial contrast imaging; arrow localizing an arterially enhancing lesion in the tail of the pancreas.

(ACTH) or the corticotropin-releasing hormone (CRH). This syndrome is usually difficult to treat with different steroid inhibitors and in the end bilateral adrenalectomy might be the solution. The ectopic Cushing's syndrome is sometimes very florid and can constitute an endocrine and metabolic emergency (14).

Conclusions

Neuroendocrine tumors can present with various types of endocrine and metabolic emergencies. They necessitate a combination of different treatment modalities to control their clinical manifestations. New agents (e.g. mTOR and TKI-based targeted therapies) can facilitate the management of hormone-related emergencies. However, an unmet need exists for additional therapies that enable more personalized therapy.

Ongoing challenges for clinicians caring for patients with NETs include the detection of tumor remnants after surgery; reliable monitoring of therapeutic efficacy; and translating research findings into clinical practice. In addition, earlier disease detection and diagnosis before metastasis may result in treatment that prevents progression to more advanced disease, which can result in the well-defined and debilitating clinical syndromes that can be associated with endocrine and metabolic emergencies.

References

1 Yao JC, Hassan M, Phan A, et al. One hundred years after "carcinoid": epidemiology of and prognostic factors for neuroendocrine tumors in 35,825 cases in the United States. *J Clin oncol.* 2008;26:3063–3072.

2 Rindi G, Kloppel G, Couvelard A, et al. TNM staging of midgut and hindgut (neuro) endocrine tumors: a consensus proposal including a grading system. *Virchows Arch.* 2007;451:757–762.

3 Bosman F, Carneiro F, Hruban RH, et al. *WHO Classification of Tumours of the Digestive System*, Lyon, France, IARC Press; 2010.

4 Strosberg JR, Cheema A, Weber JM, et al. Relapse-free survival in patients with nonmetastatic, surgically resected pancreatic neuroendocrine tumors: an analysis of the AJCC and ENETS staging classifications. *Ann Surg.* 2012;256: 321–325.

5 Strosberg J. Neuroendocrine tumours of the small intestine. *Best Pract Res Clin Gastroenterol.* 2012;26:755–773.

6 Kulke MH, Horsch D, Caplin ME, et al. Telotristat ethyl, a tryptophan hydroxylase inhibitor for the treatment of carcinoid syndrome. *J Clin Oncol.* 2017;35(1):14–23.

7 Yao JC, Shah MH, Ito T, et al. Everolimus for advanced pancreatic neuroendocrine tumors. *N Engl J Med.* 2011;364(6): 514–523.

8 Raymond E, Dahan L, Raoul JL, et al. Sunitinib malate for the treatment of pancreatic neuroendocrine tumors. *N Engl J Med.* 2011;364(6):501–513.

9 Nockel P, Babic B, Millo C, et al. Localization of insulinoma using 68Ga-DOTATATE PET/CT scan. *J Clin Endocrinol Metab.* 2017;102:195–199.

10 Oberg K. Molecular imaging radiotherapy: theranostics for personalized patient management of neuroendocrine tumors (NETs). *Theranostics.* 2012;2:448–458.

11 Bilimoria KY, Tomlinson JS, Merkow RP, et al. Clinicopathologic features and treatment trends of pancreatic neuroendocrine tumors: analysis of 9,821 patients. *J Gastrointest Surg.* 2007;11(11): 1467–1469.

12 Oberg K. Biotherapies for GEP-NETs. *Best Pract Res Clin Gastroenterol.* 2012;26:833–841.

13 Kamp K, Feelders RA, van Adrichem RC, et al. Parathyroid hormone-related peptide (PTHrP) secretion by gastroenteropancreatic neuroendocrine tumors (GEP-NETs): clinical features, diagnosis, management, and follow-up. *J Clin Endocrinol Metab.* 2014;99(9): 3060–3069.

14 Limper AH, Carpenter PC, Scheithauer B, et al. The Cushing syndrome induced by bronchial carcinoid tumors. *Ann Intern Med.* 1992;117:209–214.

29

Acute Endocrine and Metabolic Emergencies Related to Neuroendocrine Tumors

Gregory Kaltsas, Krystallenia I. Alexandraki, and Ashley B. Grossman

---

Key Points

- Neuroendocrine tumors (NETs) are considered to originate from multipotent cells scattered throughout the gastrointestinal (GI) system that belong to the diffuse endocrine system.
- NETs of the GI system were initially considered to be rare but currently constitute the second most common GI malignancy.
- A distinctive feature of these tumors is their inherent ability to synthesize, store and secrete a variety of biologically active compounds (peptides, amines) that can be metabolically active and cause characteristic clinical syndromes (i.e., functional tumors).
- Typically, tumors originating from the jejunum and ileum can secrete biologically active amines, including serotonin, prostaglandins, and tachykinins, causing the characteristic carcinoid syndrome (CS) that occurs in 20–30% of patients with hepatic metastases.
- Patients with CS are at risk for developing a life-threatening carcinoid crisis, during either minor or major surgery or other types of intervention. Patients with carcinoid crisis may have sudden changes in blood pressure, most often hypotension, sometimes combined with prolonged and excessive flushing, hyperthermia, and occasional bronchospasm.
- A distinctive feature of the majority of GI-NETs is the expression of specific somatostatin receptors (SSTRs) on their cell surface. Somatostatin analogs (SS-analogs) bind to these receptors and inhibit the secretion of vasoactive compounds, leading, to substantial symptomatic and biochemical responses in the majority of GI-NET-related secretory syndromes. Somatostatin analogs are currently the most efficient drugs inhibiting the secretion of bioactive compounds in most functional GI-NETs
- The combination of long-acting SS-analogs and the newly approved serotonin synthesis inhibitor telotristat etiprate is expected to ameliorate the symptoms of refractory CS and reduce the development of long-term sequelae.
- Intravenous octreotide is the best means to prevent and manage a carcinoid crisis and should be always considered prior to surgery and in patients undergoing diagnostic procedures, especially in the presence of extensive hepatic involvement and high 5-Hydroxyindoleacetic acid (5-HIAA) levels.

- For insulinomas, the emergency management rests on intravenous glucose plus the addition of diazoxide, octreotide, and/or pasireotide when the condition has stabilized. Pasireotide and mTOR inhibitors such as everolimus can be used alone or in combination along with other means to counteract intractable hypoglycemia.
- For gastrinomas, proton pump inhibitors (PPIs) are the essential first-line therapy.
- Cytoreductive techniques (i.e., therapy to debulk tumor) should always be considered in refractory functional syndromes aiming at reducing tumor load and the amount of the secretory component.

- Synthesis of specific receptor antagonists of the bioactive compound may be a further step forward to obtain resolution of symptoms in patients not responding to currently available therapeutic modalities.
- The main cause of morbidity and mortality in GI-NETs is mostly directly related to tumor growth and the extent of metastatic disease. However, in some patients with functioning tumors and extensive disease, control of the secretory syndrome still remains problematic, necessitating the employment of multimodality techniques, which may not always be sufficient.

Introduction

Neuroendocrine tumors (NETs) are considered to originate from multipotent cells scattered throughout the gastrointestinal (GI) system that belong to the diffuse endocrine system. A distinctive feature of these tumors is their inherent ability to synthesize, store and secrete a variety of biologically-active compounds (peptides, amines) that can be metabolically active and cause characteristic clinical syndromes (i.e., functional tumors) (1,2). Traditionally, secretory syndromes were attributed to tumors originating from the pancreas (pancreatic NETs [pNETs]) and the so-called midgut ("carcinoid") tumors, the majority of which were derived from the ileum. More recently, it has become apparent that some of these tumors are capable of secreting substances that are considered to originate from other tissues, making their diagnosis and identification difficult. Furthermore, NETs that were apparently considered to be initially non-functioning may acquire (during the course of the disease) the ability to secrete specific compounds.

Neuroendocrine tumors of the GI system were initially considered to be rare but currently constitute the second most common GI malignancy (3). Typically, tumors originating from the jejunum and ileum can secrete biologically active amines, including serotonin, prostaglandins and tachykinins, causing the characteristic carcinoid syndrome (CS) that occurs in 20–30% of patients with hepatic metastases. The classical (typical) CS is usually characterized by cutaneous flushing, gut hypermobility with diarrhea, and (less frequently) bronchospasm (1) (Figure 29-1). The syndrome may also be encountered in patients with primary ovarian lesions or bronchial carcinoids, when

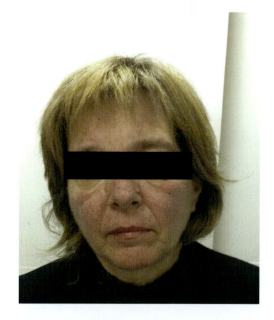

Figure 29-1 Facial flush secondary to typical carcinoid syndrome

the secretory products, mainly serotonin, exceed the capacity of inactivation by the liver or bypass the liver being released directly into the systemic circulation; this may also occasionally be seen in patients with extensive peritoneal metastases (1,4). A less common atypical CS may be found with tumors originating from the embryonic foregut, mainly lung carcinoids (4,5). Such patients present with a patchy intensely red flush, episodes of sweating, itching, cutaneous edema, bronchoconstriction, lacrimation, and cardiovascular instability in the form of hypotension (4,5). It is mostly found in patients with liver metastases and is due to the release of both histamine and serotonin. If CS remains untreated during a prolonged period, it may lead to a number of nutritional deficiencies, the development of carcinoid heart disease (CHD), and other

fibrotic changes involving the mesentery, and may be associated with increased mortality (1,6).

The majority of pNETs are non-functional but a significant number may secrete mainly peptide hormones that can originate from specific pancreatic endocrine cells or from cells that are ectopically expressed in the pancreatic parenchyma such as gastrin and serotonin secreting cells (7). The most common pNET-related secretory syndromes are shown in Table 29-1. In addition, it has recently become apparent that previously considered non-functional pNETs can during the course of the disease change their clinical phenotype and become functional (7,8). Furthermore, pNETs that originally secreted a specific hormone can change to another during the course of the disease, obscuring their clinical presentation (8,9).

Table 29-1 Functional syndromes secondary to GI-NETs (carcinoids and pNETs)

Site/type of tumor	Incidence, (New/100,000 year)	Secretory compound	Clinical syndrome
Foregut carcinoids (bronchi, thymus)	2–5	Serotonin, histamine, ACTH, GHRH, gastrin	Atypical (typical) carcinoid syndrome
Midgut (jejunum, ileum)	4–10	Serotonin, tachykinins, bradykinins	Typical carcinoid syndrome
Insulinoma	1–2	Insulin, proinsulin	Neuroglycopenia, Whipple's triad
Gastrinoma	1–1.5	Gastrin	ZES (peptic ulcer, diarrhea, epigastric pain)
VIPoma	0.2	VIP	Watery diarrhea, hypokalemia, achlorhydria (WDHA)
Glucagonoma	0.1	Glucagon	Necrolytic migratory erythema
Somatostatinoma	<0.1	Somatostatin	Gallstones, diabetes mellitus, steatorrhea, achlorhydria
PTHrPoma		PTHrP	Hypercalcemia
ACTHoma	<0.1	ACTH	Hypercortisolemia
Serotonin-secreting		Serotonin	Typical carcinoid syndrome
GHRHoma	<0.1	GHRH	Acromegaly

ACTH = Adrenocorticotrophin, GHRH = Growth hormone releasing hormone, ZES = Zollinger-Ellison Syndrome, VIP = Vasoactive intestinal-peptide, PTHrP = Parathyroid hormone-related peptide.

A distinctive feature of the majority of GI-NETs is the expression of specific somatostatin receptors (SSTRs) on their cell surface. Somatostatin analogs (SS-analogs) bind to these receptors and inhibit the secretion of vasoactive compounds, leading to substantial symptomatic and biochemical responses in the majority of GI-NET-related secretory syndromes (1,2). These agents are currently considered as first-line treatment for all functional GI-NETs; they also show anti-proliferative properties and are extensively used even for non-functional tumors, although their anti-proliferative effect on tumor growth is mainly cytostatic (4,10,11). Prior to the introduction of SS-analogs, several therapies aiming at ameliorating the symptoms rather than specifically reducing serotonin and pancreatic hormonal production from functional GI-NETs constituted the main therapeutic tools (1,2). Some of these therapies may still be used either when symptoms become refractory to SS-analogs or in combination with these agents (1,7).

Treatment with SS-analogs ameliorates the long-term sequelae of the CS and minimizes the risk of a life-threatening carcinoid crisis (i.e., sudden changes in blood pressure, most often hypotension, sometimes combined with prolonged and excessive flushing, hyperthermia, and occasional bronchospasm), induced by hypersecretion of the secretory component following a number of diagnostic and therapeutic procedures and during surgery. Initial studies used subcutaneous (SC) octreotide three-times/day, median dose 450 mcg daily, in patients with CS, and showed 70% control of both flushing and diarrhea associated with a substantial reduction of serotonin's urine metabolite 5-hydroxyindoleacetic acid (5-HIAA) (10,11). However, long-acting SS-analogs, octreotide LAR 30 mg and lanreotide autogel 120 mg administered monthly, are currently mostly employed exhibiting a mean overall symptomatic response of approximately 65–70% with minimal side effects (11,12). "Top-up" doses of 50–100 mcg (up to 1000 mcg daily) of SC octreotide can be used when symptoms are not adequately controlled with the long-acting preparations. Alternatively, the frequency or dose of long-acting SS-analog administration can be increased; doses of octreotide LAR even as high as 120 mg/month have been used without apparent major toxicity (13–16).

Although octreotide and lanreotide target mainly SSTRs 2 and 5, GI-NETs express multiple subtypes of SSTRs on their surface. Pasireotide is a multireceptor targeting SS-analog with high affinity to all SSTRs except SSTR type 4 (7). At a dose of 60 mg monthly, pasireotide LAR has not been shown to be superior to octeotide LAR 40 mg monthly in controlling CS and was associated with a higher incidence of side-effects, particularly hyperglycemia (28.3% vs. 5.3%, respectively) (17). Another agent that has been shown to have activity in controlling the symptoms of CS is interferon-α, administered in doses 3–9 MU daily (18). Interferon-α, and more recently pegylated interferon, control the symptoms of CS in 40–70% of patients (1,19). However, in clinical practice, interferon-α is less commonly used mainly due to its adverse effects profile, such as fever, fatigue, anorexia and weight loss, autoimmune diseases, and myelosuppression (1). Due to its high discontinuation rate it is considered as second-line treatment when SS-analogs are ineffective (17). There is some evidence that both compounds may exert a synergistic action (19–21).

Recently, an orally-administered serotonin synthesis inhibitor, telotristat etiprate, that does not cross the blood-brain barrier and thus has no central nervous system side-effects (because it does not deplete serotonin levels in the brain), has been shown to provide additional symptomatic control in patients with partially controlled CS with SS-analogs: it is used at doses of 250–500 mg 3-times daily (22,23). Telotristat etiprate has recently been approved by the US FDA and could offer a further therapeutic option in patients with CS refractory to SS-analogs patients particularly as it is associated with minimal side-effects (Figure 29-2). A further potential benefit of this agent is that the induced decrease in serotonin

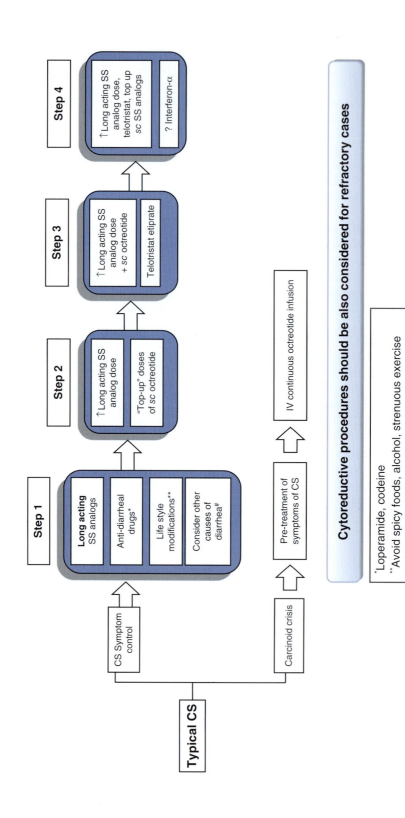

Figure 29-2 Algorithm for the management of typical carcinoid syndrome (CS) and carcinoid crisis

synthesis might reduce the onset of peritoneal and especially cardiac valvular fibrosis, which would be valuable additional therapeutic benefits (23). Anti-diarrheal agents such as loperamide and codeine phosphate can additionally be used along with avoidance of known participants, such as alcohol intake and spicy foods. Diarrhea may occasionally be the result of bacterial overgrowth from a blind enteric loop, bile acid deconjugation or exocrine pancreatic insufficiency, accordingly requiring specific treatment (1). Vitamin B supplements, to avoid niacin deficiency and the development of pellagra (dermatitis, diarrhea, and dementia) along with other fat-soluble vitamins, should be administered to avoid other nutritional deficiencies (24).

In cases where currently existing medical treatments fail to obtain adequate symptomatic relief, cytoreductive techniques (i.e., therapy to debulk tumor) including liver-directed therapies and/or surgery should be employed in order to reduce tumor load and thus the concentration of the bioactive compounds responsible for the development of these syndromes. In such cases, prophylactic administration of octreotide should be given to minimize the risk of potential life-threatening carcinoid crises.

Specific Tumors and Situations

Carcinoid Syndrome (CS)

Patients with CS are at risk for developing a life-threatening carcinoid crisis during diagnostic and/or interventional procedures such as arterial embolization, radiofrequency ablation, and endoscopic procedures; or during surgery (minor or major procedures) due to excessive amounts of hormonal secretion (25). Patients with extensive hepatic metastases and high urinary 5-HIAA levels are those at higher risk of developing a crisis that may occur even in patients with apparent non-functional tumors (26). Induction of anesthesia or tumor manipulation during surgery can provoke a crisis manifested as alterations in blood pressure,

mostly hypotension, along with prolonged and excessive flushing, hyperthermia, bronchospasm, and rarely a hypertensive crisis (25, 27). Occasionally, the crisis may be obscured by the presence of non-specific symptoms, and patients become unstable post-operatively, or fail to recover after surgery (28). Acute intravenous (IV) administration of octreotide has been reported to provide rapid reversal of a carcinoid crisis, and has largely replaced the use of other drugs for acute treatment. Pre-operative prophylactic treatment is recommended with IV octreotide, at an initial dose of 50 mcg/h starting 12 hours before and continued at least 48 hours after the operation with dose titration; doses up to 500 mcg/h may need to be administered (25, 26, 28). However, even in this setting very rare cases of crisis despite adequate octreotide cover may still occur. Pre-treatment with long-acting SS-analogs minimizes but does not eliminate the risk of such a crisis occurring. Indeed, theoretically, once the vasoactive mediators have been released, then subsequent octreotide might not be expected to be effective other than inhibiting further release. In such cases, combination treatment with histamine receptor (HR) antagonists, both H1R (e.g., loratadine) and H2R (e.g., ranitidine), at maximum administered doses along with glucocorticoids, such as prednisolone at 60 mg doses, can also be administered since histamine release and its peripheral actions are not completely blocked by SS analogs. In contrast to previous notions, inotropic support should be given in cases of intractable hypotension (25).

> ## Case Study
>
> A 56-year-old woman presented with a 3-year history of diarrhea and flushing and, recently developed shortness of breath (Figure 29-1). Initially flushing episodes lasted for a few minutes involving the upper part of her body and resolving spontaneously, and were attributed to alcohol intake and concurrent treatment with gliclazide (sulfonylurea). Because her diarrhea increased

in frequency and volume, a series of investigations were undertaken that revealed no obvious underlying pathology. On clinical examination she was tachypneic and tachycardic and had a 30 mmHg blood pressure postural drop. On auscultation there was a pan-systolic murmur, more prominent on inspiration, bilateral ankle edema, and her jugular venous pressure was elevated exhibiting prominent "v" waves. Her chest was clear but her abdomen was distended and on examination she was found to have an enlarged "knobbly" liver and ascites.

Following resuscitation and treatment of her heart failure the patient underwent computerized tomography (CT) imaging of the chest, abdomen, and pelvis. Several irregular hepatic lesions involving both hepatic lobes with areas of calcification and necrosis and enlarged abdominal lymph nodes were noted, although no localized primary lesion was identified. Subsequent investigations with conventional tumor markers, upper and lower GI endoscopy, and 18-FDG-PET/CT scan failed to identify a primary tumor. Following a hepatic biopsy the patient developed profuse diarrhea and became hemodynamically unstable necessitating transfer and treatment to the intensive care unit. On further consultation she was noted to have high urine 5-HIAA levels.

What Do You Think the Provisional Diagnosis Is and What Emergency Treatment Is Indicated?

The provisional diagnosis of CS with embedded carcinoid crisis was made and treatment with octreotide was initiated, leading to stabilization of her condition and improvement of her symptoms. This case is representative of the natural history of an undiagnosed small intestinal NET, and the potential life-threatening development of a carcinoid crisis following a diagnostic procedure such as hepatic biopsy. The delay in diagnosis is attributed to the lack of tumor-specific symptoms, the absence of highly sensitive and specific biomarkers that could be used to identify early stage

disease; and the good performance status of the patient even in the presence of extensive disease. The development of CHD results from non-metabolized secretory substances, mainly serotonin, leading to fibrosis particularly of right-sided cardiac valves (our patient demonstrated right-heart failure with clinical evidence of significant tricuspid regurgitation, the tricuspid valve is affected in >95% patients with CHD). A low threshold for further cardiac work-up should be utilized in patients with the carcinoid syndrome, employing NT-proBNP measurements and echocardiography, or cardiac magnetic resonance imaging (MRI), since the reported incidence of different grades of cardiac involvement could be as high as 50%. However, more recent studies suggest that the prevalence of CHD has decreased in the last decades to about 20%, probably due to the use of SS-analogs.

The present case further highlights the diagnostic pitfalls occurring from overlapping clinical manifestations seen in other GI pathologies and the lack of highly sensitive and specific biomarkers that could be used to identify early stage disease. The good performance status of the patients, even in the presence of extensive disease, signifies the importance of increased awareness by managing clinicians due to the increased morbidity and mortality that can arise from delayed diagnosis or even misdiagnosis, and the delay in appropriate potentially life-saving therapeutic intervention.

Pancreatic NETs: Insulinomas

The most common functional pNET is the insulinoma which, in the majority of cases, is diagnosed early when disease is usually localized. However, control of hypoglycemia may be problematic in approximately 10% of insulinomas that may exhibit distant metastases (1). The management of intractable hypoglycemia in this setting includes the administration of concentrated forms of IV glucose, along with intramuscular glucagon, and potassium replacement may be required as a rescue procedure. Diazoxide, which suppresses insulin secretion from insulinoma cells via an effect on the ATP-sensitive potassium (KATP) channels, has been extensively used at doses 50–300 mg/day (max dose up to 600 mg/day). Treatment with long-acting SS-analogs has been used in patients with insulinomas, but these drugs may worsen hypoglycemia in approximately 50% of the cases when tumors lack SSTR2 and 5 expression and as glucagon secretion is also inhibited; however, when the presence of SSTRs has been documented either by an octreotide test dose or a positive somatostatin receptor scintigraphy (SRS), these drugs may be of value.

Two relatively new drugs need particularly to be considered (7,29). The multiligand SS-analog pasireotide causes hyperglycemia in approximately 30% of cases, and in this context may be more efficacious than first generation SS-analogs in counteracting hypoglycemia. This notion needs to be explored further as currently there are limited data (30). The mTOR pathway plays a significant role in pNET progression and also in glucose homeostasis, enhancing insulin secretion and increased glucose utilization. Recently, the mTOR inhibitor everolimus, used for the management of progressive GI-NETs, seems to exert a specific hyperglycemic effect and can be a useful tool in cases of metastatic insulinomas (29,31). In a recent study, everolimus was found to be superior to other treatments in achieving a median period of glucose control of 6.5 months irrespective of its effect on tumor growth (32). A speculative mode of action is a dual effect inhibiting insulin secretion by the tumor and causing concomitant insulin resistance (32), although the latter effect appears to be less important. Nevertheless, in terms of emergency management, IV glucose either as a bolus or preferably by slow infusion remains the mainstay of treatment.

Pancreatic NETs: Gastrinomas

The Zollinger-Ellison syndrome (ZES) occurs as a result of gastrin hypersecretion,

mostly from duodenal and pancreatic NETs and may be secondary to multiple endocrine neoplasia syndrome 1 (MEN1) in up to 25% of cases (33). Such patients present with multiple peptic ulcers resistant to treatment, ulcers that are found in uncommon locations, and diarrhea secondary to the intestinal exposure of high volume of highly acidic gastric content. Currently, proton-pump inhibitors (PPIs) are considered the first-line treatment and are potent inhibitors of gastric hypersecretion, and can obtain resolution of symptoms in the majority of patients (34). Doses of up to 80 mg of omeprazole may be required; this can be administered once daily due to its long half-life of 3–4 days. In the acute setting, IV administration of 80 mg of pantoprazole given 8-hourly is efficient in obtaining rapid control of acid hypersecretion lasting for up to 7 days (34,35). Somatostatin analogs can also be used in refractory cases, starting with SC or IV octreotide at a dose of 50–100 mcg per hour, ideally as a continuous infusion. The recently synthesized orally administered gastrin receptor antagonist, netazepide, has a rapid and prolonged mode of action and could be an alternative option in refractory cases when readily available (36).

Pancreatic NETs: VIPomas

Patients with VIPomas present with excessive diarrhea, up to 20 liters per day, associated with severe fluid and electrolyte (mainly potassium and bicarbonate) loss, with subsequent development of marked asthenia, cramps leading to tetany and cardiac alterations and even sudden death (1,2). Hypokalemia is often severe (K levels <2.5 mmol/L, losses >400 mmol/day), paradoxically associated with low bicarbonate levels due to severe intestinal loss; this results in severe hyperchloremic acidosis. Hypophosphatemia and hypomagnesemia may also occur, while a number of patients have associated hypercalcemia. Somatostatin analogs can obtain a substantial reduction of VIP levels and control of diarrhea in most cases; in refractory cases previously employed medications such as glucocorti-coids, clonidine, and loperamide can also be used (1). It has recently been suggested that the multipotent tyrosine kinase (TKI) inhibitor sunitinib may exert a particular effect in VIP-secreting pNETs irrespective of its effect on tumor growth and can also be used as an adjuvant therapy (37). In an emergency situation, a continuous octreotide infusion should be started, at around 1000 mcg per 24 h, and additionally it would be useful to add in prednisolone at a dose of 60 mg daily, tapering down rapidly in response to symptom control. It is also mandatory to keep up with fluid losses for this "pancreatic cholera" with normal saline, accepting that such fluid loss can be massive.

Pancreatic NETs: Glucagonomas

Glucagonomas characteristically present with weight loss, diabetes, cheilosis, and diarrhea, and a characteristic rash named necrolytic migratory erythema (NME) (38). This dermatitis-looking lesion typically evolves over 7–14 days, initially as small erythematous lesions in the groin that can also involve the perineum, lower extremities, and peri-oral regions. Serum glucagon levels do not correlate with the presence or the severity of the rash, which is associated with fatty acid, zinc, and amino-acid deficiencies. Other common manifestations are psychiatric disorders and an increased incidence of thromboembolism in up to 30% of cases (1). Patients should be vigorously treated with SS-analogs (as above), amino-acid infusion, and antibiotics that lead to healing of the rash, albeit without effect on the diabetes (38). The diabetes should be treated in the usual fashion, but should improve as glucagon levels fall. As these patients have a particular predisposition for thromboembolism, prophylactic high-dose of low molecular weight heparin should be also administered.

Pancreatic NETs: Somatostatinomas

Somatostatinomas may occur as massive islet cell tumors arising from the body of the pancreas, duodenal somatostatinomas are usually small and may be multiple, and can occur in a context of neurofibromatosis type 1 or mosaic gain-of-function mutations of HIF-2α. Symptoms related to excessive secretion of somatostatin from a pNET are found in a minority of such tumors and include hyperglycemia, cholelithiasis, diarrhea, steatorrhea, and hypochlorhydria. Paradoxically, it has been suggested that these patients respond promptly to SS-analog administration (1). They are rarely troublesome as an emergency presentation.

Syndromes Related to Ectopic Hormonal Secretion

Particular attention should be paid in the presence of diverse clinical phenotypes secondary to the secretion of ectopically-produced vasoactive compounds (39). Occasionally the substances secreted by GI-NETs are not directly related to the tissue of origin and the corresponding clinical syndromes are related to these ectopically secreted compounds. Appreciation of the presence of such syndromes is highly relevant; if the clinical presentation is not identified, it may delay the diagnosis of the underlying neoplasia and lead to increased morbidity and mortality. In patients with uncontrolled hormonal syndrome due to ectopic hormone secretion, hepatic artery embolization or chemoembolization and/or debulking surgery can be discussed.

Adrenocorticotropic hormone (ACTH) secretion leading to Cushing's syndrome has mostly been encountered with lung NETs, but can occasionally be seen with GI tumors. Drugs aiming at controlling the hormonal secretion, either at the tumor level (somatostatin analogs, cabergoline), the adrenals (metyrapone, ketoconazole, O,p'-DDD) or rarely the glucocorticoid receptor, markedly reduce the morbidity and potential mortality if the hypercortisolism remains untreated. In refractory cases IV etomidate has successfully been used but requires intensive monitoring.

Hypersecretion of ectopic parathyroid hormone-related peptide (PTHrP) secretion by metastatic NET seems to be exclusively associated with metastatic pancreatic NETs and has a major clinical impact because poorly controlled hypercalcemia is associated with increased morbidity and mortality. In such cases and other rarer syndromes, early diagnosis and management are essential.

Conclusions

Functional secretory syndromes from GI-NETs were considered to be rare but are currently increasingly being recognized, and also exhibit a diversity of symptoms. Occasionally, these syndromes can manifest as life-threatening emergencies. Long-acting somatostatin analogs, such as octreotide and lanreotide, are currently the first-line treatment in these hormonal syndromes due to their anti-secretory effects and favorable side-effect profile. In an emergency situation they should be given as SC or IV infusions; a starting IV infusion of octreotide would be 100 mcg per hour, with dose titration until symptom control is obtained. Intravenous fluids and correction of electrolyte disorders are important in the treatment of dehydration and electrolyte and metabolic imbalances, along with previously employed anti-diarrheal drugs and newly evolving agents. Octreotide IV infusion should also routinely be employed to avoid excessive secretion of vasoactive compounds during invasive and surgical procedures. Effective surgical and medical management of the underlying NETs is important for long-term syndrome control.

References

1 Kaltsas GA, Besser GM, Grossman AB. The diagnosis and medical management of advanced neuroendocrine tumors. *Endocr Rev.* 2004;25(3):458–511.

2 Modlin IM, Oberg K, Chung DC, et al. Gastroenteropancreatic neuroendocrine tumours. *Lancet Oncol.* 2008;9(1):61–72.

3 Lepage C, Bouvier AM, Faivre J. Endocrine tumours: epidemiology of malignant digestive neuroendocrine tumours. *Eur J Endocrinol.* 2013;168(4):R77–83

4 Tomassetti P, Migliori M, Lalli S, Campana D, Tomassetti V, Corinaldesi R. Epidemiology, clinical features and diagnosis of gastroenteropancreatic endocrine tumours. *Ann Oncol.* 2001;12 Suppl 2:S95–S99.

5 Papadogias D, Makras P, Kossivakis K, Kontogeorgos G, Piaditis G, Kaltsas G. Carcinoid syndrome and carcinoid crisis secondary to a metastatic carcinoid tumour of the lung: a therapeutic challenge. *Eur J Gastroenterol Hepatol.* 2007;19(12):1154–1159.

6 Grozinsky-Glasberg S, Grossman AB, Gross DJ. Carcinoid heart disease: from pathophysiology to treatment—"something in the way it moves." *Neuroendocrinology.* 2015;101(4):263–273.

7 Dimitriadis GK, Weickert MO, Randeva HS, Kaltsas G, Grossman A. Medical management of secretory syndromes related to gastroenteropancreatic neuroendocrine tumours. *Endocr Relat Cancer.* 2016;23(9):R423–R436.

8 Crona J, Norlén O, Antonodimitrakis P, Welin S, Stålberg P, Eriksson B. Multiple and secondary hormone secretion in patients with metastatic pancreatic neuroendocrine tumours. *J Clin Endocrinol Metab.* 2016;101(2):445–452.

9 Nahmias A, Grozinsky-Glasberg S, Salmon A, Gross DJ. Pancreatic neuroendocrine tumors with transformation to insulinoma: an unusual presentation of a rare disease. *Endocrinol Diabetes Metab Case Rep.* 2015;2015:150032.

10 Kvols LK, Martin JK, Marsh HM, Moertel CG. Rapid reversal of carcinoid crisis with a somatostatin analogue. *N Engl J Med*. 1985;313(19):1229–1230.

11 Modlin IM, Pavel M, Kidd M, Gustafsson BI. Somatostatin analogues in the treatment of gastroenteropancreatic neuroendocrine (carcinoid) tumours. *Aliment Pharmacol Ther*. 2010;31(2): 169–188.

12 O'Toole D, Ducreux M, Bommelaer G, et al. Treatment of carcinoid syndrome: a prospective crossover evaluation of lanreotide versus octreotide in terms of efficacy, patient acceptability, and tolerance. *Cancer*. 2000;88(4): 770–776.

13 Anthony L, Vinik AI. Evaluating the characteristics and the management of patients with neuroendocrine tumors receiving octreotide LAR during a 6-year period. *Pancreas*. 2011;40(7): 987–994.

14 Ferolla P, Faggiano A, Grimaldi F, et al. Shortened interval of long-acting octreotide administration is effective in patients with well-differentiated neuroendocrine carcinomas in progression on standard doses. *J Endocrinol Invest*. 2012;35(3):326–331.

15 Strosberg J, Weber J, Feldman M, Goldman J, Almhanna K, Kvols L. Above-label doses of octreotide-LAR in patients with metastatic small intestinal carcinoid tumors. *Gastrointest Cancer Res*. 2013;6(3):81–85.

16 Strosberg JR, Benson AB, Huynh L, et al. Clinical benefits of above-standard dose of octreotide LAR in patients with neuroendocrine tumors for control of carcinoid syndrome symptoms: a multicenter retrospective chart review study. *Oncologist*. 2014;19(9):930–936.

17 Wolin EM, Jarzab B, Eriksson B, et al. Phase III study of pasireotide long-acting release in patients with metastatic neuroendocrine tumors and carcinoid symptoms refractory to available somatostatin analogues. *PubMed Commons Drug Des Devel Ther*. 2015;9:5075–5086.

18 Oberg K. Interferon in the management of neuroendocrine GEP-tumors: a review. *Digestion*. 2000;62(Suppl.1):92–97.

19 Janson ET, Oberg K. Long-term management of carcinoid syndrome: treatment with octreotide alone and in combination with alpha-interferon. *Acta Oncol*. 1993;32:225–229.

20 Faiss S, Pape UF, Böhmig M, et al., International Lanreotide and Interferon Alfa Study Group. Prospective, randomized, multicenter trial on the antiproliferative effect of lanreotide, interferon alfa, and their combination for therapy of metastatic neuroendocrine gastroenteropancreatic tumors. *J Clin Oncol*. 2003;21(14):2689–2696.

21 Arnold R, Rinke A, Klose KJ, et al. Octreotide versus octreotide plus interferon-alpha in endocrine gastroenteropancreatic tumors: a randomized trial. *Clin Gastroenterol Hepatol*. 2005;3(8):761–771.

22 Kulke MH, O'Dorisio T, Phan A, et al. Telotristat etiprate, a novel serotonin synthesis inhibitor, in patients with carcinoid syndrome and diarrhea not adequately controlled by octreotide. *Endocr Relat Cancer*. 2014;21(5):705–714.

23 Pavel M, Hörsch D, Caplin M, et al. Telotristat etiprate for carcinoid syndrome: a single-arm, multicenter trial. *J Clin Endocrinol Metab*. 2015;100(4):1511–1519.

24 Fiebrich HB, Van Den Berg G, Kema IP, et al. Deficiencies in fat-soluble vitamins in long-term users of somatostatin analogue. *Aliment Pharmacol Ther*. 2010;32(11–12):1398–1404.

25 Kaltsas G, Caplin M, Davies P, et al., all other Antibes Consensus Conference participants. ENETS Consensus Guidelines for the Standards of Care in Neuroendocrine Tumors: Pre- and Perioperative Therapy in Patients with Neuroendocrine Tumors. *Neuroendocrinology*. 2017;105:245–254.

26 Mancuso K, Kaye AD, Boudreaux JP, et al. Carcinoid syndrome and perioperative anesthetic considerations. *J Clin Anesth*. 2011;23(4):329–341.

27 Condron ME, Pommier SJ, Pommier RF. Continuous infusion of octreotide combined with perioperative octreotide bolus does not prevent intraoperative carcinoid crisis. *Surgery.* 2016;159(1):358–365.

28 Seymour N, Sawh SC. Mega-dose intravenous octreotide for the treatment of carcinoid crisis: a systematic review. *Can J Anaesth.* 2013;60(5):492–499.

29 de Herder WW, van Schaik E, Kwekkeboom D, Feelders RA. New therapeutic options for metastatic malignant insulinomas. *Clin Endocrinol (Oxf).* 2011;75(3):277–284.

30 Tirosh A, Stemmer SM, Solomonov E, et al. Pasireotide for malignant insulinoma. *Hormones (Athens).* 2016 Jan 6. [Epub ahead of print].

31 Kulke MH, Bergsland EK, Yao JC. Glycemic control in patients with insulinoma treated with everolimus. *N Engl J Med.* 2009;360(2):195–197.

32 Bernard V, Lombard-Bohas C, Taquet MC, et al. Efficacy of everolimus in patients with metastatic insulinoma and refractory hypoglycemia. *Eur J Endocrinol.* 2013;168(5):665–674.

33 Ito T, Igarashi H, Jensen RT. Zollinger-Ellison syndrome: recent advances and controversies. *Curr Opin Gastroenterol.* 2013;29(6):650–661.

34 Jensen RT, et al. ENETS Consensus Guidelines for the Management of Patients with Digestive Neuroendocrine Neoplasms: Functional Pancreatic Endocrine Tumor Syndromes. *Neuroendocrinology.* 2012;95:98–119.

35 Lew EA, Pisegna JR, Starr JA, et al. Intravenous pantoprazole rapidly controls gastric acid hypersecretion in patients with Zollinger-Ellison syndrome. *Gastroenterology.* 2000;118(4):696–704.

36 Fossmark, R., Sordal, O., Jianu, C.S. et al. Treatment of gastric carcinoids type 1 with the gastrin receptor antagonist netazepide (YF476) results in regression of tumours and normalisation of serum chromogranin A. *Aliment Pharmacol Ther.* 2012;36,1067–1075.

37 de Mestier L, Walter T, Brixi H, Lombard-Bohas C, Cadiot G. Sunitinib achieved fast and sustained control of VIPoma symptoms. *Eur J Endocrinol.* 2015;172(1):K1–K3.

38 Kindmark H, Sundin A, Granberg D, et al. Endocrine pancreatic tumors with glucagon hypersecretion: a retrospective study of 23 cases during 20 years. *Med Oncol.* 2007;24(3):330–337.

39 Kaltsas G, Androulakis II, de Herder WW, Grossman AB. Paraneoplastic syndromes secondary to neuroendocrine tumours. *Endocr Relat Cancer.* 2010;17(3):R173–193.

Part IX

Glucose Disorders

Introduction

Emergency Management of Glucose Disorders

Gerry Rayman

Key Points

- Diabetes is a common disorder estimated in 2015 to affect 415 million people, with a global prevalence of 8.8%. By 2040, this is predicted to rise to 10.4% and affect 642 million people.
- The increasing prevalence is a particular issue for inpatient hospital care as the prevalence of diabetes in the inpatient setting is even greater than in the community: the UK National Diabetes Inpatient Audit (NaDIA) in 2010 found the number of hospital beds occupied by people with diabetes was 14.6%; by 2015 this had increased to 16.8% and it is estimated that by 2020 it will reach 20%. Indeed, in many UK hospitals, it has already reached 30%, a rate already exceeded in parts of the United States.
- In addition, other patients may develop transient hyperglycemia detected during admission that normalizes after discharge, so-called "stress hyperglycemia."
- More than 90% of adult inpatients with diabetes have type 2 diabetes, but over 30% are insulin treated, which adds a greater complexity to their inpatient management. Good inpatient glycemic control in insulin-treated patients is achieved less than 40% of the time and one in ten patients experiences a severe hypoglycemia (blood glucose <3 mmol/L [54 mg/dL]) episode during their hospital stay.
- There is now broad agreement that inpatient hypoglycemia and hyperglycemia are associated with adverse outcomes, including increased morbidity and mortality. Whether these associations are related to the quality of glycemic management or simply to the severity of illness is at present not clear.
- Achieving good glycemic control during hospitalization presents a significant challenge to both specialist and non-specialist healthcare practitioners. Subsequently, systems need to be in place to train and support staff in the care of people with diabetes in hospital.
- In the last few years, there has been increased interest in advancing inpatient diabetes care to prevent the not infrequent harms of hypoglycemia, hospital-acquired foot ulceration, diabetic ketoacidosis and hyperglycemic hyperosmolar state, as well as to reduce the length of stay.

Introduction

Diabetes is a common disorder estimated in 2015 to affect 415 million people, with a global prevalence of 8.8%. By 2040, this is predicted to rise to 10.4% and affect 642 million people (1). The increasing prevalence is a particular issue for inpatient hospital care as the prevalence of diabetes in the inpatient setting is even greater than in the community. In the UK, the prevalence of diabetes in the general population was estimated to be 6.2% in 2015 (1). The UK National Diabetes Inpatient Audit (NaDIA) in 2010 found the number of hospital beds occupied by people with diabetes was 14.6%; by 2015, this had increased to 16.8% (2), and it is estimated that by 2020 it will reach 20%. Indeed, in many UK hospitals, it has reached 30% (2), a rate already exceeded in parts of the United States (3). In addition, other patients may develop transient hyperglycemia detected during admission that normalizes after discharge, so-called "stress hyperglycemia." Both diabetes and hyperglycemia are common and are associated with increased risk of complications among hospitalized patients.

More than 90% of adult inpatients with diabetes have type 2 diabetes, but over 30% are insulin treated, which adds a greater complexity to their inpatient management (2). Good inpatient glycemic control in insulin-treated patients is achieved less than 40% of the time and one in ten patients experiences a severe hypoglycemia (blood glucose <3 mmol/L [54 mg/dL]) episode during their hospital stay (2). There is now broad agreement that inpatient hypoglycemia and hyperglycemia are associated with adverse outcomes, including increased morbidity and mortality (4–7). Whether these associations are related to the quality of glycemic management or simply to the severity of illness is at present not clear.

To date, much attention has focused on the management of glycemia in the intensive care unit where initial studies suggested that very "tight glycemic control" reduced morbidity and mortality (8,9). Subsequent studies have not supported these findings and indeed suggest that "tight control" may be associated with greater mortality, possibly related to increased frequency of hypoglycemia (10,11). As the vast majority of diabetes admissions are not to critical care units, these studies are not helpful in informing us of the glycemic target ranges which should be safely aimed for and the most effective means of achieving these targets in patients admitted to non-critical care units where intensity of glucose monitoring is less, as is patient to nursing and medical staff ratio. This has led to a number of consensus documents suggesting a more moderate approach to glycemic control (12–15).

For a variety of reasons, achieving good glycemic control during hospitalization presents a significant challenge. These include changes in the patient's daily routine, the size and timing of their meals, reduction in carbohydrate intake from emesis or interruption of enteral feeding, periods of fasting for procedures, the effect of stress associated with illness and/or surgery, and alteration in insulin sensitivity due to use of new medications such as steroids. Since over 90% of patients with diabetes are admitted for reasons unrelated to diabetes (e.g., pneumonia or a fracture), they will be cared for by non-diabetes specialist staff who may not be familiar with insulin dose adjustment or proper prescribing, the need to tailor diabetes medications during illness (e.g., stopping sodium–glucose co-transporter 2 [SGLT-2] inhibitors and reviewing the risk of continuing metformin), and the effective management of hypoglycemia and hyperglycemia. Added to this, new classes of diabetes medications, new combinations of existing medications and biosimilar and concentrated insulins with new names have made diabetes management more complex, presenting a significant challenge the non-specialist.

For these reasons systems need to be in place to train and support non-specialist staff in the care of people with diabetes in hospital. This need led to the formation in the UK of the Joint British Diabetes Societies for Inpatient Care group (JBDS) in 2009, bringing together diabetes specialists from a variety of organizations, including the Association of British Clinical Diabetologists (ABCD), Diabetes UK and the Diabetes Inpatient Specialist Nurse Group. The main purpose of this group is to provide guidance based on evidence and consensus on inpatient management. Similarly, in the United States, an association of diabetes specialists has been formed termed PRIDE, the Planning Research in In-patient Diabetes consortium, which also aims to give guidance and to direct research into aspects of inpatient diabetes care (16).

The following chapters in Part IX offer state-of-the-art updates on the management of inpatient diabetes by renowned experts, many of whom are members of the JBDS and PRIDE groups and have contributed to or written the guidelines. These updates include the management of inpatient glycemia, the management of glycemic crises, including hypoglycemia, diabetic ketoacidosis (DKA) and hyperglycemic hyperosmolar state (HHS). Management of patients in special situations, such as during enteral and parenteral feeding and steroid therapy, is also addressed, as is the management of patients on subcutaneous insulin pumps, concentrated insulins, patients with renal insufficiency and patients with acute coronary syndrome, stroke, and heart failure. Finally, there is a chapter on diabetic foot disease, which presents very specific problems in diabetes. In addition to the importance of good metabolic control, there is a need to coordinate multiple aspects of the patient's care, which include infection control, surgical debridement, vascular intervention, and the management of the numerous medical complications which are common in these patients, such as renal insufficiency, anemia, and heart failure. Chapters on the important topics of perioperative diabetes and hyperglycemia management and diabetes in pregnancy are covered in other Parts.

In summary, in the last few years there has been increased interest in advancing inpatient diabetes care to prevent the not infrequent harms of hypoglycemia, hospital acquired foot ulceration, DKA and HHS as well as to reduce the length of stay. The evolving use of new technologies to improve in-hospital diabetes care includes electronic insulin prescribing, continuous glucose monitoring (17), as well as automated systems that deliver safer patient care. For example, a fully automated closed-loop ("artificial pancreas") system in both type 1 and type 2 diabetes patients in the inpatient setting has been tested in proof of concept studies (18). However, much work remains to be done before this system can be rolled out to non-specialist inpatient teams and especially in the emergency setting (19). The following chapters will be of considerable interest and importance to all those involved in delivering inpatient diabetes care.

References

1 Ogurtsova K, da Rocha Fernandes J, Huang Y, Linnenkamp U, Guariguata L, Cho N, Cavan D, Shaw J, Makaroff L. IDF Diabetes Atlas: global estimates for the prevalence of diabetes for 2015 and 2040. *Diabetes Res Clin Pract.* 2017:128;40–50.

2 NHS Digital. National Diabetes Inpatient Audit (NaDIA)—2016. 8 March 2017. www.digital.nhs.uk/pubs/nadia2016. 10 March 2017.

3 Meng YY, Pickett M, Babey SH, Davis AC, Goldstein H. Diabetes tied to a third of California hospital stays, driving health care costs higher. Los Angeles: UCLA Center for Health Policy Research and California Center for Public Health Advocacy; 2014. http://healthpolicy. ucla.edu/publications/search/pages/ detail.aspx?PubID=1278 on 27 September 2015.

4 Umpierrez GE, Isaacs SD, Bazargan N, You X, Thaler LM, Kitabchi AE. Hyperglycemia: an independent marker of in-hospital mortality in patients with undiagnosed diabetes. *J Clin Endocrinol Metab*. 2002;87(3):978–982.

5 Nirantharakumar K, Marshall T, Kennedy A, Narendran P, Hemming K, Coleman JJ. Hypoglycaemia is associated with increased length of stay and mortality in people with diabetes who are hospitalized. *Diabet Med*. 2012;29(12):445–448.

6 Mendez CE, Mok KT, Ata A, Tanenber RJ, Calles-Escandon J, Umpierrez GE. Increased glycemic variability is independently associated with length of stay and mortality in noncritically ill hospitalized patients. *Diabetes Care*. 2013;36:4091–4097.

7 Umpierrez GE, Smiley D, Jacobs S, et al. Randomized study of basal-bolus insulin therapy in the inpatient management of patients with type 2 diabetes undergoing general surgery (RABBIT 2 surgery). *Diabetes Care*. 2011;34:256–261.

8 Furnary AP, Zerr KJ, Grunkemeier GL, Starr, A. Continuous intravenous insulin infusion reduces the incidence of deep sternal wound infection in diabetic patients after cardiac surgical procedures. *Ann Thorac Surg*. 1999;67:352–360; discussion 360–362.

9 van den Berghe G, Wouters P, Weekers F, et al. Intensive insulin therapy in critically ill patients. *N Engl J Med*. 2001;345: 1359–1367.

10 Preiser JC, Devos P, Ruiz-Santana S, et al. A prospective randomised multi-centre controlled trial on tight glucose control by intensive insulin therapy in adult intensive care units: the Glucontrol study. *Intensive Care Med*. 2009;35:1738–1748.

11 Finfer S, Chittock DR, Su SY, et al., NICE-SUGAR Study Investigators. Intensive versus conventional glucose control in critically ill patients. *N Engl J Med*. 2009;360:1283–1297.

12 Qaseem A, Humphrey LL, Chou R, Snow V, Shekelle P, Clinical Guidelines Committee of the American College of Physicians. Use of intensive insulin therapy for the management of glycemic control in hospitalized patients: a clinical practice guideline from the American College of Physicians. *Ann Intern Med*. 2011;154: 260–267.

13 Umpierrez GE, Hellman R, Korytkowski MT, et al., Endocrine Society. Management of hyperglycemia in hospitalized patients in non-critical care setting: an Endocrine Society Clinical Practice Guideline. *J Clin Endocrinol Metab*. 2012;97:16–38.

14 Jacobi J, Bircher N, Krinsley J, et al. Guidelines for the use of an insulin infusion for the management of hyperglycemia in critically ill patients. *Crit Care Med*. 2012;40:3251–3276.

15 Moghissi ES, Korytkowski MT, DiNardo M, et al., American Association of Clinical Endocrinologists. American Diabetes Association. American Association of Clinical Endocrinologists and American Diabetes Association consensus statement on inpatient glycemic control. *Diabetes Care*. 2009;32:1119–1131.

16 Draznin B, Gilden J, Golden SH, Inzucchi SE, PRIDE investigators. Pathways to quality inpatient management of hyperglycemia and diabetes: a call to action. *Diabetes Care*. 2013;36:1807–1814.

17 Wallia A, Umpierrez GE, Nasraway SA, Klonoff DC, PRIDE Investigators. Round table discussion on inpatient use of continuous glucose monitoring at the international Hospital Diabetes Meeting. *J Diabetes Sci Technol*. 2016 10:1174–1181.

18 Thabit H, Hartnell S, Allen JM, et al. Closed loop insulin delivery in inpatients with type 2 diabetes: a randomised, parallel-group trial. *Lancet Diabetes Endocrinol*. 2017;5:117–124.

19 Rayman G. Closer to closing the loop on inpatient glycaemia. *Lancet Diabetes Endocrinol*. 2017;5:81–83.

30

Management of Diabetes and/or Hyperglycemia in Non-Critical Care Hospital Settings

Rodolfo J. Galindo and Guillermo E. Umpierrez

Key Points

- Hyperglycemia in hospitalized patients is associated with adverse outcomes, including increased mortality, morbidity, length of stay, and other complications.
- Hyperglycemia in hospitalized patients can be seen in three main scenarios: (a) patients with previously known diabetes; (b) patients with undiagnosed diabetes at admission; and (c) patients with stress-induced hyperglycemia. The latter two groups can be differentiated by measuring glycosylated hemoglobin (HbA1c) on admission (also important to assess glycemic control and to tailor the treatment regimen at discharge).
- The risk of mortality and complications correlates with the severity of hyperglycemia, with higher risk in patients without a history of diabetes.
- Numerous studies have shown that improved glycemic control during hospitalization decreases the rate of complications in critical and non-critical care settings.
- Insulin administration is the preferred way to control hyperglycemia in hospitalized patients. In addition, incretin-based therapies using dipeptidyl peptidase (DPP)-4 inhibitors (with or without insulin) may also be of value in this setting.

- However, hypoglycemia is the main limiting factor of insulin therapy and glycemic control. Thus, the overall goal of inpatient glycemic management focuses on treating hyperglycemia to individualized glycemic targets associated with reduction/prevention of complications while avoiding hypoglycemia and its associated morbidity.
- Standardized order sets, promoting the use of scheduled basal insulin ± standing prandial (bolus) insulin *or* oral DPP4-inhibitors in specific scenarios, is key in managing inpatient hyperglycemia. Correctional/supplemental insulin per sliding scale can be added as needed to any of the above regimes.
- Transition to an outpatient setting requires planning and coordination. Patients with acceptable pre-admission diabetes control may be discharged on their pre-hospitalization treatment regimen. Patients with suboptimal control should have more intensified therapy.
- Implementing personalized algorithms is the future of inpatient hyperglycemic management in non-critical care hospital settings.

Endocrine and Metabolic Medical Emergencies: A Clinician's Guide, Second Edition. Edited by Glenn Matfin.
© 2018 John Wiley & Sons Ltd. Published 2018 by John Wiley & Sons Ltd.

Introduction

Hyperglycemia in hospitalized patients can be seen in three main scenarios: (a) patients with previously known diabetes;(b) patients with undiagnosed diabetes at admission; and (c) patients with stress hyperglycemia (1). The association between inpatient hyperglycemia in hospitalized patients with and without diabetes and poor clinical outcomes, such as increased mortality, morbidity, length of stay, infections and overall number of complications, is well established (2–4). This association is well documented not only with admission glycemic status but also with the mean in-hospital blood glucose level (5,6). Notably, the risk of complications and mortality correlates to the severity of hyperglycemia (3,4). In addition, numerous studies have also shown that complication rates decrease with improved glycemic control during the hospital stay (7). However, hypoglycemia is the main limiting factor of insulin therapy and glycemic control (8–11). Thus, the overall goal of inpatient glycemic management focuses on treating hyperglycemia to glycemic targets associated with reduction/prevention of complications while avoiding hypoglycemia and its associated morbidity. This chapter reviews the definition, prevalence, and outcomes of hyperglycemia and hypoglycemia in different clinical situations in non-critically ill patients and outlines practical protocols for the management of hyperglycemia in patients with stress hyperglycemia and diabetes admitted to general medicine and surgery services.

Inpatient Hyperglycemia and Hypoglycemia: A Brief Definition

In the non-critically ill hospitalized population, the American Diabetes Association (ADA), the American Association of Clinical Endocrinologists (AACE), and the Endocrine Society have defined *inpatient hyperglycemia* as a blood glucose (BG) ≥140 mg/dL (7.8 mmol/L) on admission or at any time during the hospitalization in patients with or without diabetes (12–14). *Inpatient hypoglycemia* is defined as BG <70 mg/dL (3.9 mmol/L) and severe hypoglycemia as BG <40 mg/dL (2.2 mmol/L) (12–14).

Stress-induced hyperglycemia refers to a transient elevation of BG occurring during acute illnesses (e.g., anesthesia, surgery, infections), that resolves spontaneously after the acute insult dissipates (Figure 30-1). This disorder may occur in patients with or without diabetes, and imposes a higher risk of mortality and complications in patients without a history of diabetes (i.e., new onset and stress-induced hyperglycemia) compared to those with a known diagnosis of diabetes (2,5,15). The Endocrine Society (13), AACE (12), and ADA (14) define stress hyperglycemia as any BG concentration >140 mg/dL (7.8 mmol/L) without evidence of previous diabetes and a glycosylated hemoglobin (HbA1c) <6.5% (48 mmol/mol). Although stress hyperglycemia typically resolves as the acute illness or surgical stress abates (15,16), it is important to identify and follow these patients as 40–60% of patients admitted with new or stress-related hyperglycemia had confirmed diabetes at 1 year (17). To assess carbohydrate metabolism status after discharge in patients with history of stress hyperglycemia, national guidelines endorsed the use of HbA1c over oral glucose tolerance test (12,13).

Measurement of an HbA1c is recommended in all patients with diabetes and in patients without diabetes with persistent hyperglycemia (BG >140 mg/dL [7.8 mmol/L]) during hospitalization. HbA1c levels provide the opportunity to differentiate patients with stress hyperglycemia from those with diabetes who were previously undiagnosed, as well as to identify patients with known diabetes who would benefit from intensification of their glycemic management after discharge (13,18–20). However, clinicians should be aware that HbA1c testing in the hospital has significant limitations in the presence of hemoglobinopathies, recent transfusion, severe hepatic, renal and

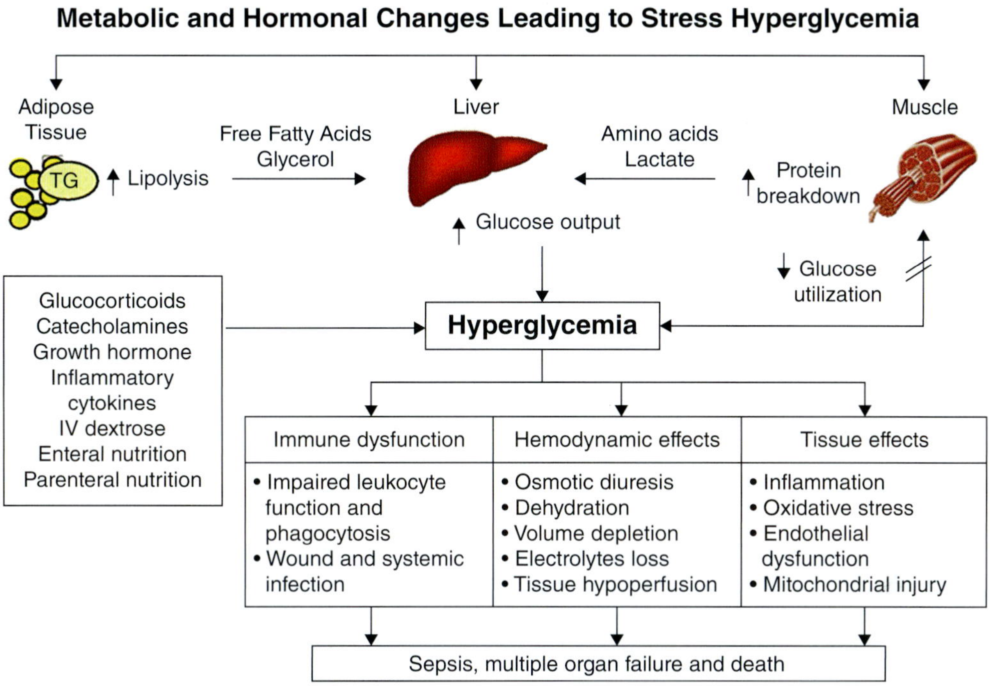

Metabolic and Hormonal Changes Leading to Stress Hyperglycemia

Figure 30-1 Pathophysiology of hyperglycemia and its complications in hospitalized patients
TG = Triglycerides.

liver disease, and iron deficiency anemia (21,22).

Prevalence of Hyperglycemia and Hypoglycemia in Non-Critical Care Settings

Data from the Centers for Diseases Control and Prevention (CDC) reported that a total of 29.1 million adults had diabetes in the USA in 2014, representing ~12% of the US adult population. Adult patients with diabetes are more frequently (up to three-fold) hospitalized than patients without diabetes (23). It is estimated that approximately 23% of adults discharged from US hospitals in 2012 had a diagnosis of diabetes, accounting for 8–9 million discharges with an annual cost of $124 billion (24,25). Observational studies have reported a prevalence of hyperglycemia ranging from 32–38% in community hospitals (2,26,27), 30–44% of patients admitted with acute coronary syndromes

or heart failure (28,29), and 80% of patients after cardiac surgery (30,31).

Hypoglycemia, as an inherent result of intensive insulin therapy, is commonly seen in hospitalized patients treated for hyperglycemia. Based on point-of-care (POC) glucose data, a national survey of 575 hospitals reported an incidence of hypoglycemia (BG <70 mg/dL [3.9 mmol/L]) of 5.7% patient-days in non-critically ill patients (32). Data from several randomized control trials (RCTs) in non-critically ill inpatients have reported a prevalence of hypoglycemia (BG <70 mg/dL [3.9 mmol/L]) and severe hypoglycemia of 10–32% (7,33,34) and 2–4%, respectively (11).

Hyperglycemia and Outcomes in Non-Critical Care Settings

In non-critically ill patients admitted to general medicine and surgery services, hyperglycemia has been associated with increased risk of infections and complications (2,4,35,36). Several mechanisms explain the detrimental effects of hyperglycemia (Figure 30-1) (18). Hyperglycemia causes osmotic diuresis that leads to hypovolemia, decreased glomerular filtration rate, and pre-renal azotemia. Hyperglycemia is associated with impaired leukocyte function, including decreased phagocytosis, impaired bacterial killing, and chemotaxis, leading to hospital infections and poor wound healing. In addition, acute hyperglycemia results in the activation of nuclear factor kB (NF-kB), the production of proinflammatory cytokines, and oxidative stress, leading to increased vascular permeability and mitochondrial dysfunction. Furthermore, hyperglycemia impairs endothelial function by suppressing the formation of nitric oxide and impairing endothelium-dependent, flow-mediated dilation.

In a prospective study of 2471 patients admitted for community-acquired pneumonia (4), the mortality rate was 13% in those with admission glucose levels >200 mg/dL (11.1 mmol/L) and 9% in those with admission levels ≤200 mg/dL (11.1 mmol/L). Similarly, those patients with admission glucose >200 mg/dL (11.1 mmol/L) also had a higher rate of inhospital complications (29% vs 22%). In a retrospective study of 348 patients with acute exacerbation of chronic obstructive pulmonary disease and respiratory tract infection, the relative risk of death was 2.1 in those with a BG of 126–160 mg/dL (7–8.9 mmol/L), and 3.4 for those with a BG of >162 mg/dL (9.0 mmol/L) compared to patients with a BG of 108 mg/dL (6.0 mmol/L) (37). Furthermore, each 18 mg/dL (1 mmol/L) increase in BG was associated with a 15% increase in the risk of an adverse clinical outcome (defined as death or length of stay of >9 days).

In general surgery patients, the development of hyperglycemia is also associated with increased risk for adverse outcomes. Patients with glucose levels of 110–200 mg/dL (6.0–11.1 mmol/L) and those with glucose levels of >200 mg/dL (11.1 mmol/L) had, 1.7-fold and 2.1-fold increased mortality compared to those with glucose levels <110 mg/dL (6.0 mmol/L), respectively (38). Another study in general surgery showed an increase in post-operative infection rate by 30% for every 40 mg/dL (2.2 mmol/L) rise in post-operative BG level >110 mg/dL (6.0 mmol/L) (39). Similarly, several recent studies and a recent meta-analysis in general non-cardiac surgery have reported an association between perioperative hyperglycemia and increased post-operative infection rates in patients with diabetes (36,40,41). In the RABBIT Surgery trial, a RCT in general surgery patients comparing treatment with a basal bolus insulin regimen to sliding-scale insulin (i.e., short-acting insulin correction coverage only with no basal dosing) reported improvement of glycemic control and significant reduction in a composite of complications including wound infection, pneumonia, acute kidney injury, and bacteremia (7).

Patients with stress hyperglycemia have been associated with a higher risk of poor outcomes and complications, compared to patients with previously diagnosed diabetes (2,42–44). In a systematic review of 54 stroke studies, it was shown that higher admission glucose was associated with less favorable outcome and more symptomatic intracranial hemorrhage (44). A study of general hospital admissions reported that patients with newly recognized hyperglycemia had a longer length of hospital stay and higher admission rate to an intensive care unit (ICU), and were less likely to be discharged to home, frequently requiring transfer to a transitional care unit or nursing home facility (2). A study of perioperative hyperglycemia after noncardiac general surgery showed that the risk of death increased in proportion to perioperative glucose levels; however, this association was significant only for patients without a history of diabetes (p = 0.008) compared with patients with known diabetes (p = 0.748) (41).

Table 30-1 Factors contributing to inpatient hypoglycemia in adults with diabetes (18)

- Medications: insulin, sulfonylureas, glinides, quinolones
- Intensive glycemic control
- Inappropriate insulin dosing and medication errors
- Poor coordination of insulin administration and food delivery
- Interruption of enteral nutrition or parenteral nutrition infusion
- Hypoglycemia unawareness
- Renal insufficiency
- Liver failure
- Severe illness, sepsis
- Dementia
- Frailty
- Medical and surgical procedures

Reproduced with permission from the American Diabetes Association.

Hypoglycemia and Outcomes in Non-Critical Care Hospital Settings

Although intensive insulin therapy is the standard of care in hospitals, it is commonly associated with hypoglycemia (9,10) (Table 30-1). Hypoglycemia has been associated with adverse cardiovascular outcomes, such as prolonged QT intervals, ischemic electrocardiogram changes/angina, arrhythmias, sudden death, and increased inflammation (45–49). Notably, the relationship between mortality and glycemic control in hospitalized patients with acute coronary syndrome follows a U-shape curve (49–51). However, recent studies have provided us with controversial results on the association between hypoglycemia and increased risk of mortality. Boucai et al., after a detailed analysis based on the etiological cause of hypoglycemia, reported that spontaneous hypoglycemia, as a marker of disease severity, was associated with worse clinical outcomes and higher mortality than iatrogenic hypoglycemia in hospitalized patients (47). However, Akirov et al. recently reported that the development of hypoglycemia, either spontaneously or as

the result of insulin therapy, was associated with increased mortality in hospitalized non-critically ill patients (52).

Hypoglycemia has been associated with increases in C-reactive protein and proinflammatory cytokines (TNFα, IL-1β, IL-6, and IL-8), markers of lipid peroxidation, reactive oxygen species, and leukocytosis (53,54). In addition, acute hypoglycemia creates a prothrombotic state, with increased levels of vasoconstrictors, platelet aggregation, endothelial dysfunction and vasoconstriction, abnormal cardiac repolarization, as well as catecholamine-induced cardiovascular changes, such as increase in heart rate, angina, and myocardial infarctions, all contributing to increased mortality (53,55).

Glycemic Variability

Glycemic variability in the critical care setting has been linked to increased mortality (56–59). Outside of the ICU, there is limited information on the association of glycemic variability and hospital-related outcomes. Studies on glycemic variability in non-critical care settings are limited by lack of patient-level data in some studies; lack of consensus on definition or metrics for glycemic variability; and reliance on POC testing from observational studies. Experimental evidence for an effect of variability on oxidative stress, endothelial dysfunction and cellular apoptosis suggests that vascular injury could be a plausible explanation for the impact of glycemic variability (56–59). In a single center, retrospective study of 748 patients having discharge diagnosis of congestive heart failure showed the median glycemic variability index was higher in non-survivors than in survivors (18.1 versus 6.82, p = 0.0003) (60). In a prospective study of 276 medical and surgical patients receiving total parenteral nutrition (TPN), glycemic variability was significantly higher in deceased patients than non-deceased patients (SD: 48 ± 25 vs. 34 ± 18 mg/dL [2.7 ± 1.4 vs. 1.9 ± 1 mmol/L]; delta change: 75 ± 39 vs. 51 ± 29 mg/dL

[4.2 ± 2.2 vs. 2.8 ± 1.6 mmol/L], both p <0.01) (61). Notably, this association was limited to patients without a history of diabetes. In a retrospective study of 935 admissions to general medicine or surgical services involving 620 patients, the 90-day risk of death increased by 10% with each 10 mg/dL (0.55 mmol/L) increment in SD of glucose (risk ratio [RR] 1.10 [95%CI 1.04–1.16], p <0.001) and by 21% with each 10% point increment in CV of glucose (RR 1.21 [1.07–1.35], p = 0.002) (62).

Management of Inpatient Hyperglycemia in Non-Critically Ill Hospitalized Patients

The implementation of computerized protocols for the management of hyperglycemia and hypoglycemia has been shown to improve glycemic control in hospitals. Thus, several hospitals have created standardized protocols for identifying and treating patients with hyperglycemia that are in line with current guidelines (Figure 30-2 and Figure 30-3). These protocols should be simple and user-friendly, identify patients who require initiation or modification of insulin therapy, address requirements for insulin infusion, and determine the consultation and educational needs of patients.

As a standard-of-care, every patient with known diabetes admitted to the hospital, regardless of the reason for admission, should have a plan for hyperglycemia management with a proactive approach upon admission, rather than a reactive response to elevation of BG. This plan should include an inpatient and discharge-planning component. By developing this proactive management plan for inpatients and discharge, we can avoid the common scenario of clinical inertia and lack of anti-diabetic regimen adjustment at discharge (63).

Common situations to avoid with a patient admitted with diabetes are: (a) neglecting the management of inpatient hyperglycemia or starting insulin sliding scale alone (i.e., fast-, rapid-, or short-acting insulin correction coverage only with no basal dosing) until hyperglycemia develops (reactive approach);

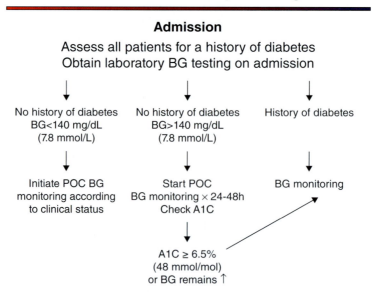

Diagnosis and monitoring of hyperglycemia and diabetes in the hospital setting

Admission
Assess all patients for a history of diabetes
Obtain laboratory BG testing on admission

| No history of diabetes BG<140 mg/dL (7.8 mmol/L) | No history of diabetes BG>140 mg/dL (7.8 mmol/L) | History of diabetes |

Initiate POC BG monitoring according to clinical status | Start POC BG monitoring × 24-48h Check A1C | BG monitoring

A1C ≥ 6.5% (48 mmol/mol) or BG remains ↑

Figure 30-2 Diagnosis, recognition and monitoring of hyperglycemia and diabetes in the hospital setting (13) POC = Point-of-care; BG = Blood glucose; A1C = HbA1c.

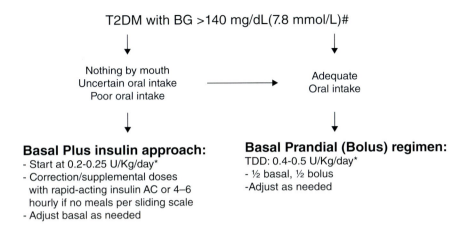

T2DM with BG >140 mg/dL(7.8 mmol/L)#

Nothing by mouth
Uncertain oral intake
Poor oral intake

Adequate
Oral intake

Basal Plus insulin approach:
- Start at 0.2-0.25 U/Kg/day*
- Correction/supplemental doses
  with rapid-acting insulin AC or 4–6
  hourly if no meals per sliding scale
- Adjust basal as needed

Basal Prandial (Bolus) regimen:
TDD: 0.4-0.5 U/Kg/day*
- ½ basal, ½ bolus
- Adjust as needed

BG target: Fasting and pre-meal BG between 140-180 mg/dL (7.8-10 mmol/L); For high-risk groups consider initiating insulin BG>180 mg/dL (10 mmol/L) or as per individualized targets and goals
*Reduce Basal insulin to 0.1-0.15 U/kg; or TDD Basal Prandial to 0.2-0.3 U/kg in patients aged ≥70 or creatinine ≥2.0 mg/dL (or eGFR <45 ml/min)

Figure 30-3 Initial insulin therapy in non-critically ill hospitalized patients with type 2 diabetes
AC = pre-meals; TDD = Total daily dose.

(b) continuing the patient's home diabetes treatment while addressing other acute issues; (c) failure to modify outpatient treatment regimens during hospitalization and discharge; and (d) withholding hyperglycemia therapy due to fear of hypoglycemia.

The Endocrine Society, AACE and ADA clinical guidelines recommended targeting a glucose level <140 mg/dL (7.8 mmol/L) before meals and a random glucose levels <180 mg/dL (10 mmol/L) for the majority of non-ICU patients (12,13). However, during the past three years, the ADA Standard of Care has recommended a target BG between 140 and 180 mg/dL (7.8–10 mmol/L) for most patients in non-ICU and ICU settings (14).

Subcutaneous (SC) insulin is the recommended treatment of choice for hyperglycemia management in non-critical hospital settings (12,13). A physiologic and proactive approach should include a calculation of the patient's total daily dose (TDD) insulin requirements, based on (a) body weight; (b) prior outpatient total insulin requirements; or (c) prior insulin utilization

during the hospitalization. To meet the daily insulin requirements, SC insulin regimens should cover the patient's basal requirements (i.e., prevents hyperglycemia during fasting states) and nutritional needs (i.e., prandial insulin, also referred to as nutritional or bolus insulin, is given before meals as fast-, rapid-, or short-acting (regular) insulin to prevent post-meal hyperglycemia). In addition, correction-dose or supplemental insulin is given to correct hyperglycemia when the glucose is above the target goal. The same insulin formulation is given together with prandial insulin (1,12,13). The TDD is a measure that comprises basal and prandial insulin.

Basal insulin requirements may be achieved with once-daily administration of a long-acting insulin analog (e.g., glargine, detemir, degludec) or with twice-daily administration of the intermediate-acting neutral protamine Hagedorn (NPH) insulin. Rapid-acting insulin analogs (e.g., lispro, aspart, or glulisine) or short-acting regular human insulin may be used to meet nutritional needs and to provide correctional insulin coverage. The use of the insulin sliding scale alone is ineffective and is not recommended in patients with diabetes. During recent years, newer formulations of ultra-long acting basal insulins have been approved for the management of diabetes, including glargine U300 and degludec U100 and U200. In addition, rapid-acting lispro U200 and fast-acting insulin aspart U100 are available in many countries. To our knowledge, no trials have studied the safety and efficacy of these insulin formulations in the inhospital setting.

The starting TDD insulin dose is 0.4–0.5 units per kg of body weight (Figure 30-3), with lower doses (0.2–0.3 units/kg) recommended for the elderly, patients with renal insufficiency (glomerular filtration rate <60 ml/min), or patients with history or at risk of hypoglycemia (18). Patients with adequate oral intake should receive a basal prandial (bolus) regimen dividing half as basal and half as prandial before meals. Patients with inadequate oral intake or who will be NPO (nil per oral) should receive basal insulin (0.2–0.25 units/kg/day) without scheduled prandial insulin. Lower basal insulin doses (0.1–0.15 units/kg) are recommended for the elderly, patients with renal insufficiency (glomerular filtration rate <60 ml/min), or patients with a history of or at risk of hypoglycemia (18). Rapid-acting insulin analogs or short-acting insulin are given to provide correctional/supplemental insulin coverage for BG >140–180 mg/dL (7.8–10 mmol/L) before meals or 4–6 hourly if no meals are given. In a RCT comparing basal-bolus insulin regimen to pre-mixed insulin (70/30) in the management of inpatient hyperglycemia, there were no differences in glycemic control, but the use of pre-mixed insulin was associated with significant risk of hypoglycemia (64). Despite the simplicity, a pre-mixed human insulin regimen should be avoided in patients with poor nutritional intake, surgery, and with multiple comorbidities in patients with type 2 diabetes (64).

The RABBIT Surgery trial, a multicenter RCT, compared the efficacy and safety of basal bolus insulin regimen to sliding-scale insulin (SSI) in patients with type 2 diabetes undergoing general surgery (65). Study outcomes included differences in daily BG levels and a composite of post-operative complications, including wound infection, pneumonia, respiratory failure, acute renal failure, and bacteremia. Patients were randomized to receive basal bolus regimen with glargine and glulisine at a starting dose of 0.5 unit/kg/day or SSI given 4 times/day. The basal bolus regimen resulted in significant improvement in BG control and in a reduction in the frequency of the composite outcome. The results of this trial indicate that treatment with glargine once daily plus rapid-acting insulin before meals improves glucose control and reduces hospital complications compared to SSI in general surgery patients with type 2 diabetes.

Personalized Hyperglycemia Management in Non-Critical Care Settings: A New Paradigm

The recently reported Basal Plus trial (66) recruited 375 patients with type 2 diabetes treated with diet, oral antidiabetic agents or low-dose insulin (≤0.4 unit/kg/day) to receive a basal bolus regimen with glargine once daily and glulisine before meals; a basal plus regimen with glargine once daily and supplemental doses of glulisine for correction of hyperglycemia (>140 mg/dL [7.8 mmol/L]) per sliding scale; or SSI. This RCT reported that the basal plus arm resulted in similar improvement in glycemic control and in the frequency of hypoglycemia compared to a standard basal bolus regimen. In addition, treatment with basal bolus and basal plus resulted in fewer treatment failures than treatment with SSI. Thus, in insulin-naïve patients or in those receiving low-dose insulin on admission (less than 0.4 units/kg/day), as well as patients with reduced oral intake, the use of a basal plus regimen is an effective alternative to basal bolus. If needed, patients with persistent hyperglycemia or with regular caloric intake

Treatment of non-critically ill hospitalized patients with type 2 diabetes

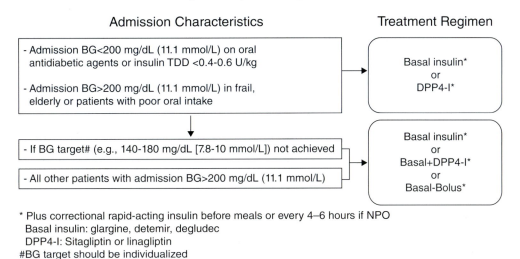

Figure 30-4 Personalized treatment approach of non-critically ill hospitalized patients with type 2 diabetes (34,81).

could be moved up to a basal bolus regimen (Figure 30-4).

Hospital Use of Incretin Therapy in Non-Critical Care Settings

The use of oral antidiabetic agents was not recommended in previous guidelines because of the lack of safety and efficacy studies in the inpatient setting (1,67). There are major limitations to the use of most oral antidiabetic agents, including the slow onset of action, which may not allow rapid dose adjustment to meet the changing needs of the acutely ill patient and risk of hypoglycemia with insulin secretagogues (68). Sulfonylureas may increase the risk of hypoglycemia in the hospitalized patient with poor appetite or ordered dietary restrictions. In addition, when inhibiting ATP-sensitive potassium channels, sulfonylurea therapy may inhibit ischemic pre-conditioning, leading to worsening cardiac and cerebral ischemia (69,70). A large number of patients have one or more contraindications to the use of metformin upon admission (71,72), including acute congestive heart failure, renal or liver

dysfunction, or hypoperfusion, which may increase the risk of lactic acidosis (73). The use of thiazolidinediones is limited as they can increase intravascular volume and may precipitate or worsen congestive heart failure and peripheral edema (72,74–76). The sodium–glucose cotransporter 2 (SGLT2) inhibitors, a class of oral antidiabetic agents that decrease concentrations of plasma glucose by inhibiting proximal tubular reabsorption in the kidney, have been shown to be effective in reducing HbA1c by 0.6–1.0% (7–13 mmol/mol) with a low risk of hypoglycemia. These agents, however, have been associated with increased risk of urinary and genital tract infections and dehydration and are contraindicated in patients with impaired renal function. In addition, an association has been reported between the use of SGLT2 inhibitors and the development of diabetic ketoacidosis among patients with type 1 and type 2 diabetes (14). These potential side effects make the use of SGLT2 inhibitors less attractive in acutely ill hospitalized patients with hyperglycemia (18).

However, the results of several clinical studies have shown that incretin-based therapy is an attractive option for use in hospital given its proven efficacy and low risk of hypoglycemia (34,77–80). A multi-center RCT determined differences in glycemic control between treatment with sitagliptin alone or in combination with basal insulin in general medicine and surgery patients with type 2 diabetes (78). In this pilot study, general medicine and surgery patients with a BG between 140 and 400 mg/dL (7.8–22.2 mmol/L) treated with diet, oral antidiabetic drugs or low-dose insulin (≤0.4 U/kg/day) were randomized to sitagliptin once daily; sitagliptin and basal insulin; or basal bolus insulin. All groups received correction/supplemental doses of rapid-acting insulin lispro before meals and bedtime for BG >140 mg/dL (7.8 mmol/L). Patients in the sitagliptin group received a single daily dose of 50–100 mg based on kidney function. In patients with mild-moderate hyperglycemia (<180 mg/dL [10 mmol/L]), the use of sitagliptin plus supplemental (correction) doses or in combination with basal insulin resulted in no significant differences in mean daily BG, frequency of hypoglycemia, or in the number of treatment failures compared to the basal bolus regimen.

The recently reported SITA-HOSPITAL study, a multicenter, non-inferiority, RCT compared the combination of oral sitagliptin plus basal insulin to the more labor-intensive basal-bolus insulin regimen in patients with type 2 diabetes admitted to general medicine and surgery services in five academic institutions in the US (34,78). A total of 279 patients, between 18 and 80 years of age, previously treated with oral anti-diabetic agents or low-dose insulin (<0.6 U/kg/d) were enrolled. The use of oral sitagliptin plus a single basal insulin dose resulted in similar glycemic control, hypoglycemia rate, hospital length-of-stay, treatment failures or hospital complications (including acute kidney injury or pancreatitis) compared to a standard basal bolus regimen (34). The use of sitagliptin plus basal insulin was associated with significant reduction in TDD insulin and in fewer insulin injections compared to the basal bolus approach (34,78).

Despite basal-bolus insulin regimen being widely used in hospitals, we now know that it may not be a "one-size-fits-all" choice. The innovative SITA-HOSPITAL trial represents a new step in the future of inpatient hyperglycemia management, with emphasis on more personalized approaches for specific populations. For instances, patients with mild hyperglycemia (<180–200 mg/dL [10–12 mmol/L), high risk for hypoglycemia, poor oral intake, frail elderly patients, insulin-naïve or insulin-experienced patients but on low-dose before admission may need a more personalized approach (34,78,81).

Recommendations After Hospital Discharge

Despite evidence showing that clinical inertia is common during hospital discharge of patients with diabetes, few studies have focused on the optimal management of hyperglycemia after hospital discharge. Griffith et al. showed that more than 60% of hospitalized patients with previously uncontrolled diabetes (based on admission HbA1c) were discharged with no change in their previous anti-diabetic regimen (13,82).

The Endocrine Society inpatient guidelines for the management of non-ICU patients with diabetes (13) recommended that patients with diabetes and hyperglycemia should have an HbA1c measured to assess pre-admission glycemic control and to tailor treatment regimen at discharge.

In a recent RCT by Umpierrez et al., a hospital discharge algorithm based on admission HbA1c was tested. Patients admitted with an HbA1c <7% (53 mmol/mol) were discharged on the same pre-admission diabetes therapy (non-insulin agents or same dose insulin); patients with HbA1c between 7–9% (53–75 mmol/mol) were discharged on their pre-admission oral anti-diabetic agents plus 50% of hospital basal insulin dose; and those with A1c >9% (75 mmol/mol) were discharged on basal bolus insulin or the combination of metformin plus basal insulin at 80% of hospital dose. The overall mean HbA1c showed significant improvement in all patients, from 8.7% (±2.5) [71.6 mmol/mol] on admission, to 7.9 (±1.7) at 4 weeks, to 7.3% (±1.5) [56 mmol/mol] at 12-weeks follow-up. Clinicians should be aware that the use of basal and basal prandial (bolus) insulin regimens was associated with ~30% risk of hypoglycemia within 3 months after discharge (63). Following this trial, unless the patient was taking insulin before admission, we usually reserve the use of basal insulin for patients with HbA1c above 7.5% (60 mmol/mol) or 8% (64 mmol/mol), in particular, in elderly patients, patients with reduced caloric intake or in subjects with impaired kidney function.

Conclusions

Hyperglycemia is a common finding in non-critically ill patients with and without diabetes. Observational and randomized controlled studies indicate that improvement in glycemic control results in lower rates of hospital complications and mortality. Standardized order sets, promoting the use of scheduled basal insulin ± standing prandial (bolus) insulin *or* oral DPP4-inhibitors in specific scenarios, is key in managing inpatient hyperglycemia. Correctional/supplemental insulin per sliding scale can be added as needed to any of the above regimes. Implementing personalized algorithms is the future of inpatient hyperglycemic management in non-critical care hospital settings.

References

1 Clement S, Braithwaite SS, Magee MF, et al. Management of diabetes and hyperglycemia in hospitals. *Diabetes Care.* 2004;27(2):553–591.

2 Umpierrez GE, Isaacs SD, Bazargan N, You X, Thaler LM, Kitabchi AE. Hyperglycemia: an independent marker of in-hospital mortality in patients with undiagnosed diabetes. *J Clin Endocrinol Metab.* 2002;87(3):978–982.

3 Fish LH, Weaver TW, Moore AL, Steel LG. Value of postoperative blood glucose in predicting complications and length of stay after coronary artery bypass grafting. *Am J Cardiol.* 2003;92(1):74–76.

4 McAlister FA, Majumdar SR, Blitz S, Rowe BH, Romney J, Marrie TJ. The relation between hyperglycemia and outcomes in 2,471 patients admitted to the hospital with community-acquired pneumonia. *Diabetes Care.* 2005;28(4):810–815.

5 Falciglia M, Freyberg RW, Almenoff PL, D'Alessio DA, Render ML. Hyperglycemia-related mortality in critically ill patients varies with admission diagnosis. *Critical Care Med.* 2009;37(12):3001–3009.

6 Krinsley JS. Association between hyperglycemia and increased hospital mortality in a heterogeneous population of critically ill patients. *Mayo Clin Proc.* 2003;78(12):1471–1478.

7 Umpierrez GE, Smiley D, Jacobs S, et al. Randomized study of basal-bolus insulin therapy in the inpatient management of patients with type 2 diabetes undergoing general surgery (RABBIT 2 surgery). *Diabetes Care.* 2011;34(2):256–261.

8 The effect of intensive treatment of diabetes on the development and progression of long-term complications in insulin-dependent diabetes mellitus. The Diabetes Control and Complications Trial Research Group. *N Engl J Med.* 1993;329(14):977–986.

9 Cryer PE. Hypoglycemia: still the limiting factor in the glycemic management of diabetes. *Endocr Pract.* 2008;14(6): 750–756.

10 Cryer PE. The barrier of hypoglycemia in diabetes. *Diabetes.* 2008;57(12):3169–3176.

11 Farrokhi F, Klindukhova O, Chandra P, et al. Risk factors for inpatient hypoglycemia during subcutaneous insulin

therapy in non-critically ill patients with type 2 diabetes. *J Diabetes Sci Technol.* 2012;6(5):1022–1029.

12 Moghissi ES, Korytkowski MT, DiNardo M, et al. American Association of Clinical Endocrinologists and American Diabetes Association consensus statement on inpatient glycemic control. *Diabetes Care.* 2009;32(6):1119–1131.

13 Umpierrez GE, Hellman R, Korytkowski MT, et al. Management of hyperglycemia in hospitalized patients in non-critical care setting: an Endocrine Society Clinical Practice Guideline. *J Clin Endocr Metab.* 2012;97(1):16–38.

14 American Diabetes Association. 14. Diabetes care in the hospital. *Diabetes Care.* 2018;41(Suppl 1):S144–S151.

15 Dungan KM, Braithwaite SS, Preiser JC. Stress hyperglycaemia. *Lancet.* 2009;373(9677):1798–1807.

16 McDonnell ME, Umpierrez GE. Insulin therapy for the management of hyperglycemia in hospitalized patients. *Endocrinology Metab Clin N Am.* 2012;41(1):175–201.

17 Greci LS, Kailasam M, Malkani S, et al. Utility of HbA(1c) levels for diabetes case finding in hospitalized patients with hyperglycemia. *Diabetes Care.* 2003;26(4):1064–1068.

18 Umpierrez GE, Pasquel FJ. Management of inpatient hyperglycemia and diabetes in older adults. *Diabetes Care.* 2017;40:509–517.

19 Ainla T, Baburin A, Teesalu R, Rahu M. The association between hyperglycaemia on admission and 180-day mortality in acute myocardial infarction patients with and without diabetes. *Diabetic Medicine* 2005;22(10):1321–1325.

20 Norhammar A, Tenerz A, Nilsson G, et al. Glucose metabolism in patients with acute myocardial infarction and no previous diagnosis of diabetes mellitus: a prospective study. *Lancet.* 2002;359(9324):2140–2144.

21 Saudek CD, Derr RL, Kalyani RR. Assessing glycemia in diabetes using self-monitoring blood glucose and hemoglobin A1c. *JAMA.* 2006;295(14):1688–1697.

22 International Expert Committee report on the role of the A1C assay in the diagnosis of diabetes. *Diabetes Care.* 2009;32(7):1327–1334.

23 Harris MI. Medical care for patients with diabetes. Epidemiologic aspects. *Ann Intern Med.* 1996;124(1 Pt 2):117–122.

24 Jiang HJ, Stryer D, Friedman B, Andrews R. Multiple hospitalizations for patients with diabetes. *Diabetes Care.* 2003;26(5):1421–1426.

25 Donnan PT, Leese GP, Morris AD, Diabetes A, Research in Tayside SMMUC. Hospitalizations for people with type 1 and type 2 diabetes compared with the nondiabetic population of Tayside, Scotland: a retrospective cohort study of resource use. *Diabetes Care.* 2000;23(12):1774–1779.

26 Cook CB, Kongable GL, Potter DJ, Abad VJ, Leija DE, Anderson M. Inpatient glucose control: a glycemic survey of 126 U.S. hospitals. *J Hosp Med.* 2009;4(9):E7–E14.

27 Levetan CS, Passaro M, Jablonski K, Kass M, Ratner RE. Unrecognized diabetes among hospitalized patients. *Diabetes Care.* 1998;21(2):246–249.

28 Kosiborod M, Rathore SS, Inzucchi SE, et al. Admission glucose and mortality in elderly patients hospitalized with acute myocardial infarction: implications for patients with and without recognized diabetes. *Circulation.* 2005;111(23):3078–3086.

29 Kosiborod M, Inzucchi SE, Spertus JA, et al. Elevated admission glucose and mortality in elderly patients hospitalized with heart failure. *Circulation.* 2009;119(14):1899–1907.

30 Schmeltz LR, DeSantis AJ, Thiyagarajan V, et al. Reduction of surgical mortality and morbidity in diabetic patients undergoing cardiac surgery with a combined intravenous and subcutaneous insulin glucose management strategy. *Diabetes Care.* 2007;30(4):823–828.

31 van den Berghe G, Wouters P, Weekers F, et al. Intensive insulin therapy in critically ill patients. *N Engl J Med.* 2001;345(19):1359–1367.

32 Swanson CM, Potter DJ, Kongable GL, Cook CB. Update on inpatient glycemic control in hospitals in the United States. *Endocr Pract.* 2011;17(6):853–861.

33 Umpierrez GE, Smiley D, Zisman A, et al. Randomized study of basal-bolus insulin therapy in the inpatient management of patients with type 2 diabetes (RABBIT 2 trial). *Diabetes Care.* 2007;30(9):2181–2186.

34 Pasquel FJ, Gianchandani R, Rubin DJ, et al. Efficacy of sitagliptin for the hospital management of general medicine and surgery patients with type 2 diabetes (Sita-Hospital): a multicentre, prospective, open-label, non-inferiority randomised trial. *Lancet Diabetes Endocrinol.* 2017;5(2):125–133.

35 Montori VM, Bistrian BR, McMahon MM. Hyperglycemia in acutely ill patients. *JAMA* 2002;288(17):2167–2169.

36 Murad MH, Coburn JA, Coto-Yglesias F, et al. Glycemic control in non-critically ill hospitalized patients: a systematic review and meta-analysis. *J Clin Eendocr Metab.* 2012;97(1):49–58.

37 Baker EH, Janaway CH, Philips BJ, et al. Hyperglycaemia is associated with poor outcomes in patients admitted to hospital with acute exacerbations of chronic obstructive pulmonary disease. *Thorax.* 2006;61(4):284–289.

38 Pomposelli JJ, Baxter JK, 3rd, Babineau TJ, et al. Early postoperative glucose control predicts nosocomial infection rate in diabetic patients. *J Parenter Enteral Nutr.* 1998;22(2):77–81.

39 Ramos M, Khalpey Z, Lipsitz S, et al. Relationship of perioperative hyperglycemia and postoperative infections in patients who undergo general and vascular surgery. *Ann Surg.* 2008;248(4):585–591.

40 Kwon S, Thompson R, Dellinger P, Yanez D, Farrohki E, Flum D. Importance of perioperative glycemic control in general surgery: a report from the Surgical Care and Outcomes Assessment Program. *Ann Surg.* 2013;257(1):8–14.

41 Frisch A, Chandra P, Smiley D, et al. Prevalence and clinical outcome of hyperglycemia in the perioperative period in noncardiac surgery. *Diabetes Care.* 2010;33(8):1783–1788.

42 Capes SE, Hunt D, Malmberg K, Gerstein HC. Stress hyperglycaemia and increased risk of death after myocardial infarction in patients with and without diabetes: a systematic overview. *Lancet.* 2000;355(9206):773–778.

43 Capes SE, Hunt D, Malmberg K, Pathak P, Gerstein HC. Stress hyperglycemia and prognosis of stroke in nondiabetic and diabetic patients: a systematic overview. *Stroke.* 2001;32(10):2426–2432.

44 Desilles JP, Meseguer E, Labreuche J, et al. Diabetes mellitus, admission glucose, and outcomes after stroke thrombolysis: a registry and systematic review. *Stroke.* 2013;44(7):1915–1923.

45 Gill GV, Woodward A, Casson IF, Weston PJ. Cardiac arrhythmia and nocturnal hypoglycaemia in type 1 diabetes: the "dead in bed" syndrome revisited. *Diabetologia.* 2009;52(1):42–45.

46 Desouza C, Salazar H, Cheong B, Murgo J, Fonseca V. Association of hypoglycemia and cardiac ischemia: a study based on continuous monitoring. *Diabetes Care.* 2003;26(5):1485–1489.

47 Boucai L, Southern WN, Zonszein J. Hypoglycemia-associated mortality is not drug-associated but linked to comorbidities. *Am J Med.* 2011;124(11): 1028–1035.

48 Garg R, Hurwitz S, Turchin A, Trivedi A. Hypoglycemia, with or without insulin therapy, is associated with increased mortality among hospitalized patients. *Diabetes Care.* 2013;36(5):1107–1110.

49 Kosiborod M, Inzucchi SE, Goyal A, et al. Relationship between spontaneous and iatrogenic hypoglycemia and mortality in patients hospitalized with acute myocardial infarction. *JAMA.* 2009;301(15): 1556–1564.

50 Pinto DS, Skolnick AH, Kirtane AJ, et al. U-shaped relationship of blood glucose with adverse outcomes among patients with ST-segment elevation myocardial infarction. *J Am Coll Cardiol.* 2005;46(1): 178–180.

51 Svensson AM, McGuire DK, Abrahamsson P, Dellborg M. Association between hyper- and hypoglycaemia and 2 year all-cause mortality risk in diabetic patients with acute coronary events. *Eur Heart J.* 2005;26(13):1255–1261.

52 Akirov A, Grossman A, Shochat T, Shimon I. Mortality among hospitalized patients with hypoglycemia: insulin-related and non-insulin related. *J Clin Endocrin Metab.* 2016:jc20162653.

53 Desouza CV, Bolli GB, Fonseca V. Hypoglycemia, diabetes, and cardiovascular events. *Diabetes Care.* 2010;33(6):1389–1394.

54 Razavi Nematollahi L, Kitabchi AE, Stentz FB, et al. Proinflammatory cytokines in response to insulin-induced hypoglycemic stress in healthy subjects. *Metab.* 2009;58(4):443–448.

55 Rana OA, Byrne CD, Greaves K. Intensive glucose control and hypoglycaemia: a new cardiovascular risk factor? *Heart.* 2014;100:21–27.

56 Krinsley JS. Glycemic variability: a strong independent predictor of mortality in critically ill patients. *Critical Care Med.* 2008;36(11):3008–3013.

57 Brownlee M, Hirsch IB. Glycemic variability: a hemoglobin A1c-independent risk factor for diabetic complications. *JAMA.* 2006;295(14):1707–1708.

58 Hirsch IB, Brownlee M. Should minimal blood glucose variability become the gold standard of glycemic control? *J Diabetes Complications.* 2005;19(3): 178–181.

59 Monnier L, Mas E, Ginet C, et al. Activation of oxidative stress by acute glucose fluctuations compared with sustained chronic hyperglycemia in patients with type 2 diabetes. *JAMA.* 2006;295(14):1681–1687.

60 Dungan KM, Binkley P, Nagaraja HN, Schuster D, Osei K. The effect of glycaemic control and glycaemic variability on mortality in patients hospitalized with congestive heart failure. *Diabetes/Metabolism Research and Reviews.* 2011;27(1):85–93.

61 Farrokhi F, Chandra P, Smiley D, et al. Glucose variability is an independent predictor of mortality in hospitalized patients treated with total parenteral nutrition. *Endocr Pract.* 2013:1–17.

62 Mendez CE, Mok KT, Ata A, Tanenberg RJ, Calles-Escandon J, Umpierrez GE. Increased glycemic variability is independently associated with length of stay and mortality in noncritically ill hospitalized patients. *Diabetes Care.* 2013;36(12):4091–4097.

63 Umpierrez GE, Reyes D, Smiley D, et al. Hospital discharge algorithm based on admission HbA1c for the management of patients with type 2 diabetes. *Diabetes Care.* 2014;37(11):2934–2939.

64 Bellido V, Suarez L, Rodriguez MG, et al. Comparison of basal-bolus and premixed insulin regimens in hospitalized patients with type 2 diabetes. *Diabetes Care.* 2015;38(12):2211–2216.

65 Umpierrez E, Smiley D, Jacobs S, et al. RAndomized study of Basal Bolus Insulin Therapy in the inpatient management of patients with type 2 diabetes undergoing general surgery (RABBIT 2 Surgery). *Diabetes.* 2010;59(Suppl 1).

66 Umpierrez GE, Smiley D, Hermayer K, et al. Randomized study comparing a basal bolus with a basal plus correction insulin regimen for the hospital management of medical and surgical patients with type 2 diabetes: basal plus trial. *Diabetes Care.* 2013.

67 Gupta T, Hudson M. Update on glucose management among noncritically ill patients hospitalized on medical and surgical wards. *J Endocrine Soc.* 2017;1:247–259.

68 Levetan CS, Magee MF. Hospital management of diabetes. *Endocrinol Metab Clin North Am.* 2000;29(4):745–770.

69 Terzic A, Jahangir A, Kurachi Y. Cardiac ATP-sensitive K+ channels: regulation by intracellular nucleotides and K+ channel-opening drugs. *Am J Physiol.* 1995;269(3 Pt 1):C525–C545.

70 Tomai F, Crea F, Gaspardone A, et al. Ischemic preconditioning during coronary

angioplasty is prevented by glibenclamide, a selective ATP-sensitive K+ channel blocker. *Circulation*. 1994;90(2): 700–705.

71 Horlen C, Malone R, Bryant B, et al. Frequency of inappropriate metformin prescriptions. *Jama*. 2002;287(19): 2504–2505.

72 Calabrese AT, Coley KC, DaPos SV, Swanson D, Rao RH. Evaluation of prescribing practices: risk of lactic acidosis with metformin therapy. *Arch Intern Med*. 2002;162(4):434–437.

73 Pasquel FJ, Klein R, Adigweme A, et al. Metformin-associated lactic acidosis. *Am J Med Sci*. 2015;349:263–267.

74 Delea TE, Edelsberg JS, Hagiwara M, Oster G, Phillips LS. Use of thiazolidinediones and risk of heart failure in people with type 2 diabetes: a retrospective cohort study: response to karter et Al. *Diabetes Care*. 2004;27(3):852–853.

75 Delea TE, Edelsberg JS, Hagiwara M, Oster G, Phillips LS. Use of thiazolidinediones and risk of heart failure in people with type 2 diabetes: a retrospective cohort study. *Diabetes Care*. 2003;26(11): 2983–2989.

76 Nesto RW, Bell D, Bonow RO, et al. Thiazolidinedione use, fluid retention, and congestive heart failure: a consensus statement from the American Heart Association and American Diabetes Association. *Diabetes Care*. 2004;27(1): 256–263.

77 Schwartz SS, DeFronzo RA, Umpierrez GE. Practical implementation of incretin-based therapy in hospitalized patients with type 2 diabetes. *Postgrad Med*. 2015;127(2): 251–257.

78 Umpierrez GE, Gianchandani R, Smiley D, et al. Safety and efficacy of sitagliptin therapy for the inpatient management of general medicine and surgery patients with type 2 diabetes: a pilot, randomized, controlled study. *Diabetes Care*. 2013;36(11):3430–3435.

79 Umpierrez GE, Korytkowski M. Is incretin-based therapy ready for the care of hospitalized patients with type 2 diabetes?: Insulin therapy has proven itself and is considered the mainstay of treatment. *Diabetes Care*. 2013;36(7):2112–2117.

80 Umpierrez GE, Schwartz S. Use of incretin-based therapy in hospitalized patients with hyperglycemia. *Endocr Pract*. 2014;20(9):933–944.

81 Nauck MA, Meier JJ. Sitagliptin plus basal insulin: simplifying in-hospital diabetes treatment? *Lancet Diabetes Endocrinol*. 2017;5(2):83–85.

82 Griffith ML, Boord JB, Eden SK, Matheny ME. Clinical inertia of discharge planning among patients with poorly controlled diabetes mellitus. *J Clin Endocrin Metab*. 2012;97(6):2019–2026.

31

Hypoglycemia

Elizabeth M. Lamos, Lisa M. Younk, and Stephen N. Davis

Key Points

- Hypoglycemia represents one of the most common endocrine emergencies that clinicians are likely to routinely encounter.
- Hypoglycemia is one of the most frequent endocrine emergencies in individuals with diabetes mellitus. However, hypoglycemia in non-diabetic individuals is relatively rare.
- In both persons with and without diabetes, acute hypoglycemia is associated with increased morbidity and in some individuals even death.
- Hypoglycemia is a significant cost burden and is the major limiting factor for short- and long-term improved glycemic control in persons with diabetes.
- The threshold value for the definition of hypoglycemia in persons with diabetes remains debated. The International Hypoglycemia Study Group defined hypoglycemia thresholds as a plasma glucose level of $\leq$70 mg/dL (3.9 mmol/L), and this is now considered a hypoglycemia alert value, indicating a need for correction with fast-acting carbohydrates and/or dose adjustment of glucose-lowering medications. A plasma glucose level of <54 mg/dL (3.0 mmol/L) is considered to be the threshold for clinically significant hypoglycemia, indicating serious, clinically important hypoglycemia.
- Subclasses of hypoglycemia include severe, symptomatic, asymptomatic, probable, and pseudo-hypoglycemia. Severe hypoglycemia is defined as hypoglycemia resulting in the requirement of assistance of another individual to administer rescue therapy.
- Most recommend documentation of Whipple's triad (i.e., low plasma glucose, symptoms or signs consistent with hypoglycemia and resolution of those symptoms after the plasma glucose has been raised) to confirm hypoglycemia, especially in persons without diabetes.
- In healthy humans, multiple mechanisms have evolved to defend against falling plasma glucose. A coordinated interplay of insulin inhibition and release of the powerful counter-regulatory hormones, including glucagon and epinephrine, form the acute defense against hypoglycemia. Sympathetic nervous system responses are also important.
- Consequently, hypoglycemia manifests as an array of autonomic (i.e., palpitations, tremor, sweating, pallor, and anxiety) and neuroglycopenic (i.e., behavior changes, fatigue, seizure, loss of consciousness) signs and symptoms. The glucose threshold for the generation of autonomic signs and symptoms is plastic in nature but is typically ~60 mg/dL (3.3 mmol/L).

Endocrine and Metabolic Medical Emergencies: A Clinician's Guide, Second Edition. Edited by Glenn Matfin.
© 2018 John Wiley & Sons Ltd. Published 2018 by John Wiley & Sons Ltd.

- Failure of these protective sympathoadrenal mechanisms can lead to severe, unimpeded hypoglycemia. In cases of recurring episodes of hypoglycemia, the threshold for initiation of counter-regulatory hormone responses is reduced to a lower plasma glucose level and hormone responses become blunted. Patients also develop hypoglycemia unawareness, in which symptoms are delayed and blunted and may be unrecognizable to the individual.
- Collectively, the reduction of hormonal and symptom responses to recurring episodes of hypoglycemia are part of a disorder termed hypoglycemia-associated autonomic failure (HAAF), the presence of which further increases the risk of severe hypoglycemia.

- HAAF may be reversible in 2–3 weeks with scrupulous avoidance of hypoglycemia. Glycemic targets should be reviewed to prevent severe hypoglycemia and preserve awareness.
- Hypoglycemia in individuals with or without diabetes should be managed quickly with the same algorithm to avoid adverse morbidity and mortality.
- Most commonly seen in individuals with diabetes, the evaluation of individuals without diabetes is more complex and requires a careful history and laboratory evaluation to discern the underlying etiology.
- Ultimately, education is the key to prevention and early intervention of hypoglycemia.

Introduction

Hypoglycemia represents one of the most common endocrine emergencies that clinicians are likely to routinely encounter. Relatively rare in non-diabetic individuals, hypoglycemia frequently occurs in persons with diabetes (1). In both type 1 diabetes (T1DM) and type 2 diabetes (T2DM), acute hypoglycemia is associated with increased morbidity and in some individuals even death. Hypoglycemia is a significant cost burden and is the major limiting factor for short- and long-term improved glycemic control (2,3). Hypoglycemia in persons without diabetes often presents a complex diagnostic challenge. The definition, mechanism(s), diagnostic pathways, and acute management of hypoglycemia in persons with and without diabetes in outpatient and inpatient settings will be discussed.

Definition of Hypoglycemia

The threshold value for the definition of hypoglycemia remains debated. Endocrine Society guideline recommendations for all individuals cite any glucose concentration below which symptoms are evident (4). A 2013 workgroup report from the American Diabetes Association (ADA) and the Endocrine Society defines iatrogenic hypoglycemia in patients with diabetes as the glucose level that exposes the individual to potential harm (5). Most recently, a joint position statement from the ADA and the European Association for the Study of Diabetes (EASD) defined hypoglycemia thresholds recommended by the International Hypoglycemia Study Group (6). A plasma glucose level of ≤70 mg/dL (3.9 mmol/L) is now considered a hypoglycemia alert value, indicating a need for correction with fast-acting carbohydrates and/or dose adjustment of glucose-lowering medications. A plasma glucose level of <54 mg/dL (3.0 mmol/L) is considered to be the threshold for clinically significant hypoglycemia, indicating serious, clinically important hypoglycemia. This is also the threshold recommended for reporting hypoglycemia events in future clinical trials of glucose-lowering medications. These thresholds have been adopted by the ADA in its 2018 guidelines (3). Subclasses of hypoglycemia include severe, symptomatic, asymptomatic, probable and pseudo-hypoglycemia (Table 31-1). Severe

Table 31-1 Classification of hypoglycemia in individuals with diabetes (5)

Severe	Requiring the assistance of another individual to administer rescue therapy
Symptomatic	Typical symptoms, plasma glucose ≤70 mg/dL (≤3.9 mmol/L)
Asymptomatic	No symptoms, plasma glucose ≤70 mg/dL (≤3.9 mmol/L)
Probable	Typical symptoms, no plasma glucose available
Pseudo-hypoglycemia	Typical symptoms, plasma glucose >70 mg/dL (>3.9 mmol/L)

Reproduced with permission from the Endocrine Society.

hypoglycemia is defined as hypoglycemia resulting in the requirement of assistance of another individual to administer rescue therapy (5).

Most recommend documentation of Whipple's triad (i.e., low plasma glucose, symptoms or signs consistent with hypoglycemia and resolution of those symptoms after the plasma glucose has been raised) to confirm hypoglycemia, especially in persons without diabetes (7). This allows clinicians to reduce unnecessary evaluation and potential harm in those situations where Whipple's triad is not observed. However, in an individual diagnosed and treated for diabetes, the probability of hypoglycemia is high, and treatment should be initiated without deferring evaluation even when plasma glucose is unavailable for documentation.

Epidemiology

Hypoglycemia occurs predominantly in patients with T1DM or T2DM treated with insulin and/or an insulin secretagogue. In a large one-year study that included more than 8500 people with diabetes, 7.1% of persons with T1DM and 7.3% with insulin-treated T2DM experienced at least one episode of severe hypoglycemia (1). In the same study, the incidence of severe hypoglycemia in T2DM patients treated with sulfonylureas was 0.8% per year. Older individuals are at increased risk for hypoglycemia. Large randomized controlled trials of intensive glycemic therapy in T2DM patients, including ACCORD (8) and ADVANCE (9), reported progressive increases in risk of ~3% per year with advancing age. In addition, the T1D Exchange study in T1DM patients demonstrated a 12-month frequency of severe hypoglycemia of 19% in patients aged ≥65 years (10). In pregnant women with diabetes, severe hypoglycemia increases nearly 3-fold during the first trimester compared to pre-pregnancy, with rates of hypoglycemia declining with each successive trimester, from 5.3 to 2.4 to 0.5 events per patient-year in the first, second and third trimesters, respectively (11). For critically ill patients treated with intensive insulin therapy in the intensive care unit (ICU), rates of hypoglycemia range from 2.1–11.5 % (12).

In the USA, from 1993 to 2005, ~5 million emergency room visits were due to hypoglycemic events, 25% of which led to hospitalization (13). This is especially common in an increasing population of elderly patients with diabetes, where hospital admissions for severe hypoglycemia were 2-fold higher than admissions for hyperglycemia among nearly 34 million Medicare beneficiaries in patients with T2DM aged 85 years and older compared with younger (65–84 years old) beneficiaries (14). Overall, hypoglycemia in patients treated with insulin is associated with a 2-fold increase in hospitalizations and emergency room visits for any reason (15). Hypoglycemia is also common in hospitalized elderly patients and is associated with poor outcomes including increased mortality (either directly or as a marker of more severe underlying diseases) (15). Hypoglycemia confers a large financial burden, with annual excess medical expenditures of $3,200 per person for care directly related to hypoglycemia. Absenteeism and use of short-term disability compensation are also drastically increased (16).

Reports suggest that 2–13% of deaths in patients with T1DM can be attributed to hypoglycemia (4,17). Hypoglycemia may be involved in "dead in bed" syndrome, perhaps through cardiac conduction system effects, as continuous electrocardiographic (ECG) monitoring has revealed sinus bradycardia, atrial and ventricular ectopic beats, and P-wave abnormalities, as well as significant QT-interval prolongation during episodes of spontaneous nocturnal hypoglycemia (18, 19). Under controlled insulin-induced hypoglycemia, bradycardia, ventricular ectopic beats, ST-segment depression, and T-wave flattening were also observed in a portion of subjects with T2DM (20). A retrospective analysis revealed that QT prolongation was present in 50% and 60% of patients with T1DM and T2DM, respectively, presenting to the emergency department with severe hypoglycemia (defined as hypoglycemic symptoms that could not be resolved by the patient and required emergency medical assistance) (21). In a separate retrospective study, QT prolongation was found to be more likely during episodes of severe hypoglycemia occurring in the morning (4 a.m. to 10 a.m.) versus other times of the day (22).

Long-term cardiovascular damage may also be attributed to hypoglycemia, as single and repeated hypoglycemic events induce acute inflammation, oxidative stress, leukocytosis, endothelial dysfunction, and prothrombogenic and atherogenic mechanisms (23–25). A history of repeated mild and severe hypoglycemia has also been associated with increased inflammation, endothelial dysfunction, and intima-media thickness and reduced flow-mediated arterial dilatation (26). In large glycemic intervention trials, hypoglycemia was associated with increased hazards ratios for major macro- and microvascular events and cardiovascular-related and all-cause mortality (9,27). Additionally, the NICE-SUGAR trial demonstrated that critically-ill patients who are intensively controlled had an increased risk of moderate to severe hypoglycemia and an increased risk of death (28).

Glucose Measurements

The accuracy of measured glucose samples should be considered when evaluating acute hypoglycemia. Plasma glucose samples are up to 15% higher than mixed venous whole blood glucose (BG) samples (29). Thus, knowing if a BG meter is providing blood or plasma values is important for interpretation, as the lower limit of normal would be approximately 60 mg/dL (3.3 mmol/L) for a mixed venous whole BG sample. Additionally, mixed venous BG values can be considerably lower than arterial or capillary levels. Thus, under high physiologic insulinemia, a venous plasma glucose value in an insulin-sensitive individual can be up to 25 mg/dL (1.5 mmol/L) lower than an arterial level, thereby resulting in a spuriously low level.

Many other factors can influence the accuracy of glucose sampling. Glucose meters can be imprecise, especially at low BG levels (29). The correct calibration of the meter should always be ensured, especially if the BG reading is low but the individual lacks corresponding symptoms. Additional confounding factors include: collection in a non-fluoride and/or oxalate containing tube (BG can decrease by 10–20 mg/dL/hr [0.5–1 mmol/L/hr] at room temperature), long duration until sample is tested, high triglyceride content, altitude, temperature, humidity, and hemoglobin level (30).

Physiology of Glucose Metabolism

In healthy humans, multiple mechanisms have evolved to defend against a falling plasma glucose. A coordinated interplay of insulin inhibition and release of the powerful counter-regulatory hormones, including glucagon and epinephrine, form the

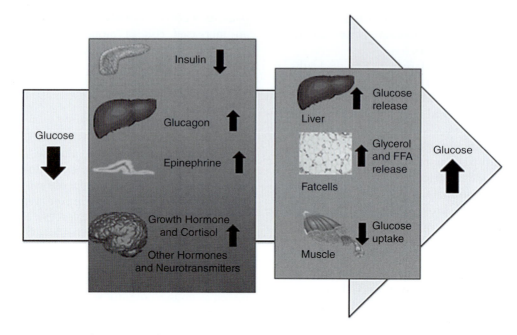

Figure 31-1 Normal counter-regulatory hormonal and metabolic responses to declining blood glucose level.

acute defense against hypoglycemia. Cortisol and growth hormone (GH) have a limited role in the homeostatic (counter-regulatory) response to acute hypoglycemia. However, chronic deficiencies of cortisol and/or GH can present as hypoglycemic emergencies (Figure 31-1) (31).

Post-prandial glucose levels are maintained by nutrient entry from the gut. In the post-absorptive state, plasma glucose is maintained by the balance of glucose release from the liver (initially glycogenolysis and then gluconeogenesis) and uptake by peripheral tissues (predominantly peripheral muscle). Hepatic glucose production is acutely regulated by the inhibitory action of insulin and the stimulatory signals of glucagon and the autonomic nervous system (ANS). Peripheral glucose uptake is regulated by insulin levels, degree of insulin resistance, and catecholamine levels (predominantly epinephrine). Glucagon has a very limited effect, if at all, on influencing peripheral glucose uptake.

As glucose levels fall, the first counter-regulatory response is to inhibit endogenous insulin release. This occurs at plasma glucose levels below 80 mg/dL (4.5 mmol/L). At ~70 mg/dL (3.9 mmol/L), the powerful anti-insulin counter-regulatory hormones (glucagon, epinephrine, cortisol, GH) are released "in concerto." In conjunction with reduced insulin levels, increasing glucagon levels stimulate hepatic glycogenolysis and gluconeogenesis. Epinephrine has a complementary and multifaceted role in the defense against hypoglycemia by stimulating hepatic glucose production (initially via glycogenolysis, then gluconeogenesis from the liver and kidney), adipose tissue lipolysis, and skeletal muscle glycogenolysis and proteolysis, while inhibiting glucose uptake by insulin-responsive tissues. The combined adrenomedullary and direct neural ANS effects on lipolysis are an additional important counter-regulatory mechanism. In fact, lipolysis provides ~25% of the defense against a falling glucose by providing glycerol and free fatty acids (FFA) as substrate and energy, respectively, for gluconeogenesis. Furthermore, elevated FFA levels provide an alternative fuel substrate for muscle, thereby preserving circulating glucose. The "threshold" level of norepinephrine release during a falling plasma glucose is difficult to determine. Hyperinsulinemia, even during euglycemic conditions, will stimulate ANS activity and norepinephrine release. If hypoglycemia is prolonged (>4 hours), then GH and cortisol begin to play a role in the counter-regulatory metabolic defense. Both can stimulate hepatic glucose production (gluconeogenesis) and inhibit glucose uptake. However, the contribution of both of these hormones is only about 20% to that of epinephrine.

Hypoglycemia manifests as an array of autonomic (i.e., palpitations, tremor, sweating, pallor and anxiety) and neuroglycopenic (i.e., behavior changes, fatigue, seizure, loss of consciousness) signs and symptoms (Figure 31-2). The glucose threshold for the generation of autonomic signs and symptoms is plastic in nature but is typically ~60 mg/dL (3.3 mmol/L). Neuroglycopenic signs and symptoms arising from a central nervous system glucose deficit occur at lower BG levels ~50 mg/dL (2.8 mmol/L). It should be noted

that hunger, per se, is a poor symptom discriminator for hypoglycemia. The origins of autonomic signs and symptoms are complex but sympathoadrenal output appears to be the primary driver. Epinephrine is responsible for ~20–25% of the symptoms of hypoglycemia, suggesting that a large portion of signs and symptoms arise from sympathetic neural activation (32). The ability to recognize hypoglycemic symptoms within oneself is known as hypoglycemia awareness. Autonomic signs and symptoms are the indicators most recognizable to the patient, but the specific combination of symptoms experienced during a hypoglycemic episode varies inter- and intra-individually.

Hormonal counter-regulatory responses and hypoglycemic symptoms occur at similar thresholds in men and women, but in women, peak counter-regulatory hormone levels are lower (33,34). The reason for these gender differences is not well understood, but increased levels of estrogen may play an important role (35).

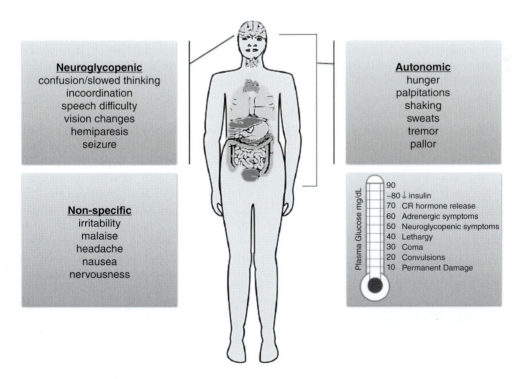

Figure 31-2 Symptoms and signs of hypoglycemia.
CR: counter-regulatory

Pathophysiology of Glucose Metabolism in Diabetes

In T1DM and insulin-deficient T2DM individuals, there are a number of pathophysiologic defects that reduce the counterregulatory response to hypoglycemia. These include:

- *First defense*: Inhibition of endogenous insulin secretion is lost in patients with absolute insulin deficiency (i.e., T1DM and longer-duration T2DM patients who are dependent on insulin therapy). Absolute insulin deficiency precludes a physiologic mechanism to reduce insulin levels, leaving the diabetic individual defenseless to previously dosed long-acting insulin or residual insulin within the subcutaneous (SC) depot, which will sustain circulating insulin levels in the face of a falling BG. Residual, albeit impaired, insulin secretion in shorter-duration T2DM provides a buffer against decreasing BG levels, as insulin secretion can still be physiologically inhibited.
- *Secondary defense*: After a duration of about 5 years, there is a loss of glucagon response to hypoglycemia in T1DM. It is postulated that the glucagon response may be lost either as a result of a signaling defect within the pancreatic alpha cell due to a lack of a reduction in endogenous insulin and/or ANS input. However, alpha cells in T1DM are present in normal number and size and respond appropriately to other physiologic stress (i.e., exercise, amino acids). Without adequate glucagon secretion, the usual rapid response (10–15 minutes) of glucose production from the liver is reduced. Glycogenolysis and later gluconeogenesis (if glycerol, lactate, pyruvate and amino acids are available) may also be impaired.
- *Third defense*: A reduction of epinephrine response occurs. The ability to promote glucose recovery from hypoglycemia is dependent upon epinephrine-mediated beta-adrenergic mechanisms in the glucagon deficient state (36). This is especially prominent after antecedent hypoglycemia or associated with classic diabetic autonomic neuropathy. Without adequate epinephrine stimulation, hepatic glycogenolysis and later hepatic and renal gluconeogenesis are impaired. Stimulation of lipolysis is also consequently blunted, reducing available FFA and glycerol and maintaining reliance on circulating glucose. The inhibitory effect of epinephrine on skeletal muscle glucose uptake is lost and hypoglycemia can be extended.
- *Signs and symptoms*: Symptom responses become blunted together with reduced hormonal counter-regulatory responses (37). Reduced epinephrine levels are a factor, but reduced sympathetic neural outflow may also be implicated. Importantly, autonomic symptoms are initiated at progressively lower BG levels, and therefore autonomic and neuroglycopenic symptom thresholds become compressed, allowing less time to recognize and appropriately respond to a low blood glucose level before cognitive dysfunction ensues.

Failure of these protective mechanisms can lead to severe, unimpeded hypoglycemia. In cases of recurring episodes of hypoglycemia, the threshold for initiation of counter-regulatory hormone responses is reduced to a lower plasma glucose level and hormone responses become blunted. A blunted epinephrine response increases the risk of iatrogenic hypoglycemia 25-fold (38). Patients also develop hypoglycemia unawareness, in which symptoms are delayed and blunted and may be unrecognizable to the individual. Hypoglycemia unawareness, affecting ~20-25% of T1DM patients (39) and increasingly recognized in T2DM (40), elevates the risk of severe hypoglycemia six-fold.

Collectively, the reduction of hormonal and symptom responses to recurring episodes of hypoglycemia (or other stressors that stimulate autonomic activation) is part of a disorder termed hypoglycemia-associated autonomic failure (HAAF) (41), the presence of which further increases the risk of severe hypoglycemia

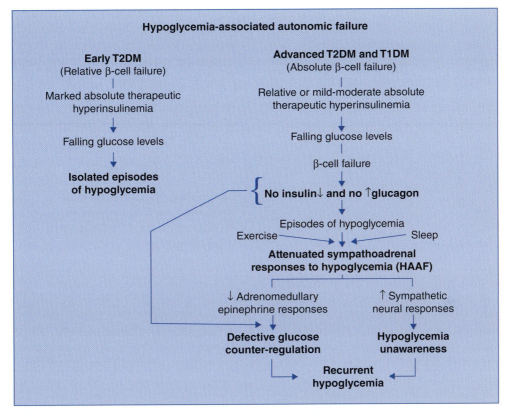

Figure 31-3 Hypoglycemia-associated failure (HAAF) in the pathogenesis of iatrogenic hypoglycemia in diabetes. Reproduced with permission from John Wiley & Sons, Ltd.

(Figure 31-3). HAAF develops independently of the presence of classic diabetic autonomic neuropathy and is not intrinsic to the diabetic state, as the syndrome can be induced in healthy non-diabetic individuals subjected to recurrent bouts of hyperinsulinemic hypoglycemia (42). Mild antecedent hypoglycemia <70 mg/dL (3.9 mmol/L) is sufficient to induce blunted glucagon and epinephrine responses to hypoglycemia on the following day. Deeper levels of hypoglycemia (60 and 52 mg/dL [3.3 and 2.9 mmol/L]) have more widespread effects, additionally reducing norepinephrine and GH levels as well as endogenous glucose production and lipolysis in response to next day hypoglycemia (43). Temporally, even very short periods of hypoglycemia (i.e., 5–30 minutes) cause substantial blunting of hormonal responses to subsequent hypoglycemia (44). Related components of HAAF include exercise and sleep. Prolonged low to moderate endurance exercise blunts counter-regulatory responses to subsequent hypoglycemia (45), while, reciprocally, antecedent hypoglycemia blunts counter-regulatory responses to exercise (46). In either scenario, the patient is exposed to a greater risk of developing hypoglycemia. During sleep, counter-regulatory responses to and awareness of hypoglycemia are delayed and reduced (47), and prolonged nocturnal hypoglycemia is a common occurrence (48). Furthermore, nocturnal hypoglycemia blunts responses to next-day hypoglycemia (49). HAAF likely arises through multiple adaptive mechanisms which are comprehensively reviewed elsewhere (41).

A number of interventions have been shown to at least partially rescue counter-regulatory responses to hypoglycemia. First, strict avoidance of hypoglycemia by relaxing glycemic targets and educating patients about preventive strategies can help to recover hypoglycemia awareness and epinephrine responses (50). Experimental pharmacologic interventions that enhance responses to hypoglycemia and/or minimize blunting effects of antecedent hypoglycemia include fluoxetine and sertraline (selective-serotonin reuptake inhibitors), naloxone (opioid receptor blocker), and diazoxide (suppresses insulin secretion via ATP-sensitive K+ channel opening mechanisms) (51).

Age Considerations

Compared to their younger counterparts, older people with diabetes are at increased risk of severe hypoglycemia, especially in cases of longer duration diabetes and limited residual insulin secretion (52). Although controversial, some data suggests that this may be a result of delayed initiation of hormonal responses and/or symptoms (lower BG levels are required to stimulate counter-regulatory responses) (53) or reduced symptom scores in the face of a normal hormonal response (54,55). Reduced perception of milder hypoglycemia may occur with aging in general, as similar impairments were found in older individuals with and without T2DM (53). Regular education regarding symptom identification and treatment options is crucial in this population as well as ongoing assessment of cognitive function (56).

Case Study

A 78-year-old man with a 19-year history of T2DM complicated by chronic kidney disease (CKD) stage 3A (eGFR 58 ml/min) and microalbuminuria returns for evaluation. He is currently taking metformin 1 g twice daily and sitagliptin 50 mg daily. Blood pressure is 134/70, 75 kg, BMI is 24 kg/m². Exam is unremarkable. His last HbA1c was 7.7% (60 mmol/mol) and basal insulin was initiated at 0.2 units/kg or 15 units before bedtime. He now reports average fasting capillary BG levels between 93–135 mg/dL

(5.2–7.5 mmol/L). His current HbA1c is 6.5% (48 mmol/mol). On further questioning, he reports waking in the middle of the night 2–3 times per week with hunger and sweats. He does not check his BG during these episodes, but will often eat a small sandwich. He reports similar symptoms after the lunch meal and this prevents him from an afternoon walk. He is very happy with his blood glucose control.

Do You Think His Current HbA1c Is an Appropriate Target in View of His Age/Longevity of Diabetes/and Other Factors?

This case illustrates the untoward effects of over-aggressive blood glucose treatment in elderly patients. An HbA1c goal in an older patient with mild CKD could reasonably be individualized and considered <7.5–8% (59–64 mmol/mol). This could be an opportunity to discuss in detail dietary and lifestyle changes that could improve the blood glucose levels without additional medical therapy. The addition of basal insulin, whilst effective and started at a relatively low dose, increases the risk of hypoglycemia (as it did in this patient).

Additionally, this is a very good opportunity to educate the patient on signs and symptoms of hypoglycemia and instruction on validating symptoms with a BG; and the appropriate treatment for hypoglycemia. This case illustrates that although a fasting BG of <135 mg/dL (7.5 mmol/L) may be acceptable in this patient, it is reflective of the small meal being eaten in the middle of the night to treat symptoms of what we suspect is a nocturnal hypoglycemia (which should either be confirmed with SMBG at the time of the episode or occasional 3 a.m. BG levels).

Management of Hypoglycemia

Most cases of hypoglycemia in patients with diabetes are self-diagnosed and

Table 31-2 Management of mild, self-diagnosed and treated hypoglycemia

1. Take 15–20 grams of carbohydrate:
   - 3-4 glucose tablets;
   - 4 oz (1/2 cup) of fruit juice;
   - 6 oz (1/2 can) of regular soda.
2. Retest and wait 15 minutes.
3. Recheck blood glucose.
4. Repeat steps 1–3 if blood glucose still less than 80 mg/dL (4.4 mmol/L).
5. If blood glucose remains less than 70 mg/dL (3.9 mmol/L) after 30–45 minutes or 3 cycles, contact clinician.
6. Once blood glucose is > 80 mg/dL (4.4 mmol/L), give long-acting complex carbohydrate.

addressed at home, without intervention of a medical provider. Initial treatment generally consists of 15–20 grams of simple carbohydrate to ameliorate the symptoms of mild hypoglycemia (Table 31-2, Figure 31-4). For a measured blood glucose of <50 mg/dL (2.8 mmol/L), 20–30 grams of carbohydrate should be considered. If the person is treated with an alpha-glucosidase inhibitor, only pure glucose gel or tablets should be taken, as this drug class inhibits absorption of other forms of carbohydrate. It is unknown how effective oral glucose supplementation is in the setting of delayed gastric emptying, for example with gastroparesis or with medications that delay gastric emptying like glucagon-like peptide-1 (GLP-1) agonists, anti-cholinergic, and narcotics. Foods containing fats should not be ingested when treating for hypoglycemia, as fats delay absorption of glucose. Blood glucose should be measured 15 minutes after consuming carbohydrate, and additional carbohydrate should be ingested if hypoglycemia or hypoglycemic symptoms persist. Glucagon kits can be prescribed to patients with diabetes, and friends, family members or co-workers

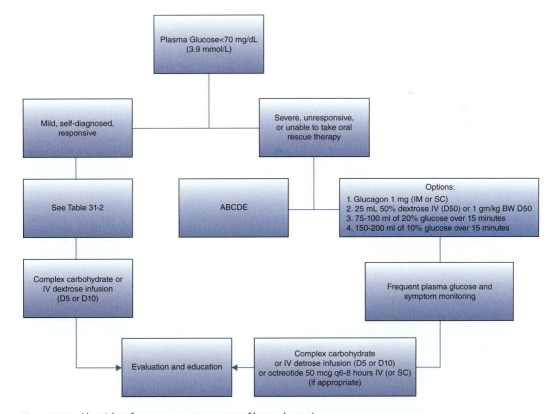

Figure 31-4 Algorithm for acute management of hypoglycemia
ABCDE = Airway; Breathing; Circulation; Disability (i.e. conscious level) and Exposure (i.e. examination and evaluation); BW = body weight; IM = intramuscular; IV = intravenous; SC = subcutaneous

can be trained to administer glucagon (1 mg) SC or intramuscularly (IM), if the patient is unable or unwilling to ingest glucose orally. The effects of glucagon, which acts through stimulation of hepatic glycogenolysis, are delayed by approximately 10 minutes from time of injection and are only inducible in those with available glycogen stores. Of note, family members or responders should avoid sublingual placement of carbohydrates (i.e., hard candy) in an unconscious or impaired individual as this can increase the risk for aspiration. After resolution of hypoglycemia, a full meal or complex snack should be consumed as an insulin depot may still be active and to restore glycogen stores. Pseudohypoglycemia in the setting of regimen intensification in an individual with previously uncontrolled glucose levels should be treated with ~5 grams of carbohydrates to avoid over-correction and the individual should receive reassurance that they will adapt to improved glycemic control in about 3–4 weeks.

Severe hypoglycemia requiring assistance of a second or third party should be assessed and addressed in the hospital setting. Initial assessment and management should begin with the ABCDEs (Airway; Breathing; Circulation; Disability [i.e., conscious level]; and Exposure [i.e., examination and evaluation]) (Figure 31-4). Consideration should always be given to other acute medical conditions that may mimic or coincide with hypoglycemia (e.g., acute coronary syndrome, acute ischemic stroke, sepsis, and shock). However, rapid recognition of a low glucose is imperative as prolonged severe hypoglycemia can result in irreversible brain damage, cardiovascular strain, and death (25,57).

The majority of protocols for emergency medical responders indicate the use of 25 g of 50% dextrose in water (D50), although some protocols indicate D10 (10% dextrose) or provide both D10 and D50 as treatment options (58). IM glucagon is used in the setting of lack of intravenous (IV) access. Patients hospitalized for hypoglycemia can be initially managed with IV infusion of 25 g of D50 or 1 g/kg of body weight D50. D50 is an irritant and delivery through a large gauge port and vein, followed by a saline flush, is preferable. Alternatively, D20 (20% dextrose) or D10 are less irritating and can be administered via a peripheral vein in a proportionally larger volume. In fact, use of D10 and D20 glucose solutions are now the preferred preparation recommended in the United Kingdom for inpatient IV glucose resuscitation (Figure 31-4) (59).

As in self-treated patients, once euglycemia is attained, a meal or a snack including carbohydrate and protein should be ingested to prevent a recurrent episode of hypoglycemia. If oral intake is not an option, D5 or D10 can be infused to maintain euglycemia. Parenteral or enteric feeding may be considered in individuals to replenish glycogen stores as clinically indicated. In cases of sulfonylurea-induced hypoglycemia, glucose administration can actually stimulate continued insulin secretion, and the somatostatin analog octreotide, 50–100 mcg administered IV or SC every 8 hours, can be used to inhibit insulin secretion and prevent recurring hypoglycemia in this setting (60). Exogenous administration of long-acting and ultra-long-acting insulin (e.g., U100/U200 insulin degludec; U300 insulin glargine), resulting in persistent hypoglycemia, will require the administration of infused dextrose or continuous carbohydrate ingestion till the duration of insulin action is surpassed.

Individuals with malnutrition or suspected long-term alcohol use should receive thiamine (100 mg IV) to reduce the risk for Wernicke's encephalopathy (61). These individuals may also benefit from enteral or parenteral feeding due to reduced glycogen stores. When adrenal crisis is suspected, administration of IV saline solution and glucocorticoids with IV hydrocortisone 50–100 mg IV will provide glucocorticoid, mineralocorticoid, and vascular support (62). Hydrocortisone can be transitioned to oral therapy once the individual is stabilized.

In the case of suspected inborn errors of metabolism (Table 31-3), specific

Table 31-3 Inborn errors of metabolism causing hypoglycemia (63)

Fasting hypoglycemia	
Glycogen storage disorders	Types I, III, O, Fanconi-Bickel (GLUT 2)
Defect in fatty acid oxidation	CPT1, VLCAD, MCAD, SCHAD, LCHAD, HMG-CoA synthase and lyase
Gluconeogenesis	fructose 1,6-bisphosphatase
Post-prandial hypoglycemia	
Non-insulinoma pancreatogenic hypoglycemia syndrome	Mutations in SUR1, Kir6.2, SCHAD, GDH, glucokinase, MCT1 (also associated with exercise induced hypoglycemia); UCP2
Congenital disorders of glycosylation	Types 1a, 1b, 1d
Inherited fructose intolerance	

CPT = carnitine palmitoyltransferase, GDH = glutamate dehydrogenase; GLUT 2 = Glucose transporter 2; HMG = 3-hydroxy-3-methyl-glutary; LCHAD = long-chain 3 hydroxyacyl-Co-A dehydrogenase; MCAD = medium-chain acyl-CoA dehydrogenase; MCT = monocarboxylate transporter; SCHAD = short chain L-3-hydroxyacyl-Co-A dehydrogenase; UCP = mitochondrial uncoupling protein; VLCAD = very long-chain acyl-CoA dehydrogenase.

treatments may be indicated (63). For example, fructose elimination is the treatment for inherited fructose intolerance; carnitine supplementation and/or avoidance of fasting and maintenance of glucose levels during stress in mitochondrial fatty acid oxidation disorders; and avoidance of stress, frequent meals (especially overnight), and the use of uncooked starch supplementation in glycogen storage diseases.

Blood glucose measurements should be repeated every 15–30 minutes for at least 2 hours, or longer depending on the etiology, following resolution of hypoglycemia (3,4). Symptoms and signs of hypoglycemia should resolve once euglycemia is achieved and maintained. However, alternative diagnosis (i.e., stroke, delirium, drug overdose) should be considered if symptoms persist despite euglycemia.

Etiology

Once an individual and the serum glucose have been stabilized, evaluation of the underlying etiology is imperative to reduce the risk of future episodes of hypoglycemia and, in the case of non-diabetes-associated hypoglycemia, to ultimately treat the underlying condition (Table 31-4). The focus of investigation is markedly different in those individuals with diabetes and those with non-diabetes-associated hypoglycemia.

Non-Hospitalized Individuals

All outpatient encounters with individuals with diabetes should address hypoglycemia. Patients with diabetes (T1DM or T2DM) with frequent and/or severe hypoglycemia that is treated outside of the hospital require an extensive review of treatment regimen and adherence, timing and frequency of hypoglycemia, timing and frequency of hypoglycemia to medication administration (especially in those treated with insulin and insulin secretagogues or treatments that are in combination with either), new medications (such as indomethacin, non-selective beta-blockers and antibiotics like trimethoprim-sulfamethoxazole), and alcohol use. An individual should provide the glucose value at which they first feel hypoglycemic symptoms or signs. It is important to recognize that antihyperglycemic agents that are not routinely associated with hypoglycemia (i.e., GLP-1 agonists, dipeptidyl-dipeptidase-4 [DPP-4] inhibitors,

Table 31-4 Etiologies and possible mechanisms of hypoglycemia

Increased insulin
- Exogenous insulin
- Sulfonylurea
- Meglitinides
- Quinine
- Trimethoprim-sulfamethoxazole
- Alcohol
- Insulinoma
- Insulin or insulin receptor antibodies (autoimmune)

Impaired gluconeogenesis/glycogenolysis
- Salicylates
- Beta-adrenergic blockers
- Hepatic failure
- Renal failure
- Alcohol

Counter-regulatory failure
- Autonomic dysfunction
- Exercise
- Addison's disease
- Pan-hypopituitarism
- Growth hormone deficiency
- Hypothyroidism

Increased insulin sensitivity
- Exercise
- Weight loss
- Fasting

Increased glucose utilization/peripheral tissue uptake
- Exercise
- Sepsis

Complex mechanisms
- Mesenchymal tumors (IGF-2)
- Islet cell hyperplasia
- Inborn errors of metabolism

Beta cell toxicity
- Pentamidine

Decreased insulin clearance
- Renal failure

Reactive hypoglycemia
- Idiopathic
- Dumping syndrome (including post-bariatric surgery)

IGF-2 = Insulin-like growth factor-2.

thiazolidinediones [TZD], acarbose, metformin, sodium glucose co-transporter 2 [SGLT2] inhibitors), may result in unanticipated hypoglycemic events when combined with insulin and/or sulfonylureas (64). A detailed exercise or weight loss history can elucidate why particular patients may be more insulin-sensitive. Social situations like Ramadan fasting may necessitate temporary changes to an individual's diabetic regimen or the addition of a continuous glucose monitor (CGM) for improved glucose monitoring (65). Food insecurity should also be assessed. Patients with T1DM may require additional structured education on carbohydrate counting and review of the often complex regimens that accompany insulin pump therapy. New or worsening neuropathy may be a red flag to indicate evaluation of autonomic dysfunction and hypoglycemic unawareness. Progressive renal disease may lead to decreased clearance of insulin or sulfonylureas and their metabolites (i.e., glyburide [glibenclamide]) (66). An increased risk for adrenal insufficiency and thyroid disease may prompt appropriate evaluation in individuals with T1DM (67).

A meta-analysis (CONTROL) based on a number of large studies investigating the effect of tight glycemic control in T2DM patients has shown a small effect on reducing the risk of major cardiovascular disease within 5 years of intensification of therapy (68). As expected, microvascular benefits were also evident. However, the meta-analysis (CONTROL) suggested that overall intensive glycemic control caused about twice the number of severe hypoglycemic events than the microvascular and macrovascular events it prevented. In addition, one of the component studies (ACCORD) demonstrated that intensive glycemic control was associated with increased mortality (although increased mortality was not seen overall in the CONTROL meta-analysis) and a higher frequency of hypoglycemia (68,69). These findings and recommendations from ADA/EASD should always prompt the provider to review and individualize treatment goals based on age and comorbidities, while taking into account the established microvascular and macrovascular benefits of improved glycemic control (68,70). Implementation of flexible insulin regimens, increased frequency of self-monitoring of blood glucose (SMBG), and CGM should be considered, such as investigated in the Dose Adjustment for Normal Eating (DAFNE) trial (71). A switch to insulin pump therapy may be considered in individuals with T1DM (or T2DM with absolute insulin deficiency) with frequent hypoglycemia. Use of insulin pump therapy has been shown to improve glycemic control while reducing the rate of hypoglycemia (72,73).

The dangerous condition of hypoglycemic unawareness is prevalent in patients with absolute insulin deficiency (i.e., T1DM or long-duration T2DM) and can lead to a vicious cycle of hypoglycemia (Figure 31-3). There can be a substantial fear of nocturnal hypoglycemia and the associated "dead in bed" syndrome that precludes adequate treatment and achievement of glycemic goals. Review of basal regimens and bedtime glucose monitoring may be necessary. Newer basal insulins, such as insulin U300 glargine and insulin degludec (U100/U200), appear to reduce nocturnal hypoglycemia in T2DM and T1DM (74,75). The role of CGM and/or insulin pumps in persons with type 1 or type 2 diabetes, including those with significant issues with hypoglycemia were recently reviewed in an Endocrine Society 2016 guideline (76). The use of CGM to alert individuals or close third-parties to a rapidly falling glucose and/or use of low glucose suspension thresholds on insulin pumps to automatically halt insulin delivery can reduce nocturnal hypoglycemia. The low-glucose suspend technology will automatically pause insulin delivery from the insulin pump for up to 2 hours when an individual does not respond to the present low glucose alarm. In a recent study in T1DM patients using a low glucose suspend feature on the insulin pump, nocturnal hypoglycemia was reduced by 31.8% compared with controls (77). Sensor-augmented insulin pump therapy also reduces glycemic variability and achieves improved glycemic

goals compared to multi-daily injections without an increased rate of hypoglycemia (76,78). Accuracy of CGM systems, especially at lower BG levels, continues to improve (79). More recently, a number of pilot studies have shown that insulin pumps and CGM work well as part of a closed-loop ("artificial pancreas") system in both type 1 and type 2 diabetes patients, in both the inpatient and outpatient settings. These initial studies hold promise of patients with diabetes spending more "time in (glycemic) range" without hypoglycemia.

Scrupulous avoidance of hypoglycemia by changing target glucoses and toleration of a higher threshold of average glucose for as little as 3 weeks can help improve symptom awareness to hypoglycemia in individuals with T1DM and T2DM (41).

Exercise

Exercise is a significant component of the larger diabetes treatment plan. However, exercise-associated hypoglycemia can prevent individuals from embracing this beneficial intervention. Exercise-associated hypoglycemia can occur within minutes to several hours post-exercise (80). Thus, patient education regarding the timing of exercise to insulin/secretagogue administration, carbohydrate ingestion and frequent glucose monitoring before, during and after exercise are necessary to address this risk.

Alcohol

Alcohol consumption can block the release of hepatic glucose stores, leading to hypoglycemia. Fasting, sustained physical exercise, malnutrition, and medication administration (i.e., insulin or insulin secretagogues) are precipitating factors (81). Alcohol can cause hypoglycemia up to 24 hours after ingestion. Recommendations from the ADA include limited alcohol consumption, increasing non-alcohol hydration (i.e., water, tonic water), and avoidance of using alcohol carbohydrates in carbohydrate counting and maintaining carbohydrate intake while consuming alcohol. Increased frequency of SMBG may be necessary and should be performed prior to bedtime (3).

Other Activities

Specific recommendations should be provided to individuals at risk for hypoglycemia or in whom one is evaluating for hypoglycemia regarding driving and recreational activities like scuba diving. Driving restrictions have recently been relaxed in Europe and the USA for individuals with diabetes (82). However, individuals with diabetes should not drive if they have hypoglycemic unawareness or recent severe hypoglycemia (i.e., within the last 12 months). They should receive regular diabetes education and evaluation. Prior to driving, SMBG should be checked and rechecked at 1–2 hour intervals. Drivers should wait at least 45 minutes to drive after BG has returned to normal and a fast-acting supply of carbohydrates should always be available.

Pregnancy

Maternal hypoglycemia during pregnancy is a risk factor for newborns small for gestational age, which in turn is associated with increased long-term risks, such as development of diabetes, coronary artery disease, and hypertension (83). Post-absorptive BG tends to decline in non-diabetic women during pregnancy by ~10 mg/dL (0.55 mmol/L), with a reported mean of 71 mg/dL (4.1 mmol/L) (84), although BG measurements <70 mg/dL (3.9 mmol/L) are not abnormal. Therefore, recommendations for target pre-meal, post-prandial and average daily BG levels in pregnant women with diabetes are <95 mg/dl (5.3 mmol/L), <140 mg/dL (7.8 mmol/L) and <120 mg/dL (6.7 mmol/L), respectively, with a target HbA1c 6.0–6.5% (42–48 mmol/mol) (3). Reports generally indicate that hormonal counter-regulatory responses to hypoglycemia are impaired during pregnancy (85), but risk of severe hypoglycemia is related to a history of severe

hypoglycemia, hypoglycemia unawareness, >10 years' diabetes duration, larger total daily dose of insulin, and HbA1c <6.5% (<48 mmol/mol) (11). Recommendations for reducing the risk of hypoglycemia include educating pregnant women regarding recognizing and treating of hypoglycemia, SMBG and CGM, maintaining an available supply of carbohydrate snacks, and timing exercise, food consumption, and insulin dosing. Additionally, intensified glycemic control prior to pregnancy may help reduce risk, while relaxing glycemic targets is recommended for women reporting impaired awareness (3,84).

Case Study

A 28-year-old female with a 2-year history of T1DM is interested in fertility planning. She has been advised to aggressively treat her BG levels to target an HbA1c of <6.5% (48 mmol/mol). Multi-daily injection insulin therapy was stopped and she is on a combination of insulin pump and continuous glucose monitoring (CGM). In the office, her HbA1c is 5.9% (41 mmol/mol) and she is very happy and would like to stop her oral birth control pill.

On review of her CGM download, she has significant glucose variability and spends >15% of recorded time with a BG <70 mg/dL (3.9 mmol/L). Her BG range is 45–350 mg/dL (2.5–19.4 mmol/L). She has suspended the low glucose alert alarm on the CGM. She reports that she has had two specific times in the last month with a BG <50 mg/dL (2.8 mmol/L) in which she has had no symptoms. It is taking more time and more carbohydrate to normalize her BG levels than previously.

Would You Agree with the Patient that She Should Stop Her Contraceptive Now and Try and Get Pregnant?

This case illustrates hypoglycemic unawareness. An improvement in overall average

BG was at the expense of significant hypoglycemia. It is reasonable to consider relaxing her glycemic control to achieve a 2- to 3-week period of active avoidance (zero tolerance) of hypoglycemia. Using the CGM technology (i.e., re-activating the low- and high-glucose level alarms) appropriately may also help.

This is not the correct time to encourage pregnancy. Although her HbA1c is at the target range for pregnancy, her frequent and severe hypoglycemia may be a risk factor for fetal complications. In addition, she is at increased risk for severe hypoglycemia during a potential pregnancy due to her history of severe hypoglycemia, long duration of diabetes, and current HbA1c.

Hospitalized Individuals

The preceding discussion of the evaluation of hypoglycemia in the outpatient individual with diabetes should be a component of the assessment of the inpatient person with diabetes with hypoglycemia. A detailed medication history and reconciliation are imperative especially in the elderly with greater likelihood of polypharmacy. This should include the individual's outpatient diabetic regimen, and if this was continued, adjusted, and/or altered as an inpatient. Hypoglycemic events can be prevented with improved coordination of patient transfer within the hospital setting and at discharge. Systematic verification processes (preferably including electronic prescribing and administration resources) for insulin administration, especially with use of U500 regular insulin and other concentrated insulins (e.g., U200; U300) can identify incorrect prescriptions and administration errors (86,87). Hypoglycemia can occur when there is failure to recognize or adjust insulin regimens based on available BG data. Continuation of prandial insulin or insulin secretagogue therapy in individuals who are not eating or have been placed on a diet restriction should be identified and corrected, as should insulin therapy in patients in whom parenteral or enteral feeding is interrupted. There is a limited role for non-insulin glucose-lowering agents in the inpatient setting. Concomitant malnourishment, renal or hepatic disease, sepsis, malignancy and rapid withdrawal of glucocorticoid therapy may alter peripheral glucose uptake, gluconeogenesis and glycogenolysis, and medication clearance (88). The challenges posed with the use of insulin in hospitalized patients occur throughout all areas of this care setting. For example, the UK 2016 National Diabetes Inpatient Audit (NaDIA) revealed that almost half (46%) of inpatients treated with insulin had an error (i.e., prescription or medication management) related to insulin therapy (89). In addition, 1 in 5 inpatients (20%) with diabetes had a hypoglycemic episode during their hospital stay, with almost 1 in 12 (8%) having severe hypoglycemia (89). For inpatients with type 1 diabetes, almost a quarter (27%) of inpatients had a severe hypoglycemic episode during their hospital stay (89).

All hospitalized patients with diabetes benefit from a structured diabetes care plan, ideally supervised by specialists (90). As recommended by the ADA, glycemic goals should be tailored to the patient, surgical versus medical status, and level of acuity. Most critically ill patients managed in an intensive care unit (ICU) or similar setting, should aim for BG levels from 140–180 mg/dL (7.8–10 mmol/L); and less-intensive patients should aim for pre-meal BG levels <140 mg/dL (7.8 mmol/L) and random BG levels <180 mg/dL (10 mmol/L) if they can be achieved safely (i.e., without excessive risk of hypoglycemia). The use of IV insulin infusion in critically ill patients is the most effective method for controlling BG (91). Validated written or computerized algorithms should be employed for adjustments to IV insulin infusion rate based on fluctuations in BG (90). The Endocrine Society has recommended that non-ICU patients benefit from structured basal and/or nutritional/correction with rapid-acting insulin (92).

Non-Diabetic Individuals

Non-diabetes-associated hypoglycemia is essentially a failure of endogenous glucose production to match high rates of glucose utilization. An extensive history, physical, and laboratory review should be undertaken to identify drug-induced hypoglycemia, hormonal deficiencies, critical illness, and/or reactive hypoglycemia. Mechanisms of drug-induced hypoglycemia include exogenous hyperinsulinemia, impaired gluconeogenesis, and increased insulin secretion (93). By extension, trials off these offending agents should be attempted. Alcohol use or abuse should also be documented. Hormonal deficiencies such as adrenal insufficiency (primary, secondary, or post-surgical Cushing's disease patients) and hypopituitarism can lead to failure of glucose counter-regulation. A plasma cortisol at the time of hypoglycemia may not be sufficient to diagnose adrenal insufficiency and should be followed by a formal short ACTH stimulation test (62). Hypothyroidism may be associated with abnormalities in the hypothalamic-pituitary-adrenal axis leading to hypoglycemia (94). Growth hormone deficiency is a rare cause of hypoglycemia. Sepsis can lead to increased glucose uptake whereas hepatic failure or severe malnutrition is associated with impaired gluconeogenesis and glycogenolysis. The kidney is responsible for 25–50% of total gluconeogenesis and individuals with advanced renal disease may present with hypoglycemia.

A childhood history of inherited metabolic disorders can also alert potential associations (i.e., hereditary fructose intolerance or multiple endocrine neoplasia [MEN] syndromes) or the risk for polyglandular syndromes (i.e., adrenal insufficiency, hypothyroidism, type 1 diabetes) (95). A number of inborn errors of metabolism can present with hypoglycemia (Table 31-3) (63).

This is usually the result of impaired gluconeogenesis and the inability to rely on ketone bodies for alternative fuel. Adult presentations of these disorders are usually less frequent and severe than the presentations observed in children. Hypoglycemia associated with encephalopathy, neurologic defects, multi-organ involvement and even death should raise one's suspicion of an inborn error of metabolism. Appropriate evaluation should include blood lactate, pyruvate, FFA, glycerol, ketones, amino acid profile, carnitine, acyl carnitine, and a galactosemia screen. Urine tests should include organic acids and carnitine (63).

Post-Bariatric Surgery

With a history of reactive or post-prandial hypoglycemia, documentation of recent bariatric or gastric surgery is helpful. As many as 30% of individuals in the post-gastric bypass population may experience asymptomatic hypoglycemia, however, a small group are actually hospitalized (1%) (96). When the different types of gastric bypass surgery (restrictive versus malabsorptive) were evaluated, the rapid delivery of nutrients to the lower gut (by virtue of excluding the proximal gut), appears to be the critical element in the manifestation of severe hypoglycemia (97). The mechanisms by which this occurs remain poorly understood. Reactive hypoglycemia results in inappropriate hyperinsulinemia and GLP-1 release that usually occurs within 4 hours of an ingested mixed-meal (98). The contribution of pancreatic islet nesidioblastosis; the contribution of GLP-1 action to beta cell proliferation; and/or association of post-bariatric hypoglycemia with insulinoma are also reported (99). Mixed-meal testing (over 5 hours) can be supportive to the diagnosis (4), and treatment can include surgery (i.e., partial pancreatectomy in the case of nesidioblastosis although many patients experience repeat hypoglycemia post-procedure, likely due to diffuse β-cell changes throughout the pancreas), dietary modifications (i.e., long-acting carbohydrate sources or small frequent meals), and/or pharmaceutical treatment (i.e., alpha-glucosidase inhibitor, calcium channel blockers, diazoxide, or somatostatin analogs such as octreotide, lanreotide, or pasireotide) (100).

Rare Etiologies

In individuals without historical or physical findings that elucidate the etiology of hypoglycemia and who satisfy Whipple's triad, it is reasonable to perform diagnostic differentiation of endogenous and exogenous hyperinsulinemia from other causes. At the time of hypoglycemia, plasma glucose, insulin, C-peptide, proinsulin, beta-hydroxybutyrate, and an oral sulfonylurea screen that includes glinides should be obtained. Following the lab draw, administering glucagon IV and subsequent 30-minute plasma glucose can evaluate hepatic glycogen stores. Critical diagnostic values are plasma insulin of ≥3 μU/mL (18 pmol/L), C-peptide ≥0.6 ng/mL (0.2 nmol/L) and proinsulin of ≥5 pmol/L when the plasma glucose is <55 mg/dL (3 mmol/L). A beta-hydroxybutyrate level ≤2.7 mmol/L and an increase of at least 25 mg/dL (1.4 mmol/L) of plasma glucose after glucagon stimulation indicate normal glycogen stores. The patterns of specific laboratory findings and associated diagnoses can be found in the Endocrine Guidelines for evaluation and management of adult hypoglycemic disorders (4). Obtaining insulin antibodies will identify those with insulin autoimmune-mediated hypoglycemia (i.e., one of the mechanisms of hypoglycemia are insulin antibodies directly stimulating the insulin receptor). Rarely, insulin receptor antibodies make a diagnosis (101). Treatment of autoimmune hypoglycemia with immunosuppressant therapy is variably effective, but the disease may be self-limiting. Non-islet cell tumors, such as large mesenchymal tumors or hepatocellular tumors, may secrete insulin-like growth factor-2 (IGF-2), which cross-reacts with the insulin receptor and/or increases glucose utilization due to the large size of the tumor. Surgery, radiation, or chemotherapy can often resolve hypoglycemia in these cases, but

medical therapy (as described above) can be utilized.

Recreating certain circumstances may help in obtaining the laboratory evaluation, such as timing with early morning, fasting or postprandial symptoms. Some patients can tolerate an overnight fast and others may require a formal 72-hour inpatient fast. Most patients with an insulinoma will meet diagnostic criteria in less than 72 hrs (102). Diagnosis of an insulinoma may be complicated. Because an insulin-sensitive individual, under high physiologic insulinemia, can have spuriously low venous plasma glucose, evaluation of insulinoma should be performed with a 72-hour fast rather than a 3-hour oral glucose tolerance test. They are often small (<1 cm) and negative imaging should not exclude the diagnosis. When traditional localization studies such as computed tomography (CT); magnetic resonance imaging (MRI); selective arterial secretagogue injection (SASI); and ultrasound (both standard and intraoperative) fail to identify a suspected insulinoma, newer imaging modalities which target somatostatin receptors such as ^{68}Ga-DOTATATE positron emission tomography (PET)/CT scanning may be considered as an adjunct imaging study when all of the standard imaging modalities are negative and especially when a focused or minimally invasive surgical approach is planned (103). Treatment of benign insulinoma is surgical resection. Treatment of malignant and/or metastatic insulinoma can include surgery and/or other cytoreductive therapies; and/or pharmaceutical treatments (e.g., diazoxide; somatostatin analogs such as octreotide, lanreotide, or pasireotide; or targeted therapies such as sunitinib or everolimus).

Lastly, evaluation of an otherwise healthy individual with hypoglycemia requires some consideration of malicious or surreptitious abuse of insulin or insulin secretagogue therapy or accidental inappropriate medication administration. This may be as simple as sending the urine sulfonylurea screen or close inspection of pills (medication reconciliation).

Case Study

An otherwise healthy 54-year-old man complains of intermittent episodes of sweats, jitters, and nausea for the last 6 months. He has a history of hypertension and pre-diabetes. These episodes are random, but reports that exercise can provoke symptoms. He was initially going to the gym up to 5 times per week but has now stopped because these episodes scare him. The episodes are often relieved by eating. His blood pressure is 135/82 mmHg, HR 75 bpm, BMI 29 kg/m². He has gained 8 lbs since he stopped going to the gym. His exam is unremarkable.

HbA1c is 5.5% (37 mmol/mol), Thyroid function tests are normal. AM cortisol is 20 μg/dL (550 nmol/L). Capillary BG during three different episodes are 72, 82 and 101 mg/dL (4, 4.6, and 5.6 mmol/L respectively). He is unable to obtain serum blood samples during these episodes because the symptoms are too intense and he is uncomfortable driving to the laboratory. Fasting blood glucose after an overnight fast is normal and sulfonylurea screen is negative. A diagnostic (professional or retrospective) continuous glucose monitor (CGM) demonstrates a BG level of 45 mg/dL (2.5 mmol/L) during a recorded episode, but is not confirmed with a serum sample.

He is admitted for a 72-hour fasting protocol. At 18 hours his capillary BG is 58 mg/dL (3.2 mmol/L) and a serum BG is 49 mg/dL (2.7 mmol/L). Insulin level at this time is 4.2 μU/mL (normal <3), proinsulin is 7 pmol/L (normal <5), C-peptide is 1.1 nmol/L (normal <0.2).

Beta-hydroxybutyrate is 0.6 mmol/L (normal >2.7). Glucagon is administered and BG rises to 92 mg/dL (5.1 mmol/L).

How Would You Interpret the 72-Hour Fasting Results?

This case illustrates the complexity in evaluating and diagnosing hyperinsulinemic hypoglycemia. Identifying Whipple's triad can be difficult. Utilizing alternative diagnostic technology can be helpful, such as a CGM. In situations of high suspicion, one must pursue a gold standard 72-hour fast. Most hyperinsulinemic hypoglycemia will declare itself within 24–48 hours of the 72-hour fast.

Critical diagnostic values are symptoms, signs, or both when the plasma glucose is <54 mg/dL (3 mmol/L), plasma insulin of ≥3 μU/mL (18 pmol/L), C-peptide ≥0.6 ng/mL (0.2 nmol/L) and proinsulin of ≥5 pmol/L document endogenous hyperinsulinism. A beta-hydroxybutyrate level ≤2.7 mmol/L and an increase of at least 25 mg/dL (1.4 mmol/L) of plasma glucose after glucagon stimulation (the latter showing intact glycogen stores) indicate mediation of the hypoglycemia by insulin (4).

Additional testing should include a screen for oral hypoglycemic agents, inspection of current medications, and insulin antibody testing. If these additional tests are negative, appropriate localizing imaging for an insulinoma should be pursued.

Conclusions

Acute hypoglycemia is a common endocrine emergency that requires prompt treatment and evaluation. Individuals with or without diabetes should be managed quickly with the same algorithm to avoid adverse morbidity and mortality. Most commonly seen in individuals with diabetes, an assessment of multiple factors including regimen, comorbid conditions and education is necessary. The evaluation of individuals without diabetes is more complex and requires a careful history and potentially laboratory evaluation to discern the underlying etiology. Ultimately, education is the key to prevention and early intervention.

Acknowledgments

This work was supported by the following grants: 5-R01-DK-069803, 5-P01-HL-056693, JDF-12001-828.

References

1 Leese GP, Wang J, Broomhall J, Kelly P, Marsden A, Morrison W, Frier BM, Morris AD. DARTS/MEMO Collaboration frequency of severe hypoglycemia requiring emergency treatment in type 1 and type 2 diabetes: a population-based study of health service resource use. *Diabetes Care*. 2003;26(4): 1176–1180.

2 The Diabetes Control and Complications Trial Research Group. Hypoglycemia in the diabetes control and complications trial. *Diabetes*. 1997;46(2):271–286.

3 American Diabetes Association. Standards of medical care in diabetes – 2018. *Diabetes Care* 41(Suppl 1):S1–S159.

4 Cryer PE, Axelrod L, Grossman AB, et al. Endocrine Society Evaluation and management of adult hypoglycemic disorders: an Endocrine Society Clinical Practice Guideline. *J Clin Endocrin Metab*. 2009;94(3):709–728.

5 Seaquist ER, Anderson J, Childs B, et al., American Diabetes Association. Endocrine Society Hypoglycemia and diabetes: a report of a workgroup of the American Diabetes Association and the Endocrine Society. *J Clin Endocrinol Metab*. 2013;98(5):1845–1859.

6 International Hypoglycaemia Study Group. Glucose concentrations of less than 3.0 mmol/L (54 mg/dL) should be reported in clinical trials: a joint position statement of the American Diabetes Association and the European Association for the Study of Diabetes. *Diabetes Care*. 2017;40(1):155–157.

7 Whipple A. The surgical therapy of hyperinsulinism. *J Int Chir*. 1938;3: 237–276.

8 Miller ME, Bonds DE, Gerstein HC, et al., ACCORD Investigators. The effects of baseline characteristics, glycaemia treatment approach, and glycated haemoglobin concentration on the risk of severe hypoglycaemia: post hoc epidemiological analysis of the ACCORD study. *BMJ*. 2010;340:b5444.

9 Zoungas S, Patel A, Chalmers J, et al., ADVANCE Collaborative Group. Severe hypoglycemia and risks of vascular events and death. *N Engl J Med*. 2010;363(15): 1410–1418.

10 Weinstock RS, Xing D, Maahs DM, et al., T1D Exchange Clinic Network. Severe hypoglycemia and diabetic ketoacidosis in adults with type 1 diabetes: results from the T1D exchange clinic registry. *J Clin Endocrinol Metab*. 2013;98(8):3411–3419.

11 Nielsen LR, Pedersen-Bjergaard U, Thorsteinsson B, Johansen M, Damm P, Mathiesen ER. Hypoglycemia in pregnant women with type 1 diabetes: predictors and role of metabolic control. *Diabetes Care*. 2008;31(1):9–14.

12 Mukherjee E, Carroll R, Matfin G. Endocrine and metabolic emergencies: hypoglycaemia. *Ther Adv Endocrinol Metab*. 2011;2(2):81–93.

13 Ginde AA, Espinola JA, Camargo CA, Jr. Trends and disparities in U.S. emergency department visits for hypoglycemia, 1993-2005. *Diabetes Care*. 2008;31(3): 511–513.

14 Lipska KJ, Ross JS, Wang Y, et al. National trends in US hospital admissions for hyperglycemia and hypoglycemia among medicare beneficiaries, 1999 to 2011. *JAMA Intern Med*. 2014;174(7): 1116–1124.

15 Umpierrez GE, Pasquel FJ. Management of inpatient hyperglycemia and diabetes in older adults. *Diabetes Care*. 2017;40: 509–517.

16 Brod M, Christensen T, Thomsen TL, Bushnell DM. The impact of non-severe hypoglycemic events on work productivity and diabetes management. *Value Health*. 2011;14(5):665–671.

17 Awoniyi O, Rehman R, Dagogo-Jack S. Hypoglycemia in patients with type 1 diabetes: epidemiology, pathogenesis, and prevention. *Curr Diab Rep*. 2013;13(5): 669–678.

18 Gill GV, Woodward A, Casson IF, Weston PJ. Cardiac arrhythmia and nocturnal

hypoglycaemia in type 1 diabetes–the 'dead in bed' syndrome revisited. *Diabetologia*. 2009;52(1):42–45.

19 Robinson RT, Harris ND, Ireland RH, Macdonald IA, Heller SR. Changes in cardiac repolarization during clinical episodes of nocturnal hypoglycaemia in adults with type 1 diabetes. *Diabetologia*. 2004;47(2):312–315.

20 Lindstrom T, Jorfeldt L, Tegler L, Arnqvist HJ. Hypoglycaemia and cardiac arrhythmias in patients with type 2 diabetes mellitus. *Diabet Med*. 1992;9(6):536–541.

21 Tsujimoto T, Yamamoto-Honda R, Kajio H, et al. Vital signs, QT prolongation, and newly diagnosed cardiovascular disease during severe hypoglycemia in type 1 and type 2 diabetic patients. *Diabetes Care*. 2014;37(1):217–225.

22 Tsujimoto T, Yamamoto-Honda R, Kajio H, et al. High risk of abnormal QT prolongation in the early morning in diabetic and non-diabetic patients with severe hypoglycemia. *Ann Med*. 2015;47(3):238–244.

23 Razavi Nematollahi L, Kitabchi AE, Stentz FB, et al. Proinflammatory cytokines in response to insulin-induced hypoglycemic stress in healthy subjects. *Metabolism*. 2009;58(4): 443–448.

24 Gogitidze JN, Hedrington MS, Briscoe VJ, Tate DB, Ertl AC, Davis SN. Effects of acute hypoglycemia on inflammatory and pro-atherothrombotic biomarkers in individuals with type 1 diabetes and healthy individuals. *Diabetes Care*. 2010;33(7):1529–1535.

25 Wright RJ, Newby DE, Stirling D, Ludlam CA, Macdonald IA, Frier BM. Effects of acute insulin-induced hypoglycemia on indices of inflammation: putative mechanism for aggravating vascular disease in diabetes. *Diabetes Care*. 2010;33(7):1591–1597.

26 Gimenez M, Gilabert R, Monteagudo J, et al. Repeated episodes of hypoglycemia as a potential aggravating factor for preclinical atherosclerosis in subjects with type 1 diabetes. *Diabetes Care*. 2011;34(1): 198–203.

27 Bonds DE, Miller ME, Bergenstal RM, et al. The association between symptomatic, severe hypoglycaemia and mortality in type 2 diabetes: retrospective epidemiological analysis of the ACCORD study. *BMJ*. 2010;340:b4909.

28 NICE-SUGAR Study Investigators, Finfer S, Liu B, Chittock DR, et al. Hypoglycemia and risk of death in critically ill patients. *N Engl J Med*. 2012;367(12):1108–1118.

29 Sacks DB, Arnold M, Bakris GL, et al. Guidelines and recommendations for laboratory analysis in the diagnosis and management of diabetes mellitus. *Clin Chem*. 2011;57(6):e1–e47.

30 Sacks DB, Arnold M, Bakris GL, et al., National Academy of Clinical Biochemistry. Position statement executive summary: Guidelines and recommendations for laboratory analysis in the diagnosis and management of diabetes mellitus. *Diabetes Care*. 2011;34(6):1419–1423.

31 Cryer PE, Davis SN, Shamoon H. Hypoglycemia in diabetes. *Diabetes Care*. 2003;26(6):1902–1912.

32 Aftab Guy D, Sandoval D, Richardson MA, Tate D, Davis SN. Effects of glycemic control on target organ responses to epinephrine in type 1 diabetes. *Am J Physiol Endocrinol Metab*. 2005;289(2): E258–E265.

33 Davis SN, Shavers C, Costa F. Differential gender responses to hypoglycemia are due to alterations in CNS drive and not glycemic thresholds. *Am J Physiol Endocrinol Metab*. 2000;279(5): E1054–E1063.

34 Davis SN, Fowler S, Costa F. Hypoglycemic counterregulatory responses differ between men and women with type 1 diabetes. *Diabetes*. 2000;49(1):65–72.

35 Sandoval DA, Ertl AC, Richardson MA, Tate DB, Davis SN. Estrogen blunts neuroendocrine and metabolic responses to hypoglycemia. *Diabetes*. 2003;52(7): 1749–1755.

36 Cryer PE, Gerich JE. Relevance of glucose counterregulatory systems to patients with diabetes: critical roles of glucagon and epinephrine. *Diabetes Care.* 1983;6(1):95–99.

37 Ryder RE, Owens DR, Hayes TM, Ghatei MA, Bloom SR. Unawareness of hypoglycaemia and inadequate hypoglycaemic counterregulation: no causal relation with diabetic autonomic neuropathy. *BMJ.* 1990;301(6755): 783–787.

38 White NH, Skor DA, Cryer PE, Levandoski LA, Bier DM, Santiago JV. Identification of type I diabetic patients at increased risk for hypoglycemia during intensive therapy. *N Engl J Med.* 1983;308(9):485–491.

39 Geddes J, Schopman JE, Zammitt NN, Frier BM. Prevalence of impaired awareness of hypoglycaemia in adults with type 1 diabetes. *Diabet Med.* 2008;25(4):501–504.

40 Schopman JE, Geddes J, Frier BM. Prevalence of impaired awareness of hypoglycaemia and frequency of hypoglycaemia in insulin-treated type 2 diabetes. *Diabetes Res Clin Pract.* 2010;87(1):64–68.

41 Cryer PE. Mechanisms of hypoglycemia-associated autonomic failure in diabetes. *N Engl J Med.* 2013;369(4):362–372.

42 Davis MR, Shamoon H. Counterregulatory adaptation to recurrent hypoglycemia in normal humans. *J Clin Endocrinol Metab.* 1991;73(5):995–1001.

43 Davis SN, Shavers C, Mosqueda-Garcia R, Costa F. Effects of differing antecedent hypoglycemia on subsequent counterregulation in normal humans. *Diabetes.* 1997;46(8):1328–1335.

44 Davis SN, Mann S, Galassetti P, et al. Effects of differing durations of antecedent hypoglycemia on counterregulatory responses to subsequent hypoglycemia in normal humans. *Diabetes.* 2000;49(11): 1897–1903.

45 Sandoval DA, Guy DL, Richardson MA, Ertl AC, Davis SN. Effects of low and moderate antecedent exercise on counterregulatory responses to subsequent hypoglycemia in type 1 diabetes. *Diabetes.* 2004;53(7): 1798–1806.

46 Galassetti P, Tate D, Neill RA, Richardson A, Leu SY, Davis SN. Effect of differing antecedent hypoglycemia on counterregulatory responses to exercise in type 1 diabetes. *Am J Physiol Endocrinol Metab.* 2006;290(6):E1109–E1117.

47 Banarer S, Cryer PE. Sleep-related hypoglycemia-associated autonomic failure in type 1 diabetes: reduced awakening from sleep during hypoglycemia. *Diabetes.* 2003;52(5): 1195–1203.

48 Juvenile Diabetes Research Foundation Continuous Glucose Monitoring Study Group. Prolonged nocturnal hypoglycemia is common during 12 months of continuous glucose monitoring in children and adults with type 1 diabetes. *Diabetes Care.* 2010;33(5): 1004–1008.

49 Veneman T, Mitrakou A, Mokan M, Cryer P, Gerich J. Induction of hypoglycemia unawareness by asymptomatic nocturnal hypoglycemia. *Diabetes.* 1993;42(9):1233–1237.

50 Cranston I, Lomas J, Maran A, Macdonald I, Amiel SA. Restoration of hypoglycaemia awareness in patients with long-duration insulin-dependent diabetes. *Lancet.* 1994;344(8918):283–287.

51 Briscoe VJ, Ertl AC, Tate DB, Davis SN. Effects of the selective serotonin reuptake inhibitor fluoxetine on counterregulatory responses to hypoglycemia in individuals with type 1 diabetes. *Diabetes.* 2008;57(12):3315–3322.

52 Amiel SA, Dixon T, Mann R, Jameson K. Hypoglycaemia in type 2 diabetes. *Diabet Med.* 2008;25(3):245–254.

53 Meneilly GS, Cheung E, Tuokko H. Altered responses to hypoglycemia of healthy elderly people. *J Clin Endocrinol Metab.* 1994;78(6):1341–1348.

54 Brierley EJ, Broughton DL, James OF, Alberti KG. Reduced awareness of hypoglycaemia in the elderly despite an intact counter-regulatory response. *QJM*. 1995;88(6):439–445.

55 Bremer JP, Jauch-Chara K, Hallschmid M, Schmid S, Schultes B. Hypoglycemia unawareness in older compared with middle-aged patients with type 2 diabetes. *Diabetes Care*. 2009;32(8):1513–1517.

56 Kirkman MS, Briscoe VJ, Clark N, et al. Diabetes in older adults. *Diabetes Care*. 2012;35(12):2650–2664.

57 Graveling AJ, Frier BM. Impaired awareness of hypoglycaemia: a review. *Diabetes Metab*. 2010;36 Suppl 3:S64–S74.

58 Rostykus P, Kennel J, Adair K, et al. Variability in the treatment of prehospital hypoglycemia: a structured review of EMS protocols in the United States. *Prehosp Emerg Care*. 2016;20(4):524–530.

59 Joint British Diabetes Societies for Inpatient Care Group. *The Hospital Management of Hypoglycemia in Adults with Diabetes Mellitus* (revised 2013). 2nd ed. London: Diabetes UK.

60 Dougherty PP, Klein-Schwartz W. Octreotide's role in the management of sulfonylurea-induced hypoglycemia. *J Med Toxicol*. 2010;6(2):199–206.

61 Schabelman E, Kuo D. Glucose before thiamine for Wernicke encephalopathy: a literature review. *J Emerg Med*. 2012;42(4):488–494.

62 Bornstein SR, Allolio B, Arlt W, et al. Diagnosis and treatment of primary adrenal insufficiency: an Endocrine Society Clinical Practice Guideline. *J Clin Endocrinol Metab*. 2016;101:364–389.

63 Douillard C, Mention K, Dobbelaere D, Wemeau JL, Saudubray JM, Vantyghem MC. Hypoglycaemia related to inherited metabolic diseases in adults. *Orphanet J Rare Dis*. 2012;7:26–1172–7–26.

64 Stein SA, Lamos EM, Davis SN. A review of the efficacy and safety of oral antidiabetic drugs. *Expert Opin Drug Saf*. 2013;12(2):153–175.

65 Khalil AB, Beshyah SA, Abu Awad SM, et al. Ramadan fasting in diabetes patients on insulin pump therapy augmented by continuous glucose monitoring: an observational real-life study. *Diabetes Technol Ther*. 2012;14(9):813–818.

66 Abe M, Okada K, Soma M. Antidiabetic agents in patients with chronic kidney disease and end-stage renal disease on dialysis: metabolism and clinical practice. *Curr Drug Metab*. 2011;12(1):57–69.

67 Hardy KJ, Burge MR, Boyle PJ, Scarpello JH. A treatable cause of recurrent severe hypoglycemia. *Diabetes Care*. 1994;17(7):722–724.

68 Zoungas S, Abraira C, Anderson RJ, et al. Effects of intensive glucose control on microvascular complications in patients with type 2 diabetes: a meta-analysis of individual participant data from randomized controlled trials. *Lancet Diabetes Endocrinol*. 2017;5:431–437.

69 Action to Control Cardiovascular Risk in Diabetes Study Group, Gerstein HC, Miller ME, Byington RP, et al. Effects of intensive glucose lowering in type 2 diabetes. *N Engl J Med*. 2008;358(24): 2545–2559.

70 Inzucchi SE, Bergenstal RM, Buse JB, et al. Management of hyperglycemia in type 2 diabetes, 2015: a patient-centered approach: Update to a position statement of the american diabetes association and the european association for the study of diabetes. *Diabetes Care*. 2015;38(1): 140–149.

71 Hopkins D, Lawrence I, Mansell P, et al. Improved biomedical and psychological outcomes 1 year after structured education in flexible insulin therapy for people with type 1 diabetes: The U.K. DAFNE experience. *Diabetes Care*. 2012;35(8):1638–1642.

72 Bailey TS, Zisser HC, Garg SK. Reduction in hemoglobin A1C with real-time continuous glucose monitoring: results from a 12-week observational study. *Diabetes Technol Ther*. 2007;9(3): 203–210.

73 Fatourechi MM, Kudva YC, Murad MH, Elamin MB, Tabini CC, Montori VM. Clinical review: hypoglycemia with intensive insulin therapy: a systematic

review and meta-analyses of randomized trials of continuous subcutaneous insulin infusion versus multiple daily injections. *J Clin Endocrinol Metab*. 2009;94(3): 729–740.

74 Ratner RE, Gough SC, Mathieu C, et al. Hypoglycaemia risk with insulin degludec compared with insulin glargine in type 2 and type 1 diabetes: a pre-planned meta-analysis of phase 3 trials. *Diabetes Obes Metab*. 2013;15(2): 175–184.

75 Ritzel R, Roussel R, Bolli GB, et al. Patient-level meta-analysis of the EDITION 1, 2 and 3 studies: glycaemic control and hypoglycaemia with new insulin glargine 300 U/ml versus glargine 100 U/ml in people with type 2 diabetes. *Diabetes Obes Metab*. 2015;17(9): 859–867.

76 Peters AL, Ahmann AJ, Battelino T, et al. Diabetes technology – continuous subcutaneous insulin infusion therapy and continuous glucose monitoring in adults: an Endocrine Society Clinical Practice Guideline. *J Clin Endocrinol Metab*. 2016;101:3922–3937.

77 Bergenstal RM, Klonoff DC, Garg SK, et al. ASPIRE In-Home Study Group. Threshold-based insulin-pump interruption for reduction of hypoglycemia. *N Engl J Med*. 2013;369(3):224–232.

78 Bergenstal RM, Tamborlane WV, Ahmann A, et al. STAR 3 Study Group. Effectiveness of sensor-augmented insulin-pump therapy in type 1 diabetes. *N Engl J Med*. 2010;363(4): 311–320.

79 Laffel L. Improved accuracy of continuous glucose monitoring systems in pediatric patients with diabetes mellitus: results from two studies. *Diabetes Technol Ther 18 Suppl*. 2016;2:S223–S233.

80 MacDonald MJ. Postexercise late-onset hypoglycemia in insulin-dependent diabetic patients. *Diabetes Care*. 1987;10(5):584–588.

81 van de Wiel A. Diabetes mellitus and alcohol. *Diabetes Metab Res Rev*. 2004;20(4):263–267.

82 Inkster B, Frier BM. Diabetes and driving. *Diabetes Obes Metab*. 2013;15(9): 775–783.

83 Blumer I, Hadar E, Hadden DR, et al. Diabetes and pregnancy: an Endocrine Society Clinical Practice Guideline. *J Clin Endocrinol Metab*. 2013;98(11): 4227–4249.

84 Kitzmiller JL, Block JM, Brown FM, et al. Managing preexisting diabetes for pregnancy: Summary of evidence and consensus recommendations for care. *Diabetes Care*. 2008;31(5):1060–1079.

85 Ringholm L, Pedersen-Bjergaard U, Thorsteinsson B, et al. Impaired hormonal counterregulation to biochemical hypoglycaemia does not explain the high incidence of severe hypoglycaemia during pregnancy in women with type 1 diabetes. *Scand J Clin Lab Invest*. 2013;73(1):67–74.

86 Dooley MJ, Wiseman M, McRae A, et al. Reducing potentially fatal errors associated with high doses of insulin: a successful multifaceted multidisciplinary prevention strategy. *BMJ Qual Saf*. 2011;20(7):637–644.

87 Samaan KH, Dahlke M, Stover J. Addressing safety concerns about U-500 insulin in a hospital setting. *Am J Health Syst Pharm*. 2011;68(1):63–68.

88 Lansang MC, Umpierrez G. Inpatient hyperglycemia management: a practical review for primary medical and surgical teams. *Cleveland Clinic J Med*. 2016;83 (Suppl 1):S34–S43.

89 Health and Social Care Information Centre. *National Diabetes Inpatient audit (NaDIA), open data 2016*, 2017. www.digital.nhs.uk/pubs/nadia2016 (accessed April 24, 2017).

90 Moghissi ES, Korytkowski MT, DiNardo M, et al., American Association of Clinical Endocrinologists, American Diabetes Association. American Association of Clinical Endocrinologists and American Diabetes Association consensus statement on inpatient glycemic control. *Diabetes Care*. 2009;32(6):1119–1131.

91 Clement S, Braithwaite SS, Magee MF, et al., American Diabetes Association Diabetes in Hospitals Writing Committee.

Management of diabetes and hyperglycemia in hospitals. *Diabetes Care*. 2004;27(2):553–591.

92 Umpierrez GE, Hellman R, Korytkowski MT, et al., Endocrine Society. Management of hyperglycemia in hospitalized patients in non-critical care setting: an Endocrine Society Clinical Practice Guideline. *J Clin Endocrinol Metab*. 2012;97(1):16–38.

93 Murad MH, Coto-Yglesias F, Wang AT, et al. Clinical review: Drug-induced hypoglycemia: A systematic review. *J Clin Endocrinol Metab*. 2009;94(3):741–745.

94 Johnson EO, Kamilaris TC, Calogero AE, Konstandi M, Chrousos GP. Effects of short- and long-duration hypothyroidism on function of the rat hypothalamic-pituitary-adrenal axis. *J Endocrinol Invest*. 2013;36(2):104–110.

95 Betterle C, Lazzarotto F, Presotto F. Autoimmune polyglandular syndrome type 2: The tip of an iceberg? *Clin Exp Immunol*. 2004;137(2):225–233.

96 Marsk R, Jonas E, Rasmussen F, Naslund E. Nationwide cohort study of post-gastric bypass hypoglycaemia including 5,040 patients undergoing surgery for obesity in 1986-2006 in Sweden. *Diabetologia*. 2010;53(11):2307–2311.

97 Patti ME, Goldfine AB. Hypoglycaemia following gastric bypass surgery–diabetes remission in the extreme? *Diabetologia*. 2010;53(11):2276–2279.

98 Goldfine AB, Mun EC, Devine E, et al. Patients with neuroglycopenia after gastric bypass surgery have exaggerated incretin and insulin secretory responses to a mixed meal. *J Clin Endocrinol Metab*. 2007;92(12):4678–4685.

99 Carpenter T, Trautmann ME, Baron AD. Hyperinsulinemic hypoglycemia with nesidioblastosis after gastric-bypass surgery. *N Engl J Med*. 2005;353(20): 2192–2194; author reply 2192–2194.

100 Schwetz V, Horvath K, Kump P, et al. Successful medical treatment of adult nesidioblastosis with pasireotide over 3 years: a case report. *Medicine (Baltimore)* 2016;95(14):e3272.

101 Basu A, Service FJ, Yu L, Heser D, Ferries LM, Eisenbarth G. Insulin autoimmunity and hypoglycemia in seven white patients. *Endocr Pract*. 2005;11(2):97–103.

102 Service FJ, O'Brien PC. Increasing serum betahydroxybutyrate concentrations during the 72-hour fast: evidence against hyperinsulinemic hypoglycemia. *J Clin Endocrinol Metab*. 2005;90(8): 4555–4558.

103 Nockel P, Babic B, Millo C, et al. Localization of insulinoma using 68Ga-DOTATATE PET/CT scan. *J Clin Endocrinol Metab*. 2017;102:195–199.

32

Severe Hyperglycemia, Diabetic Ketoacidosis, and Hyperglycemic Hyperosmolar State

Ketan Dhatariya and Glenn Matfin

Key Points

- Emergency admissions due to hyperglycemia remain some of the most common and challenging metabolic conditions to deal with.
- Diabetic ketoacidosis (DKA) and hyperglycemic hyperosmolar state (HHS) are biochemically different conditions that require different approaches to treatment. They often occur in different age groups, and there is a need for coordinated care from the multidisciplinary team to ensure the timely delivery of the correct treatments.
- Over the last few years, the management of these conditions has changed. With DKA, it remains important to ensure that the

diagnosis is made only when all three components (the "D," the "K," and the "A") are present. In addition, the use of bedside monitoring of plasma ketone levels now drives treatment.
- With HHS, the treatment now focuses on the use of fluid rehydration in the initial phases rather than insulin treatment as the means by which glucose lowering should be achieved, with insulin only being introduced when the rate of glucose lowering levels off.
- Prevention of these states is always preferred and this requires appropriate education of patients, carers, and healthcare practitioners on an ongoing basis.

Introduction

Diabetic ketoacidosis (DKA) and hyperglycemic hyperosmolar state (HHS) are acute severe metabolic complications of uncontrolled diabetes mellitus (1). Severe hyperglycemia can escalate into the potentially fatal complications of DKA and HHS. Subsequently, these conditions demand immediate recognition and early, aggressive treatment.

Severe hyperglycemia is characterized by significant hyperglycemia (i.e., glycosylated hemoglobin [HbA1c] ≥10% [86 mmol/mol]); or fasting plasma glucose [FPG] >250 mg/dL [13.9 mmol/L]; or random plasma glucose

>300 mg/dL [16.7 mmol/L]); or when symptomatic (e.g., sudden persistent weight-loss, polyuria, and polydipsia) (2).

DKA is a complex disordered metabolic state which the American Diabetes Association (ADA) characterizes by severe hyperglycemia (i.e., plasma glucose levels >250 mg/dL [14 mmol/L]), ketonemia (ketosis), and metabolic acidosis (pH ≤ 7.3, serum bicarbonate <18 mmol/L) (1). The 2009 ADA Hyperglycemic Crises Consensus Guidelines further subdivide DKA into mild DKA (serum bicarbonate of 15–18 mmol/L, pH 7.25–7.30); moderate DKA (serum bicarbonate 10 to <15 mmol/L, pH

Endocrine and Metabolic Medical Emergencies: A Clinician's Guide, Second Edition. Edited by Glenn Matfin.
© 2018 John Wiley & Sons Ltd. Published 2018 by John Wiley & Sons Ltd.

7.00–7.24): and severe DKA (serum bicarbonate <10 mmol/L, pH <7.00) (1). More recently, the UK 2013 Joint British Diabetes Societies Inpatient (JBDS IP) Group DKA Guidelines have incorporated serum ketone levels (3-beta-hydroxybutyrate [βHBA]) in the definition of DKA (3). The measurement of βHBA for diagnosis and monitoring of DKA was also recommended in the 2011 ADA Diabetes Laboratory Guidelines (4). The rationale for the use of serum ketones over urine ketones has recently been reviewed (5). The 2013 JBDS IP Group DKA definition requires the combined presence of three biochemical abnormalities: (a) ketonemia ≥3 mmol/L or significant ketonuria (≥2+ urine ketones on standard urine sticks); (b) blood glucose >200 mg/dL (11.1 mmol/L) or known diabetes; and (c) venous (or arterial) blood bicarbonate <15 mmol/L and/or pH <7.3 (3). Recently, the ADA Consensus Guideline has been questioned because it fails to emphasize the importance of euglycemic DKA, or the importance of having all three components (the "D", the "K" and the "A") present (6). In addition, there needs to be a greater emphasis on the use of plasma ketones, rather than urine, as well as making the document clearer for those "at the front door" treating DKA in the first few hours after initial presentation (6).

DKA primarily affects persons known to have type 1 diabetes and may be the initial manifestation of previously undiagnosed type 1 diabetes in between 2% and 25% of cases (7–9). DKA most frequently results from increased insulin requirements during situations that increase the release of counter-regulatory hormones (i.e., glucagon, cortisol, epinephrine, and growth hormone) (8). When hyperglycemia initially presents in the presence of ketones or other signs of metabolic decompensation, the diagnosis of type 1 diabetes is generally straightforward (especially in children and adolescents). However, ketonemia can also be found in individuals with type 2 diabetes (i.e., ketosis-prone hyperglycemia, especially in persons of African descent), with 5–25% having DKA (10). More recently apparent, however, is the increasing risk of developing DKA, especially euglycemic DKA, in persons with type 1 and type 2 diabetes taking sodium-glucose co-transporter 2 (SGLT2) inhibitors (11).

HHS is characterized by marked hyperglycemia (blood glucose levels >600 mg/dL [33.3 mmol/L]); hyperosmolarity (plasma osmolarity >320 mOsm/kg) and dehydration; the absence of ketoacidosis; and depression of the sensorium (1). The 2012 JBDS IP Group HHS definition includes: marked hyperglycemia (>540 mg/dL [30 mmol/L]); no significant ketonemia (<3 mmol/L); no acidosis (pH >7.3, bicarbonate >15 mmol/L); hypovolemia; and osmolality usually >320 mosmol/kg (12). These guidelines also highlight that a mixed picture of HHS and DKA may occur. HHS is seen most frequently in persons with type 2 diabetes, however, approximately 20% of cases have no history of this diagnosis.

In the USA, the prevalence of DKA has risen while mortality has decreased (8, 13). This is related in part to an improved understanding of the pathophysiology of DKA together with close monitoring and correction of electrolytes. Up to 42% of DKA hospitalizations are due to re-admissions with DKA within 12 months (7, 9). Mortality rates have fallen significantly in the last 20 years from 7.96% to less than 1% (8,14,15). The mortality rate is still higher for those over 60 years old, in particular with significant comorbidities; those living in low-income countries; and among non-hospitalized patients (16). This high mortality rate illustrates the necessity of early diagnosis and the implementation of effective prevention programmes. The ready availability of cheaper insulin to all parts of the world should remain a priority (17). Cerebral edema remains the most common cause of mortality, particularly in young children and adolescents. The main causes of mortality in the adult population include severe hypokalemia (and related cardiac dysrhythmias), adult respiratory distress syndrome (ARDS), and comorbid states such as pneumonia, acute coronary syndromes (ACS) and sepsis (18). Hypokalemia and hypoglycemia were common in a large national survey of DKA management (9). However, the questions remain as to whether this finding was due to the guideline being incorrect, or incorrectly followed. There is an argument to reduce the rate of insulin infusion once the glucose concentration drops to <250 mg/dL (14 mmol/L) to prevent both of these from occurring, but this continues to be a matter of debate (19). In comparison, HHS is rare but mortality attributed to HHS is considerably higher than that attributed to DKA, with recent mortality rates of 5–20% (8).

Pathophysiology

DKA usually occurs as a consequence of absolute or relative insulin deficiency that is accompanied by an increase in counter-regulatory hormones (20). This type of hormonal imbalance enhances hepatic gluconeogenesis and glycogenolysis resulting in severe hyperglycemia (Figure 32-1). Enhanced lipolysis increases serum free fatty acids that are then metabolized as an alternative energy source in the process of ketogenesis (5). This results in the accumulation of large quantities of ketone bodies and subsequent metabolic acidosis. Acetone is a ketone, while βHBA is a hydroxy acid, and acetoacetate a ketoacid. The predominant acid in DKA is βHBA.

There are several mechanisms responsible for fluid depletion in DKA. These include osmotic diuresis due to hyperglycemia, vomiting (commonly associated with DKA) and, eventually, inability to take in fluid due to a diminished level of consciousness. Electrolyte shifts and depletion are in part related to the osmotic diuresis. Hyperkalemia and hypokalemia need particular attention.

Unlike DKA, which is a condition most frequently associated with absolute insulin deficiency, in HHS there is sufficient insulin to prevent ketogenesis, but insufficient insulin to either prevent hepatic gluconeogenesis and/or stimulate cellular glucose uptake (21). If a counter-regulatory hormone excess is also present (e.g., concomitant illness), then this leads to a further rise in blood glucose, and a subsequent osmotic diuresis. If sufficient water is not available, this leads to

dehydration and the resultant impaired renal function. The high plasma glucose causes a raised serum osmolality. The impaired renal function then leads to a further inability to excrete glucose, thus perpetuating the hyperglycemia, osmotic diuresis, volume depletion, and dehydration (22). Alterations in mental status are common with serum osmolality >330 mosmol/kg.

Etiology

DKA and HHS can be precipitated by various conditions (which can easily be remembered by the letter **I**), including **I**nsulin deficiency (i.e., diabetes presentation or failure to take enough insulin); **I**atrogenic (e.g., glucocorticoids, thiazides, and atypical antipsychotic drugs); **I**nfection (the most common precipitating factor for both DKA and HHS); **I**nflammation (e.g., acute pancreatitis, cholecystitis); **I**schemia or **I**nfarction (e.g., ACS, stroke, bowel); and **I**ntoxication (e.g., alcohol, cocaine).

Few studies have assessed factors associated with DKA in adults with type 1 diabetes. However, the T1D Exchange clinic registry at 70 US endocrinology centers recently performed a cross-sectional analysis including 7012 participants with type 1 diabetes (23). Higher frequencies of DKA were associated with lower socio-economic status (p <0.001); and higher HbA1c levels (p <0.001), with 21.0% of those with HbA1c ≥10.0% having an event in the past 12 months. Notably, the frequency was no higher in insulin pump users than injection users, an important finding because DKA is a potential risk with pump infusion failure. Further work has shown that, in the USA, fragmentation of care (i.e., admission to more than one hospital) was more likely to be associated with recurrent DKA and those patients had a higher mortality (24).

Diagnostic Considerations

The diagnostic criteria of severe hyperglycemia, DKA, and HHS are outlined in the

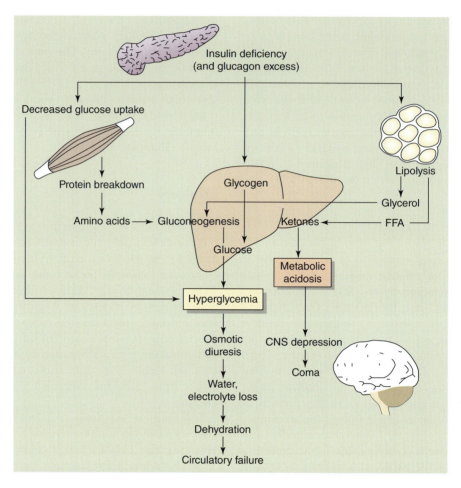

Figure 32-1 Mechanisms of diabetic ketoacidosis (DKA). DKA is associated with insulin deficiency and high levels of glucagon, catecholamines, and other counter-regulatory hormones. Increased levels of glucagon and the catecholamines lead to mobilization of substrates for gluconeogenesis and ketogenesis by the liver. Gluconeogenesis in excess of that needed to supply glucose to the brain and other glucose-dependent tissues (which may depend on insulin) produces a rise in blood glucose levels. Mobilization of free fatty acids (FFAs) from triglyceride stores in adipose tissue (due to increased lipolysis resulting from insulin deficiency) leads to accelerated ketone production and ketosis.

Introduction. However, the diagnosis of DKA should not be made until all three criteria are met (i.e., the "D", the "K" and the "A").

The initial laboratory evaluation of patients should include a determination of plasma glucose, blood urea nitrogen (BUN) or urea, creatinine, electrolytes, serum osmolality, serum ketones, urinalysis, baseline venous (or arterial) blood gases, complete (full) blood count with differential, and ESR or CRP (if indicated). An electrocardiogram (ECG), chest X-ray, and urine and blood cultures should also be considered where comorbidity

is possible. Other investigations are performed as warranted by the clinical situation (e.g., cardiac troponins, serum lactate, appropriate imaging, toxicology, and drug screen).

Point of care testing equipment should be used to measure the plasma concentrations of βHBA, because this is the direct marker of disease severity. The anion gap is calculated by subtracting the sum of chloride $[Cl^-]$ and bicarbonate $[HCO3^-]$ concentration from the uncorrected measured (see below) sodium $[Na^+]$ concentration: $[Na^+] - ([Cl^-] + [HCO3^-])$. A normal anion gap is between 7 and 9 mmol/L and an anion gap >10–12 mmol/L indicates the presence of increased anion gap metabolic acidosis (although UK guidelines also add [K^+] to [Na^+] before subtracting anions, hence abnormal value is higher [>16]). While arterial blood gas (ABG) is the most accurate method of assessing ventilation and acid-base status, venous blood gas (VBG) is preferred to ABG for bicarbonate and pH measurements because the differences in arterial and venous pH (e.g., venous pH only 0.03 lower than arterial), bicarbonate and potassium measurements are not large enough (in either direction) to alter management (25,26).

The admission serum sodium is usually low or normal, despite water loss (renal and gut) because of an intracellular–extracellular fluid shift. To assess the severity of sodium and water deficit, serum sodium may be corrected by adding 1.6 mmol/L to the measured serum sodium for each 100 mg/dL (5.6 mmol/L) of glucose above 100 mg/dL (5.6 mmol/L) up to 440 mg/dL (~24 mmol/L) (27). For glucose levels >440 mg/dL (~24 mmol/L), serum sodium may be further corrected by adding 4 mmol/L to the measured serum sodium for each 100 mg/dL (5.6 mmol/L) glucose above this threshold. A more simple approach is to divide measured serum glucose (in mmol/L) by 4; and add this number to measured serum sodium level to obtain the corrected serum sodium level. Serum potassium levels may also be low, normal, or elevated, despite total body potassium depletion resulting from protracted polyuria and vomiting (1).

On admission, leukocytosis with cell counts in the 10,000–15,000 mm^3 range is the rule in DKA and is generally attributed to stress and may not be indicative of an infection. However, leukocytosis with cell counts >25,000 mm^3 may designate infection and appropriate evaluation is indicated.

Hyperamylasemia has been reported in 21–79% of patients with DKA; however, there is little correlation between the presence, degree, or isoenzyme type of hyperamylasemia (e.g., salivary amylase can also be increased in DKA) and the presence of gastrointestinal symptoms (nausea, vomiting, and abdominal pain) or pancreatic imaging studies. A serum lipase determination may be beneficial in the differential diagnosis of pancreatitis; however, lipase can also be elevated in DKA in the absence of pancreatitis.

Not all patients with ketoacidosis have DKA. Starvation ketosis and alcoholic ketoacidosis are distinguished by clinical history and by plasma glucose concentrations that range from mildly elevated (rarely >200 mg/dL [11.1 mmol/L]) to hypoglycemia. A clinical history of previous drug abuse and intoxication should be sought.

Clinical Signs and Features

The process of HHS usually evolves over several days to weeks, whereas the evolution of the acute DKA episode tends to be much shorter (typically <24 h). For both DKA and HHS, the classical clinical picture includes a history of polyuria, polydipsia, weight loss, visual changes, vomiting, dehydration, weakness, and mental status change. Physical findings may include increased rate and depth of respiration in DKA (i.e., Kussmaul's breathing) with the odor of acetone, tachycardia, and hypotension. Assessment of fluid status encompasses subjective observations (skin turgor, mucous membranes, and cerebral dysfunction), objective measurements (blood pressure, pulse, postural measurements, body weight), and laboratory measurements (serum sodium, serum osmolality, BUN, hematocrit, and urine osmolality). Severe hypovolemia may manifest as tachycardia (pulse >100 bpm) and/or hypotension (systolic blood pressure <100 mmHg). Each has its limitations particularly on initial assessment where previous comparator data may not be available.

Mental status can vary from full alertness to profound lethargy or coma, with the latter more frequent in HHS. Acute impairment in cognitive function may be associated with dehydration but is not specific to the condition and is not necessarily present.

Alterations in mental status are common with serum osmolality over 330 mosmol/kg. Focal neurologic signs (hemianopia and hemiparesis), positive Babinski reflexes, aphasia, visual hallucinations, seizures (focal or generalized), and coma may also be features of HHS. Because HHS more frequently occurs in older people, the neurological findings may be mistaken for a stroke. Because of the increasing frequency of diabetes (both diagnosed and undiagnosed) or stress-related hyperglycemia, and with the harms associated with increased glucose concentrations, glucose should be measured in all unwell patients presenting to the hospital.

Although infection is a common precipitating factor for both DKA and HHS, patients can be normothermic or even hypothermic primarily because of peripheral vasodilation. Nausea, vomiting, diffuse abdominal pain are frequent in patients with DKA (>50%) but are uncommon in HHS. Further evaluation is necessary if this complaint does not resolve with resolution of dehydration and metabolic acidosis.

Management of Severe Hyperglycemia, DKA, and HHS

Successful treatment of severe hyperglycemia, DKA, and HHS requires the correction of dehydration, hyperglycemia, and electrolyte imbalances; identification of comorbid precipitating events; and above all, frequent patient monitoring.

Acute Intervention

Once severe hyperglycemia, DKA, or HHS is recognized, the patient should be managed in an appropriate location. This could be in the outpatient setting (e.g., rapid access clinic) for selected cases of severe hyperglycemia and mild DKA. However, the majority of patients will be hospitalized and managed in an emergency care setting such as emergency department, acute medical unit (AMU) or equivalent, as well as more advanced step-up facilities such as high dependency unit (HDU), or intensive care unit (ICU). As

with all acute medical patients, prompt assessment and management of the ABCDEs should occur (i.e., Airway; Breathing; Circulation; Disability [i.e., conscious level]; and Exposure [i.e., examination]). Other markers of DKA and HHS severity should be assessed and recorded (Table 32-1).

General Supportive Care

Supportive care includes inserting large bore intravenous (IV) cannulae and starting appropriate IV fluid resuscitation, electrolyte replacement, nutritional support, continuous cardiac monitoring, and pulse oximetry. Co-incident comorbidities should be treated appropriately. It is also imperative to exclude unknown pregnancy by performing a pregnancy test in appropriate patient.

Hyperglycemia bundle: Due to the increased risk of arterial and venous thromboembolism (VTE), all patients with DKA or HHS should receive low molecular weight heparin (LMWH) for the full duration of admission unless contraindicated. HHS (and some DKA) patients are also at high risk of pressure ulceration. An initial foot assessment should be undertaken and heel protectors applied in those with neuropathy, peripheral arterial disease (PAD), a history of previous ulceration, or lower limb deformity. The feet should be re-examined daily. Consider an NG tube with airway protection to prevent aspiration if Glasgow Coma Scale (GCS) score is <12 or if the patient is excessively vomiting. Consider urinary catheterization if the patient is incontinent, if there is difficulty monitoring urine output (minimum urine output should be no less than 0.5 ml/kg/hr), or if the patient is anuric (i.e., not passed urine by 60 minutes).

Hyperglycemia-Specific Therapy

Severe Hyperglycemia

Healthcare providers are concerned by the risk of severe hyperglycemia during acute illness in persons with diabetes, especially those treated with insulin therapy. Prevention of hyperglycemia, and their management

Table 32-1 Markers of severity in DKA (3) and HHS (12). After a diagnosis of DKA or HHS has been made, the presence of any of the following during the admission should prompt a swift senior review and/or indicate admission to a High Dependence Unit (HDU) environment.

Marker of severity	DKA (JBDS IP Group 2013)	HHS (JBDS IP Group 2012)
Mental status	GCS <12 or abnormal AVPU	GCS <12 or abnormal AVPU
Oxygen saturation	<92% on air (assuming normal baseline respiratory function)	<92% on air (assuming normal baseline respiratory function)
Venous/arterial pH	pH <7.1	pH <7.1
Potassium	Hypokalemia (<3.5 mmol/L) or Hyperkalemia (>6 mmol/L)	Hypokalemia (<3.5 mmol/L) or Hyperkalemia (>6 mmol/L)
Systolic blood pressure	<90 mmHg	<90 mmHg
Pulse	>100 or <60 bpm	>100 or <60 bpm
Urine output	<0.5 mls/kg/hr or other evidence of acute kidney injury (AKI)	<0.5 mls/kg/hr or other evidence of acute kidney injury (AKI)
Blood ketones	>6 mmol/L	>1 mmol/L
Bicarbonate level	<5 mmol/L	
Anion gap	>16 mmol/L*	
Sodium		>160 mmol/L
Osmolality		>350 mosm/kg
Miscellaneous		Hypothermia Acute or serious comorbidity (e.g., ACS, heart failure, or stroke)

GCS = Glasgow Coma Scale; AVPU = (Alert, Voice, Pain, Unresponsive) scale.
*Equivalent to >12 mEq/L for USA anion gap calculation (USA equation does not add [K$^+$] to [Na$^+$] before subtracting anions).

with a step-by-step procedure (generally referred to as "sick-day" rules) when they eventually occur, are integral to diabetes management. Blood glucose concentrations normally increase during illness because of the release of stress hormones. Thus, sick-day rules should be initiated. The instructions include maintaining usual food plan, non-insulin therapies, and/or insulin regimen whenever possible. When possible, low-caloric oral fluid intake should be increased as appropriate. Persons with diabetes, who experience nausea or vomiting, should initiate the sick-day food plan. In patients treated with insulin, blood glucose and ketone (if available) monitoring should be carried out as recommended (e.g., every 2–4 hours). If the blood glucose concentration is >250 mg/dL (~14 mmol/L) on two consecutive tests despite following the sick day rules,

persons with diabetes are recommended to contact their clinician due to the possible need to supplement their current insulin regimen with short- or rapid-acting insulin as necessary. The individual must be instructed to contact their healthcare provider when the blood glucose is persistently raised (e.g., >300 mg/dL [16.6 mmol/L]) and/or they develop moderate to high ketonuria/ketonemia (i.e., ≥2+ urine ketones; or serum ketones ≥2.0 mmol/L). DKA or HHS can occur in this setting, thus frequent communication is necessary between clinician and the individual to prevent the situation from deteriorating further.

The most important consideration in the initial assessment of acute illness in persons with diabetes is whether the individual needs inpatient admission or can be safely managed in the community or outpatient setting (including a review in a rapid-access clinic). The majority of these "mild" situations will be managed in the community or outpatient setting. However, this decision has to take into account various factors including medical (e.g., severity of metabolic decompensation, associated comorbidities, presence of confusion or impaired consciousness) and social issues (e.g., whether the patient lives alone or has adequate family support, whether there are reliable communication channels between healthcare provider and person with diabetes and/or caregivers). Inpatient admission can be considered when: (a) there is severe and prolonged hyperglycemia; (b) there is the presence of high (urinary ketones ≥2+) for more than 6 hours, or a single plasma ketone concentration on a point of care meter of ≥3.0 mmol/L; (c) there is vomiting, diarrhea, and/or abdominal pain; (d) there is inadequate phone contact between healthcare provider and person with diabetes and/or caregiver; or (e) at the discretion of the clinician and/or according to local practice guidelines.

DKA and HHS

The 2009 ADA Hyperglycemic Crises Consensus and the JBDS-IP Guidelines remain the predominant protocols of choice for the management of patients with DKA and HHS (1, 28). The protocols from the ADA guideline are summarized in Figure 32-2 (1). The overall goals in treating DKA are to improve circulatory volume and tissue perfusion, decrease blood glucose, and correct the acidosis and electrolyte imbalances. These objectives usually are accomplished through the administration of low-dose (0.1 unit/kg/hour) insulin and IV fluid and electrolyte replacement solutions. An initial loading dose of short-acting or rapid-acting insulin may be needed if there is a delay in setting up an IV insulin infusion, followed by a fixed rate intravenous insulin infusion (FRIII) or equivalent (i.e., continuous intravenous insulin infusion [CII]) (28). Frequent point-of-care tests should be used to monitor blood glucose, venous pH, and βHBA concentrations. Near patient testing for βHBA

is now readily available for the monitoring of the abnormal metabolite allowing for a shift away from using glucose levels to drive treatment decisions in the management of DKA. Frequent laboratory measurements of creatinine, and serum electrolyte levels should be done to guide fluid and electrolyte replacement. It is important to replace fluid and electrolytes and correct pH while bringing the blood glucose concentration to a normal level. Too rapid a drop in blood glucose may cause hypoglycemia (although there is debate as to whether this is due to the protocols not being followed, or of the rate of intravenous insulin infusion being too high) (19). A sudden change in the osmolality of extracellular fluid can also occur when blood glucose levels are lowered too rapidly, and this can cause cerebral edema. Serum potassium levels often fall as acidosis is corrected and potassium moves from the extracellular into the intracellular compartment, but again, this may be due to the rate of insulin infusion being too high as glucose concentrations drop (19). Thus, it is usually necessary to add potassium to the IV infusion.

Identification and treatment of the underlying cause, such as infection, are also important. During treatment of DKA, hyperglycemia is corrected faster than ketoacidosis. The mean duration of treatment until blood glucose is <250 mg/dL (~14 mmol/L) and ketoacidosis (pH >7.30; bicarbonate >18 mmol/L) is corrected is between 6 and 12 hours, respectively (9). Once the plasma glucose is approx. <200 mg/dL (11.1 mmol/L), 10% dextrose should be added to replacement fluids to allow continued insulin administration until ketonemia is controlled while at the same time avoiding hypoglycemia. For DKA occurring in individuals with type 2 diabetes (i.e., ketosis-prone hyperglycemia), the initial management is similar to standard DKA (4).

Until recently there was no easily available assay for ketone bodies, hence capillary glucose, venous pH and bicarbonate were used to diagnose and monitor response to treatment in DKA. Some of the major recommendations of the 2013 JBDS IP

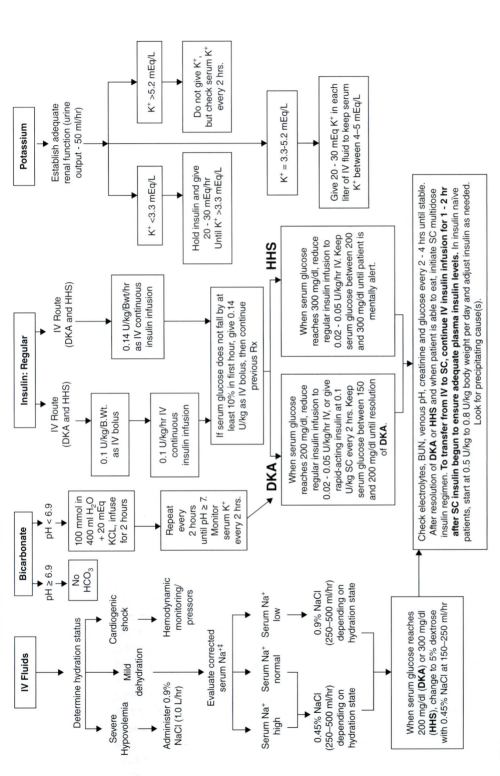

Figure 32-2 Protocol for management of adult patients with DKA or HHS

DKA diagnostic criteria: blood glucose >250 mg/dL (13.8 mmol/L), arterial pH ≤7.3, bicarbonate <15 mEq/l (15 mmol/L), and moderate ketonuria or ketonemia. HHS diagnostic criteria: serum glucose >600 mg/dL (33.3 mmol/L), arterial pH >7.3, serum bicarbonate >15 mEq/L, and minimal ketonuria and ketonemia. †15–20 ml/kg/h; ‡serum Na should be corrected for hyperglycemia (for each 100 mg/dL [5.6 mmol/L] >glucose 100 mg/dL (5.6 mmol/L), add 1.6 mEq/L (1.6 mmol/L) to sodium value for corrected serum value). Bwt = body weight; IV = intravenous; SC = subcutaneous.

<u>Fixed rate intravenous insulin infusion (FRIII)</u>

Adult guidelines for managing
Diabetic KetoAcidosis (DKA) (18 yrs and over)

Name:...

NHS/Hosp Number:....................

DOB:...

Discuss with Medical Team on call for advice and **Refer to Diabetes Team**

Diagnosis of DKA	Request ITU review if any of the following are present:
• Glucose >11 mmo/L (200 mg/dL) or known diabetes • pH <7.3 +/- HCO3 < 15 mmol/L • Ketonemia ≥3 mmol/L or ketonuria > 2+	• pH ≤7.1 or not improving after 2 hours • Persistent low systolic BP <100 mmHg • Urine output <0.5 ml/kg/hour for 3 hours • Glasgow Coma Scale (GCS) <12 or falling or abnormal AVPU Scale • Blood ketones >6 mmol/L • HCO3 <5 mmol/L • Hypokalemia on admission (under 3.5 mmol/L) • ALL pregnant patients suspected of DKA

0 - 60 minutes - DIAGNOSE, RESUSCITATE & START TREATMENT

Investigations	Management	Monitoring
• FBC, U&E (inc. serum potassium & bicarbonate), LFT • Venous blood gas for pH HCO3 glucose electrolytes • ECG • Chest x-ray • Infection screen (if indicated)	• **Start 1 litre 0.9% saline over 1 hour** via volumetric pump • **Start IV insulin fixed rate** based on body weight **0.1 unit/kg of body weight/hour** (correct severe hypokalemia before insulin initiated) • **Potassium replacement -** If > 5.5 mmol/L = NO potassium If 3.5–5.5 mmol/L - need 20–40 mmol/L If < 3.5 mmol/L - needs 40 mmol/L over 1–2 hours with cardiac monitoring (maintain between 3.5–5.5 mmol/L) **If eGFR <15 ml/min discuss with Renal team before adding potassium** (Typical fluid deficit is 100 ml/kg of body weight Aim to correct over 24–48 hours) • Prescribe prophylactic heparin - if no contra-indications	• Hourly capillary blood glucose • Hourly capillary blood ketones • Cardiac monitoring • Baseline & hourly BP, pulse, respirations • Pulse oximetry • Neurological observations • Strict fluid input/output (Aiming to reduce blood glucose by 3 mmol/L/hr, reduce blood ketones by 0.5 mmol/L/hr & increase HCO3 by 3 mmol/L/hr)

60 minutes - 6 hours - RE-ASSESS PATIENT & MONITOR RESPONSE to TREATMENT

Investigations	Management	Monitoring

• 2-hourly serum potassium & bicarbonate
• Venous blood gas for pH HCO3
	• IVI 0.9% saline 1 litre over 2 hours
	      then 1 litre over 2 hours
	      then 1 litre over 4 hours
	• Continue IV insulin at fixed rate
	• Potassium replacement if needed
	• **Once blood glucose <14 mmol/L (250 mg/dL), start IVI 10% glucose at 125 ml/hour**
	• BUT continue 0.9% saline hydration fluids, adjust rate if concern over fluid overload
	• **Continue basal insulins - Glargine (U100 or U300), Detemir, Degludec, NPH (e.g., Insuman Basal, Insulatard, Humulin I) - if usually taken**
		• Hourly capillary blood glucose
		• Hourly capillary blood ketones
		• Cardiac monitoring
		• Hourly BP, pulse, respirations
		• Pulse oximetry
		• Neurological observations
		• Strict fluid input/output

6–24 hours - IMPROVING/RESOLVING BIOCHEMICAL PARAMETERS

Investigations	Management	Monitoring

• U&E at 6 hours and 12 hours - (more frequently if potassium low)	• IVI 0.9% saline 1 litre over 4 hours
	      then 1 litre over 6 hours
	      then 1 litre over 6 hours
	• Continue IV insulin at fixed rate
	• Potassium replacement if needed
	• Add in IVI 10% glucose once blood glucose < 14 mmol/L (250 mg/dL)
		(As above)

RESOLUTION OF DKA = Blood ketones <0.6 mmol/L + HCO3 >15 mmol/L + pH >7.3

IMPORTANT – if patient not eating & drinking yet and ketones <0.6 mmol/L, switch to variable rate intravenous insulin infusion (VRIII)

Figure 32-3 Generic example of UK adult guidelines for managing diabetic ketoacidosis (DKA).

DISCONTINUATION of FRIII

Points to consider:
- If DKA resolved (ketones <0.6 mmol/L) but NOT eating & drinking yet, switch to variable rate intravenous insulin infusion (VRIII)
- Discontinue FRIII at MEALTIME
- If previously taking subcutaneous insulin, restart usual insulin & refer to Diabetes Team for titration advice

For new diagnosis:
- Add up total insulin in last 24 hours (if blood glucose stable) and reduce by 30%, then
  Divide this total daily dose by 5 and give ⅕ with each meal as rapid acting insulin and ⅖ as basal insulin pre-bed (e.g. Detemir or Glargine)
  OR for twice daily insulin, divide this total daily dose by 3 and give ⅔ with breakfast and ⅓ with evening meal (e.g. Insuman Comb 25, Novomix 30 or Humalog Mix 25)
  Continue FRIII for 30–60 mins after first subcutaneous injection of short- or rapid-acting insulin at meal-time

Subcutaneous insulin pump - reconnect the pump, start normal basal rate, give a mealtime bolus then stop infusions 1 hour later
- Continue to monitor blood glucose pre-meal and before bed to ensure readings remain stable

For advice, contact the Diabetes Team

Figure 32-3 (*Continued*)

Group DKA Guidelines (see Figure 32-3 for representative FRIII and DKA patient flowchart) include:

1. Aim to treat the cause of the acidosis (i.e., ketonemia). Subsequently, bedside ketone monitors should be used to measure βHBA, because this is the direct marker of disease severity. The resolution of DKA depends upon the suppression of ketonemia, and measurement of blood ketones now represents best practice in monitoring the response to treatment (29–32).

2. Insulin is given as a standard dose per kg until the ketones are cleared. A weight-based, FRIII via an infusion pump should be used. Fifty units of short-acting insulin or rapid-acting insulin made up to 50 ml with 0.9% sodium chloride solution (resulting concentration of insulin is 1 unit per ml). The initial starting dose of a fixed dose per kg body weight (0.1 units per kg per hour [i.e., 7 units per hour for a 70 kg individual]) enables rapid blood ketone clearance. The fixed rate may be adjusted if the metabolic targets are not met (i.e., reduction of the blood ketone concentration by at least 0.5 mmol/L/hour; increase in venous bicarbonate concentrations by at least 3 3 mmol/L/hour); or reduction capillary blood glucose by at least 50 mg/dL/hour [3 mmol/L/hour]). The insulin infusion rate is increased by 1.0 unit/hr increments hourly until the ketones are falling at target rates (also check infusion set for leaks and connection problems).There is no need to give a bolus dose of insulin as long as the FRIII is set up promptly. Only use a variable-rate IV insulin infusion (VRIII) with 10% dextrose when the blood glucose is <250 mg/dL (~14 mmol/L).

3. Subcutaneous injections of long-acting insulin should be continued if the patient is already using these agents. They provide background insulin when the FRIII is discontinued, and should avoid excess length of stay. This does not obviate the need for giving short-acting or rapid-acting insulin before discontinuing the FRIII. Most units experienced in managing DKA now also continue intermediate-acting insulin (NPH) if that is what the patient normally uses. The FRIII is thus a "top-up" on the (inadequate) background insulin already circulating. Patients presenting with newly diagnosed type 1 diabetes should be given long-acting insulin (or NPH insulin, depending on local policy) at a dose of 0.25 units/kg subcutaneously once daily to mitigate against rebound ketosis when they are taken off the FRIII (33,34).

Table 32-2 Recommended rate of fluid replacement in DKA assuming the individual has normal baseline cardiovascular reserve (3). Potassium levels needs careful monitoring and replacement as per Table 32-3

Fluid	Volume
0.9% sodium chloride 1 L	1000 ml over 1st hour
0.9% sodium chloride 1 L with potassium chloride	1000 ml over next 2 hours
0.9% sodium chloride 1 L with potassium chloride	1000 ml over next 2 hours
0.9% sodium chloride 1 L with potassium chloride	1000 ml over next 2 hours
0.9% sodium chloride 1 L with potassium chloride	1000 ml over next 4 hours
0.9% sodium chloride 1 L with potassium chloride	1000 ml over next 4 hours

Re-assessment of cardiovascular status at 12 hours is mandatory, further fluid may be required

Reproduced with permission from John Wiley & Sons, Ltd.

4. Use 0.9% sodium chloride solution for resuscitation, not colloid. If the systolic blood pressure (BP) is <90 mmHg, consider causes other than fluid depletion, such as heart failure, sepsis, etc. Give 500 ml of 0.9% sodium chloride solution over 10–15 minutes and repeat if necessary (i.e., fluid challenge). If there has been no improvement in BP, call for urgent senior help. If the systolic BP is >90 mmHg, use the typical recommendations outlined in Table 32-2. More cautious fluid replacement should be considered in young people aged 18–25 years, the elderly, pregnant ladies, those with heart or renal failure (also consider HDU and/or central line). Reduce the rate of fluid replacement in the elderly/cardiac disease/mild-moderate DKA (e.g., bicarbonate >10 mmol/L). More rapid infusion increases risk of ARDS and cerebral edema.

5. Measure venous blood gas for pH, bicarbonate and potassium at 60 minutes, 2 hours and 2 hourly thereafter.

6. Keep potassium between 4.5 and 5.5 mmol/L (Table 32-3). Hypokalemia

Table 32-3 Recommended rate of potassium replacement in DKA and HHS assuming the individual has normal baseline renal function (3)

Potassium level in first 24 hours (mEq/L [mmol/L])	Potassium replacement in mEq/L (mmol/L) of infusion solution
Over 5.5	Nil
3.5–5.5	40 mEq/L (40 mmol/L)
Below 3.5	Senior review because additional potassium needs to be given

and hyperkalemia are life-threatening conditions and are common in DKA (9).

7. Avoid hypoglycemia. If the glucose falls below 250 mg/dL (~14.0 mmol/L), commence 10% dextrose given at 125 mls/hour alongside the 0.9% sodium chloride solution. This provides the substrate for the insulin and also helps avoid hypoglycemia if the FRIII is still required to drive down the ketones and acidosis.

8. Bicarbonate should not generally be given because it may worsen intracellular acidosis, and it may precipitate cerebral edema, particularly in children and adolescents (35,36).

9. Hypophosphatemia and hypomagnesemia are common in DKA and HHS, however, routine replacement is not recommended, unless associated with significant malnutrition.

10. It is expected that by 24 hours the ketonemia (<0.6 mmol/L) and acidosis (venous bicarbonate >15 mmol/L; venous pH >7.3) should have resolved. Continue IV fluids if the patient is not eating and drinking. If the patient is not eating and drinking and there is no ketonemia, move to a VRIII. Transfer to subcutaneous insulin if the patient is eating and drinking normally. Ensure that the subcutaneous insulin is started before the IV insulin is discontinued. Ideally give the subcutaneous short-acting or rapid-acting insulin at a meal and discontinue IV insulin one hour later.

11. Where available, the diabetes inpatient team should ideally be involved as early as is practical after admission.

Unlike DKA, specific guidelines on the management of the HHS in adults are uncommon and often there is little to differentiate them from the management of DKA. However, HHS is different from DKA and treatment requires a different approach. The person with HHS is often elderly, frequently with multiple comorbidities but always very sick. Even when specific hospital guidelines are available, adherence to and use of these are variable among inpatient teams. The major goals of treatment of HHS are to gradually and safely normalize the osmolality; replace fluid and electrolyte losses; and normalize blood glucose. Other goals includes identifying and treating the underlying cause; prevent arterial or venous thrombosis; prevent other potential complications (e.g., cerebral edema); and prevent foot ulceration. The UK JBDS IP group has produced some specific guidance for the management of HHS (12).

Some of the major recommendations of the 2012 JBDS IP group HHS guidelines include:

1. Measure or calculate osmolality (2x Na [mEq/L] + glucose [mg/dL)]/18 + BUN [mg/dL]/2.8; or (2x Na [mmol/L] + glucose [mmol/L] + urea [mmol/L]) frequently to monitor the response to treatment.

2. The aim of the initial therapy is expansion of the intra and extravascular volume and to restore peripheral perfusion. The fluid replacement of choice is 0.9% sodium chloride. Measurement or calculation of osmolality should be undertaken every hour initially and the rate of fluid replacement adjusted to ensure a positive fluid balance sufficient to promote a gradual decline in osmolality. Urinary fluid losses may be considerable due to osmotic diuresis which may persist for hours as glucose concentrations slowly decrease. The fall in osmolality with the lowering of blood glucose and shift of water into the intracellular space inevitably results in a rise in serum

sodium. This is not necessarily an indication to give hypotonic solutions (so-called "isotonic" 0.9% sodium chloride is relatively hypotonic compared to the serum) especially if the person remains clinically hypovolemic. An initial rise in serum sodium concentration is common and must be interpreted in the context of what is happening to tonicity (effective osmolality). Provided plasma glucose is declining at a safe rate, for example, no more than 90 mg/dL/hr (5 mmol/L/hr), this will be accompanied by a rise in serum sodium, but a fall in osmolality. Serum sodium concentrations should be frequently monitored, and the concentration of sodium in fluids adjusted to promote a gradual decline in corrected serum sodium. An optimal rate of decline in serum sodium of 0.5 mmol/L per hour has been recommended for hypernatremic dehydration. The rate of fall of plasma sodium should not exceed 10–12 mmol/L per day. The aim of treatment should be to replace approximately 50% of estimated fluid loss within the first 12 hr and the remainder in the following 12 hours, although this will, in part, be determined by the initial severity, and the degree of renal impairment and associated comorbidities, which may limit the speed of correction.

3. If significant ketonemia is present (βHBA >1 mmol/L), this indicates relative hypoinsulinemia and insulin should be started at time zero. If significant ketonemia is not present (βHBA <1 mmol/L), insulin should not be started. Fluid replacement alone with 0.9% sodium chloride will result in a drop in blood glucose, and because most patients with HHS are insulin-sensitive, there is a risk of lowering the osmolality precipitously. Insulin treatment prior to adequate fluid replacement may result in cardiovascular collapse as water moves out of the intravascular space, with a resulting decline in intravascular volume. Lack of appropriate decline in serum glucose with rehydration should prompt reassessment and evaluation of

renal function. Insulin may be started at this point, or if already in place the infusion rate increased (increased by 1 unit/hr). The recommended insulin dose is an FRIII given at 0.05 units per kg per hour (e.g., 4 units/hour in an 80 kg person). A fall of glucose at a rate of up to 90 mg/dL/hr (5 mmol/L/hr) is ideal.

4. Avoid hypoglycemia. A blood glucose target of between 180 and ~270 mg/dL (10 and 15 mmol/L) is a reasonable goal in the first 24 hours. If the blood glucose falls below 250 mg/dL (~14 mmol/L), commence 10% dextrose at 125 ml/h and continue the 0.9% sodium chloride solution.

5. Potassium replacement. This is the same as DKA and the same principles can be applied using Table 32-3.

6. Complete normalization of electrolytes and osmolality may take up to 72 hours.

7. Assess for any complications of treatment (e.g., fluid overload, cerebral edema, osmotic demyelination syndrome, such as a deteriorating conscious level).

8. Because of the increased risk of arterial and venous thromboembolism, all patients should receive prophylactic LMWH for the full duration of admission unless contraindicated. Consideration should be given to extending prophylaxis beyond the duration of admission in HHS patients deemed to be at high risk.

9. Discharge planning: because many of these patients have multiple comorbidities, recovery will largely be determined by their previous functional level and the underlying precipitant of HHS. IV insulin can usually be discontinued once they are eating and drinking but their fluids may be required for longer if intake remains inadequate. Many patients may require conversion to subcutaneous insulin treatment. For patients with previously undiagnosed diabetes or who were well controlled on oral agents, switching from insulin to the appropriate non-insulin therapy should be considered after a period of stability.

10. Where available, the diabetes inpatient team should ideally be involved as early as is practical after admission.

Treatment of Precipitating Illness

For both DKA and HHS, consider any precipitating causes and treat appropriately.

DKA in Pregnancy

DKA is a medical emergency during pregnancy and can be complicated by fetal loss rates as high as 10–25%. The incidence is 1–3%. During pregnancy, there is an accelerated maternal response to starvation and this predisposes women with diabetes mellitus to DKA. DKA occurs at lower glucose levels in pregnancy. In one series, 4 out of 11 patients presented in DKA with blood glucose <200 mg/dL (11.1 mmol/L). Several factors contribute to the occurrence of DKA in the setting of near euglycemia in pregnancy, including an increased flux of glucose from the maternal circulation to the fetus and placenta possibly by means of an increase in the glucose transporter GLUT-1, the accelerated starvation state of pregnancy contributing to ketonuria, and a lowered renal threshold for glucose leading to enhanced glycosuria due to reduced tubular reabsorption capacity. In addition, higher progesterone levels in pregnancy induce a respiratory alkalosis that results in a compensatory metabolic acidosis which reduces buffering capacity. Prompt evaluation for DKA should occur in the setting of nausea, vomiting, abdominal discomfort, limited oral intake, or fever and hyperglycemia. Common precipitants during pregnancy include infection (especially urinary tract infections), hyperemesis gravidarum, new onset of type 1 or occasionally type 2 diabetes (ketosis-prone hyperglycemia) occurring in pregnancy, insulin omission, insulin pump malfunction or catheter occlusion in women using CSII (insulin pump), glucocorticoid use to induce fetal lung maturity, and the use of terbutaline (to prevent pre-term labor). The diagnosis and treatment algorithm of DKA in pregnancy is similar to non-pregnant cases (although euglycemic DKA can occur, resulting in early addition of dextrose to insulin to reduce ketone levels). The management of DKA requires close maternal and fetal monitoring. Prompt management and adherence to standard guidelines are essential (3).

Conclusions

Severe hyperglycemia, DKA, and HHS are medical emergencies that demand immediate recognition and treatment. However, prevention of these states is always preferred and this requires appropriate education of patients, carers, and healthcare practitioners on an ongoing basis. In addition, effective inpatient management of persons with diabetes is critical. The challenges posed with the use of insulin in hospitalized patients occur throughout all areas of this care setting. For example, the UK 2016 National Diabetes Inpatient Audit (NaDIA) revealed that 1 in 25 of patients with type 1 diabetes developed DKA in hospital (4%) after under-treatment with insulin (37). Around 1 in 500 inpatients with type 2 diabetes developed HHS during their hospital stay (0.2%). It is important to record all hospital-acquired DKA and HHS as serious incidents and undertake appropriate root cause analysis.

References

1 Kitabchi AE, Umpierrez GE, Miles JM, Fisher JN. Hyperglycemic crises in adult patients with diabetes. *Diabetes Care.* 2009;32(7):1335–1343.

2 American Diabetes Association. Standards of medical care in diabetes – 2018. *Diabetes Care* 41(Suppl 1):S1–S159.

3 Dhatariya K, Savage M, Kelly T, et al. Joint British Diabetes Societies Inpatient Care Group. The management of diabetic ketoacidosis in adults. 2nd edn. Update: September 2013. http://www.diabetologists-abcd.org.uk/JBDS/JBDS.htm. 2013.

4 Sacks DB, Arnold M, Bakris GL, et al. Guidelines and recommendations for laboratory analysis in the diagnosis and management of diabetes mellitus. *Diabetes Care.* 2011;34(6):e61–e99.

5 Dhatariya K. Blood ketones: measurement, interpretation, limitations and utility in the management of diabetic ketoacidosis. *Rev Diabet Stud.* 2016;13(4):217–225.

6 Dhatariya KK, Umpierrez GE. Guidelines for management of diabetic ketoacidosis: time to revise? *Lancet Diabetes Endocrinol.* 2017;5(5):321–323.

7 Edge JA, Nunney I, Dhatariya KK. Diabetic ketoacidosis in an adolescent and young adult population in the UK in 2014: a national survey comparison of management in paediatric and adult settings. *Diabetic Med.* 2016; 33(10):1352–1359.

8 Umpierrez G, Korytkowski M. Diabetic emergencies: ketoacidosis, hyperglycaemic hyperosmolar state and hypoglycaemia. *Nat Rev Endocrinol.* 2016;12(4):222–232.

9 Dhatariya KK, Nunney I, Higgins K, Sampson MJ, Iceton G. A national survey of the management of diabetic ketoacidosis in the UK in 2014. *Diabetic Med.* 2016;33(2):252–260.

10 Smiley D, Chandra P, Umpierrez GE. Update on diagnosis, pathogenesis and management of ketosis-prone Type 2 diabetes mellitus. *Diabetes Manag (Lond).* 2011;1(6):589–600.

11 Peters AL, Buschur EO, Buse JB, et al. Euglycemic diabetic ketoacidosis: a potential complication of treatment with sodium-glucose cotransporter 2 inhibition. *Diabetes Care.* 2015;38(9):1687–1693.

12 Scott A, on Behalf of the Joint British Diabetes Societies (JBDS) for Inpatient

Care. Management of hyperosmolar hyperglycaemic state in adults with diabetes. *Diabetic Med.* 2015;32(6): 714–724.

13 Centers for Disease Control and Prevention. *Diabetes Public Health Resource: Hospitalisation for Diabetic Ketoacidosis.* http://www.cdc.gov/diabetes/statistics/dkafirst/. 2016. (accessed May 9, 2017).

14 Wang J, Williams DE, Narayan KM, Geiss LS. Declining death rates from hyperglycemic crisis among adults with diabetes, U.S., 1985–2002. *Diabetes Care.* 2006;29(9):2018–2022.

15 Lin SF, Lin JD, Huang YY. Diabetic ketoacidosis: comparisons of patient characteristics, clinical presentations and outcomes today and 20 years ago. *Chang Gung Med J.* 2005;28(1):24–30.

16 Otieno CF, Kayima JK, Omonge EO, Oyoo GO. Diabetic ketoacidosis: risk factors, mechanisms and management strategies in sub-Saharan Africa: a review. *E Afr Med J.* 2005;82(12 (Suppl)): S197–S203.

17 Greene JA, Riggs KR. Why is there no generic insulin? Historical origins of a modern problem. *N Eng J Med.* 2015;372(12):1171–1175.

18 Hamblin PS, Topliss DJ, Chosich N, Lording DW, Stockigt JR. Deaths associated with diabetic ketoacidosis and hyperosmolar coma, 1973–1988. *Med J Aust.* 1989;151(8):441–442.

19 Varadarajan M, Patel M, Kakkar N, et al. Are the results from the 2014 UK national survey on the management of diabetic ketoacidosis applicable to individual centres? *Diabetes Res Clin Pract.* 2017;127:140–146.

20 Matfin G. Diabetes mellitus and the metabolic syndrome. In: Porth CM, Matfin G. eds. *Pathophysiology: Concepts of Altered Health States.* Philadelphia, PA: Lippincott Williams & Wilkins; 2008: 1047–1077.

21 Barwell ND, McKay GA, Fisher M. Drugs for diabetes: part 7 insulin. *Br J Cardiol.* 2011;18:224–228.

22 English P, Williams G. Hyperglycaemic crises and lactic acidosis in diabetes mellitus. *Postgrad Med J.* 2004;80(943): 253–261.

23 Weinstock RS, Xing D, Maahs DM, et al. Severe hypoglycemia and diabetic ketoacidosis in adults with type 1 diabetes: results from the T1D Exchange Clinic Registry. *J Clin Endocrinol Metab.* 2013;98(8):3411–3419.

24 Mays JA, Jackson KL, Derby TA, et al. An evaluation of recurrent diabetic ketoacidosis, fragmentation of care, and mortality across Chicago, Illinois. *Diabetes Care.* 2016;39(10):1671.

25 Herrington WG, Nye HJ, Hammersley MS, Watkinson PJ. Are arterial and venous samples clinically equivalent for the estimation of pH, serum bicarbonate and potassium concentration in critically ill patients? *Diabetic Med.* 2012;29(1): 32–35.

26 Ma OJ, Rush MD, Godfrey MM, Gaddis G. Arterial blood gas results rarely influence emergency physician management of patients with suspected diabetic ketoacidosis. *Acad Emerg Med.* 2003;10(8):836–841.

27 Verbalis JG, Goldsmith SR, Greenberg A, et al. Diagnosis, evaluation, and treatment of hyponatremia: Expert panel recommendations. *Am J Med.* 2013; 126(Suppl):S1–S42.

28 Savage MW, Dhatariya KK, Kilvert A, et al. Joint British Diabetes Societies Guideline for the management of diabetic ketoacidosis. *Diabetic Med.* 2011;28(5): 508–515.

29 Sheikh-Ali M, Karon BS, Basu A, et al. Can serum beta-hydroxybutyrate be used to diagnose diabetic ketoacidosis? *Diabetes Care.* 2008;31(4):643–647.

30 Bektas F, Eray O, Sari R, Akbas H. Point of care blood ketone testing of diabetic patients in the emergency department. *Endocr Res.* 2004;30(3):395–402.

31 Khan AS, Talbot JA, Tieszen KL, et al. Evaluation of a bedside blood ketone sensor: the effects of acidosis, hyperglycaemia and acetoacetate on sensor

performance. *Diabetic Med*. 2004;21(7): 782–785.

32 Wallace TM, Matthews DR. Recent advances in the monitoring and management of diabetic ketoacidosis. *QJM*. 2004;97(12):773–780.

33 Hsia E, Seggelke S, Gibbs J, et al. Subcutaneous administration of glargine to diabetic patients receiving insulin infusion prevents rebound hyperglycemia. *J Clin Endocrinol Metab*. 2012;97(9):3132–3137.

34 George S, Dale J, Stanisstreet D. A guideline for the use of variable rate intravenous insulin infusion in medical inpatients. *Diabetic Med*. 2015;32(6): 706–713.

35 Hale PJ, Crase JE, Nattrass M. Metabolic effects of bicarbonate in the treatment of diabetic ketoacidosis. *Br Med J*. 1984;290(6451):1035–1038.

36 Chua HR, Schneider A, Bellomo R. Bicarbonate in diabetic ketoacidosis: a systematic review. *Ann Intensive Care*. 2013;1(23).

37 Health and Social Care Information Centre. *National Diabetes Inpatient Audit (NaDIA), Open Data 2016*, 2017. www.digital.nhs.uk/pubs/nadia2016 (accessed April 24, 2017).

33

Short-Term Intensive Insulin Therapy in Patients with Newly Presenting Type 2 Diabetes

Wen Xu, David Owens, and Jianping Weng

Key Points

- Type 2 diabetes mellitus (T2DM) is a complex, chronic metabolic disorder characterized by two major pathophysiological defects, i.e., insulin resistance and pancreatic beta-cell dysfunction.
- However, the natural history of T2DM is primarily determined by the progressive deterioration of pancreatic beta-cell function, a pathological process that continues over time.
- In recent years, temporary administration of short-term intensive insulin (STII) therapy early in the course of T2DM has been a strategy of considerable interest to try to arrest or alter this natural history. STII offers the possibility of preserving beta-cell function and inducing a long-term, drug-free period of diabetes remission in newly presenting persons with T2DM.
- The concept of "diabetes in remission" has received renewed interest in view of the beneficial effects of bariatric (metabolic) surgery in persons with T2DM, which can induce diabetes remission in up to 95% of patients.

- Diabetes in remission has been defined by an ADA Consensus Statement: partial remission is hyperglycemia below diabetes diagnostic thresholds for at least one year; complete remission is normal glycemic measures of at least one year's duration; and prolonged remission is complete remission of at least five years' duration. It is an encouraging concept because it implies that the natural course of T2DM may be partially or even completely reversed.
- Clinicians in the precision medicine era of patient care are in the position to apply the most appropriate therapy for personalized or individualized treatment approaches.
- Knowledge of STII and other short-term intensive intervention therapies (including diet and intensive lifestyle changes) are of relevance to clinicians who manage patients presenting with newly-diagnosed and possibly even established T2DM, and highlights a treatment paradigm shift that focuses on reversing the disease (i.e., inducing diabetes remission) rather than simply controlling progressive hyperglycemia.

Introduction

Type 2 diabetes mellitus (T2DM) is a complex, chronic metabolic disorder, the pathophysiology of which is driven by two main co-existing defects, i.e., target-cell resistance to the activity of insulin (insulin resistance), and relative insulin secretion insufficiency by the pancreatic beta-cell (beta-cell dysfunction) to overcome the insulin insensitivity.

The relative contribution of these main defects varies between individuals. However, the natural history of T2DM is primarily determined by the progressive deterioration of pancreatic beta-cell function, a pathological process that continues over time. As a consequence, the typical clinical course of this disease consists of the sequential addition of anti-hyperglycemic preparations over time, followed ultimately by insulin therapy when functional beta-cell capacity deteriorates to the point at which glycemic control can no longer be achieved without exogenous insulin supplementation. At this point in the progressive course of T2DM, insulin therapy is generally continued indefinitely thereafter.

It is widely acknowledged that glycemic control in T2DM is suboptimal worldwide, and that evidence from several geographic areas demonstrates that glycosylated hemoglobin (HbA1c) is often high at the time of initial presentation (1,2). For example, among 1256 newly diagnosed T2DM patients in two managed care databases in the USA, 66% had an HbA1c >7% (53 mmol/mol) in the 180 days prior to first medication, and nearly one-quarter (23%) had an HbA1c ≥9.0% (75 mmol/mol) (1). In another population-based sample from Denmark of 1136 newly diagnosed persons with T2DM (i.e., single fasting, whole blood glucose ≥126 mg/dL [7.0 mmol/L] or plasma glucose [FPG] ≥144 mg/dL [8.0 mmol/L]), only 8.5% had an HbA1c ≤7.4% (57 mmol/mol) (2).

The importance of normalizing blood glucose early after diagnosis and induce long-term benefits (i.e., "metabolic memory" or legacy effect) was firmly established by the United Kingdom Prospective Diabetes Study (UKPDS) (3), and as several recent reviews demonstrate, further supporting evidence continues to accrue (4,5). However, timely initiation of therapy alone is insufficient to ensure that the pathophysiological processes in T2DM are adequately interrupted. Expert guidelines address the importance of selecting a therapy that is not only appropriately intensive but also timely, so as to minimize avoidable glycemic exposure (6,7). In recent years, temporary administration of short-term intensive insulin (STII) therapy early in the course of T2DM has been a strategy of considerable interest. Short-term intensive insulin therapy for recently diagnosed T2DM patients offers the potential to restore beta-cell function and induce remission of hyperglycemia (i.e., maintenance of normoglycemia without use of anti-diabetic medication). STII therapy has been demonstrated to improve residual beta-cell function and thereby stabilize the disease process in its very early stages, proving to be of value in the treatment of newly presenting T2DM (8,9). Benefits of early intensive insulin therapy include marked reductions in glucose toxicity, restoration of beta-cell responsiveness and insulin sensitivity, and even reduction in hyperglucagonemia, representing remission of the disease processes in many instances (9,10). Recent basic research suggested the potential mechanism of such benefits: beta-cell dedifferentiation to endocrine progenitor-like cells during stress-induced hyperglycemia, and strictly normalizing blood glucose could induce dedifferentiated cells' re-differentiation to mature beta-cells and hence restoration of drug responsivity (11,12).

In the AACE/ACE (American Association of Clinical Endocrinologists/American College of Endocrinology) comprehensive type 2 diabetes management algorithm 2018, insulin is recommended for T2DM patients presenting with symptoms and an HbA1c >9.0% (75 mmol/mol) (6). The Global Partnership for Effective Diabetes Management model also refers to the temporary use of insulin for newly diagnosed T2DM adults with HbA1c >9% (75 mmol/mol), but fails to elaborate further, neither strongly endorsing or refuting the STII therapy concept (13). In addition, the American Diabetes Association (ADA)/European Association for the Study of Diabetes (EASD) consensus statement recommends initial insulin therapy as an option when HbA1c ≥9% (75 mmol/mol), and definite consideration with HbA1c ≥10–12% (86–108 mmol/mol), and also mentions that it may be possible to taper off insulin once initial glucotoxicity is reversed and to consider transfer to other types of non-insulin therapies (7). Based on the accumulating evidence, an expert group advocated to endorse the concept of STII therapy as an option for some patients with T2DM at the time of diagnosis (14). Notably, the latest Israeli guidelines suggested considering immediate, sometimes short-term, insulin treatment for patients with HbA1c >9% (75 mmol/mol) or in a symptomatic patient based on current evidence which reinforces the importance and safety of early STII and the ability of such treatment to decrease glucotoxicity and lipotoxicity and to preserve beta-cell function (15,16). This is the first expert guidelines to include STII therapy as an option. Several issues are worthy of being explored to help the optimal use of STII therapy in clinical practice, such as the target population and biomarkers, follow-up treatment regimen, generalizability to primary care, education of patients and providers, etc. In this chapter, we briefly discuss developments and clinical experience in the current understanding of STII therapy of T2DM.

Clinical Evidence of STII Therapy in Newly Presenting T2DM

There is a wide range of evidence currently available supporting the use of STII therapy in newly diagnosed T2DM. Our group have repeatedly shown that following STII therapy, many subjects are able to achieve and sustain prolonged diabetes remissions (periods of euglycemia) despite having discontinued all anti-hyperglycemic medications. In addition, numerous formal clinical studies have demonstrated that STII therapy (delivered via either continuous subcutaneous insulin infusion [CSII] or multiple daily injections [MDI]) can quickly normalize glycemic control, improve beta-cell function, and restore first-phase insulin secretion in newly diagnosed T2DM (9,17–21) (Table 33-1). Moreover, recent studies have demonstrated that STII can reduce post-challenge

hyperglucagonemia, indicating the improvement of α cell function (10,22). STII therapy has also been favorably assessed in a recent meta-analysis (23), as well as in review articles, where it has either been the focus of the review (24) or been discussed along with other treatment options as a new therapeutic approach (5).

The largest and most robust clinical trial of STII therapy enrolled 382 newly diagnosed persons with T2DM at nine centers in China and randomized them to either insulin (CSII or MDI) or oral anti-hyperglycemic therapy (9). Baseline assessments showed similar beta-cell function and insulin resistance in the three groups. Therapies were titrated to fasting and post-prandial glucose targets after each of the three main meals, and continued until normoglycemia was achieved for two consecutive weeks. Two days following cessation of treatment, the first-phase insulin secretion was increased in all three groups in response to intravenous glucose. Remission rates at 1 year were higher in the two insulin-treated groups (51.1% CSII, 44.9% MDI) than in the oral therapy group (26.7%). Furthermore, the increase in the first-phase insulin response was maintained at 1 year in the two insulin-treated groups, but declined in the group allocated to oral medication (Figure 33-1).

A meta-analysis performed including this trial and those of six other smaller trials of STII therapy, involving 839 participants was performed (23). This meta-analysis further underscored the robustness of the evidence supporting STII therapy where 46% of patients were seen to remain in drug-free remission after 12 months. All but one study showed an improvement in beta-cell function, as assessed by Homeostasis Model Assessment-Beta-cell function (HOMA-B), and all but one study showed a decrease in insulin resistance, as assessed by HOMA-Insulin Resistance (HOMA-IR). In the pooled data analysis, the proportion of patients in drug-free remission was 66.2% at 3 months, 58.9% at 6 months, 46.3% at 12 months, and 42.1% at 24 months (Figure 33-2).

Table 33-1 Characteristics of STII studies included in a meta-analysis (23)

	Year of publication	Sample size	design	IIT regimen	IIT duration (days)	Baseline mean age (years)	Baseline proportion of men (%)	Base line mean BMI (kg/m²)	Baseline HbA1c (%)	Total follow-up after IIT (months)	Evaluation of Glycemic remission
Li Y et al. (8)	2004	126	Interventional; one arm	CSII	14	48.6(11.6)	61.9%	25.1(3.6)	10.0% (1.9)	24	Yes
Chen H et al. (25)	2007	138	Interventional; one arm	CSII	14	45.8(7.0)	62.3%	25.4(3.4)	11.9% (2.0)	0	No
Zhao Q et al. (26)	2007	120	Interventional; one arm	CSII	14	47.0(12.0)	83.3%	24.0(3.0)	Not available	0	No
Chen H et al. (27)	2008	22	Randomized controlled trial; one arm long-term IIT; one arm on short-term IIT	MDI	14	58.7(16.0)	77.3%	27.7(6.5)	11.7% (1.9)	0	No
Weng J et al. (9)	2008	251	Randomized controlled trial; two arms on IIT	CSII or MDI	14	50.0(10.5)	67.3%	24.7(2.8)	9.7% (2.3)	12	Yes
Chen A et al. (28)	2012	118	Interventional; one arm	CSII	14–21	51.6(10.2)	66.0%	25.0(3.0)	11.0% (2.1)	12	Yes
Liu L et al. (29)	2012	64	Interventional; one arm	CSII	14	49.3(9.5)	68.7%	25.5(3.5)	11.0% (1.8)	3	Yes

Data are mean (SD) unless otherwise stated.

IIT = intensive insulin therapy; CSII = continuous subcutaneous insulin infusion; MDI = multiple daily injections; BMI = body-mass index; HbA1c = glycated hemoglobin. Reproduced with permission from Elsevier.

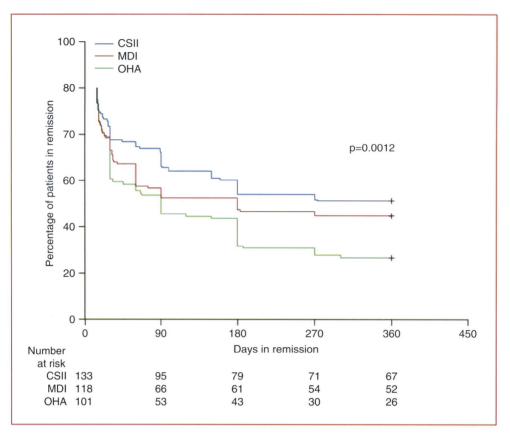

Figure 33-1 Percentage of patients with newly diagnosed type 2 diabetes treated with short-term continuous subcutaneous insulin infusion (CSII), multiple daily injections (MDI) and oral anti-hyperglycemic agents (OHA) in remission along with time (9)

Not all newly diagnosed T2DM subjects have experienced improved beta-cell function or achieved long-term remission following cessation of STII therapy (30), although any therapy that reduces glucotoxicity is likely to improve measures of pancreatic beta-cell response (31). Therefore, a critical requirement is to be able to identify those individuals most likely to achieve sustained preservation of beta-cells following STII by phenotypic characteristics and/or other biomarkers in order to personalize treatment approaches. Numerous predictors of long-term remission of hyperglycemia have previously been identified in clinical studies (23). Many of these predictors include markers of glycemic control. In the meta-analysis discussed above, the presence at baseline of lower FPG and higher body mass index (BMI) were significantly associated with STII remission (21). Mechanistically, it is possible that once STII therapy is implemented, elimination of detrimental effects of glucotoxicity on existing beta-cell mass provides more capacity to improve endogenous insulin secretion. With respect to other specific characteristics and biomarkers, studies have indicated that improved beta-cell response and elimination of hyperglycemia can also be predicted by shorter diabetes duration (32,33), increased 1,5-anhydroglucitol (a validated short-term marker of glycemic control) (29), preserved late-phase insulin secretion (24), FPG (29,32,34), 2h post-breakfast plasma glucose (32) measured after cessation of STII treatment, and the presence

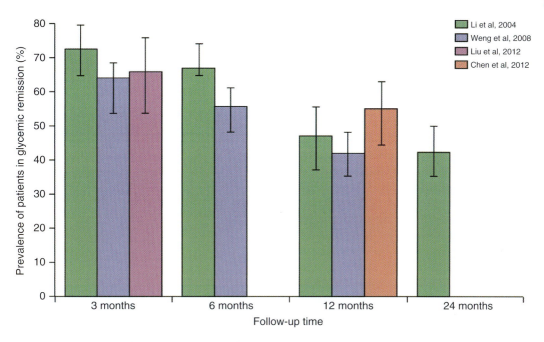

Figure 33-2 Prevalence of participants in drug-free glycemic remission during follow-up after short-term intensive insulin therapy, by study. Bars are 95% CIs (23).

of a higher HbA1c prior to STII therapy (21). The explanation for the latter finding is unclear, but that some persons with higher HbA1c at diagnosis may have a greater residual beta-cell function that is masked by glucotoxicity.

As suggested above, one problem with assessing the potential for remission in an individual with T2DM is that beta-cell function is influenced by a combination of factors that are potentially reversible with treatment (e.g., glucotoxicity, lipotoxicity) as well as intrinsic functional deficits that are not improved by treatment (23). The relative contribution of these two sets of factors (reversible and irreversible) will vary within each person. This raises the question relating to the use of beta-cell function at baseline to predict remission. As has been shown in clinical trials, when beta-cell function is an outcome, it is important to first remove the confounding effect of having differential amounts of reversible components (23,24). Removing these confounding effects prior to randomization is essential if the mechanism

of action by which STII therapy improves beta-cell function (e.g., beyond elimination of glucotoxicity) is to be elucidated. Several other possible mechanisms have been proposed, including a decrease in tumor-necrosis factor (TNF)-alpha which may contribute to the positive effect of STII therapy on beta-cells (25). In another study, evidence implies that decreased visceral fat and increased skeletal muscle mass following insulin treatment may be associated with the observed improvements in beta-cell function (35). The liver is central to the pathogenesis of T2DM, with hepatic glucose production being tightly regulated by portal-insulin concentration (36). Hepatic insulin resistance occurs because of impaired insulin signaling in the liver, impairment of lipolysis resulting in excess free fatty acids, and elevated plasma glucagon levels, which all facilitate gluconeogenesis and hyperglycemia. Improvement in hepatic insulin resistance [HOMA-IR] in response to STII was shown to be necessary to achieve reversibility of beta-cell dysfunction (21).

Clinical Practice of STII Therapy in Newly Presenting T2DM

There is as yet no consensus about the most appropriate threshold (e.g., HbA1c) for initiating STII treatment or about how long to maintain STII therapy after normalization of blood glucose. Due to the novelty of STII therapy and potential reservations among clinicians, it may be advisable to recommend STII therapy for those with an HbA1c >9.0% (75 mmol/mol) and FPG >200 mg/dL [11.1 mmol/L] (6,23). Using a more familiar and practical threshold for starting insulin therapy might facilitate acceptance until more definitive data from larger comparative studies are published, even though benefit could also be seen in patients with lower HbA1c at baseline (37). However, it is important to note that STII therapy would involve a basal–bolus approach which is more intense than the basal-only treatment as an initial regimen recommended by the ADA/EASD or AACE/ACE guidelines. With respect to optimal duration of treatment, future clinical studies are needed to examine time to failure of remission as it appears to vary according to the duration of STII therapy. Although the meta-analysis of STII therapy provides some guidance about time to failure, those data must be used cautiously as the studies were heterogeneous (23). Additionally, it would be important to know how the timing of initiating STII therapy with respect to disease diagnosis might affect beta-cell preservation and recovery.

The optimal treatment regimen following discontinuation of STII therapy also remains to be determined. Despite the benefits of a remission period free of drug therapy, it is possible that the optimal regimen would include some form of ongoing pharmacological treatment (in addition to lifestyle changes). To clarify this, one option would be to start with STII therapy and then to randomize the persons with T2DM to standard therapy or metformin or alternative non-insulin therapies (e.g., incretin-based therapy, such as glucagon-like 1 receptor [GLP-1] agonists or dipeptidyl peptidase-4 [DPP-4] inhibitors) and compare time to remission failure. One clinical study randomized 51 patients with T2DM to daily subcutaneous liraglutide or placebo injection after 4 weeks of STII. The results showed that liraglutide provides robust enhancement of beta-cell function that was sustained over 48 weeks but lost – two weeks after cessation of therapy (37).

There is a substantial educational need among healthcare providers with respect to STII therapy, due to very limited clinical experience even among endocrinologists. However, healthcare practitioners should be aware that this is a viable option for certain groups of newly diagnosed persons with T2DM. A key difference, as well as potential advantage which needs to be appreciated, when using insulin early at the time of diagnosis of T2DM is that the comparatively greater existing beta-cell mass should allow the use of lower insulin doses while still achieving the desired level of glucose control, with the added benefit of a low risk of hypoglycemia (since the residual beta-cells ultimately modulate the amount of endogenous insulin secreted, insulin secretion is inhibited in response to hypoglycemia). Consistent with this concept, the improvement in beta-cell function in response to STII is associated with decreased glycemic variability (38). Indeed, rates of hypoglycemia tend to be low when applying STII early in the course of type 2 diabetes (39). Much, of course, depends on the competence of the healthcare team and the recipient's behavior and preconceptions about insulin therapy. Nevertheless, despite these considerations, it is quite feasible with experience to use STII therapy in an ambulatory setting.

Education in insulin initiation and intensification is also very important for clinicians and patients alike. Although reluctance to initiate insulin treatment in T2DM is well described (40), other studies have shown that insulin administration issues become less of a concern once patients gain familiarity with insulin therapy and experience the clinical benefits (41). Indeed, several studies have now demonstrated that insulin can be well accepted as initial therapy, particularly once patients are well informed and understand the advantages (18,42,43). Positive attitudes have also been seen to correlate well with improved glycemic control (42). One study of 34 patients with insulin-naïve T2DM commenced a course of STII therapy for 4–8 weeks to determine eligibility for a clinical trial (43). Quality of life and treatment satisfaction were assessed at baseline and after completion of the STII. There were statistically significant improvements on the following items in the Medical Short-Form 36 (SF-36): physical functioning (P = 0.009), general health (P = 0.03), and mental health (P = 0.04). The Diabetes Quality of Life (DQOL) instrument also showed significant improvements in diabetes worry (P = 0.006) and treatment satisfaction (P = 0.007). In another study, insulin was used in conjunction with metformin in 63 newly diagnosed, treatment-naïve T2DM patients (18). Results indicated that 97% were satisfied with their insulin treatment. In another trial of newly diagnosed persons, insulin plus metformin was initiated for a 3-month lead-in period prior to randomization to further treatment of continuing insulin plus metformin or triple oral therapy (metformin, pioglitazone, and glyburide [glibenclamide]) for 36 months (42). All of the subjects randomized to insulin were willing to continue, and there were no differences in treatment satisfaction between the two groups. In future clinical diabetes trials, STII therapy may be a useful pre-randomization method of improving glycemic function (23). There is a real possibility that because the recipients will be satisfied with the results and clinical benefits, that, post-trial they may request to resume using insulin therapy, finding it much easier and better tolerated than expected.

From a practical perspective, there are some logistical issues that are potential barriers to achieving broader introduction and acceptance of the use of STII therapy. Endocrinologists, who may be the most comfortable at initiating this treatment regimen in T2DM, are usually managing patients well beyond the stage of being newly, or even recently, diagnosed except for maybe those presenting with a hyperglycemic emergency. By contrast, primary care physicians, who are more likely to make the initial diagnosis, are unlikely to initiate STII therapy themselves due to inadequate training and infrastructure (e.g., lack of diabetes educators), and also limited consultation time with patients (especially in the ambulatory setting). There are also other logistical issues such as inadequate number and access to endocrinologists in many countries. From a public health standpoint, overall increasing numbers of persons with T2DM represent a huge challenge for diabetes management, especially as a significant proportion remain undiagnosed (e.g., approximately 8 million out of a total of 29 million persons with T2DM in the USA are undiagnosed). If the diagnosis is undetected or significantly delayed, it may be that these persons are unlikely to benefit from STII therapy due to the availability of insufficient residual beta-cell function (although patients with higher HbA1c responded better to STII therapy). This problem is even more likely to be an issue in many low- and middle-income countries around the world due to limited public health infrastructure and robust access to insulin and monitoring tools. A better understanding of the cost-effectiveness of STII is clearly warranted. Other unique challenges include those individuals with T2DM who believe that insulin is only for the very severely ill and that using insulin represents a lifetime commitment. Another issue to be mindful of is that because the studies so far have been conducted predominantly in Asian populations, there is a perception that STII therapy is not applicable to other ethnic groups. However, a study conducted in multiple ethnic groups has shown that STII therapy can also be efficacious in non-Asian populations (21).

With respect to health economics, a modeling study to show how STII therapy could reduce medical costs would be beneficial in promoting acceptance. In addition, a long-term study to demonstrate that remission secondary to STII therapy could reduce the microvascular complications of diabetes would be very helpful. Logically, one would expect that improved beta-cell function could result in better long-term glycemic control and health, although the details of how this would translate into cost savings are not entirely clear. Once STII therapy is clearly defined and a consensus is reached, it should be possible to construct the health economic models using available data. It would be worthwhile reviewing existing data on diabetes remission and prediction that could be used to show the potential cost savings.

Conclusions

STII therapy offers the possibility of preserving beta-cell function and inducing a long-term, drug-free period of diabetes remission in newly presenting persons with T2DM. The concept of "Diabetes in remission" (44) has received renewed interest in view of the beneficial effects of bariatric (metabolic) surgery on glucose metabolism and beta-cell function, and can induce diabetes remission in up to 95% of patients (44). Diabetes in remission has been defined by an ADA Consensus Statement: partial remission is hyperglycemia below diabetes diagnostic thresholds for at least one year; complete remission is normal glycemic measures of at least one year's duration; and prolonged remission is complete remission of at least five years' duration (45). It is an encouraging concept because it implies that the natural course of T2DM may be partially or even completely reversed.

A recent study used a combination of oral medications, insulin, and lifestyle therapy (termed "short-term intensive metabolic" strategy) to treat both newly and established T2DM patients intensively for 2–4 months. They found that up to 40% of participants were able to stay in diabetes remission three months after stopping diabetes medications (46). The authors concluded that "the findings support the notion that T2DM can be reversed, at least in the short term –

not only with bariatric surgery, but with medical approaches." This study had several important features compared with previous studies (47). First, lifestyle therapy aiming to achieve and maintain ≥5% weight reduction was integrated with medications, which was proven to be an acceptable short-term intensive intervention with high adherence. Second, participants with not only newly diagnosed but also established diabetes were included. Third, various durations of the same combination interventions were adopted to evaluate the impact of the time effect on remission. Consequently, the results from this trial provide new evidence for diabetes remission in T2DM. This study, along with others, strongly supports the concept of diabetes remission induced by intensive interventions in some T2DM patients. Accordingly, it is time to reconsider the initiation strategy when treating patients with T2DM (47). However, the recently published DiRECT study in primary care (48), suggests that we should reconsider not just treatment initiation in T2DM, but also later on in the course of diabetes. This study demonstrated that compared with standard care in T2DM (mean diagnosis duration 6 years), withdrawal of antidiabetic drugs and total diet replacement with very low calorie diet (~825–850 kcal/day) for 3–5 months, followed by diet reintroduction and lifestyle changes, showed that at 12 months almost half of participants achieved diabetic remission (HbA1c <6.5% [<48 mmol/mol]) off all antidiabetic drugs.

We believe that clinicians in the precision medicine era of patient care are in a position to apply the most appropriate therapy for personalized or individualized treatment approaches. Knowledge of STII and other short-term intensive intervention therapies (e.g., diet and intensive lifestyle changes) are of relevance to clinicians who manage patients presenting with newly-diagnosed and possibly even established T2DM, and highlights a treatment paradigm shift that focuses on reversing the disease (i.e., inducing diabetes remission) rather than simply controlling progressive hyperglycemia.

References

1 Brouwer ES, West SL, Kluckman M, et al. Initial and subsequent therapy for newly diagnosed type 2 diabetes patients treated in primary care using data from a vendor-based electronic health record. *Pharmacoepidemiol Drug Saf.* 2012;21: 920–928.

2 Veloso AG, Siersma V, Heldgaard PE, de Fine Olivarius N. Patients newly diagnosed with clinical type 2 diabetes mellitus but presenting with HbA1c within normal range: 19-year mortality and clinical outcomes. *Prim Care Diabetes.* 2013;7: 33–38.

3 Stratton IM, Adler AI, Neil HA, et al. Association of glycaemia with macrovascular and microvascular complications of type 2 diabetes (UKPDS 35): prospective observational study. *BMJ.* 2000;321:405–412.

4 Hanefeld M, Bramlage P. Insulin use early in the course of type 2 diabetes mellitus: the ORIGIN trial. *Curr Diab Rep.* 2013;13: 342–349.

5 Owens DR. Clinical evidence for the earlier initiation of insulin therapy in type 2 diabetes. *Diabetes Technol Ther.* 2013;15: 776–785.

6 Garber AJ, Abrahamson MJ, Barzilay JI, et al. Consensus statement by the American Association of Clinical Endocrinologists and American College of Endocrinology on the Comprehensive Type 2 Diabetes Management Algorithm – 2018 executive summary. *Endocr Pract.* 2018;24:91–120.

7 Inzucchi SE, Bergenstal RM, Buse JB, et al. Management of hyperglycaemia in type 2 diabetes, 2015: a patient-centred approach: update to a position statement of the American Diabetes Association and the European Association for the Study of Diabetes. *Diabetologia.* 2015;58:429–442.

8 Li Y, Xu W, Liao Z, Yao B, et al. Induction of long-term glycemic control in newly diagnosed type 2 diabetic patients is associated with improvement of beta-cell function. *Diabetes Care.* 2004;27: 2597–2602.

9 Weng J, Li Y, Xu W, et al. Effect of intensive insulin therapy on beta-cell function and glycaemic control in patients with newly diagnosed type 2 diabetes: a multicentre randomised parallel-group trial. *Lancet.* 2008;371:1753–1760.

10 Kramer C K, Zinman B, Choi H, Retnakaran R. Effect of short-term intensive insulin therapy on post-challenge hyperglucagonemia in early type 2 diabetes. *J Clin Endocrinol Metab.* 2015; 100:2987–2995.

11 Talchai C, Xuan S, Lin HV, Sussel L, Accili D. Pancreatic beta cell dedifferentiation as a mechanism of diabetic beta cell failure. *Cell.* 2012;150:1223–1234.

12 Wang Z, York NW, Nichols CG, Remedi MS. Pancreatic beta cell dedifferentiation in diabetes and redifferentiation following insulin therapy. *Cell Metab.* 2014;19: 872–882.

13 Bailey CJ, Aschner P, Del Prato S, LaSalle J, Ji L, Matthaei S, Global Partnership for Effective Diabetes M. Individualized glycaemic targets and pharmacotherapy in type 2 diabetes. *Diab Vasc Dis Res.* 2013; 10:397–409.

14 Weng J, Retnakaran R, Ariachery CA, et al. Short-term intensive insulin therapy at diagnosis in type 2 diabetes: plan for filling the gaps. *Diabetes Metab Res Rev.* 2015;31: 537–544.

15 Mosenzon O, Pollack R, Raz I. Treatment of type 2 diabetes: from "guidelines" to "position statements" and back: recommendations of the Israel National Diabetes Council. *Diabetes Care.* 2016;39 Suppl 2:S146–S153.

16 Raz I, Mosenzon O. Early insulinization to prevent diabetes progression. *Diabetes Care.* 2013;36 Suppl 2:S190–S197.

17 Ilkova H, Glaser B, Tunckale A, Bagriacik N, Cerasi E. Induction of long-term glycemic control in newly diagnosed type 2

diabetic patients by transient intensive insulin treatment. *Diabetes Care*. 1997; 20:1353–1356.

18 Lingvay I, Kaloyanova PF, Adams-Huet B, Salinas K, Raskin P. Insulin as initial therapy in type 2 diabetes: effective, safe, and well accepted. *J Investig Med*. 2007; 55:62–68.

19 Chon S, Oh S, Kim SW, Kim JW, Kim YS, Woo JT. The effect of early insulin therapy on pancreatic beta-cell function and long-term glycemic control in newly diagnosed type 2 diabetic patients. *Korean J Intern Med*. 2010;25:273–281.

20 Retnakaran R, Qi Y, Opsteen C, Vivero E, Zinman B. Initial short-term intensive insulin therapy as a strategy for evaluating the preservation of beta-cell function with oral antidiabetic medications: a pilot study with sitagliptin. *Diabetes Obes Metab*. 2012;12:909–915.

21 Kramer CK, Choi H, Zinman B, Retnakaran R. Determinants of reversibility of beta-cell dysfunction in response to short-term intensive insulin therapy in patients with early type 2 diabetes. *Am J Physiol Endocrinol Metab*. 2013;305:E1398–1407.

22 Zhang B, Chen YY, Yang ZJ, Wang X, Li GW. Improvement in insulin sensitivity following intensive insulin therapy and association of glucagon with long-term diabetes remission. *J Int Med Res*. 2016; 44:1543–1550.

23 Kramer CK, Zinman B, Retnakaran R. Short-term intensive insulin therapy in type 2 diabetes mellitus: a systematic review and meta-analysis. *Lancet Diabetes Endocrinol*. 2013;1:28–34.

24 Xu W, Weng J. Current role of short-term intensive insulin strategies in newly diagnosed type 2 diabetes. *J Diabetes*. 2013;5:268–274.

25 Chen H, Ren A, Hu S, Mo W, Xin X, Jia W. The significance of tumor necrosis factor-alpha in newly diagnosed type 2 diabetic patients by transient intensive insulin treatment. *Diabetes Res Clin Pract*. 2007;75:327–332.

26 Zhao QB, Wang HF, Sun CF, Ma AQ, Cui CC. [Effect of short-term intensive treatment with insulin pump on beta cell function and the mechanism of oxidative stress in newly diagnosed type 2 diabetic patients]. *Nan Fang Yi Ke Da Xue Xue Bao*. 2007;27:1878–1879.

27 Chen HS, Wu TE, Jap TS, Hsiao LC, Lee SH, Lin HD. Beneficial effects of insulin on glycemic control and beta-cell function in newly diagnosed type 2 diabetes with severe hyperglycemia after short-term intensive insulin therapy. *Diabetes Care*. 2008;31:1927–1932.

28 Chen A, Huang Z, Wan X, et al. Attitudes toward diabetes affect maintenance of drug-free remission in patients with newly diagnosed type 2 diabetes after short-term continuous subcutaneous insulin infusion treatment. *Diabetes Care*. 2012;35: 474–481.

29 Liu L, Wan X, Liu J, Huang Z, Cao X, Li Y. Increased 1,5-anhydroglucitol predicts glycemic remission in patients with newly diagnosed type 2 diabetes treated with short-term intensive insulin therapy. *Diabetes Technol Ther*. 2012;14:756–761.

30 Retnakaran R, Yakubovich N, Qi Y, Opsteen C, Zinman B. The response to short-term intensive insulin therapy in type 2 diabetes. *Diabetes Obes Metab*. 2010;12: 65–71.

31 Chiasson JL. Early insulin use in type 2 diabetes: what are the cons? *Diabetes Care*. 2009;32 Suppl 2:S270–S274.

32 Xu W, Li YB, Deng WP, Hao YT, Weng JP. Remission of hyperglycemia following intensive insulin therapy in newly diagnosed type 2 diabetic patients: a long-term follow-up study. *Chin Med J (Engl)*. 2009;122:2554–2559.

33 Kramer CK, Zinman B, Choi H, Retnakaran R. Predictors of sustained drug-free diabetes remission over 48 weeks following short-term intensive insulin therapy in early type 2 diabetes. *BMJ Open Diabetes Res Care*. 2016;4:e000270.

34 Liu J, Liu J, Fang D, Liu L, et al. Fasting plasma glucose after intensive insulin therapy predicted long-term glycemic control in newly diagnosed type 2 diabetic patients. *Endocr J*. 2013;60:725–732.

35 Son JW, Jeong HK, Lee SS, et al. The effect of early intensive insulin therapy on body fat distribution and beta-cell function in newly diagnosed type 2 diabetes. *Endocr Res*. 2013;38:160–167.

36 Del Prato S, Marchetti P. Beta- and alpha-cell dysfunction in type 2 diabetes. *Horm Metab Res*. 2004;36: 775–781.

37 Retnakaran R, Kramer CK, Choi H, Swaminathan B, Zinman B. Liraglutide and the preservation of pancreatic beta-cell function in early type 2 diabetes: the LIBRA trial. *Diabetes Care*. 2014;37: 3270–3278.

38 Kramer CK, Choi H, Zinman B, Retnakaran R. Glycemic variability in patients with early type 2 diabetes: the impact of improvement in beta-cell function. *Diabetes Care*. 2014;37:1116–1123.

39 Retnakaran R, Zinman B. Short-term intensified insulin treatment in type 2 diabetes: long-term effects on beta-cell function. *Diabetes Obes Metab*. 2012;14 Suppl 3:161–166.

40 Polonsky WH, Hajos TR, Dain MP, Snoek FJ. Are patients with type 2 diabetes reluctant to start insulin therapy? An examination of the scope and underpinnings of psychological insulin resistance in a large, international population. *Curr Med Res Opin*. 2011; 27:1169–1174.

41 Casciano R, Malangone E, Ramachandran A, Gagliardino JJ. A quantitative assessment of patient barriers to insulin. *Int J Clin Pract*. 2011;65:408–414.

42 Lingvay I, Legendre JL, Kaloyanova PF, Zhang S, Adams-Huet B, Raskin P. Insulin-based versus triple oral therapy for newly diagnosed type 2 diabetes: which is better? *Diabetes Care*. 2009;32:1789–1795.

43 Opsteen C, Qi Y, Zinman B, Retnakaran R. Effect of short-term intensive insulin therapy on quality of life in type 2 diabetes. *J Eval Clin Pract*. 2012;18:256–261.

44 Hillson R. Diabetes in remission. *Practical Diabetes*. 2017;34:78–80.

45 Buse JB, Caprio S, Cefalu WT, et al. How do we define cure of diabetes? *Diabetes Care*. 2009;32:2133–2135.

46 McInnes N, Smith A, Otto R, et al. Piloting a remission strategy in type 2 diabetes: results of a randomized controlled trial. *J Clin Endocrinol Metab*. 2017;102: 1596–1605.

47 Weng J. Piloting a remission strategy in type 2 diabetes: results of a randomized controlled trial. PracticeUpdate website. http://www.practiceupdate.com/content/piloting-a-remission-strategy-in-type-2-diabetes/50898/65/8/1 (accessed June 4, 2017).

48 Lean MEJ, Leslie WS, Barnes AC, et al. Primary care-led weight management for remission of type 2 diabetes (DiRECT): an open-label, cluster-randomised trial. *Lancet* 2017. DOI: http://dx.doi.org/10.1016/S0140-6736(17)33102-1 (accessed December 15, 2017).

34

Management of Concentrated Insulins in Acute Care Settings

Nuha El Sayed, Megan J. Ritter, and Alissa R. Segal

Key Points

- Standard insulin preparations are 100 units/mL (i.e., U100 insulin). They have been used therapeutically for many years, and are the most common insulins used in acute care settings.
- More recently, several new insulins have become available in concentrations other than the standard U100 formulation (i.e., U200 and U300).
- These newer insulin formulations may extend the duration of basal activity and/or allow for the delivery of more insulin per volume. Decreasing insulin injection volume may be particularly valuable in insulin-resistant patients who require increased doses of insulin, as this may improve treatment adherence and effectiveness.
- However, use of these concentrated insulins may lead to medication errors by both providers and patients.
- Although the concentrated insulins will infrequently be utilized within hospital or urgent care settings, it is important to understand the differences with these therapies and how they may impact the care of patients transitioning between care systems into or out of these settings.
- Use of regular (human) insulin at the concentration 500 units/mL (i.e., U500) has significantly increased over the years, primarily due to the increase in obesity and associated insulin resistance. In obese and other insulin-resistant patients, the higher U500 insulin concentration results in an activity profile more similar to a pre-mixed short- and intermediate-acting insulin (i.e., onset of action of 30–45 minutes, peak pharmacodynamic action at 7–8.5 hours, and duration of action of 11.5 hours).
- Concentrated formulations of both rapid-acting insulin lispro (U200); and ultra-long acting degludec (U200), are considered bioequivalent when compared to their standard formulations (U100) in pharmacodynamic evaluations.
- Increasing the concentration of insulin glargine from the standard U100 to U300 (300 units/mL) formulation results in extending both the duration and time to onset (i.e., changed from long-acting to ultra-long-acting insulin).
- The challenges posed with the use of insulin occur throughout all areas of the acute care setting. Patients who require concentrated formulations of insulin in outpatient settings pose additional complications to these difficult transitions across care systems.
- Use of standardized practices and education tools provide a base for the safe care of patients using insulin (both standard and concentrated formulations) as they transition acute healthcare settings.

Endocrine and Metabolic Medical Emergencies: A Clinician's Guide, Second Edition. Edited by Glenn Matfin.
© 2018 John Wiley & Sons Ltd. Published 2018 by John Wiley & Sons Ltd.

Introduction

Over the last few years, there has been a rapid expansion of the options available for insulin therapy. These therapies may extend the duration of basal activity (Figure 34-1) and/or allow for the delivery of more insulin per volume, but they also may lead to medication errors by both providers and patients. One of the situations that places patients using insulin at increased risk is when they are transitioning between care into or out of the hospital. Although the newer insulins will infrequently be utilized within hospital or urgent care settings, it is important to understand the differences with these therapies and how they may impact the care of patients transitioning between care systems into or out of these settings. This chapter will briefly review the newer insulin options and address common situations during transitions in care and hospitalizations when using any type of concentrated insulin.

Table 34-1 Concentrated insulins for subcutaneous use

Insulin	Concentration
Degludec (Tresiba™)	200 units/mL (U200)
Glargine (Toujeo™)	300 units/mL (U300)
Lispro (Humalog™)	200 units/mL (U200)
Regular (Humulin™)	500 units/mL (U500)

Background to Concentrated Insulins

Four insulins are now available in concentrations other than the standard 100 units/mL (i.e., U100 insulin) (Table 34-1). Historically, higher concentrations of insulin made it possible to treat patients with significant insulin resistance (generally defined as needing >200 units/day or >2 units/kg insulin), but also heightened the risk of

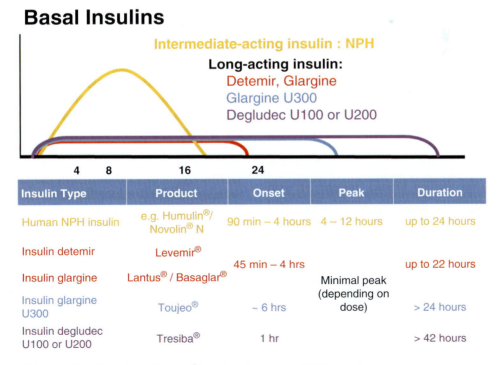

Figure 34-1 Basal insulin options. Basaglar® is an insulin glargine U100 biosimilar.

insulin-related medication errors (1). Use of regular (human) insulin at the concentration 500 units/mL (i.e., U500 insulin) has significantly increased over the years, primarily due to an increase in obesity and associated insulin resistance. In obese and other insulin-resistant patients, the higher insulin concentration results in an activity profile more similar to a pre-mixed short- and intermediate-acting insulin (i.e., onset of action of 30–45 minutes, peak pharmacodynamic action at 7–8.5 hours, and duration of action of 11.5 hours) (1,2). Clinical trials and experience have demonstrated the ability to safely use this concentration of insulin dosed either twice or thrice daily before meals in ambulatory populations (3,4). To improve the safe use of this agent, dedicated administration devices (insulin syringe and disposable pen calibrated for 500 units/mL concentration) have become available in some markets (5,6). However, these devices are not universally available. Careful use of U500 insulin without these devices can still be achieved.

Insulin Lispro and Degludec are both available in concentrations of 200 units/mL (i.e., U200 insulin). Insulin lispro (U100 insulin) has an onset of action of within 15 minutes, peak effects in 30–90 minutes, and rapid clearance within 5 hours of the initial injection (7), making it an ideal rapid-acting (prandial and correction) insulin used in both outpatient and inpatient settings. Insulin degludec forms multihexamers after the subcutaneous injection from which monomers slowly dissociate (8). This process results in a protracted activity profile with a duration of action greater than 42 hours (i.e., ultra-long-acting insulin) (9). Limited data are available regarding the use of insulin degludec in hospital settings (10). Concentrated formulations of both insulin lispro (U200 insulin) and degludec (U200 insulin) are considered be bioequivalent when compared to their standard formulations in pharmacodynamic evaluations (11,12). Thus, they are expected to have the same activity profile, but deliver twice the number of units in the same volume of injection. The two concentrations

of insulin degludec also demonstrated similar effects in an ambulatory population when compared in a clinical trial (13).

The other higher concentration insulin for consideration is insulin glargine, which is formulated in a concentration of 300 units/mL (i.e., U300 insulin). Increasing the concentration of insulin glargine from 100 units/ml (U100) to 300 units/mL (U300) formulation resulted in extending both the duration and time to onset (i.e., changed from long-acting to ultra-long-acting insulin). These factors lead to smoother activity extended up to 33 hours (14). This concentration of insulin glargine demonstrated similar effects with a lower incidence of hypoglycemic events, primarily nocturnal, when compared to the standard concentration in patients with both type 1 and type 2 diabetes within the ambulatory setting in the EDITION series of trials (15–20). An upcoming clinical trial is evaluating the use of this concentrated insulin in hospitalized patients (21).

The challenges posed with the use of insulin in hospitalized patients occur throughout all areas of this care setting (22). For example, the UK 2016 National Diabetes Inpatient Audit (NaDIA) revealed that almost half (46%) of inpatients treated with insulin had an error (i.e., prescription or medication management) related to insulin therapy (23). Patients who require concentrated formulations of insulin in outpatient settings pose additional complications to these difficult transitions. Most of the information regarding the use of concentrated insulins is from the use of regular (human) insulin at a concentration of 500 units/mL (U500). This is due to a couple of reasons. First, this insulin has been available in animal forms since 1952 and human since 1997 (4), whereas the newer concentrated insulin formulations were not available until earlier this decade. Second, all of the newer concentrated insulins are only available in disposable insulin pens, which enable dosing using actual insulin units (24–26). Administration using only these devices decreases the chance of dosing errors during administration, as well as after communication of the actual doses during care transitions, however, insulin pens are not often used in hospital settings. Concentrated regular U500 insulin is still available in a vial, as well as in a disposable insulin pen (6). To avoid errors due to use of concentrated insulins, institutions can implement strict policies and education programs.

Admission

Processes to avoid errors should start upon the point at which patients enter the care system. This section provides guidance on handling patients who enter acute health care systems on concentrated insulins. There is little data on the newer concentrated insulins to utilize in the formation of this information, thus most is drawn from concentrated regular insulin (U500) and standard insulin concentrations (U100). Providers need to be familiar with the various concentrated insulins' basic pharmacodynamics and kinetics and if not comfortable with this, should immediately request consultations by endocrinology or their pharmacy department for patients entering their care who require these insulins.

There are guidelines and studies that provide weight-based insulin dosing algorithms or adjustments based on glucose or HbA1c (A1C) levels (27–31). Thus, the determination of the initial insulin regimen should adjust the outpatient dosage based on the glucose control pre-admission and at admission, as well as a thorough evaluation of the patient. The glucose control assessment should include an A1C checked on all patients with known diabetes (if not performed in prior 3 months) or suspected to have diabetes (an A1C above 9% [75 mmol/mol] warrants re-evaluation of home regimen) and review pre-admission hypoglycemia frequency, severity, timing, and unawareness (28). The clinical evaluation should include assessment of the patient's clinical situation and upcoming treatment plans, along with consideration of the patient's ability to accurately report, administer, and adhere to their outpatient insulin regimen. The dosage of insulin required during the hospitalization may be higher or lower than that required by a patient as an outpatient (27,32,33). Table 34-2 contains a selection of the reasons why a patient may require a higher or lower insulin dose (27,32,33). For example, patients requiring concentrated regular insulin (U500) as outpatients were converted to standard concentrations of insulin with more than a 50% dose reduction likely to accommodate for a significant reduction in nutritional intake (33,34). Frequent glucose monitoring is crucial to allow for early detection of any alterations in metabolic control (28).

Table 34-2 Clinical considerations for insulin dose requirements (27,32,33)

Increased insulin requirements	Reduced insulin requirements
Infections and sepsis	Nil per oral (NPO) status
High HbA1c on admission	Acute renal failure
Use of steroids	Acute liver failure
New use of atypical antipsychotics	Frequent hypoglycemia as an outpatient
Stress of acute illness	Non adherence to diabetes management as an outpatient
Use of total parenteral nutrition (TPN)	
Use of glucose containing IV fluids	Reduced appetite
Dietary causes	Use of high doses of long acting insulins incorrectly as an outpatient to cover prandial glycemia
Bed rest especially in previously active patients	

Table 34-3 Dose conversion of regular (U500) concentrated insulin

U500 insulin dose (actual units)	U100 (units markings)	Tuberculin syringe (volume in mL)
25	5	0.05
50	10	0.1
75	15	0.15
100	20	0.2
125	25	0.25
150	30	0.3
175	35	0.35
200	40	0.4
225	45	0.45
250	50	0.5
275	55	0.55
300	60	0.6
325	65	0.65
350	70	0.7
375	75	0.75
400	80	0.8
425	85	0.85
450	90	0.9
475	95	0.95
500	100	1
Actual units	Divide by 5	Divide by 500

Dose (actual units)/5 = unit markings on U100 insulin syringe.
Dose (actual units)/500 = mL markings on a tuberculin syringe.

Concentrated insulins are not always included in an institution's formulary. In this case, the outpatient insulin dosage must also be converted to those on formulary. In general, insulin doses can be converted unit for unit after determination of the accurate dosage. Concentrated insulins administered using the disposable insulin pens are dosed in actual units, so no dose conversion is necessary (6,24–26). Careful inquiry regarding the administration device when using concentrated regular (U500) insulin is necessary. Although in some cases actual units are used for the dosing of this insulin (when using the disposable insulin pen specifically calibrated for U500 or U500 insulin syringe), in others, this insulin is dosed using "insulin marks" on a U100 insulin syringe or milliliters using volumetric syringes (Table 34-3) (4,6). In addition, concentrated insulins may be administered using continuous subcutaneous insulin infusion. As there are currently no insulin pump programs that are calibrated for concentrated insulins, careful inquiry into the dosage, as well as the type of insulin, administered using an insulin pump must be completed when a patient is admitted who uses an insulin pump as an outpatient.

During Hospitalization

There are many different reasons why patients on concentrated insulins enter an acute care setting. Data is limited on regimen adjustments for concentrated insulins while in acute care settings. Guidance on how to approach the care of these patients may vary based on those reasons and the anticipated length of their stay. There are general considerations and policies that may assist providers in enhancing the likelihood of appropriate and safe care of these patients.

In the acute care setting, glycemic control may sometimes be best achieved with an intravenous (IV) continuous insulin infusion (CII, also known as a variable rate IV insulin infusion [VRIII]) using an effective and safe protocol (preferably using validated written or computerized physician order entry [CPOE]) (28). The short half-life of IV insulin (<15 minutes) allows flexibility in adjusting the infusion rate in the event of unpredicted changes in nutrition or the patient's health. It is expected that if the patient was taking long-acting or ultra-long-acting basal insulin (including insulin degludec U100/U200; and concentrated insulin glargine U300) prior to admission, then this should be continued if these products are available. Continuation of the background subcutaneous (SC) insulin prevents rebound hyperglycemia when the IV insulin is stopped. At this point when transitioning from IV insulin to SC insulin, it is important to administer the short-, rapid-, or fast-acting insulin at least 30 minutes prior to stopping IV insulin (although fast-acting insulin aspart has even faster onset than usual rapid-acting insulins); and the basal component at an appropriate interval prior to stopping insulin infusion dependent on the formulations' pharmacodynamics, the interval for: U100 basal insulin formulations is at least 2 hours, concentrated insulin glargine (U300) 6 hours is preferred, and insulin degludec (U100 and U200) is 2–4 hours.

Planned Short Hospital Stays and Elective Procedures

Inpatient glycemic management recommendations are generally based on the nature and extent of the procedure, the outpatient insulin regimen, and the state of metabolic control before hospitalization/surgery (35,36). Knowledge of the insulins' peak activity and duration of action is essential to determine the adjustment prior to procedures or periods when patients may have no nutritional intake. The duration of the action of insulin degludec (U100/U200) and of concentrated insulin glargine (U300) is longer than other basal insulins; whereas concentrated regular insulin (U500) has both bolus and basal activity (2,12,14). Information on the type of diabetes, the insulin used, when the previous dose was taken and the duration of time that the patient will have limited nutritional intake must be considered when determining adjustment or whether to hold doses prior to and during procedures (27,37). In general, for concentrated insulin glargine (U300) or insulin degludec (U100/U200) in patients with type 2 diabetes, a dose reduction of 20–50% of their home regimen should be considered, however, for patients with type 1 diabetes, a dose reduction of 20% is suggested (38). Concentrated prandial insulins (i.e., insulin lispro U200) should be held and only corrective doses should be used. Correction doses with a rapid-acting (or fast-acting) analog every 4 hours, or with standard concentration regular short-acting insulin every 6 hours, should be used for those patients who are NPO status (31,39–42). Treating providers must write the correction order for one time only, so that it is not repeated without re-evaluation of the clinical situation which may require a change in insulin dose or regimen. Providers should also notify the pharmacy with planned or unplanned NPO status.

Extended or Nonelective Stays

The care of patients in the acute setting is often very fluid and needs to be guided by the measures necessary to both achieve the institution's and the patient's glycemic goals, prevent hypoglycemia, and decrease or eliminate the likelihood of medication errors (4,43–45). As mentioned before, correct ordering practices should be followed, pharmacists should continue to ascertain that insulin dosage, route, and frequency are accurate. Verification of the administration devices, whether syringes or pens, should be done at every dose administration. Concentrated insulins should always be stored in bins clearly labeled "High-Risk." The bin should bear a "High Risk" warning sticker as well as a laminated notification card labeled "For Sterile Products Area Use Only." Storage outside the pharmacy is not advised.

Concentrated insulins should always be administered using their designated administration devices (disposable insulin pens or syringe), if available. If those devices for any concentrated insulin (except for concentrated regular insulin) are not available, the patient's insulin requirements should be converted to the appropriate standard concentration insulin formulation(s) available. If designated devices are not available for concentrated regular U500 insulin, preparation of concentrated insulin doses in clinical settings should be prepared by a pharmacist. All doses should be prepared by converting the actual units of insulin to the volume required for administration using a 1 mL tuberculin (TB) safety needle syringe (or U100 insulin syringe if this is the local standard of care). Prepared syringes should not have any overfill and the syringes should contain the needle.

Consistent use of a TB syringe with concentrated regular U500 insulin is recommended, with total doses expressed in terms of both units and volume (e.g., 200 units [0.4 mL]) (43,45). Each syringe should be given a 24-hour expiration date. Each syringe should be dispensed with a High-Risk medication sticker. To ensure timely availability of concentrated regular U500 insulin syringes, the pharmacy should deliver the drug to the patient care unit at least 2 hours prior to the scheduled time of administration. The pharmacists should modify the due times in the dosing schedule and multidose vials should never be dispensed to the floor.

Prior to administration of the first dose of concentrated insulin, communication between the pharmacist and nurse should occur. The pharmacist and registered nurse (RN) caring for the patient should review the clinician order, concentrated insulin dose, route, and administration frequency. Prior to each administration of concentrated insulin, two RNs must perform an independent double-check, which is documented in the chart (46). Once components of the ordered medication are verified as correct, the RN may administer the dose subcutaneously. Nurses should not be permitted to alter the amount of concentrated insulin to be administered. Any changes to a patient's regimen must be reordered by the prescriber and a new dosage must be prepared and dispensed by pharmacy. Nurse-to-nurse communication should occur at each shift change. Any prescribed changes to the scheduled administration times must be communicated to the pharmacist. Use of these processes when using concentrated insulins will reduce the chances of medication errors (Table 34-4).

Once patient and/or caregivers are capable, consider inpatient diabetes education to improve and/or assess outpatient care and patient's ability for self-care and insulin administration. Table 34-5 contains suggested topics for diabetes education (47,48).

Table 34-4 Processes that help reduce concentrated insulin errors

- Pharmacist verification processes
- Proper storage and labeling practices
- Standardized prescribing, preparation, dispensing, and administration protocols
- Nursing education and training in proper administration and double-checking procedures

Discharge

In preparation for patients transitioning out of acute care settings, there are several steps to take to ensure patients are best able to care for their diabetes upon discharge, that can be standardized via policy and procedures at each institution, including self-management education, receipt of supplies and/or prescriptions for all necessary medications and supplies, and appropriate follow-up appointments scheduled (27,49). Institutions should have standard discharge educational materials to provide to patients and/or caregivers (27,28,50).

Table 34-5 Suggested topics for discharge education tools

Basic Diabetes Survival Skills
- Glucose monitoring
- Medication administration
- Recognition of hypoglycemia and hyperglycemia
- Hypoglycemia treatment
- Basic meal planning
- Sick day rules

Insulin Education
- Name(s)
- Type(s) and action profile(s)
- Doses
- Timing
- Storage
- Insulin pen and pen needle use
- Insulin vial and syringe use
- Injection site selection and rotation
- Safe sharps disposal

Advanced Skills (if applicable)
- Insulin pump management
- Carbohydrate counting

Table 34-6 Reasons for adjustment of pre-admission and hospital insulin dosage upon discharge (27,28,51)

Increased insulin requirements	Reduced insulin requirements
High HbA1c on admission	HbA1c at or near patient-specific target on admission
Use of steroids	Initiation or re-initiation of non-insulin agents
New use of atypical antipsychotics	Frequent hypoglycemia as an outpatient or inpatient
Increased nutritional intake (compared to hospitalization or pre-admission)	Non-adherence to diabetes management as an outpatient
	Expected continued reduced dietary intake
Continued bed rest (related to bed rest-induced insulin resistance)	Use of high doses of long-acting insulins incorrectly as an outpatient to cover prandial glycemia

There is limited data on how or whether to convert patients back to their concentrated insulin regimens after discharge. An assessment of the insulin requirements during hospitalization, admission assessment of pre-hospitalization glycemic control (A1C), changes to their health status resulting from their hospitalization, and immediate post-discharge clinical plans need to be considered when determining the discharge insulin plans (Table 34-6) (27,28,51). Prescriptions or orders should be provided to the patients for their insulin regimen and appropriate monitoring supplies. These prescriptions should be carefully worded to limit medication errors (4). It is important to remember that all designated administration devices for concentrated insulins (including disposable insulin pens and syringes) are dosed using actual units of insulin, so no dose conversion needs to be made for the concentration (6,24–26). If concentrated regular U500 insulin is being prescribed, the use of the specific U500 disposable insulin pen or the U500 insulin syringe is recommended (5,6). If these designated devices are not available, suggestions for the wording used for prescriptions to reduce confusion and prevent errors can be found in Table 34-7 (4). Careful reassessment post-discharge is important for maintaining glycemic control and reinforcing education. Most guidelines recommend identification of the specific provider the patient will be reassessed by, and to schedule that reassessment within 1 month post-discharge, but ideally in the first week or two (27,28).

Table 34-7 Suggestions for concentrated insulin prescriptions to avoid errors (4,6)

Always include:
- Insulin dose in actual units
- Frequency
- Administration device

Example prescriptions of concentrated regular insulin

If prescribing a concentrated insulin to be administered using a designated administration device,
- Inject 50 units subcutaneous 3 times daily before meals using U500 insulin syringe

If designated administration device(s) are not available

For patients using U100 syringes:
- Draw up 10 unit marks using a U100 syringe (which equals 50 units of U500) 3 times daily before meals

For patients using tuberculin syringes:
- Draw up 0.1 mL using a tuberculin syringe (which equals 50 units of U500) 3 times daily before meals

Conclusions

The use of concentrated insulins increases the complexity of the care of patients. Providers and acute care staff need to be knowledgeable about the differences and similarities in the variety of insulins (both concentrated and standard formulations [including biosimilar U100 versions of insulin glargine and insulin lispro]). Use of standardized practices and education tools provide a base for the safe care of patients using insulin as they transition acute health care settings.

References

1 Church TJ, Haines ST. Treatment approach to patients with severe insulin resistance. *Clin Diabetes*. 2016;34(2):97–104.

2 de la Pena A, Ma X, Reddy S, Ovalle F, Bergenstal RM, Jackson JA. Application of PK/PD modeling and simulation to dosing regimen optimization of high-dose human regular U-500 insulin. *J Diabetes Sci Technol*. 2014;8(4):821–829.

3 Hood RC, Arakaki RF, Wysham C, et al. Two treatment approaches for human regular U-500 insulin in patients with type 2 diabetes not achieving adequate glycemic control on high-dose U-100 insulin therapy with or without oral agents: a randomized, titration-to-target clinical trial. *Endocr Pract*. 2015;21(7):782–793.

4 Segal AR, Brunner JE, Burch FT, Jackson JA. Use of concentrated insulin human regular (U-500) for patients with diabetes. *Am J Health Syst Pharm*. 2010;67: 1526–1535.

5 Institute for Safe Medication Practices. U-500 syringe approved by FDA. In: *ISMP Medication Safety Alert*. Horsham, PA: Institute for Safe Medication Practices; 2016.

6 Humulin R. U-500 [package insert]. Indianapolis, IN: Lilly USA, LLC; 2016.

7 Wilde MI, McTavish D. Insulin lispro: a review of its pharmacological properties and therapeutic use in the management of diabetes mellitus. *Drugs*. 1997;54:597–614.

8 Jonassen I, Havelund S, Hoeg-Jensen T, Steensgaard DB, Wahlund P-O, Ribel U. Design of the novel protraction mechanism of insulin degludec, an ultra-long-acting basal insulin. *Pharm Res*. 2012;29: 2104–2114.

9 Heise T, Nosek L, Bøttcher SG, Hastrup H, Haahr H. Ultra-long-acting insulin degludec has a flat and stable glucose-lowering effect in type 2 diabetes. *Diabetes Obes Metab*. 2012;14:944–950.

10 Bulisani MGP, de Almeida MFO, Abdon CM, Moreno ACS, Fonseca MIH, Genestreti PRR. In-hospital experience with insulin degludec (IDeg). *Diabetol Metabol Synd*. 2015;7(Suppl 1):A90.

11 de la Pena A, Seger M, Soon D, et al. Bioequivalence and comparative pharmacodynamics of insulin lispro 200 U/mL relative to insulin lispro (Humalog) 100 U/mL. *Clin Pharmacol Drug Dev*. 2016;5(1):69–75.

12 Korsatko S, Deller S, Koehler G, et al. A comparison of the steady-state pharmacokinetic and pharmacodynamic profiles of 100 and 200 u/ml formulations of ultra-long-acting insulin degludec. *Clin Drug Investig*. 2013;33:515–521.

13 Bode BW, Chaykin LB, Sussman AM, et al. Efficacy and safety of insulin degludec 200 u/ml and insulin degludec 100 u/ml in patients with type 2 diabetes (BEGIN: COMPARE). *Endocr Pract*. 2014;20: 785–791.

14 Becker RH, Dahmen R, Bergmann K, Lehmann A, Jax T, Heise T. New insulin glargine 300 units/mL provides a more even activity profile and prolonged glycemic control at steady state compared with insulin glargine 100 units/mL. *Diabetes Care*. 2014; 38: 637–643.

15 Dailey G, Lavernia F. A review of the safety and efficacy data for insulin glargine 300 units/ml, a new formulation of insulin glargine. *Diabetes Obes Metab*. 2015; 17(12):1107–1114.

16 Riddle MC, Bolli GB, Ziemen M, et al. New insulin glargine 300 units/ml versus glargine 100 units/ml in people with type 2 diabetes using basal and mealtime insulin: glucose control and hypoglycemia in a 6-month randomized controlled trial (EDITION 1). *Diabetes Care*. 2014;37: 2755–2762.

17 Yki-Jarvinen H, Bergenstal RM, Bolli GB, et al. Glycaemic control and hypoglycaemia with new insulin glargine 300 u/ml versus insulin glargine 100 u/ml in people with type 2 diabetes using basal insulin and oral antihyperglycaemic drugs: the EDITION 2

randomized 12-month trial including 6-month extension. *Diabetes Obes Metab.* 2015;17:1142–1149.

18 Bolli GB, Riddle MC, Bergenstal RM, et al. New insulin glargine 300 U/ml compared with glargine 100 U/ml in insulin-naïave people with type 2 diabetes on oral glucose-lowering drugs: a randomized controlled trial (EDITION 3). *Diabetes Obes Metab.* 2015;17(4):386–394.

19 Home PD, Bergenstal RM, Bolli GB, et al. New insulin glargine 300 units/ml versus glargine 100 units/ml in people with type 1 diabetes: a randomized, phase 3a, open-label clinical trial (EDITION 4). *Diabetes Care.* 2015;38:2217–2225.

20 Ritzel R, Roussel R, Bolli GB, et al. Patient-level meta-analysis of the EDITION 1, 2 and 3 studies: glycaemic control and hypoglycaemia with new insulin glargine 300 U/ml versus glargine 100 U/ml in people with type 2 diabetes. *Diabetes Obes Metab.* 2015;17(9):859–867.

21 Emory University. Glargine U300 Hospital Trial. In: ClinicalTrials.gov [Internet]. Bethesda (MD): National Library of Medicine (US). 2000- [2017 March 1]. http://clinicaltrials.gov/show/NCT03013985 NLM Identifier: NCT03013985.

22 Cobaugh DJ, Maynard G, Cooper L, Kienle PC, et al. Enhancing insulin-use safety in hospitals: practical recommendations from and ASHP Foundation expert consensus panel. *Am J Health-Syst Pharm.* 2013;70: 1404–1413.

23 Health and Social care information Centre. *National Diabetes Inpatient audit (NaDIA), Open Data 2016,* 2017. www.digital.nhs.uk/pubs/nadia2016 (accessed April 16, 2017).

24 Humalog [package insert]. Indianapolis, IN: Eli Lilly & Co.; 2015.

25 Toujeo [package insert]. Bridgewater, NJ: Sanofi-Aventis US LLC; 2015.

26 Tresiba [package insert]. Plainsboro, NJ: Novo Nordisk, Inc; 2015.

27 Umpierrez GE, Hellman R, Korytkowski MT, Kosiborod M, Maynard GA, Montori VM, Seley JJ, Van den Berghe G. Management of hyperglycemia in hospitalized patient in non-critical care setting: an endocrine society clinical practice guideline. *J Clin Endocrinol Metab.* 2012;97(1):16–38.

28 American Diabetes Association. 14. Diabetes Care in the Hospital. *Diabetes Care.* 2018;41(Suppl 1):S144–S151.

29 Umpierrez GE, Smiley D, Hermayer K, et al. Randomized study comparing a basal-bolus with a basal plus correction insulin regimen for the hospital management of medical and surgical patients with type 2 diabetes. *Diabetes Care.* 2013;36:2169–2174.

30 Umpierrez GE, Smiley D, Jacobs S, et al. Randomized study of basal bolus insulin therapy in the inpatient management of patients with type 2 diabetes undergoing general surgery (rabbit surgery). *Diabetes Care.* 2011;34:256–261.

31 Umpierrez GE, Hor T, Smiley D, et al. Comparison of inpatient insulin regimens with detemir plus aspart versus neutral protamine Hagedorn plus regular in medical patients with type 2 diabetes. *J Clin Endocrinol Metab.* 2009;94:564–569.

32 Kienle PC, Maynard G, Kulasa K, Weber R. Insulin safety webinar slides May 2014: Ten ways to prevent insulin-use errors in your hospital. http://www.ashpfoundation.org/ MainMenuCategories/Advancing Practice/Insulin-Use-Safety-Recommendations (accessed March 4, 2017).

33 Palladino CE, Eberly ME, Emmons JT, Tannock LR. Management of U-500 insulin users during inpatient admissions within a veterans affairs medical center. *Diabetes Res Clin Pract.* 2016;114:32–36.

34 Paulus AO, Colburn JA, True MW, et al. Evaluation of total daily dose of glycemic control for patients taking U-500 regular insulin admitted to the hospital. *Endocr Pract.* 2016;22:1187–1191.

35 Sato H, Carvalho G, Sato T, Lattermann R, Matsukawa T, Schricker T. The association

of preoperative glycemic control, intraoperative insulin sensitivity, and outcomes after cardiac surgery. *J Clin Endocrinol Metab*. 2010;95:4338–4344.

36 Dagogo-Jack S, Alberti KG. Management of diabetes mellitus in surgical patients. *Diabetes Spectrum*. 2002;15:44–48.

37 Dhatariya K, Levy N, Kilvert A, et al. Diabetes UK position statements and care recommendations: NHS diabetes guideline for the perioperative management of the adult patient with diabetes. *Diabetic Med*. 2012;29(4):420–433.

38 Takeishi S, Mori A, Fushimi N, et al. Evaluation of safety of insulin degludec on undergoing total colonoscopy using continuous glucose monitoring. *J Diabetes Investig*. 2016;7:374–380.

39 Clement S, Braithwaite SS, Magee MF, et al. Management of diabetes and hyperglycemia in hospitals. *Diabetes Care*. 2004;27:553–591.

40 Umpierrez GE, Smiley D, Zisman A, et al. Randomized study of basal-bolus insulin therapy in the inpatient management of patients with type 2 diabetes (Rabbit 2 Trial). *Diabetes Care*. 2007;30:2181–2186.

41 Kosiborod M, Inzucchi SE, Goyal A, et al. Relationship between spontaneous and iatrogenic hypoglycemia and mortality in patients hospitalized with acute myocardial infarction. *J Am Med Asso*. 2009;301: 1556–1564.

42 Noschese ML, DiNardo MM, Donihi AC, et al. Patient outcomes after implementation of a protocol for inpatient insulin pump therapy. *Endocr Pract*. 2009;15:415–424.

43 Food and Drug Administration. Potential signals of serious risks/new safety information identified from the Adverse Event Reporting System (AERS) between January–March 2008. www.fda.gov/Drugs/ GuidanceComplianceRegulatory Information/Surveillance/AdverseDrug Effects/ucm085914.htm (accessed April 16, 2017).

44 Hellman R. A systems approach to reducing errors in insulin therapy in the inpatient setting. *Endocr Pract*. 2004;10(suppl 2):100–108.

45 Cohen MR, Smetzer JL. ISMP medication error report analysis: insulin concentrate U-500. *Hosp Pharm*. 2007;42:887.

46 Nguyen H-T, Nguyen T-D, Haaijer-Ruskamp FM, Taxis K. Errors in preparation and administration of insulin in two urban Vietnamese hospitals: an observational study. *Nurs Res*. 2014;63(1): 68–72.

47 Corl DE, Guntrum PL, Graf L, Suhr LD, Thompson RE, Wisse BE. Inpatient diabetes education performed by staff nurses decreases readmission rates. *AADE in Practice*. 2015;3(2):19–23.

48 Healy SJ, Black D, Harris C, Lorenz A, Dungan KM. Inpatient diabetes education is associated with less frequent hospital readmission among patients with poor glycemic control. *Diabetes Care*. 2013; 2960–2967.

49 Schnipper JL, Magee M, Larsen K, Inzucchi SE, Maynard G. Society of hospital medicine glycemic control task force summary: practical recommendations for assessing the impact of glycemic control efforts. *J Hosp Med*. 2008;3(S5):66–75.

50 American Association of Clinical Endocrinologists. AACE diabetes resource center. resources.aace.com (accessed March 1, 2017).

51 Umpierrez GE, Reyes D, Smiley D, et al. Hospital discharge algorithm based on admission HbA1c for the management of patients with type 2 diabetes. *Diabetes Care*. 2014;37:2934–2939.

35

Management of Insulin Pumps in Hospitalized Patients

Bithika M. Thompson, Patricia A. Mackey, and Curtiss B. Cook

Key Points

- Continuous subcutaneous insulin infusion (CSII) therapy (also known as insulin pump therapy), is employed to treat patients with diabetes mellitus.
- While most frequently seen in the outpatient setting, insulin pump technology is now encountered by clinicians in various other clinical scenarios not originally intended for CSII use. This includes CSII therapy increasingly being used in the hospital setting.
- Despite managing their insulin pump therapy effectively in the ambulatory setting, many patients may not be aware of potential problems associated with continued pump usage in the hospital; especially in the setting of acute illness when blood glucose levels are expected to change rapidly (e.g., decreased nutritional intake, infection, changes in kidney function, steroids).
- Inpatient practitioners may encounter three possible situations when someone on an outpatient CSII program is admitted to the hospital. First, the clinical situation may permit ongoing patient self-management of the CSII program from admission to discharge without interruption in therapy. Second, the patient's status may necessitate early disconnection from the device. The pump may or may not be restarted prior to discharge

depending on the clinical course. Third, the patient may be admitted to the hospital and may not perform CSII self-management at all throughout their hospitalization. This last scenario may either occur because of the patient's choice, clinical status, or because the institution simply does not permit CSII therapy.

- If CSII therapy is discontinued for other than a short period of time (e.g., for a radiological procedure), then insulin treatment should be replaced by a multiple daily injection (MDI) program or continuous insulin infusion (CII, also known as variable-rate intravenous insulin infusion [VRIII]) depending on the clinical circumstances.
- Hospitals that do not allow CSII therapy should have a formal process in place to transfer the patient to MDI or CII (VRIII) as needed. It is also important that safe and effective transition from MDI or CII (VRIII) back to CSII also occurs as part of ongoing care and discharge planning.
- A key factor in minimizing errors and adverse events when using CSII in-hospital is a collaborative relationship between the patient and hospital staff. In addition, because of the continuous advances in diabetes devices and technologies, adequate ongoing education of all key stakeholders about insulin pumps and other evolving technologies is warranted.

Endocrine and Metabolic Medical Emergencies: A Clinician's Guide, Second Edition. Edited by Glenn Matfin.
© 2018 John Wiley & Sons Ltd. Published 2018 by John Wiley & Sons Ltd.

Introduction

Continuous subcutaneous insulin infusion (CSII) therapy (also known as insulin pump therapy), is employed to treat patients with diabetes mellitus. An estimated 400,000 patients in the USA use CSII for management of their diabetes (1). Data from the Type 1 Diabetes Exchange looking at over 16,000 participants with type 1 diabetes reported that 60% were using an insulin pump in 2014. Use of insulin pumps among patients with type 2 diabetes is also increasing (2). While most frequently seen in the outpatient setting, insulin pump technology is now encountered by clinicians in various other clinical scenarios not originally intended for use. The number of hospitalizations associated with diabetes in the USA is increasing, and diabetes is associated with greater odds of requiring a hospitalization, a higher risk of needing multiple hospitalizations, and results in longer hospital stays than in patients without diabetes (3–8). Therefore, healthcare professionals should expect to see patients with CSII increasingly in the hospital setting, and will be confronted with how to manage CSII therapy when the patient on CSII requires hospitalization.

While information on the number of hospitalizations associated with diabetes is available, there is no data on hospital discharges occurring among CSII users. Nonetheless, many patients on insulin pumps are likely hospitalized for reasons other than their diabetes, and many of these patients may be doing very well on their technology as outpatients. Patients can become frustrated when they are asked to transfer their diabetes self-management to hospital staff who may be less knowledgeable about diabetes than the patient. However, patients capable and comfortable with CSII use in the ambulatory setting may not be aware of potential problems associated with continued pump usage in the hospital; especially in the setting of acute illness when blood glucose levels are expected to change rapidly (e.g., decreased nutritional intake, infection, changes in kidney function, steroids). Empowering patients to make

decisions in areas where they have demonstrated competency in the outpatient setting could alleviate some of that distress, and make them more involved in their care without jeopardizing their outcome.

Inpatient self-management of CSII can be defined as a process whereby patients, in collaboration with the hospital staff and if not contraindicated, are allowed to remain on their insulin pump. Studies have shown that patients proficient in CSII use often request to continue use of CSII during hospitalization and report high patient satisfaction (86%) when they are allowed to do so (9). Some institutions have published guidelines on inpatient CSII self-management (9–12). Recent reports confirm that with proper patient selection, individuals treated with insulin pumps can successfully transition their treatment from the outpatient to the inpatient environment (9,13–16).

There are potential safety issues with using CSII technology in the hospital (e.g., pump malfunction or unrecognized disconnection). Given the issues associated with self-management of CSII in the hospital, the lack of familiarity of inpatient practitioners with the technology, and the ensuing angst on the part of hospital staff when such patients are encountered, a process for transitioning outpatient insulin pumps into the inpatient setting and subsequent self-management should be clearly described in an institutional policy. This chapter provides suggestions for use of CSII in the hospital, reviews available published data on their use in the inpatient setting, and highlights particular scenarios which may be encountered with patients on CSII.

Contexts of Inpatient CSII Therapy

Inpatient practitioners may encounter three possible situations when someone on an outpatient CSII program is admitted to the hospital. First, the clinical situation may permit ongoing self-management of the CSII program from admission to discharge without interruption in therapy. Second, the patient's status may necessitate early disconnection from the device. The pump may or may not be restarted prior to discharge depending on the clinical course. Third, the patient may be admitted to the hospital and may not perform CSII self-management at all throughout their hospitalization. This last scenario may either occur because of the patient's choice, clinical status, or because the institution simply does not permit CSII therapy. Regardless of the reasons, if CSII therapy is discontinued for other than a short period of time (e.g., for a radiological procedure), then insulin treatment should be substituted with a multiple daily injection (MDI) program or continuous insulin infusion (CII, also known as variable-rate intravenous insulin infusion [VRIII]) depending on the clinical circumstances. Hospitals who do not allow CSII therapy should have a formal process in place to transfer the patient to MDI or CII (VRIII) as needed.

General Considerations

CSII users are likely to represent only a small subset of patients with diabetes in the hospital. Therefore, institutional guidelines for CSII self-management should exist within a larger framework of already established policies and procedures for inpatient diabetes care that also includes recognition and treatment of hypoglycemia, point-of-care (POC) glucose testing, and subcutaneous or CII (VRIII) administration. Several institutions have published a framework for management, but there are currently no consensus guidelines regarding transitioning the patient on CSII therapy from the ambulatory to the acute care setting. The American Diabetes Association (ADA) simply indicates that a policy and procedures should be in place without providing specifics (17). The Joint Commission advises that if insulin pump therapy is allowed, that a policy should be developed for determining whether patients will continue to use their insulin pump therapy while hospitalized. The policy should include a list of contraindications for

continuation of a patient's insulin pump therapy, and responsibilities on the part of the staff and patient (18).

In the authors' institution, a process for use of CSII in the hospital was first published in 2005 (Figure 35-1) (10). The institutional guidelines and procedures for inpatient insulin pumps usually have three general components: (a) contraindications for CSII self-management within the hospital; (b) an agreement signed by the patient detailing the conditions for CSII use in the hospital; and (c) procedures to guide the hospital staff in managing the insulin pump after admission. Patients selected for inpatient self-management should already be on a CSII program as outpatients. Patients can initially continue the rates of basal and dose of meal-time insulin in a manner similar to their outpatient practice. However, changes in the pump settings during the hospitalization may be appropriate based on the patient's glycemic status and their ongoing clinical situation. It is also important to note that hospitalized patients may reside in other areas of the country, and therefore their current pump setting times may reflect that of their own local time zone. The transition to an alternate insulin regimen should take place whenever safety parameters set in place for the patient seem to be at risk of being breached by the patient's CSII management. If transitioned to subcutaneous insulin injections from CSII, carbohydrate counting may be a preferable method for determining the meal-time insulin doses. The process involving CSII self-management in the hospital requires continuous evaluation to ascertain its continued safety and efficacy.

Contraindications to Inpatient CSII Self-Management

The proper selection of patients for this protocol is the critical first step in ensuring its success (Table 35-1). The service managing the patient's diabetes should be the

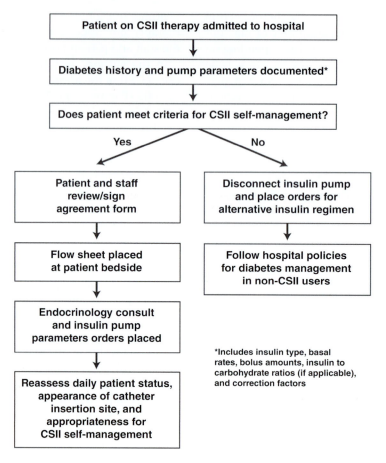

Figure 35-1 Care process model outlining steps to transition a patient on outpatient continuous subcutaneous insulin infusion (CSII) therapy to the hospital. The model assumes that other diabetes care policies (e.g., recognition and management of hypoglycemia, point-of-care glucose testing, insulin administration) are already in place. For examples of a patient agreement, flow sheet, and order set, see (10,13).

one deciding if CSII therapy is suitable for that individual. If the patient presents to the Emergency Room with an insulin pump that is determined to be malfunctioning, or anything that impairs the patient's ability to self-manage CSII therapy, such as an altered sensorium, that should prompt a change to an alternative insulin therapy. The authors' institution does permit a family member to assist with managing the patient's insulin pump if the patient cannot, contingent upon that person being available to come to the bedside 24 hours a day. Changes in the patient's clinical status that are deemed to be posing a major stress on glycemic control (e.g.,

liver failure, renal failure, frequent hypoglycemic events or severe hyperglycemia) or otherwise place the patient at risk (e.g., suicidal tendencies) should lead to reconsideration of CSII self-management. Hyperglycemia during critical illness or due to diabetic ketoacidosis (DKA)/hyperglycemic hyperosmolar state (HHS) is best managed with CII until the episode is resolved. Discontinuation of therapy is also recommended if the patient does not wish to cooperate with the hospital staff, is unable to provide the necessary insulin pump supplies, or otherwise does not meet the requirements as detailed in the patient agreement form.

Table 35-1 Suggested contraindications for CSII self-management in the hospital

- Patient with altered state of consciousness
- Presence of diabetic ketoacidosis (DKA)/hyperglycemic hyperosmolar state (HHS) at admission
- Critically ill patient requiring intensive care or other major stresses on glycemic control
- Patient at risk for suicide
- Inability of the patient to participate in CSII management, or if the patient is unable to identify a family member who is knowledgeable and competent with the insulin pump function who can remain at the bedside to assist with the pump management
- Patient's refusal to agree with conditions of CSII self-management, or patient's preference to use alternate therapy during the hospitalization
- Other circumstances identified by the physician primarily responsible for the individual's care in the hospital

Table 35-2 Suggested elements to be included in any hospital-based CSII self-management patient agreement form

- Change the infusion set every 48–72 hours or as needed, allow staff to intermittently assess infusion site
- Provide own insulin pump supplies (including CGM if patient wears this also)
- Show staff basal rates and bolus amounts*
- Agree to let staff perform point-of-care glucose testing using institution's glucometer
- Report symptoms of low or high blood sugar to the staff
- Report any pump problems
- Understanding that a family member may assist with the operation of the insulin infusion pump on condition that they must remain in the hospital during the entire hospital stay
- The pump may be discontinued and a different insulin delivery given for any of the following:
  - Doctor's order
  - Changes in judgment
  - Changes in level of awareness or consciousness
  - Any x-ray procedure
  - Other reasons deemed necessary by medical staff

CSII = Continuous subcutaneous insulin infusion.
*Recorded on a flow sheet kept at bedside (see (7) for sample agreement and flow sheet)

Patient Agreement

To assure safety and optimal medical management during hospital-based CSII management, the patient should recognize and acknowledge their responsibility in the process. At the authors' institution this is achieved via an agreement that the patient or their representative reviews and signs. There are some basic elements that should be considered to be included in any such agreement (Table 35-2).

The patient should already be accustomed to changing the catheter infusion set every 48–72 hours, and this requirement should be no different in the hospital setting. Additionally, it is unlikely that inpatient formularies are going to stock supplies for the various CSII devices on the market, and the patient should therefore agree to have their own on-hand. In some cases, the patient's brand of insulin may not be on the hospital formulary, and they will either have to provide their own or agree to the hospital substitution. Many patients have POC glucose measurement technology that communicates directly with the pump. Nonetheless, because hospitals have standardized technology that often communicates with their laboratory information system for purposes of tracking and quality control, the patient should still agree to let staff perform measurements using the organization's glucometer. Daily communication with the staff on blood glucose readings, pump parameters, and insulin boluses is essential. The patient (or their proxy) should keep track of basal rates and meal-time boluses. A provided bedside flow sheet is an empowering tool, in that the patient can complete it, and maintain it at their bedside. Is useful for tracking glucose levels, basal rates, and bolus amounts, and it allows a quick review when staff visits the patient's bedside. The patient should agree to report any issues with pump function or symptoms of hyperglycemia/hypoglycemia to the staff. Finally, the patient should be made aware that there may be circumstances when it may be best to terminate CSII self-management and disconnect the pump.

Admission/Post-admission Procedures

A diabetes history should be obtained by the physician and non-physician hospital staff who are performing the admission, and use of CSII therapy should be documented in the medical record (Figure 35-1). The type of insulin pump, date of last infusion site change, type of insulin used, and the insulin pump parameters (basal rates, bolus amounts, insulin carbohydrate ratios, correction factors) are recommended documentation. Contraindications to CSII self-management are assessed, and if none are present, the patient can be offered the option of continuing insulin pump therapy in the hospital. If CSII therapy is contraindicated, then the device should be disconnected and an alternative insulin therapy ordered. Considering the enormous cost of insulin pumps, the disconnected device should be given to a family member at bedside to take back home so it is not misplaced, being mindful that patients are frequently away from their hospital room for tests, and sometimes moved to different rooms throughout their hospital stay, based on their acuity and level of care needed at the time.

If both patient and staff find no contraindications to CSII self-management, the agreement is reviewed and signed by the patient and countersigned by one of the hospital staff, the flow sheet is placed at the bedside, and the corresponding orders are placed. The format of these orders will vary according to the nature of the electronic (or alternative) ordering process. If access to one is available, an endocrinologist should be consulted to provide support to the patient and inpatient staff. Daily assessment and engagement with the patient are necessary, including examination of the insulin pump catheter site and the flow sheet, to identify problems and establish any changes in the patient's status that might warrant cessation of CSII self-management.

Practical Experience with Inpatient CSII Self-Management

Safety data on inpatient CSII use and effectiveness in controlling hyperglycemia are limited, but suggest that in properly selected patients, successful transition from outpatient to inpatient insulin pump therapy is possible. Noschese and colleagues examined glycemic and safety data in 50 consecutive CSII-treated patients admitted to their hospital between 2004 and 2006. Only two minor events were noted (one pump malfunction and one catheter infusion site problem). Patient satisfaction with their inpatient pump experience was generally high (9).

Kannan et al. reported on 51 hospital admissions of patients using CSII aimed at studying the relationship between a patient's knowledge of their insulin pump and glucose control during the inpatient period. In this study, three groups of patients were identified: (a) those who did not require any inpatient diabetes education and continued on CSII (group A); (b) those who received education and then continued on CSII (group B); and (c) those in whom continued CSII use was felt to be inappropriate and who were transitioned to MDI insulin (group C). There were no statistically significant differences in mean blood glucose and frequency of hyperglycemic and hypoglycemic events between those patients who received inpatient education (group B) vs. those who did not (group A). This study suggests that even when minor educational gaps are identified in this population, if addressed, patients are able to continue use of their insulin pump in an effective and safe manner (19).

In sequential publications with ever increasing sample sizes, authors have been reporting on institutional experience with transitioning insulin pump users from their outpatient-based therapy to the hospital setting, detailing compliance with required procedures, evaluating glycemic control, and assessing safety among those patients conducting inpatient CSII self-management (13–15). The most recent analysis comprised 136 patients totaling 253 hospitalizations between 2006 and 2011 – the largest reported series to date (16). By the time of this last assessment, three subsets of patients had been identified. The "pump on" group (164/253 or 65%) comprised hospitalized patients who met the criteria for CSII self-management and continued until discharge. "Pump off" patients (38/253 or 15%) did not meet the conditions for inpatient CSII use and had therapy discontinued at admission and remained off even at the time of discharge. "Intermittent pump" cases (50/253 or 20%) were either those cases whose CSII therapy was continued at admission but then stopped during their hospitalization because of changing clinical circumstances, or patients whose CSII was stopped at admission but then restarted when their clinical status improved and they satisfied institutional criteria for use of the devices. Thus, most cases were able to continue CSII self-management throughout their hospital course (16). In addition, it was found that compliance with the necessary procedures (e.g., placing appropriate orders, completion of patient agreement and endocrinology consult) was high. Mean POC glucose was not significantly different between cases who remained on CSII and those for whom it was discontinued (p>0.1), but episodes of severe hyperglycemia (>300 mg/dL [16.7 mmol/L]) and hypoglycemia (<40 mg/dL [2.2 mmol/L]) were significantly less common among individuals who continued to perform CSII self-management. In this entire case series, only one adverse event occurred when an infusion catheter kinked, resulting in correctable nonfatal hyperglycemia that was recognized and corrected. No pump site infections, mechanical pump failures, or episodes of DKA were observed among patients remaining on therapy (16).

Although uncommon, insulin pump malfunctions and failures have been reported during hospitalization. Fauld et al. describe two cases of the "runaway pump" phenomenon in which patients received an unsolicited bolus of insulin. In both cases the malfunction resulted in severe hypoglycemia (20).

Continuous Glucose Monitoring Systems

Continuous glucose monitoring (CGM) systems provide real-time, continuous glucose data. Modern CGM technology is now often integrated with the CSII device, with data transmitted to a mobile device. Thus, some patients admitted with insulin pumps may also have associated CGM devices. Institutional policies on inpatient insulin pump use in the hospital should now have provisions for CGM devices. A recent consensus conference could not find specific evidence for the safety or benefit of CGM use in the hospital, and concluded that further study was needed (21). In the authors' institution, patients are allowed to wear their CGM, however, any treatment decisions regarding glucose management must be made via POC testing performed by hospital staff using hospital-approved devices.

Specific Scenarios

The summary above provides a framework for transitioning outpatient CSII into the hospital. However, it does not provide guidance for situations that might arise once the patient has been hospitalized. In particular, the process described up to now does not provide guidance for situations where transitions of care might be needed once the patient is in the hospital. The following case studies provide some examples and suggestions on how to approach special scenarios that might arise.

Case Study: Transitioning CSII Therapy during Procedures

A 76-year-old man with a 40-year history of type 1 diabetes on CSII was admitted for chest pain. On admission, standard procedures to allow continued use of the insulin pump were followed and he remained on therapy. A cardiac catheterization was planned. Prior to the procedure, the insulin pump was turned off. No blood glucose values were documented in the catheterization lab. Following the procedure, the patient was returned to the nursing unit, the pump remained off, and no alternative insulin orders were provided. Over the next 5 hours the pump remained off, the glucose steadily rose to over 500 mg/dL (28 mmol/L), requiring treatment with CII.

The above case illustrates the need to have a process in place for transitioning CSII therapy across all areas within the hospital. To address this gap in care, a process (with accompanying orders) was put in place (Figure 35-2). Briefly, if the insulin pump is to be continued, glucose monitoring has to occur. If the device is to be disconnected, alternative insulin orders need to be placed, and the frequency of glucose monitoring may need to be adjusted. Essential for success is effective hand-off (handover) communication across the different units informing the next team of the status of the insulin pump.

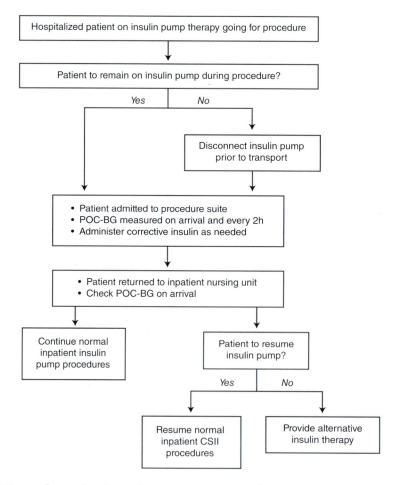

Figure 35-2 Process for transitioning patients using continuous subcutaneous insulin infusion (CSII) therapy in the hospital to procedural areas

Case Study: Transition from CSII to MDI

A 60-year-old man with type 2 diabetes for 30 years on CSII was admitted for chest pain. Multiple procedures were anticipated and his appetite was poor. After discussion with his health team, he did not feel confident in managing his insulin pump under these circumstances and preferred to be managed with subcutaneous insulin injections instead. If the patient is not comfortable remaining on CSII therapy during the hospitalization, then the device should be disconnected and an alternative insulin therapy ordered. For non-critically ill patients a course of long-acting or intermediate-acting insulin combined with a short- or rapid-acting insulin given with meals is most effective to control hyperglycemia, supplemented by correction doses for high glucose values when needed (22). The initial pump settings can be used to determine the doses of long- and short-acting insulin. The 24-hour basal amount on the insulin pump is equivalent to the long-acting insulin dose. The pump should be discontinued 2 hours after the first injection of basal insulin. Meal insulin and correction doses should be given according to the insulin to carbohydrate ratio and the insulin sensitivity factor on the insulin pump respectively. If the institution does not allow for patient carbohydrate counting, a set short-acting insulin dose can be given for meals with a consistent pre-determined carbohydrate amount.

Case Study: Transition from CII to CSII

A 45-year-old woman with long-standing type 1 diabetes complicated by end-stage renal disease requiring a renal transplant was admitted with DKA. She had undergone a renal transplant the month prior and was using her insulin pump at home. On admission, the pump was disconnected and she was treated with CII. After resolution of the DKA, she wished to resume her insulin pump treatment. A patient normally on CSII may require transition to CII during the hospital stay. Common reasons for this may be in the post-operative setting, while critically ill (intubated and/or on vasopressors), for treatment of DKA on admission, or readmission for rejection of the transplanted organ, which then usually requires large doses of steroids. Once the patient's glucose has reached a steady state, and she is clinically stable, and cognitively able to use the insulin pump, she can then be transitioned back to CSII. On transition, the insulin pump should be connected with the basal rate infusing for 2 hours prior to stopping the IV insulin infusion. This is necessary given the slow absorption of insulin from the subcutaneous pump site. Allowing the pump to run for 2 hours prior to stopping the IV infusion allows a subcutaneous depot to develop.

Use of CSII in the Perioperative Period

There are no data on how many patients on CSII treatment require surgical procedures each year. However, as use of CSII increases, it is likely that this scenario will become increasingly common. The perioperative period consists of a series of transitions including admission to the preoperative area, transfer to the operating room, surgery, transfer to recovery and then discharge to either home or to the inpatient setting. Each of these transitions has the potential for a gap in insulin pump therapy to occur. Potential safety concerns include lack of staff awareness of the insulin pump, inadequate glucose monitoring leading to missed hyperglycemia and/or hypoglycemia, inadvertent dislodgement or disconnection of the insulin pump, failure to move the insertion site out of the surgical field, and trauma to the insulin pump during the perioperative period of care. Given these safety concerns, if institutions are going to permit use of insulin pumps during surgery, there must be procedures in place to ensure patient safety.

When confronted with the patient using CSII undergoing surgery, the surgical and anesthesiology teams have the option of either disconnecting patients from their devices and providing alternative therapy or allowing continued use of the device. In emergent situations (e.g., life-threatening trauma), it is likely more effective to disconnect the pump and manage with CII (VRIII) intraoperatively. With elective surgeries, three options exist for the perioperative management of patients using CSII: (a) continuation of CSII (with supplemental IV or subcutaneous insulin if needed); (b) converting from CSII to CII (VRIII); or (c) suspending CSII and substituting with intermittent correction insulin. Continuation of CSII has been advocated during elective surgery in the Society for Ambulatory Anesthesia Consensus Statement (23). As with other aspects of use of this technology in the hospital, a process should

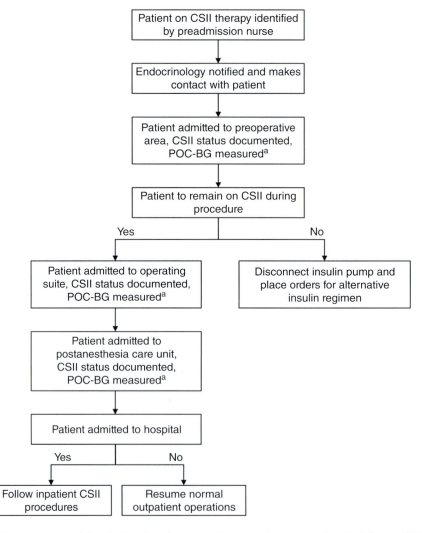

Figure 35-3 Care process model outlining steps for use continuous subcutaneous insulin infusion (CSII) therapy in the perioperative period (26). [a]POC-BG to be measured at least hourly.
Reproduced with permission from SAGE.

be put in place to assure proper selection of candidates for use and steps to assure safety.

Emerging data indicate that insulin pumps can be safely allowed in the operating room and may provide glucose control similar to CII (24–26). In a retrospective analysis of four centers in Italy of 68 pregnant women using CSII, glucose control was assessed at the time of delivery. The primary aim of the study was to evaluate the safety and efficacy of CSII during delivery in pregnant women with type 1 diabetes. A secondary outcome was the need to transition to IV insulin due to metabolic decompensation. In this analysis, 56–85% of women underwent Cesarean section while on CSII. The study showed no difference in mean blood glucose according to delivery procedure (cesarean section vs. vaginal delivery). In addition, none of the women required transition to CII (25).

In an attempt to provide a more structured approach to ensure patient safety, a care process model (Figure 35-3) was developed and implemented by the authors that allowed CSII treatment to be transitioned through the different segments of perioperative care. A recent review indicated that the new process did result in improved glucose monitoring, and no adverse events were seen (26). Other institutions have instituted glycemic management protocols to guide processes for same day surgery. Similarly, they have noted that these protocols are both safe and effective for use in clinical practice (27).

Limitations of Guidelines

The suggestions outlined here are geared towards transitioning adults from outpatient to non-critically ill inpatient CSII use, and are not intended for the hospitalized pediatric population. There has been some interest in the literature about allowing use in the hospitalized pediatric population, but no data on safety of the devices in this population is available (28). Furthermore, these guidelines do not apply to application of CSII therapy *de novo* in the hospital as a means to control inpatient hyperglycemia (29,30).

Conclusions

Individuals whose diabetes is managed via CSII may require hospitalization. While these are low frequency events in comparison to the total number of hospitalizations, they are high visibility when they are admitted. Available data suggest that in properly selected patients and with appropriate guidelines in place; most patients on outpatient CSII therapy can safely transition treatment to the hospital setting. A key factor in minimizing errors and adverse events in these situations is a collaborative relationship between the patient and hospital staff. In addition, because of the continuous advances in diabetes devices and technologies, adequate ongoing education of all key stakeholders about insulin pumps and other evolving tools is warranted.

References

1 Anonymous. Research and markets: US insulin delivery devices market: an analysis. http://www.businesswire.com/news/home/20110825005874/en/Research-Markets-Insulin-Delivery-Devices-Market-Analysis (accessed April 19, 2017).

2 Miller KM, Foster NC, Beck RW, et al. Current state of type 1 diabetes treatment in the U.S.: updated data from the T1D Exchange Clinic Registry. *Diabetes Care*. 2015;38(6):971–978.

3 Centers for Disease Control and Prevention. Hospitalizations for diabetes as any listed diagnosis. http://www.cdc.gov/diabetes/statistics/dmany/index.htm. (accessed March 22, 2017).

4 Rosenthal M, Fajardo M, Gilmore S, Morley JE, Naliboff BD. Hospitalization and mortality of diabetes in older adults. *Diabetes Care*. 1998;21:231–235.

5 Donnan PT, Leese GP, Morris AD, Research in Tayside SMMU, Collaboration.

Hospitalizations for people with Type 1 and Type 2 diabetes compared with the nondiabetic population of Tayside, Scotland: a retrospective cohort study of resource use. *Diabetes Care.* 2000;23(12): 1774–1779.

6 Jiang HJ, Stryer D, Friedman B, Andrews R. Multiple hospitalizations for patients with diabetes. *Diabetes Care.* 2003;26(5): 1421–1426.

7 Bo S, Ciccone G, Grassi G, et al. Patients with type 2 diabetes had higher rates of hospitalization than the general population. *J Clin Epidemiol.* 2004;57: 1196–1201.

8 Dungan KM. The effect of diabetes on hospital readmissions. *J Diabetes Science Tech.* 2012;6(5):1045–1052.

9 Noschese ML, DiNardo MM, Dohini AC, et al. Patient outcomes after implementation of a protocol for inpatient insulin pump therapy. *Endocr Pract.* 2009; 15:415–424.

10 Cook CB, Boyle ME, Cisar NS, et al. Use of continuous subcutaneous insulin infusion (insulin pump) therapy in the hospital setting: proposed guidelines and outcome measures. *Diabetes Educator.* 2005;31: 849–857.

11 Dalton MF, Klipfel L, Carmichael K. Safety issues: use of continuous subcutaneous insulin infusion (CSII) pumps in hospitalized patients. *Hospital Pharmacy.* 2006;41:956–969.

12 Lee SW, Im R, Magbual R. Current perspectives on the use of continuous subcutaneous insulin infusion in the acute care setting and overview of therapy. *Crit Care Nurs Q.* 2004;27:172–184.

13 Leonhardi BJ, Boyle ME, Beer KA, et al. Use of continuous subcutaneous insulin infusion (insulin pump) therapy in the hospital: a review of one institution's experience. *J Diabetes Sci Technol.* 2008; 2(6):948–962.

14 Bailon RM, Partlow BJ, Miller-Cage V, et al. Continuous subcutaneous insulin infusion (insulin pump) therapy can be safely used in the hospital in select patients. *Endocrine Prac.* 2009;15:24–29.

15 Nassar AA, Partlow BJ, Boyle ME, Castro JC, Bourgeois PB, Cook CB. Outpatient to inpatient transition of insulin pump therapy: successes and continuing challenges. *J Diabetes Science Technol.* 2010;4(4):863–872.

16 Cook CB, Beer KA, Seifert KM, Boyle ME, Mackey P, Castro JC. Transitioning insulin pump therapy from the outpatient to the inpatient setting: a review of 6 years' experience with 253 cases. *J Diabetes Science Technol.* 2012;6(5):995–1002.

17 American Diabetes Association. Diabetes care in the hospital. *Diabetes Care.* 2018;41 (Suppl. 1):S144–S151.

18 Joint Commission on Accreditation of Healthcare Organizations. http://www. jointcommission.org/certification/ inpatient_diabetes.aspx (accessed March 25, 2017).

19 Kannan S, Satra A, Calogeras E, Lock P, Lansang MC. Insulin pump patient characteristics and glucose control in the hospitalized setting. *J Diabetes Sci Technol.* 2014;8(3):473–478.

20 Faulds ER, Wyne KL, Buschur EO, McDaniel J, Dungan K. Insulin pump malfunction during hospitalization: two case reports. *Diabetes Technol Ther.* 2016;18(6):399–403.

21 Wallia A, Umpierrez GE, Rushakoff RJ, et al. Consensus statement on inpatient use of continuous glucose monitoring. *J Diabetes Science Technol.* in press.

22 Umpierrez GE, Hellman R, Korytkowski MT, et al. Management of hyperglycemia in hospitalized patients in non-critical care setting: an Endocrine Society Clinical Practice Guideline. *J Clin Endocrin & Metab.* 2012;97(1):16–38.

23 Joshi GP, Chung F, Vann MA, et al. Society for Ambulatory Anesthesia consensus statement on perioperative blood glucose management in diabetic patients undergoing ambulatory surgery. *Anesthesia & Analgesia.* 2010;111:1378–1387.

24 Corney SM, Dukatz T, Rosenblatt S, et al. Comparison of insulin pump therapy (continuous subcutaneous insulin infusion) to alternative methods for perioperative

glycemic management in patients with planned postoperative admissions. *J Diabetes Sci Technol*. 2012;6(5):1003–1015.

25 Fresa R, Visalli N, Di Blasi V, et al. Experiences of continuous subcutaneous insulin infusion in pregnant women with type 1 diabetes during delivery from four Italian centers: a retrospective observational study. *Diabetes Technol Ther*. 2013;15(4):328–334.

26 Mackey PA, Thompson BM, Boyle ME, et al. Insulin pump therapy use during surgery: an update on a quality initiative. *J Diabetes Science Technol*. 2015;9: 1299–1306.

27 Sobel SI, Augustine M, Donihi AC, Reider J, Forte P, Korytkowski M. Safety and efficacy of a peri-operative protocol for patients with diabetes treated with continuous subcutaneous insulin infusion who are admitted for same-day surgery. *Endocr Pract*. 2015;21(11):1269–1276.

28 Einis SB, Mednis GN, Rogers JE, Walton DA. Cultivating quality: a program to train inpatient pediatric nurses in insulin pump use. *Am J Nursing*. 2011;111(7):51–55.

29 Lee I-T, Liau Y-J, Lee W-J, Huang C-N, Sheu WHH. Continuous subcutaneous insulin infusion providing better glycemic control and quality of life in Type 2 diabetic subjects hospitalized for marked hyperglycemia. *J Evaluation in Clin Prac*. 2010;16(1):202–205.

30 Bodur HA, Saygili E, Saygili S, Doganay LH, Yesil S. Continuous infusion of subcutaneous compared to intravenous insulin for tight glycaemic control in medical intensive care unit patients. *Anaesthesia & Intensive Care*. 2008;36(4): 520–527.

36

Management of Diabetes and/or Hyperglycemia during Enteral and Parenteral Nutrition

Aidar R. Gosmanov and Niyaz R. Gosmanov

Key Points

- Hyperglycemia is frequently observed in hospitalized patients receiving specialized nutritional support.
- It is reported that up to 30% of patients receiving enteral nutrition (EN) and more than 50% of patients receiving parenteral nutrition (PN) have blood glucose levels above suggested inpatient glycemic targets.
- Pathogenesis of hyperglycemia during nutrition support is complex.
- Capillary blood glucose monitoring should be initiated for all patients starting EN or PN.
- The development of hyperglycemia during nutrition support is associated with increased risk of complications and mortality.
- There are no prospective randomized control trials conducted in this group of patients; therefore, our approach to managing hyperglycemia in patients on specialized

nutritional support largely relies on recommendations by professional societies.
- The glycemic strategies should also follow common sense in selecting appropriate therapeutic approaches that not only control hyperglycemia but also have low hypoglycemia risk.
- Insulin therapy should be considered for blood glucose more than 180 mg/dL (10 mmol/L).
- Frequent reassessment of patients' clinical status is critical not only to help maintain adequate glycemic control but also to prevent hypoglycemia.
- Future studies are needed to determine safe and beneficial glycemic targets in patients receiving specialized nutrition support as well as to determine optimal therapeutic strategies.

Introduction

Malnutrition, common in hospitalized patients, is associated with longer length of stay, poorer outcomes and survival, and increased cost of care. In general, the nutritional assessment, indications for nutrition support, and estimate of nutrition requirements for critically ill patients with hyperglycemia are similar to those of non-diabetic patients (1). The need for nutritional support in malnutrition is a reflection of

---

the timing and extent of recent (previous 3–6 months) unintentional weight loss, the degree of depletion of energy stores (in turn dependent on baseline energy stores (or body mass index [BMI]), the presence or absence of clinical markers of stress, and the anticipated time that the patient will be unable to meet nutritional requirements orally. There is no gold standard for assessing nutrition status and the accuracy of nutrition assessment methods as a true marker of nutrition status has never been validated. Studies that have demonstrated a beneficial influence of nutritional support on clinical outcome have provided nutrition for a minimum of 1 week. Because there is no evidence that shorter duration nutrition support provides benefit, the Society of Critical Care Medicine (SCCM) and American Society for Parenteral and Enteral Nutrition (ASPEN) joint guidelines state that parenteral nutrition (PN, which is a solution of intravenous (IV) nutrition compounded to include macronutrients [protein, dextrose, fat]; micronutrients [electrolytes, minerals, trace elements, vitamins]; and water) should not be given unless anticipated need is for ≥7 days (2). Enteral nutrition (EN, liquid nutritional formulation is given through a tube [i.e., "tube feeding"] into the stomach or small bowel), rather than PN, should be used in patients with a functioning gastrointestinal tract.

From a general internal medical perspective, it is important to monitor for the presence of the refeeding syndrome which is a collection of metabolic derangements that can occur during refeeding in patients who are starved or severely malnourished. Metabolic derangements in electrolytes, minerals (especially hypophosphatemia), and water-soluble vitamins are common and may be mild or severe. Organ compromise can manifest as pulmonary, cardiac, neuromuscular, and hematologic complications. Appropriate monitoring includes daily weight, fluid balance, and signs of oedema until stable. Levels of serum potassium, phosphorus, and magnesium should be measured daily, and any deficiencies replaced. Thiamine should be administered. Overfeeding and excess PN volume and sodium should be avoided.

Hyperglycemia is frequently observed in hospitalized patients receiving specialized nutritional support. It is reported that up to 30% of patients receiving EN and more than 50% of patients receiving PN have blood glucose (BG) levels above suggested inpatient glycemic targets (1). Of note, there are no prospective randomized control trials (RCTs) conducted in this group of patients; therefore, our approach to managing hyperglycemia in patients on specialized nutritional support should rely on most recent recommendations by the professional societies (2, 3). The glycemic strategies should also follow common sense in selecting appropriate therapeutic approaches that not only control hyperglycemia but also have low hypoglycemia risk.

Common causes of hyperglycemia in hospitalized patients include inadequate insulin dosing, overfeeding, medications, as well as stress, inflammation, and infection. Pathogenesis of hyperglycemia during nutrition support is complex. Elevation of BG occurs as the result of upregulation of pathways responsible for increased glucose production and reduced glucose utilization by peripheral tissues (1). In addition, excessive delivery of glucose and gluconeogenic substrates via the enteral or parenteral route in hospitalized patients can also contribute to hyperglycemia. In general, diabetic patients experiencing inpatient hyperglycemia are at higher risk of complications and mortality (3), though evidence is lacking if interventions designed to reduce hyperglycemia do improve clinical outcomes, at least in non-critically ill patients (4). The evidence from retrospective and observational studies is clear that hyperglycemia is a frequent complication of EN and PN in both diabetic and non-diabetic patients (5), and that the development of hyperglycemia (and hypoglycemia resulting from attempts to correct hyperglycemia) during nutrition support increases the risk of complications and mortality (6).

Glycemic Goals in Patients Receiving Enteral and Parenteral Nutrition

Management of hyperglycemia in patients receiving specialized nutrition support is complicated by therapeutic inertia, a multitude of accompanying patient comorbidities (e.g., in acute stroke patients needing EN, greater fear of inducing hypoglycemia), and by the lack of well-designed RCTs addressing potential harms of hyperglycemia and glycemic goals during nutrition support. In the majority of non-critically ill patients, the pre-meal BG target should be between 100–140 mg/dL (5.6–7.8 mmol/L) and random BG below 180 mg/dL (10 mmol/L), provided that these targets can be safely achieved (3). Target BG levels between 140–180 mg/dL (7.8–10 mmol/L) is recommended in critically ill patients (7). The ASPEN recommends a BG goal of 140–180 mg/dL (7.8–10 mmol/L) for adult patients receiving EN and PN (2). It is reasonable to advise higher BG targets for patients prone to hypoglycemia and/or with multiple comorbidities, while more stringent glycemic goals are recommended in patients with stable glucose trends. Pending the results of prospective RCTs, several observational and intervention studies in intensive care unit (ICU) patients have suggested that a BG goal between 110–150 mg/dL (6–8.3 mmol/L) is associated with better clinical outcomes in patients receiving nutrition support (1,8).

Managing Hyperglycemia in Patients During Specialized Nutrition Support

Any patient who is unable to consume adequate nutrients orally (≥60% nutrition needs) for at least 5 days in the ICU or 7–14 days in the general ward should be a candidate for specialized nutrition support (9). Current evidence and opinions in the field argue for delayed and permissive underfeeding (e.g., giving 75% of basal energy requirements in overweight or obese patients, especially in those with hyperglycemia and/or hypertriglyceridemia) of hospitalized diabetes patients by providing no more than 15–25 calories/kg/day with suggested average carbohydrate content in the formulas of ~150 grams/day (10–13). Both EN and PN have been proven effective in preventing the adverse effects of starvation and malnutrition in hospitalized patients. However, EN is preferred to PN in clinical practice for many reasons, including higher rates of hyperglycemia and infections with the PN use (5). Strategies for managing hyperglycemia in patients requiring specialized nutrition support should consider modifications in the content of feedings as well as the initiation of safe and effective pharmacological therapies to reduce BG levels (Figure 36-1). For patients receiving EN or PN feedings who require insulin should be divided into basal, nutritional, and correctional components. This is particularly important for patients with type 1 diabetes mellitus who should continue a minimum of basal insulin therapy (i.e., nutritional and correction insulin requirements depending on clinical status) in the hospital delivered subcutaneously (SC) or IV regardless whether nutritional support is initiated or not.

Patients Receiving Enteral Nutrition

Specific strategies to control hyperglycemia during EN therapy should include the assessment of caloric needs, evaluation of composition of nutrition support formulas, and safe use of pharmacologic agents (Figure 36-1 and Table 36-1).

Standard enteral formulas contain 1–2 cal/ml and, in general, consist of protein, lipid in the form of long-chain triglycerides, and carbohydrates. In contrast to the standard formulas in which carbohydrates provide 55–60% of total calories, newer diabetic specific formulas (DSFs) have lower carbohydrate content and contain dietary fiber (10–15 g/L) and fructose. In studies conducted in ambulatory non-acutely ill patients with diabetes, the use of DSFs has been

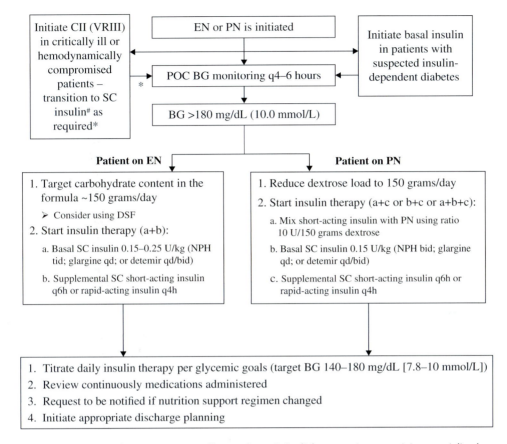

Figure 36-1 Approach to the management of hyperglycemia in diabetes patients receiving specialized nutrition support

The total daily dose (TDD) of insulin used during CII (VRIII) can help inform TDD of SC insulin if patient transitioned. For example, the total dose of insulin administered in the last 6 hours of the CII (VRIII) is divided by 6 to calculate the hourly dose of insulin. This is then multiplied by 20 (not 24, to reduce risk of hypoglycemia) to estimate patient's SC insulin requirement. This dose can then be divided into basal (e.g., 30–50% of calculated TDD) +/- bolus as needed.

POC = point of care; BG = blood glucose; EN = enteral nutrition; PN = parenteral nutrition; DSF = diabetic specific formula; SC = subcutaneous; CII = continuous insulin infusion (also known as variable-rate intravenous insulin infusion [VRIII]).

shown to reduce hyperglycemia (by approximately 20–30 mg/dL [1.1–1.7 mmol/L] post-prandial rise), improve hemoglobin A1c and lower insulin requirements, compared to the standard high carbohydrate formulas (1). However, so far, there is no evidence that the use of DSFs in hospitalized patients with diabetes can result in significant improvements of glycemic control and improve clinical outcomes compared to the treatment with standard EN formulas (2,14).

It is important to recognize that EN may cause bacterial colonization of the stomach, high gastric residual volumes with subsequent risk of aspiration pneumonia, and diarrhea. In addition, unanticipated dislodgement of feeding tubes or temporary discontinuation of nutrition due to nausea or for diagnostic testing may result in increased risk of hypoglycemic events in patients treated with insulin or with oral hypoglycemic agents (OHAs).

Table 36-1 Glucose management unique to EN for patients with diabetes mellitus or hyperglycemia (2).

- Tube feeding can be administered into the stomach or the small bowel. Tube feeding in the stomach can be continuous or intermittent. Often, continuous feeding is used in critically ill patients and intermittent (gravity) feeding is used in medically stable patients. By contrast, jejunal feeding should always be continuous (nocturnal or 24-hour infusion). The format of the feeding regimen has a major impact on the design of insulin management programs.
- Increases in the tube feeding infusion rate should be avoided until adequate glucose control has been achieved by appropriate insulin management.
- For patients with hyperglycemia without prior diagnosis of diabetes and no prior use of insulin or oral diabetic agents, initially recommend treatment with short-acting insulin until tube feeding is well tolerated. This minimizes the risk of hypoglycemia which may result from continued SC absorption of intermediate-acting NPH (isophane) insulin following unexpected discontinuation of tube feeding, because of tube feeding intolerance. Once the tube feeding infusion rate has reached 30–40 ml/hr, the use of intermediate-acting insulin is generally safe.
- Gravity administration: The BG concentration should be checked immediately before each feeding and no sooner than 4 hours after the end of the prior feeding. Thus, feedings should be spaced a minimum of 4 hours apart. Although some patients receiving gravity feedings can be managed with once or twice daily intermediate-acting insulin alone, others will need combined intermediate and short-acting insulin therapy.
- Continuous feeding over 12 hours: Generally use this EN form for patients on home tube feeding. Most patients will require only a once-daily administration of intermediate-acting insulin (alone or combined with a short-acting insulin preparation) prior to the onset of tube feeding.
- Continuous feeding over 24 hours: Scheduled administration of intermediate-acting insulin, usually given every 8 hours, may be required. Use of intermediate-acting rather than long-acting insulin is preferred. If the feeding tube is removed or dislodged, the potential for prolonged hypoglycemia is greater if long-acting insulin is used. Also, reliance on intermediate insulin requires a more frequent dose-adjustment than use of long-acting insulin, resulting in the potential for more rapid achievement of glucose control.
- For hospitalized diabetic subjects treated with once or twice daily SC intermediate-acting insulin (with or without short-acting insulin), begin by providing one-half of the patient's total pre-admission morning insulin as a morning intermediate-acting insulin SC dose. Similarly, one-half of the patient's total pre-admission evening insulin may be provided as an evening intermediate-acting insulin SC dose.
- For patients with type 1 diabetes treated with long-acting insulin for basal insulin needs, generally continue their long-acting SC insulin at the pre-admission dose. Adhere to a rapid-acting SC insulin algorithm for the management of hyperglycemia above the patient's glucose goal range.
- An insulin infusion should be initiated for severe hyperglycemia or if glucose goals cannot be achieved with SC insulin. At this point, reassessment of caloric provision also is indicated. Permissive underfeeding should be considered.
- For patients on tube feeding, the most common cause of hypoglycemia is unexpected discontinuation of tube feedings.

SC = subcutaneous; BG = blood glucose; EN = enteral nutrition.
Reproduced with permission from SAGE.

One prospective RCT evaluated the effectiveness of different insulin regimens in managing hyperglycemia in hospitalized patients receiving EN (15). In this study, 50 patients with and without a history of diabetes and BG levels above 140 mg/dL (7.8 mmol/L) were randomized to receive either a standard therapy consisting of a "sliding scale" regular (short-acting) insulin or a long-acting insulin glargine administered once daily. The investigators showed that initiation of insulin glargine is an effective strategy to manage hyperglycemia during EN. Patients with diabetes required a total daily dose (TDD) of 0.61±0.28 units/kg/day. The hypoglycemic efficacy of insulin glargine in diabetes patients receiving EN was also shown in retrospective studies (16). Insulin detemir can also be used every 12 hours in this setting. Other insulin regimens consisting of NPH (i.e., isophane, intermediate-acting) insulin administered every 8–12 hours (17) or biphasic insulin 70/30 given twice (e.g., 50% of TDD given with each injection) or preferably thrice daily (18) have also been shown to be effective in managing diabetes patients on enteral feeding. The incidence of hypoglycemia reported in these retrospective studies varied between 0.9–1.4%. There is a tremendous need in future prospective studies to evaluate the risk-benefit profile of insulin therapy, including rates of hypoglycemia in patients receiving EN.

The initial approach in calculating insulin TDD for diabetes patient on continuous EN should rely on a weight-based equation. Starting a TDD insulin regimen using formula 0.3–0.5 U/kg (the basal insulin component should be 50% TDD, i.e., 0.15–0.25 U/kg [Figure 36-1]) is effective and safe for the majority of non-critically ill diabetes patients (19). We also suggest that, if hospitalized diabetes patients with well-managed hyperglycemia on pre-existing basal insulin therapy are started on EN, providers should consider a 25–50% increase in insulin dose via basal insulin optimization or via the initiation of scheduled rapid-acting (every 4 hours) or short-acting (every 6 hours) insulin injections using an insulin-to-carbohydrate ratio ranging between 1:10 to 1:15. The rationale for the conservative approach to insulin intensification in these patients is justified by the fact that it may take several days to achieve the desired nutrition goals due to the potential gastrointestinal intolerance during early optimization of enteral feeding.

Diabetes mellitus can affect the entire gastrointestinal tract. Significant diabetic gastroparesis is often present in patients with long-standing type 1 diabetes. The diagnosis should be suspected from the patient's history, and requires exclusion of other factors capable of slowing gut motility. Demonstration of delayed gastric emptying establishes the diagnosis of gastroparesis. Accurate diagnosis of diabetic gastroparesis is important, as it avoids the erroneous attribution of gastrointestinal symptoms to tube feeding or to other factors capable of slowing gut motility. Most patients with diabetic gastroparesis intolerant of gastric feedings are able to tolerate isoosmolar jejunal tube feedings when initiated at a low rate and advanced slowly. Parenteral nutrition should be used only if patients fail a reasonable trial of tube feeding.

Patients Receiving Parenteral Nutrition

The use of PN has been shown to improve nutritional status and lower hospital complications in critically ill patients (5). However, excessive glucose administration during PN may have metabolic disadvantages and result in gut mucosal atrophy, overfeeding, hyperglycemia, an increased risk of infectious complications, and increased mortality in critically ill patients (5). The development of hyperglycemia during PN in the hospital has been independently associated with higher rates of mortality and hospital complications (1). Therefore, prevention and correction of hyperglycemia via modification of nutrient composition and/or by insulin administration should be strongly considered during the PN therapy.

The timing of the PN initiation in critically ill patients should be considered as an initial strategy in reducing the risk of complications associated with PN. In a large multicenter study (20) that compared the early initiation of nutrition support with IV dextrose (20% solution) on ICU day 1, followed by EN plus PN on day 2; versus late initiation of nutrition support consisting of IV dextrose (5% solution) on day 1, EN on day 2, and PN on day 8; it was shown that withholding PN until day 8 resulted in significantly less ICU infections, shorter course of organ dysfunction, a shorter ICU stay, and reduced healthcare costs.

Total daily caloric target range for most adults in the ICU can vary between 15–25 kcal/kg (10). In critical illness, improved glycemic indices were achieved if a hypocaloric PN formula (15 kcal/kg/day) was prescribed to diabetes patients who were expected to stay in the ICU for more than 3 days (12). The macronutrient composition of the PN should consist of 2–3 g/kg/day of glucose (the only carbohydrate in PN formulations), 0.7–1.5 g/kg/day of lipid emulsions, and 1.3–1.5 g/kg/day of amino acids calculated per ideal body weight (1). Dextrose administration rate in PN below 4 mg/kg/min is preferred in critically ill patients because glucose infusion at higher rates is associated with increased incidence of hyperglycemia and insulin use (21,22). Therefore, one approach to reduce the development of hyperglycemia during PN therapy is to lower the amount of infused dextrose to 150 g/day, a glucose load that is sufficient in meeting the metabolic demands of the brain and basic cellular functions (23). In fact, in non-diabetic patients, a glucose load of 1.8±1.3 g/kg/day in PN is associated with improved mortality compared with receiving dextrose infusion rates of 2.6±1.4 g/kg/day in ICU (24). Collectively, it may be reasonable to limit the dextrose load in PN to 150–200 g/day, although prospective RCTs are needed to determine if the differences in glucose load rates improve clinical outcomes in critically ill patients with diabetes.

The increased rate of PN-associated complications may also be related to the type of lipid solutions used. The FDA-approved soybean oil-based lipid emulsion with a high content of linoleic acid and ω-6 polyunsaturated fatty acids may be detrimental. Due to its high content of linoleic acid, soybean-based lipid emulsions might promote the generation of arachidonic acid-derived eicosanoids and exaggerate the inflammatory response during stress and trauma (25). The efficacy and safety of lipid emulsion with lower linoleic acid content by partly replacing soybean oil with olive oil have been compared with the PN containing standard soybean oil-based lipid emulsion in 100 medical and surgical ICU patients. There was no difference in the rates of infectious and non-infectious complications, length of ICU or hospital stay, or glycemic control in critically ill patients (26).

Insulin is the treatment of choice to control hyperglycemia during PN (Figure 36-1; Figure 36-2; Table 36-2). Both SC and IV insulin have been shown to be effective in managing hyperglycemia in these patients (22,27). In critically ill or hemodynamically compromised patients, treatment with IV continuous insulin infusion (CII, also known as variable-rate intravenous insulin infusion [VRIII]) is preferred, as it allows frequent dose adjustments to control glucose values. Several studies have shown that adding insulin to the PN mixture (where this is accepted practice) is clinically safe and effective in controlling hyperglycemia during total PN. The initiation of therapy by adding insulin at the ratio of 1 unit of insulin per 10–15 grams of dextrose (i.e., 10 units per 100 or 150 grams dextrose) in patients with diabetes receiving PN should be an effective initial step to control hyperglycemia (1). In patients with marked insulin resistance, PN insulin requirements may reach an insulin to carbohydrate ratio of 1 unit:4 grams (28).

In non-critically ill patients with diabetes receiving PN, the daily basal insulin administration can be considered as an alternative approach to control hyperglycemia in hospitalized diabetes patients (29). It is not infrequent that the PN administration mode can be cyclic or overnight and can even be interrupted for other reasons, which places diabetes patient at risk for hyperglycemia due to the discontinuation of the insulin administered via PN. Furthermore, in some cases, the diabetes history is unknown and it might be difficult initially to rule out the presence of truly insulin-dependent diabetes in the hospital setting. Therefore, weight-based administration of basal insulin in addition to the insulin added to the PN formulation can, in our opinion, prevent the unexpected deterioration of glycemic control should the PN (containing insulin) delivery be temporarily discontinued.

Lipid Management Issues Unique to PN

A number of studies suggest that the administration of IV fat emulsions (IVFEs) is responsible for the increased infection rates commonly observed with PN use, and some

Management of Hyperglycemia in (Total) Parenteral Nutrition

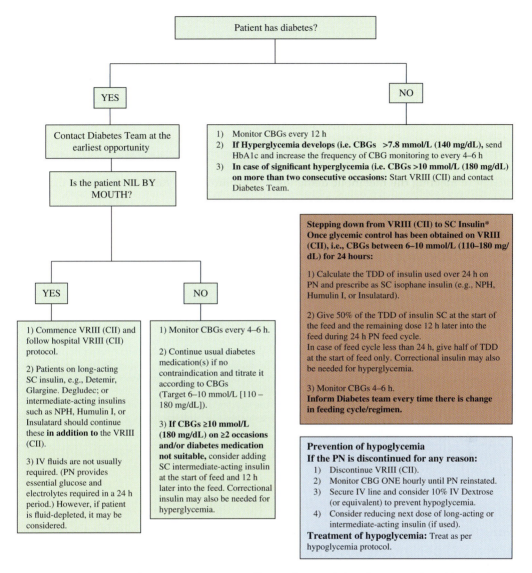

Figure 36-2 Generic UK guidance on management of hyperglycemia in (total) parenteral nutrition. In the UK, adding short-acting (regular) insulin directly to the PN formulation is generally not accepted practice. CBG = capillary blood glucose; PN = parenteral nutrition; SC = subcutaneous; CII = continuous insulin infusion (also known as variable-rate intravenous insulin infusion [VRIII]).

suggest this occurs because of an impairment of the immune function (29). It is not known whether hypertriglyceridemia, a common occurrence in PN-fed patients and exacerbated by the administration of IVFEs, is a factor in impaired immune function. Nonetheless, it is important to check a triglyceride level 1–2 days post-initiation of an IVFE. If the triglyceride values are >300 mg/dL (3.4 mmol/L), the IVFE dose should be reduced or stopped and a hypocaloric regimen should usually be employed, since isocaloric fat-free feeding can lead to worsening of hypertriglyceridemia (29).

Table 36-2 Glucose management unique to PN for patients with diabetes mellitus or hyperglycemia (2,11,27).

- A BG level should be measured before initiation of PN. Avoid overfeeding and limit PN dextrose to 150–200 grams on the first day of nutrition support.
- Recommend measuring BG levels in all patients the first and second morning following initiation of PN. The frequency of subsequent monitoring should be individualized. For patients with established diabetes or significant hyperglycemia, measure BG levels two to four times per day until glucose values are stable. Subsequently, glucose levels are checked twice daily.
- The majority of diabetic patients require insulin coverage when dextrose is infused. For patients previously treated with insulin or oral diabetic agents or patients with two consecutive BG values greater than 150 mg/dL (8.3 mmol/L), generally add 0.1 units of short-acting (regular) insulin per gram of dextrose (e.g., 20 units/liter of D 20% [200 g/L]. This ratio of insulin to dextrose is unlikely to cause hypoglycemia and thus minimizes the need to waste a bag of PN. If the patient has end-stage renal disease or severe depletion, initially add 0.05 units per gram. This approach automatically implies a proportional change in PN insulin when the PN dextrose content is increased or decreased.
- If the PN is discontinued, it is important to remember that the PN insulin also will be stopped. The advantage of this approach is that the infusion of dextrose and insulin are linked; if the infusion is interrupted for any reason, the administration of insulin is also stopped.
- If needed, supplemental SC short-acting insulin or IV insulin infusion is administered according to established algorithms.
- If over a 24-hour period BG values consistently exceed the desired goal range, increase the PN insulin each day by 0.05 units of short-acting (regular) insulin per gram of dextrose to a maximum of 0.2 units of insulin per gram of dextrose.
- At this point, reassessment of caloric provision is indicated. Permissive underfeeding should be considered.
- The PN dextrose content should not be increased until the glucose values of the previous 24-hour period are in the goal range.
- If the patient develops hypoglycemia, management should be as per hypoglycemia treatment protocol.
- A substantial (~50%) reduction of insulin in the subsequent PN admixture is generally indicated, unless the concurrent SC insulin administration contributed to the episode of hypoglycemia. This approach should decrease the incidence of subsequent hypoglycemia.
- The incidence of symptomatic hypoglycemia after the sudden discontinuation of continuous PN is uncommon if satisfactory glucose control has been achieved (i.e., glucose levels <160 mg/dL [8.9 mmol/L]).

SC = subcutaneous; BG = blood glucose; PN = parenteral nutrition.

Hospital Discharge Diabetes Management Options for Patients Receiving Specialized Nutrition Support

Following recovery from an acute illness, a few patients may still require the continuation of specialized nutrition even after discharge from the hospital. In the case of the patients receiving EN, it may not be unreasonable to reassess the hyperglycemia therapy once the patient becomes more clinically stable. This is particularly true for the patients who were transitioned from continuous enteral feedings to bolus feeding 3–4 times a day. Some of the patients who are thought to have residual ß-cell function, based on the diabetes history and the amount of inpatient insulin used, can be started on OHAs in an attempt to de-escalate the insulin regimen. In our experience, type 2 diabetes patients whose total insulin requirements are less than 40–50 units/day can safely be started on OHAs. Insulin secretagogues and dipeptidyl peptidase 4 (DPP4) inhibitors may be used to augment endogenous insulin production while patients are under close observation in the hospital. Metformin therapy provides many benefits to type 2 diabetes patients; special liquid or powder metformin formulations to allow delivery via the enteral feeding tube can be tried but can be expensive (30). Crushing OHAs is not advised,

Table 36-3 Preventing and managing hypoglycemia in patients receiving EN and PN. Dextrose 10% or 20% equivalent doses can be given instead of 50% (less irritant to veins).

1. **Prevention of hypoglycemia:**
   - EN is interrupted:
     - o Start IV 10% Dextrose infusion 50 mL/hr
     - o Consider reducing next dose of long-acting insulin
     - o Increase frequency of BG monitoring
   - PN is interrupted:
     - o Increase frequency of BG monitoring
   - Reduce dose of scheduled insulin if:
     - o Renal insufficiency
     - o Discontinuation or reduction in steroids
     - o Discontinuation of vasopressors
     - o Decrease in carbohydrate delivery rate
2. **Management of hypoglycemia:**
   - Request from the pharmacy 10% Dextrose infusion bag to be available in the unit
   - If BG<70 mg/dL (3.9 mmol/L):
     - o Administer IV 25–50 mL of Dextrose 50% (use 1 mg Glucagon intramuscularly if there is no IV access present)
     - o If repeat BG is <70 mg/dL (3.9 mmol/L) in 15 minutes, repeat dextrose IV push and start IV 10% Dextrose infusion 50 mL/hr
     - o If repeat BG is ≥70 mg/dL (4.0 mmol/L) in 15 minutes, measure BG in 1 hour and repeat treatment until BG is >100 mg/dL (5.6 mmol/L)
   - Reduce or hold next dose of scheduled insulin injection and review cause of hypoglycemia

BG = blood glucose; EN = enteral nutrition; PN = parenteral nutrition; IV = intravenous.

given the unpredictable medication absorption and potential tube blockage. The use of OHAs without medication crushing can be beneficial for patients who can swallow while receiving EN. In the authors' opinion, the addition of an extended-release secretagogue and/or a DPP4 inhibitor can replace the prandial insulin or reduce long-acting insulin dose if the latter is used as a monotherapy in carefully selected type 2 diabetes mellitus patients.

Hypoglycemia in Patients Receiving Specialized Nutrition Support

The development of hypoglycemia has been shown to be associated with the increased risk of complications, the length of hospital stay, and mortality. In addition, fear of hypoglycemia in hospitalized patients remains a major barrier in achieving the optimal glycemic control in the inpatient setting. Patients who receive EN or PN are at higher risk for hypoglycemia as clinical manifestations of declining BG levels are blunted in these patients. Hypoglycemia can develop due to an excess of insulin dose, the abrupt reduction or discontinuation of nutrition support, recovery from an acute illness, the titration of glucocorticosteroids or vasopressors, and progressive organ failure. Strategies that would prevent and address hypoglycemia in patients during specialized nutrition support involve approaches that are pertinent to the management of hypoglycemia in general as well as would reflect the specifics of potential comorbidities in this patient population (Table 36-3).

Case Study

A 70-year-old man with a recent history of total pancreatectomy for chronic painful pancreatitis was admitted to a surgical ward for management of intractable nausea and vomiting. After the surgery, his diabetes was managed at home by injections of insulin glargine 12 units daily and rapid-acting insulin (aspart) with meals, using a ratio of 1 unit to 15 grams of carbohydrates. On admission, he was afebrile and nor-motensive, his weight was 60 kg (BMI was 21 kg/m^2). Laboratory evaluation was significant for normal white blood cell count, random plasma glucose of 189 mg/dL (10.5 mmol/L) and serum creatinine of 1.2 mg/dL (106 μmol/L) which corresponded to eGFR of 60 ml/min/1.73m^2. The primary surgical team started total parenteral nutrition (TPN) with fat emulsion at 75 ml/hr continuously; the total daily dextrose content in the TPN was 160 grams. The diabetes team was consulted for the management of his diabetes.

Considering the patient's age, mild renal insufficiency, and his highly insulin-sensitive state, we initiated capillary blood glucose measurements every 4 hours and injections of insulin glargine 10 units/daily, along with very sensitive supplemental rapid-acting insulin (aspart) given every 4 hours. During the course of the hospitalization, the insulin glargine dose was not changed and his blood glucose levels ranged between 100 and 200 mg/dL (5.5–11.1 mmol/L). Following 3 days of TPN administration, his gastrointestinal symptoms resolved. He was successfully discharged home while being able to tolerate oral intake.

Are There Any Specific Glycemic Targets for Hospitalized Patients with Diabetes Receiving Specialized Nutritional Support?

Current data suggest that the optimal daily carbohydrate requirements in hospitalized patients with diabetes, who receive specialized nutritional support, is 150 grams. There is no clear systematic evidence guiding clinicians to effectively manage hyperglycemia in patients receiving enteral or parenteral nutrition. Until such evidence becomes available, routine therapeutic strategies to control diabetes in hospitalized patients should be used as described elsewhere. Similarly, glycemic goals in these patients should be in accord with the common recommendations for glycemic targets in non-critically ill and critically ill patients with diabetes.

Conclusions

The need for nutrition support requires an assessment of the patient's nutrient intake, body fat and protein stores, severity of illness, and anticipated duration of inadequate volitional oral intake. When possible, EN rather than PN should be used in patients requiring nutrition support. Hyperglycemia is common in patients receiving specialized nutritional support (Table 36-4). The development of hyperglycemia during EN and PN is independently associated with adverse clinical outcome and mortality, at least in the acute care setting. There have been only a few small prospective trials that have addressed glycemic targets and outcomes in this patient population; these trials mostly focused on hospitalized patients with diabetes. Our approach to the management of hyperglycemia in the hospitalized patient receiving specialized nutrition support, shown in Figure 36-1. We recommend that capillary BG monitoring be initiated for patients with diabetes starting EN or PN. Insulin therapy should be initiated for BG more than 180 mg/dL (10 mmol/L). Providers may also consider reduction in carbohydrate content in order to lower the BG concentration. Frequent reassessment of patients' clinical status is critical, not only to help maintain adequate glycemic control but also to prevent hypoglycemia. Future studies are needed to determine safe and beneficial glycemic targets in patients receiving specialized nutrition support as well as to determine optimal therapeutic strategies.

Acknowledgments

The current authors wish to acknowledge the contributions to the previous edition by Molly McMahon and John Miles, upon which portions of this chapter are based.

Table 36-4 Insulin dosing for EN and PN (adapted from American Diabetes Association 2018 recommendations) (31)

Situation	Basal/Nutritional	Correctional
Continuous EN feeding	*Basal:* Continue prior basal or, if none, calculate from TDD (30–50%); or consider 5 units NPH/detemir every 12 h SC; or 10 units glargine/degludec daily SC	*Correctional:* Short-acting (regular) insulin every 6 h SC; or rapid-acting insulin every 4 h SC for hyperglycemia
	Nutritional: Short-acting (regular) insulin every 6 h SC; or rapid-acting insulin every 4 h SC; start with 1 unit per 10–15 g of carbohydrate or calculate from TDD (50–70%); Adjust daily	
Bolus EN feeding	*Basal:* Continue prior basal or, if none, calculate from TDD (30–50%); or consider 5 units NPH/detemir every 12 h SC; or 10 units glargine/degludec daily SC	*Correctional:* Short-acting (regular) insulin every 6 h SC; or rapid-acting insulin every 4 h SC for hyperglycemia
	Nutritional: Short-acting (regular) insulin or rapid-acting insulin every SC before each feeding, starting with 1 unit per 10–15 g of carbohydrate; Adjust daily	
PN feeding	Add Short-acting (regular) insulin to PN IV solution, starting with 1 unit per 10 g of carbohydrate; Adjust daily	*Correctional:* Short-acting (regular) insulin every 6 h SC; or rapid-acting insulin every 4 h SC for hyperglycemia

EN = enteral nutrition; PN = parenteral nutrition; IV = intravenous; TDD = total daily (insulin) dose; SC = subcutaneous.

References

1 Gosmanov AR, Umpierrez GE. Management of hyperglycemia during enteral and parenteral nutrition therapy. *Curr Diab Rep.* 2013;13:155–162.

2 McMahon MM, Nystrom E, Braunschweig C, et al. A.S.P.E.N. clinical guidelines: nutrition support of adult patients with hyperglycemia. *JPEN J Parenter Enteral Nutr.* 2013;37:23–36.

3 Umpierrez GE, Hellman R, Korytkowski MT, et al. Management of hyperglycemia in hospitalized patients in non-critical care setting: an Endocrine Society Clinical Practice Guideline. *J Clin Endocrinol Metab.* 2012;97:16–38.

4 Murad MH, Coburn JA, Coto-Yglesias F, et al. Glycemic control in non-critically ill hospitalized patients: a systematic review and meta-analysis. *J Clin Endocrinol Metab.* 2012;97:49–58.

5 Ziegler TR. Parenteral nutrition in the critically ill patient. *N Engl J Med.* 2009; 361:1088–1097.

6 Pasquel FJ, Spiegelman R, McCauley M, et al. Hyperglycemia during total parenteral nutrition: an important marker of poor outcome and mortality in hospitalized patients. *Diabetes Care.* 2010;33:739–741.

7 Moghissi ES, Korytkowski MT, DiNardo M, et al. American Association of Clinical Endocrinologists and American Diabetes Association consensus statement on inpatient glycemic control. *Endocr Pract.* 2009;15:353–369.

8 Marik PE, Preiser JC. Toward understanding tight glycemic control in the

ICU: a systematic review and metaanalysis. *Chest*. 2010;137:544–551.

9 Cresci G. Targeting the use of specialized nutritional formulas in surgery and critical care. *JPEN J Parenter Enteral Nutr*. 2005; 29:S92–S95.

10 Marik PE, Hooper MH. Normocaloric versus hypocaloric feeding on the outcomes of ICU patients: a systematic review and meta-analysis. *Intensive Care Med*. 2016;42:316–323.

11 Mundi MS, Nystrom EM, Hurley DL, McMahon MM. Management of parenteral nutrition in hospitalized adult patients. *JPEN J Parenter Enteral Nutr*. 2016;41(4): 535–549.

12 Petros S, Horbach M, Seidel F, Weidhase L. Hypocaloric vs normocaloric nutrition in critically ill patients: a prospective randomized pilot trial. *JPEN J Parenter Enteral Nutr*. 2016;40:242–249.

13 Rugeles S, Villarraga-Angulo LG, Ariza-Gutierrez A, et al. High-protein hypocaloric vs normocaloric enteral nutrition in critically ill patients: a randomized clinical trial. *J Crit Care*. 2016:35:110–114.

14 Mesejo A, Montejo-Gonzalez JC, Vaquerizo-Alonso C, et al. Diabetes-specific enteral nutrition formula in hyperglycemic, mechanically ventilated, critically ill patients: a prospective, open-label, blind-randomized, multicenter study. *Crit Care*. 2015;19:390.

15 Korytkowski MT, Salata RJ, Koerbel GL, et al. Insulin therapy and glycemic control in hospitalized patients with diabetes during enteral nutrition therapy: a randomized controlled clinical trial. *Diabetes Care*. 2009;32:594–596.

16 Fatati G, Mirri E, Del Tosto S, et al. Use of insulin glargine in patients with hyperglycaemia receiving artificial nutrition. *Acta Diabetologica*. 2005;42: 182–186.

17 Cook A, Burkitt D, McDonald L, Sublett L. Evaluation of glycemic control using NPH insulin sliding scale versus insulin aspart sliding scale in continuously tube-fed patients. *Nutrition Clinical Pract*. 2009; 24:718–722.

18 Hsia E, Seggelke SA, Gibbs J, et al. Comparison of 70/30 biphasic insulin with glargine/lispro regimen in non-critically ill diabetic patients on continuous enteral nutrition therapy. *Nutrition Clinical Pract*. 2011;26:714–717.

19 Gosmanov AR. A practical and evidence-based approach to management of inpatient diabetes in non-critically ill patients and special clinical populations. *J Clin Transl Endocrinol*. 2016;6:1–6.

20 Casaer MP, Mesotten D, Hermans G, et al. Early versus late parenteral nutrition in critically ill adults. *N Engl J Med*. 2011; 365:506–517.

21 Ahrens CL, Barletta JF, Kanji S, et al. Effect of low-calorie parenteral nutrition on the incidence and severity of hyperglycemia in surgical patients: a randomized, controlled trial. *Crit Care Med*. 2005;33:2507–2512.

22 McCowen KC, Bistrian BR. Hyperglycemia and nutrition support: theory and practice. *Nutr Clin Pract*. 2004;19:235–244.

23 McClave SA, Martindale RG, Vanek VW, et al. Guidelines for the Provision and Assessment of Nutrition Support Therapy in the Adult Critically Ill Patient: Society of Critical Care Medicine (SCCM) and American Society for Parenteral and Enteral Nutrition (A.S.P.E.N.). *JPEN J Parenter Enteral Nutr*. 2009;33:277–316.

24 Lee H, Koh SO, Park MS. Higher dextrose delivery via TPN related to the development of hyperglycemia in non-diabetic critically ill patients. *Nutr Res Pract*. 2011;5:450–454.

25 Gosmanov AR, Umpierrez GE. Medical nutrition therapy in hospitalized patients with diabetes. *Curr Diab Rep*. 2012;12: 93–100.

26 Umpierrez GE, Spiegelman R, Zhao V, et al. A double-blind, randomized clinical trial comparing soybean oil-based versus olive oil-based lipid emulsions in adult medical-surgical intensive care unit patients requiring parenteral nutrition. *Crit Care Med*. 2012;40:1792–1798.

27 McMahon MM. Management of parenteral nutrition in acutely ill patients with hyperglycemia. *Nutr Clin Pract*. 2004; 19:120–128.

28 Valero MA, Leon-Sanz M, Escobar I, et al. Evaluation of nonglucose carbohydrates in parenteral nutrition for diabetic patients. *Eur J Clin Nutr*. 2001;55:1111–1116.

29 Hakeam HA, Mulia HA, Azzam A, Amin T. Glargine insulin use versus continuous regular insulin in diabetic surgical noncritically ill patients receiving parenteral nutrition: randomized controlled study. *J Parenter Enteral Nutr*. 2016;41(7):1110–1118.

30 JBDS Glycaemic management during the inpatient enteral feeding of stroke patients with diabetes (Aug 2012). https://www. diabetes.org.uk/Professionals/Position-statements-reports/Specialist-care-for-children-and-adults-and-complications/ Glycaemic-management-during-the-inpatient-enteral-feeding-of-stroke-patients-with-diabetes/ (accessed May 2017).

31 American Diabetes Association. Diabetes care in the hospital. *Diabetes Care*. 2018;41 (Suppl. 1):S144–S151.

37

Management of Diabetes and/or Hyperglycemia in Hospitalized Patients with Renal Insufficiency

Glenn Matfin

Key Points

- Acute kidney injury (AKI) and chronic kidney disease (CKD) are frequently encountered in hospitalized patients with diabetes and/or hyperglycemia.
- AKI and CKD are important risk factors for hypoglycemia, if these patients are treated with sulfonylureas and/or insulin. Common reasons include decreased insulin clearance, reduced elimination of non-insulin glucose-lowering therapies, reduced renal gluconeogenesis, gastroparesis, increased glycemic variability, hypoglycemic unawareness, improved insulin sensitivity following initiation of renal replacement therapy, and decreased food intake due to poor appetite or lack of timely access to food.
- Current inpatient diabetes guidelines generally recommend avoiding certain non-insulin agents for hospitalized patients, and using intravenous insulin ($\pm$ subcutaneous [SC] basal insulin); or SC basal insulin ($\pm$ nutritional/correction insulin).
- Patients with diabetes and CKD/end-stage renal disease [ESRD]) are known to have decreased insulin requirements and a specific approach for insulin dosing in this population of hospitalized patients is needed to minimize the incidence of hypoglycemia.
- Many insulin-treated patients with type 2 diabetes and CKD stop or need less insulin as kidney disease progresses (known as "burnt out" type 2 diabetes). Similarly, insulin total daily dose (TDD) in persons with type 1 diabetes may also decrease dramatically in CKD/ESRD.
- Glycosylated hemoglobin (HbA$_{1C}$) values are often unreliable in patients with CKD/ESRD; close monitoring by capillary blood glucose testing is recommended during hospitalization.
- An individualized approach to glycemic control is always recommended. However, optimal management of diabetes patients with CKD/ESRD (many of whom have other significant comorbidities) should focus on reducing hypoglycemia risk and takes precedence over meeting strict blood glucose targets.
- Knowledge about which non-insulin glucose-lowering agent(s) can be used effectively and safely for this population in the inpatient setting is important.
- Metformin-associated lactic acidosis (MALA) although rare ($\sim$5–10 cases per 100,000 patient-years), mortality rate remains high ($\sim$50%). MALA may result from metformin accumulation with eGFR <30 ml/min (i.e., AKI and/or advanced CKD), and/or metformin overdose. Metformin should be used cautiously in CKD stage 3B (i.e. eGFR 30–45 ml/min), and is contraindicated in CKD stages 4 and 5 (i.e. eGFR <30 ml/min).

Endocrine and Metabolic Medical Emergencies: A Clinician's Guide, Second Edition. Edited by Glenn Matfin.
© 2018 John Wiley & Sons Ltd. Published 2018 by John Wiley & Sons Ltd.

- Diabetic ketoacidosis (DKA) in advanced CKD or dialysis patients may differ in the clinical and laboratory presentation and the treatment, compared with DKA in non-advanced CKD patients.

- Timely nephrology referral for diabetes patients presenting with AKI and/or CKD can be useful if there is uncertainty regarding renal diagnosis and/or acute/chronic management.

Introduction

Acute kidney injury (AKI), previously known as acute renal failure, encompasses a wide spectrum of injury to the kidneys. The definition of AKI is constantly evolving but usually involves sudden and temporary loss of kidney function. The diagnosis of AKI currently focuses on monitoring serum creatinine levels and derived estimated glomerular filtration rates (eGFR), with or without urine output. AKI is seen in 13–20% of all people admitted to hospital. Most patients with AKI will be managed (at least initially) by a non-renal specialist. AKI tends to be under-diagnosed, under-reported, yet is associated with recurrent AKI hospitalization (23–35% within 1 year) and increased mortality rate (~50% in patients requiring kidney replacement therapy) (1). Major complications of AKI includes volume overload, electrolyte disorders, uremic complications, and drug toxicity. Management includes specific treatments according to underlying cause and supportive treatment to prevent and manage complications. AKI is now recognized as major risk factor for the development of chronic kidney disease (CKD) and other poor health outcomes.

CKD (also known as chronic renal failure/insufficiency) is much more prevalent than AKI, affecting 15% of the US adult general population (1). The definition of CKD also focuses on serum creatinine levels and derived eGFR (preferably calculated with CKD-EPI formula); and kidney damage detected predominantly through urinary albumin excretion estimated by urine albumin/creatinine ratio (ACR), although other renal abnormalities on pathological, urine, blood, or imaging tests can be included (Table 37-1). In addition, persistence of abnormalities in the estimated glomerular filtration rate (eGFR) and/or ACR for at least 3 months or

longer is required for CKD diagnosis. Development of CKD is characterized by a progression from stages 1–5 (Table 37-1). Risk factors for CKD progression include hypertension, glycemia, and albuminuria. AKI and CKD can co-exist in patients resulting in acute-on-chronic deterioration in renal function. Advanced CKD usually relates to CKD stages 4–5 (although stage 3B can also have significant metabolic and other systemic consequences). CKD stage 5 occurs when eGFR <15 ml/min, and is further sub-divided into end-stage renal disease (ESRD) for those patients treated with dialysis or transplant; and kidney (renal) failure for the remainder not treated with these modalities. Diabetes remains the leading cause of CKD (CKD

Table 37-1 Stages of chronic kidney disease (CKD)

Stage	Estimated GFR (eGFR)	Description
1	>90 ml/min	Kidney damage* with normal or increased eGFR
2	60–89 ml/min	Kidney damage* with mildly decreased eGFR
3A	45–59 ml/min	Mildly to moderately decreased eGFR
3B	30–44 ml/min	Moderately to severely decreased eGFR
4	15–29 ml/min	severely decreased eGFR
5	<15 ml/min or renal replacement therapy (i.e., transplant or dialysis)	Kidney failure or end-stage renal disease (ESRD)

*Kidney damage is defined as persistent microalbuminuria or other abnormalities on pathological, urine, blood, or imaging tests (and can also be present in CKD stages 3–5).
GFR = Glomerular Filtration Rate.

due to diabetes is also known as diabetic kidney disease or diabetic nephropathy) and accounts for ~50% ESRD in the developed world (2). Consequently, many individuals with CKD also have diabetes (~40%) (1).

The numbers of inpatients with diabetes continues to grow (e.g., 17% in the UK; and more than 20% in the USA) (3). The UK's National Diabetes Inpatient Audit (NaDIA) projects that the numbers of hospital beds occupied by persons with diabetes will increase to nearly 20% by 2020; in many hospitals it already exceeds 30% (4). In addition, other patients may develop transient hyperglycemia detected during admission that normalizes after discharge, so-called "stress hyperglycemia" (i.e., HbA1c on admission will be normal or pre-diabetes range) (5). Taken together, the numbers of people in-hospital with either diabetes or transient hyperglycemia are high, with a prevalence of between 32–38% on general wards; and between 28–80% of patients with critical illness or undergoing cardiac surgery.

AKI and CKD are frequently encountered in hospitalized patients with diabetes or hyperglycemia (6). AKI and CKD are important risk factors for hypoglycemia, especially if these patients are treated with sulfonylureas and/or insulin (2,6–8). Under normal conditions, renal glucose release accounts for 20–40% of overall gluconeogenesis and, in conditions such as fasting and hypoglycemia, can increase 2- to 3-fold. In patients with renal insufficiency, decreased renal gluconeogenesis, lack of gluconeogenic substrates with decreased food intake or lack of timely access to food, increased glycemic variability, decreased renal degradation and excretion of insulin, decreased elimination of other glucose-lowering therapies, improved insulin sensitivity following initiation of renal replacement therapy, and impairment of counter-regulatory hormonal responses, can all lead to hypoglycemia (2,9). Recent studies have reported that the increased mortality rates associated with inpatient hypoglycemia may not be caused directly by hypoglycemia *per se* but may instead be due to the association between hypoglycemia

and more severe underlying illnesses such as advanced CKD/ESRD (9,10).

Current inpatient diabetes guidelines generally recommend avoiding certain non-insulin agents for hospitalized patients, and using intravenous (IV) insulin (± subcutaneous [SC] basal insulin); or SC basal insulin (± nutritional/correction insulin) (4,11). The sole use of the SC "sliding scale" insulin (i.e., short-, rapid-, or fast-acting insulin correction coverage only with no basal dosing) in the in-hospital setting is strongly discouraged (4,11).

Patients with diabetes and advanced CKD (especially ESRD), are known to have decreased insulin requirements and a specific approach for insulin dosing in this population of hospitalized patients is needed to minimize the incidence of hypoglycemia. In the early years after diagnosis of diabetes, therapy is aimed at "normalizing" glycemic control (while minimizing the risk of hypoglycemia) and inducing metabolic memory in order to decrease the risk of long-term microvascular (including diabetic kidney disease) and macrovascular complications (12,13). An individualized approach to glycemic control is always recommended. However, optimal management of diabetes patients with CKD/ESRD (many of whom have other significant comorbidities, especially cardiovascular disease) should generally focus on reducing hypoglycemia risk and this takes precedence over meeting strict blood glucose (BG) targets. The aims of insulin therapy in diabetes patients on maintenance hemodialysis are to improve the quality of life and avoid the extremes of hypo- and hyperglycemia. Inherent risks, including severe hypoglycemia and increased cardiovascular risk, should be considered when formulating therapeutic strategies in this setting (12,13). In addition, knowledge about which non-insulin glucose-lowering agent(s) can be used safely and effectively for this population in-hospital is also important (2,8,10).

Diabetic ketoacidosis (DKA) in advanced CKD or dialysis patients may differ in the clinical and laboratory presentation and in the treatment, compared with DKA in non-advanced CKD patients.

Diabetes, Hypoglycemia, and Chronic Kidney Disease

Diabetes is the leading cause of CKD and ESRD, and the combination of CKD and diabetes is commonly encountered in clinical practice (1). Unfortunately, the combination of diabetes and CKD is also associated with increased morbidity and mortality, mainly due to increased cardiovascular risk (14).

In patients with diabetes and CKD/ESRD, glycosylated hemoglobin (HbA_{1C}) values are often unreliable for many reasons (e.g., increased red blood cell turnover or recent blood transfusions can "falsely" decrease HbA_{1C}; while iron deficiency, common in hemodialysis patients, leads to increased HbA_{1C} which is reversed by iron replacement therapy). Consequently, close monitoring by capillary BG testing is recommended during hospitalization (4,11). However, despite this, there is still a significant correlation between HbA_{1C} and survival in CKD and ESRD; increased mortality is associated with either HbA_{1C} <7% (53 mmol/mol) or >8% (64 mmol/mol) as compared with 7–8% (53–64 mmol/mol) (15–17). The finding of an increased mortality associated with HbA_{1C} <6–7% (42–53 mmol/mol) is particularly important in light of the increased incidence of hypoglycemia in CKD/ESRD patients.

In a study of hypoglycemia among 243,222 patients cared for by the US Veterans Health Administration, the rate of BG <70 mg/dL (3.9 mmol/L) was 10.72 per 100 patient-months in patients with diabetes and eGFR <60 ml/min per 1.73 m² as compared with 5.33 per 100 patient-months in patients with diabetes and normal renal function after adjustment for age, race, and other comorbidities (18). Approximately 57% of 2,040,206 glucose measurements collected in this database were from patients during hospitalization. Mortality within one day of the hypoglycemic episode was increased in all patients with CKD, OR 1.85 for BG 60–69 mg/dL (3.3–3.8 mmol/L), OR 4.10 for BG 50–59 mg/dL (2.8-3.2), and OR 6.09 for BG <50 mg/dL (2.8 mmol/L) (all p <0.0001). Thus hypoglycemia is a potential threat (or marker) of increased mortality to inpatients with diabetes, including those with CKD/ESRD (9,10).

Insulin Therapy in Patients with Diabetes and/or Hyperglycemia in CKD/ESRD

Current guidelines generally recommend using insulin therapy as opposed to non-insulin therapies in the inpatient setting (4,11). Regardless of the form of insulin regimen chosen (IV and/or SC insulin) to treat diabetes or hyperglycemia, caution is needed for patients with CKD/ESRD. Optimizing individualized glycemic control requires an understanding of the altered pharmacokinetics and pharmacodynamics of insulin as well as many other factors in this setting.

Insulin Clearance in Advanced CKD/ESRD

Multiple alterations in insulin and glucose metabolism occur in CKD/ESRD. Since endogenous insulin is secreted via the portal vein, the liver metabolizes ~50% of insulin in the first pass. The kidney plays a secondary role in the metabolism of endogenous insulin but will clear ~65% of insulin reaching it. In contrast, exogenous insulin is absorbed systemically, and thus the kidney plays a primary role in the metabolism of injected therapeutic insulin (19). After GFR <20 ml/min, renal clearance of insulin is dramatically reduced (20). Other factors in ESRD that mitigate diabetes and increase the risk for hypoglycemia include decreased renal gluconeogenesis, anorexia, weight loss, and protein malnutrition (8,21).

Insulin Requirements in CKD/ESRD

When patients with diabetes are followed from the onset of overt nephropathy to ESRD, their insulin requirements decrease by 38% from 0.72 units/kg/day to 0.45 units/kg/day in type 1 diabetes; and by 51% from 0.68 units/kg/day to 0.33 units/kg/day in type 2 diabetes (22). Many patients with type 2 diabetes progress to needing no therapy for hyperglycemia after developing ESRD, a phenomenon known as "burnt out" type 2 diabetes (23). For example, around 65% of dialysis patients have HbA_{1C} <7% (53 mmol/mol), and 35% HbA_{1C} <6% (42 mmol/mol). These levels have no prognostic benefit in this population and an appropriate review of insulin and/or non-insulin therapies and glycemic targets should be undertaken.

Insulin Sensitivity in CKD/ESRD

There are significant changes in insulin sensitivity and glycemic control in patients with type 2 diabetes and ESRD when these parameters were compared before and after hemodialysis treatment. Continuous glucose monitoring (CGM) in 19 subjects found that mean BG was 226 ± 101 mg/dL (12.5 ± 5.6 mmol/L) in the 24 hours prior to dialysis but dropped to 176 ± 68 mg/dL (9.8 ± 3.8 mmol/L) in the 24 hours after dialysis (24). Asymptomatic hypoglycemia was more common after dialysis. A study using the euglycemic clamp technique demonstrated a 25% reduction in basal insulin requirements on the day after dialysis as compared with the day before dialysis, with no difference in mealtime insulin needs (25).

A study evaluating insulin glargine and glulisine (i.e., basal-bolus) in non-critically ill hospitalized subjects with type 2 diabetes and advanced CKD (mean eGFR 31 ml/min) included 107 subjects not yet requiring dialysis (26). They were randomized to an insulin total daily dose (TDD) of 0.5 units/kg vs. 0.25 units/kg, 50% of the TDD was given daily as insulin glargine (basal), and subjects who were eating also received one-sixth of the TDD as insulin glulisine with each meal (bolus). Doses were titrated daily based on pre-meal and bedtime BG measurements. Mean HbA_{1C} on admission was 8% (64 mmol/mol); and 76% of patients were treated with insulin prior to admission. Mean BG was the same for both insulin dose groups on day 1 (196 ± 62 mg/dL [10.9 ± 3.4 mmol/L]) and decreased to mean 174 ± 49 mg/dL (9.7 ± 2.7 mmol/L) in both groups on subsequent days. Although the glucose-lowering effect of the different insulin doses was no different, there was a

50% reduction in the frequency of hypoglycemia in the lower dose group.

New Insulin Therapies in CKD/ESRD

Based on limited clinical experience and research evidence for newer insulin formulations (e.g., ultra-long acting insulin U100/U200 degludec and U300 glargine; rapid-acting insulin U100/U200 lispro; and fast-acting insulin aspart), dose adjustments for patients with CKD/ESRD on these agents should be based on patient response as advised for traditional insulin compounds (i.e., short- and rapid-acting; intermediate; and long-acting insulins) in this setting (2). With respect to the new fixed-ratio combinations of basal insulin and glucagon-like peptide-1 (GLP-1) analogs (e.g., insulin degludec combined with liraglutide; and insulin glargine with lixisenatide), which are administered together in a single injection, the limiting factor from a renal perspective is the GLP-1 component (i.e., lixisenatide caution CKD stage 4 and avoid in stage 5; whereas, liraglutide can be used in all CKD stages [limited experience in stage 5]).

Non-Insulin Therapies in Patients with Diabetes and/or Hyperglycemia in CKD/ESRD

Intensive glycemic control with the goal of achieving near-normoglycemia has been shown in large prospective randomized studies to delay the onset and progression of diabetic nephropathy (i.e., albuminuria and reduced eGFR) in patients with type 1 diabetes and type 2 diabetes (5,13). Some glucose-lowering medications also have beneficial effects on the kidney that are direct (i.e., not mediated through glycemia). For example, sodium-glucose co-transporter 2 (SGLT2) inhibitors (a class of oral anti-diabetic agents that decrease BG by inhibiting proximal tubular glucose reabsorption in the kidney), also reduce intraglomerular pressure, albuminuria and slow GFR loss through mechanisms

Table 37-2 Non-insulin therapies for type 2 diabetes mellitus in CKD

Class/name	Usual dosing range	Safe in CKD?	Dose modification for CKD
Sulfonylureas			
Glyburide	1.25–10 mg/day	No	Avoid in stages 3–5
Glipizide	2.5–20 mg/day	With caution	No dose modification needed
Glimepiride	1-6 mg/day	With caution	Initiate conservatively (e.g., 1 mg/day)
Gliclazide	40–320 mg/day	With caution	No dose modification needed
Glinides			
Repaglinide	0.5–2 mg with meals	With caution	Stage 4–5 Initiate 0.5 mg with meals
Nateglinide	60–120 mg with meals	With caution	Stage 4–5 Initiate 60 mg with meals
Metformin	500–2000 mg/day	With caution	Full dose in stages 1–3A
			50% reduced dose in stage 3B
			Avoid in stages 4–5
Pioglitazone	15–45 mg/day	Yes	No dose modification needed
DPP-4 Inhibitors			
Sitaglipin	100 mg/day	Yes	Full dose in stages 1–2
			50 mg/day in stage 3
			25 mg/day in stages 4–5
Saxagliptin	5 mg/day	Yes	Full dose if eGFR >50
			2.5 mg/day if eGFR ≤50
Linagliptin	5 mg/day	Yes	Full dose
Alogliptin	25 mg/day	Yes	Full dose in stages 1–2
			12.5 mg/day in stage 3
			6.25 mg/day in stages 4–5
Vildagliptin	50 mg twice daily	Yes	50 mg once daily in stages 3–5
GLP-1 agonists			
Exenatide	10 mcg BID	With caution	Full dose in stages 1–3
			Avoid in stages 4–5
Exenatide XR	2 mg/once weekly	With caution	Full dose in stages 1–3
			Avoid in stages 4–5
Liraglutide	0.6–1.8 mg/day	With caution	Full dose in stages 1–5
			Limited experience severe CKD
Lixisenatide	10–20 mcg/daily	With caution	Full dose in stages 1–3
			Avoid in stages 4–5
Semaglutide	0.5–1 mg/once weekly	With caution	Full dose in stages 1–5
			Limited experience severe CKD
Dulaglutide	0.75–1.5 mg/once weekly	With caution	Full dose in stages 1–5
			Limited experience severe CKD
Alpha glucosidase inhibitors			
Acarbose	25–50 mg with meals	With caution	Limit to stages 1–3 only
Miglitol	25–50 mg with meals	With caution	Limit to stages 1–3 only

(continued)

Table 37-2 (*Continued*)

Class/name	Usual dosing range	Safe in CKD?	Dose modification for CKD
SGLT-2 inhibitor			
Canagliflozin	100–300 mg/day	With caution	Full dose in stages 1–2
			100 mg/day if eGFR 45–59 ml/min
			Avoid if eGFR <45 ml/min
Dapagliflozin	10 mg/day	With caution	Full dose in stages 1–2
			Avoid in stages 3–5
Empagliflozin	10–25 mg/day	With caution	Full dose in stages 1–2
			10 mg/day if eGFR 45–60 ml/min
			Avoid if eGFR <45 ml/min
			(contraindicated eGFR <30 ml/min)
Ertugliflozin	5–15 mg/day	With caution	Full dose in stages 1–2
			Avoid in stages 3–5

DPP-4 = Dipeptidyl peptidase-4; eGFR = estimated Glomerular Filtration Rate; GLP-1 = Glucagon-like peptide-1; SGLT-2 = Sodium-glucose co-transporter 2; XR = extended release.

that appear independent of glycemia (27). Although the glucose-lowering effects of SGLT2 inhibitors are blunted with reduced eGFR (Table 37-2), the renal (28) and cardiovascular benefits (29) of empagliflozin, compared with placebo, were not reduced among trial participants in a large cardiovascular outcome study (EMPA-REG) with baseline eGFR 30–59 mL/min/1.73 m^2, compared with participants with baseline eGFR ≥60 mL/min/1.73 m^2. More recently, canagliflozin also reduced cardiovascular outcomes and the progression of albuminuria and a composite 40% reduction in eGFR, renal replacement therapy or renal death, compared to placebo (30). These beneficial kidney effects may be related to osmotic diuresis and hemodynamic factors induced by SGLT2 inhibitors, although several other putative mechanisms are being explored (e.g. increased tubuloglomerular feedback) (27). Similarly, glucagon-like peptide-1 (GLP-1) receptor agonists (31) and dipeptidyl peptidase-4 (DPP-4) inhibitors also have direct effects on the kidney and have been reported to improve renal outcomes compared with placebo.

However, several non-insulin glucose-lowering therapies are best avoided in hospitalized patients, including those with AKI and/or CKD/ESRD, decompensated heart failure, hypoperfusion or shock, acute/chronic pulmonary disease, or for those given IV contrast. Many non-insulin medications used to treat diabetes are affected by reduced kidney function, resulting in prolonged drug exposure and increased risk of hypoglycemia in patients with AKI and/or CKD/ESRD. Currently available non-insulin therapies for type 2 diabetes (some of these agents are also used off-label as adjunctive treatments in type 1 diabetes) and their safety in various stages of CKD are shown in Table 37-2.

It is important to recognize that if non-insulin glucose-lowering therapies are discontinued in the in-hospital (or even community/outpatient) setting, that BG monitoring should be intensified as patients may become severely hyperglycemic and insulin therapy may be needed (at least temporarily). For patients with acute and/or chronic renal insufficiency, severe hyperglycemia resulting from holding/discontinuing glucose-lowering therapies can further aggravate AKI or CKD/ESRD due to dehydration and hypotension. In addition, it is critical to discontinue/hold/review any nephrotoxic drugs frequently used by patients with diabetes, such as angiotensin converting enzyme (ACE) inhibitors, angiotensin receptor blockers (ARBs), mineralocorticoid antagonists, diuretics, and non-steroidal anti-inflammatory drugs (NSAIDs) for patients presenting with AKI or CKD/ESRD. The risks/benefits IV contrast in this setting is also important to consider. In addition, statins can rarely cause statin-induced rhabdomyolysis which can lead to AKI and/or worsening CKD. The continual use of these drugs or alternatives should be reviewed as part of ongoing care and discharge planning.

Metformin

Metformin is the current gold standard treatment for patients with type 2 diabetes and is generally safe and effective (5,13). Metformin accumulates in renal impairment, but is not nephrotoxic. The US prescribing information for metformin was recently revised to reflect its safety in patients with eGFR $\geq$30 ml/min/1.73 m^2 (5). The Food and Drug Administration (FDA) also recommended the use of eGFR instead of serum creatinine to guide treatment. Revised FDA guidance states that metformin is contraindicated in patients with an eGFR <30 mL/min/1.73 m^2; eGFR should be monitored while taking metformin; the benefits and risks of continuing treatment should be reassessed when eGFR falls <45 mL/min/1.73 m^2 (i.e., CKD stage 3B or worse); metformin should not be initiated for patients with an eGFR <45 mL/min/1.73 m^2; and metformin should be temporarily discontinued at the time of or before IV iodinated contrast imaging procedures in patients with eGFR 30–60 mL/min/1.73 m^2 (e.g., one scheduled metformin dose can be held before contrast; reinstate 24 hours later if patient is eating and drinking and eGFR >60 ml/min [or patient is back to an acceptable baseline eGFR]).

Suggested metformin dosing for patients with CKD stage 3A (i.e., eGFR 45–59 ml/min), no metformin dose modification needed; for patients with CKD stage 3B (i.e., eGFR 30–44 ml/min), lower metformin dose (i.e., no more than 1g/day); and CKD stages 4 or 5, discontinue metformin (32). In patients with AKI, metformin should be discontinued and re-initiation reviewed as part of ongoing care and discharge planning.

However, metformin should be used cautiously in the in-hospital setting because of possible fluctuations in renal function and cardiorespiratory compromise during an acute hospital admission. Adverse events include nausea, vomiting, diarrhea, and contrast-related complications. The most serious adverse effect is the development of metformin-associated lactic acidosis (MALA), although this is a very rare occurrence with approximately 5–10 cases per 100,000 patient-years, mortality rate for MALA approaches 50% (32–34). Metformin, along with other drugs in the biguanide class, increases plasma lactate levels in a plasma concentration-dependent manner by inhibiting mitochondrial respiration predominantly in the liver (however, metformin has about 24-times less reported incidents of lactic acidosis than phenformin, which is a more powerful inhibitor of mitochondrial respiration). Elevated plasma metformin concentrations (as occur in individuals with renal impairment) and a secondary event or condition that further disrupts lactate production or clearance (e.g., cirrhosis, sepsis, or hypoperfusion) are typically necessary to cause MALA (34). MALA occurs when there is an imbalance between increased lactate production and impaired metabolism/reduced clearance. If concerned about MALA, lactate levels can be measured (plasma lactate <3.5 mmol/L is generally safe) and other assessments and investigations performed as needed. MALA may result from metformin accumulation with eGFR <30 ml/min (i.e., AKI and/or advanced CKD), and/or metformin overdose. This results in: (a) impaired mitochondrial function leading to reduced gluconeogenesis and glycogenolysis and increased glycolysis; and (b) activation of the anaerobic metabolism in the intestine (32). Multi-system organ failure can result, including cardiac (decreased cardiac output and hypotension, arrhythmias); respiratory (pulmonary edema); and central nervous system (delirium, coma) events.

Lactic acidosis has been divided into two categories: Type A lactic acidosis results from the accumulation of lactate via glycolysis in the absence of oxygen; Type B lactic acidosis occurs during conditions when lactate production is increased at a time when clearance of lactic acid by oxidation or gluconeogenesis is reduced. MALA is a form of Type B (nonhypoxic) lactic acidosis and is generally characterized by blood pH<7.35; very high lactate levels (>15 mmol/L); large anion gap (>20 mmol/L); and renal insufficiency (eGFR <30 ml/min) (35). Hypoglycemia at presentation of MALA is rare (metformin is an insulin sensitizer). Toxic levels of metformin can cause pancreatitis. Emergency management of MALA includes discontinuing metformin, and managing patient in intensive care unit setting. Hemofiltration treats the severe metabolic acidosis and AKI, and also removes metformin (35).

Sulfonylureas

Sulfonylureas are drugs that stimulate endogenous insulin secretion by pancreatic beta cells. These agents can cause hypoglycemia. Commonly used sulfonylureas include glyburide [glibenclamide], which has a long half-life and is known to accumulate in renal insufficiency and thus should be avoided for diabetes patients with CKD stages 3–5 (36). Glimepiride can also accumulate in CKD stages 4–5, but can be used cautiously in this group (e.g., starting conservatively with 1 mg/day) (2). Gliclazide is widely used outside the USA, and offers numerous dose alternatives which can be helpful practically (including the inpatient setting). Gliclazide presents a lower risk of severe hypoglycemia than glibenclamide and glimepiride, but should also be used cautiously in CKD stages 4–5 with lower starting doses being considered (2). Glipizide is metabolized by the liver into several inactive metabolites, and its clearance and elimination half-life are not affected by a reduction in eGFR, so dose adjustments are not necessary in patients with CKD although initiate conservatively

at 2.5 mg/day to avoid hypoglycemia (which can occur in this setting due to many factors and not just decreased drug clearance). Therefore, glipizide is the preferred sulfonylurea in patients with CKD (although glimepiride; or small doses of gliclazide [e.g., 40 mg once or twice daily] can be utilized with careful titration and constant vigilance).

Sulfonylureas work quickly (within 24–48 h) so may be of value in the treatment of some non-decompensated hyperglycemic states. However, all sulfonylureas should be used with extreme caution in the in-hospital setting where the timing of meals is frequently disrupted and other patient- and hospital-related factors can predispose to increased risk of hypoglycemia (4,13).

SGLT2 Inhibitors

The glucose-lowering effects of SGLT2 inhibitors are blunted with reduced eGFR. Empagliflozin and canagliflozin are approved eGFR >45 ml/min with dose adjustment in CKD stage 3A (Table 37-2). In contrast, dapagliflozin can only be used with eGFR >60 ml/min. However, the renal (i.e., slower progression of kidney disease and less renal events including need for renal replacement therapy) and cardiovascular (i.e., decreased cardiovascular death and reduction in heart failure hospitalization) benefits of empagliflozin, compared with placebo, were not reduced among trial participants in a large cardiovascular outcome study with baseline eGFR 30–59 mL/min/1.73 m^2, compared with participants with baseline eGFR ≥60 mL/min/1.73 m^2 (28,29). Similar beneficial cardiovascular and renal findings were seen with canagliflozin in the CANVAS program (30).

SGLT2 inhibitors are associated with a number of adverse events, including dehydration, AKI, urinary tract infections, and diabetic ketoacidosis (DKA, including euglycemic) (12,13). Increased risk of leg and foot amputations (mostly affecting the toes) was seen in two large studies with canagliflozin (30), a FDA black box warning has been added to canagliflozin to describe this risk. SGLT2 inhibitors should be avoided in severe illness when ketone bodies are present and during prolonged fasting and surgical procedures (37). When initiating SGLT2 inhibitors in persons using diuretics (or vice versa), it is important to reduce the diuretic dose and monitor kidney function in order to prevent dehydration and potential AKI or exacerbation of CKD. Until safety and effectiveness are established, SGLT2 inhibitors are not generally recommended for routine in-hospital use (37).

GLP-1 Agonists

GLP-1 receptor agonists also have direct effects on the kidney and have been reported to improve renal and cardiovascular outcomes (i.e., once-daily liraglutide, and once-weekly semaglutide) compared with placebo (31). GLP-1 agonist adverse events include nausea, vomiting, and dehydration, which can result in AKI and/or acute exacerbation of CKD. Until safety and effectiveness are established, GLP-1 agonists are not generally recommended for routine in-hospital use (4).

DPP-4 Inhibitors

DPP-4 inhibitors (which enhance circulating concentrations of active GLP-1) are approved for use with or without dose reduction in CKD (Table 37-2). DPP-4 inhibitors are used in the in-hospital setting. Sitagliptin has shown efficacy and safety in both a pilot and more definitive study of patients with mild-moderately severe type 2 diabetes in the inpatient setting. Sitagliptin (using renal dosing) in combination with basal insulin was non-inferior in controlling glycemia versus basal-bolus insulin regimen in medical and surgical patients (38). Sitagliptin (± basal insulin) may be especially useful for elderly inpatients (9). In comparison, saxagliptin and alogliptin have not been widely studied in the in-hospital setting. They should also be discontinued in patients who develop heart failure on starting either of these two agents (more common in patients with established

heart or kidney disease) or are contraindicated with existing heart failure (which is very prevalent in persons with diabetes, especially with CKD/ESRD and associated cardiovascular comorbidities) (5).

Diagnosis and Management of Diabetic Ketoacidosis in Advanced CKD/ESRD

DKA in advanced CKD or dialysis patients may differ in the clinical and laboratory presentation and the treatment, compared with DKA in non-advanced CKD patients (39). DKA is infrequent in dialysis patients but it has been increasingly encountered due to the rising prevalence of diabetes-related ESRD.

Metabolic acidosis is usually present in dialysis-associated DKA. The average reported serum bicarbonate and anion gap (AG) in dialysis-dependent patients with DKA were 12.0 ± 4.6 mmol/L and 27.2 ± 6.4 mEq/L, respectively (40). Rarely, metabolic acidosis can be masked by concomitant metabolic alkalosis from exposure to a high bicarbonate dialysate during hemodialysis. Mixed acid base disorder in this case can produce normal or minimally reduced serum bicarbonate; nevertheless, a high AG will be present in DKA and serves as a clue for DKA. Additionally, AG in ESRD patients can be elevated in the absence of DKA because of the accumulation of organic acids and reduced acid secretion from kidney failure. However, AG >20 mEq/L (>20 mmol/L) is not typical of ESRD alone, and should prompt the search for additional causes of AG metabolic acidosis, such as DKA.

It is important to note that no prospective studies have systematically evaluated strategies assessing treatment and resolution of DKA in dialysis patients; therefore, the diagnosis of DKA and monitoring for its resolution should be done in close collaboration with a nephrologist (39). Insulin administration is a mainstay and frequently the only treatment required for DKA management in dialysis patients (40). Clinically, dialysis patients usually present with minimal or no signs of volume depletion, and often have signs of extracellular volume expansion, such as lower extremity and pulmonary edema and elevated blood pressure (39). The absence of volume depletion is explained by the lack of osmotic diuresis when residual renal function is severely reduced or absent. It is believed that, in dialysis patients with DKA, overall intracellular volume is preserved and extracellular volume remains normal to increased (41). Therefore, ESRD patients often do not require IV fluids in the absence of a clinical history of extracellular fluid loss, such as vomiting, diarrhea, or excessive insensible losses. If evidence for intravascular volume depletion is present, judicious administration of small boluses of normal saline (i.e., 250 mL) with close monitoring of respiratory and hemodynamic parameters is required (39). Infrequently, severe DKA can lead to pulmonary edema due to hyperglycemia-associated interstitial hypertonicity. Pulmonary edema in DKA usually responds to administration of insulin alone (41); in severe cases, acute dialysis may be required.

Reduced glomerular filtration rate, insulinopenia, and hypertonicity result in a positive potassium balance, placing ESRD patients with DKA at high risk for hyperkalemia (42). Hyperkalemia is typically more severe in dialysis patients compared with non-dialysis patients for the same levels of hyperglycemia and can be life-threatening (42). Consequently, routine potassium replacement is not indicated unless plasma potassium level is <3.3 mmol/L (39). Insulin is typically the only treatment necessary for hyperkalemia in dialysis-dependent patients with DKA. Severe hyperkalemia requires electrocardiographic monitoring for signs of cardiac toxicity. The potassium measurement level should be repeated 2 hours post-procedure to monitor for its intracellular rebound after hemodialysis.

The role of hemodialysis in the treatment of DKA is controversial and has not been systematically studied in ESRD patients. Severe pulmonary edema and hyperkalemia are two main indications for acute hemodialysis in DKA. Emergent dialysis in patients with DKA without clear indications can cause rapid decrease of serum tonicity, which can present a potential concern for neurological complications in ESRD patients (39).

Practical Management of Diabetes and/or Hyperglycemia in CKD/ESRD

How should the various clinical and research findings described impact the care of patients with diabetes and/or hyperglycemia and CKD during hospitalization? Practical suggestions for successful management of diabetes in patients with CKD/ESRD are outlined in Table 37-3.

The presence of CKD/ESRD affects the risks and benefits of intensive glycemic control (there is a lag time of at least 2 years in type 2 diabetes to over 10 years in type 1 diabetes for the effects of intensive glycemic control to manifest as improved eGFR outcomes in earlier CKD and practically no benefit in advanced CKD/ESRD) and a number of specific glucose-lowering medications. The aim of insulin therapy in diabetes patients on maintenance hemodialysis is to improve the quality of life and avoid the extremes of hypo- and hyperglycemia. HbA_{1C} should be measured in all inpatients with hyperglycemia or a history of diabetes if a recent result is not available. (5,11) Targeting HbA_{1C} between 7.0–7.9% (53–63 mmol/mol) is associated with the lowest mortality in dialysis patients. Patients' diabetes treatment regimen should be adjusted at the time of hospital discharge if the HbA_{1C} is either too low (e.g., <7% [53 mmol/mol]) or too high (e.g., >8% [64 mmol/mol]) depending on the patients' individualized glycemic goals (5). Many dialysis patients with diabetes, treated with insulin or a sulfonylurea, will have inpatient HbA_{1C} <7% (53 mmol/mol). It is important to recognize that these patients have

Table 37-3 Practical suggestions for improving insulin safety in diabetes patients with CKD/ESRD

1. Elderly patients may have a substantial decrease in GFR despite having a mild elevation in serum creatinine (less muscle mass). Despite this reservation, always incorporate eGFR into dosing of non-insulin therapies and into weight-based initiation of insulin dosing.

2. • 0.5 units/kg/day (0.2–0.3 units/kg/day aged >70 years) is a commonly recommended TDD for initiation of in-hospital insulin therapy in type 2 diabetes patients: 50% long-acting insulin; and 50% rapid- or fast-acting insulin split into three meals.
   • Alternatively, if basal insulin alone is initiated (intermediate NPH or long-acting) 0.1–0.2 units/kg/day (± non-insulin therapies).

3. • Reduce the TDD for initiation of in-hospital insulin therapy in type 2 diabetes patients to 0.25 units/kg/day in patients with eGFR <45 ml/min (CKD stages 3B–4); if eGFR <15ml/min (CKD stage 5) reduce TDD 0.2 units/kg/day in order to reduce the frequency of hypoglycemia. Divide TDD 50% long-acting insulin; and 50% rapid- or fast-acting.
   • If basal insulin alone given (intermediate NPH or long-acting), reduce starting dose to 0.1–0.15 units/kg/day (± non-insulin therapies) if eGFR <45 ml/min (CKD stages 3B–5).

4. If intermediate-acting NPH insulin is used in patients with ESRD, once daily AM dosing will usually suffice; PM dosing increases the risk of next AM hypoglycemia and is usually not needed.

5. Hypoglycemia in insulin-treated patients occurs most frequently between 0200 and 0700 hours, a time window largely regulated by the dose of long-acting insulin.
   a) Decrease the dose of basal insulin once or twice weekly (or as often as needed) by at least 10–20% if the nocturnal/fasting BG* level is <100 mg/dL (5.6 mmol/L).
   b) Increase the dose of basal insulin once or twice weekly (or as often as needed) by at least 10–20% if the fasting BG* level is >200 mg/dL (11.1 mmol/L).
   c) Avoid the temptation to give "correction" doses of rapid- or fast-acting insulin at bedtime if BG* is moderately elevated. The most common outcome is nocturnal/fasting hypoglycemia.
   d) Reduce the dose of basal insulin by 25% (or as needed) on hemodialysis days in ESRD. Other insulin doses during and following dialysis (i.e., on "dialysis day") may also need decreasing by 10–15% (i.e., rapid-acting or pre-mixed insulin).

6. Titrate doses of rapid- or fast-acting insulin down by 10–20% if pre-lunch, pre-dinner, or bedtime BG* levels are <100 mg/dL (5.6 mmol/L) or up by 10–15% if >200 mg/dL (11.1 mmol/L). All hospitalized patients treated with insulin must have a BG* level >140 mg/dL (7.8 mmol/L) before going to sleep for the night. Recheck BG level on all patients with bedtime BG <140 mg/dL (7.8 mmol/L) within 1–2 hours and consider bedtime snack as needed (uncorrected).

7. 20 min post-meal dosing of rapid- or fast-acting insulin and last minute reduction or holding of meal-time insulin when meal ingestion is poor or absent are successful strategies to reduce post-prandial hypoglycemia.

8. Discharge recommendations for patients with ESRD and type 2 diabetes: the role of inpatient HbA_{1C}*:
   a) When HbA_{1C} <8% (64 mmol/mol) – reduce/stop sulfonylurea therapy because of the increased risk of hypoglycemia.
   b) When HbA_{1C} <7% (53 mmol/mol) – reduce/stop rapid- or fast-acting insulin.
   c) When HbA_{1C} <6% (42 mmol/mol) – reduce/stop all anti-diabetic therapy.
   d) When HbA_{1C} >8% (64 mmol/mol) and anti-diabetic therapy is needed, DPP-4 inhibitors, pioglitazone (watch for fluid retention), or low-dose, long-acting insulin are the safest choices.

*All glycemic targets and treatment recommendations must be individualized (12,13). In addition, inpatient glycemic targets are generally different from outpatient goals and should be used accordingly (5,11).

eGFR = estimated glomerular filtration rate; ESRD = end-stage renal disease; NPH = neutral protamine Hagedorn; TDD = total daily dose; BG = blood glucose.

significant risks for hypoglycemia and increased mortality, and their insulin regimen should be incrementally "down-titrated" (or sulfonylurea ideally discontinued) at the time of hospital discharge. Blood glucose patterns and insulin doses during the hospital stay are usually informative as to which components of an insulin regimen should be modified. Recent guidelines from the Joint British Diabetes Societies (JBDS) suggest that target HbA_{1C} in patients with diabetes on maintenance hemodialysis should be individualized, but if the patient is on a hypoglycemia-inducing treatment, it

Table 37-4 Principles of hypoglycemia management in non-diabetic and diabetic patients with CKD/ESRD. Adapted from (8).

1. **Managing acute hypoglycemia:**
   - Administer 15–20 grams of glucose *orally*
     - If repeat blood glucose is <70 mg/dL (3.9 mmol/L) in 15 minutes, repeat 15–20 grams rapid glucose ingestion followed by 10–20 grams complex or low glycemic index carbohydrate. Rapid glucose ingestion can be repeated once in 15 minutes as needed.
   - If patient is unable to tolerate *orally* or not responded to oral glucose therapy administer:
     - Intravenous (IV) dextrose 50% 25–50 mL* or, if there is no IV access present, intramuscular 1 mg glucagon
     - Intravenous 10–20% Dextrose infusion if hypoglycemia persists
   - Discontinue temporarily causative hypoglycemic agent in diabetic patient
     - Consider octreotide (IV or subcutaneously) if sulfonylurea is suspected cause, and patient not maintaining normoglycemia despite oral and/or IV glucose therapy
2. **Preventing and managing recurrent hypoglycemia:**
   - Review ("root-cause" analysis) and adjust hypoglycemic therapy in patients with diabetes
     - Consider using antidiabetic medications with low hypoglycemia risk
     - Reduce insulin dose in patients with insulin-treated diabetes
     - Refer for diabetes education as indicated
   - Optimize nutrition
   - Implement ambulatory self-monitoring of blood glucose (or CGM)
   - If the pre-dialysis blood glucose <126 mg/dL (7 mmol/L), 20–30 g of a low glycemic index carbohydrate is recommended at the beginning of the hemodialysis session to prevent further decline of blood glucose level

*Dextrose 10% or 20% equivalent doses can be given instead of 50% (less irritant to veins).

should be targeted between 7.5–8.5% (58–68 mmol/mol) (21). Reduction in treatment should be considered for patients with HbA1c <7.5% (58 mmol/mol) when on glucose-lowering agents associated with increased risk of hypoglycemia.

Prevention and optimal treatment of hypoglycemia are critical in both the inpatient (where episodes of hypoglycemia should be documented and tracked) and the outpatient setting. If hypoglycemia does occur, it should be treated promptly as detailed in Table 37-4.

Maintenance hemodialysis can independently contribute to hypoglycemic events in ESRD and glucose-free dialysate use for hemodialysis should be avoided. The UK JBDS guidelines suggest that patients on insulin should only be dialysed against a dialysate containing glucose (21). The risk of asymptomatic/symptomatic hypoglycemia is highest during the first 24 hours after dialysis, independent of caloric intake. Improved insulin sensitivity may partially explain this observation. In addition, hemodialysed subjects have greater glycemic variability due to the fact that they are dialysed on alternate days and tend to have lower BG values on dialysed days; their lowest readings are usually after their dialysis session. BG values are higher on non-dialysed days as glucose accumulates in the blood, despite receiving similar glucose-lowering medication. Proper adjustment of the dose of hypoglycemic agents, especially the reduction of insulin doses during and immediately following dialysis (i.e., on the dialysis day), avoidance of missed meals, and self-monitoring BG (or CGM) may lower the risk of hypoglycemia (8,21). Capillary BG should also be checked pre- and post-dialysis. If the pre-dialysis BG <126 mg/dL (7 mmol/L), 20–30g of a low glycemic index carbohydrate is recommended at the beginning of the hemodialysis session to prevent a further decline in the BG level.

In certain situations, it is important to recognize the possibility of "non-diabetic" causes of hypoglycemia in patients with diabetes and CKD/ESRD (8). The etiology of hypoglycemia in non-diabetic ESRD patients can be grouped into conditions associated with decreased or undetectable insulin levels, and those with inappropriately high

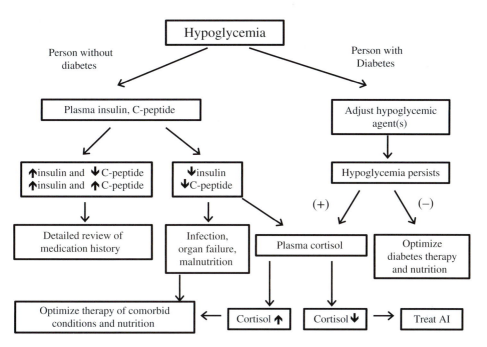

Figure 37-1 Algorithm for the diagnostic approach to hypoglycemia in advanced CKD/ESRD patients. Adapted from (8). AI = Adrenal insufficiency

insulin concentration (Figure 37-1). Malnutrition, alcohol abuse, organ failure, infections, drugs, and/or adrenal insufficiency are among frequently encountered clinical states in which hypoglycemia is most likely to be associated with hypoinsulinemia. Importantly, in clinical practice, hypoglycemia in non-diabetic ESRD is often multifactorial and triggered by more than one event. A review of medical history and a physical examination are necessary to identify early clues suggesting potential etiologies of hypoglycemia in ESRD and appropriate prevention and treatment are warranted (8).

Peritoneal dialysis exposes patients to a high glucose load via the peritoneum, which can worsen insulin resistance. Intraperitoneal administration of insulin during peritoneal dialysis provides a more physiologic effect than SC administration: it prevents fluctuations of the BG and the formation of insulin antibodies. But insulin requirements are often higher owing to a dilutional effect and to insulin binding to the plastic surface of the dialysis fluid reservoir (43). Peritonitis (which can be recurrent) can be a major

complication of peritoneal dialysis and should be managed emergently.

Hemodialysis patients with diabetes are at high risk of developing foot ulcers (due to multiple factors including diabetic and uremic neuropathy, peripheral arterial disease, arterial calcification, and endothelial dysfunction) (14). The heels of all patients with diabetes should therefore be protected with a suitable pressure-relieving device during hemodialysis. All patients with diabetes on dialysis should also have their feet inspected at least weekly; and should have regular review by the podiatry team (21);

Deciding to withdraw from renal replacement therapy is recognized as a common cause of death in ESRD patients in the USA, the UK, and many other countries (44,45). This is more common in older people, those with chronic or progressive comorbidities, and people who are becoming increasingly dependent. This multidisciplinary patient-centred decision should involve the patient, family members, and all relevant stakeholders. Treatment should focus on symptom control (45).

Referral to a Nephrologist

Consider referral to nephrology when there is uncertainty about the etiology of kidney disease (i.e., AKI or CKD); difficult management issues (e.g., anemia, secondary hyperparathyroidism, metabolic bone disease, resistant hypertension, or electrolyte disturbances); or advanced CKD (e.g., eGFR <30 mL/min/1.73 m^2) requiring discussion of renal replacement therapy for ESRD (2,5). Early vaccination against hepatitis B virus is indicated in patients likely to progress to ESRD.

Case Study

A 72-year-old woman with a 60-year history of type 1 diabetes was admitted to a medical ward for management of epigastric pain, nausea, and vomiting, which had been present for 5 days. Her diabetes was managed at home by injections of insulin glargine 22 units daily and rapid-acting insulin (aspart) 5–10 units with meals ("guesstimates" dose). She had been on a similar insulin regimen and dosage for at least the last decade because her "sugar control was normal." She had a past medical history of autoimmune hypothyroidism on replacement thyroxine; and coronary heart disease which included aspirin therapy. On admission, she was afebrile and normotensive, her weight was 60 kg (BMI was 24 kg/m^2). Laboratory evaluation was significant for normal white blood cell count, hemoglobin 10.2 g/dL, amylase/lipase normal, TSH normal, random plasma glucose 76 mg/dL (4.2 mmol/L), and eGFR of 18 ml/min/1.73 m^2 (baseline eGFR was 20–25, CKD related to diagnosis of diabetic kidney disease). HbA1c 6.5% (48 mmol/mol). Her diabetes was initially managed with IV insulin as she could not tolerate oral intake and was fasting for endoscopy. The basal insulin dose was continued at full dose in conjunction with the IV insulin infusion. During the IV insulin infusion she got recurrent hypoglycemic episodes requiring rescue glucose therapy and holding insulin

---

infusion. The endoscopy confirmed gastritis and she was treated with proton-pump inhibitor and aspirin was switched to clopidogrel. She was then transitioned back to her usual insulin regimen and dose. Capillary BG levels varied between 50–97 mg/dL (2.8 and 5.4 mmol/L) during the next 48 hours requiring repeated glucose rescue therapies.

Do You Think Her HBA1c Is Appropriate in View of Her Age and Comorbidities?

Why is she getting recurrent hypoglycemic episodes on her usual insulin regimen? Considering the patient's age, the long duration of type 1 diabetes with existing microvascular and macrovascular complications, and her advanced CKD, her glycemic targets including HbA1c are too aggressive. Glycemic targets and management should be individualized and not "one-size fits all." Glycemic targets are fluid and should be reviewed regularly (this patient has had the same BG and HBA1c target for more than 10 years despite evolving cardiac issues and her eGFR decreasing from 38 ml/min 10 years prior). The diabetes team was consulted for the management of her diabetes and on further questioning she admitted to hypoglycemic episodes 1 or 2 times per week for at least the last year. She was quite pleased that she did not have pronounced hypoglycemic symptoms until her BG was ~50 mg/dL (2.8 mmol/L). She had had no episodes of severe hypoglycemia prior to current hospital admission. During the remaining course of the hospitalization, the insulin glargine dose was gradually decreased to 6 units daily, with aspart 1–2 units per meal administered 20 minutes into the meal (dose depending on premeal glucose values and amount eaten). Blood glucose levels ranged between 110 and 200 mg/dL (6.0–11.1 mmol/L). She had no further "hypos" during the remainder of her in-hospital stay. She was successfully discharged home, being able to tolerate oral intake and re-educated regarding optimal

BG levels and hypoglycemia prevention and management.

This lady had had frequent hypoglycemic episodes with hypoglycemic unawareness due in part to her over-insulinization. Her glycemic goals were too aggressive, and she was on excessive insulin doses, especially in view of her advanced CKD and frequent hypos. Increased mortality associated with HbA$_{1C}$ <6–7% (42–53 mmol/mol) in patients with CKD/ESRD is in part related to increased incidence of hypoglycemia. Many insulin-treated patients with type 2 diabetes and CKD stop or require less insulin as kidney disease progresses (known as "burnt out" type 2 diabetes). Similarly, the insulin total daily dose in persons with type 1 diabetes may also decrease dramatically, as in this patient. In view of her autoimmune diathesis, other causes of hypoglycemia and increased insulin sensitivity, such as adrenal insufficiency and celiac disease, should be screened for (and in this case were negative).

and/or insulin. Current in-hospital diabetes guidelines generally recommend avoiding certain non-insulin glucose-lowering agents in the inpatient setting, and using various insulin regimens. Patients with diabetes and renal insufficiency are known to have decreased insulin requirements and a specific approach for insulin dosing in this population of hospitalized patients is needed to minimize the incidence of hypoglycemia. In addition, knowledge about which non-insulin glucose-lowering agents can be used safely and effectively for the inpatient population is critical. As diabetes patients with CKD/ESRD are at high risk of cardiovascular events, the ADA 2018 (12) and AACE 2018 (13) treatment guidelines have now recommended that in patients with type 2 diabetes and established atherosclerotic CVD, glucose-lowering agents with proven CV and renal benefits (currently empagliflozin, liraglutide, semaglutide and canagliflozin) should be preferentially added to therapy when safe and reasonable to do so (12, 13).

Conclusions

AKI and CKD are frequently encountered in hospitalized patients with diabetes and/or hyperglycemia. AKI and CKD are important risk factors for hypoglycemia, if these patients are treated with sulfonylureas

Acknowledgments

The current author wishes to acknowledge the contributions to the previous edition by David Baldwin, upon which portions of this chapter are based.

References

1 Saran R, Robinson B, Abbott KC, et al. 2016 USRDS Annual Data Report: epidemiology of kidney disease in the United States. *Am J Kidney Dis.* 2017;69(3S1):A7–A8.

2 Tuttle KR, Bakris GL, Bilous RW, et al. Diabetic kidney disease: a report from an ADA consensus conference. *Diabetes Care.* 2014;37:2864–2883.

3 Anonymous. Inpatient care and diabetes: putting poor glycaemic control to bed. *Lancet Diabetes and Endocrinology.* 2017;5:770.

4 Health and Social Care Information Centre. *National Diabetes Inpatient Audit (NaDIA), Open Data 2016*, 2017. www.digital.nhs.uk/pubs/nadia2016

5 American Diabetes Association. Diabetes care in the hospital. *Diabetes Care.* 2018;41 (Suppl. 1):S144–S151.

6 Iyer SN, Tanenberg RJ Managing diabetes in hospitalized patients with chronic kidney disease. *Cleveland Clinic J Med.* 2016;83:301–310.

7 Betonico CC, Titan SMO, Correa-Giannella ML. Management of diabetes mellitus in individuals with chronic kidney disease: therapeutic

perspectives and glycemic control. *Clinics.* 2016;71:47–53.

8 Gosmanov AR, Gosmanova EO, Kovesday CP. Evaluation and management of diabetic and non-diabetic hypoglycemia in end-stage renal disease. *Nephrol Dial Transplant.* 2016;31:8–15.

9 Umpierrez GE, Pasquel FJ. Management of inpatient hyperglycemia and diabetes in older adults. *Diabetes Care.* 2017;40: 509–517.

10 Akirov A, Grossman A, Shockut T, Shimon I. Mortality among hospitalized patients with hypoglycemia: insulin related and noninsulin related. *J Clin Endocrinol Metab.* 2017;102:416–424.

11 Umpierrez GE, Hellman R, Korytkowski MT, et al. Management of hyperglycemia in hospitalized patients in non-critical care setting: an Endocrine Society Clinical Practice Guideline. *J Clin Endocrinol Metab.* 2012;97:16–38.

12 American Diabetes Association. Standards of medical care in diabetes: 2018. *Diabetes Care.* 2018;41(Suppl. 1):S1–S159.

13 Garber AJ, Abrahamson MJ, Barzilay JI, et al. Consensus statement by the American Association of Clinical Endocrinologists and American College of Endocrinology on the comprehensive Type 2 diabetes management algorithm: 2018 Executive Summary. *Endocrine Practice.* 2018;24:91–120.

14 Vanholder R, Fauque D, Glorieux G, et al. Clinical management of the uraemic syndrome in chronic kidney disease. *Lancet Diabetes Endocrinol.* 2016;4:360–373.

15 Ricks J, Molnar MZ, Kovesdy CP, et al. Glycemic control and cardiovascular mortality in hemodialysis patients with diabetes: a 6-year cohort study. *Diabetes.* 2012;61:708–715.

16 Shurraw S, Hemmelgarn B, Lin M, et al. Association between glycemic control and adverse outcomes in people with diabetes mellitus and chronic kidney disease: a population-based cohort study. *Arch Intern Med.* 2011;171:1920–1927.

17 Kalantar-Zadeh K. A critical evaluation of glycated protein parameters in advanced nephropathy: a matter of life or death: A1C

remains the gold standard outcome predictor in diabetic dialysis patients. *Diabetes Care.* 2012;35:1625–1628.

18 Moen MF, Zhan M, Hsu VD, et al. Frequency of hypoglycemia and its significance in chronic kidney disease. *Clin J Am Soc Nephrol.* 2009;4:1121–1127.

19 Iglesias P, Díez JJ. Insulin therapy in renal disease. *Diabetes Obes Metab.* 2008;10: 811–823.

20 Mak RH. Impact of end-stage renal disease and dialysis on glycemic control. *Semin Dial.* 2000;13:4–8.

21 Frankel A, Kazempour-Ardebili S. Management of adults with diabetes on the haemodialysis unit. 2016. http://www. diabetologists-abcd.org.uk/JBDS/JBDS_ RenalGuide_2016.pdf

22 Biesenbach G, Raml A, Schmekal B, Eichbauer-Sturm G. Decreased insulin requirement in relation to GFR in nephropathic Type 1 and insulin-treated Type 2 diabetic patients. *Diabet Med.* 2003;20:642–645.

23 Park J, Lertdumrongluk P, Molnar MZ, Kovesdy CP, Kalantar-Zadeh K. Glycemic control in diabetic dialysis patients and the burnt-out diabetes phenomenon. *Curr Diab Rep.* 2012;12:432–439.

24 Kazempour-Ardebili S, Lecamwasam VL, Dassanyake T, et al. Assessing glycemic control in maintenance hemodialysis patients with type 2 diabetes. *Diabetes Care.* 2009;32:1137–1142.

25 Sobngwi E, Enoru S, Ashuntantang G, et al. Day-to-day variation of insulin requirements of patients with type 2 diabetes and end-stage renal disease undergoing maintenance hemodialysis. *Diabetes Care.* 2010;33:1409–1412.

26 Baldwin D, Zander J, Munoz C, et al. A randomized trial of two weight-based doses of insulin glargine and glulisine in hospitalized subjects with type 2 diabetes and renal insufficiency. *Diabetes Care.* 2012;35:1970–1974.

27 Monica Reddy RP, Inzucchi SE. SGLT2 inhibitors in the management of type 2 diabetes. *Endocrine.* 2016;53:364–372.

28 Wanner C, Inzucchi SE, Lachin JM, et al. Empagliflozin and progression of kidney

disease in type 2 diabetes. *N Engl J Med.* 2016;375:323–334.

29 Zinman B, Wanner C, Lachin JM, et al. Empagliflozin, cardiovascular outcomes, and mortality in type 2 diabetes. *N Engl J Med.* 2015;373:2117–2128.

30 Neal B, Perkovic V, Mahaffey KW, et al. for the CANVAS Program group. Canagliglozin and cardiovascular and renal events in type 2 diabetes. *N Eng J Med.* 2017 doi: 10.1056/NEJMoa1611925.

31 Marso SP, Daniels GH, Brown-Frandsen K, et al. Liraglutide and cardiovascular outcomes in type 2 diabetes. *N Engl J Med.* 2016;375:311–322.

32 Rhee CM, Kovesdy CP, Kalantar-Zadeh K. Risks of metformin in type 2 diabetes and chronic kidney disease: lessons learned from Taiwanese data. *Nephron.* 2017;135:147–153.

33 Game F. Novel hypoglycaemic agents: considerations in patients with chronic kidney disease. *Nephron Clin Pract.* 2014;126(1):14–18.

34 DeFronzo R, Fleming GA, Chen K, et al. Metformin-associated lactic acidosis: Current perspectives on causes and risk. *Metabolism Clinical and Experimental.* 2016;65:20–29.

35 Kalanter-Zadeh K, Uppot RN, Lewandrowski KB. A 54 year-old woman with abdominal pain, vomiting, and confusion [Metformin toxicity and its management]. *N Eng J Med.* 2013;369: 374–382.

36 Holstein A, Hammer C, Hahn M, Kulamadayil NS, Kovacs P. Severe sulfonylurea-induced hypoglycemia: a problem of uncritical prescription and deficiencies of diabetes care in geriatric patients. *Expert Opin Drug Saf.* 2010; 9:675–681.

37 Dashora U, Gallagher A, Dhatariya K et al. Association of British Clinical Diabetologists (ABCD) position statement

on the risk of diabetic ketoacidosis associated with the use of sodium-glucose cotransporter-2 inhibitors. *Br J Diabetes.* 2016;16:206–209.

38 Nauck MA, Meier JJ. Sitagliptin plus basal insulin: simplifying in-hospital diabetes treatment. *Lancet Diabetes Endocrinology.* 2017;5:83–85.

39 Gosmanov AR, Gosmanova EO, Dillard-Cannon E. Management of adult diabetic ketoacidosis. *Diabetes, Metabolic Syndrome Obes.* 2014;7: 255–264.

40 Tzamaloukas AH, Rohrscheib M, Ing TS, et al. Serum potassium and acid-base parameters in severe dialysis-associated hyperglycemia treated with insulin therapy. *Int J Artif Organs.* 2005;28(3): 229–236.

41 Tzamaloukas AH, Ing TS, Siamopoulos KC, et al. Body fluid abnormalities in severe hyperglycemia in patients on chronic dialysis: review of published reports. *J Diabetes Complications.* 2008;22(1): 29–37.

42 Tzamaloukas AH, Ing TS, Siamopoulos KC, et al. Pathophysiology and management of fluid and electrolyte disturbances in patients on chronic dialysis with severe hyperglycemia. *Semin Dial.* 2008;21(5):431–439.

43 Quellhorst E. Insulin therapy during peritoneal dialysis: pros and cons of various forms of administration. *J Am Soc Nephrol.* 2002;13 (Suppl. 1):S92–S96.

44 Diabetes UK, Association of British Clinical Diabetologists, Training Research and Education for Nurses on Diabetes-UK, Institute of Diabetes for Older People. *End of Life Diabetes Care.* Available at https://www.diabetes.org.uk/end-of-life-care (accessed June 2017).

45 Schmidt RJ, Moss A. Dying on dialysis: the case for a dignified withdrawal. *Clin J Am Soc Nephrol.* 2014;9:174–180.

38

Management of Glucocorticoid-Induced Diabetes and/or Hyperglycemia

Han Na Kim and Nestoras Mathioudakis

Key Points

- Glucocorticoids (GCs) are commonly pre-scribed to treat a wide spectrum of condi-tions due to their useful anti-inflammatory and immunosuppressive effects.
- The prevalence of oral GC use in the general population is approximately 1%, with higher rates observed in older adults, and chronic use (≥5 years) in nearly one-third of patients.
- Despite their beneficial effects, GCs are the most common medication class associated with drug-induced hyperglycemia.
- Not only do GCs tend to worsen glycemic control in patients with pre-existing dia-betes, but they also commonly precipitate hyperglycemia in previously euglycemic patients.
- Glucocorticoid-induced hyperglycemia (GIH) describes hyperglycemia in patients with pre-existing diabetes; whilst glucocorticoid-induced diabetes (GID) refers to the development of diabetes in persons with previously normal glucose tolerance.
- Several factors make the management of GIH and GID particularly challenging in both inpatient and outpatient settings. Consider-ations that need to be taken into account in managing this condition include the phar-macologic action and the potency of the GC, the expected duration of use, and the base-line level of glycemic control (in GIH).

- Although evidence-based strategies for the management of GIH and GID are limited, understanding the action profile of GCs and their effects on blood glucose (BG) are paramount in identifying a manage-ment strategy to treat this common clini-cal problem that can result in hyperglycemic emergencies.
- Consequently healthcare providers should anticipate and be ready to treat hyper-glycemia prior to initiation of GCs.
- Patients who do not have pre-existing dia-betes but are at high risk of developing GID should monitor post-lunch and pre-dinner BG for the first two days of GC therapy. If all values are <140 mg/dL (7.8 mmol/L), it is rea-sonable to stop BG monitoring.
- Patients with pre-existing diabetes should monitor their BG frequently including a post-prandial check after lunch as to not miss post-prandial hyperglycemia.
- All patients should be encouraged to main-tain adequate hydration and counseled on the need to follow a lower carbohydrate diet.
- The choice of glucose-lowering therapy and management approach will depend on the baseline insulin reserve, the dose and dura-tion of GC therapy.

- Evidence for use of non-insulin therapy is scant and these medications have not been tested rigorously; however, based on the limited number of studies, clinical experience, known glycemic effect and action profile of GCs, as well as pharmacologic properties of non-insulin therapy, some patients may be able to achieve adequate glycemic control with non-insulin therapy alone.
- Agents that enhance insulin sensitivity and target post-prandial hyperglycemia are favored and options for non-insulin therapy include: metformin; short-acting sulfonylureas and glinides; dipeptidyl-peptidase (DPP)-4 inhibitors; and glucagon-like peptide-1 (GLP-1) agonists. Selection of medication should also consider the onset of action and glucose-lowering effect of individual drugs.
- There should be a low threshold to initiate insulin in patients who have sustained hyperglycemia despite maximal non-insulin therapy.
- Once-daily intermediate (NPH) insulin timed with the morning GC dose is favored during treatment with intermediate-acting GC, as its peak effect will coincide with that of the GC.
- A modified basal-bolus insulin regimen with higher proportion of bolus insulin (e.g., 70%) or twice-daily NPH can be used with twice-daily intermediate-acting or once-daily long-acting GC.

Introduction

Glucocorticoids (GCs) are commonly prescribed to treat a wide spectrum of conditions due to their useful anti-inflammatory and immunosuppressive effects. The prevalence of oral GC use in the general population is approximately 1%, with higher rates observed in older adults, and chronic use (≥5 years) in nearly one-third of patients (1,2). Despite their beneficial effects, GCs are the most common medication class associated with drug-induced hyperglycemia (3). Not only do they tend to worsen glycemic control in patients with pre-existing diabetes, but they also commonly precipitate hyperglycemia in previously euglycemic patients. Several factors make management of glucocorticoid-induced hyperglycemia particularly challenging in both inpatient and outpatient settings. Considerations that need to be taken into account in managing this condition include the pharmacologic action and potency of the glucocorticoid, the expected duration of use, and the baseline level of glycemic control. Although evidence-based strategies for management of glucocorticoid-induced hyperglycemia are limited, understanding the action profile of GCs and their effects on blood glucose (BG) are paramount in identifying a management strategy to treat this common clinical problem.

Definition

No standardized terminology exists to describe the phenomenon of worsened hyperglycemia with GC use in patients with pre-existing diabetes versus new onset hyperglycemia in patients without pre-existing diabetes. Glucocorticoid-induced hyperglycemia (GIH) or glucocorticoid-induced diabetes (GID) are often used interchangeably but some have used the term GIH to describe hyperglycemia in patients with pre-existing diabetes; and GID to refer to development of diabetes in persons with previously normal glucose tolerance. In this chapter, we will follow this distinction and use the terminologies GIH for patients with diabetes and GID for patients without pre-existing diabetes.

Prevalence

The reported prevalence of hyperglycemia with GC use varies widely in the literature. A meta-analysis of 13 observational studies that examined patients receiving GCs of variable doses and treatment duration reported rates of GIH and GID to be 18.6% and 32.3% respectively (4). In a study at a single tertiary care hospital, 64% of all inpatients and 56% of patients without diabetes on the medicine service receiving high-dose GCs for more than 2 days experienced hyperglycemia (5). The prevalence of hyperglycemia has been reported to be 39% in hospitalized patients with hematologic malignancies receiving GCs, over 40% and 15% in patients without diabetes receiving GCs for primary renal and respiratory diseases respectively (6–8). In transplant recipients, reported incidence of new onset diabetes has been highly variable (2–50%) in part due to concomitant use of immunosuppressive agents also known to impact glucose metabolism (9).

Risk Factors for the Development of GID

One of the challenges in managing hyperglycemia associated with GC therapy is that it is not always possible to predict who will develop GID since the impact of systemic GC use on an individual's glucose metabolism is variable and not all patients

develop hyperglycemia; however, dose and duration of GC use are clearly associated with higher risk (10,11). In one case-control study of close to 12,000 cases, the risk of developing GID increased with increasing the GC dose from a 2-fold increase in risk with a hydrocortisone-equivalent dose of 1–39 mg/day; 3-fold for 40–79 mg/day; 6-fold for 80–119 mg/day; and 10-fold for doses 120 mg/day or more (10). Traditional risk factors for type 2 diabetes (T2DM) have also been identified as risk factors for GID: older age, body mass index (BMI), impaired glucose tolerance, and family history of diabetes (12). Hepatitis C virus (HCV) infection, as well as the concurrent use of medications such as calcineurin inhibitors in transplant recipients and mycophenolate mofetil in patients with systemic lupus erythematosus, have also been reported to be independent risk factors for development of GID (12).

Common Glucocorticoid Regimens

There are several GC preparations of varying potency and duration of action (Figure 38-1) used for different indications. Hydrocortisone is a short-acting glucocorticoid most commonly used in the hospital at stress doses

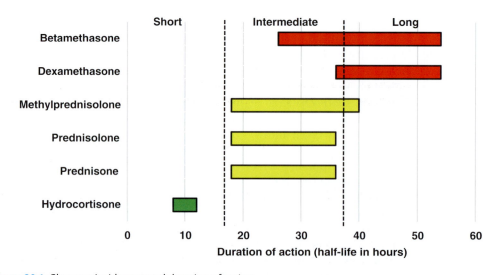

Figure 38-1 Glucocorticoid types and duration of action.

(e.g., 100 mg intravenously [IV] q8 hr or 50 mg IV q6–8 hrs) in perioperative period for adrenal insufficiency or to treat adrenal crisis and septic shock.

Prednisone and methylprednisolone are intermediate-acting GCs used widely in varying doses and duration for their anti-inflammatory and immunosuppressive properties. Some examples of their uses include acute treatment of chronic obstructive pulmonary disease (COPD) or asthma exacerbation with high dose prednisone 40–60 mg daily with or without taper; depending on the severity of the respiratory symptoms, an oral GC course may be preceded by methylprednisolone 60–125 mg, 1–4 times a day for several days. Treatment of lupus nephritis and acute transplant rejection may include high-dose pulse glucocorticoid therapy using methylprednisolone 250–1000 mg daily for 3 days.

The long-acting GC, dexamethasone, is often used for neurosurgical and oncologic conditions. For example, dexamethasone 4–8 mg IV q4–6 hours is a common regimen used to treat cerebral edema. Much higher doses can be used as part of chemotherapy regimen. The induction regimen for acute lymphocytic leukemia (ALL) includes use of dexamethasone 40 mg on days 1–4 and days 4–11. Dexamethasone is also used in palliative care or in surgical setting for the treatment of nausea at 8–20 mg doses. The intermittent use of this potent GC as an anti-nausea agent for chemotherapy can pose unique challenges in glucose management, since the management choice will need to balance the short duration of use against the potential for significant glycemic excursions.

Pathophysiology and Pattern of GIH

GIH is largely mediated through increased insulin resistance with decreased peripheral uptake of glucose by the muscle and adipose tissue, hepatic gluconeogenesis particularly in the post-prandial period and suppression of endogenous insulin production (3,13). Glucocorticoids cause significant post-prandial hyperglycemia and have less impact on fasting BG. When commonly prescribed intermediate-acting GCs, such as prednisone and prednisolone, are administered once daily in the morning, there is a gradual rise in glucose throughout the day with its peak at post-lunch and pre-dinner before returning to baseline the next morning (Figure 38-2) (7,14–16). This glycemic pattern is reflective of the GC action profile, with peak effect at 4–8 hours and duration of action lasting 12–16 hours (16).

Much less is known about effects of other GCs. One small study examining the effect of dexamethasone on glucose tolerance in healthy adults showed an increase in fasting BG after dexamethasone 8 mg, but not with 2 or 4 mg doses (17). Despite a duration of action of 36–54 hours, the hyperglycemic effect of a single dose of dexamethasone peaked at 24 hours and dissipated by 48 hours. In another study of patients receiving pulse-dose dexamethasone therapy (40 mg) in the morning for multiple myeloma, peak hyperglycemia occurred between 5–6 p.m. in both patients with and without pre-existing diabetes (18). Fasting glucose was not affected in patients without pre-existing diabetes but doubled in patients with diabetes. Finally, in healthy subjects receiving dexamethasone, the insulin level was significantly elevated at 20 hours after the GC dose suggesting a slightly different peak glycemic effect and longer duration of action compared to intermediate-acting GCs (16).

Diagnosis

There are no formal diagnostic guidelines for GIH/GID but the same American Diabetes Association (ADA) criteria used to diagnose diabetes are applicable; however, relying solely on fasting BG values may be a diagnostic pitfall since GCs largely impact the post-prandial glucose metabolism and fasting glucose values could be normal. Using HbA1c (A1C) may not be suitable in patients who have recently initiated GCs or receive

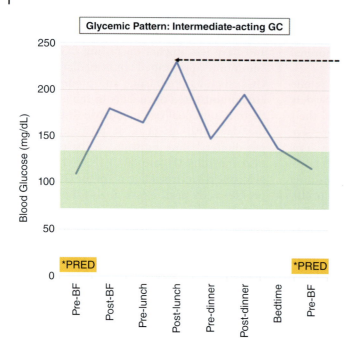

Figure 38-2 The graph illustrates a gradual rise in blood glucose during the day with peak at post-lunch and pre-dinner (arrow), with return to baseline blood glucose the following morning.
GC = glucocorticoid. BF = breakfast.
*PRED = prednisone or prednisolone administered once daily in the morning.

only a brief course of therapy. Thus, the most practical and useful diagnostic criterion is a random glucose >200 mg/dL (11.1 mmol/L). Post-prandial glucose is likely the most sensitive measure in detecting GIH and some studies recommend monitoring post-lunch or pre-dinner glucose values for the first 2–3 days of treatment in patients receiving GCs in the morning and considering treatment if pre-prandial and post-prandial glucose levels are ≥140 mg/dL (7.8 mmol/L) and ≥200 mg/dL (11.1 mmol/L) respectively (3).

Associated Adverse Outcomes

Uncontrolled hyperglycemia with GC use may not only result in dehydration, renal impairment and acute kidney injury (AKI), and unnecessary hospitalizations but studies of various patient populations have shown association with several serious adverse outcomes. In patients with acute exacerbations of COPD receiving GCs, risk of death and length of stay increased with increasing BG levels (19). In a recent retrospective study of patients with hematologic malignancies receiving systemic GC therapy, the maximum glucose level was predictive of the hospital length of stay for patients without pre-existing diabetes (6). Furthermore, in a study of patients with acute graft-versus-host disease, early hyperglycemia with GC treatment was associated with decreased overall survival (20). Other studies of patients with hematologic malignancies have shown associations between hyperglycemia and increased risk of infection, toxicity from chemotherapy, graft-versus-host disease and mortality (6,21–24). Hyperglycemia has been found to be associated with shorter overall survival in patients with brain tumor, and in solid organ transplant patients with increased major cardiac events and graft failure (25–27). Thus, identification of patients at high risk of developing hyperglycemia, early diagnosis and timely implementation of effective treatment strategy are crucial in caring for patients receiving GCs.

Treatment Options

Evidence to guide pharmacologic management strategies for GIH/GID is very limited. There have not been any large randomized controlled trials evaluating different treatment strategies or glucose-lowering therapies. There are a few small studies that have investigated the effectiveness of various insulin regimens and there are even fewer studies examining the role of different non-insulin glucose-lowering therapies. Some of these studies were conducted in healthy subjects, which also limit the generalizability of the inferences to patients with glucose intolerance or baseline diabetes. Furthermore, there have been no head-to-head trials comparing various non-insulin therapies, and to our knowledge, no studies evaluating the role of newer concentrated insulins or sodium–glucose co-transporter 2 (SGLT-2) inhibitors exist. Thus, our proposed management recommendations are based on limited evidence, known pathophysiology, pharmacologic properties of various glucose-lowering therapies, expert opinion, and personal clinical experience.

Non-Insulin Glucose-Lowering Therapies

Depending on baseline insulin reserve, dose and duration of GC therapy, some patients may be able to achieve satisfactory glycemic control through titration of non-insulin glucose-lowering agents; however, there should be a low threshold to initiate insulin in patients who have sustained or severe hyperglycemia, despite maximal non-insulin therapy, given that evidence for use of non-insulin therapy is scant and these medications have not been tested rigorously.

Metformin

In a recent double-blind, placebo-controlled trial of 34 patients without pre-existing diabetes receiving at least 4 weeks of prednisone (median dose 30–35 mg), subjects treated with metformin (850 mg twice daily) had no change in glucose tolerance compared to placebo at 4 weeks (28). Since GCs significantly reduce hepatic insulin sensitivity, in theory, metformin should be at the foundation of management for GIH (29); however, metformin has a slow onset of action and may not be suitable for use in short courses of GC therapy. Concurrent use of a potent, faster-acting glucose-lowering medication,

such as sulfonylurea (SU) or meglitinides (glinides) may be needed in combination with metformin for patients with marked hyperglycemia; in these cases, in addition to alleviating insulin resistance, increasing endogenous insulin production may be required. In patients already on insulin therapy, maximizing metformin to improve insulin sensitivity may minimize overall insulin requirements and reduce the risk of hypoglycemia and weight gain.

Insulin Secretagogues

The evidence supporting the use of SUs is limited to glimepiride. Treatment with glimepiride in chronic prednisolone use (initially 20–40 mg/day then 5–10 mg daily for more than a year) reversed β-cell dysfunction and improved A1C by about 2% (26 mmol/mol) after 8 weeks of treatment (30). Successful use of nateglinide has also been described in the literature to treat post-prandial hyperglycemia seen with prednisolone therapy (31).

Mechanistically, insulin secretagogues, such as SUs or glinides, are attractive options as they counteract the β-cell dysfunction seen with GC treatment; however, some SUs have a long action profile that may not match the duration of the hyperglycemia anticipated with intermediate-acting GCs, and patients can be at risk of fasting hypoglycemia, especially during GC dose taper. On the other hand, glinides have an immediate onset and short duration of action, and could be useful to target post-prandial hyperglycemia without significantly increasing the risk of fasting hypoglycemia.

Overall, insulin secretagogues may have a role in the treatment of modest hyperglycemia or in patients who are against injectable medications. When an insulin secretagogue is used, the provider should select a shorter-acting agent and time the administration with the expected peak effect of the GC. For example, prednisone given in the morning is expected to result in a peak BG around lunch time, with declining BG values throughout the rest of the day (Figure 38-2). A longer acting SU, such as glyburide or glimepiride, could predispose to fasting hypoglycemia in such patients, whereas a shorter-acting SU, like glipizide or gliclazide (or a glinide) given with breakfast or lunch would have less potential to do so.

Thiazolidinediones (TZD)

In a small study (n = 7) of patients with long-standing GID, treatment with troglitzone 400 mg/day for 5–8 weeks significantly improved A1C and post-prandial glucose values but this specific medication has been taken off the market due to associated hepatic injury (32). Given limited evidence of TZD (e.g. pioglitazone) use with GCs and known serious adverse effects, such as congestive heart failure and fragility fractures, we do not recommend their use for this indication.

Dipeptidyl Peptidase (DPP)-4 Inhibitors

A study investigating sitagliptin with high dose prednisolone failed to show benefit at 2 weeks despite improvement in β-cell function in patients with metabolic syndrome and no pre-existing diabetes (33). On the other hand, a study by Ohashi et al. demonstrated a positive effect with alogliptin (34). In patients with hyperglycemia from high dose prednisolone therapy without pre-existing diabetes, 3 weeks of alogliptin treatment lowered 2-hr post-prandial glucose level by ~35 mg/dL (~2 mmol/L). Despite conflicting evidence, their immediate onset of action and targeted post-prandial effect, DPP-4 inhibitors may be reasonable to use in patients without pre-existing diabetes and modest hyperglycemia from GCs.

Glucagon-like peptide (GLP)-1 Agonists

GLP-1 agonists improve glycemic control through multiple mechanisms including enhanced glucose-dependent insulin release, the suppression of post-prandial glucagon secretion and slowed gastric emptying. In a small randomized, placebo-controlled study in healthy subjects given prednisolone 80 mg daily, exenatide prevented post-prandial hyperglycemia and β-cell dysfunction compared to placebo (35). Although GLP-1 agonists have not been rigorously studied in patients receiving GCs with diabetes or at high risk of developing diabetes, their

mechanism of action targeting post-prandial hyperglycemia serves as an advantage for this indication; however, for patients without pre-existing diabetes, initiation of an injectable medication for a condition that may be short-lived may be an unattractive option (especially with the associated gastrointestinal side-effects).

SGLT-2 Inhibitors

To our knowledge, no studies have been conducted investigating the role of SGLT-2 inhibitors in GIH; however, given their fast onset of action, there may be a role for their use in select patients with moderate hyperglycemia who are averse to injectable therapy (although may exacerbate dehydration and AKI risk associated with GCs).

Insulin

Almost all patients with advanced diabetes treated with GCs will require initiation or intensification of an insulin regimen. Furthermore, insulin should be initiated in patients with sustained hyperglycemia on maximal non-insulin therapy. Various insulin preparations are available but selection of an insulin therapy or regimen will depend in part on the duration of action and the dosing interval of the GC.

NPH

NPH given once daily in the morning is the preferred insulin regimen for coverage of intermediate-acting GCs since NPH peak effect will coincide with that of the GC (Figure 38-3). This insulin type can be used as monotherapy or in combination with pre-existing long-acting insulin or basal-bolus regimen (long-acting and short-, rapid- or fast-acting insulins) to mainly counteract post-prandial hyperglycemia. When NPH is used in combination with pre-existing insulin regimen, no changes are necessary to baseline insulin regimen, and NPH dose is simply added and timed with the GC.

A recommended starting dose of NPH is 0.1 units/kg per 10-mg equivalent of prednisone with maximum initial dose of

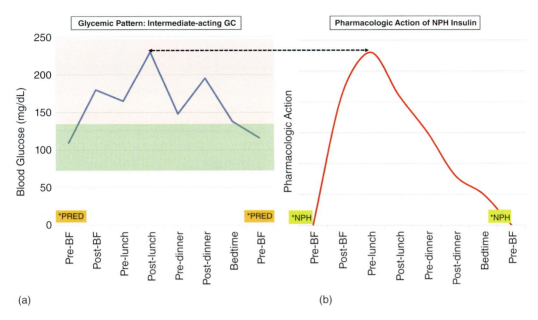

Figure 38-3 Mirrored profile of NPH insulin and glycemic pattern resulting from use of intermediate-acting glucocorticoid (GC). Figure 38-3(b) shows the peak effect of NPH insulin at 4–8 hours, coinciding with the peak blood glucose rise, and decline in action after 16 hours coinciding with return of blood glucose to normal levels in the overnight fasting state. The shaded green area indicates normal glucose range (71–140 mg/dL [4–7.8 mmol/L]) and the red area indicates hyperglycemia.
BF = breakfast, *PRED = administration of prednisone or prednisolone. *NPH = administration of NPH insulin.

0.4 units/kg for doses 40 mg or above as proposed by Clore and Thurby-Hay (16). For example, an initial NPH dose for a 70-kg patient starting 40 mg of prednisone in the morning would be 28 units (0.4 units/kg × 70 kg) and should be given at the time of the prednisone dose. If a patient is receiving intermediate-acting GC twice daily or long-acting GC once daily, the total daily dose of NPH is calculated the same way but administered in two divided doses.

Basal-Bolus Insulin Regimen

For patients receiving intermediate-acting GC twice daily or long-acting GC once daily, an alternative strategy is using a basal-bolus insulin (BBI) regimen since a more sustained hyperglycemia may be seen throughout the day (Figure 38-4). We recommend using a long-acting (e.g., glargine, detemir) and rapid-acting insulin (aspart, lispro, glulisine) with a dosing regimen that is disproportionately higher in prandial coverage to accommodate the post-prandial

hyperglycemic effect of GCs. A recommended starting total daily dose is typically 0.5–0.6 units/kg/day with a 30% of the dose as basal insulin and 70% of the dose as bolus insulin.

Insulin Pumps

Management for a patient on an insulin pump is similar to using injection BBI. Due to increased insulin resistance and exaggerated hyperglycemia seen post-prandially with GC use, the insulin-to-carb ratio and insulin sensitivity factor will need adjustment. The morning basal rate may need to be increased as well, but overall basal rates may remain the same unless sustained hyperglycemia is seen throughout the day based on the type and dosing interval of the GC.

Concentrated Insulins

Some patients may develop severe insulin resistance in the setting of GC use, requiring large amount of insulin. In

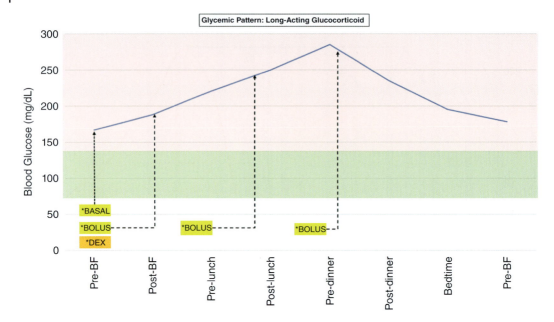

Figure 38-4 Mirrored profile of basal-bolus insulin regimen and glycemic effect resulting from use of long-acting glucocorticoid. The graph shows that both fasting and post-prandial glucose readings are elevated following use of a long-acting glucocorticoid, with peak hyperglycemia occurring around 5–6 p.m. Basal insulin targets the fasting hyperglycemia, while bolus insulin targets post-prandial hyperglycemia (timing of insulin represented by position of yellow boxes, whereas major associated glycemic target represented by arrows). The shaded green area indicates the normal glucose range (71–140 mg/dL [4–7.8 mmol/L]) and the red area indicates hyperglycemia.
BF = breakfast, *DEX = dexamethasone. *BASAL = long-acting insulin (e.g., glargine, detemir); *BOLUS = rapid-acting insulin (e.g., aspart, lispro, glulisine).

such circumstances, to ensure the reliable absorption of injected insulin and avoid patient discomfort, concentrated insulins such as U200, U300, or U500 insulin may be considered. When titrating an existing regimen of U500 insulin, providers should be mindful that this particular type of insulin has an onset of action close to regular (human) insulin but a duration of action that is intermediate between regular and NPH insulin (36). To avoid prescription or user error, use of an U500 pen or an U500 specific syringe is recommended (when available) (37,38).

Premixed Insulin
Premixed insulins (e.g., human NPH/regular; and analog aspart protamine/aspart, or lispro protamine/lispro) are generally not useful for management of GID/GIH because of their inherent inflexibility in dosing.

Insulin Titration
Regardless of which insulin regimen is selected, BG must be monitored frequently (pre-meal [also reflects previous post-prandial BG excursion] and bedtime) and insulin doses may need to be titrated on a daily basis to maintain adequate control. Typically 10–20% dose adjustments are recommended but more aggressive dose increases of 20–50% may be needed in the setting of GC use. For most patients, a BG target of 80–130 mg/dL (4.4–7.2 mmol/L) pre-meal and <180 mg/dL (10 mmol/L) post-prandial is recommended. However, these glycemic goals should be individualized and adjusted based on age and risk of hypoglycemia (e.g., 90–150 mg/dL [5–8.3 mmol/L] pre-meal and <200 mg/dL [11.1 mmol/L] post-prandial for the elderly) (39).

Adjusting Insulin with a Glucocorticoid Taper
When a GC dose is tapered (a reduction in daily dose by at least 15%), a pre-emptive

adjustment in insulin dose is necessary to avoid hypoglycemia. The amount of insulin reduction is dictated by the glycemic pattern over the past 24 hours and the anticipated GC dose decrease. If NPH is being used, one can adjust the dose using the previously described rule of 0.1 units/kg per 10-mg equivalent of prednisone or decrease the dose by 10–20% if most BG values fall within the target range. For a BBI regimen, basal and bolus insulins may need to be adjusted separately depending on the degree of glycemic control for fasting versus pre-meal values. Generally, 10–20% dose adjustments are recommended but more aggressive dose changes may be necessary based on the degree of glycemic derangements.

General Management Approach

All patients with or without pre-existing diabetes should be advised to follow a lower carbohydrate diet, considering that GCs exaggerate the hyperglycemia response to carbohydrate intake. In addition, adequate hydration should be encouraged.

Glucocorticoid-Induced Diabetes (GID)

For patients without pre-existing diabetes on a short-course of GCs (e.g., <7 days) and no alarming symptoms, it may be reasonable to withhold pharmacologic therapy as hyperglycemia would be expected to resolve after discontinuation of the GC. Patients, however, should adhere to low carbohydrate diet and ensure adequate hydration.

On the other hand, for patients who will be on GCs long-term, we recommend an approach to management dictated by degree of post-prandial (especially post-lunch) hyperglycemia based on the known glycemic effect of GCs. For modest but sustained post-prandial hyperglycemia (<200 mg/dL [11.1 mmol/L]), consideration may be made to start metformin and/or a mild glucose-lowering medication, such as a DPP-4 inhibitor or SGLT-2 inhibitor

(Figure 38-5). GLP-1 agonists are also an option for patients who are not averse to injectable therapy. If patients experience sustained hyperglycemia on maximal doses of oral or non-insulin agents, NPH insulin should be started.

For patients with sustained and severe hyperglycemia (post-prandial glucose ≥200 mg/dL [11.1 mmol/L]), metformin should be started to improve insulin sensitivity along with NPH. In patients who are not in favor of starting insulin, given the longer onset of action of metformin, a faster-acting glucose-lowering medication will likely also need to be started. Options include: glinides, short-acting sulfonylureas (glipizide, gliclazide), and/or daily GLP-1 agonists (Table 38-1).

Glucocorticoid-Induced Hyperglycemia (GIH)

For patients with diabetes treated with non-insulin agents, it may be possible to achieve satisfactory glycemic control through the titration of existing non-insulin agents or through the addition of new medications; however, providers should have a low threshold to initiate insulin therapy for patients with sustained hyperglycemia on maximal non-insulin agents.

In non-insulin-requiring patients with modest hyperglycemia (post-prandial glucose <200 mg/dL [11.1 mmol/L]), it is recommended that metformin therapy be maximized as tolerated to improve insulin sensitivity. If the patient is not already taking a medication that targets post-prandial hyperglycemia, options include the addition of a DPP-4 inhibitor, an SGLT-2 inhibitor, a daily GLP-1 agonist, or an insulin secretagogue (preferably a glinide or short-acting SU). The choice of these agents will depend on the expected duration of GC use and the degree of hyperglycemia (Figure 38-6). For patients on maximal non-insulin agents and yet with sustained hyperglycemia, initiation of insulin is recommended with the choice of regimen determined by GC type and dosing interval.

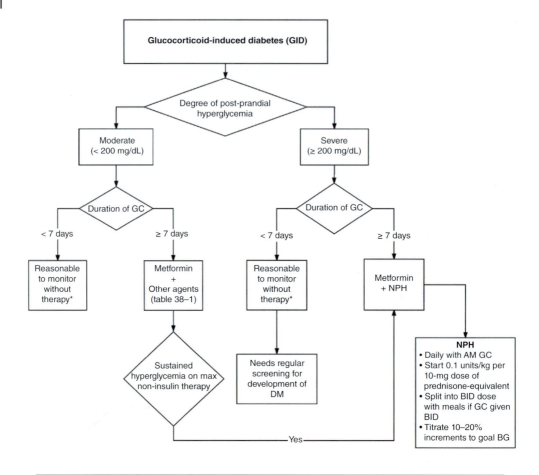

Figure 38-5 Recommended approach to management of GID.

Table 38-1 Onset of action and glycemic efficacy of various glucose-lowering therapies.

	Glycemic efficacy	
	Less potent (A1C lowering <1% [13 mmol/mol])	More potent (A1C lowering ≥1% [13 mmol/mol])
Slow (days–weeks)		Metformin
		Pioglitazone
		GLP-1 RA
Fast (hours)	Alpha glucosidase inhibitors	Sulfonylureas
	DPP-4 inhibitors	Glinides
	SGLT-2 inhibitors	Basal insulin
	Pramlintide	Intermediate-acting insulin
		Rapid-acting insulin
		Concentrated insulin

Onset of action (row label spanning both "Slow" and "Fast" rows)

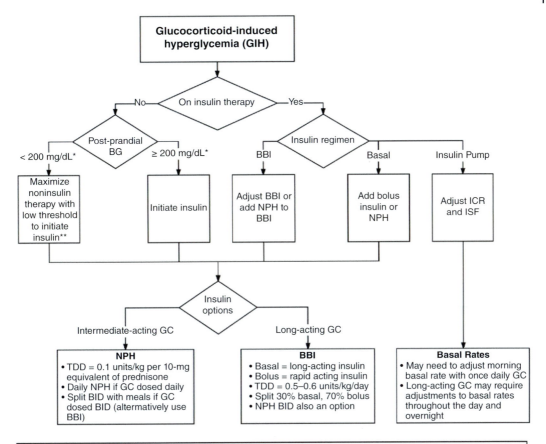

Figure 38-6 Recommended approach to management of GIH.

Case Study: Patient with T2DM on Oral Glucose-Lowering Therapy Receiving Low Dose Prednisone

A 56-year-old woman with T2DM is started on prednisone 15 mg daily for new diagnosis of polymyalgia rheumatica. She takes metformin 1000 mg bid and glipizide 5 mg bid without episodes of hypoglycemia. On prednisone, her home BG readings were fasting 110 mg/dL (5.6 mmol/L), pre-lunch 145 mg/dL (8 mmol/L), pre-dinner 171 mg/dL (9.5 mmol/L). She weighs 78 kg (BMI 32 kg/m²).

What Are Possible Management Options?

She has moderate hyperglycemia on low dose prednisone. It may be possible to achieve better glycemic control with the addition of non-insulin therapy that targets post-prandial hyperglycemia. She is already on the maximum dose of metformin and short-acting SU. A trial with a DPP-4 inhibitor or a GLP-1 agonist may be considered but if the patient is not against injectable therapy, a GLP-1 agonist may be tried first, given more potent glucose lowering effect compared to a DPP-4 inhibitor. A GLP-1 agonist may also help counteract the weight gain effect of GC therapy.

If a short trial of noninsulin glucose-lowering therapy fails, insulin should be initiated quickly. NPH can be used at a starting dose of 12 units (0.15 units/kg/day) timed with morning prednisone dose.

Case Study: Patient with Poorly Controlled T2DM on Oral Glucose-Lowering Therapy Starting on Dexamethasone

A 52-year-old overweight woman with poorly controlled T2DM (A1C 9.2% [78 mmol/mol]) is started on scheduled dexamethasone as part of chemotherapy. She takes glyburide/metformin 5/500 mg daily and receives dexamethasone 12 mg IV once a week on two out of every three weeks. She weighs 80 kg (BMI 28 kg/m^2) and has a normal renal function. Her home BG readings showed pre-breakfast average of 187 mg/dL (10.4 mmol/L), pre-lunch 196 mg/dL (10.9 mmol/L) and pre-dinner 224 mg/dL (12.4 mmol/L).

What Are the Possible Management Options?

Given severe hyperglycemia at baseline, insulin therapy is indicated but concurrently metformin should be maximized to 1000 mg bid to increase insulin sensitivity, and we recommend stopping glyburide due to long duration of action and risk of hypoglycemia.

One option is to use a BBI regimen using long-acting insulin (e.g., glargine, detemir) and rapid-acting insulin (aspart, lispro, glulisine). A starting total daily dose of 40 units (0.5 units/kg/day × 80 kg) is recommended with a 30% basal (12 units) and 70% bolus split (9 units with each meal). The insulin dose can then be adjusted based on the degree of BG control.

The glycemic impact of dexamethasone is expected to last for 48 hours and the patient should be advised to decrease insulin doses preemptively if glycemic control is reasonable. For example, the strategy in Table 38-2 can be used.

Table 38-2 Insulin dosage and timing

	Long-acting insulin dose	Rapid-acting insulin dose
Day of chemotherapy	12 units	9 units with meals
Day # 2	12 units	9 units
Day # 3	11 units	7 units
Day # 4	11 units	7 units
Day # 5	10 units	5 units
Day # 6	10 units	5 units
Day # 7	9 units	3 units
Day of chemotherapy	12 units	9 units

Another approach is using NPH twice daily. The dexamethasone dose needs to be converted to a prednisone equivalent dose (dexamethasone 12 mg = prednisone 75 mg), then a starting dose can be estimated by using the rule 0.4 units/kg/day corresponding to 32 units per day. This is administered in two divided doses with meals (i.e., 16 units bid). The insulin dose should be titrated based on the glucose response to therapy and empirically decreased after two days of dexamethasone use in a similar fashion as outlined above.

Case Study: Patient with Poorly Controlled T2DM on BBI Starting Once Daily Prednisone

A 53-year-old woman with T2DM on insulin has a flare-up of her rheumatoid arthritis and is started on prednisone 40 mg daily. She takes metformin 1000 mg bid, glargine 42 units at bedtime, aspart 16 units with meals, and a correctional scale. Her A1C is 8.6% (71 mmol/mol). She weighs 90 kg (BMI 32 kg/m^2) and her renal function is normal.

What are Possible Approaches to Treatment?

One approach is to adjust the existing BBI to cover the predominantly post-prandial hyperglycemia. Her TDD of insulin is 90 units but, given inadequate baseline control, a 10% increase in her TDD is reasonable (~100 units) which can be then redistributed to 30% basal (30 units) and 70% bolus (23 units with meals).

Alternatively, NPH can be added to the existing basal bolus regimen. A starting dose of 36 units (0.4 unit/kg/day) once daily timed with morning prednisone is reasonable. NPH should be adjusted further based on glucose response.

Conclusions

Providers should anticipate and be ready to treat hyperglycemia prior to initiation of GCs. Patients who do not have pre-existing diabetes but are at high risk of developing GID should be monitored for post-lunch and pre-dinner BG for the first two days of glucocorticoid therapy. If all values are <140 mg/dL (7.8 mmol/L), it is reasonable to stop monitoring. Patients with pre-existing diabetes should monitor their BG frequently, including a post-prandial check after lunch so to not miss post-prandial hyperglycemia. All patients should be encouraged to maintain adequate hydration and counseled on the need to follow a lower carbohydrate diet. The choice of therapy and the management approach will depend on the baseline insulin reserve, the dose and the duration of the GC therapy. Evidence for use of non-insulin therapy is scant and these medications have not been tested rigorously; however, based on the limited number of studies, clinical experience, the known glycemic effect and action profile of GCs as well as pharmacologic properties of non-insulin therapy, some patients may be able to achieve adequate glycemic control with non-insulin therapy alone. Agents that enhance insulin sensitivity and target post-prandial hyperglycemia are favored, and options for non-insulin therapy include: metformin, short-acting SU and glinides, DPP-4 inhibitors, and GLP-1 agonists. The selection of medication should also consider the onset of action and the glucose-lowering effect of individual drugs. There should be a low threshold to initiate insulin in patients who have sustained hyperglycemia despite maximal non-insulin therapy. Choice of insulin therapy will depend on the duration of action of the GC and dosing interval. Once-daily intermediate-acting NPH insulin timed with the morning GC dose is favored during treatment with intermediate-acting GC, as its peak effect will coincide with that of the GC. A modified BBI regimen with a higher proportion of bolus insulin (70%) or twice-daily NPH can be used with twice-daily intermediate-acting or once-daily long-acting GC.

References

1 van Staa TP, Leufkens HG, Abenhaim L, Begaud B, Zhang B, Cooper C. Use of oral corticosteroids in the United Kingdom. *QJM*. 2000;93:105–111.

2 Overman RA, Yeh JY, Deal CL. Prevalence of oral glucocorticoid usage in the United States: a general population perspective. *Arthritis Care Res (Hoboken)*. 2013;65:294–298.

3 Perez A, Jansen-Chaparro S, Saigi I, Bernal-Lopez MR, Miñambres I, Gomez-Huelgas R. Glucocorticoid-induced hyperglycaemia. *J Diabetes*. 2014;6:9–20.

4 Liu XX, Zhu XM, Miao Q, Ye HY, Zhang ZY, Li YM. Hyperglycemia induced by glucocorticoids in nondiabetic patients: a meta-analysis. *Ann Nutr Metab*. 2014;65:324–332.

5 Donihi AC, Raval D, Saul M, Korytkowski MT, DeVita MA. Prevalence and predictors of corticosteroid-related hyperglycemia in hospitalized patients. *Endocr Pract*. 2006;12:358–362.

6 Healy SJ, Nagaraja HN, Alwan D, Dungan KM. Prevalence, predictors, and outcomes of steroid-induced hyperglycemia in hospitalized patients with hematologic malignancies. *Endocrine*. 2017;56:90–97.

7 Uzu T, Harada T, Sakaguchi M, et al. Glucocorticoid-induced diabetes mellitus: prevalence and risk factors in primary renal diseases. *Nephron Clin Pract*. 2007;105:c54–57.

8 Kim SY, Yoo CG, Lee CT, et al. Incidence and risk factors of steroid-induced diabetes in patients with respiratory disease. *J Korean Med Sci*. 2011;26:264–267.

9 Montori VM, Basu A, Erwin PJ, Velosa JA, Gabriel SE, Kudva YC. Posttransplantation diabetes: a systematic review of the literature. *Diabetes Care*. 2002;25:583–592.

10 Gurwitz JH, Bohn RL, Glynn RJ, Monane M, Mogun H, Avorn J. Glucocorticoids and the risk for initiation of hypoglycemic therapy. *Arch Intern Med*. 1994;154:97–101.

11 Jeong IK, Oh SH, Kim BJ, et al. The effects of dexamethasone on insulin release and biosynthesis are dependent on the dose and duration of treatment. *Diabetes Res Clin Pract*. 2001;51:163–171.

12 Hwang JL, Weiss RE. Steroid-induced diabetes: a clinical and molecular approach to understanding and treatment. *Diabetes Metab Res Rev*. 2014;30:96–102.

13 Delaunay F, Khan A, Cintra A, et al. Pancreatic beta cells are important targets for the diabetogenic effects of glucocorticoids. *J Clin Invest*. 1997;100:2094–2098.

14 Fong AC, Cheung NW. The high incidence of steroid-induced hyperglycaemia in hospital. *Diabetes Res Clin Pract*. 2013;99:277–280.

15 Burt MG, Roberts GW, Aguilar-Loza NR, Frith P, Stranks SN. Continuous monitoring of circadian glycemic patterns in patients receiving prednisolone for COPD. *J Clin Endocrinol Metab*. 2011;96:1789–1796.

16 Clore JN, Thurby-Hay L. Glucocorticoid-induced hyperglycemia. *Endocr Pract*. 2009;15:469–474.

17 Abdelmannan D, Tahboub R, Genuth S, Ismail-Beigi F. Effect of dexamethasone on oral glucose tolerance in healthy adults. *Endocr Pract*. 2010;16:770–777.

18 Véber O, Wilde A, Demeter J, Tamás G, Mucsi I, Tabák AG. The effect of steroid pulse therapy on carbohydrate metabolism in multiple myeloma patients: a randomized crossover observational clinical study. *J Endocrinol Invest*. 2014;37:345–351.

19 Baker EH, Janaway CH, Philips BJ, et al. Hyperglycaemia is associated with poor outcomes in patients admitted to hospital with acute exacerbations of chronic obstructive pulmonary disease. *Thorax*. 2006;61:284–289.

20 Stauber MN, Aberer F, Oulhaj A, et al. Early hyperglycemia after initiation of glucocorticoid therapy predicts adverse outcome in patients with acute graft-versus-host disease. *Biol Blood Marrow Transplant*. 2017.

21 Jung SH, Jang HC, Lee SS, et al. The impact of hyperglycemia on risk of severe

infections during early period of induction therapy in patients with newly diagnosed multiple myeloma. *Biomed Res Int.* 2014;2014:413149.

22 Ali NA, O'Brien JM, Blum W, et al. Hyperglycemia in patients with acute myeloid leukemia is associated with increased hospital mortality. *Cancer.* 2007;110:96–102.

23 Gebremedhin E, Behrendt CE, Nakamura R, Parker P, Salehian B. Severe hyperglycemia immediately after allogeneic hematopoietic stem-cell transplantation is predictive of acute graft-versus-host disease. *Inflammation.* 2013;36:177–185.

24 Brunello A, Kapoor R, Extermann M. Hyperglycemia during chemotherapy for hematologic and solid tumors is correlated with increased toxicity. *Am J Clin Oncol.* 2011;34:292–296.

25 Liu H, Liu Z, Jiang B, et al. Prognostic significance of hyperglycemia in patients with brain tumors: a meta-analysis. *Mol Neurobiol.* 2016;53:1654–1660.

26 Thomas MC, Mathew TH, Russ GR, Rao MM, Moran J. Early peri-operative glycaemic control and allograft rejection in patients with diabetes mellitus: a pilot study. *Transplantation.* 2001;72:1321–1324.

27 Ganji MR, Charkhchian M, Hakemi M, et al. Association of hyperglycemia on allograft function in the early period after renal transplantation. *Transplant Proc.* 2007;39:852–854.

28 Seelig E, Meyer S, Timper K, et al. Metformin prevents metabolic side effects during systemic glucocorticoid treatment. *Eur J Endocrinol.* 2017;176:349–358.

29 Petersons CJ, Mangelsdorf BL, Jenkins AB, et al. Effects of low-dose prednisolone on hepatic and peripheral insulin sensitivity, insulin secretion, and abdominal adiposity in patients with inflammatory rheumatologic disease. *Diabetes Care.* 2013;36:2822–2829.

30 Kasayama S, Tanaka T, Hashimoto K, Koga M, Kawase I. Efficacy of glimepiride for the treatment of diabetes occurring during glucocorticoid therapy. *Diabetes Care.* 2002;25:2359–2360.

31 Ito S, Ogishima H, Kondo Y, et al. Early diagnosis and treatment of steroid-induced diabetes mellitus in patients with rheumatoid arthritis and other connective tissue diseases. *Mod Rheumatol.* 2014;24:52–59.

32 Willi SM, Kennedy A, Brant BP, Wallace P, Rogers NL, Garvey WT. Effective use of thiazolidinediones for the treatment of glucocorticoid-induced diabetes. *Diabetes Res Clin Pract.* 2002;58:87–96.

33 van Genugten RE, van Raalte DH, Muskiet MH, et al. Does dipeptidyl peptidase-4 inhibition prevent the diabetogenic effects of glucocorticoids in men with the metabolic syndrome? A randomized controlled trial. *Eur J Endocrinol.* 2014;170:429–439.

34 Ohashi N, Tsuji N, Naito Y, et al. Alogliptin improves steroid-induced hyperglycemia in treatment-naïve Japanese patients with chronic kidney disease by decrease of plasma glucagon levels. *Med Sci Monit.* 2014;20:587–593.

35 van Raalte DH, van Genugten RE, Linssen MM, Ouwens DM, Diamant M. Glucagon-like peptide-1 receptor agonist treatment prevents glucocorticoid-induced glucose intolerance and islet-cell dysfunction in humans. *Diabetes Care.* 2011;34:412–417.

36 de la Peña A, Riddle M, Morrow LA, et al. Pharmacokinetics and pharmacodynamics of high-dose human regular U-500 insulin versus human regular U-100 insulin in healthy obese subjects. *Diabetes Care.* 2011;34:2496–2501.

37 Cohen MR, Smetzer JL. Pen device for U-500 insulin; tamper-resistant seals; dispelling myths about ISMP. *Hosp Pharm.* 2016;51:279–283.

38 Drug Safety and Availability. FDA approves a dedicated syringe to be used with Humulin R U-500 insulin. Center for Drug Evaluation and Research, 2016. https://www.fda.gov/Drugs/DrugSafety/ucm510318.htm.)

39 American Diabetes Association. Glycemic targets. *Diabetes Care* 2018;41:S55–S64.

39

Management of Diabetes and/or Hyperglycemia in Acute Coronary Syndrome, Acute Stroke, and Acute Heart Failure

Miles Fisher

Key Points

- The importance of cardiovascular disease (CVD) in diabetes mellitus is well established. CVD is a common cause of morbidity and mortality in persons with diabetes.
- The modern multifaceted management of type 2 diabetes, with a focus on the treatment of hypertension and the use of statins, has reduced the prevalence of atherosclerotic CVD, and where previously this was increased 4–6-fold compared to non-diabetic subjects, this is now around double.
- Intensive insulin therapy reduced mortality following myocardial infarction in the DIGAMI study, but these results have not been replicated in any other study or in meta-analysis.
- Cardiology treatment for acute coronary syndromes (ACS) builds on the same principles as in people without diabetes and includes dual antiplatelet therapy, fondaparinux, or low molecular weight heparin (LMWH), reperfusion or revascularization with percutaneous coronary interventions (PCI), angiotensin-converting enzyme inhibitors (ACEI) or angiotensin receptor blockers (ARB), beta-blockers, and high-dose statin therapy.
- Recommendations in guidelines on the management of hyperglycemia following ACS do not routinely recommend intensive intravenous insulin infusions unless clinically indicated.
- Intensive insulin therapy following an acute stroke has not demonstrated any reduction in mortality or disability and is not routinely recommended as it increases hypoglycemia.
- Patients with acute stroke can be treated to maintain a blood glucose concentration between 5 and 15 mmol/L (90–270 mg/dL) with close monitoring to avoid hypoglycemia.
- Pioglitazone reduced events in non-diabetic subjects with insulin resistance following a recent stroke, but is not recommended in routine clinical practice because of fluid retention and an increase in fractures.
- There are no studies on the management of hyperglycemia following acute heart failure.
- Cardiology treatment for acute heart failure builds on the same principles as in people without diabetes and includes ACEI or ARB, beta-blockers, mineralocorticoid antagonists, ivabradine if heart rate is raised, and diuretics for symptom relief.
- Metformin should be withheld during acute heart failure episodes, then restarted once the patient is stable. Metformin appears safe in patients with chronic heart failure, pioglitazone should be avoided, and sodium-glucose co-transporter-2 (SGLT-2) inhibitors may be of some benefit.

Endocrine and Metabolic Medical Emergencies: A Clinician's Guide, Second Edition. Edited by Glenn Matfin.
© 2018 John Wiley & Sons Ltd. Published 2018 by John Wiley & Sons Ltd.

- The ADA 2018 and AACE 2018 treatment guidelines have now recommended that in patients with type 2 diabetes and established atherosclerotic CVD, glucose-lowering agents with proven CV benefit (currently empagliflozin, liraglutide and canagliflozin) should be preferentially added to lifestyle therapy and metformin when reasonable to do so. It is anticipated that the newly-approved semaglutide (which also has CVD benefits), will be be added to this list in future updates.

Introduction

The importance of cardiovascular disease (CVD) in diabetes mellitus is well established. CVD is a common cause of morbidity and mortality in people with diabetes. The modern multifaceted management of type 2 diabetes, with a focus on the treatment of hypertension and the use of statins, has reduced the prevalence of atherosclerotic CVD, and where previously this was increased 4–6-fold compared to non-diabetic subjects, this is now around double (1,2).

Not all patients with diabetes develop CVD and patients with diabetes can be classified according to increasing cardiovascular (CV) risk and mortality from CVD as:

1. No known vascular disease.
2. Stable coronary artery disease (i.e., angina) or cerebrovascular disease (i.e., strokes and transient ischemic attacks [TIAs]).
3. Acute coronary syndromes (ACS, i.e., ST-and non-ST-elevation MI [STEMI or NSTEMI respectively], and unstable angina).
4. Chronic heart failure (highest risk group with one-year mortality 30–40%).

When looked at from a vascular perspective, diabetes is common in patients admitted to coronary care units and acute stroke units, and when patients with diagnosed diabetes are excluded, around one-third of remaining patients in these units have newly-diagnosed diabetes and one-third have pre-diabetes. This proportion is likely to increase as the prevalence of diabetes increases in the population related to reduced physical activity and increasing obesity.

The metabolic and endocrine response to acute illness includes the release of counter-regulatory hormones which can provoke and worsen hyperglycemia. Emergency treatment with insulin following myocardial infarction (MI) to try and reduce mortality is an intervention that has been tested for over 40 years, with mixed and conflicting results.

This chapter examines the evidence for the treatment of hyperglycemia in patients with ACS, acute stroke, and acute heart failure. The evidence that long-term treatment with intensive glycemic control or with specific anti-diabetes drugs might reduce recurrent events in patients that have survived the acute episode is also examined.

Acute Coronary Syndromes

Definitions and Pathophysiology

Acute coronary syndromes describe a spectrum of disorders including STEMI, NSTEMI and unstable angina. The diagnosis is based on a history of chest pain, electrocardiogram (ECG) changes, and measurement of biochemical markers of cardiac damage. Myocardial infarction occurs following plaque rupture with thrombosis and myocardial ischemia. A total occlusion of the coronary artery leads to STEMI, where the best treatment is an emergency percutaneous coronary intervention (PCI). A partial occlusion leads to NSTEMI. Myocardial infarction is detected by measuring increases in troponin levels as a biomarker of myocardial necrosis, while in unstable angina, troponin is not increased.

People with diabetes are more likely to have a NSTEMI compared to non-diabetic subjects. The clinical presentation in people with diabetes is more likely to be atypical or painless, leading to delays in presentation and treatment. All of the modern cardiology treatments used for the initial management of ACS are of proven benefit in people with diabetes, including PCI, dual antiplatelet therapy, low molecular weight heparin (LMWH) or fondaparinux, and beta-blockers. Serious complications such as re-infarction and heart failure are more common in people with diabetes, and despite the use of modern treatments, the mortality is doubled.

The increased mortality has been attributed to factors present before the acute event:

- more widespread and distal coronary artery disease;
- impaired fibrinolysis;
- autonomic neuropathy;
- diabetic cardiomyopathy.

And also attributable to factors immediately following the infarction:

- increased insulin resistance;
- increased uptake and beta-oxidation of fatty acids by the myocardium.

Intensive Treatment of Hyperglycemia

The metabolic effects of intravenous (IV) insulin following MI include:

- the lowering of blood glucose;
- the reduction of free fatty acids which may be toxic or arrhythmogenic;
- a switch to aerobic metabolism in the myocardium which might be protective;
- increasing potassium entry into the myocardium, which may improve function.

Other effects of insulin that may be beneficial include:

- an antithrombotic/fibrinolytic effect;
- reduced platelet aggregation;
- an anti-inflammatory effect;

- reduced reperfusion injury;
- increased myocardial blood flow.

Several studies over a period of 20 years have examined the effects of intensive IV insulin following MI in people with known diabetes and/or in patients with hyperglycemia at the time of MI (i.e., newly diagnosed diabetes or "stress hyperglycemia"). These have been divided into two groups:

- studies with a glycemic focus, where insulin has been given to try and normalize hyperglycemia (e.g., DIGAMI, DIGAMI 2, HI-5, HEART2D, BIOMArCS 2) (3–8);
- studies with an insulin focus, where insulin had been administered for its effect in supressing free fatty acids, stimulating potassium uptake, and enhancing glycolysis (IMMEDIATE) (9).

These studies are summarized in Table 39-1.

The DIGAMI study tested the hypothesis that intensive IV insulin followed by intensive subcutaneous (SC) insulin would reduce mortality following STEMI in patients with admission blood glucose (BG) > 11.0 mmol/L (200 mg/dL) (3). Some 620 subjects were recruited through Swedish coronary care units and the principal outcome was the mortality at a mean of 3.4 years follow-up. The BG in response to IV insulin was significantly reduced at 24 hours, and glycosylated hemoglobin (HbA1c) in response to SC insulin was significantly reduced at 3 months. Total mortality was reduced at 1 year and 3.4 years. The 20 years follow-up data were published in 2014, and by then 89% of patients in the intensive treatment group were dead compared to 91% in the control group. The mean follow-up was 7.8 years, and it was estimated that intensive therapy had prolonged survival by 2.3 years (4).

These results could not be replicated in the later DIGAMI 2 (5), and HI-5 studies (6), and a recent meta-analysis combining DIGAMI, DIGAMI 2 and HI-5 showed no significant effect on mortality, heart failure, arrhythmias or re-infarction rates, but a significant increase in hypoglycemia

Table 39-1 Studies of insulin therapy following acute coronary syndromes

Study	Subjects	Intervention	Primary outcome	Comments
DIGAMI	620 patients with acute myocardial infarction and BG > 11.0 mmol/L (200 mg/dL)	Intensive IV insulin followed by intensive SC insulin vs. conventional management	Significant reduction in total mortality	
DIGAMI 2	1253 patients with acute myocardial infarction and type 2 diabetes or BG > 11.0 mmol/L (200 mg/dL)	Intensive IV insulin plus intensive SC insulin vs. intensive IV insulin alone vs. conventional management	No difference in total mortality	Study halted because of under-recruitment and futility
HI-5	240 patients with acute myocardial infarction and BG > 7.8 mmol/L (140 mg/dL)	IV insulin/dextrose infusion aiming for BG < 10.0 mmol/L (180 mg/dL) vs. conventional management	No effect on mortality	Reduced re-infarction and heart failure within 3 months
HEART2D	1115 patients with type 2 diabetes and acute myocardial infarction	SC basal insulin vs, SC prandial insulin	No difference in cardiovascular outcomes	Stopped for lack of efficacy on differences in fasting and post-prandial blood glucose
BIOMArCS 2	294 patients with ACS and BG 7.8–16.0 mmol/L (140–288 mg/dL)	Intensive IV insulin vs. conventional management	No effect on Troponin T as a measure of infarct size	Increased mortality with intensive IV insulin
IMMEDIATE	871 patients with suspected ACS	Out of hospital infusion of glucose-insulin-potassium (GIK) vs dextrose infusion	No effect on the progression to ACS	Reduced composite of cardiac arrest and in-hospital mortality

IV = intravenous; SC = subcutaneous; BG = blood glucose; ACS = acute coronary syndromes

(10). DIGAMI 2 recruited 1253 subjects with suspected acute MI and either previously diagnosed diabetes or an admission BG >11.0 mmol/L (200 mg/dL). Patients were randomized to intensive IV insulin followed by intensive SC insulin; intensive IV insulin without subsequent intensive SC insulin, and conventional management throughout. The study was under-recruited, glycemic differences were slight, and DIGAMI 2 was halted because of futility, with negative results.

The HI-5 study recruited 240 subjects with acute MI and either known diabetes or a BG >7.8 mmol/L (140 mg/dL). Subjects were randomized to receive either insulin/dextrose infusion therapy for at least 24 hours to maintain a BG <10 mmol/L (180 mg/dL), or conventional therapy, so the intervention was less intensive than in DIGAMI and DIGAMI 2. No effect was demonstrated on total mortality, although post hoc analysis suggested possible benefit in subjects whose BG was maintained below 8.0 mmol/L (144 mg/dL).

Three other studies on glycemic management following acute MI are worthy of mention. The HEART2D trial was performed in

Table 39-2 Guidelines for management of hyperglycemia in ACS (11,12,14,51)

NICE 2011 CG130	SIGN 148 2016	ESC/EASD 2013	CDA 2013
• Manage hyperglycemia in patients admitted to hospital for an ACS by keeping BG levels <11.0 mmol/L (200 mg/dL) while avoiding hypoglycemia. In the first instance, consider a dose-adjusted insulin infusion (i.e., variable-rate IV insulin infusion [VRIII]) with regular monitoring of BG levels. • Do not routinely offer intensive insulin therapy (i.e., an IV infusion of insulin and glucose with or without potassium) to manage hyperglycemia (BG >11.0 mmol/L [200 mg/dL]) in patients admitted to hospital for an ACS unless clinically indicated.	• Patients with confirmed ACS and diabetes mellitus or marked hyperglycemia (>11.0 mmol/L [200 mg/dL]) should have immediate BG control aiming for a target BG of 7.0–10.9 mmol/L (126–200 mg/dL) • Instituting an insulin and glucose infusion should not delay institution of time-dependent interventions such as primary PCI.	• Insulin-based glucose control should be considered in ACS patients with significant hyperglycemia (>10 mmol/L [>180 mg/dL]) with the target adapted to co-morbidities • Glycemia control, that may be accomplished by different glucose-lowering agents, should be considered in patients with diabetes mellitus and ACS	• Patients with acute myocardial infarction and BG >11.0 mmol/L (200 mg/dL) on admission may receive glycemic control in the range of 7.0–10.0 mmol/L (126–180 mg/dL), followed by strategies to achieve recommended glucose targets long-term. • Insulin therapy may be required to achieve these targets. • A similar approach may be taken to this with diabetes and admission BG <11.0 mmol/L (200 mg/dL).

patients with type 2 diabetes following an acute MI and compared the use of basal insulin versus prandial insulin. That trial was also stopped early as the pre-specified BG targets were not reached, the separation of BG between the groups was slight, and there was no difference in CV outcomes (7).

The BIOMArCS 2 study was a single center, open label, randomized controlled trial comparing the effects of intensive IV insulin versus conventional treatment in 294 subjects with an ACS and BG 7.8–16.0 mmol/L (140–288 mg/dL), and compared intensive IV insulin, aiming for normoglycemia, with conventional management (8). The median BG was lower in the intensive treatment group and there was no difference in primary endpoint of Troponin T at 72 hours. Alarmingly there was a significant increase in deaths in the intensive group (8 deaths versus 1 death, p = 0.04), as well as in severe hypoglycemia, and this increase in

mortality persisted for a mean of 5 years of follow-up.

Finally, the IMMEDIATE trial examined the effects of glucose-potassium-insulin (GKI) administered out of hospital by paramedics in 871 patients with suspected ACS (9). The primary endpoint was progression to confirmed MI within 24 hours and this was not changed by the intervention. A secondary composite of cardiac arrest or in-hospital mortality was reduced, especially in patients with STEMI.

Guidelines

Trying to incorporate the results of these conflicting and largely negative studies into a meaningful guideline for clinical practice has been challenging, and it is not surprising that differing recommendations have been made (11–14). Some recent recommendations from the guidelines are included in

Table 39-2 as examples. Interestingly, the American Diabetes Association (ADA) does not have any recent specific recommendation on the management of hyperglycemia following ACS.

Longer-term Management of Diabetes Following Recent Myocardial Infarction

Following the rosiglitazone controversy, where rosiglitazone was suspected to be associated with an increase in non-fatal myocardial infarctions (15), the cardiovascular safety of new glucose-lowering drugs must be demonstrated before receiving a license from the Food and Drug Administration (FDA) and the European Medicines Agency (EMA). This usually includes a dedicated randomized-controlled CV outcome trial (CVOT), and the primary endpoint is either major adverse CV events (MACE), a composite of nonfatal MI, nonfatal stroke, or CV death, or MACE plus hospitalization for unstable angina. The study design is usually events-driven, so including subjects with a recent ACS is one way of quickly reaching the number of required events.

EXAMINE was a double-blind placebo-controlled trial which compared alogliptin and placebo following ACS (acute MI or unstable angina requiring hospitalization) in 5380 patients with type 2 diabetes (Table 39-2) (16). Treatment with the dipeptidyl peptidase (DPP)-4 inhibitor alogliptin was commenced within 15–90 days of the ACS for a median duration of 18 months. The primary MACE endpoint occurred in 305 (11.3%) patients in the alogliptin group and 316 (11.8%) patients in the placebo group, indicating that alogliptin was non-inferior but not superior to placebo.

A similar study design was used in the ELIXA trial which compared the glucagon-like peptide-1 (GLP-1) agonist lixisenatide with placebo in 6088 patients with type 2 diabetes who had been hospitalized for MI or unstable angina within the previous 180 days (mean 72 days from index case until randomization) (17). The primary endpoint of MACE plus hospitalization for unstable

angina occurred in 406 patients (13.4%) in the lixisenatide group and 399 patients (13.2%) in the placebo group, indicating that lixisenatide was non-inferior but not superior to placebo.

Longer-Term Management of Diabetes Following Myocardial Infarction

The small metformin subgroup in UKPDS, which included overweight patients with recently diagnosed diabetes, but excluded patients with recent MI or heart failure, demonstrated a significant reduction in MI and total mortality during the study (18). As this benefit was not demonstrated in larger groups treated with sulfonylureas or insulin, it was concluded that metformin was reducing CV events through mechanisms other than glucose-lowering. Support for CV benefits of metformin comes from the SPREAD-DIMCAD trial, where metformin-treated patients with existing CVD had less a reduction in recurrent CV events compared to patients on glipizide (19), and from the "Hyperinsulinemia: the Outcome of its Metabolic Effects" (HOME) study, where metformin reduced a secondary composite macrovascular endpoint (20).

PROactive was the first double-blind, placebo-controlled, randomized-controlled trial to examine the effects of a specific anti-diabetes drug, pioglitazone, on hard CV endpoints in patients with diabetes and existing atherosclerotic vascular disease (21) (Table 39-3). This was performed before the FDA requirements were introduced. Nearly half of the subjects (47%) had a previous MI. The results of the study were controversial at that time. First, the primary endpoint which included peripheral vascular events and interventions was not significantly reduced but the main secondary endpoint of CV death, MI and stroke were significantly reduced by pioglitazone. Second, an increase in heart failure was seen with pioglitazone, and the mechanism of this increase was uncertain at that time. A detailed post-hoc analysis of the 2445 patients who had a previous MI at baseline showed a significant

Table 39-3 Results of cardiovascular outcome trials (53)

Study	Intervention	Effect on MACE/MACE plus	Effect on myocardial infarctions	Effect on strokes	Effect on heart failure
PROactive	Pioglitazone	Reduced MACE	Non-significant reduction	Non-significant reduction	Increased HFH
RECORD	Rosiglitazone	No effect	No effect	No effect	Increased HFH
SAVOR-TIMI	Saxagliptin	No effect	No effect	No effect	Increased HFH
EXAMINE	Alogliptin	No effect	No effect	No effect	Increased HFH in subgroup
TECOS	Sitagliptin	No effect	No effect	No effect	No effect
ELIXA	Lixisenatide	No effect	No effect	No effect	No effect
EXSCEL	Exenatide extended release	No effect	No effect	No effect	No effect
ACE	Acarbose	No effect	No effect	No effect	No effect
EMPA-REG OUTCOME	Empagliflozin	Reduced MACE	Non-significant reduction	Non-significant increase	Reduced HFH
CANVAS Program	Canagliflozin	Reduced MACE	Non-significant reduction	Non-significant reduction	Reduced HFH
LEADER	Liraglutide	Reduced MACE	Non-significant reduction	Non-significant reduction	No effect
SUSTAIN-6	Semaglutide	Reduced MACE	Non-significant reduction	Reduced strokes	No effect
ORIGIN	Glargine	No effect	No effect	No effect	No effect
DEVOTE	Degludec or Glargine	No effect	No effect	No effect	No effect

MACE = Major adverse CV events; HFH = Heart failure hospitalization

19% relative risk reduction in a composite of cardiac endpoints including ACS and cardiac death (22).

In the ORIGIN trial, basal insulin glargine was compared to placebo in a large group of people with short-duration diabetes or pre-diabetes. Some 66% of subjects had prior CVD, and 34% had prior MI (23). Glargine treatment had no effect on MACE (CV death, MI, stroke) or on a composite CV outcome, but, as expected, hypoglycemia increased.

Most of the FDA-mandated CVOTs have included substantial numbers of subjects with previous myocardial infarctions, MI has been included in the primary MACE endpoint, and the results of effects on MI have been included as pre-specified secondary endpoints. We have the results of two other safety CVOTs with the DPP-4 inhibitors, saxagliptin (SAVOR-TIMI) (24) and sitagliptin (TECOS) (25). The results have been disappointing but not unexpected, as DPP-4 inhibitors have no significant effects on CV risk factors. All three showed neutral effects on the primary endpoint which was either MACE (SAVOR-TIMI, EXAMINE) or MACE plus hospitalization for unstable angina (TECOS) (Table 39-3).

EMPA-REG OUTCOME was a large safety CVOT in 7020 people with type 2 diabetes and existing CVD (26). It compared the SGLT-2 inhibitor empagliflozin 10 mg; empagliflozin 25 mg; and placebo in addition to usual standards of care, and nearly half of the participants were on insulin. Nearly half of the patients had a prior MI, a quarter had a previous coronary artery bypass graft (CABG), a quarter had a history of stroke, and a fifth had peripheral arterial disease. One quarter had a baseline estimated glomerular filtration rate (eGFR) between 30 and 60 ml/min/1.73m^2, and 10% had heart failure so this was a very high-risk group of subjects.

The results were remarkable, as empagliflozin was superior to placebo in reducing major adverse coronary events (CV death, nonfatal MI, nonfatal stoke) and reduced total mortality by 32%. The effects were the same for both doses of empagliflozin. Hospitalization for heart failure was also significantly reduced by a third. The reduction in non-fatal myocardial infarctions as a secondary endpoint was not statistically significant (Table 39-3).

Since then, two safety CVOTs with GLP-1 receptor agonists have demonstrated a significant reduction in MACE compared to placebo. In LEADER, liraglutide reduced MACE was compared to placebo in a group of 9340 diabetic patients (27). Some 82% had prior CVD and 31% prior MI. The reduction in non-fatal myocardial infarctions as a secondary endpoint was not statistically significant. In SUSTAIN-6, semaglutide reduced MACE compared to placebo (28). Some 83% had prior CVD and 32% prior MI. Again the reduction in non-fatal myocardial infarctions as a secondary endpoint was not statistically significant.

More recently, the SGLT-2 inhibitor canagliflozin was compared to placebo in the CANVAS program (29). These two trials integrated data from 10,142 participants; 66% had a history of CVD. Canagliflozin

reduced MACE compared to placebo. The reduction in secondary endpoints of death from CV causes, nonfatal MI and nonfatal stroke was not statistically significant. However, similar to the EMPA-REG OUTCOME study, hospitalization for heart failure was significantly reduced by more than a third. Progression of albuminuria and a composite 40% reduction in eGFR, renal replacement therapy or renal death was also observed compared to placebo. Unfortunately, the canagliflozin group had an increased risk of amputation primarily at the level of the toe or metatarsal.

In the recent DEVOTE CVOT, the ultra-long basal insulin degudec was compared to an active control of long-acting basal insulin glargine in patients with type 2 diabetes and high CV risk (30). Insulin degudec was non-inferior to glargine treatment, and both had no significant effect on MACE (CV death, MI, stroke) or on component CV outcomes (confirming the previous CVD findings for glargine in the ORIGIN trial).

Does Intensive Glycemia Control Reduce Myocardial Infarctions?

The DCCT in people with type 1 diabetes, and UKPDS, ADVANCE, ACCORD and VADT in people with type 2 diabetes, all attempted to address whether intensive glycemic control reduced CV events including myocardial infarctions (31–35) (Table 39-4). No significant reduction in composite CV events was demonstrated at the end of the intervention in any of these studies, and ACCORD was stopped prematurely at 3.5 years because of an increase in total mortality, particularly sudden CV deaths (Table 39-3). It is noteworthy, however, that in ACCORD there was a statistically significant reduction in myocardial infarctions at the end of the 5-year treatment phase but an increase in total mortality. These overall negative results were not unexpected as BG is a less important risk factor for the development of CVD than hypertension or cholesterol (1), so even if a wide separation

Table 39-4 Results of studies of intensive glycemic management on microvascular outcomes, macrovascular outcomes and total mortality

Study	Effect on microvascular complications	Effect on macrovascular complications	Effect on total mortality
DCCT	Reduced retinopathy, nephropathy, neuropathy	No effect on major cardiovascular and peripheral vascular events	No effect
UKPDS	Reduced microvascular endpoints	No effect on myocardial infarctions	No effect
ACCORD	Reduced retinopathy, nephropathy, neuropathy	No effect on major adverse cardiovascular events (MACE)	Increased Mortality
ADVANCE	Reduced nephropathy	No effect on MACE	No effect
VADT	Reduced albuminuria progression	No effect on major cardiovascular events	No effect

in HbA1c could be safely obtained, it would take a long time for the CV benefit to accrue. Serious concerns with the intensive glycemic treatment used in ACCORD are the rapid escalation of therapies, the early use of large doses of insulin, massive weight gain, and frequent hypoglycemia.

Meta-analysis of individual subject data from UKPDS, ACCORD, ADVANCE and VADT demonstrated a significant reduction in myocardial infarctions and major CV events, but no difference in stroke, heart failure or mortality comparing intensive and less intensive glycemic control (36). The main side-effect of intensive therapy was an increase in hypoglycemia.

At the end of these intervention studies the subjects returned to routine diabetes care. The clear reduction in microvascular events with intensive control was adopted into routine care and glycemic control improved in the subjects who had been receiving conventional therapy. Glycemic control deteriorated outside the supported study environment in subjects, who had previously been in the intensive control groups. Within one year of finishing the intervention study, HbA1c concentrations were similar in the two groups.

Longer-term epidemiological follow-up has been performed in each of these studies, and a clear pattern of CV benefit has emerged (Table 39-5) (37–41). In DCCT/EDIC we

Table 39-5 Results of epidemiologic follow-up of studies of intensive glycemic management on microvascular outcomes, macrovascular outcomes and total mortality

Study	Effect on microvascular complications	Effect on macrovascular complications	Effect on total mortality
DCCT/EDIC	Reduced retinopathy, nephropathy, neuropathy	Reduced MACE	Reduced mortality
UKPDS-PTM	Reduced microvascular disease	Reduced myocardial infarctions	Reduced mortality
ACCORDION	Reduced retinopathy	No effect on MACE	No longer increased
ADVANCE-ON	Reduced end-stage renal disease	No effect on MACE	No effect
VADT	Not available	Reduced major cardiovascular events	No effect

now have 30 years of total follow-up, which has demonstrated a significant 33% reduction in total mortality, a 32% reduction in MACE (MI, stroke, CV death) and a 30% reduction in CV events (MI plus CV death) (37).

UKPDS post-trial monitoring (PTM) with 20 years of total follow-up has shown reductions in myocardial infarctions and total mortality both in the group of overweight patients treated with metformin, and in the group previously treated intensively with sulfonylureas or insulin. (38). Shorter overall follow-up of the VADT (10 years) has shown a significant reduction in the primary outcome of major CV events (heart attack, stroke, new or worsening congestive heart failure, amputation for ischemic gangrene, or CV-related death) with MI and heart failure being the commonest outcomes (39). By contrast, shorter follow-up of the ADVANCE study in ADVANCE-ON demonstrated no significant effect on CV events (40). Even in the epidemiological follow-up of ACCORD in ACCORDION, the excess increase in total mortality that was seen during 3.5 years of intensive treatment was reduced by returning to conventional control, so that there was no difference in total mortality after a total of 9 years of follow-up and the increase in CV deaths was obtunded (41).

Collectively the results of these studies confirm the long-term benefits of intensive glycemic control in reducing CV events, particularly myocardial infarctions, and suggest that the method of obtaining intensive control should be based on the packages of care used in UKPDS, ADVANCE or VADT.

Strokes and TIAs

Definitions and Pathophysiology

Previously a stroke was defined as the sudden onset of loss of neurological function due to infarction or hemorrhage in the nervous system lasting longer than 24 hours, and a transient ischemic attack (TIA) if the symptoms lasted less than 24 hours. The current definition of stroke is acute dysfunction lasting more than 24 hours, or of any duration if computed tomography (CT) or magnetic resonance imaging (MRI) shows infarction or ischemia relevant to the symptoms. TIA has been redefined as focal dysfunction lasting less than 24 hours with no evidence of infarction on imaging. The risk of stroke is more than doubled in people with diabetes, mortality is increased, and functional outcomes are worse than non-diabetic subjects with stroke. It was previously thought that the pattern of strokes that is seen in people with diabetes was different, with more lacunar strokes, but some recent epidemiological studies have not demonstrated any clear link between diabetes and any subtype of stroke.

Immediate Treatment of Hyperglycemia

Patients with hyperglycemia following an acute stroke have worse outcomes than patients whose glucose remains in the normal range, including an increase in mortality, worse stroke severity, and greater functional impairment. This occurs both in subjects treated with thrombolytic therapy and those who do not receive this treatment. Acute hyperglycemia increases plasminogen activator type 1 and hyperglycemia delays reperfusion of the ischemic penumbra in patients treated with tissue plasminogen activator (tPA) thrombolytic therapy, decreases tPA-induced recanalization rates, and is associated with a reduced rate of desirable clinical outcomes. Following on the model for the treatment of MI with IV insulin, there have been several studies that have examined the effects of intensive insulin therapy on stroke outcomes.

The results have recently been the subject of a recent Cochrane Review and are disappointing (42). Eleven randomized controlled trials were identified involving only 791 subjects in the intervention groups and 792 in the control groups. The separation in BG was slight, with a mean BG of 6.7 mmol/L (121 mg/dL) in the intervention groups and 7.3 mmol/L (131 mg/dL) in the control groups, which were either placebo or less intensive insulin. No difference was observed in mortality, dependency, or final neurological deficit. There was an increase in hypoglycemia in the intervention group. There were no differences in the results when the subjects were divided into people with and without diabetes.

The authors concluded that there was no benefit from IV insulin, but an increased risk of symptomatic and asymptomatic hyperglycemia. An obvious deficiency is the small number of subjects in these studies. The ongoing SHINE study will compare conventional SC insulin with intensive IV insulin in 1400 subjects with an acute ischemic stroke and will add considerably to the available data (43).

Long-Term Management of Diabetes Following a Stroke

Some 19% of subjects in PROactive had a previous stroke at baseline, and a post-hoc subgroup analysis of subjects with a previous stroke showed a highly significant 47% relative risk reduction in further strokes, which occurred in 6% of the pioglitazone group and 10% of the placebo group (44). The Insulin Resistance Intervention after Stroke (IRIS) trial examined the use of pioglitazone 45 mg versus placebo in 3876 patients with insulin resistance but without diabetes and a recent ischemic stroke or TIA (45). Insulin resistance was assessed using the homeostasis model assessment of insulin resistance (HOMA-IR) index, i.e., an estimate of beta cell function and insulin sensitivity calculated using fasting BG and insulin values.

There was a significant reduction in the primary composite outcome of fatal or non-fatal stroke or MI in the pioglitazone group compared with the placebo group (9% vs 11.8%; HR, 0.76). The incidence of a new diagnosis of diabetes was also reduced with 73 (4%) cases in the pioglitazone group compared with 149 (8%) cases in the placebo group (HR, 0.48). Analysis of fatal and non-fatal strokes as a secondary outcome showed a numerical reduction that did not reach significance, and the same was seen for fatal and non-fatal MI.

The numbers of subjects with baseline cerebrovascular disease in the FDA-mandated CVOTs are much less than the numbers with a previous MI, and stroke has occurred less frequently than MI as a secondary endpoint in these studies. There have been no statistically significant effects on recurrent stroke, with the exception of the SUSTAIN-6 trial with semaglutide (28) where non-fatal stroke occurred in 1.6% of the semaglutide group and 2.7% of the placebo group (hazard ration 0.61, p = 0.04) (Table 39-3). The mechanism of benefit is unknown, and may relate to modification of the progression of atherosclerosis.

Heart Failure

Immediate Treatment

Heart failure is a common end-stage vascular complication of diabetes, particularly in people who have survived previous myocardial infarctions. It is also common for patients with heart failure to develop diabetes, related to the counter-regulatory hormone increases and insulin resistance that accompany heart failure. During episodes of acute heart failure, hyperglycemia worsens, and is an indicator of a poor prognosis. Detailed literature review has failed to identify any studies on intensive insulin therapy during acute heart failure, and this is an area that is worthy of further study. One concern would be fluid overload, and any intensive treatment regimen would probably require a combination of insulin, concentrated dextrose, and potassium. In the absence of any definitive evidence, a low dose variable rate insulin infusion can be used in the acute stages.

Previously the use of metformin was contraindicated in patients with heart failure because of concerns about the development of lactic acidosis. This is no longer the case, and cohort studies suggest that diabetic patients with chronic heart failure who are treated with metformin have a better survival than those treated with comparators, often sulfonylureas. There was an attempt to formally study metformin versus placebo in a randomized controlled trial in diabetic patients with chronic heart failure but this was halted because of futility. Hypoxia and acidosis can occur during acute heart failure, so it is prudent to withhold metformin until the acute heart failure is treated and to restart it prior to discharge.

Long-Term Management

Meta-analysis of the intensive glycemic studies (UKPDS, ACCORD, ADVANCE, VADT) has not shown any overall reduction in the development of heart failure, and the number of subjects in these studies who had heart failure at baseline was very small, so underpowered for any possible subgroup analysis (46). Further research on glitazones identified that there was an increased renal retention of sodium and water, unmasking undiagnosed heart failure, and pioglitazone is contraindicated in patients with heart failure NYHA stage I-IV. Information on heart failure events from the PROactive study and other studies is included in Table 39-3.

When the first FDA-mandated studies on DPP-4 inhibitors were presented, an unexpected finding was an increase in heart failure hospitalization (HFH). A significant increase in HFH was demonstrated with saxagliptin in SAVOR-TIMI, and with alogliptin in a subgroup of the EXAMINE study. No increase was seen in the TECOS study with sitagliptin. Further publications on heart failure events in these three studies have given conflicting results (47–49). Post-hoc analysis of SAVOR-TIMI showed the significant increase occurred in patients taking saxagliptin with no previous history of heart failure (2.3% vs 1.7%; HR, 1.3; p = 0.03). No significant difference in HFH was seen in patients with heart failure at baseline. In EXAMINE, heart failure was present in 1501 patients at baseline (28%), and pre-dated the index ACS event in approximately 60% of these patients. Post-hoc subgroup analysis of patients with no history of heart failure at baseline showed alogliptin was associated with an increased risk of HFH with 43 (2.2%) events in the alogliptin group compared with 24 (1.3%) events in the placebo group (HR,

1.76; p = 0.026). There was no significant difference seen for patients with heart failure at baseline. Further analysis of TECOS comparing subjects with heart failure at baseline showed no significant difference in HFH with 97 (7.4%) events in the sitagliptin group and 94 (7.0%) events in the placebo group (HR, 1.03; p = 0.86). Clinically it would be prudent to avoid saxagliptin or alogliptin in patients with previous heart failure, and to withdraw any DPP-4 inhibitor if a patient is hospitalized with heart failure.

When the EMPA-REG OUTCOME trial was published as well as reductions in atherosclerotic endpoints, there was a significant reduction in HFH. Some 10% of subjects at baseline were recorded as having clinical heart failure, but this was not characterized by biochemical or imaging modalities. The separation in HFH was seen early in the study. Post-hoc analysis of heart failure in EMPA-REG OUTCOME showed that consistent effects of empagliflozin were observed across subgroups defined by baseline characteristics, including patients with versus those without heart failure, and across categories of medications to treat diabetes and/or heart failure (50). Empagliflozin improved other heart failure outcomes, including hospitalization for or death from heart failure. The mechanism of the benefit is unknown, and several metabolic and hemodynamic hypotheses have been suggested. Studies have been started examining the use of SGLT-2 inhibitors in patients with chronic heart failure, with and without diabetes, with characterization of ejection fraction at baseline, to see if similar reductions in HFH would be obtained in a pure heart failure population (DAPA-HF and EMPEROR HF).

Similarly to empagliflozin in the EMPA-REG OUTCOME trial, canagliflozin showed reductions in atherosclerotic endpoints as well as a significant reduction in HFH in the CANVAS program (29). Some 14% of subjects at baseline were recorded as having clinical heart failure, but this was not characterized by biochemical or imaging modalities. The separation in HFH was seen early in the study similar to findings in EMPA-REG OUTCOME trial.

No significant effect, either beneficial or harmful, on HFH was seen with lixisenatide in ELIXA, liraglutide in LEADER, or semaglutide in SUSTAIN-6 (Table 39-3).

Conclusions

Hyperglycemia is a common occurrence in patients admitted with ACS, acute stroke, and acute heart failure, and is associated with a poor prognosis. Meta-analysis of studies using intensive insulin therapy following ACS and acute stroke has demonstrated no benefits, and in one study of insulin following ACS, there was an increase in mortality. There is a continuing need for large, prospective, randomized trials of intensive IV (and/or SC) insulin therapy following these common cardiovascular emergencies.

National guidelines for the management of hyperglycemia following ACS vary in recommendations (Table 39-2), so the clinician should adopt the relevant guideline for that area, and it would be helpful if this could be endorsed by acute physicians, hospitalists, cardiologists, and diabetologists. Many stroke guidelines do not make any recommendation on the management of hyperglycemia, so local discussion among key clinicians is also necessary. In the longer term, more intensive managment of hyperglycemia may reduce further myocardial infarctions and strokes, and some individual treatments may offer particular benefits. There is no evidence of benefit when these are started at the time of the acute event, and diabetes treatments should be reviewed when the patient is next seen by their diabetes care provider. However, the ADA 2018 treatment guidelines have now recommended that in patients with type 2 diabetes and established atherosclerotic CVD, glucose-lowering agents with proven CV benefit (currently empagliflozin, liraglutide and canagliflozin) should be preferentially added to lifestyle therapy and metformin when reasonable to do so (52). It is anticipated that the newly-approved semaglutide (which also has CVD benefits), will be be added to this list in future updates.

References

1 Emerging Risk Factors Collaboration. Diabetes mellitus, fasting blood glucose concentration, and risk of vascular disease: a collaborative meta-analysis of 102 prospective studies. *Lancet.* 2010;375: 2215–2222.

2 Rawshani A, Rawshani A, Franzen S, et al. Mortality and cardiovascular disease in type 1 and type 2 diabetes: Sweden. *N Engl J Med.* 2017;376:1407–1418.

3 Malmberg K for the DIGAMI (Diabetes mellitus, Insulin Glucose Infusion in Acute Myocardial Infarction) Study Group. Prospective randomised study of intensive insulin treatment on long-term survival after acute myocardial infarction in patients with diabetes mellitus. *BMJ.* 1997;314:1512–1515.

4 Ritsinger V, Malmberg K, Martensson A, et al. Intensified insulin-based glycaemic control after myocardial infarction: mortality during 20 year follow-up of the randomised Diabetes Mellitus Insulin Glucose Infusion in Acute Myocardial Infarction (DIGAMI 1) trial. *Lancet Diabetes Endocrinol.* 2014;2:627–633.

5 Malmberg K, Ryden L, Wedel H, et al. for the DIGAMI 2 Investigators. Intense metabolic control by means of insulin in patients with diabetes mellitus and acute myocardial infarction (DIGAMI 2): effects on mortality and morbidity. *Eur Heart J.* 2005;26:650–661.

6 Cheung NW, Wong VW, McLean M. The Hyperglycemia: Intensive Insulin Infusion in Infarction (HI-5) study. *Diabetes Care.* 2006;29:765–770.

7 Raz I, Wilson PWF, Strojek K, et al. Effects of prandial versus fasting glycemia on cardiovascular outcomes in type 2 diabetes:

the HEART2D trial. *Diabetes Care.* 2009;32:381–386.

8 de Mulder M, Umans VA, Cornel JH, et al. Intensive glucose regulation in hyperglycemic acute coronary syndrome: results of the randomized BIOMarker study to identify the acute risk of a coronary syndrome-2 (BIOMArCS-2) glucose trial. *JAMA Intern Med.* 2013;173:1896–1904.

9 Selker HP, Beshansky JR, Sheehan PR, et al. Effect of out-of-hospital administration of intravenous glucose, insulin, and potassium (GIK) in patients with suspected acute coronary syndromes: the IMMEDIATE randomized controlled trial. *JAMA.* 2012;307:1925–1933.

10 Chatterjee S, Sharma A, Lichstein E, Mukherjee D. Intensive glucose control in diabetics with an acute myocardial infarction does not improve mortality and increases risk of hypoglycaemia - a meta-regression analysis. *Current Vascular Pharmacology.* 2013;11: 100–104.

11 NICE. *Hyperglycaemia in Acute Coronary Syndromes.* Clinical guideline CG130. NICE. 2011. https://www.nice.org.uk/ Guidance/CG130.

12 SIGN 148. Acute coronary syndrome. A national clinical guideline. 2016. www.sign.ac.uk/assets/sign148.pdf

13 Ryden L, Grant PJ, Anker SD, et al. ESC guidelines on diabetes, pre-diabetes, and cardiovascular diseases developed in collaboration with the EASD. *Eur Heart J.* 2013;34:3035–3087.

14 Canadian Diabetes Association Clinical Guidelines Expert Committee. Management of acute coronary syndromes. *Can J Diabetes.* 2013;37:S119–S123.

15 Nissen SE, Wolski K. Effect of rosiglitazone on myocardial infarction and death from cardiovascular causes. *N Engl J Med.* 2007;356:2457–2471.

16 White WB, Cannon CP, Heller SR et al. for the EXAMINE investigators. Alogliptin after acute coronary syndrome in patients with type 2 diabetes. *N Engl J Med.* 2013;369;1327–1335.

17 Pfeffer MA, Clagett B, Diaz R, et al. for the ELIXA investigators. Lixisenatide in patients with type 2 diabetes and acute coronary syndrome. *N Engl J Med.* 2015;373:2247–2257.

18 UK Prospective Diabetes Study (UPDS) Group. Effect of intensive blood-glucose control with metformin on complications in overweight patients with type 2 diabetes (UKPDS 34). *Lancet.* 1998;352:854–865.

19 Kooy A, de Jager J, Lehert P, et al. Long-term effects of metformin on metabolism and microvascular and macrovascular disease in patients with type 2 diabetes. *Arch Intern Med.* 2009;169: 616–625.

20 Hong J, Zhang Y, Lai S, et al. on behalf of the SPREAD-DIMCAD investigators. Effects of metformin versus glipizide on cardiovascular outcomes in patients with type 2 diabetes and coronary artery disease. *Diabetes Care.* 2013;36:1304–1311.

21 Dormandy JA, Charbonnel B, Eckland DA, et al. on behalf of the PROactive investigators. Secondary prevention of macrovascular events in patients with type 2 diabetes in the PROactive Study (PROspective pioglitazone Clinical Trial in macroVascular Events): a randomised controlled trial. *Lancet.* 2005;36: 1279–1289.

22 Erdmann E, Dormandy JA, Charbonnel B, et al. on behalf of the PROActive investigators. The effect of pioglitazone on recurrent myocardial infarction in 2,455 patients with type 2 diabetes and previous myocardial infarction. *J Am Coll Cardiol.* 2007;49:1772–1780.

23 ORIGIN trial investigators. Basal insulin and cardiovascular and other outcomes in dysglycemia. *N Engl J Med.* 2012;367: 319–328.

24 Scirica BM, Bhatt DL, Brunwald E, et al. for the SAVOR-TIMI steering committee and investigators. Saxagliptin and cardiovascular outcomes in patients with type 2 diabetes mellitus. *N Engl J Med.* 2013;369:1317–1326.

25 Green JB, Bethel MA, Armstrong PW, et al. for the TECOS study group. Effect of

sitagliptin on cardiovascular outcomes in type 2 diabetes. *N Engl J Med*. 2015;373: 232–242.

26 Zinman B, Wanner C, Lachin JM, et al. for the EMPA-REG OUTCOME investigators. Empagliflozin, cardiovascular outcomes, and mortality in type 2 diabetes. *N Engl J Med*. 2015;373:2117–2128.

27 Marso SP, Daniels GH, Brown-Frandsen K, et al. on behalf of the LEADER Trial investigators. Liraglutide and cardiovascular outcomes in type 2 diabetes. *N Engl J Med*. 2016;375:311–322.

28 Marso SP, Bain SC, Consoli A, et al. for the SUSTAIN-6 investigators. Semaglutide and cardiovascular outcomes in patients with type 2 diabetes. *N Engl J Med*. 2016;375: 1834–1844.

29 Neal B, Perkovic V, Mahaffey KW, et al. for the CANVAS Program group. Canagliglozin and cardiovascular and renal events in type 2 diabetes. *N Engl J Med*. 2017. doi: 10.1056/NEJMoa1611925.

30 Marso SP, McGuire DK, Zinman B, et al. for the DEVOTE Study Group. Efficacy and safety of degludec versus glargine in type 2 diabetes. *N Engl J Med*. 2017. doi: 10.1056/NEJMoa1615692.

31 Diabetes Control and Complications Trial (DCCT) Research group. Effect of intensive diabetes management on macrovascular events and risk factors in the Diabetes Control and Complications Trial. *Am J Cardiol*. 1995;75:894–903.

32 UK Prospective Diabetes Study (UKPDS) Group. Intensive blood-glucose control with sulphonylureas or insulin compared with conventional treatment and risk of complications in patients with type 2 diabetes (UKPDS 33). *Lancet*. 1998;352: 837–853.

33 ADVANCE Collaborative Group. Intensive blood glucose control and vascular outcomes in patients with type 2 diabetes. *N Engl J Med*. 2008;358:2560–2572.

34 Action to Control Cardiovascular Risk in Diabetes Study Group. Effects of intensive glucose lowering in type 2 diabetes. *N Engl J Med*. 2008;358:2545–2559.

35 Duckworth W, Abraira C, Moritz T, et al. for the VADT investigators. Glucose

control and vascular complications in veterans with type 2 diabetes. *N Engl J Med*. 2009;360:129–139.

36 Turnbull FM, Abraira C, Anderson RJ, et al. Intensive glucose control and macrovascular outcomes in type 2 diabetes. *Diabetologia*. 2009;52:2288–2298.

37 The DCCT/EDIC Study Research group. Intensive diabetes treatment and cardiovascular outcomes in type 1 diabetes: the DCCT/EDIC study 30-year follow-up. *Diabetes Care*. 2016;39:686–693.

38 Holman RR, Paul SK, Bethel MA, Mathews DR, Neil HAW. 10-year follow-up of intensive glucose control in type 2 diabetes. *N Engl J Med*. 2008;359:1577–1589.

39 Hayward RA, Reaven PD, Wiitala WI, et al. for the VADT investigators. Follow-up of glycemic control and cardiovascular outcomes in type 2 diabetes. *N Engl J Med*. 2015;372:2197–2206.

40 Zoungas S, Chalmers J, Neal B, et al. for the ADVANCE-ON Collaborative Group. Follow-up of blood-pressure lowering and glucose control in type 2 diabetes. *N Engl J Med*. 2014;371:1392–1406.

41 Accord Study Group Writing Committee. 9-year effects of 3.7 years of intensive glycemic control on cardiovascular outcomes. *Diabetes Care*. 2016;39: 701–708.

42 Belloliol MF, Gilmore RM, Ganti L. Insulin for glycaemic control in acute iscahemic stroke (rview). *Cochrane Database Syst Rev*. 2014;1:cd005346.

43 Bruno A, Durkalski VL, Hall CE, et al. The Stroke Hyperglycemia Insulin Network Effort (SHINE) trial protocol: a randomized, blinded, efficacy trial of standard vs. intensive hyperglycemia management in acute stroke. *Int J Stroke*. 2014;9:246–251.

44 Wilcox R, Bousser M-J, Bettridge J, et al. for the PROactive investigators. Effects of pioglitazone in patients with type 2 diabetes with and without previous stroke. *Stroke*. 2007;38:856–873.

45 Kernan WN, et al. for the IRIS Trial investigators. Pioglitazone after ischemic stroke or transient ischemic attack. *N Engl J Med*. 2016;374:1321–1331.

46 Castagno D, Baird-Gunning J, Jhund PS, et al. Intensive glycemic control has no impact on the risk of heart failure in type 2 diabetic patients: evidence from a 37,229 patient meta-analysis. *Am Heart J.* 2011;162:938–948.

47 Scirica BM, Braunwald E, Raz I, et al. Heart failure, saxagliptin, and diabetes mellitus: observations from the SAVOR-TIMI 53 randomized trial. *Circulation.* 2014;130:1579–1588.

48 Zannad F, Cannon CP, Cushman WC, et al. Heart failure and mortality outcomes in patients with type 2 diabetes taking alogliptin versus placebo in EXAMINE: a multicentre, randomised, double-blind trial. *Lancet.* 2015;385:2067–2076.

49 McGuire DK, Van de Werf F, Armstrong PW, et al. Association between sitagliptin use and heart failure hospitalization and related outcomes in type 2 diabetes mellitus: secondary analysis of a randomized clinical trial. *JAMA Cardiol.* 2016; 1:126–135.

50 Fitchett D, Zinmann B, Wanner C, et al. on behalf of the EMPA-REG OUTCOME trial investigators. Heart failure outcomes with empaglflozin in patients with type 2 diabetes at high cardiovascular risk: results of the EMPA-REG OUTCOME trial. *Eur Heart J.* 2016;37:1526–1534.

51 European Society for Cardiology/European Association for Study of Diabetes: ESC/EASD. 2013. https://www.escardio.org/Guidelines/Clinical-Practice-Guidelines/Diabetes-Pre-Diabetes

52 American Diabetes Association. 9. Cardiovascular Disease and Risk Management. *Diabetes Care.* 2018;41(Suppl 1):S86–S104.

53 Cefalu WT, Kaul S, Gerstein HC, et al. Cardiovascular Outcomes Trials in Type 2 Diabetes: Where Do We Go From Here? Reflections From a Diabetes Care Editors' Expert Forum. *Diabetes Care.* 2018;41:14–31.

40

Acute Diabetic Foot

Glenn Matfin

Key Points

- Foot problems are among the most common and feared complication of diabetes mellitus and are now the leading diabetes-related cause of hospitalization, as well as the major cause of lower extremity amputations.
- Diabetic foot problems have a significant financial impact on healthcare systems, increased in-hospital occupancy and length of stay.
- The UK 2016 National Diabetes Inpatient Audit (NaDIA) revealed that almost 1 in 10 inpatients (9%) with diabetes had active foot disease on admission. Almost 1 in 20 inpatients was admitted directly for active foot disease (4%). Worryingly, 1 in 75 patients with diabetes developed a new foot lesion during their in-hospital stay (1.4%).
- All persons with diabetes should be screened for risk of foot problems on at least an annual basis: those with risk factors require regular podiatry, patient education, and instruction in foot self-care
- The most common foot complication is skin ulceration, which is usually secondary to diabetes-related peripheral neuropathy (with loss of protective sensation) and less often related to peripheral arterial disease, or both.
- A diabetic foot ulcer can be defined as a localized injury to the skin and/or underlying tissue, below the ankle, in a person with diabetes. The lifetime risk of a person with diabetes developing a foot ulcer is 10–25%.
- Up to 85% of lower limb amputations are preceded by foot ulcers.
- Persons with diabetes who have an amputation have a 5-year survival rate of only 30%. Most of the excess morbidity and mortality in these patients is related to cardiovascular disease, and emphasizes the need for good diabetes and cardiovascular risk management.
- Most foot ulcers should heal if pressure is removed from the ulcer site, the arterial circulation is sufficient, and infection is managed and treated aggressively.
- More recently, treatment with the glucose-lowering sodium-glucose co-transporter-2 (SGLT-2) inhibitor, canagliflozin, has been associated with an increase in lower limb amputations (usually affecting the mid-foot and toes) and now has a FDA "black box" warning in the USA. This may be a SGLT-2 class effect but more information is needed (although empagliflozin date are reassuring). Prescribers should consider stopping therapy with SGLT-2 inhibitors if patients with diabetes develop significant foot complications such as infections or diabetic foot ulcers.
- Any person with diabetes with a warm unilateral swollen foot without ulceration should be presumed to have an acute Charcot neuroarthropathy (CN) until proven otherwise.

Endocrine and Metabolic Medical Emergencies: A Clinician's Guide, Second Edition. Edited by Glenn Matfin.
© 2018 John Wiley & Sons Ltd. Published 2018 by John Wiley & Sons Ltd.

- The general principles for in-hospital foot care in people with diabetes should apply to all admissions, not just those with active foot disease. These measures include taking a specific foot history and an inspection of the feet, looking for evidence of neuropathy, ischemia, ulceration, inflammation and/or infection, deformity, or CN.
- The feet of persons with diabetes should be inspected daily during the hospital stay and new problems that are identified should be managed in conjunction with the specialist diabetic foot multidisciplinary team (or equivalent).
- Appropriate ongoing education of patients and healthcare providers about the importance of prevention and early recognition of diabetes-related foot problems is critical.

Introduction

Foot problems are among the most common and feared complication of diabetes mellitus and are now the leading diabetes-related cause of hospitalization, as well as the major cause of lower extremity amputations. Diabetic foot problems have a significant financial impact on healthcare systems, with increased in-hospital occupancy and length of stay. It has been estimated that ~£1 in every £150 spent by the National Health Service (NHS) in England is on diabetes-related foot disease (1), although more recent figures suggest it could be an even higher proportion costing £1 billion overall (total NHS budget £120 billion) (2). It has also been estimated that worldwide, foot ulcers develop in 9.1 million to 26.1 million people with diabetes annually; and that a diabetes-related amputation of the lower limb occurs every 30 seconds (3).

The most common foot complication is skin ulceration, which is usually secondary to diabetes-related peripheral neuropathy (with loss of protective sensation) and less often related to peripheral arterial disease (PAD), or both. A diabetic foot ulcer (DFU) can be defined as a localized injury to the skin and/or underlying tissue, below the ankle, in a person with diabetes. The lifetime risk of a person with diabetes developing a foot ulcer is 15–25%, although when additional data are considered, between 19% and 34% of persons with diabetes are likely to be affected (4).

About half of DFUs are clinically infected at presentation, and these wounds are at substantially increased risk of various adverse outcomes. Infection is best defined as an invasion and multiplication of microorganisms in host tissues that induce a host inflammatory response, usually followed by tissue destruction. Infection is usually the final precipitating cause of lower extremity amputations, the risk of which is 23 times higher in persons with diabetes than those without. Over 85% of lower extremity amputations in persons with diabetes are preceded by foot ulceration (4). Overall, persons with diabetes who have an amputation have a 5-year survival rate of only 30%, whereas those on renal replacement therapy have 74% mortality just 2 years after amputation (2,4). Most of the excess morbidity and mortality in these patients is related to cardiovascular (CV) disease, and emphasizes the need for good diabetes and CV risk management (5). Another serious, but less common, complication of diabetic neuropathy is Charcot neuroarthropathy (CN), which can lead to foot deformities and ulceration.

The general principles for in-hospital foot care in people with diabetes should apply to all admissions, not just those with active foot disease. These measures include taking a specific foot history and an inspection of the feet, looking for evidence of neuropathy, ischemia, ulceration, inflammation, and/or infection, deformity, or CN (6). It is important to take the shoes, socks, and any dressings off the feet to inspect any underlying wounds, ensuring that pressure areas are healthy. The feet should be inspected daily during the hospital stay and new problems that are identified should be managed ideally in conjunction with the specialist diabetic foot multidisciplinary team (which should include timely access to podiatrist, diabetologist, vascular and orthopedic surgeon, interventional radiologist, tissue viability nurse, infectious disease/microbiologist, diabetes educator/nurse, and orthotist). The acute diabetic foot includes any foot wound present on admission; any newly acquired foot wound picked up on daily whole foot checks (see Table 40-1, for an example of daily foot assessment for all patients with diabetes during hospitalization); suspected CN; any unexplained erythema, discoloration or swelling; and a cold pale foot (Figure 40-1).

The UK 2016 National Diabetes Inpatient Audit (NaDIA) revealed that almost 1 in 10 inpatients (9%) with diabetes had active foot disease on admission (7). Almost 1 in 20 inpatients was admitted directly for active foot disease (4%). Worryingly, 1 in 75 patients with diabetes developed a new foot lesion during their in-hospital stay (1.4%).

Understanding the management of these severe diabetic foot complications is key, as most foot infections and other problems are preventable, or at least treatable (8).

Prevention of Diabetes Foot Complications

Vascular complications are a major cause of morbidity and mortality in diabetic patients. These result from interactions between systemic metabolic abnormalities such as hyperglycemia, dyslipidemia, genetic and epigenetic modulators, and local tissue responses to toxic metabolites. In addition, other factors such as smoking are important risk factors.

Macrovascular complications, such as PAD, and microvascular complications, such as peripheral and autonomic neuropathy (9), are common, and both are important in the pathophysiology of diabetic foot problems (Figure 40-2). For example, motor nerve dysfunction results in disturbances in posture and balance that can lead to increased pressures within the foot (Figure 40-3); loss of

sensory perception results in inability to feel pain, thus inhibiting any preventative action from being taken; loss of autonomic function in the lower limbs leads to loss of sweating and hence dry skin that can predispose to infection; and autonomic dysregulation can alter microvascular flow leading to arteriovenous "shunting," with resultant tissue hypoxia and paradoxically warm feet. The other major pathology in addition to neuropathy and ischemia is infection. Infection can proceed rapidly and the end-stage of tissue death is quickly reached. Thus, the window of opportunity for intervention is limited and is often missed (10).

Optimal management of glycemic control, hypertension, dyslipidemia, smoking cessation, weight management, use of antiplatelet agents, and addressing other modifiable risk factors are important to prevent or slow any progression of these and other vascular complications (10,11).

More recently, treatment with the glucose-lowering sodium-glucose co-transporter-2 (SGLT-2) inhibitor, canagliflozin, has been associated with an increase in lower limb amputations (usually affecting the mid-foot and toes) in two large clinical trials. This may be a SGLT-2 class effect but more information is needed (although empagliflozin data is reassuring). The canagliflozin-prescribing information now has a FDA "black box" warning regarding this risk. Amputations occurred about twice as often as in the control group. The risk for lower limb amputations occurred in 3–7.5 patients per 1000 over a year's time. Prescribers should consider stopping therapy with this agent (and likely other SGLT-2 inhibitors if used) in patients with diabetes who develop significant foot complications such as infection or DFU.

Screening

Most foot complications are potentially preventable. The first step in prevention is identifying the "at-risk" population during the comprehensive foot evaluation. This should be performed at least annually in all

Table 40-1 Generic example of UK in-hospital daily foot assessment chart for persons with diabetes

	Affix patient label here First name: Last name: Hospital Number: NHS Number: DOB:
Ward: Consultant:	

This chart is a
DAILY FOOT ASSESSMENT for <u>all</u> Patients with Diabetes

ON ADMISSION, RN to perform **Ipswich Touch Test** to check for loss of sensation

IPSWICH TOUCH TEST

- Ask patient to close their eyes
- Confirm right & left sides with patient
- Inform patient that you will touch their toes and they should say 'left' or 'right' when they feel the touch
- VERY LIGHTLY touch tips of toes for 1-2 seconds, as illustrated in the sequence shown
- Toe sequence = 1.right big, 2.right little, 3.left big, 4.left little, 5.right middle, 6. Left middle
- Record the results by circling **Y** if touch was felt and **N** if not

Two or more negatives = abnormal sensation
= HIGH RISK
DATE TEST COMPLETED...............................

CARE PLAN
1. **Nurse on Airwave** if required
2. **Reduce pressure** of feet resting on floor, stool or end of bed
3. **Daily foot inspection,** include checking between the toes & underneath the feet
4. **Use heel protectors,** BUT if any pressure damage to heels offload using Repose boots or pillows
5. **Update whole foot status** on check box (below). DO THIS DAILY, plus Waterlow
6. **Emollient** - twice daily use of urea-based heel balm to prevent drying & cracking of feet
7. **Deterioration** – consider if this is an acute Diabetic foot problem and refer if necessary.

If acute foot problem noted please refer

Two or more negatives = sensation is abnormal.
PLEASE FOLLOW CARE PLAN

Subject's right foot, your left side

Subject's left foot, your right side

The foot is **HIGH RISK** if <u>any</u> of the following apply, therefore follow **CARE PLAN**

One or less negatives = sensation is normal

Previous ulcer / amputation	☐
Deformity such as Charcot	☐
Known peripheral artery disease	☐
Cognitive impairment	☐
Impaired consciousness	☐
Stroke	☐
Renal Failure / Dialysis	☐
Visual impairment	☐
Known or suspected neuropathy	☐

The ACUTE diabetic foot SHOULD BE referred IMMEDIATELY to the Diabetes Foot team. Contact details overleaf. (see Ward Referral for Diabetes Podiatry form for criteria)

INSPECT FEET DAILY and update status (below)

EVERY DAY complete **FOOT STATUS** below. This is in addition to the Waterlow & Skin Bundle

WHOLE FOOT STATUS – can be completed by nurse or HCA

Circle below to show whether feet are healthy or unhealthy and then initial. If unhealthy, contact Tissue Viability & Podiatry

DATE:																
Healthy	R	L	R	L	R	L	R	L	R	L	R	L	R	L
Unhealthy	R	L	R	L	R	L	R	L	R	L	R	L	R	L

Unhealthy = discoloration, red, mottled, black, cracked skin

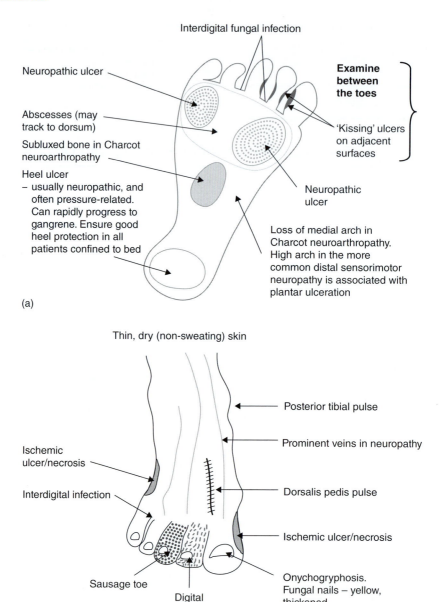

Interdigital fungal infection

Neuropathic ulcer

Examine between the toes

Abscesses (may track to dorsum)

Subluxed bone in Charcot neuroarthropathy

Heel ulcer
– usually neuropathic, and often pressure-related. Can rapidly progress to gangrene. Ensure good heel protection in all patients confined to bed

'Kissing' ulcers on adjacent surfaces

Neuropathic ulcer

Loss of medial arch in Charcot neuroarthropathy. High arch in the more common distal sensorimotor neuropathy is associated with plantar ulceration

(a)

Thin, dry (non-sweating) skin

Posterior tibial pulse

Prominent veins in neuropathy

Ischemic ulcer/necrosis

Interdigital infection

Dorsalis pedis pulse

Ischemic ulcer/necrosis

Sausage toe

Digital gangrene

Onychogryphosis. Fungal nails – yellow, thickened

(b)

Figure 40-1 Clinical features of the neuropathic and ischemic foot, and associated lesions. (a) Plantar view. (b) Dorsal view. Remove dressings. Document all findings including completing daily foot inspection chart (Table 40-1). In patients with extensive ulceration, document with medical photography as soon as possible. Reproduced with permission from John Wiley & Sons, Ltd.

adults with diabetes. Detailed foot assessment may occur more often in "at-risk" patients. In addition, all patients with diabetes should have their feet inspected at every visit (including inpatient admission). The risk of ulcers or amputation is increased in people with the following risk factors: poor glycemic control; peripheral neuropathy with loss of protective sensation (LOPS); cigarette smoking; foot deformities; Charcot foot; pre-ulcerative callus or corn; PAD; history of foot ulcer; previous amputation; visual impairment; and diabetic kidney disease especially patients on dialysis (6,9,10).

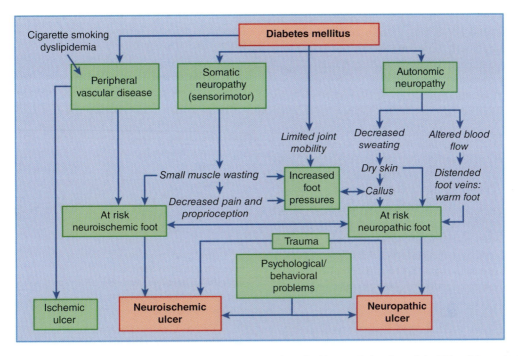

Figure 40-2 Pathways to foot ulceration in diabetes. Reproduced with permission from John Wiley & Sons, Ltd.

Foot examination should include general inspection of skin integrity, and musculoskeletal deformities. Vascular assessment should include inspection and palpation of pedal pulses, capillary refill, foot

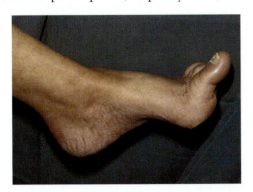

Figure 40-3 High-risk neuropathic foot demonstrating high-arch, prominent metatarsal heads, clawing of toes, and callus under first metatarsal head. The characteristic clawing seen in motor nerve dysfunction is due to the differential loss of strength between the extensor muscles and the flexor muscles leading to areas of high plantar pressures (leading to callus and increased risk of ulcer) and an increased risk of the dorsal aspects of the toes rubbing against the inside of the toe box of a shoe. Reproduced with permission from John Wiley & Sons, Ltd.

temperature, and ankle-brachial pressure index (as indicated). Neurological exam is designed to identify LOPS rather than early neuropathy. LOPS (large-fiber function) indicates the presence of distal sensorimotor polyneuropathy and is a risk factor for diabetic foot ulceration and amputation. The 10-g monofilament is the most useful test to diagnose LOPS. This should be done on four sites on each foot. At least one other assessment (pinprick or temperature [small-fiber function], vibration or ankle reflexes [large-fiber function]) should be performed (6,9,10). Any of the five tests can be used to identify LOPS, although at least two of these should be performed at screening exam. One or more abnormal tests would suggest LOPS, while at least two normal (and no abnormal) tests would rule out LOPS. In the UK, the Ipswich touch test is widely used (Table 40-1).

Management of High-Risk Patients

All patients with diabetes and particularly those with high-risk foot conditions (i.e., history of ulcer or amputation, deformity, LOPS, and/or PAD) and their families should be educated about risk factors and appropriate management. Appropriate footwear (including orthotist review) and footwear behaviors at home (and also in the hospital setting) should be outlined. Regular podiatry review as needed is important and clear instructions on how and when to access urgent/emergency foot care is critical. The recent UK National Diabetes Foot Care Audit (NDFA) 2014–2016 (2), which captured data on 11,000 people with acute foot ulcers, showed that one-third of ulcer episodes self-referred for expert assessment. Unfortunately, two-fifths (40%) of ulcer episodes referred by a clinician (i.e., those patients who did not self-refer) had an interval of two or more weeks to first expert assessment (2).

Classification and Diagnosis

Over the past three decades, several schemes for classification of the most common diabetic foot complications have been published. In 2004, guidelines specifically devoted to diabetic foot infections (DFI), including an infection-related classification scheme, were published by multidisciplinary panels of experts from the Infectious Diseases Society of America (IDSA) and the International Working Group on the Diabetic Foot (IWGDF); IDSA were updated in 2012 and the IWGDF (the "infection" part of the **PEDIS** classification: **P**erfusion, **E**xtent, **D**epth, **I**nfection and **S**ensation) in 2016 (12,13). These guidelines have been validated in several studies. The IDSA/IWGDF scheme for defining infection and classifying its severity is shown in Table 40-2. In addition, the IDSA guidelines provided answers to 10 key questions (Table 40-3), along with the evidence supporting the recommendations and a grading of the quality and strength of the recommendations. A key feature is that DFIs are diagnosed clinically, based on the presence of clinical signs and symptoms of inflammation (i.e., redness, warmth, swelling, pain or tenderness) or purulent secretions, not by the results of cultures of wounds. For stage 1 (uninfected)

Table 40-2 IDSA/IWGDF diabetic foot infection severity classification scheme (13). Reproduced with permission from John Wiley & Sons, Ltd.

Clinical description	IDSA	IWGDF
Uninfected		
Wound without purulence and no systemic or local symptoms or signs of infection	Uninfected	1
Infected		
Infection is limited to skin or superficial subcutaneous tissues: ≥2 manifestations of inflammation (purulence or erythema, pain, tenderness, warmth, or induration); any cellulitis or erythema extends ≤2 cm around ulcer*, and no local complications or systemic illness	Mild	2
Infection involving structures deeper than the skin and subcutaneous tissues. Patient who is systemically well and metabolically stable but has ≥2 cm erythema*; lymphangitis spread beneath fascia; deep tissue abscess; gangrene; muscle, tendon, joint, or bone involvement	Moderate	3
Any foot infection with the systemic inflammatory response syndrome (SIRS) manifested by ≥2 of the following: • Temperature >38°C (100.4°F) or <36°C (96.8°F) • Heart rate >90 bpm • Respiratory rate >20 breaths/minute or PaCO$_2$ <32 mmHg • White blood cell count >12 × 10^9/L or <4 × 10^9/L or >10% immature cells (bands)	Severe	4

Systemic toxicity may also present with anorexia, chills, hypotension, confusion, vomiting, acidosis, hyperglycemia, and/or azotemia. The presence of critical limb ischemia may increase the level of severity

*In any direction, from the rim of the wound.

Table 40-3 The 10 key questions posed and answered in the IDSA diabetic foot infection (DFI) guidelines (12). Reproduced with permission from Oxford University Press.

I. **In which diabetic patients with a foot wound should I suspect infection, and how should I classify it?**
Every foot wound in a diabetic patient should be considered as possibly infected, particularly if the patient is at high risk due to the presence of peripheral neuropathy or arterial disease.

The classification by the IDSA/IWGDF (see Table 40-2) defines and rates the severity of infection.

II. **How should I assess a patient presenting with a DFI?**
Clinicians should assess the patient at three different levels: first, the patient as a whole; then the affected limb; and, finally, the wound. Assess for neuropathy, vasculopathy, and infection.

III. **When and from whom should I request a consultation for a patient with a DFI?**
Outpatients and inpatients with a DFI should benefit from a multidisciplinary foot care team. If not available, the clinicians in charge of the patient should attempt to coordinate obtaining and deploying the advice of all the key specialists required.

The UK NICE diabetic foot care pathway recommends that all inpatients with diabetes should be assessed within 24 hours for foot issues, and, if found, should be referred for prompt review by a multidisciplinary foot care team within 24 hours (8,13).

IV. **Which patients with a diabetic foot infection should I hospitalize, and what criteria should they meet before I discharge them?**
Hospitalization should be considered in case of severe infection, moderate infection and complications (e.g., peripheral artery disease) and for those who cannot or would not comply with an outpatient treatment regimen.

V. **When and how should I obtain specimen(s) for culture from a patient with a diabetic foot wound?**
Only for wounds presenting evidence of infection. Clinicians should obtain appropriate specimens for aerobic and anaerobic culture. The samples should be taken before starting empirical antibiotic therapy. After careful cleaning and wound debridement, obtain the sample from deep tissue by biopsy or curettage or by aspiration of purulent secretions, if at all possible.

VI. **How should I initially select, and when should I modify, an antibiotic regimen for a DFI?**
Select an empiric regimen based on the likeliest pathogens and known local antibiotic sensitivity patterns and consider modifying it based on the clinical response to treatment and the results of culture and sensitivity tests.

The choice of an empiric antibiotic regimen should also be based on the severity of the infection (Table 40-4) and other factors (Table 40-5).

VII. **When should I consider imaging studies to evaluate a DFI, and which should I select?**
Order plain radiographs for all patients with a new DFI to look for bony abnormalities, soft tissue gas, or radio-opaque foreign bodies. Advanced imaging tests may be needed in some instances, such as MRI, SPECT/CT and PET.

VIII. **How should I diagnose and treat osteomyelitis of the foot in a patient with diabetes?**
In any infected, deep, or large foot ulcer, particularly if the lesion is chronic or overlies a bony prominence, consider the possibility of osteomyelitis. When a definitive diagnosis of osteomyelitis is required, clinicians should obtain a bone specimen for microbiological and histopathological evaluation. Treating osteomyelitis almost always requires antibiotic therapy, which may be effective alone but is often combined with at least some surgical resection of necrotic and infected bone.

IX. **In which patients with a DFI should I consider surgical intervention, and what type of procedure may be appropriate?**
Many DFI require some type of surgical procedure and a surgeon should evaluate most moderate, and all severe (especially potentially limb-threatening, see Table 40-4), DFI, if possible. Emergency amputation is rarely needed except in life-threatening infections or with extensive tissue necrosis. An elective amputation may be appropriate in several situations, such as irreversible loss of limb function, recurrence of the wound despite adequate preventive management, or the need for an unacceptably prolonged or intensive hospital management.

X. **What types of wound care techniques and dressings are appropriate for diabetic foot wounds?**
Adequate management of a wound should include proper cleansing, followed by debridement of callus and necrotic tissue and pressure offloading.

severity, it is important to rule-out other causes of an inflammatory response of skin such as trauma, gout, acute CN, fracture, thrombosis and venous stasis (13).

Other classification systems are available including SINBAD and Wagner score system. SINBAD is recommended by the UK National Institute for Health and Care Excellence (NICE) (8). Ulcer severity is recorded using the SINBAD scoring system, which scores an ulcer between 0 (least severe) and 6 (most severe) depending on how many of the six SINBAD elements are present. The six **SINBAD** elements are: **S**ite (on hindfoot) – ulcer penetrates the hindfoot (rear of the foot); **I**schemia – impaired circulation in the foot; **N**europathy – LOPS in the foot; **B**acterial infection – signs of bacterial infection of the foot (e.g., redness, swelling, heat, discharge); **A**rea (≥ 1 cm^2) – ulcer covers a large surface area (1 cm^2 or more); and **D**epth (to tendon or bone) – ulcer penetrates to tendon or bone. An ulcer with a SINBAD score of 3 or above is classed as a severe ulcer. An ulcer with a SINBAD score of less than 3 is classed as a less severe ulcer. In the recent UK National Diabetes Foot Care Audit (NDFA) 2014–2016 (2), almost half (46%) of ulcer episodes were graded severe (SINBAD score ≥ 3) at first expert assessment.

Management of Diabetic Foot Infections

Evaluation

Clinicians assessing a patient presenting with a DFI should consider the problem at three levels: (a) the whole patient (e.g., cognitive, metabolic and fluid status); (b) the affected limb (e.g, presence of neuropathy and vascular insufficiency); and, finally, (c) the wound. The clinician should measure the vital signs, palpate for pedal pulses, check for peripheral neuropathy and debride and probe any open wounds. Special attention should be paid to detecting crepitus, bullae, new onset tenderness or anesthesia, rapidly advancing cellulitis or gangrenous tissue (Table 40-4 and Figure 40-4). The presence of any of these findings should prompt rapid

Table 40-4 Signs of a possibly imminently limb-threatening infection (IDSA guidelines 2012 [12]) with some examples demonstrated in Figure 40-4. Reproduced with permission from Oxford University Press.

- Evidence of systemic inflammatory response syndrome (SIRS)
- Rapid progression of infection
- Extensive necrosis or gangrene
- Crepitus on examination or tissue gas on imaging
- Extensive ecchymoses or petechiae
- Bullae, especially hemorrhagic
- New onset wound anesthesia
- Pain out of proportion to clinical findings
- Recent loss of neurologic function
- Critical limb ischemia
- Extensive soft tissue loss
- Extensive bony destruction, especially midfoot/hindfoot
- Failure of infection to improve with appropriate therapy

In clinical settings in which advanced healthcare is not available, lesser degrees of infection severity may make an infection limb-threatening.

consultation with an experienced foot surgeon. In addition to basic hematology and blood chemistry tests, virtually all patients with a foot wound should have a plain radiograph of the foot to look for the presence of gas, a foreign body or bone lesions. Where clinical circumstances or the findings on plain x-ray suggest a more sensitive or specific imaging test is needed, magnetic resonance imaging (MRI) is generally best (14). Typical indications for MRI of the diabetic foot include: suspicion of deep infection (e.g., necrotizing fasciitis, deep abscess); as an aid to diagnosing CN; establishing the extent of osteomyelitis when plain X-ray is equivocal or even negative; and when trying to diagnose mid-foot and metatarsal fractures that are not clear-cut on plain X-ray.

Classifying the severity of a DFI is important as it helps determine which patients may require hospitalization and broad-spectrum, intravenous (IV) antibiotic therapy, which is usually required for severe infections but rarely for mild (or many moderate) infections. DFIs also may require inpatient management when they are associated with critical limb ischemia, have not responded to

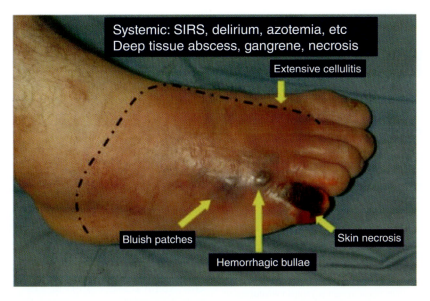

Figure 40-4 Diabetic foot infection with rapidly spreading soft tissue infection demonstrating characteristics of a serious soft tissue infection (Table 40-4) requiring urgent surgical exploration.

outpatient therapy or when social or psychological issues do not allow management in the outpatient setting. A severe DFI requires rapid evaluation (especially for vascular status), attention to any metabolic disorders and consideration for appropriate surgical procedures. Similarly, the presence of a deep soft tissue abscess or osteomyelitis also requires surgical evaluation.

Multidisciplinary Teams and Clinical Pathways

Early and continued care provided by a multidisciplinary team has been repeatedly shown to be associated with better outcomes in inpatient, as well as outpatient, settings and to reduce likelihood of major lower extremity amputation. The key criterion for membership is less the specific specialty of the members than their expertise and interest (6, 15). Multidisciplinary teams meeting together at the bedside may be optimal, but when this is not possible teams may be set up to communicate by telemedicine, teleconference, or email (15). Several recent DFI guidelines address the critical role of multidisciplinary teams, which have, unfortunately, largely been established only

in large hospitals in resource-rich countries (12,16,17). However, even in resource-rich countries the existence and appropriate referral to multidisciplinary foot teams may be deficient. For example, in the UK 2016 National Diabetes Inpatient Audit (NaDIA), despite the fact that inpatient multidisciplinary foot teams lead to better outcomes, almost one quarter of hospital sites involved in the audit did not have a multidisciplinary foot team. In addition, in defiance of the national NICE guidelines on diabetic foot clinical care pathway (8), fewer than one-third (30%) of inpatients with diabetes had a specific diabetic foot exam within 24 hours (Table 40-1). Despite these undesirable deficits in care, having a robust diabetic foot care pathway with clear antibiotic protocols in place enables the majority of patients in the hospital setting to get immediate appropriate treatment with a clear plan of action.

Antibiotic Therapy

Clinically uninfected wounds do not need to be cultured, as there is no evidence that treating colonization with antibiotics will improve wound healing or prevent infection. Infected wounds, however, virtually always

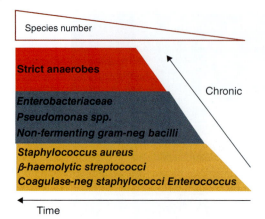

Figure 40-5 Schematic diagram showing how the microbiology of the DFU develops over time. The colonizing bacterial species are dependent on the chronicity of the ulcer and the age of the wound. Species numbers increase resulting in the evolution from a monomicrobial to a polymicrobial community (18). Reproduced with permission from John Wiley & Sons, Ltd.

require antibiotic therapy. Effective DFI treatment requires an understanding of the formation and composition of the DFU microbiota (i.e., bacteria associated with infection) (18). Obtaining a tissue sample for culture from any clinically infected wound, preferably before initiating empirical antibiotic therapy, is a crucial step toward ensuring an appropriate agent is selected. Wound specimens should be taken only after careful cleaning and debriding. Specimens of deep tissue obtained by biopsy or curettage, or aspirations of purulent secretions are more apt to grow the true pathogens and less likely to yield colonizing microorganisms. Swabs should be avoided (12). Blood cultures are rarely positive, except in patients with evidence of systemic sepsis.

The choice of empiric antibiotic(s) should be based on the severity of the infection, consideration of the most likely pathogens (Figure 40-5) (18), and local knowledge of their probable antibiotic susceptibility pattern (Table 40-5). Additional considerations include whether or not the patient has had any recent antibiotic therapy, if he has any allergies or comorbidities, which agents have been shown to be effective in DFI, cost and convenience of the drugs and any formulary restrictions. Suggested guidance on selecting antibiotic therapy is shown in Table 40-6. For a patient with a mild or moderate DFI, who has not had any prior recent antibiotic treatment, empirically selecting an oral agent targeting only aerobic gram-positive cocci (especially *Staphylococcus aureus* or streptococci) is usually sufficient. When the infection is chronic, or the patient has been treated with antimicrobials, aerobic gram-negative organisms often join the gram-positives. In cases of severe infection, empirical antibiotic therapy should be administrated parenterally and should be broad-spectrum, covering staphylococci, streptococci and commonly reported gram-negatives. Obligate anaerobes are almost always part of a mixed infection and usually one accompanied by gangrene or ischemia. These patients should be referred emergently to a multidisciplinary diabetic foot team (or equivalent) (10).

Initial empiric antibiotic choices may need to be adapted based on the results of culture and sensitivity tests. If the patient is clinically responding, it may not be necessary to cover all isolates, especially relatively avirulent organisms (e.g., coagulase-negative staphylococci or enterococci) isolated from a suboptimal wound specimen. The clinician should attempt to narrow unnecessarily broad-spectrum therapy whenever possible and consider switching from parenteral to oral therapy when the patient's general clinical condition and wound infection have improved. Antibiotic therapy need only be given until resolution of the infectious signs and symptoms and not prolonged until the complete healing of the wound. The usual duration needed for soft tissue infection is 1 to 2 weeks (13).

Surgical Interventions

Surgical procedures are needed for most severe infections and for many moderate and some mild infections. These may range from minor bedside debridement or incision and drainage, performed at the bedside or in the clinic, to major operative procedures (e.g., drainage of abscess, bone resection) that are done in the operating theater. Surgery

Table 40-5 Factors that may influence the choice of an antibiotic regimen for diabetic foot infections (specific agents, route of administration and duration of therapy) from IWGDF guidelines 2016 (13). Reproduced with permission from John Wiley & Sons, Ltd.

Infection-related	Pathogen-related	Patient-related	Drug-related
Clinical severity of the infection (Table 40-2)	Likelihood of non-gram-positive cocci etiologic agent(s)	Allergies to antibiotics	Safety profile (frequency and severity of adverse effects)
History of antibiotic therapy within previous 3 months	History of colonization or infection with multi-drug-resistant organisms (MDROs)	Impaired immunological status	Drug interactions potential
Presence of bone infection (presumed or proven)	Local rates of antibiotic resistance	Patient treatment preferences	Frequency of dosing
		Patient adherence to therapy	Formulary availability/restrictions
		Renal or hepatic insufficiency	Cost considerations (acquisition and administration)
		Impaired gastrointestinal absorption	Approval for indication
		Arterial insufficiency in affected limb	Likelihood of inducing *C. difficile* disease or antibiotic resistance
		Exposure to environment with high risk of MDROs or unusual pathogens	Published efficacy data

should not be delayed in cases of life- or limb-threatening infections, such as extensive soft tissue necrosis or gas gangrene. Consider a surgical exploration when there are systemic signs of infection that are not responding, or there is local evidence suggesting a deep infection. All wounds require daily inspection and some will need serial debridement. If conservative surgical management has not resolved the infection or left the patient with a non-function foot, or if there is recurrence of the ulcers despite appropriate preventive treatment, an elective amputation may be the best option. Efforts should be made to make this at as low an anatomical level as possible. Patients with evidence of limb ischemia should undergo vascular evaluation; if blood flow is inadequate (based on transcutaneous oxygen measurements or other appropriate studies), consider early revascularization by open surgery or an endovascular approach (19).

Additional Care

Antibiotics and surgery are necessary, but not sufficient, to cure DFI. Concomitant with these specific treatments clinicians must also manage metabolic disorders (principally hyperglycemia) and comorbidities, such as CV disease or advanced chronic kidney disease (CKD stages 4–5) (Figure 40-6). If the patient is on the SGLT-2 inhibitor, canagliflozin (and likely other members of the SGLT-2 class), this should be stopped in patients with diabetes who develop significant foot complications such as DFI or DFU. Wounds should be covered with properly selected dressings (largely dependent on whether they are predominantly dry or exudative) and any pressure on the wound must be adequately off-loaded (15). Effective off-loading is also an important aspect of the successful clinical management of DFU. The total contact cast (TCC) and other

Table 40-6 Suggested empiric antibiotic recommendations based on clinical severity for diabetic foot infections (DFI)

Grade of Infection (PEDIS[1])	Signs/symptoms	First antibiotic Choice	Alternative	Notes	Duration	Investigations	Referral route
Mild	Two or more signs of inflammation, e.g. pus, pain, warmth, induration. Infection limited to skin or subcutaneous tissue and spreads no more than 2 cm from any ulcer margin. No systemic signs of infection e.g. abscess or suspected osteomyelitis.	Oral flucloxacillin 1 g QDS	Oral clarithromycin 500 mg BD	If known to be an MRSA carrier, consider empirical MRSA treatment with a suitable oral antibiotic such as doxycycline	1–2 weeks	Tissue sample by curettage or scraping with a scalpel blade after debridement of the wound and washing with water is preferable to superficial swab. If there is pus, needle aspiration yields the most suitable specimen.	Outpatient referral to MDT foot team
Moderate	Systemically well patient who has any of: • Cellulitis extending >2 cm from the ulcer margin • Lymphangetic streaking • Spread beneath the deep fascia including local abscess • Suspected osteomyelitis	Oral co-amoxiclav 625 mg TDS	Oral levofloxacin 500 mg OD or BD and clindamycin 300–450 mg QDS	If the patient is a known MRSA Carrier ADD empirical IV teicoplanin or PO doxycycline AND PO rifampicin. When MRSA is excluded, the anti-MRSA treatment can be stopped. Suspect osteomyelitis in any ulcer with visible bone or bone that can be easily probed and if an ulcer fails to heal after 6 weeks of appropriate wound care and offloading.	Typically 2–4 weeks for non bone infections Treat osteomyelitis for at least six weeks	As above suspected osteomyelitis: X-ray and repeat 2–4 weeks. If osteomyelitis still suspected MRI. If bone biopsy is required, this should be an operative or radiological procedure under local anaesthesia. Microbiological and histological examination can be carried out. White cell counts and CRP lack specificity. Lytic bone on X-ray is likely to represent osteomyelitis especially if there are progressive changes over time with no other reason for lytic osteoarthropathy.	Outpatient referral to MDT foot team *or* Inpatient assessment and initiation of treatment

| Severe | IV Pip/ tazobactam plus teicoplanin | Teicoplanin, PO/IV Levofloxacin and Metronidazole | If MRSA is excluded as a causative organism the teicoplanin can be stopped | 2–4 weeks | Inpatient assessment and initiation of treatment |

Management of residual infection after minor or major amputation

What is left after amputation debridement	First antibiotic Choice	Alternative	Duration
All infected tissue removed	Stop surgical prophylaxis <72 hours	Stop surgical prophylaxis <72 hours	<72 hours
Residual infected **soft** tissue ONLY	Co-amoxiclav 625 mg TDS PO	Oral levofloxacin 500 mg OD or BD and clindamycin 300–450 mg QDS	2–4 weeks
Residual infected **VIABLE** bone	As above	As above	6 weeks
Residual dead **NONVIABLE** bone (Why has dead bone been retained, can this not be removed?)	As above	As above	Review at a minimum of 12 weeks

IV = Intravenous; PO = Oral; TDS = three times a day; QDS = four times a day; MRSA = Methicillin-resistant *Staphylococcus aureus*; CRP = C-reactive protein; Pip= piperacillin.
[1] See Table 40-2.

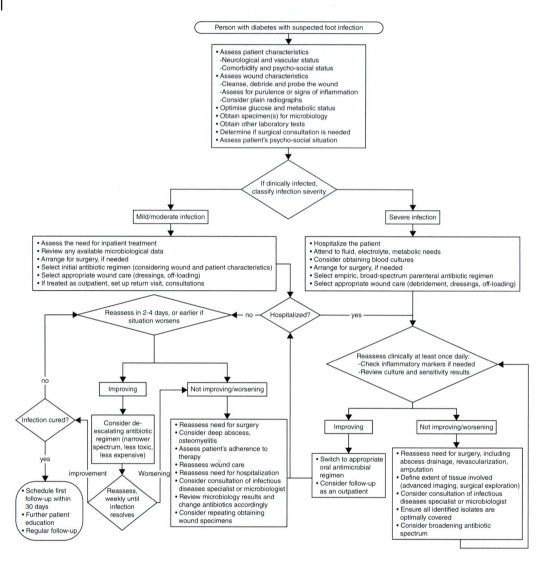

Figure 40-6 Overview of the approach to the management of patients with diabetic foot infections. Reproduced with permission from John Wiley & Sons, Ltd.

non-removable devices are most effective because they avoid the problem of patient non-adherence to using the device. Contra-indications to using a TCC are acute infection, limb ischemia, deep ulcers, and draining wounds. Uncomplicated plantar ulcers should heal in 6–8 weeks with adequate off-loading (20). Hyperbaric oxygen (HBO) therapy is defined as the inhalation of 100% oxygen at pressures greater than sea level. HBO has been shown to improve formation of granulation tissue, improve leukocyte function, stimulate angiogenesis, and promote vasoconstriction that reduces edema (21,22).

Although HBO has been used as an adjunct for healing DFU for decades and despite many clinical trials, its efficacy remains a matter of debate (23–25). A Cochrane Systematic Review concluded that HBO led to an increased rate of ulcer healing at short-term follow-up (6 weeks) but not longer-term follow-up (1 year) and did not appear to reduce the major amputation rate (26). Because the function of leukocytes may be altered in patients with diabetes, administering granulocyte-colony stimulating factor (G-CSF) has been evaluated for DFI in several studies. A Cochrane Review reported on studies of the effects of administering various types of adjunctive G-CSF compared with a placebo or no growth factor in patients with DFI. They concluded there was no evidence of increased rates of infection cure or wound healing with adjunctive G-CSF, but there was a reduced need for surgical procedures, especially amputations, and a reduced length of hospital stay (27). More recently, the US FDA have approved the first shock wave device (i.e. the Dermapace system) to treat DFU. The external shock wave system mechanically stimulates the wound and should be used with standard ulcer care.

Admission Criteria for Diabetic Foot Infection

Assess severity of infection using IDSA/IWGDF (or similar) classification (Table 40-2).

Consider admitting (Table 40-7) the following patients:

1. All patients with a severe infection.
2. Patients with a moderate infection with complicating features (e.g., severe PAD or lack of home support), or who require urgent surgical debridement (e.g., deep collections) or are unable to comply with the required outpatient treatment regimen.
3. Patients with critical limb ischemia.
4. Dialysis patients (risk of rapid progression and systemic infection).
5. Patients who do not meet any of these criteria, but are failing to improve with outpatient therapy, may also need to be hospitalized.
6. Patients whose glycemic control has decompensated to the point that it is now an acute problem in its own right.

Osteomyelitis

Osteomyelitis is apparent at presentation in about 20% of cases of all DFI, but in over 60% of severe infections. Its clinical manifestations can vary depending on the site involved, the extent of the infection, the causative pathogen(s), the involvement of soft tissue and the vascular status. Suspect osteomyelitis in a patient with an infected, large or deep wound, particularly if the ulcer is chronic, or if there is a swollen, erythematous ("sausage") toe. The probe-to-bone test is a valuable diagnostic tool when correctly performed (with a sterile blunt metal probe, after wound debridement) and interpreted (based on the likelihood of osteomyelitis) (13). For patients with a low pre-test probability of osteomyelitis, a negative test substantially reduces the likelihood of osteomyelitis (28). When the pre-test probability of osteomyelitis is high, a positive test has a high predictive value for osteomyelitis (29).

Imaging for osteomyelitis generally begins with plain-x rays, but these have a relatively low sensitivity (for acute infection) and specificity. The main issue is differentiating osteomyelitis from noninfectious CN (30). Serial plain films over time may be useful for diagnosis and follow-up. Computed tomography (CT) scans or nuclear medicine imaging, e.g., with ^{99tm}TC-methylene diphosphonate, are more sensitive, but relatively non-specific (31). Among the advanced imaging tests, MRI is currently the best technique, not only for the diagnosis of bone infection but also to appreciate deep soft tissue or sinus tract involvement. The few available studies of newer procedures such as single-photon emission CT (SPECT)/CT and positron-emission tomography (PET) combined with MRI suggest they may be more accurate than MRI alone (14).

The generally accepted criterion standard for diagnosing osteomyelitis remains obtaining a specimen of bone (either at surgery or percutaneously) for the combination of microbiological culture and histopathological evaluation (32,33). This approach is not always needed, but is particularly useful when there is diagnostic uncertainty, uninterpretable cultures or a non-response to empirical antibiotic therapy. A probable diagnosis of bone infection is reasonable if there are positive results on a combination of diagnostic tests, such as probe-to-bone, serum inflammatory markers, plain X-rays, MRI or radionuclide scanning (13).

Table 40-7 Characteristics suggesting a more serious diabetic foot infection and potential indications for hospitalization (13)

Findings suggesting a more serious diabetic foot infection	
Wound specific	
Wound	Penetrates to subcutaneous tissues (e.g., fascia, tendon, muscle, joint and bone)
Cellulitis	Extensive (>2 cm), distant from ulceration or rapidly progressive
Local signs	Severe inflammation or induration, crepitus, bullae, discoloration, necrosis or gangrene, ecchymoses or petechiae and new anesthesia
General	
Presentation	Acute onset/worsening or rapidly progressive
Systemic signs	Fever, chills, hypotension, confusion and volume depletion
Laboratory tests	Leukocytosis, very high C-reactive protein or erythrocyte sedimentation rate, severe/worsening hyperglycemia, acidosis, new/worsening azotemia and electrolyte abnormalities
Complicating features	Presence of a foreign body (accidentally or surgically implanted), puncture wound, deep abscess, arterial or venous insufficiency, lymphedema, immunosuppressive illness or treatment
Current treatment	Progression while on apparently appropriate antibiotic and supportive therapy

Factors suggesting hospitalization may be necessary

- Severe infection (see Table 40-4)
- Metabolic or hemodynamic instability
- Intravenous therapy needed (and not available/appropriate as outpatient)
- Diagnostic tests needed that are not available as outpatient
- Critical foot ischemia present
- Surgical procedures (more than minor) required
- Failure of outpatient management
- Patient unable or unwilling to comply with outpatient-based treatment
- Need for more complex dressing changes than patient/caregivers can provide
- Need for careful, continuous observation

Osteomyelitis is generally treated with antibiotic therapy, either alone or combined with surgery to removed necrotic and infected bone. The duration of antibiotic therapy for osteomyelitis remains controversial, but depends on whether or not necrotic bone has been resected and probably does not need to exceed 6 weeks (Table 40-6) (13,34). A trial of antibiotic therapy alone can be undertaken in selected cases; several retrospective studies (35,36) and one recent prospective study show a remission rate of 60–70% (37). Surgical resection may allow a reduced hospital stay, a shorter duration of antibiotic treatment, and a higher remission rates, but can be associated with operative and post-operative complications.

Necrotizing Fasciitis

Necrotizing fasciitis is a life-threatening, rapidly progressive invasive soft tissue infection involving subcutaneous fat and deep fascia layers (38). The rapid tissue necrosis often leads to systemic sepsis, toxic-shock like syndrome and multi-organ failure. The mortality of necrotizing fasciitis is reported to be 15–30%. Necrotizing fasciitis in diabetic patients is usually polymicrobial and most often involves both aerobic organisms (especially streptococci, staphylococci,

Enterobacteriaceae) and obligate anaerobes (usually *Bacteroides* species, peptostreptococci). Less commonly infection may be monomicrobial, usually with β-hemolytic streptococci or staphylococci (39). Gas gangrene is a less common separate entity that is usually caused by *Clostridium* species.

Necrotizing fasciitis typically begins as an area of inflamed, swollen skin, with or without a history of recent local trauma. Although diagnosis in the early stages may be difficult, it is important to differentiate more common skin infections, such as erysipelas, cellulitis or soft tissue abscess, from the more dangerous necrotizing fasciitis. In necrotizing fasciitis, pain may be disproportionately severe compared to the limited visible extent of infection. Conversely, as infection progresses, there may be new onset local anesthesia, presumably related to necrosis of nerve fibers. Necrotizing fasciitis can be accompanied by fever and crepitus, but spontaneous drainage and pus are usually not present. As the infection progresses, bullae, petechiae, ecchymoses, purplish coloration, and skin lesions resembling deep burns may develop. Necrotizing fasciitis can involve almost any part of the body (classically involving the perineum in persons with diabetes, termed Fournier's gangrene), including the foot in cases with pre-existing ulcers. Scoring systems using clinical findings and blood tests, as well as CT, may aid in suspected necrotizing fasciitis, but direct examination of the involved tissues is usually necessary to make a definitive diagnosis (39).

Using multivariable analysis, one study of patients with necrotizing fasciitis found that the presence of diabetes was associated with a significantly increased risk of amputation, as were other selected underlying conditions and evidence of cutaneous gangrene on admission (40). Similarly, factors found to be associated with significantly increased mortality include underlying conditions, advanced or very young age, or evidence of sepsis (40).

Treatment of necrotizing fasciitis requires rapid fluid and electrolyte corrections, hemodynamic stabilization, support for failing organ systems and appropriate parenteral antibiotic therapy. Several different regimens of antibiotics have been recommended, and the choice may depend on local/national guidelines. In general, consider broad-spectrum agents, such as piperacillin-tazobactam, or carbapenems, often with concomitant clindamycin, or vancomycin if methicillin-resistant *Staphylococcus aureus* (MRSA) is suspected (Table 40-6). In addition, early aggressive surgical debridement (often repeated to ensure all necrotic tissue has been removed) is usually necessary. Delayed or inadequate operative debridement may be associated with increased mortality rates. In a few cases an experienced surgeon may decide that urgent ablative surgery may not be needed; in such cases frequent, careful follow-up is mandatory. Various adjunctive treatments, including HBO, have been used but the efficacy of each is unclear (13).

Charcot Neuroarthropathy

Charcot neuroarthropathy is a non-infectious condition affecting bone, joints, and soft tissues of the foot and ankle. The exact pathogenesis remains unclear, but available evidence suggests that it is caused by a combination of peripheral neuropathy, PAD, unrecognized or untreated injury, and continued repetitive trauma (41,42). In addition, other potential contributory factors include reduced bone density (the RANK/RANKL system is important in aberrant bone resorption which may be modulated tumor necrosis factor alpha), non-enzymatic collagen glycation, and excessive local inflammation accompanied by increases in various cytokines (e.g., tumor necrosis factor alpha, interleukin 1 beta) (43).

In the acute phase a Charcot foot is erythematous, indurated, and painful and may be mistaken for gout, deep venous thrombosis, cellulitis or a sprain (42). In the chronic phase CN is associated with subluxations and fractures, especially of the midfoot (Lisfranc injury), causing substantial deformity

(Figure 40-7). The estimated prevalence of CN among persons with diabetes is 7.5% with an incidence of about 0.2%, but the true figure is probably higher as many cases remain undiagnosed (44,45). CN is indirectly a potentially limb- and even life-threatening condition because the resultant foot deformities lead to high pressures, recurrent ulcerations, and potentially lower extremity amputation (46). In the recent UK National Diabetes Foot Care Audit (NDFA) 2014–2016 (2), 3% of all new ulcers were associated with active or possibly active Charcot foot disease. In addition, 4% of all new ulcers were associated with previous, inactive Charcot foot disease.

CN can be classified by anatomical localization, clinical stage, or natural history. Pain is often minimal or absent, due to the sensory neuropathy, and pedal pulses are usually present (43). Plain radiographs are the first-line imaging method, but they can be normal for up to three weeks after the start of the acute episode. Typical early radiographic findings include subtle fractures and dislocations, while in later stages features "pencil in cup" deformity of the metatarsophalangeal joints or talocalcaneal dislocation are common (47). In the absence of characteristic findings, MRI can provide a non-invasive and sensitive diagnostic tool in the evaluation of soft tissue and bone marrow abnormalities (48–50). Nuclear medicine studies, e.g., three-phase bone scans with technetium-99m (^{99m} Tc), provide an alternative technique when MRI is unavailable or contraindicated (13,51). As with osteomyelitis, bone scans have a high sensitivity for early CN but lack specificity. Monitoring of skin temperatures may also be of value.

The management of active CN consists mainly of immediate pressure offloading, optimally with a TCC (52), which should be replaced after ~3 days, then changed every week to permit examination of the foot. Casting is usually needed for 3–6 months, or until there is a resolution of the swelling and warmth and evidence of healing on X-rays or MRI. After resolution of the acute episode the most appropriate type of device will depend on the level of deformities. For patients with a minor foot deformity, consider prefabricated footwear with extra depth and a stiff rocker bottom walking sole as appropriate, while for moderate deformity, consider a custom-made shoe associated with custom-molded, full contact insoles. In situations where there are severe foot deformities or ankle involvement, a removable Charcot Restraint Orthotic Walker (CROW) is useful. Close monitoring is also required after an acute episode for all stages (53).

In cases of CN refractory to offloading and immobilization, or when ulcers fail to heal, surgical treatment is generally beneficial to prevent severe deformity or joint instability. It is preferable to delay the surgery after the acute phase of CN to avoid the risk of secondary infection or mechanical failure. In cases of a bony prominence that leads to ulcers that cannot be accommodated with prosthetics or orthotics, exostectomy is usually required. When there is abnormal plantar pressure distribution, consider an Achilles tendon lengthening or gastrocnemius tendon reduction to decrease forefoot pressure and improve alignment of the ankle and hindfoot to the midfoot and forefoot. In cases of recurrent ulcers, arthrodesis may be helpful. If these procedures fail to stabilize the foot, an amputation may be required.

Various medical therapies, such as bisphosphonates, have been tried for the management of acute CN. In some studies bisphosphonate treatment has reduced skin temperature and bone turnover, but the long-term efficacy, particularly in preventing the occurrence of ulcerations and deformities, remains unclear (54). Early identification and management of acute CN are necessary to avoid the rapid progression towards permanent foot deformation and its associated devastating complications (Figure 40-7).

Peripheral Arterial Disease (PAD)

PAD is present in about half of patients with a DFU and is an independent risk factor for limb loss in diabetes (55). Identifying

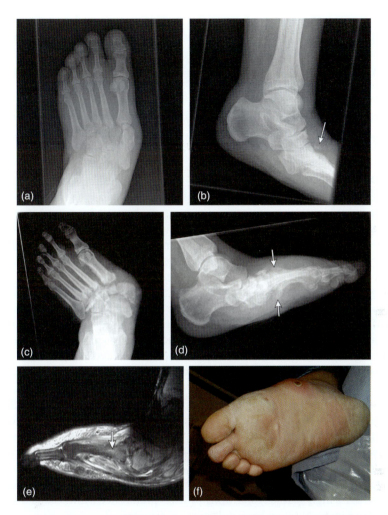

Figure 40-7 Charcot neuroarthropathy. Male, Type 2 diabetes, aged 72, known neuropathy. He injured his foot about 7 months ago before presenting to the specialist podiatry team; he had noticed increasing deformity of the foot, and then developed an ulcer, ultimately 5 cm in diameter over the medial aspect of the tarsometatarsal joint of the great toe. Ulceration with notable foot deformity should alert to a combination of Charcot neuroarthropathy and osteomyelitis. (a) and (b) Anteroposterior and lateral radiographs of the left foot showing the classical radio graphic triad of a Charcot foot: (1) dislocation of the 2nd and 3rd tarsometatarsal joints (Lisfranc joint); (2) early destruction of the tarsometatarsal and intermetatarsal joints; and (3) new heterotopic bone formation (arrow). (c), (d): radiographs 6 months later. (c) and (d) Anteroposterior and lateral radiographs with increasing foot deformity with severe dislocation of all the tarsometatarsal joints, progressive destruction of the tarsometatarsal and intermetatarsal joints and exuberant new heterotopic bone formation (arrows). (e) MRI showing early osteomyelitis in the proximal 1st metatarsal indicated by bone marrow edema (arrow). (f) Male, aged 36, Type 1 Diabetes 15 years. He twisted his ankle, but continued to walk on it for 2 weeks because of loss of pain sensation. Typical Charcot foot appearance: flattened arches and medial displacement of the navicular with secondary ulceration from footwear. Reproduced with permission from John Wiley & Sons, Ltd.

PAD can be challenging in these patients as the signs and the symptoms may be masked (or mimicked) by co-existing distal symmetrical polyneuropathy. All patients presenting with a foot ulcer should undergo at least a basic evaluation of the vascular status of the lower extremities. This should include a history (specifically targeting claudication, rest pain and any previous vascular assessments and interventions) and palpation of pedal (dorsalis pedis and posterior tibial) pulses. Patients without palpable pedal pulses or with clinical signs of ischemia should be evaluated with a hand-held Doppler device to assess for the presence of pulses, their waveforms (mono-, bi- or tri-phasic) and to measure ankle brachial index (ABI). ABI is the first-line screening and diagnostic test for lower extremity PAD, and is also a strong marker of generalized atherosclerosis and CVD risk. If these examinations are inconclusive, consider measuring the transcutaneous pressure of oxygen ($TcPO_2$) or toe-brachial index (TBI) (56). An ABI <0.6 (normal ABI 1.0–1.4; borderline 0.9–0.99; abnormal <0.9 or >1.4 [higher value associated with arterial stiffening due to medial arterial calcification]), a $TcPO_2$ <40 mmHg or toe pressure <30 mmHg suggest clinically significant ischemia, with a low probability of wound healing (57).

A vascular surgeon or angiologist should assess patients with signs, symptoms or Doppler evidence of clinically significant PAD. Among radiological evaluations of PAD, duplex ultrasound is the first imaging modality of choice; when revascularization is considered, most consider intra-arterial digital subtraction angiography optimal (especially for below knee arterial disease) because of its high spatial resolution. Although it allows concomitant endovascular therapy during the procedure, it can provoke contrast-induced nephropathy, allergic reactions or severe hematomas. Other radiological procedures, such as contrast-enhanced magnetic resonance angiography (MRA) or CT angiography (CTA) can also be used (58,59).

The decision on when to revascularize a patient with an ulcerated foot remains complex (58,59). Considerations should include the probability of wound healing without revascularization compared with the potential benefits and risks of a revascularization procedure. Patients with good skin perfusion ($TcPO_2$ >40 mmHg), relatively mild PAD (ABI ≥0.6) and a small wound can usually be treated initially by optimal wound care and a period of 6 weeks of observation.

Patients who present with more severe PAD, especially if associated with a foot infection and large ulceration, usually benefit from early revascularization. A new classification system (**WIfI**) has been proposed as the initial assessment of all patients with ischemic rest pain or wounds (including DFU) (59). The three primary factors that contribute to the 1 year risk of limb threat (i.e., amputation) are: **W**ound (**W**), **I**schemia (**I**), and foot **I**nfection (**fI**). Revascularization should always be discussed (if feasible) as its suitability is increased (i.e., higher risk of amputation) with more severe stages (except clinical stage 5, which signifies an unsalvageable foot [most often because of wound extent or severity of infection]). The clinician must then choose between open bypass surgery and endovascular interventions. Although there are several published cases series using each procedure, there are no randomized controlled clinical trials comparing the two techniques in patients with ischemic DFU. Available data and systematic suggest the outcomes are similar and there is insufficient evidence to recommend one method of revascularization over another (60). Selecting a treatment strategy relies on issues such as the extent and the site of the disease, the patient's associated comorbidities, and the preferences and skills of the available operators.

Overall management of PAD includes optimizing glycemic control, hypertension, dyslipidemia, smoking cessation, use of antiplatelet agents, exercise, weight loss, and addressing other modifiable risk factors that are important to prevent or slow any progression of PAD and other vascular complications for which the patient is at increased risk (the SGLT-2 inhibitor, empagliflozin, was recently shown to decrease major adverse CV events in patients with PAD) (11).

Discharge Planning

Prior to being discharged, a patient with a DFU should be clinically stable; have had any urgently needed surgery performed; have achieved acceptable glycemic control; be able to manage (on his/her own or with help) at the designated discharge location; and have a well-defined plan that includes an appropriate antibiotic regimen to which he/she will adhere; an off-loading scheme (if needed); specific wound care instructions; and appropriate outpatient follow-up. Remind the patient to come back if the infection worsens or other foot complication develops.

Conclusions

Foot ulcerations complicated by infection are a major and growing problem for patients with diabetes. These disorders largely result from peripheral neuropathy and/or PAD and are associated with severe consequences if they are not properly managed. DFI is often an epiphenomenon, reflecting poor glycemic control and is associated with increased morbidity and mortality. In the past decades many studies have been published that have allowed experts to develop robust recommendations and guidelines for management of DFI and CN. Perhaps the most important task to undertake now is to develop a multidisciplinary team infrastructure to permit optimal care for these complications with appropriate ongoing education of patients and healthcare providers about the importance of prevention and early recognition of diabetes-related foot problems (13). The use of new remote sensing technology (e.g., dermal thermography scanning, hyperspectral imaging, and skin perfusion pressure) to identify people at risk of developing foot ulceration in an attempt to allow early intervention and prevention of foot ulcers is also potentially on the horizon (18).

Acknowledgments

The current author wishes to acknowledge the contributions to the previous edition by Ben Lipsky, Karim Gariani and Ilker Uckay, upon which portions of this chapter are based.

References

1 Kerr M. *Foot Care for People with Diabetes: The Economic Case for Change*, 2012. https://www.diabetes.org.uk/Documents/nhs-diabetes/footcare/footcare-for-people-with-diabetes.pdf (accessed April 24, 2017).

2 Health and Social Care Information Centre. *National Diabetes Foot Care Audit Report 2014–2016*, 2017. www.digital.nhs.uk/pubs/ndfa1516 (accessed April 24, 2017).

3 Ogurtsova K, da Rocha Fernandes J, Huang Y, et al. IDF Diabetes Atlas: global estimates for the prevalence of diabetes for 2015 and 2040. *Diabetes Research and Clinical Practice*. 2017;128;40–50.

4 Armstrong DG, Boulton AJ, Bus SA. Diabetic foot ulcers and their recurrence. *N Engl J Med*. 2017;376:2367–2375.

5 Morbach S, Furchert H, Gröblinghoff U, et al. Long-term prognosis of diabetic foot patients and their limbs: amputation and death over the course of a decade. *Diabetes Care*. 2012;35(10):2021–2027.

6 Wukich DK, Armstrong DG, Attinger CE, et al. Inpatient management of diabetic foot disorders: a clinical guide. *Diabetes Care*. 2013;36(9):2862–2871.

7 Health and Social care information Centre. *National Diabetes Inpatient Audit (NaDIA), Open Data 2016*, 2017. www.digital.nhs.uk/pubs/nadia2016 (accessed April 24, 2017).

8 National Institute for Health and Care Excellence. *Diabetic Foot Problems: Prevention and Management. NICE Guideline NG19*, 2016.

https://www.nice.org.uk/guidance/ng19 (accessed April 24, 2017).

9   Pop-Busui R, Boulton AJM, Feldman EL, et al. Diabetic neuropathy: a position statement by the American Diabetes Association. *Diabetes Care.* 2017;40:136–154.

10 Edmunds M. The benefits of working together in diabetic foot care for the vulnerable patient. *Practical Diabetes.* 2016;33:29–33.

11 American Diabetes Association 2018 Standards of medical care in diabetes – 2018. *Diabetes Care.* 2018;41(Suppl 1): S1–S159.

12 Lipsky BA, Berendt AR, Cornia PB, et al. Infectious Diseases Society of America clinical practice guideline for the diagnosis and treatment of diabetic foot infections. *Clin Infect Dis.* 2012;54(12):e132–173.

13 Lipsky BA, Aragon-Sanchez J, Diggle M, et al. IWGDF guidance on the diagnosis and management of foot infections in persons with diabetes. *Diabetes Metab Res Rev.* 2016;32 (Suppl 1):45–74.

14 Israel O, Sconfienza LM, Lipsky BA. Diagnosing diabetic foot infection: the role of imaging and a proposed flow chart for assessment. *Q J Nucl Med Mol Imaging.* 2013;57(1):1–13.

15 Armstrong DG, Bharara M, White M, et al. The impact and outcomes of establishing an integrated interdisciplinary surgical team to care for the diabetic foot. *Diabetes Metab Res Rev.* 2012;28(6):514–518.

16 Lazzarini PA, O'Rourke SR, Russell AW, Derhy PH, Kamp MC. Standardising practices improves clinical diabetic foot management: the Queensland Diabetic Foot Innovation Project, 2006–09. *Aust Health Rev.* 2012;36:8–15.

17 Nather A, Siok Bee C, Keng Lin W, et al. Value of team approach combined with clinical pathway for diabetic foot problems: a clinical evaluation. *Diabet Foot Ankle.* 2010;1:1–5.

18 Clokie M, Greenway AL, Harding K, et al. New horizons in the understanding of the causes and management of diabetic foot disease: report from the 2017 Diabetes UK Annual Professional Conference Symposium. *Diabet. Med.* 2017;34, 305–315.

19 Hingorani A, LaMuraglia GM, Henke P, et al. The management of diabetic foot: a clinical practice guideline by the Society for Vascular Surgery in collaboration with the American Podiatric Medical Association and the Society for Vascular Medicine. *J Vasc Surg.* 2016;63:3S–21S.

20 Cavanagh PR, Bus SA. Off-loading the diabetic foot for ulcer prevention and healing. *J Vasc Surg.* 2010;52(3 Suppl): 37S–43S.

21 Hunt TK, Pai MP. The effect of varying ambient oxygen tensions on wound metabolism and collagen synthesis. *Surg Gynecol Obstet.* 1972;135(4): 561–567.

22 Hunt TK, Linsey M, Grislis H, Sonne M, Jawetz E. The effect of differing ambient oxygen tensions on wound infection. *Ann Surg.* 1975;181(1):35–39.

23 Liu R, Li L, Yang M, Boden G, Yang G. Systematic review of the effectiveness of the hyperbaric oxygenation therapy in the management of chronic diabetic foot ulcers. *Mayo Clin Proc.* 2013;88(2): 166–175.

24 Margolis DJ, Gupta J, Hoffstad O, et al. Lack of effectiveness of hyperbaric oxygen therapy for the treatment of diabetic foot ulcer and the prevention of amputation: a cohort study. *Diabetes Care.* 2013;36(7): 1961–1966.

25 Berendt AR. Counterpoint: hyperbaric oxygen for diabetic foot wounds is not effective. *Clin Infect Dis.* 2006;43(2): 193–198.

26 Kranke P, Bennet MH, Martyn-St James M, Schnabel A, Debus SE. Hyperbaric oxygen therapy for chronic wounds. *Cochrane Database Syst Rev.* 2012;4:CD004123.

27 Cruciani M, Lipsky BA, Mengoli C, de Lalla F. Granulocyte-colony stimulating factors as adjunctive therapy for diabetic foot infections. *Cochrane Database Syst Rev.* 2013;17;8.

28 Butalia S, Palda VA, Sargeant RJ, Detsky AS, Mourad O. Does this patient with

diabetes have osteomyelitis of the lower extremity? *JAMA*. 2008;299(7):806–813.

29 Aragón-Sánchez J, Lipsky BA, Lázaro-Martínez JL. Diagnosing diabetic foot osteomyelitis: is the combination of probe-to-bone test and plain radiography sufficient for high-risk inpatients? *Diabet Med*. 2011;28(2):191–194.

30 Ertugrul BM, Lipsky BA, Sayk O. Osteomyelitis or Charcot neuro-osteoarthropathy? Differentiating these disorders in diabetic patients with a foot problem. *Diabetic Foot & Ankle*. 2013. DOI:10.3402/dfa.v4i0.21855.

31 Uçkay I, Aragón-Sánchez J, Lew D, Lipsky BA. Diabetic foot infections: what have we learned in the last 30 years? *International J Infectious Diseases*. 2015;40:81–91.

32 Hatzenbuehler J, Pulling TJ. Diagnosis and management of osteomyelitis. *Am Fam Physician*. 2011;84(9):1027–1033.

33 Berendt AR, Peters EJ, Bakker K, et al. Diabetic foot osteomyelitis: a progress report on diagnosis and a systematic review of treatment. *Diabetes/Metabolism Res Rev*. 2008;24 (Suppl 1):S145–S161.

34 Lazzarini L, Lipsky BA, Mader JT. Antibiotic treatment of osteomyelitis: what have we learned from 30 years of clinical trials? *Int J Infect Dis*. 2005;9(3): 127–138.

35 Pittet D, Wyssa B, Herter-Clavel C, Kursteiner K, Vaucher J, Lew PD. Outcome of diabetic foot infections treated conservatively: a retrospective cohort study with long-term follow-up. *Arch Intern Med*. 1999;159(8):851–856.

36 Jeffcoate WJ, Lipsky BA. Controversies in diagnosing and managing osteomyelitis of the foot in diabetes. *Clin Infect Dis*. 2004;39 Suppl 2:S115–S122.

37 Lázaro-Martínez J, Aragón-Sánchez J, García-Morales E. Antibiotics versus conservative surgery for treating diabetic foot osteomyelitis: a randomized comparative trial. *Diabetes Care*. 2014;37(3): 789–795.

38 Jallali NJ. Necrotising fasciitis: its aetiology, diagnosis and management. *Wound Care*. 2003;12(8):297–300.

39 Stevens DL, Bryant AE. Necrotizing soft-tissue infections. *N Engl J Med*. 2017;377:2253–2265.

40 Dworkin MS, Westercamp MD, Park L, McIntyre A. The epidemiology of necrotizing fasciitis including factors associated with death and amputation. *Epidemiol Infect*. 2009;137: 1609–1614.

41 Rogers LC, Frykberg RG, Armstrong DG, et al. The Charcot foot in diabetes. *Diabetes Care*. 2011;34(9):2123–2129.

42 Wukich DK, Sung W, Wipf SA, Armonstrong DG. The consequence of complacency: managing the effects of unrecognized Charcot feet. *Diabet Med*. 2011;28:195–198.

43 Papanas N, Maltezos E. Etiology, pathophysiology and classifications of the diabetic Charcot foot. *Diabet Foot Ankle*. 2013;4(10).

44 Rathur RM, Boulton AM. Recent advances in the diagnosis and management of diabetic neuropathy. *J Bone Joint Surg Br*. 2005;87-B:1605–1610.

45 Gouveri E, Papanas N. Charcot osteoarthropathy in diabetes: a brief review with an emphasis on clinical practice. *World J Diabetes*. 2011;2(5):59–65.

46 van Baal J, Hubbard R, Game F, Jeffcoate W. Mortality associated with acute Charcot foot and neuropathic foot ulceration. *Diabetes Care*. 2010;33(5):1086–1089.

47 Rajbhandari SM, Jenkins RC, Davies C, Tesfaye S. Charcot neuroarthropathy in diabetes mellitus. *Diabetologia*. 2002;45:1085–1096.

48 Kapoor A, Page S, Lavalley M, Gale DR, Felson DT. Magnetic resonance imaging for diagnosing foot osteomyelitis: a meta-analysis. *Arch Intern Med*. 2007;167(2):125–132.

49 Zampa V, Bargellini I, Rizzo L, et al. Role of dynamic MRI in follow-up of acute Charcot foot in patients with diabetes mellitus. *Skeletal Radiol*. 2011;40: 991–999.

50 Schlossbauer T, Mioc T, Sommerey S, Kessler SB, Reiser MF, Pfeifer KJ. Magnetic

Resonance Imaging in Early Stage Charcot Arhtropathy- correlation of imaging findings and clinical symptoms. *Eur J Med Res*. 2008;13:409–414.

51 Prandini N, Beretta F. *Radionuclide Imaging of Infection and Inflammation Nuclear Medicine Imaging of Diabetic Foot*. New York: Springer; 2013: 253–269.

52 Van der Ven A, Chapman CB, Bowker JH. Charcot neuroarthropathy of the foot and ankle. *J Am Acad Orthop Surg*. 2009;17: 562–571.

53 Milne TE, Rogers JR, Kinnear EW. Developing an evidence-based clinical pathway for the assessment, diagnosis and management of acute Charcot Neuro-Arthropathy: a systematic review. *Journal of Foot and Ankle Research*. 2013;6(1):30.

54 Richard JL, Almasri M, Schuldiner S. Treatment of acute Charcot foot with bisphosphonates: a systematic review of the literature. *Diabetologia*. 2012;55(5): 1258–1264.

55 Prompers L, Huijberts M, Apelqvist J, et al. High prevalence of ischaemia, infection and serious comorbidity in patients with diabetic foot disease in Europe: baseline results from the Eurodiale study. *Diabetologia*. 2007;50(1):18–25.

56 Schaper NC, Andros G, Apelqvist J, et al. Diagnosis and treatment of peripheral arterial disease in diabetic patients with a foot ulcer: a progress report of the International Working Group on the Diabetic Foot. *Diabetes Metab Res Rev*. 2012;28(Suppl 1):218–224.

57 Kalani M, Brismar K, Fagrell B, Ostergren J, Jörneskog G. Transcutaneous oxygen tension and toe blood pressure as predictors for outcome of diabetic foot ulcers. *Diabetes Care*. 1999;22(1):147–151.

58 Barrett C, et al. 2016 AHA/ACC Guideline on the Management of Patients With Lower Extremity Peripheral Artery Disease: Executive Summary. *Journal of the American College of Cardiology* 2017;69:e71–e126.

59 Aboyans V, Ricco JB, Bartelink ML, et al. Treatment of Peripheral Arterial Diseases, in collaboration with the European Society for Vascular Surgery (ESVS). *European Heart Journal*, ehx095, https://doi.org/10.1093/eurheartj/ehx095

60 Hinchliffe RJ, Andros G, Apelqvist J, et al. A systematic review of the effectiveness of revascularization of the ulcerated foot in patients with diabetes and peripheral arterial disease. *Diabetes Metab Res Rev*. 2012;28(Suppl 1):179–217.

Part X

Sodium Disorders

Introduction

Emergency Management of Sodium Disorders

Richard H. Sterns

Key Points

- Human cells dwell in salt water, their well-being depends on the ability of the body to regulate the salinity of the extracellular environment. By controlling water intake and excretion, the osmoregulatory system normally keeps the plasma sodium concentration between 135 and 142 mmol/L. Failure of the system to regulate within this range exposes to hypotonic or hypertonic stress.
- The term "tonicity" describes the effect of plasma on cells; hypotonicity makes cells swell and hypertonicity makes them shrink.

- Hypernatremia always indicates hypertonicity; hyponatremia usually indicates hypotonicity.
- Although all cells are affected, clinical manifestations of hyponatremia and hypernatremia are primarily neurologic, and rapid changes in plasma sodium concentrations in either direction can cause severe, permanent, and sometimes lethal brain injury.
- Because the brain adapts to an abnormal plasma sodium level, excessive or over rapid correction of a chronic disturbance can be injurious and should be avoided.

Normally, our cells thrive in a properly salted extracellular environment, provided by an osmoregulatory system that keeps the plasma sodium concentration between 135 and 142 mmol/L. When that system fails or is overwhelmed, cellular well-being rests in the hands of the treating physician. High or low extracellular sodium levels are detrimental to all cells, particularly those in the brain, and the brain may be permanently damaged by sudden changes in the plasma sodium concentration (1).

The serious consequences of disordered osmoregulation have been understood for nearly a century (2,3). Sadly, even though we know what untreated hypo- and hypernatremia can do to the brain, we lack reliable data on the frequency of these neurological complications; published accounts are limited to individual case reports or case series derived from consultations that sought to explain an adverse outcome. Likewise, despite an expanding understanding of why brain damage occurs when chronically abnormal plasma sodium concentrations are corrected too rapidly, current recommendations for therapeutic limits are based on surprisingly meager data. Finally, even when clinicians think they know what their therapeutic targets should be, they often miss the mark, and must rely on anecdotal evidence on what measures best achieve correction goals.

Endocrine and Metabolic Medical Emergencies: A Clinician's Guide, Second Edition. Edited by Glenn Matfin.

Fueled, in part, by the absence of definitive data, there has been a great deal of controversy regarding the proper treatment of severe hyponatremia (4). When it was first reported that central pontine and extrapontine myelinolysis (now, often called "the osmotic demyelination syndromes") were complications of rapid correction of hyponatremia, a therapeutic dilemma emerged. Because many experts believed that the serum sodium concentration had to be raised above 120 or even 128 mmol/L to ensure survival and avoid hypoxic brain damage,

it appeared that patients with extremely low serum sodium concentrations would be harmed by treatment that was either too slow or too fast. This conundrum led to the complaint that clinicians treating severe hyponatremia were "damned if they do and damned if they don't" and the joking suggestion that the treatment of hyponatremia must be "unsafe at any speed" (4,5).

Although we do need better evidence, a convincing body of experimental and observational data has now led to a near consensus among experts that, hopefully, puts

Table X-1 Treatment of symptomatic hyponatremia

Duration	Several hours	1–2 days	Unknown or >2 days
Clinical setting	Self-induced water intoxication • Psychosis • Exercise • Ecstasy*	Parenteral fluids, especially postoperative	Develops outside the hospital in patients drinking conventional amounts of fluid
Symptoms and signs before Rx	Headache, nausea, vomiting, delirium, seizures, risk of respiratory arrest, neurogenic pulmonary edema and brain herniation	Headache, nausea, vomiting, delirium, seizures, risk of respiratory arrest, neurogenic pulmonary edema and brain herniation	Malaise, fatigue, confusion, cramps, falls, seizures relatively uncommon (10% when serum Na < 110 mmol/L)
Brain damage	Brain herniation pre-Rx (no risk of post-Rx osmotic demyelination)	Brain herniation pre-Rx (little, if any risk of post-Rx osmotic demyelination)	Post-Rx Osmotic demyelination (little if any risk of pre-Rx brain herniation)
Risk factors for permanent brain damage	Unknown	Women and young children account for most reported deaths	• Na ≤ 105 mmol/L • Hypokalemia • Alcoholism • Malnutrition • Liver disease
Rx goals	Urgently increase 4–6 mmol/L with 100 ml bolus of 3% saline x 3 if needed	4–6 mmol/L within 6 hours with 100 ml bolus of 3% saline x 3 if needed	4–6 mmol/L per day (or within 6 hrs for severe symptoms), 100 ml bolus of 3% saline for seizures, repeated if needed
Rx limit if Serum Na < 120 mmol/L	No limit defined	• 10–12 mmol/L/day • 18 mmol/L/48 hrs	• 10–12 mmol/L/day • 18 mmol/L/48 hrs • 8 mmol/L/day if high risk of osmotic demyelination
Re-lowering Serum Na for overcorrection	Unnecessary	Probably unnecessary	Recommended if high risk of osmotic demyelination

*Ecstasy denotes use of 3,4-Methylenedioxymethamphetamine.
Rx = treatment of hyponatremia.

this conundrum to rest (6). If symptoms are severe, or if there is concern about life-threatening cerebral edema with impending herniation, all agree that hypertonic saline should be urgently infused to promptly raise the serum sodium by approximately 4–6 mmol/L. That means that no matter how acute the disturbance, how severe the symptoms, or how low the serum sodium concentration, there should be no compelling need to correct hyponatremia by more than 6 mmol/L in a single day. There is also a consensus that too much correction of hyponatremia can cause osmotic demyelination, but minor disagreements remain as to where the "stop sign" should be placed: 8 mmol/L, 10 mmol/L or 12 mmol/L in a single day and/or 16 mmol/L, 18 mmol/L or 20 mmol/L in 48 hours (4,7). Despite the remaining uncertainty, clinicians no longer need to make a "Sophie's choice" between inadequate and excessive therapy.

Long before the association between rapid correction of chronic hyponatremia and osmotic demyelination was reported, rapid correction of chronic hypernatremia was known to cause rehydration seizures and cerebral edema in infants (8). There have been no reports of this complication in adults. Because it is now known that a rapid onset of severe hypernatremia can cause osmotic demyelination, a new therapeutic dilemma has emerged. Re-lowering the serum sodium concentration can prevent osmotic demyelination after rapid correction of hyponatremia in experimental animals and it seems to be well tolerated in hyponatremic patients who have been inadvertently overcorrected (9). Does that mean that rapid correction of hypernatremia will also prevent osmotic demyelination? And, if it does, might the benefit of rapid correction of hypernatremia in adults exceed the risk of cerebral edema?

Tables X-1 and X-2 summarize commonly accepted guidelines for the treatment of symptomatic hyponatremia and hypernatremia (1). Let us hope that the coming years bring us new evidence to put our treatment of plasma sodium disorders on firmer ground.

Table X-2 Treatment of symptomatic hypernatremia

Duration	Several hours	1-2 days	Unknown or >2 days
Clinical setting	Acute salt poisoning	Unreplaced water losses from diabetes insipidus or osmotic diuresis	Develops slowly in patients who are able to concentrate their urine
Symptoms and signs before Rx	Seizures, coma, fever	Lethargy, coma	Lethargy, confusion
Brain damage	Cerebral hemorrhage	Osmotic demyelination caused by rapid onset of hypernatremia	Post-Rx cerebral edema
Risk factors for permanent brain damage	Unknown	Unknown	Only reported in infants
Rx goals	Rapid correction to 145 mmol/L	Normalization of serum Na within 24 hours	10 mmol/L/day
Rx limit	No limit defined	No limit defined	• 1 mmol/L/hour • 10–12 mmol/L/day
Re-raising Serum Na for overcorrection	Unnecessary	Unnecessary	Recommended for cerebral edema or seizures (only reported in infants)

Rx = treatment of hypernatremia.

References

1 Sterns RH. Disorders of plasma sodium: causes, consequences, and correction. *N Engl J Med*. 2015.372:55–65.

2 Weed LH, McKibben PS. Experimental alteration of brain bulk. *Am J Physiology–Legacy Content*. 1919;48(4): 531–558.

3 Rowntree LG. Water intoxication. *Arch Int Med*.1923;32(2):157–174.

4 Sterns RH, Nigwekar SU, Hix JK. The treatment of hyponatremia. *Sem Nephr*. Vol. 29. No. 3. Philadelphia, PA: WB Saunders, 2009.

5 Berl T. Treating hyponatremia: damned if we do and damned if we don't. *Kidney Int*. 1990;37:1006–1018.

6 Hoorn EJ, Zietse R. Diagnosis and treatment of hyponatremia: compilation of the guidelines. *J Am Soc Nephrology*. 2017;28(5):1340–1349.

7 Verbalis JG, et al. Diagnosis, evaluation, and treatment of hyponatremia: expert panel recommendations. *Am J Med*. 2013;126(10)): S1–S42.

8 Hogan GR, et al. Pathogenesis of seizures occurring during restoration of plasma tonicity to normal in animals previously chronically hypernatremic. *Pediatrics*. 1969;43(1):54–64.

9 Sterns, RH, Hix JK. Overcorrection of hyponatremia is a medical emergency. *Kidney Int*. 2009;76(6);587–589.

41

Emergency Management of Acute and Chronic Hyponatremia

Joseph G. Verbalis

Key Points

- Severely symptomatic hyponatremia does not occur often, but its importance lies in the high morbidity and mortality rates characteristic of this metabolic disorder.
- Symptoms of hyponatremia correlate both with the magnitude and rate of decrease in the serum [Na$^+$] and with the chronicity of the hyponatremia. The development of neurological symptoms also depends on the age and sex of the patient.
- Acute hyponatremia is defined as ≤48 hrs duration; while chronic hyponatremia as >48 hrs duration.
- Evaluation and treatment of symptomatic hyponatremia in hospitalized patients should be initiated promptly in order to provide symptom relief and prevent or minimize the many adverse outcomes that have been independently associated with this disorder.
- Severe hyponatremia generally is defined by a lower serum [Na$^+$] (typically <125 mmol/L) and with symptoms indicating significant neurological dysfunction, such as coma, obtundation, seizures, respiratory distress, and unexplained vomiting. The typical duration of these cases is short and generally represents a more acute form of hyponatremia, but even more chronic forms of hyponatremia can have significant neurological symptomatology and occasionally life-threatening manifestations.

- It is important to assess the severity of the hyponatremia because most treatment algorithms use the severity of hyponatremia, as determined by the degree of neurological symptoms, to determine the initial therapy as opposed to the absolute level of serum [Na$^+$] alone.
- Consideration of treatment options should always include an evaluation of the benefits as well as the potential toxicities of any therapy, and must be individualized for each patient. It should always be remembered that sometimes simply stopping treatment with an agent that is associated with hyponatremia is sufficient to correct low [Na$^+$].
- Acute hyponatremia presenting with severe neurological symptoms is life-threatening, and should be treated promptly with hypertonic solutions, typically 3% saline, as this represents the most reliable method to quickly raise the serum [Na$^+$]. No active hyponatremia therapy (e.g., vaptans) should be administered until at least 24 hours following successful increases in serum [Na$^+$] using hypertonic saline.
- Hypovolemic patients with mild or moderate symptoms should be treated with solute repletion, either via isotonic (0.9%) saline infusion or oral sodium replacement.

Endocrine and Metabolic Medical Emergencies: A Clinician's Guide, Second Edition. Edited by Glenn Matfin.
© 2018 John Wiley & Sons Ltd. Published 2018 by John Wiley & Sons Ltd.

- It is imperative that all patients undergoing active treatment of symptomatic hyponatremia should have frequent monitoring of serum [Na$^+$] and ECF volume status to ensure that the serum [Na$^+$] does not exceed the limits of safe correction. Monitoring urine output is also important.
- The recommended maximal daily rate of serum [Na$^+$] change is 10–12 mmol/L/24 h or 18 mmol/L/48 h to prevent *osmotic demyelination syndrome* (ODS) in chronic hyponatremia (or lower rates if high risk of ODS). If this is rate is exceeded, especially in patients with high risk of ODS, re-lowering serum [Na$^+$] with hypotonic fluids (with or without desmopressin) should be considered. In acute symptomatic hyponatremia, serum [Na$^+$] can be corrected to a normal level quickly because the patient is not at risk for ODS.

Introduction

Severely symptomatic hyponatremia does not occur often, but its importance lies in the high morbidity and mortality rates characteristic of this metabolic disorder. Most cases of severely symptomatic hyponatremia occur when the hyponatremia has developed acutely, but even more chronic forms of hyponatremia can have significant neurological symptomatology and occasionally life-threatening manifestations

Table 41-1 Common clinical causes of symptomatic hyponatremia in hospitalized patients.

Acute hyponatremia (≤48 h duration):

- Water intoxication from psychogenic polydipsia (typically in schizophrenic patients) or excessive forced water ingestion (fraternity hazing)
- Exercise-associated hyponatremia (marathons, ultramarathons and similar prolonged endurance exercise activities)
- Post-operative hyponatremia
- 3,4-methylenedioxymethamphetamine ("Ecstasy")

Chronic hyponatremia (>48 h duration):

- Syndrome of inappropriate antidiuretic hormone secretion (SIADH; all etiologies)
- Drug-induced hyponatremia (particularly SSRI antidepressants)
- Hypovolemic hyponatremia (all etiologies, but particularly thiazide-induced hyponatremia)
- Heart failure
- Cirrhosis
- Nephrotic syndrome
- Renal failure

(Table 41-1). Several recent reviews have proposed comprehensive recommendations by expert panels for the evaluation and treatment of all types and etiologies of hyponatremia (1,2); this chapter will not reiterate those recommendations, but rather will focus on the evaluation and treatment of symptomatic hyponatremia in hospitalized patients that should be initiated promptly in order to provide symptom relief and prevent or minimize the many adverse outcomes that have been independently associated with this disorder (3–5). Determining appropriate treatment choices entails first understanding the classification of different types of hyponatremia and how this relates to the wide spectrum of symptoms of hyponatremia, their pathogenesis, and the morbidity and mortality associated with this important metabolic disorder.

Classification of Hyponatremia by Plasma Tonicity, Extracellular Fluid Volume Status, and Severity

Hyponatremia can be classified in a variety of manners. The first is generally by plasma *tonicity*. Patients with hyponatremia can be hypotonic, isotonic, or hypertonic in terms of their plasma tonicity, which depends on the relationship of the plasma osmolality to the serum sodium concentration ([Na$^+$]). In the most common form, hypotonic hyponatremia, serum [Na$^+$] and plasma osmolality are both low. Examples of this form of hyponatremia include the syndrome of inappropriate antidiuretic hormone secretion (SIADH), heart failure, and cirrhosis. It is important clinically to differentiate hypotonic hyponatremia from isotonic and hypertonic hyponatremia. Isotonic hyponatremia occurs when the serum [Na^+] is low but the plasma osmolality is normal. This can be seen in hyperglycemia and conditions that are called *pseudohyponatremia* because of hyperlipidemia or hyperproteinemia. Hypertonic hyponatremia also has a low serum [Na^+], but in this case, plasma osmolality is high rather than low. This can be seen with severe hyperglycemia with dehydration, as well as with the use of some osmotic agents such as mannitol. These distinctions are important because only hypotonic hyponatremia causes a shift of water from the extracellular fluid (ECF) into cells along osmotic gradients; therefore, it is the only type of hyponatremia that results in alterations of the water balance between the intracellular fluid (ICF) and ECF compartments.

Once it is confirmed that a patient has hypotonic hyponatremia with a low plasma osmolality, the next level of classification is to determine the ECF volume status of the patient. Patients with hypotonic hyponatremia can be hypovolemic with a decreased ECF volume, euvolemic with a normal clinically determined ECF volume, or hypervolemic with an expanded ECF volume. Hypovolemic patients have the typical signs of volume depletion. The usual causes include gastrointestinal, renal, or cutaneous fluid losses, diuretic therapy, and rarely cerebral salt wasting and primary adrenal insufficiency. In contrast, euvolemic hyponatremia is characterized by an absence of any clinical signs of ECF volume depletion or expansion. Typically, the blood urea nitrogen (BUN):creatinine ratio is normal or low, the serum uric acid is low, and the urine sodium is elevated or reflects dietary sodium intake. This is the pattern encountered with SIADH; other less common causes include nonsteroidal anti-inflammatory drug (NSAID) use, primary adrenal insufficiency, severe hypothyroidism (i.e., myxedema), exercise-associated hyponatremia, low solute intake, and polydipsia. Finally, hypervolemic hyponatremia patients are those who have edema, ascites, pulmonary congestion, or edema-forming disorders that typically include heart failure, cirrhosis, kidney failure, and the nephrotic syndrome. Classification by clinically determined ECF volume status is important because this determination dictates the next steps in terms of both diagnostic and treatment decisions.

Finally, hyponatremia can also be classified by severity, which is indicated mainly by neurological symptomatology (Table 41-2). Severe hyponatremia generally is defined by a lower serum [Na^+] (typically <125 mmol/L) and with symptoms indicating significant neurological dysfunction, such as coma, obtundation, seizures, respiratory distress, and unexplained vomiting. The typical

Table 41-2 Classification of hyponatremia according to severity of presenting symptoms

	Serum sodium	Neurological symptoms	Typical duration of hyponatremia
Severe	<125 mmol/L	Vomiting; seizures; obtundation; respiratory; distress; coma	Acute (<24–28 h)
Moderate	<130 mmol/L	Nausea; confusion; disorientation; altered mental status; unstable gait/falls	Intermediate or chronic (>24–48 h)
Mild	<135 mmol/L	Headache; irritability; difficulty concentrating; altered mood; depression	Chronic (several days to many weeks/months)

duration of these cases is short and it generally represents a more acute form of hyponatremia (Table 41-1). Moderate hyponatremia is also characterized by a low serum [Na$^+$]; however, the serum [Na$^+$] is generally not quite as low as in severe hyponatremia (although it can be), and generally is in the range of <130 mmol/L. The neurological symptoms of moderate hyponatremia, while still present, are not as marked as with severe hyponatremia and include altered mental status, disorientation, confusion, unexplained nausea, unstable gait, and increased falls. Typically these patients have a duration of hyponatremia that is intermediate or chronic, usually greater than 24–48 hours but generally not weeks or months in duration. Finally, mild hyponatremia can have any serum [Na$^+$], including up to 134 mmol/L and is characterized by very mild and often non-specific neurological symptoms including difficulty concentrating, irritability, altered mood, depression, and unexplained headache. Typically patients with this level of severity of hyponatremia have been hyponatremic for several days to many weeks to months; so mild hyponatremia typically is a manifestation of chronic hyponatremia. As explained in the next section, the severity of neurological symptoms is more dependent on the degree of brain adaptation to the hyponatremia than on the level of serum [Na$^+$]; that is why in the serum [Na$^+$] column in Table 41-2, there is a wide range of [Na$^+$] values that can encompass the various severity levels of hyponatremia. It is important to assess the severity of the hyponatremia because most treatment algorithms use the severity of hyponatremia, as determined by the degree of neurological symptoms, to determine the initial therapy.

Hyponatremia Symptoms, Morbidity, and Mortality

Symptoms of hyponatremia correlate both with the magnitude and rate of decrease in the serum [Na$^+$] and with the chronicity of the hyponatremia. Most clinical manifestations of hyponatremia usually begin at serum [Na$^+$] <130 mmol/L. Although gastrointestinal symptoms often occur early, the majority of the manifestations are neurological, including lethargy, confusion, disorientation, obtundation and seizures, often described as *hyponatremic encephalopathy* (6). Many of the symptoms of hyponatremic encephalopathy are caused by cerebral edema. In its most severe form, the cerebral edema can lead to tentorial herniation; in such cases, death can occur as a result of brainstem compression with respiratory arrest. The cerebral edema can also cause a neurogenic pulmonary edema and hypoxemia (7), which can in turn increase the severity of brain swelling (8). The most severe life-threatening clinical features of hyponatremic encephalopathy are generally seen in cases of acute hyponatremia, defined as <48 hrs in duration, but in most cases <24 hrs in duration (Table 41-1). The development of neurological symptoms also depends on the age and sex of the patient, and the magnitude and acuteness of the process. Elderly persons and young children with hyponatremia are most likely to develop severe neurological symptoms. In some studies, neurologic complications also appear to occur more frequently in menstruating women (8).

The observed central nervous system symptoms of severe hyponatremia are most likely related to the cellular swelling and cerebral edema that result from acute lowering of ECF osmolality, which leads to movement of water into cells. Such cerebral edema occasionally causes brain herniation, as has been noted in postmortem examination of both humans and experimental animals. The increase in brain water is, however, much less marked than would be predicted from the decrease in tonicity were the brain to operate as a passive osmometer. The volume regulatory responses that protect against cerebral edema, and which occur to varying degrees throughout the body, have been extensively studied and reviewed (9); studies of rats demonstrate a prompt loss of both electrolyte and organic osmolytes from the

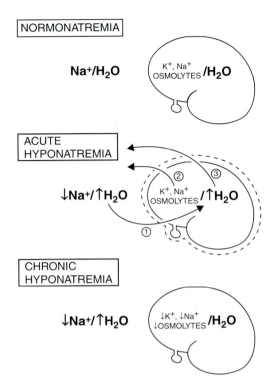

NORMONATREMIA

Na^+/H_2O

$\overset{K^+, Na^+}{OSMOLYTES}/H_2O$

ACUTE
HYPONATREMIA

$\downarrow Na^+/\uparrow H_2O$

$\overset{K^+, Na^+}{OSMOLYTES}/\uparrow H_2O$

CHRONIC
HYPONATREMIA

$\downarrow Na^+/\uparrow H_2O$

$\overset{\downarrow K^+, \downarrow Na^+}{\downarrow OSMOLYTES}/H_2O$

Figure 41-1 Schematic diagram of brain volume adaptation to hyponatremia. Under normal conditions brain osmolality and extracellular fluid (ECF) osmolality are in equilibrium (top panel); for simplicity, the predominant intracellular solutes are depicted as K^+ and organic osmolytes, and the extracellular solute as Na^+). Following the induction of ECF hypoosmolality, water moves into the brain (middle panel) in response to osmotic gradients producing brain edema (dotted line, #1). However, in response to the induced swelling, the brain rapidly loses both extracellular and intracellular solutes (middle panel, #2). As water losses accompany the losses of brain solute, the expanded brain volume then decreases back toward normal (middle panel, #3). If hypoosmolality is sustained, brain volume eventually normalizes completely and the brain becomes fully adapted to the ECF hyponatremia (bottom panel).

brain after the onset of hyponatremia (10) (Figure 41-1). The rate at which the brain restores the lost electrolytes and osmolytes when hyponatremia is corrected is also of pathophysiologic importance. Na^+ and Cl^- recover quickly and even overshoot normal brain contents; however, the re-accumulation of osmolytes is considerably delayed (11). This process is likely to account for the more

marked cerebral dehydration that accompanies the correction in experimental animals previously adapted to chronic hyponatremia (12).

The mortality of acute symptomatic hyponatremia has been noted to be as high as 55%, and as low as 5% (13,14). The former reflects the observation of few symptomatic hyponatremic patients in a consultative setting, the latter the estimate from a broad-based literature survey. The mortality associated with chronic hyponatremia is generally lower, and has been reported to be between 14% and 27% (15,16). The actual contribution of the hyponatremia to the observed mortality in hyponatremic patients remains uncertain. In a survey of hospitalized hyponatremic patients (serum $[Na^+]$ <128 mmol/L), 46% had central nervous system symptoms and 54% were asymptomatic (17). However, the authors judged that the hyponatremia was the cause of the symptoms in only 31% of the symptomatic patients. In this subgroup of symptomatic patients, the mortality was no different from that of asymptomatic patients (9–10%). In contrast, the mortality of patients whose central nervous system symptoms were not caused by hyponatremia was high (64%), suggesting that the mortality of these patients is more often due to the associated disease than to the electrolyte disorder itself. This is in agreement with the early report of Anderson et al. (18), who noted a 60-fold increase in mortality in hyponatremic patients over that of normonatremic control subjects, but in the hyponatremic patients, death frequently occurred after the serum $[Na^+]$ was returned toward normal and was generally felt to be due to progression of severe underlying diseases. These and other studies suggest that hyponatremia may be more an indicator of severe disease and poor prognosis, rather than a causal factor contributing to mortality. However, in opposition to this presumption, an increasing number of studies indicate that even mild hyponatremia is an independent predictor of higher mortality across a wide variety of disorders, including patients with acute ST elevation myocardial infarctions, heart failure and liver disease (5,19), as well as all hospitalized medical (3) and surgical (20) patients. In support of this view, a meta-analysis of studies in which a subset of patients had a correction of hyponatremia showed a significantly decreased risk ratio for mortality in the corrected patients (21). Consequently, the degree to which hyponatremia actually causes adverse outcomes rather than simply being associated with underlying co-morbidities remains uncertain at the present time (22).

In contrast to acute hyponatremia, chronic hyponatremia is much less symptomatic. The major reason for the profound differences between the symptoms of acute and chronic hyponatremia is now well understood to be due to the process of *brain volume regulation* described above (23) (Table 41-2). Despite this powerful adaptation process, chronic hyponatremia is frequently associated with varying degrees of neurological symptomatology, albeit usually milder and more subtle in nature. Even in patients adjudged to be "asymptomatic" by virtue of a normal neurological exam, accumulating evidence suggests that there may be previously unrecognized adverse effects as a result of chronic hyponatremia. In one study, 16 patients with hyponatremia secondary to SIADH in the range of 124–130 mmol/L demonstrated a significant gait instability that normalized after correction of the hyponatremia to normal ranges (24). The functional significance of the gait instability was illustrated in a study of 122 patients with a variety of levels of hyponatremia, all judged to be "asymptomatic' at the time of visit to an emergency department (ED). These patients were compared with 244 age-, sex-, and disease-matched controls also presenting to the ED during the same time period. Researchers found that 21% of the hyponatremic patients presented to the ED because of a recent fall, compared to only 5% of the controls; this difference was highly significant and remained so after multivariable adjustment (24). Consequently, this study clearly documented an increased incidence of falls in so-called "asymptomatic" hyponatremic patients. These findings have

been verified in a retrospective analysis of 2370 geriatric patients admitted for trauma to a large US hospital that showed that hyponatremia was associated with a 1.81 odds ratio for presenting with a fall, which was greater than any other risk factor for falls except age ≥ 85 years (25). The clinical significance of the gait instability and fall data have been indicated by multiple independent studies that have demonstrated increased rates of bone fractures in patients with hyponatremia (4,26–29). More recently published studies have shown that hyponatremia is associated with increased bone loss in experimental animals and a significant increased odds ratio for osteoporosis of the femoral neck (OR, 2.85; 95% CI 1.03–7.86, p < 0.01) in humans over the age of 50 in the NHANES III database (30). These findings have been confirmed in an analysis of 2.9 million electronic health records that demonstrated a significantly increased odds ratio for fractures in patients with chronic hyponatremia (OR, 3.97; 95% CI 3.59–4.39, p < 0.001), and even greater in patients with chronic persistent hyponatremia (OR, 12.09; 95% CI 9.34–15.66, p < 0.001) (31). Thus, the major clinical significance of chronic hyponatremia may lie in the increased morbidity and mortality associated with falls and fractures in our elderly population.

Treatment of Symptomatic Hyponatremia: General Principles

Correction of hyponatremia is associated with markedly improved neurological outcomes in patients with severely symptomatic hyponatremia. In a retrospective review of patients who presented with severe neurological symptoms and serum $[Na^+]$ <125 mmol/L, prompt therapy with isotonic or hypertonic saline resulted in a correction in the range of 20 mmol/L over several days and neurological recovery in almost all cases; in contrast, in patients who were treated with fluid restriction alone, there was very little correction over the study period (<5 mmol/L over 72 h), and the neurological outcomes were much worse, with most of these patients either dying or entering a persistently vegetative state (32). Consequently, based on this and similar retrospective analyses, prompt therapy to rapidly increase the serum [Na$^+$] represents the standard-of-care for treatment of patients presenting with severe life-threatening neurological symptoms of hyponatremia.

Brain herniation, the most dreaded complication of hyponatremia, is seen almost exclusively in patients with acute hyponatremia (usually <24 hours) or in patients with intracranial pathology (33–35). In postoperative patients and in patients with self-induced water intoxication associated with marathon running, psychosis, or use of "ecstasy" (methylenedioxy-N-methamphetamine or MDMA), nonspecific symptoms like headache, nausea, and vomiting or confusion can rapidly progress to seizures, respiratory arrest, and ultimately death or to a permanent vegetative state as a complication of severe cerebral edema (36). Hypoxia from non-cardiogenic pulmonary edema and/or hypoventilation can exacerbate brain swelling caused by the low serum [Na$^+$] (7,8). Seizures can complicate both severe chronic hyponatremia and acute hyponatremia. Although usually self-limited, hyponatremic seizures may be refractory to anticonvulsants.

As discussed earlier, chronic hyponatremia is much less symptomatic as a result of the process of brain volume regulation. Because of this adaptation process, chronic hyponatremia is arguably a condition that clinicians feel they may not need to be as concerned about, which has been reinforced by the common usage of the descriptor "asymptomatic hyponatremia" for many such patients. However, as discussed previously, it is clear that many such patients very often do have neurological symptoms, even if milder and more subtle in nature (24). Consequently, all patients with hyponatremia who manifest any neurological symptoms that could possibly be related to the hyponatremia should be considered candidates for treatment of the hyponatremia, regardless of the chronicity of the hyponatremia or the level of serum [Na$^+$]. An additional reason to treat even asymptomatic hyponatremia effectively is to prevent a lowering of the serum [Na$^+$] to more symptomatic and dangerous levels during treatment of underlying conditions (e.g., increased fluid administration via parenteral nutrition, treatment of heart failure with loop diuretics).

Currently Available Therapies for Treatment of Symptomatic Hyponatremia

Conventional management strategies for hyponatremia range from saline infusion and fluid restriction to pharmacologic measures to adjust fluid balance. Although the number of available treatments for hyponatremia is large, some are not appropriate for correction of symptomatic hyponatremia because they work too slowly or inconsistently to be effective in hospitalized patients (e.g., demeclocycline, mineralocorticoids). Consideration of treatment options should always include an evaluation of the benefits as well as the potential toxicities of any therapy, and must be individualized for each patient (37). It should always be remembered that sometimes simply stopping treatment with an agent that is associated with hyponatremia is sufficient to correct a low serum [Na$^+$].

Hypertonic Saline

Acute hyponatremia presenting with severe neurological symptoms is life-threatening, and should be treated promptly with hypertonic solutions, typically 3% NaCl ([Na$^+$] = 513 mmol/L), as this represents the most reliable method to quickly raise the serum [Na$^+$]. A continuous infusion of hypertonic NaCl is usually utilized in inpatient settings. Various formulae have been suggested to calculate the initial rate of infusion of hypertonic solutions (33), but until now there has been no consensus regarding optimal infusion rates of 3% NaCl. One of the simplest methods to estimate an initial 3% NaCl infusion rate utilizes the following relationship (37):

Patient's weight (kg) ×
desired correction rate (mmol/L/h)
= infusion rate of 3% NaCl (mL/h)

Depending on individual hospital policies, the administration of hypertonic solutions may require special considerations (e.g., placement in the ICU, use of central intravenous [IV] catheters, sign-off by a consultant, etc.), which each clinician needs to be aware of to optimize patient care.

An alternative option for more emergent situations is administration of a 100 mL bolus of 3% NaCl, repeated twice if there is no clinical improvement at 10 min intervals, which has been recommended by a consensus conference organized to develop guidelines for prevention and treatment of exercise-induced hyponatremia, an acute and potentially lethal condition (38), and adopted as a general recommendation by an expert panel (1). Injecting this amount of hypertonic saline IV raises the serum [Na$^+$] by an average of 2–4 mmol/L, which is well below the recommended maximal daily rate of change of 10–12 mmol/L/24 h or 18 mmol/L/48 h to prevent osmotic demyelination syndrome (ODS) (39). Because the brain can only accommodate an average increase of approximately 8% in brain volume before herniation occurs, quickly increasing the serum [Na$^+$] by as little as 2–4 mmol/L in acute hyponatremia can effectively reduce brain swelling and intracranial pressure (40).

Isotonic Saline

The treatment of choice for depletional hyponatremia (i.e., hypovolemic hyponatremia) is isotonic saline ([Na$^+$] = 154 mmol/L) to restore ECF volume and ensure adequate organ perfusion. This initial therapy is appropriate for patients who either have clinical signs of hypovolemia, or in whom a spot urine Na$^+$ concentration is <20–30 mmol/L (1). However, this

therapy is generally ineffective for dilutional hyponatremias such as SIADH (41), and continued inappropriate administration of isotonic saline to a euvolemic patient may worsen their hyponatremia (42,43), and/or cause fluid overload. Although isotonic saline may improve the serum [Na$^+$] in some patients with hypervolemic hyponatremia, their volume status will generally worsen with this therapy, so unless the neurological symptoms are severe, isotonic saline should be avoided.

Fluid Restriction

For patients with chronic hyponatremia, fluid restriction has been the most popular and most widely accepted treatment. When SIADH is present, fluids should generally be limited to 500–1000 mL/24 h. Because fluid restriction increases the serum [Na$^+$] largely by under-replacing the excretion of fluid by the kidneys, some have advocated an initial restriction to 500 ml less than the 24-hour urine output (44). When instituting a fluid restriction, it is important for the nursing staff and the patient to understand that this includes all fluids that are consumed, not just water (Table 41-3). Generally the water

Table 41-3 General recommendations for employment of fluid restriction and predictors of the increased likelihood of failure of fluid restriction (1)

General recommendations

- Restrict *all* intake that is consumed by drinking, not just water
- Aim for a fluid restriction that is 500 mL/d *below* the 24-h urine volume
- Do *not* restrict sodium or protein intake unless indicated

Predictors of the likely failure of fluid restriction

- High urine osmolality (>500 mOsm/kg H$_2$O)
- Sum of the urine Na$^+$ and K$^+$ concentrations exceeds the serum Na$^+$ concentration
- 24-h urine volume <1,500 mL/d
- Increase in serum Na$^+$ sodium concentration <2 mmol/L/d in 24–48 h on a fluid restriction of ≤1 L/d

content of ingested food is not included in the restriction because this is balanced by insensible water losses (perspiration, exhaled air, feces, etc.), but caution should be exercised with foods that have high fluid concentrations (such as fruits and soups). Restricting fluid intake can be effective when properly applied and managed in selected patients, but serum [Na$^+$] are generally increased only slowly (1–2 mmol/L/d) even with severe fluid restriction (41). In addition, this therapy is often poorly tolerated because of an associated increase in thirst leading to poor compliance with long-term therapy. However, it is economically favorable, and some patients do respond well to this option.

Fluid restriction should not be used with hypovolemic patients, and is particularly difficult to maintain in hospitalized patients with very elevated urine osmolalities secondary to high arginine vasopressin (AVP) levels; if the sum of urine Na$^+$ and K$^+$ exceeds the serum [Na$^+$], most patients will not respond to a fluid restriction since an electrolyte-free water clearance will be difficult to achieve (45–47). This and other known predictors of failure of fluid restriction are summarized in Table 41-3; the presence of any of these factors in hospitalized patients with symptomatic hyponatremia makes this less than ideal as an initial therapy. In addition, fluid restriction is not practical for some patients, particularly including patients in intensive care settings who often require administration of significant volumes of fluids as part of their therapies. Consequently, such patients are candidates for more effective pharmacological or saline treatment strategies.

Arginine Vasopressin Receptor Antagonists

Conventional therapies for hyponatremia, although effective in specific circumstances, are suboptimal for many different reasons, including variable efficacy, slow responses, intolerable side effects, and serious toxicities. But perhaps the most striking deficiency of most conventional therapies is that most of these therapies do not directly target the underlying cause of most dilutional hyponatremias, namely inappropriately elevated plasma arginine vasopressin (AVP) levels. A new class of pharmacological agents, vasopressin receptor antagonists, also known as "vaptans," that directly block AVP-mediated receptor activation have recently been approved for treatment of euvolemic (in the USA and the EU) and hypervolemic (in the USA) hyponatremia (48).

Conivaptan is FDA-approved for euvolemic and hypervolemic hyponatremia in hospitalized patients. It is available only as an IV preparation and is given as a 20-mg loading dose over 30 min, followed by a continuous infusion of 20 or 40 mg/d (49). Generally, the 20-mg continuous infusion is used for the first 24 hours to gauge the initial response. If the correction of serum [Na$^+$] is felt to be inadequate (e.g., < 5 mmol/L), then the infusion rate can be increased to 40 mg/d. Therapy is limited to a maximum duration of 4 days because of drug-interaction effects with other agents metabolized by the CYP3A4 hepatic isoenzyme. Importantly, for conivaptan and all other vaptans, it is critical that the serum [Na$^+$] concentration is measured frequently during the active phase of correction of the hyponatremia – a minimum of every 6 to 8 hours for conivaptan but more frequently in patients with risk factors for ODS (37). If the correction exceeds 10–12 mmol/L in the first 24 hours, the infusion should be stopped and the patient monitored closely. Consideration should be given to administering sufficient water, either orally or as IV 5% dextrose in water, to avoid a correction of > 12 mmol/L/d. The maximum correction limit should be reduced to 8 mmol/L over the first 24 hours in patients with risk factors for ODS (1) (Figure 41-2, Table 41-4). The most common side effects of conivaptan include headache, thirst, and hypokalemia (50).

Tolvaptan, an oral vasopressin receptor antagonist, is also FDA-approved for the treatment of euvolemic and hypervolemic hyponatremia. In contrast to conivaptan, the availability of tolvaptan in tablet form

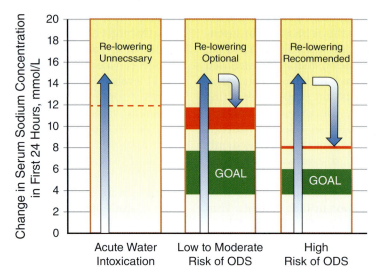

Figure 41-2 Recommended goals (green) and limits (red) for correction of hyponatremia based on risk of producing ODS, and recommendations for re-lowering of serum sodium concentration ([Na$^+$]) to goals for patients presenting with serum [Na$^+$] < 120 mmol/L who exceed the recommended limits of correction in the first 24 hours (1).
ODS = osmotic demyelination syndrome.

allows both short- and long-term use (51). Similar to conivaptan, tolvaptan treatment must be initiated in a hospital setting so that the rate of correction can be monitored carefully. In the USA, patients with a serum [Na$^+$] <125 mmol/L are eligible for therapy with tolvaptan as primary therapy; if the serum [Na$^+$] is ≥125 mmol/L, tolvaptan therapy is only indicated if the patient has symptoms that could be attributable to the hyponatremia and the patient is

resistant to attempts at fluid restriction (52). In the EU, tolvaptan is approved only for the treatment of euvolemic hyponatremia, but any symptomatic euvolemic patient is eligible for tolvaptan therapy regardless of the level of hyponatremia or response to previous fluid restriction. The starting dose of tolvaptan is 15 mg on the first day, and the dose can be titrated to 30 mg and 60 mg at 24-hour intervals if the serum [Na$^+$] remains < 135 mmol/L or the increase in serum [Na$^+$] has been < 5 mmol/L in the previous 24 hours. As with conivaptan, it is essential that the serum [Na$^+$] concentration is measured frequently during the active phase of correction of the hyponatremia at a minimum of every 6–8 h, particularly in patients with risk factors for ODS. Goals and limits for safe correction of hyponatremia and methods to compensate for overly rapid corrections are the same as described previously for conivaptan (Figure 41-2). One additional factor that helps to avoid overly rapid correction with tolvaptan is the recommendation that fluid restriction not be used during the active phase of correction, thereby allowing the

Table 41-4 Factors conferring increased risk of osmotic demyelination syndrome (ODS) that necessitate slower correction of hyponatremia (1)

High risk of osmotic demyelination syndrome:
- Serum sodium concentration ≤105 mmol/L
- Hypokalemia*
- Alcoholism*
- Malnutrition*
- Advanced liver disease*

---

*Unlike the defined level of serum sodium concentration, neither the precise level of the serum potassium concentration nor the degree of alcoholism, malnutrition, or liver disease that alters the brain's tolerance to an acute osmotic stress have been rigorously defined.

patient's thirst to compensate for an overly vigorous aquaresis. Common side effects of tolvaptan include dry mouth, thirst, increased urinary frequency, dizziness, nausea, and orthostatic hypotension (51,52).

Vaptans are not indicated for treatment of hypovolemic hyponatremia, since simple volume expansion would be expected to abolish the nonosmotic stimulus to AVP secretion and lead to a prompt aquaresis. Furthermore, inducing increased renal fluid excretion via either a diuresis or an aquaresis can cause or worsen hypotension in such patients. This possibility has resulted in the labeling of these drugs as contraindicated for hypovolemic hyponatremia (37). Importantly, clinically significant hypotension was not observed in either the conivaptan or tolvaptan clinical trials in euvolemic and hypervolemic hyponatremic patients. Although vaptans are not contraindicated with decreased renal function, these agents generally will not be effective if the serum creatinine is >3.0 mg/dL (265 μmol/L).

Urea

Urea has been described as an alternative oral treatment for SIADH and other hyponatremic disorders. The mode of action is to correct hypoosmolality not only by increasing solute-free water excretion but also by decreasing urinary sodium excretion. Doses of 15–60 g/d are generally effective; the dose can be titrated in increments of 15 g/d at weekly intervals as necessary to achieve normalization of the serum [Na$^+$]. It is advisable to dissolve the urea in orange juice or some other strongly flavored liquid to camouflage the bitter taste. Even if completely normal water balance is not achieved, it is often possible to allow the patient to maintain a less strict regimen of fluid restriction while receiving urea. The disadvantages associated with the use of urea include poor palatability (though newer flavored preparations have recently become available), the development of azotemia at higher doses, and the unavailability of a convenient or FDA-approved form of the agent. Data suggest that blood urea

concentrations may double during treatment (53), but it is important to remember that this does not represent renal impairment.

Reports of retrospective, uncontrolled studies suggest that the use of urea has been effective in treating SIADH in patients with hyponatremia due to subarachnoid hemorrhage and in critical care patients (54), and case reports have documented success in infants with chronic SIADH (55) and the nephrogenic syndrome of inappropriate antidiuresis (56). More recent evidence from a short study in a small cohort of SIADH patients suggests that urea may have a comparable efficacy to vaptans in reversing hyponatremia due to chronic SIADH (57).

Furosemide and NaCl

The use of furosemide (20–40 mg/d) coupled with a high salt intake (200 mmol/d), which represents an extension of the treatment of acute symptomatic hyponatremia (58) to the chronic management of euvolemic hyponatremia, has also been reported to be successful in small series of patients (59). However, the efficacy of this approach to correct symptomatic hyponatremia both promptly and within accepted goals limits (Figure 41-2) is unknown.

Efficacy of Different Treatments to Correct Hyponatremia

There have been no adequately powered randomized controlled trials to compare the efficacy and safety of different treatments utilized to correct hyponatremia. However, results of a prospective observational study in a large number of hospitalized patients in the USA and the EU provide useful data about the success rates of different therapies in euvolemic hyponatremic patients (60,61) (Table 41-5). In this study, "success" was defined by three different criteria: (a) the least stringent was an increase in serum [Na$^+$] of at least 5 mmol/L; (b) the next was correction to a serum [Na$^+$] of ≥ 130 mmol/L; and (c) the most stringent was correction to a normal serum [Na$^+$] of ≥ 135 mmol/L. As seen

Table 41-5 Success rates of therapies for hyponatremia in hospitalized patients with SIADH in the Hyponatremia Registry (61)

Diagnosis and treatment	$\Delta[Na^+] \geq 5$ mmol/L (%)	$[Na^+] \geq 130$ mmol/L (%)	$[Na^+] \geq 135$ mmol/L (%)
SIADH, no Rx (n = 168)	41	45	20
SIADH, FR (n = 625)	44	29	10
SIADH, NS (n = 384)	36	20	4
SIADH, tolvaptan (n = 183)	78	74	40
SIADH, 3% NaCI (n = 78)	60	25	13

Rx = treatment; FR = fluid restriction; NS = normal saline; 3% NaCL = 3% saline.

in Table 41-5, only 3% NaCl and tolvaptan had success rates significantly >50% for the least stringent criterion, and only tolvaptan achieved this level for the next most stringent criteria and a significantly higher rate for the most stringent criteria of normalization of the serum [Na⁺]. Of particular note, fluid restriction, the most frequently prescribed therapy in the Hyponatremia Registry patients, achieved a correction of serum [Na⁺] in only 44% of patients treated with this therapy, and isotonic saline in only 36% of patients.

Hyponatremia Treatment Guidelines Based on Symptom Severity

Although various authors have published recommendations on the treatment of hyponatremia (1,2,33,35,37,62–64), no standardized treatment algorithms have yet been universally accepted. For most treatment recommendations, the initial evaluation includes an assessment of the ECF volume status of the patient, since treatment recommendations differ in hypovolemic, euvolemic, and hypervolemic hyponatremic patients. A synthesis of expert opinion recommendations for treatment of hyponatremia is illustrated in Figure 41-3. This algorithm is based primarily on the neurological symptomatology of

hyponatremic patients rather than the serum [Na⁺] or on the chronicity of the hyponatremia, the latter of which is often difficult to ascertain. A careful neurological history and assessment should always be done to identify potential causes for the patient's symptoms other than hyponatremia, although it will not always be possible to exclude an additive contribution from the hyponatremia to an underlying neurological condition. In this algorithm, patients are divided into three groups based on their presenting symptoms (Table 41-2): mild, moderate, and severe:

- *Level 3 symptoms* include coma, obtundation, seizures, respiratory distress or arrest, and unexplained vomiting, and usually imply a more acute onset or worsening of hyponatremia requiring immediate active treatment. Therapies that will quickly raise serum [Na⁺] are required to reduce cerebral edema and decrease the risk of potentially fatal brain herniation.
- *Level 2 symptoms*, which are more moderate, include altered mental status, disorientation, confusion, unexplained nausea, gait instability, and falls. These symptoms can be either chronic or acute, but allow more time to elaborate a deliberate approach to choice of treatment.
- *Level 1 symptoms* range from minimal symptoms such as difficulty concentrating, irritability, altered mood, depression,

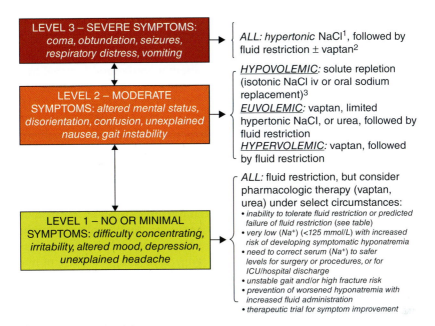

Figure 41-3 Algorithm for treatment of patients with hypotonic hyponatremia based on their presenting symptoms. The arrows between the symptom boxes indicate movement of patients between different symptom levels.
HYPOVOLEMIC, hypovolemic hyponatremia; **EUVOLEMIC**, euvolemic hyponatremia; **HYPERVOLEMIC**, hypervolemic hyponatremia; **ALL**, all types of hypotonic hyponatremia.
[1]Some authors recommend simultaneous treatment with desmopressin to limit speed of correction.
[2]No active therapy should be started within 24 h of hypertonic saline to decrease the chance of overly rapid correction of [Na+] and risk of ODS.
[3]With isotonic NaCl infusion, serum [Na+] and urine output must be followed closely to prevent overly rapid correction and risk of ODS due to a secondary water diuresis. Table in figure refers to Table 41-3. Modified from (78).

and unexplained headache, to a virtual absence of discernible symptoms, and indicate that the patient may have chronic or slowly evolving hyponatremia. These symptoms necessitate a cautious approach, especially when patients have underlying co-morbidities.

Patients with severe symptoms (Level 3) should be treated with hypertonic (3%) NaCl as first-line therapy, followed by fluid restriction with or without vaptan therapy. Because overly rapid correction of serum [Na+] occurs in >10% of patients treated with hypertonic NaCl (43,65), such patients are at risk for ODS unless carefully monitored. For this reason, some authors have proposed simultaneous treatment with desmopressin to reduce

the rate of correction to only that produced by the hypertonic NaCl infusion itself (66,67). Whether sufficient clinical data eventually prove that this approach is both effective and safe in larger numbers of patients remains to be determined. Only a single case of ODS has been reported in a patient receiving tolvaptan alone as monotherapy, but this patient was allowed to reach severely hypernatremic levels (68). In addition, two abstracts have been reported where ODS occurred when vaptans were used directly following hypertonic saline administration within the same 24-hour period (1). Consequently, no active hyponatremia therapy should be administered until at least 24 hours following successful increases in serum [Na+] using hypertonic NaCl.

The choice of treatment for patients with moderate symptoms (Level 2) will depend on their ECF volume status (Figure 41-3). Hypovolemic patients should be treated with solute repletion, either via isotonic NaCl infusion or oral sodium replacement (1). Euvolemic patients, typically with SIADH, will benefit from vaptan therapy, limited hypertonic saline administration, or in some cases urea, where available. This can then be followed by fluid restriction or long-term vaptan therapy when the etiology of the SIADH is expected to be chronic (1). In hypervolemic patients with heart failure, vaptans are usually the best choice since fluid restriction is rarely successful in this group, saline administration can cause fluid retention with increased edema, and urea can lead to ammonia build-up in the gastrointestinal tract if hepatic function is impaired. Although moderate neurological symptoms can indicate that a patient is in an early stage of acute hyponatremia, they more often indicate a chronically hyponatremic state with sufficient brain volume adaptation to prevent marked symptomatology from cerebral edema. Since most patients with moderate hyponatremic symptoms have a more chronic form of hyponatremia, recommendations for goals and limits of correction should be followed closely (Figure 41-2), and close monitoring of these patients in a hospital setting is warranted until the symptoms improve or stabilize.

Patients with no or minimal symptoms should be managed initially with fluid restriction, although treatment with pharmacologic therapy, such as vaptans or urea, may be appropriate for a wide range of specific clinical conditions (Figure 41-2), foremost of which is a failure to improve the serum [Na$^+$] despite reasonable attempts at fluid restriction, or the presence of clinical characteristics associated with poor responses to fluid restriction (Table 41-3).

A special case is when spontaneous correction of hyponatremia occurs at an undesirably rapid rate as a result of the onset of a water diuresis. This can occur following cessation of desmopressin therapy in a patient who has become hyponatremic, replacement of glucocorticoids in a patient with adrenal insufficiency, replacement of solutes in a patient with diuretic-induced hyponatremia, or spontaneous resolution of transient SIADH. Brain damage from ODS can clearly ensue in this setting if the preceding period of hyponatremia has been of sufficient duration (usually ≥48 hrs) to allow brain volume regulation to occur. If the previously discussed correction parameters have been exceeded and the correction is proceeding more rapidly than planned (usually because of continued excretion of hypotonic urine), the pathological events leading to demyelination can be reversed by administration of hypotonic fluids, with or without desmopressin. Efficacy of this approach is suggested both from animal studies (69) as well as case reports in humans (35,70) even when patients are overtly symptomatic (71). However, re-lowering the serum [Na$^+$] after an initial overly rapid correction is only strongly recommended in patients who are at high risk of ODS (Table 41-4), and is considered optional in patients with low to moderate risk of ODS and unnecessary in patients with acute water intoxication (Figure 41-2).

Although this classification is based on presenting symptoms at the time of initial evaluation, it should be remembered that in some cases patients initially exhibit more moderate symptoms because they are in the early stages of worsening hyponatremia. In addition, some patients with minimal symptoms are prone to develop more symptomatic hyponatremia during periods of increased fluid ingestion. In support of this, approximately 70% of 31 patients presenting to a university hospital with symptomatic hyponatremia and a mean serum [Na$^+$] of 119 mmol/L had pre-existing "asymptomatic" hyponatremia as the most common risk factor identified (72). Consequently, therapy of hyponatremia should also be considered to prevent progression from lower to higher levels of symptomatic hyponatremia, particularly in patients with a past history of repeated presentations for symptomatic hyponatremia.

Case study

A 75-year-old female was admitted for symptomatic hyponatremia with a serum $[Na^+] = 123$ mmol/L. She has a several years history of mild chronic hyponatremia, but recently has experienced confusion and dizziness. She was euvolemic on clinical exam, and was not taking antidepressants or diuretics. After 3 days on a confirmed 1,000 ml/d fluid restriction, the patient is still symptomatic and complains of thirst. Laboratory data on day 3 are: serum $[Na^+] = 126$ mmol/L (normal 135–145), serum $[K^+] = 4.0$ mmol/L (normal 3.5–5.0), plasma osmolality = 265 mOsm/kg H_2O (normal 285–300), urine osmolality = 535 mOsm/kg H_2O, urine $[Na^+] = 45$ mmol/L, urine $[K^+] = 70$ mmol/L, plasma glucose = 99 mg/dL (normal 65–100) [5.6 mmol/L], BUN = 18 mg/dL (normal 8–21), serum creatinine = 0.8 mg/dL (normal 0.8–1.3), serum TSH = 3.5 mcu/mL (normal 0.5–5.0), plasma cortisol = 18 μg/dL (500 nmol/L).

Does This Fit with a Diagnosis of SIADH and Is Fluid Restriction Likely to Be Successful?

This patient meets the criteria for SIADH, so the initial choice of fluid restriction was reasonable. However, she has three parameters that predict likely failure of her current fluid restriction: (a) urine osmolality >500; (b) a urine:plasma electrolyte ratio = 0.91 (i.e., 45 + 70/126); and (c) failure to increase serum $[Na^+]$ by at least 2 mmol/L/d on a 1,000 ml/d fluid restriction (Table 41-3). While tightening the fluid restriction to 500–800 ml/d would likely result in an improved serum $[Na^+]$ (i.e., urine:plasma electrolyte ratio <0.5, fluid restriction up to 1000 ml/d is recommended; 0.5–1.0, up to 500 ml/d preferred; and >1.0, 0 ml fluid restriction is needed which is not an option), the patient is already thirsty and has an elevated BUN/Cr ratio >20 indicating early volume contraction, so this would not be a viable option. Isotonic saline is not indicated for treatment of hyponatremia due to SIADH, and the high urine:plasma electrolyte ratio increases the risk of possible further lowering of the serum $[Na^+]$ using this therapy. Hypertonic saline would be effective at increasing the serum $[Na^+]$, but would not be necessary since the patient does not have severe neurological symptoms (e.g., seizures, obtundation, coma, respiratory distress), and would not be a viable long-term treatment for chronic hyponatremia. Urea would also likely be effective in increasing the serum $[Na^+]$, but lacks evidence-based data on the time required to do so and may be difficult to obtain in a hospital setting in the USA. Consequently, a vaptan offers the most reliable option for a prompt increase in serum $[Na^+]$ to relieve the patient's neurological symptoms, with a 76% efficacy of tolvaptan to raise the serum $[Na^+] \geq 5$ mmol/L. The major teaching point of this case is not to persist more than 1–2 days with a fluid restriction that is predicted to fail, or has failed, but rather move quickly to more effective therapies (see Figure 41-3).

Monitoring the Serum $[Na^+]$ in Hyponatremic Patients

The frequency of serum $[Na^+]$ monitoring is dependent on both the severity of the hyponatremia and the therapy chosen. In all hyponatremic patients, neurological symptomatology should be carefully assessed very early in the diagnostic evaluation to define the symptomatic severity of the hyponatremia and to determine whether the patient requires more urgent therapy. All patients undergoing active treatment with hypertonic saline for level 3 or 2 symptomatic hyponatremia should have frequent monitoring of serum $[Na^+]$ and ECF volume status (every 2-4 hours) to ensure that the serum $[Na^+]$ does not exceed the limits of safe correction during the active phase of correction (37), since overly rapid correction of serum $[Na^+]$ will increase the risk of ODS (73). Patients treated with vaptans for level 2 or 3 symptoms should have serum [Na$^+$] monitored every 6–8 hours during the active phase of correction, which will generally be the first 24–48 hours of therapy. All patients undergoing treatment for hyponatremia should have their urine output monitored as well, since production of large volumes of dilute urine (i.e., an *aquaresis*) constitutes a warning sign that the serum [Na$^+$] will correct more rapidly than predicted; this is particularly important for patients with hypovolemic hyponatremia being treated with isotonic or hypertonic NaCl since normalization of ECF volume will decrease elevated plasma AVP levels (1). Active treatment with hypertonic saline or vaptans should be stopped when the patient's symptoms are no longer present, a safe serum [Na$^+$] (usually >120 mmol/L) has been achieved, or the rate of correction has reached maximum limits of 10–12 mmol/L within 24 h or 18 mmol/L within 48 hours (37;39), or 8 mmol/L over any 24 h period in patients at high risk of ODS (Table 41-4). Some authors have recommended the more cautious limits of 8 mmol/L in any 24 h period for all hyponatremic patients regardless of duration of hyponatremia or risk of ODS (2;74). In patients with a stable level of serum [Na$^+$] treated with fluid restriction or therapies other than hypertonic saline, measurement of serum [Na$^+$] daily is generally sufficient, since levels will not change that quickly in the absence of active therapy or large changes in fluid intake or administration.

Case Study

A healthy 25-year-old female just completed her first marathon race. She felt ill toward the end of the race, but was able to walk back to her hotel unassisted. Six hours later, her roommate noticed that she was not making sense. She was taken to the nearby ED where she was found to be disoriented and confused but without focal neurological deficits. Vital signs were stable except for an increased respiratory rate to 32 and the patient was euvolemic by clinical exam. Laboratory data from the ED are: serum [Na$^+$] = 122 mmol/L (normal 135–145), serum [K$^+$] = 3.6 mmol/L (normal 3.5–5.0), plasma osmolality = 254 mOsm/kg H$_2$O (normal 285–300), urine osmolality = 412 mOsm/kg H$_2$O, urine [Na$^+$] = 50 mmol/L, plasma glucose = 120 mg/dL (normal 65–100) [6.8 mmol/L], BUN = 12 mg/dL (normal 8–21), serum creatinine = 0.8 mg/dL (normal 0.8–1.3).

What Is the Likely Cause of the Hyponatremia?

This patient has exercise-associated hyponatremia (EAH), which is almost always due to retention of water consumed during or after endurance events relative to the fluid lost via sweating and renal excretion. EAH has been shown to be associated with inappropriate AVP levels, likely of multifactorial origin. Because this is an acute hyponatremia that developed in <24 h (Table 41-1), the patient is at risk for cerebral edema from movement of water into the brain along osmotic gradients. In order to prevent tentorial herniation with brainstem compression and respiratory arrest, acute treatment is clearly indicated. The only therapy that can be depended upon to increase the serum [Na$^+$] within minutes is 3% NaCl; no other therapy can be relied upon to do this as quickly. An initial bolus of 100 ml will begin to reverse the osmotic gradient pulling water into the brain, and decrease the intracranial pressure. In the medical area of an endurance event, repeated boluses of 3% NaCl are recommended to correct hyponatremia, but in a hospital setting it would be more efficacious to begin a continuous infusion following the initial bolus. The serum [Na$^+$] should be monitored frequently (every 1–2 h initially) to ensure correction of hyponatremia, but the patient is not at risk for ODS since this is an acute not a chronic hyponatremia. Therefore, the correction does not need to be interrupted once an increase of serum [Na$^+$] of 10–12 mmol/L has occurred, and can be corrected to a normal serum [Na$^+$] quickly (see Figure 41-2). The major teaching point of this case is that acute hyponatremias with neurological dysfunction should be treated quickly with therapies proven to increase the serum [Na$^+$] with high reliability.

Common Clinical Questions about the Therapy of Symptomatic Hyponatremia

1. *What is the best method to assess the ECF volume status in patients who appear euvolemic by clinical examination?* In most cases the urine sodium concentration is the best discriminator of effective ECF volume (75,76). Although various authors have proposed different cut-off values for this measure, most agree that a urine sodium <20–30 mmol/L is low and indicates hypovolemia. An exception is patients with heart failure or cirrhosis, who have a low urine sodium because of renal hypoperfusion despite ECF volume expansion.

2. *Can the urine sodium be used in patients on diuretic therapy?* The urine sodium should always be measured prior to initiating therapy in symptomatic patients. If the urine sodium is low, it indicates hypovolemia unless the patient has heart failure or cirrhosis. If the urine sodium is >30 mmol/L, it cannot be determined whether this is due to a contracted ECF volume or to the diuretic until the effect of the diuretic therapy has dissipated (generally 24 h). Alternatives are measurement of the fractional urine uric acid excretion (76), although it usually takes more than 24 h to obtain results of this measurement, or a limited trial infusion of isotonic NaCl to see if the serum [Na$^+$] improves (1).

3. *What is the best initial therapy of hyponatremia in patients in whom the ECF volume is indeterminate?* If the patient has severe hyponatremia by symptoms, infusion of hypertonic NaCl is indicated and will correct both the serum [Na$^+$] as well as expand the ECF volume. If the patient has moderately symptomatic hyponatremia, the best initial therapy is a limited trial infusion of isotonic saline to see if the serum [Na$^+$] improves (1). Generally 1–2 L (over 24 hours) will suffice to make this determination. If no improvement in serum [Na$^+$] occurs, the infusion should be discontinued, since continued infusion of isotonic NaCl in patients with SIADH can lower the serum [Na$^+$] via a process called "desalination" (42,43).

4. *Is measurement of urine sodium concentration valid in patients who have already received saline administration prior to consultation?* The urine sodium reflects the current ECF volume status of the patient. Therefore, it remains useful to differentiate hyponatremia from euvolemia even if patents have already received a saline infusion, which typically occurs in the ED, regardless of the etiology of the hyponatremia. However, once the serum [Na$^+$] begins to correct, the urine sodium is not as useful since many patients with SIADH enter a phase of sodium retention to correct the total body sodium deficiency that develops during adaptation to chronic hyponatremia (77).

5. *Should a trial of fluid restriction be performed if the patient manifests predictors of failure of fluid restriction?* The predictors of failure of fluid restriction (Table 41-3) indicate the relative likelihood of failure of fluid restriction, but not an absolute certainty. However, if fluid restriction is attempted in the presence of one or more of these predictors, the stringency should be increased to have the best chance of success (i.e., maximum fluid intake of 500–800 ml/day).

6. *Given FDA warnings, should liver function tests be monitored in patients receiving a vaptan?* Liver function abnormalities in patients receiving vaptans occurred in clinical trials of polycystic kidney disease using 3–5 times the dose of tolvaptan recommended for the treatment of hyponatremia for >3 months (1). While it is therefore appropriate to avoid tolvaptan use in

patients with known liver disease, it is not necessary to closely monitor liver function tests in patients treated with tolvaptan at FDA-approved doses (15–60 mg/day) for shorter periods (<30 days).

7. *Can tolvaptan be used for periods longer than 30 days?* As in the previous question, the recommendation that tolvaptan not be used for >30 d is based on the occurrence of liver failure in a small number of patients treated with higher doses. Therefore, the decision of how long to treat a patient should be based on a clinical determination of risk versus benefit for individual patients. However, if tolvaptan is prescribed for periods longer than 30 d, it is appropriate to monitor liver function tests every 3 months at least during the first year of therapy (1).

References

1 Verbalis JG, Goldsmith SR, Greenberg A et al. Diagnosis, evaluation, and treatment of hyponatremia: expert panel recommendations. *Am J Med*. 2013;126(10 Suppl 1):S1–S42.

2 Spasovski G, Vanholder R, Allolio B, et al. Clinical practice guideline on diagnosis and treatment of hyponatraemia. *Nephrol Dial Trans*. 2014;170:G1–G47.

3 Wald R, Jaber BL, Price LL, Upadhyay A, Madias NE. Impact of hospital-associated hyponatremia on selected outcomes. *Arch Intern Med*. 2010;170(3): 294–302.

4 Hoorn EJ, Rivadeneira F, van Meurs JB, et al. Mild hyponatremia as a risk factor for fractures: The Rotterdam Study. *J Bone Miner Res*. 2011;26:1822–1828.

5 Corona G, Giuliani C, Parenti G, et al. Moderate hyponatremia is associated with increased risk of mortality: evidence from a meta-analysis. *PLoS ONE*. 2013;8(12): e80451.

6 Fraser CL, Arieff AI. Epidemiology, pathophysiology, and management of hyponatremic encephalopathy. *Am J Med*. 1997;102:67–77.

7 Ayus JC, Varon J, Arieff AI. Hyponatremia, cerebral edema, and noncardiogenic pulmonary edema in marathon runners. *Ann Intern Med*. 2000;132(9):711–714.

8 Ayus JC, Arieff AI. Pulmonary complications of hyponatremic encephalopathy. noncardiogenic pulmonary edema and hypercapnic respiratory failure [see comments]. *Chest*. 1995;107(2):517–521.

9 Pasantes-Morales H, Franco R, Ordaz B, Ochoa LD. Mechanisms counteracting swelling in brain cells during hyponatremia. *Arch Med Res*. 2002;33(3):237–244.

10 Lien YH, Shapiro JI, Chan L. Study of brain electrolytes and organic osmolytes during correction of chronic hyponatremia: implications for the pathogenesis of central pontine myelinolysis. *J Clin Invest*. 1991;88:303–309.

11 Verbalis JG, Gullans SR. Rapid correction of hyponatremia produces differential effects on brain osmolyte and electrolyte reaccumulation in rats. *Brain Res*. 1993;606:19–27.

12 Berl T. Treating hyponatremia: damned if we do and damned if we don't. *Kidney Int*. 1990;37:1006–1018.

13 Sterns RH. Severe symptomatic hyponatremia: treatment and outcome: a study of 64 cases. *Ann Int Med*. 1987;107:656–664.

14 Berl T. Treating hyponatremia: what is all the controversy about? [see comments]. [Review]. *Ann Int Med*. 1990;113: 417–419.

15 Sterns RH. The treatment of hyponatremia: first, do no harm. *Am J Med*. 1990;88: 557–560.

16 Tierney WM, Martin DK, Greenlee MC, Zerbe RL, McDonald CJ. The prognosis of hyponatremia at hospital admission. *J Gen Intern Med*. 1986;1:380–385.

17 Baran D, Hutchinson TA. The outcome of hyponatremia in a general hospital population. *Clin Nephrol*. 1984;22:72–76.

18 Anderson RJ, Chung HM, Kluge R, Schrier RW. Hyponatremia: a prospective analysis of its epidemiology and the pathogenetic role of vasopressin. *Ann Int Med*. 1985;102:164–168.

19 Upadhyay A, Jaber BL, Madias NE. Incidence and prevalence of hyponatremia. *Am J Med*. 2006; 119(7 Suppl 1): S30–S35.

20 Leung AA, McAlister FA, Rogers SO, Jr., Pazo V, Wright A, Bates DW. Preoperative hyponatremia and perioperative complications. *Arch Intern Med*. 2012;172(19):1474–1481.

21 Corona G, Giuliani C, Verbalis JG, Forti G, Maggi M, Peri A. Hyponatremia improvement is associated with a reduced risk of mortality: evidence from a meta-analysis. *PLoS ONE*. 2015;10(4):e0124105.

22 Hoorn EJ, Zietse R. Hyponatremia and mortality: how innocent is the bystander? *Clin J Am Soc Nephrol*. 2011;6(5):951–953.

23 Verbalis JG. Brain volume regulation in response to changes in osmolality. *Neuroscience*. 2010;168(4):862–870.

24 Renneboog B, Musch W, Vandemergel X, Manto MU, Decaux G. Mild chronic hyponatremia is associated with falls, unsteadiness, and attention deficits. *Am J Med*. 2006;119(1):71.

25 Rittenhouse KJ, To T, Rogers A, et al. Hyponatremia as a fall predictor in a geriatric trauma population. *Injury*. 2015;46(1):119–123.

26 Gankam KF, Andres C, Sattar L, Melot C, Decaux G. Mild hyponatremia and risk of fracture in the ambulatory elderly. *QJM*. 2008;101(7):583–588.

27 Sandhu HS, Gilles E, DeVita MV, Panagopoulos G, Michelis MF. Hyponatremia associated with large-bone fracture in elderly patients. *Int Urol Nephrol*. 2009;41(3):733–737.

28 Kinsella S, Moran S, Sullivan MO, Molloy MG, Eustace JA. Hyponatremia independent of osteoporosis is associated with fracture occurrence. *Clin J Am Soc Nephrol*. 2010;5(2):275–280.

29 Ayus JC, Fuentes NA, Negri AL, et al. Mild prolonged chronic hyponatremia and risk of hip fracture in the elderly. *Nephrol Dial Transplant*. 2016;31(10):1662–1669.

30 Verbalis JG, Barsony J, Sugimura Y, et al. Hyponatremia-induced osteoporosis. *J Bone Miner Res*. 2010;25(3):554–563.

31 Usala RL, Fernandez SJ, Mete M, et al. Hyponatremia is associated with increased osteoporosis and bone fractures in a large US health system population. *J Clin Endocrinol Metab*. 2015;100(8):3021–3031.

32 Ayus JC. Diuretic-induced hyponatremia [editorial]. *Arch Intern Med*. 1986;146(7):1295–1296.

33 Adrogue HJ, Madias NE. Hyponatremia. *N Engl J Med*. 2000;342(21):1581–1589.

34 Sterns RH, Hix JK, Silver S. Treatment of hyponatremia. *Curr Opin Nephrol Hypertens*. 2010;19(5):493–498.

35 Sterns RH, Nigwekar SU, Hix JK. The treatment of hyponatremia. *Semin Nephrol*. 2009;29(3):282–299.

36 Arieff AI. Hyponatremia, convulsions, respiratory arrest, and permanent brain damage after elective surgery in healthy women. *N Engl J Med*. 1986;314: 1529–1535.

37 Verbalis JG, Goldsmith SR, Greenberg A, Schrier RW, Sterns RH. Hyponatremia treatment guidelines 2007: expert panel recommendations. *Am J Med*. 2007; 120(11 Suppl 1):S1–S21.

38 Hew-Butler T, Ayus JC, Kipps C, et al. Statement of the Second International Exercise-Associated Hyponatremia Consensus Development Conference, New Zealand, 2007. *Clin J Sport Med*. 2008;18(2):111–121.

39 Sterns RH, Cappuccio JD, Silver SM, Cohen EP. Neurologic sequelae after treatment of severe hyponatremia: a multicenter perspective. *J Am Soc Nephrol*. 1994;4:1522–1530.

40 Battison C, Andrews PJ, Graham C, Petty T. Randomized, controlled trial on the effect of a 20% mannitol solution and a 7.5% saline/6% dextran solution on increased intracranial pressure after brain injury. *Crit Care Med*. 2005;33(1):196–202.

41 Schwartz WB, Bennett S, Curelop S, Bartter FC. A syndrome of renal sodium

loss and hyponatremia probably resulting from inappropriate secretion of antidiuretic hormone. *Am J Med.* 1957;23:529–542.

42 Steele A, Gowrishankar M, Abrahamson S, Mazer CD, Feldman RD, Halperin ML. Postoperative hyponatremia despite near-isotonic saline infusion: a phenomenon of desalination [see comments]. *Ann Intern Med.* 1997;126(1):20–25.

43 Greenberg A, Verbalis JG, Amin AN, et al. Current treatment practice and outcomes. Report of the hyponatremia registry. *Kidney Int.* 2015;88:167–177.

44 Robertson GL. Regulation of arginine vasopressin in the syndrome of inappropriate antidiuresis. *Am J Med.* 2006;119(7 Suppl 1):S36–S42.

45 Furst H, Hallows KR, Post J, et al. The urine/plasma electrolyte ratio: a predictive guide to water restriction. *Am J Med Sci.* 2000;319(4):240–244.

46 Decaux G. The syndrome of inappropriate secretion of antidiuretic hormone (SIADH). *Semin Nephrol.* 2009;29(3): 239–256.

47 Berl T. Impact of solute intake on urine flow and water excretion. *J Am Soc Nephrol.* 2008;19(6):1076–1078.

48 Greenberg A, Verbalis JG. Vasopressin receptor antagonists. *Kidney Int.* 2006;69(12):2124–2130.

49 Vaprisol (conivaptan hydrochloride injection) prescribing information. Deerfield, IL: Astellas Pharma US, Inc., 2006.

50 Zeltser D, Rosansky S, van Rensburg H, Verbalis JG, Smith N. Assessment of the efficacy and safety of intravenous conivaptan in euvolemic and hypervolemic hyponatremia. *Am J Nephrol.* 2007;27(5):447–457.

51 Schrier RW, Gross P, Gheorghiade M et al. Tolvaptan, a selective oral vasopressin V2-receptor antagonist, for hyponatremia. *N Engl J Med.* 2006;355(20):2099–2112.

52 Otsuka Pharmaceutical Co L, Tokyo Japan. Samsca (tolvaptan) prescribing information. 2009. Pamphlet.

53 Coussement J, Danguy C, Zouaoui-Boudjeltia K, et al. Treatment of the syndrome of inappropriate secretion of antidiuretic hormone with urea in critically ill patients. *Am J Nephrol.* 2012;35(3): 265–270.

54 Decaux G, Andres C, Gankam KF, Soupart A. Treatment of euvolemic hyponatremia in the intensive care unit by urea. *Crit Care.* 2010;14(5):R184.

55 Chehade H, Rosato L, Girardin E, Cachat F. Inappropriate antidiuretic hormone secretion: long-term successful urea treatment. *Acta Paediatr.* 2012;101(1): e39–e42.

56 Levtchenko EN, Monnens LA. Nephrogenic syndrome of inappropriate antidiuresis. *Nephrol Dial Trans.* 2010;25(9):2839–2843.

57 Soupart A, Coffernils M, Couturier B, Gankam-Kengne F, Decaux G. Efficacy and tolerance of urea compared with vaptans for long-term treatment of patients with SIADH. *Clin J Am Soc Nephrol.* 2012;7(5):742–747.

58 Hantman D, Rossier B, Zohlman R, Schrier R. Rapid correction of hyponatremia in the syndrome of inappropriate secretion of antidiuretic hormone: an alternative treatment to hypertonic saline. *Ann Int Med.* 1973;78:870–875.

59 Decaux G, Waterlot Y, Genette F, Mockel J. Treatment of the syndrome of inappropriate secretion of antidiuretic hormone with furosemide. *N Engl J Med.* 1981;304:329–330.

60 Greenberg A, Verbalis JG, Amin AN, et al. Current treatment practice and outcomes: report of the hyponatremia registry. *Kidney Int.* 2015;88(1):167–177.

61 Verbalis J, Greenberg A, Burst V, et al. Diagnosing and treating the syndrome of inappropriate antidiuretic hormone secretion. *Am J Med.* 2016;129: 537.e9–537.e23.

62 Ellison DH, Berl T. Clinical practice: the syndrome of inappropriate antidiuresis. *N Engl J Med.* 2007;356(20):2064–2072.

63 Verbalis JG. Hyponatremia and hypo-osmolar disorders. In: Greenberg A,

Cheung AK, Coffman TM, Falk RJ, Jennette JC, eds. *Primer on Kidney Diseases.* Philadelphia. PA: Saunders Elsevier, 2009: 52–59.

64 Sterns RH. Disorders of plasma sodium: causes, consequences, and correction. *N Engl J Med.* 2015; 372(1):55–65.

65 Mohmand HK, Issa D, Ahmad Z, Cappuccio JD, Kouides RW, Sterns RH. Hypertonic saline for hyponatremia: risk of inadvertent overcorrection. *Clin J Am Soc Nephrol.* 2007;2(6):1110–1117.

66 Perianayagam A, Sterns RH, Silver SM, et al. DDAVP is effective in preventing and reversing inadvertent overcorrection of hyponatremia. *Clin J Am Soc Nephrol.* 2008;3(2):331–336.

67 Sterns RH, Hix JK, Silver S. Treating profound hyponatremia: a strategy for controlled correction. *Am J Kidney Dis.* 2010;56(4):774–779.

68 Malhotra I, Gopinath S, Janga KC, Greenberg S, Sharma SK, Tarkovsky R. Unpredictable nature of tolvaptan in treatment of hypervolemic hyponatremia: case review on role of vaptans. *Case Rep Endocrinol.* 2014; 2014:807054.

69 Soupart A, Penninckx R, Crenier L, Stenuit A, Perier O, Decaux G. Prevention of brain demyelination in rats after excessive correction of chronic hyponatremia by serum sodium lowering. *Kidney Int.* 1994;45:193–200.

70 Goldszmidt MA, Iliescu EA. DDAVP to prevent rapid correction in hyponatremia. *Clin Nephrol.* 2000;53(3):226–229.

71 Oya S, Tsutsumi K, Ueki K, Kirino T. Reinduction of hyponatremia to treat central pontine myelinolysis. *Neurology.* 2001;57(10):1931–1932.

72 Bissram M, Scott FD, Liu L, Rosner MH. Risk factors for symptomatic hyponatraemia: the role of pre-existing asymptomatic hyponatraemia. *Intern Med J.* 2007;37(3):149–155.

73 Sterns RH, Riggs JE, Schochet SS, Jr. Osmotic demyelination syndrome following correction of hyponatremia. *N Engl J Med.* 1986;314:1535–1542.

74 Adrogue HJ, Madias NE. Diagnosis and treatment of hyponatremia. *Am J Kidney Dis.* 2014;64(5):681–684.

75 Chung HM, Kluge R, Schrier RW, Anderson RJ. Clinical assessment of extracellular fluid volume in hyponatremia. *Am J Med.* 1987;83:905–908.

76 Fenske W, Stork S, Koschker AC et al. Value of fractional uric acid excretion in differential diagnosis of hyponatremic patients on diuretics. *J Clin Endocrinol Metab.* 2008;93(8):2991–2997.

77 Verbalis JG. Whole-body volume regulation and escape from antidiuresis. *Am J Med.* 2006;119(7 Suppl 1): S21–S29.

78 Verbalis JG. Managing hyponatremia in patients with syndrome of inappropriate antidiuretic hormone secretion. *Endocrinol Nutr.* 2010;57(Suppl 2):30–40.

42

Emergency Management of Acute and Chronic Hypernatremia

Aoife Garrahy and Christopher Thompson

Key Points

- Hypernatremia is a common condition in emergency medicine, which is associated with high morbidity, and in many conditions is a predictor of excess mortality.
- The majority of cases of hypernatremia arise secondary to inadequate water intake, often exacerbated by comorbid acute illnesses and excess fluid loss.
- However, emerging data, particularly from patients in intensive care settings, have shown that significant numbers of hypernatremic patients – up to 50% – may have increased blood volume. Hypernatremia develops due to a combination of increased renal free water clearance due to the impairment of urine-concentrating ability, along with the use of isotonic intravenous (IV) fluids.
- Diabetes insipidus (DI), which results in inappropriate hypotonic polyuria, rarely causes hypernatremia, as the intact thirst mechanism generates sufficient drinking to replace renal water losses. However, if DI is associated with adipsia, diminished conscious levels or vomiting, severe hypernatremia may occur.
- Clinical features of hypernatremia are predominantly a consequence of the shrinkage of the brain cells, and include lethargy, drowsiness, and altered mental status, progressing to seizures, coma, and death if left untreated.

- Understanding the disorders which cause hypernatremia is essential to enable prompt, correct management. It is extremely important to note that the severity of symptoms is strongly influenced by the rapidity of the development of hypernatremia: those with acute hypernatremia (<48 h) are at far higher risk than those with chronic hypernatremia (>48 h).
- When hypernatremia is acute or when severe neurological symptoms are present, immediate treatment is indicated; a contemporary review has recommended normalization of plasma sodium within 24 h of commencement of therapy for acute hypernatremia.
- In circumstances where the onset of hypernatremia is unknown, a more conservative recommended rate of correction of plasma sodium with hypotonic fluids would be a maximum of 1 mmol/L/hr to a maximum of 10–12 mmol/L/day. If hypernatremia is chronic and only slightly symptomatic then correction should take place gradually.
- When a patient with hypernatremia is hypotensive, treatment should start with isotonic IV fluids (either crystalloids or colloids) in order to restore hemodynamic stability. In all other settings, hypernatremia can be treated with hypotonic fluids administered either orally or IV.

Endocrine and Metabolic Medical Emergencies: A Clinician's Guide, Second Edition. Edited by Glenn Matfin.
© 2018 John Wiley & Sons Ltd. Published 2018 by John Wiley & Sons Ltd.

Introduction

Hypernatremia is relatively uncommon in clinical practice, and much less likely to be the source of inpatient consultation than hyponatremia (1). However, hypernatremia is often a clinical and biochemical complication of the presentation of seriously ill patients, particularly in intensive care, in the elderly, and in young children (2). In addition, in the emergency room, hypernatremia has been reported to be commoner than hyponatremia; in a retrospective review of 3182 patients presenting to the emergency department, 13% had hypernatremia, compared with 4% with hyponatremia (3).

The likelihood of developing hypernatremia increases with age and particularly with residence in long-term care. Up to 50% of residents of long-term care have been estimated to develop hypernatremia at some time (4), and in one prospective study of hospital admissions, elderly patients from nursing homes were found to have a ten-fold increased risk of hypernatremia compared with age-matched patients, who were self-caring in their own homes (5). The factors which contribute to the excess risk of hypernatremia in elderly patients are multifactorial; osmotically-stimulated thirst is attenuated in the elderly, which leads to reduced fluid intake (6). In addition, many elderly patients in long-term care institutions exhibit permanent hypernatremia, through a combination of cognitive impairment, age-related attenuation of thirst, and reduced mobility (7).

Hypernatremia is associated with cellular shrinkage due to osmotic movement of water from the intracellular to the extracellular space. Clinical features of hypernatremia are predominantly a consequence of the shrinkage of the brain cells, and include lethargy, drowsiness, and altered mental status, progressing to seizures, coma, and death if left untreated (8). Hypernatremia has a significant impact on patient morbidity and mortality if the correct management is not promptly initiated (9,10).

In this chapter, we will discuss the physiological control of water balance, the main pathologies affecting this system, and the differential diagnosis and management of hypernatremia.

The Physiological Control of Water Balance

Plasma osmolality in healthy person varies by only 1–2% in physiological conditions where there is free access to water. For this reason, clinical conditions in which hypernatremia occurs are characterized by very major abnormalities in the physiology of sodium and water balance. The accurate regulation of plasma osmolality is maintained by the homeostatic process of osmoregulation.

Changes in the tonicity of the plasma are detected by specialized osmoreceptor cells in the anterior hypothalamus (Figure 42-1). The osmoreceptor cells are solute-specific, in that they respond to stimulations by alterations in plasma sodium concentration, less so to alterations in blood urea, and not at all to perturbations in plasma glucose. Changes in plasma sodium cause the depolarization of the magnocellular osmoreceptors which are situated mainly in the organum vasulosum lamina terminalis and the subfornical organ, initiating neural signals via the nucleus medianus, to the supraoptic and paraventricular nuclei. Elevation in plasma osmolality causes depolarization of these nuclei, leading to increased synthesis of vasopressin (also known as arginine vasopressin [AVP] or antidiuretic hormone [ADH]), and secretion of vasopressin from the posterior pituitary. When plasma vasopressin concentrations rise, there is increased receptor binding in the collecting tubules of the kidneys, generating the synthesis of aquaporin-2, and the insertion of pre-formed aquaporin-2 into the luminal membrane of the collecting tubules, thus allowing the reabsorption of water, and the concentration of urine.

This homeostatic process occurs continuously to maintain plasma osmolality within

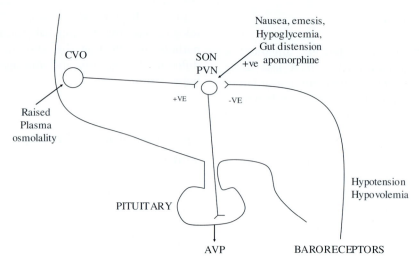

Figure 42-1 Factors governing vasopressin secretion
CVO = circumventricular organ (site of osmoreceptors); SON = supraoptic nuclei; PVN = paraventricular nuclei.

a narrow reference range, as shown in Figure 42-2. The relationship between plasma vasopressin concentration and urine osmolality is shown in Figure 42-3. If plasma concentrations are lowered by excessive ingestion of hypotonic fluid to below 280–285 mOsm/kg, the secretion of vasopressin is suppressed, and plasma concentrations of the hormone are undetectable, leading to hypotonic polyuria (11). The increase in free water

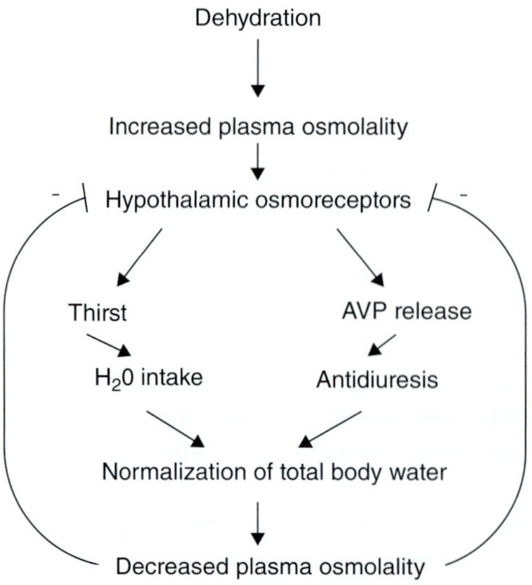

clearance allows plasma osmolality to rise into the normal range.

Although physiological control of vasopressin secretion and thirst is almost entirely osmotic, the switch-off of both is nonosmotic and is triggered by the act of drinking. In studies of healthy men who have been rendered hyperosmolar, drinking is associated with an immediate fall in plasma vasopressin and thirst, before any changes in plasma osmolality can be measured (12). The fall in plasma vasopressin following fluid intake is very rapid and suggests that a neuroendocrine reflex, stimulated by oropharyngeal distension, switches off vasopressin secretion.

Causes of Hypernatremia

There are a large number of potential causes of hypernatremia in the inpatient setting and these can be divided into six major groups:

1. Decreased water intake.
2. Excess water losses with inadequate replacement.
3. Redistribution of water from the extracellular to the intracellular space.
4. Intensive care hypernatremia.
5. Excess salt intake.
6. Hyperaldosteronism.

Figure 42-2 The regulation of plasma osmolality.

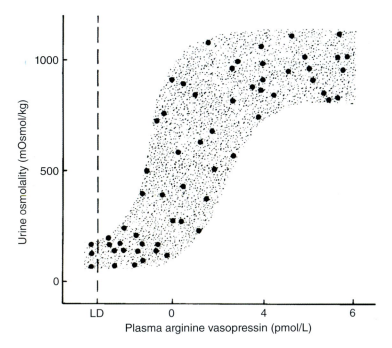

Figure 42-3 The relationship between plasma vasopressin concentration and urine osmolality.

The causes of hypernatremia contained in each group are summarized in Table 42-1, and several of these etiologies will be now be discussed in more detail.

Decreased Water Intake

Healthy individuals are vulnerable to the development of hypernatremia in circumstances where the availability of water for physiological need is insufficient. Climatic extremes, such as unusual exposure to heat or altitude need a healthy fluid intake to prevent hypernatremic dehydration. In the elderly, particularly in nursing homes, decreased cognitive awareness can attenuate the appreciation of the need for fluid intake and immobility may further compromise the ability to maintain adequate fluid intake.

Certain rare conditions are associated with loss of awareness of thirst: adipsia (13). Upwards resetting of the osmotic thresholds for both thirst and vasopressin release ("essential hypernatremia"), occurs when the osmotic threshold is over 300 mOsm/kg (normal 282–286); the stimulation of thirst

and vasopressin secretion above this threshold mitigate against the development of severe hypernatremia (14,15). Complete absence of thirst and osmotically stimulated vasopressin secretion have been reported after clipping of anterior communicating artery aneurysms, following subarachnoid hemorrhage (16); the classical presentation is a patient who develops polyuria and hypernatremia after recovery of cognition following neurosurgery. The vascular supply to the osmoreceptors is derived from small arteries arising from the anterior communicating artery and it is assumed that these vessels may be damaged during aneurysm clipping. As only the osmoreceptors are affected, these patients can produce vasopressin in response to non-osmotic stimuli such as nausea and hypotension, but not in response to hyperosmolarity (17). Neurosarcoidosis, extensive hypothalamic surgery for craniopharyngioma (16), or, rarely, pituitary macroadenoma (18), have also been reported to cause adipsia.

Patients with adipsic diabetes insipidus (DI) are much more likely to develop

Table 42-1 Causes of hypernatremia

Setting	Causes
Decreased water intake	Aging Impaired cognition Inadequate access to fluids Adipsia/Essential hypernatremia
Excess water losses with inadequate replacement	Gastrointestinal losses Fever/hyperventilation Tubing/drains/Intraoperative losses Diuretics, mannitol, vaptans, demeclocycline DKA/HHS DI
Redistribution of extracellular water to the intracellular space	Exercise Seizures
Intensive care hypernatremia	Abnormal renal water handling Isotonic/hypertonic fluids Mobilization of bone sodium stores?
Excess salt intake	Salt/seawater ingestion IV bicarbonate administration
Hyperaldosteronism	Conn's syndrome Cushing's syndrome Carbenoloxone/liquorice ingestion

DKA = diabetic ketoacidosis; HHS = hyperglycemic hyperosmolar state; DI = diabetes insipidus.

hypernatremia than patients with DI and intact thirst. A large, retrospective series reported that hypernatremia is rare in ambulatory patients with DI, unless there is co-existing adipsia (19). Hypernatremia was relatively common in DI patients, irrespective of the presence or absence of thirst, during acute admissions to hospital for intercurrent illness however, which emphasizes how important care of fluid balance is during infections or surgery for DI patients.

Case Study

A 27-year-old man presents with sudden severe headache, and is found to be hypertensive (BP 186/112), with meningism and drowsiness. A CT brain scan reveals evidence of a subarachnoid bleed and angiography identifies an aneurysm of the anterior communicating artery. The aneurysm is surgically clipped, but 24 h post op the patient has become polyuric; plasma sodium has risen from 138 to 156 mmol/L, urine is dilute (urine osmolality 102 mOsm/kg), and urine volume is 4800 mls/24 h. The patient is not cognitively impaired but expresses no sense of thirst and makes no effort to correct hypernatremia by drinking. Repeat CT brain scan reveals infarction in the anterior hypothalamus.

What Is the Likely Diagnosis and Cause?

Diabetes insipidus (DI) is diagnosed secondary to clipping of anterior communicating artery aneurysms, following subarachnoid hemorrhage. Continued polyuria (i.e., urine volume >3L/day) is controlled with oral desmopressin. Six weeks later water deprivation test confirms DI, and visual analogue scale testing reveals no sense of thirst despite hypernatremia. Adipsic DI is confirmed. The patient controls urine output with desmopressin, but remains intermittently hypernatremic due to adipsia.

Excess Water Losses with Inadequate Replacement

This describes the scenario when a patient has pathological loss of fluids and is unable to redress the deficit with adequate fluid intake. The commonest scenario is a patient who has gastroenteritis; there is excess gastrointestinal fluid loss, from vomiting and diarrhea, but the patient is unable to maintain fluid intake because of the vomiting. This inevitably leads to hypernatremic dehydration. Insensible losses from hyperventilation and sweating in pneumonia may have the same effect, especially if there is associated vomiting. The elderly are particularly prone to hypernatremia in this situation, as the attenuation in thirst with age may reduce the drive to drink. This might be contributory in conditions such as hyperglycemic hyperosmolar state (HHS), which particularly affects the elderly, and is characterized by extreme hypernatremia. Physiological studies in survivors of HHS show that they have diminished thirst and water intake in response to water deprivation, compared with age-matched control patients with type 2 diabetes (20).

Patients with DI which may be central or nephrogenic in etiology, will also result in inappropriate renal water loss. A full list of causes of DI is shown in Table 42-2. The majority of patients with DI are able to maintain a normal plasma sodium even in the absence of treatment, as their intact thirst mechanism allows them to maintain a sufficient fluid intake to compensate for excessive urinary losses (21). However, if their thirst sensation is impaired, for example through the presence of a comorbid condition such as a head injury, hypernatremia will rapidly develop (19). Hypernatremia appears anecdotally to be more common in nephrogenic DI due to lithium administration rather than cranial DI; the reasons for this are unclear (22). However, bipolar disorder is associated with cognitive impairment which may reduce patients' ability to drink appropriate volumes of water, resulting in hypernatremia

Table 42-2 Causes of diabetes insipidis (DI)

Cranial DI	
Congenital	Hereditary (X linked or AD)
	DIDMOAD
Acquired	Pituitary surgery
	Tumors (craniopharyngioma, germinoma, pinealoma, metastases)
	Traumatic brain injury
	Granuloma (TB, sarcoid, histiocytosis X)
	Infections (encephalitis, meningitis)
	Vascular disorders (Sheehan's syndrome, aneurysms, SAH)
	Hypophysitis (autoimmune, lymphocytic, drug-related)
	Idiopathic
	Pregnancy
Nephrogenic DI	
Congenital	Hereditary (X linked recessive or AD)
Acquired	Chronic kidney disease (polycystic kidneys, obstructive uropathy)
	Metabolic disease (hypercalcemia, hyokalemia)
	Drugs (lithium, demeclocycline)
	Osmotic diuresis (glucose, mannitol)
	Amyloidosis
	Myelomatosis

AD = autosomal dominant; DIDMOAD = **DI**, **D**iabetes **M**ellitus, **O**ptic **A**trophy, and **D**eafness; TB = tuberculosis.

(23); lithium itself does not have a major effect on cognition (24). In the extremely rare condition of adipsic DI, the patient has both a vasopressin secretory defect and an impaired thirst mechanism, commonly resulting in hypernatremia (16).

Demeclocycline is a tetracycline derivative which is utilized in the treatment of the syndrome of inappropriate antidiuresis (SIAD, also commonly termed syndrome of inappropriate antidiuretic hormone secretion [SIADH]); it causes nephrogenic DI in about 60% of patients for whom it is prescribed. However, the induced vasopressin resistance is not predictable and some patients may become markedly symptomatic, occasionally developing hypernatremia if access to water is compromised. Lithium therapy also causes nephrogenic DI in 30% of patients (13), with an even larger proportion of patients having attenuation of maximal urine concentrating ability (15). This effect is usually (16) but not always reversible upon stopping the medication. The vasopressin-2 receptor antagonist drugs (the vaptans), which have been used in the management of SIADH, can cause hypernatremia when used to treat SIADH (25,26). Up to 25% of patients develop hypernatremia, usually soon after initiation of therapy; retrospective studies have associated hypernatremia higher doses of the drug (>7.5mg tolvaptan) and older age of patient (27). In addition, misadministration of vaptans to patients with volume depletion may lead to profound hypernatremia (28,29).

Case Study

A 76-year-old woman is admitted as an emergency from a nursing home with three days of vomiting and diarrhea. Three other inmates have had similar, less severe, symptoms. On admission, the patient is semi-conscious, pulse 120/min, weak, BP is 92/58 and skin turgor is reduced. Bowel sounds are hyperactive. Plasma sodium is 166 mmol/L, blood urea 29 mmol/L (2–8 mmol/L) and creatinine 173 μmol/L (70–100 μmol/L). Catheterization shows low residual bladder urine volume, with urine osmolality 985 mOsm/kg. Stool cultures are negative.

What Immediate Management Is Needed?

The patient is fluid resuscitated, initially with colloids and 0.9% saline, with recovery of BP, and increased urine flow. Creatinine fell into the normal range over 60 h. Once BP was normalized, the patient was treated with intravenous 5% dextrose, with potassium supplementation, and encouraged to drink water. Plasma sodium normalized over 48 h, with improvement in conscious level and a return to normal eating and drinking.

Redistribution of Water into the Intracellular Space

The commonest cause of this type of hypernatremia (due to hypotonic fluid moving from the extracellular to the intracellular compartment) is exercise. Although exercise–induced hyponatremia is the subject of conferences and position statements, hypernatremia is significantly more common. An analysis of runners in the Boston marathon between 2001–8 showed that while 5% developed hyponatremia, a higher proportion (28%) became hypernatremic (30). The phenomenon is not confined to marathon running; an analysis of a volunteer cohort participating in the Nijmeded Four Day March, who walked 30–50 km daily for four days, showed that 5% became hyponatremic, and 16% hypernatremic. As the Marches attract 45,000 participants annually, the authors calculated that approximately 7,000 walkers could be developing hypernatremia.

Intensive Care Hypernatremia

Although the conventional teaching has been that hypernatremia is almost always a reflection of volume depletion and fluid intake inadequate for needs, there is emerging evidence from intensive care patients that a subset of patients have normovolemia or even evidence of fluid overload. Up to 50% of hypernatremic patients in intensive care have been reported to have positive fluid balance (31). There have been arguments made for impaired renal water handling (32), due to diuretics, acute kidney injury (AKI), hyperglycemia and hypokalemia as well as evidence for excess administration of intravenous (IV) sodium (33,34), but the etiology of hypernatremia in critically ill patients may be even more complex. A recent carefully conducted balance study felt that alterations in sodium/water balance, either through administration or renal handling, were insufficient to explain the full extent of hypernatremia in critically ill patients (35). The authors noted the store of osmotically inactive sodium ions in bone and other tissues, and hypothesized that the inflammatory process of critical illness could somehow mobilize this vast sodium store and contribute to hypernatremia. Whatever the etiology, calls for critical appraisal of the type of IV fluids and limitation of the duration of administration (1) seem well founded.

Excess Salt

This is much commoner in the neonatal and pediatric populations, though hypernatremia in intensive care patients may be partially attributed to salt administration against a background of impaired water retention (see above). Drinking salt water is rare. It is worth carefully considering the value of use of sodium bicarbonate administration, because of the risk of hypernatremia (36), and most modern protocols for diabetic ketoacidosis (DKA) advise against the use of this agent.

Hyperaldosteronism

Renal sodium and potassium excretion is regulated by the mineralocorticoid hormone, aldosterone. Excess aldosterone production due to an adrenal adenoma (Conn's syndrome) or bilateral adrenal hyperplasia may lead to excessive potassium loss and sodium retention (37), resulting in mild chronic hypernatremia. However, only 40% of those with excess aldosterone production have any electrolyte imbalance, and hypokalemia is commoner than hypernatremia (38). Chronic mild volume expansion also leads to upwards resetting of the osmostat such that patients with mild hypernatremia due to hyperaldosteronism do not drink large volumes of fluid to normalize their sodium levels (39). Thus, although patients with aldosterone excess may have a mild chronic hypernatremia (usually between 143 and 147 mmol/L), it does not usually lead to adverse clinical events (37).

Excess glucocorticoid production due to Cushing's syndrome may also cause hypernatremia. Hypernatremia usually occurs when grossly elevated plasma glucocorticoid concentrations overwhelm the capacity of the shuttle enzyme, 11-beta-hydroxysteroid dehydrogenase type 2, which converts cortisol to inactive cortisone at the level of the mineralocorticoid receptor, such that cortisol binds to, and activates, the mineralocorticoid receptor. This is particularly seen in those with Cushing's syndrome due to ectopic ACTH secretion (40). Liquorice and carbenoxolone may cause hypertension, hypernatremia and hypokalemia, also via inhibition of 11-beta-hydroxysteroid dehydrogenase type 2, producing apparent mineralocorticoid excess, despite normal plasma aldosterone concentrations (41,42).

Consequences of Hypernatremia

Hypernatremia has multiple adverse effects, predominantly due to the movement of water from cells to the extracellular space, leading to cell shrinkage (2,43). One of the most common and feared effects is free water shift leading to brain shrinkage, which may causes vascular rupture and permanent cognitive deficits (8). Cerebral demyelination has also been reported in severe hypernatremia (44), particularly in liver disease (45). Hypernatremia also leads to muscle weakness (46), impaired glucose utilization and insulin function (47) which may lead to hyperglycemia in the critically ill (48), an increase in venous thromboembolism risk (49), and decreased left ventricular contractility (2). The cellular shrinkage induced by hypernatremia can have catabolic effects and induce proinflammatory cytokine responses (50), which may impair lactate clearance (51). In addition, severe hypernatremia has been reported to cause rhabdomyolysis and consequent AKI (52).

In the intensive care setting, even mild hypernatremia has been shown to double mortality (53). Hypernatremia due to DI has been linked with excess mortality following both traumatic brain injury (54) and subarachnoid hemorrhage (55), and patients with adipsic DI due to surgery for craniopharyngioma have an extremely high mortality (16), due to multiple pathologies including obesity, obstructive sleep apnea, and venous thromboembolism. Cardiovascular and thromboembolic events are particularly common in those with hypernatremia due to HHS (56). Hypernatremia has also been associated with a doubling of mortality and prolonged length of stay in the intensive care unit following cardiac surgery (57). An association has been shown between mortality and hypernatremia in sepsis (58), PEG feeding (59), the elderly (5,60) and internal medicine patients (33). Propspective data in men with no definable cardiovascular disease has additionally linked hypernatremia to more frequent cardiovascular events and death (61).

Although hypernatremia is common in the Emergency Department, data have shown that no corrective action was taken in 18% of those with hypernatremia on presentation, even in the presence of severe, symptomatic hypernatremia (62). Understanding the disorders which cause hypernatremia is essential to enable prompt, correct management. It is extremely important to note that the severity of symptoms is strongly influenced by the rapidity of the development of hypernatremia: those with acute hypernatremia are at far higher risk than those with chronic hypernatremia (2,43). We will now discuss the acute and chronic management of hypernatremia.

Management of Acute Hypernatremia

Because of the excess mortality associated with hypernatremia, treatment is indicated to reduce mortality and to reverse neurological symptoms. Rapidly developing hypernatremia (<48 hours) is particularly associated with the development of neurological sequelae. The majority of cases of acute hypernatremia are simply due to water depletion, usually precipitated by an intercurrent illness, and occasionally exacerbated by poor thirst response. They therefore respond to replacement of extracellular water (63). When hypernatremia is acute or when severe neurological symptoms are present, immediate treatment is indicated; a contemporary review has recommended normalization of plasma sodium within 24 h of commencement of therapy for acute hypernatremia (64). In circumstances where the onset of hypernatremia is unknown, a more conservative recommended rate of correction of plasma sodium with hypotonic fluids would be a maximum of 1 mmol/L/hr to a maximum of 10–12 mmol/L/day. If hypernatremia is chronic and only slightly symptomatic, then correction should take place gradually (e.g., 6–8 mmol/L/day) (8,65).

When a patient with hypernatremia is hypotensive, treatment should start with isotonic IV fluids (either crystalloids or colloids) in order to restore hemodynamic stability (8). In all other settings, hypernatremia can be treated with hypotonic fluids administered either orally or IV; patients who are acutely unwell may have difficulty in consuming large volumes of oral fluids and so we recommend IV administration of either 0.45% saline or 5% dextrose hypotonic solutions. The patient's total body water deficit can be calculated prior to commencing the infusion using the following formula:

$$0.6 \times \text{lean body weight (kg)}$$
$$\times ([\text{serum sodium } /140] - 1).$$

The volume and rate of fluid replacement needed to achieve a certain rate of decline in plasma sodium concentration can be calculated using the Adrogue-Madias formula (8). However, as there is a huge variation between patients in terms of the rate of correction of plasma sodium (66), it is important to be prepared to alter the infusion fluid and the rate of administration in response to plasma sodium concentrations. We would therefore advise monitoring of plasma sodium concentration every 2 to 4 hours (65); in addition, the outcomes are likely to be improved if the patient is managed by a team who are experienced in electrolyte disorders.

There is evidence to suggest improved outcomes in patients who have active management of hypernatremia (67), however, it is important to consider the potential consequences of over-rapid correction. The consequences of over-rapid correction of hypernatremia are not as well documented as are those of over-correction of hyponatremia. Nevertheless, there are anecdotal reports of extrapontine myelinolysis associated with over-correction of hypernatremia (68). It is difficult, however, to be certain that the relationship between over-correction of hypernatremia and osmotic demyelination is causal, as demyelination has also been reported in association with hypernatremia itself (69–73). In fact, as most of the cases in the literature are associated with a rise, rather than a fall in plasma sodium concentration, the risk of osmotic demyelination could reasonably be considered a reason for more rapid reversal of hypernatremia. More information on the causality of osmotic demyelination is needed to be certain.

Patients who develop severe hypernatremic dehydration have an increased hematocrit and are at risk therefore of thrombotic complications due to the hypercoagulable state. This is well recognized in HHS, and we have also reported pulmonary thromboembolism during severe hypernatremia in adipsic DI (16). We therefore recommend the use of prophylactic anticoagulation with low molecular weight heparin in patients with vascular disease, in the elderly and in very severe dehydration. Although there is very little evidence base to support this practice, prophylactic short-term anticoagulation in at-risk patients seems sensible.

Hypernatremia caused by volume depletion due to DKA or HHS may worsen if there is over-rapid correction of hyperglycemia (74, 75); plasma sodium rises as blood glucose falls. Hypernatremia may impair patient consciousness and slow down recovery and hospital discharge. It is important therefore to monitor for the development of hypernatremia during the correction of severe hyperglycemia, particularly in the management of HHS, and slow down the rate of correction of glucose and move to hypotonic IV fluids if plasma sodium rises.

In a patient with DI, the limitation of renal free water excretion with desmopressin treatment is important. Acute onset DI is often seen in neurosurgical units; the majority of cases are transient, and respond to a single parenteral (subcutaneous or intramuscular) dose of DDAVP (synthetic, long-lasting vasopressin), which is active for 6–12 h; our policy is to re-treat only if there is development of further symptoms (76). Regular DDAVP is only prescribed if there is persistent polyuria for more than 48 h (76). Withdrawal of DDAVP prior to discharge from hospital is helpful in identifying those patients who have recovered secretion of endogenous vasopressin.

Case Study

A 64-year-old man was transferred from a general hospital to the endocrine unit. He had presented three days earlier with hyperglycemic hyperosmolar state (HHS), with plasma sodium 152 mmol/L, blood urea 26 mmol/L (2–8 mmol/L), blood glucose 91 mmol/L (1640 mg/dL) and creatinine 210 µmol/L. (80–110 µmol/L). He was treated with aggressive insulin therapy and isotonic fluids, with a fall in blood glucose to 11 mmol/L (200 mg/dL) over 36 hours. Despite switching to isotonic fluids, his plasma sodium concentration rose to 174 mmol/L, associated with decreased conscious level, and the patient was transferred to the university hospital. On arrival, he had flaccid paralysis of all limbs, and an MRI scan showed demyelination in the pons (Figure 42-4).

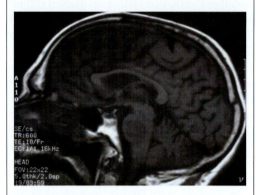

Figure 42-4 MRI brain showing osmotic demyelination in the pons

What Is the Diagnosis and Likely Cause?

Osmotic demyelination syndrome related to hypernatremia and over-rapid correction of the hyperosmolar state is the diagnosis. Plasma sodium was normalized by IV glucose/insulin/potassium infusion, supplemented by nasogastric water and hypotonic saline infusion, but quadriparesis did not reverse, and became hypertonic. The patient remains wheelchair-bound.

Management of Chronic Hypernatremia

Elderly patients in long-term care are at risk of developing chronic hypernatremia, which may worsen during acute illness. Prevention is the key, and the importance of adequate fluid intake should be emphasized to carers and nursing staff. Any non-specific decline in the patient's cognition or the development of intercurrent illness should prompt urgent electrolyte measurement.

The intact thirst mechanism generally prevents hypernatremic dehydration in DI in the outpatient setting. The treatment of choice for CDI is DDAVP, which can be administered as an intranasal spray, or, more often, orally, in 2–3 daily doses (77). The main complication is dilutional hyponatremia, and in our experience less than 3% of plasma sodium concentrations in ambulatory patients with DI are in the hypernatremic range (19).

Nephrogenic DI due to an acquired metabolic problem is best managed by addressing the underlying cause and maintaining adequate hydration while function recovers. For those patients with congenital nephrogenic DI or in whom the acquired defect is irreversible, a number of additional measures, including thiazide diuretics (hydrochlorothiazide, 25 mg/24 h); prostaglandin inhibitors, such as nonsteroidal anti-inflammatory drugs (ibuprofen, 200 mg/24 h); and dietary salt restriction can be used. All probably work through a combination of reducing glomerular filtration rate and interference with the diluting capacity of the distal nephron. Occasionally DDAVP can produce some benefit (77–79).

The diagnosis of adipsic DI presents a management dilemma, as severe hypernatremia is a particular hazard. Management requires regular DDAVP, fixed fluid intakes, which may vary with climatic conditions, and regular review for measurement of plasma sodium. Associated hypothalamic abnormalities are often seen with adipsic DI, including hypothalamic obesity and seizure disorders (16). Episodes of dehydration are often complicated by thrombotic complications, including pulmonary thromboembolism. Many patients die prematurely, due to postsurgical complications, electrolyte abnormalities or sleep apnea. The main management points are summarized in Table 42-3.

The use of demeclocycline for the treatment of SIADH can cause nephrogenic DI in up to 60% of patients for whom it is prescribed (28). Although there is no reliable way to predict those who will develop nephrogenic DI, the presence of intact thirst mechanism will prevent the development of hypernatremia unless an intercurrent illness supervenes. However, although the vaptan class of medications rarely causes hypernatremia in patients with SIADH (26), they have the potential to cause severe hypernatremia

Table 42-3 Management of adipsic diabetes insipidus

- Initial inpatient management to determine correct fluid intake and desmopressin dose, to ensure eunatremia
- Daily weights
- Fixed fluid intake, approx. 2L/day (consider weight, exercise and climate), with extra fluid below eunatremic weight
- Regular clinic review and plasma sodium measurement
- Low molecular weight heparin during periods of hypernatremic dehydration
- Screen for hypothalamic complications: sleep apnea, obesity, seizures, etc.
- Formal diet and exercise programs

if used erroneously in patients with hypovolemic hyponatremia. As clinical assessment of blood volume status is difficult (80), vaptans should only be prescribed by those with expertise in this field (28,81).

In chronic hypernatremia of any cause, the mainstay of treatment is encouragement of water intake, regular measurement of plasma sodium concentration, and regular medical or nursing review.

Conclusions

Hypernatremia is common in the emergency setting and it is associated with significant morbidity and mortality, primarily caused by cell shrinkage due to extracellular movement of water. Acute hypernatremia usually occurs due to inadequate water intake and/or excessive water loss, leading to inappropriate plasma hyperosmolality. It is often seen in elderly patients with a comorbid condition which further affects cognition and thirst, and/or insensible fluid losses. In a small number of cases, hypernatremia develops in patients with DI, who develop an intercurrent illness, such as gastroenteritis.

The mainstay of management of acute hypernatremia is rehydration with 0.45% saline or 5% dextrose, used for their high free water content when compared with isotonic saline. However, if the patient is hemodynamically unstable, isotonic saline should be used initially. Symptomatic hypernatremia may be corrected relatively rapidly; the rate of correction can reach a maximum of 1 mmol/L/hr to a maximum of 10–12 mmol/L/day; where the development of hypernatremia is known to have occurred rapidly, over 48 h or less, faster rates of correction may be considered with normalization of plasma sodium within 24 h of commencement of therapy. Chronic hypernatremia should be corrected more gradually as cerebral edema may develop if correction is over-rapid. In patients at risk of thrombotic episodes, prophylactic anticoagulation should also be considered.

References

1 Eijgelsheim M, Hoorn EJ. Hypernatraemia: balancing is challenging. *Neth J Med*. 2015;73(10):446–447.

2 Lindner G, Funk GC. Hypernatremia in critically ill patients. *J Crit Care*. 2013;28(2):216 e11–e20.

3 Arampatzis S, Exadaktylos A, Buhl D, Zimmermann H, Lindner G. Dysnatraemias in the emergency room: Undetected, untreated, unknown? *Wien Klin Wochenschr*. 2012;124(5–6): 181–183.

4 Morley JE. Dehydration, Hypernatremia, and hyponatremia. *Clinics Geriatric Med*. 2015;31(3):389–399.

5 Wolff A, Stuckler D, McKee M. Are patients admitted to hospitals from care homes dehydrated? A retrospective analysis of hypernatraemia and in-hospital mortality. *J Royal Soc Med*. 2015;108(7):259–265.

6 Miller M. Fluid and electrolyte homeostasis in the elderly: physiological changes of ageing and clinical consequences. *Baillieres Clin Endocrinol Metab*. 1997;11(2):367–387.

7 Crowe MJ, Forsling ML, Rolls BJ, Phillips PA, Ledingham JG, Smith RF. Altered water excretion in healthy elderly men. *Age Ageing*. 1987;16(5):285–293.

8 Adrogue HJ, Madias NE. Hypernatremia. *N Engl J Med*. 2000;342(20):1493–1499.

9 Kraft MD, Btaiche IF, Sacks GS, Kudsk KA. Treatment of electrolyte disorders in adult patients in the intensive care unit. *Am J Health Syst Pharm*. 2005;62(16):1663–1682.

10 Arampatzis S, Funk GC, Leichtle AB, et al. Impact of diuretic therapy-associated electrolyte disorders present on admission to the emergency department: a cross-sectional analysis. *BMC Med*. 2013;11:83.

11 Baylis PH, Thompson CJ. Osmoregulation of vasopressin secretion and thirst in health and disease. *Clin Endocrinol (Oxf)*. 1988;29(5):549–576.

12 Thompson CJ, Burd JM, Baylis PH. Acute suppression of plasma vasopressin and thirst after drinking in hypernatremic humans. *Am J Physiol*. 1987;252(6 Pt 2):R1138–1142.

13 McKenna K, Thompson C. Osmoregulation in clinical disorders of thirst appreciation. *Clin Endocrinol (Oxf)*. 1998;49(2):139–152.

14 Gill G, Baylis P, Burn J. A case of 'essential' hypernatraemia due to resetting of the osmostat. *Clin Endocrinol (Oxf)*. 1985;22(4):545–551.

15 Thompson CJ, Freeman J, Record CO, Baylis PH. Hypernatraemia due to a reset osmostat for vasopressin release and thirst, complicated by nephrogenic diabetes insipidus. *Postgrad Med J*. 1987;63(745):979–982.

16 Crowley RK, Sherlock M, Agha A, Smith D, Thompson CJ. Clinical insights into adipsic diabetes insipidus: a large case series. *Clin Endocrinol (Oxf)*. 2007;66(4):475–482.

17 Smith D, McKenna K, Moore K, et al. Baroregulation of vasopressin release in adipsic diabetes insipidus. *J Clin Endocrinol Metab*. 2002;87(10):4564–4568.

18 Sherlock M, Agha A, Crowley R, Smith D, Thompson CJ. Adipsic diabetes insipidus following pituitary surgery for a macroprolactinoma. *Pituitary*. 2006;9(1):59–64.

19 Behan LA, Sherlock M, Moyles P, et al. Abnormal plasma sodium concentrations in patients treated with desmopressin for cranial diabetes insipidus: results of a long-term retrospective study. *European J Endocrinol*. 2015;172(3):243–250.

20 McKenna K, Morris AD, Azam H, Newton RW, Baylis PH, Thompson CJ. Exaggerated vasopressin secretion and attenuated osmoregulated thirst in human survivors of hyperosmolar coma. *Diabetologia*. 1999;42(5):534–538.

21 Thompson CJ, Baylis PH. Thirst in diabetes insipidus: clinical relevance of quantitative assessment. *Q J Med*. 1987;65(246):853–862.

22 Moeller HB, Rittig S, Fenton RA. Nephrogenic diabetes insipidus: essential insights into the molecular background and potential therapies for treatment. *Endocr Rev*. 2013;34(2):278–301.

23 Manove E, Levy B. Cognitive impairment in bipolar disorder: an overview. *Postgrad Med*. 2010;122(4):7–16.

24 Wingo AP, Wingo TS, Harvey PD, Baldessarini RJ. Effects of lithium on cognitive performance: a meta-analysis. *J Clin Psychiatry*. 2009;70(11):1588–1597.

25 Schrier RW, Gross P, Gheorghiade M, et al. Tolvaptan, a selective oral vasopressin V2-receptor antagonist, for hyponatremia. *N Engl J Med*. 2006;355(20):2099–2112.

26 Berl T, Quittnat-Pelletier F, Verbalis JG, et al. Oral tolvaptan is safe and effective in chronic hyponatremia. *J Am Soc Nephrol*. 2010;21(4):705–712.

27 Hirai K, Shimomura T, Moriwaki H, et al. Risk factors for hypernatremia in patients with short- and long-term tolvaptan treatment. *European J Clin Pharm*. 2016;72(10):1177–1183.

28 Sherlock M, Thompson CJ. The syndrome of inappropriate antidiuretic hormone: current and future management options. *Eur J Endocrinol*. 2010;162 Suppl 1:S13–S18.

29 Thompson C, Hoorn EJ. Hyponatraemia: an overview of frequency, clinical presentation and complications. *Best Pract*

Res Clin Endocrinol Metab. 2012;26 Suppl 1:S1–S6.

30 Siegel AJ, d'Hemecourt P, Adner MM, Shirey T, Brown JL, Lewandrowski KB. Exertional dysnatremia in collapsed marathon runners: a critical role for point-of-care testing to guide appropriate therapy. *Am J Clin Path*. 2009;132(3):336–340.

31 Lindner G, Kneidinger N, Holzinger U, Druml W, Schwarz C. Tonicity balance in patients with hypernatremia acquired in the intensive care unit. *Am J Kidney Dis*. 2009;54(4):674–679.

32 Hoorn EJ, Betjes MG, Weigel J, Zietse R. Hypernatraemia in critically ill patients: too little water and too much salt. *Nephrol, Dial, Transplant*. 2008;23(5): 1562–1568.

33 Felizardo Lopes I, Dezelee S, Brault D, Steichen O. Prevalence, risk factors and prognosis of hypernatraemia during hospitalisation in internal medicine. *Neth J Med*. 2015;73(10):448–454.

34 Choo WP, Groeneveld AB, Driessen RH, Swart EL. Normal saline to dilute parenteral drugs and to keep catheters open is a major and preventable source of hypernatremia acquired in the intensive care unit. *J Crit Care*. 2014;29(3):390–394.

35 van IMC, Buter H, Kingma WP, Navis GJ, Boerma EC. The development of intensive care unit acquired hypernatremia is not explained by sodium overload or water deficit: a retrospective cohort study on water balance and sodium handling. *Crit Care Res Prac*. 2016;2016:9571583.

36 Ghadimi K, Gutsche JT, Ramakrishna H, et al. Sodium bicarbonate use and the risk of hypernatremia in thoracic aortic surgical patients with metabolic acidosis following deep hypothermic circulatory arrest. *Ann Card Anaesth*. 2016;19(3):454–462.

37 Young WF. Primary aldosteronism: renaissance of a syndrome. *Clin Endocrinol (Oxf)*. 2007;66(5):607–618.

38 Mulatero P, Stowasser M, Loh KC, et al. Increased diagnosis of primary aldosteronism, including surgically correctable forms, in centers from five continents. *J Clin Endocrinol Metab*. 2004;89(3):1045–1050.

39 Gregoire JR. Adjustment of the osmostat in primary aldosteronism. *Mayo Clin Proc*. 1994;69(11):1108–1110.

40 Torpy DJ, Mullen N, Ilias I, Nieman LK. Association of hypertension and hypokalemia with Cushing's syndrome caused by ectopic ACTH secretion: a series of 58 cases. *Ann N Y Acad Sci*. 2002;970:134–144.

41 Edwards CR. Renal 11-beta-hydroxysteroid dehydrogenase: a mechanism ensuring mineralocorticoid specificity. *Horm Res*. 1990;34(3–4):114–117.

42 Walker BR, Edwards CR. Licorice-induced hypertension and syndromes of apparent mineralocorticoid excess. *Endocrinol Metab Clin North Am*. 1994;23(2): 359–377.

43 Arora SK. Hypernatremic disorders in the intensive care unit. *J Intensive Care Med*. 2013;28(1):37–45.

44 Orainy IA, O'Gorman AM, Decell MK. Cerebral bleeding, infarcts, and presumed extrapontine myelinolysis in hypernatraemic dehydration. *Neuroradiology*. 1999;41(2):144–146.

45 Clark WR. Diffuse demyelinating lesions of the brain after the rapid development of hypernatremia. *West J Med*. 1992;157(5):571–573.

46 Knochel JP. Neuromuscular manifestations of electrolyte disorders. *Am J Med*. 1982;72(3):521–535.

47 Komjati M, Kastner G, Waldhausl W, Bratusch-Marrain P. Detrimental effect of hyperosmolality on insulin-stimulated glucose metabolism in adipose and muscle tissue in vitro. *Biochem Med Metab Biol*. 1988;39(3):312–318.

48 Bratusch-Marrain PR, DeFronzo RA. Impairment of insulin-mediated glucose metabolism by hyperosmolality in man. *Diabetes*. 1983;32(11):1028–1034.

49 Kamijo Y, Soma K, Hamanaka S, Nagai T, Kurihara K. Dural sinus thrombosis with severe hypernatremia developing in a patient on long-term lithium therapy. *J Toxicol Clin Toxicol*. 2003;41(4):359–362.

50 Berneis K, Ninnis R, Haussinger D, Keller U. Effects of hyper- and hypoosmolality on whole body protein and glucose kinetics in humans. *Am J Physiol*. 1999;276(1 Pt 1):E188–E195.

51 Druml W, Kleinberger G, Lenz K, Laggner A, Schneeweiss B. Fructose-induced hyperlactemia in hyperosmolar syndromes. *Klin Wochenschr*. 1986;64(13):615–618.

52 Abramovici MI, Singhal PC, Trachtman H. Hypernatremia and rhabdomyolysis. *J Med*. 1992;23(1):17–28.

53 Darmon M, Timsit JF, Francais A, et al. Association between hypernatraemia acquired in the ICU and mortality: a cohort study. *Nephrol Dial Transplant*. 2010;25(8):2510–2515.

54 Hannon MJ, Crowley RK, Behan LA, et al. Acute glucocorticoid deficiency and diabetes insipidus are common after acute traumatic brain injury and predict mortality. *J Clin Endocrinol Metab*. 2013;98(8):3229–3237.

55 Hannon MJ, Behan LA, O'Brien MM, et al. Hyponatremia following mild/moderate subarachnoid hemorrhage is due to siad and glucocorticoid deficiency and not cerebral salt wasting. *J Clin Endocrinol Metab*. 2014;99:291–298.

56 Ekpebegh C, Longo-Mbenza B. Mortality in hyperglycemic crisis: a high association with infections and cerebrovascular disease. *Minerva Endocrinol*. 2013;38(2):187–193.

57 Lindner G, Funk GC, Lassnigg A, et al. Intensive care-acquired hypernatremia after major cardiothoracic surgery is associated with increased mortality. *Intensive Care Med*. 2010;36(10):1718–1723.

58 Ni HB, Hu XX, Huang XF, et al. Risk factors and outcomes in patients with hypernatremia and sepsis. *Am J Medical Scien*. 2016;351(6):601–605.

59 Muratori R, Lisotti A, Fusaroli P, et al. Severe hypernatremia as a predictor of mortality after percutaneous endoscopic gastrostomy (PEG) placement: digestive and liver disease: *Official J Italian Society of Gastroenterology and the Italian Association for the Study of the Liver*. 2017;49(2):181–187.

60 Liber M, Sonnenblick M, Munter G. Hypernatremia and copeptin levels in the elderly hospitalized patient. *Endocrine Prac*. 2016;22(12):1429–1435.

61 Wannamethee SG, Shaper AG, Lennon L, Papacosta O, Whincup P. Mild hyponatremia, hypernatremia and incident cardiovascular disease and mortality in older men: a population-based cohort study. *Nutrit, Metab, Cardiovascular Dis*. 2016;26(1):12–19.

62 Arampatzis S, Frauchiger B, Fiedler GM, et al. Characteristics, symptoms, and outcome of severe dysnatremias present on hospital admission. *Am J Med*. 2012;125(11):1125 e1–e7.

63 Sterns RH. Hypernatremia in the intensive care unit: instant quality–just add water. *Crit Care Med*. 1999;27(6):1041–1042.

64 Rondon-Berrios H, Argyropoulos C, Ing TS, et al. Hypertonicity: clinical entities, manifestations and treatment. *World J Nephrol*. 2017;6(1):1–13.

65 Hoorn EJ, Tuut MK, Hoorntje SJ, van Saase JL, Zietse R, Geers AB. Dutch guideline for the management of electrolyte disorders - 2012 revision. *Neth J Med*. 2013;71(3):153–165.

66 Mohmand HK, Issa D, Ahmad Z, Cappuccio JD, Kouides RW, Sterns RH. Hypertonic saline for hyponatremia: risk of inadvertent overcorrection. *Clin J Am Soc Nephrol*. 2007;2(6):1110–1117.

67 Darmon M, Pichon M, Schwebel C, et al. Influence of early dysnatremia correction on survival of critically ill patients. *Shock (Augusta, Ga)*. 2014;41(5):394–399.

68 Go M, Amino A, Shindo K, Tsunoda S, Shiozawa Z. [A case of central pontine myelinolysis and extrapontine myelinolysis during rapid correction of hypernatremia]. *Rinsho shinkeigaku [Clinical Neurology]*. 1994;34(11):1130–1135. In Chinese.

69 McComb RD, Pfeiffer RF, Casey JH, Wolcott G, Till DJ. Lateral pontine and extrapontine myelinolysis associated with hypernatremia and hyperglycemia. *Clin Neuropathology*. 1989;8(6):284–288.

70 O'Malley G, Moran C, Draman MS, et al. Central pontine myelinolysis complicating treatment of the hyperglycaemic hyperosmolar state. *Ann Clin Biochemistry.* 2008;45(Pt 4):440–443.

71 Han MJ, Kim DH, Kim YH, Yang IM, Park JH, Hong MK. a case of osmotic demyelination presenting with severe hypernatremia. *Electrolyte & Blood Pressure.* 2015;13(1):30–36.

72 Aoki R, Morimoto T, Takahashi Y, Saito H, Fuchigami T, Takahashi S. Extrapontine myelinolysis associated with severe hypernatremia in infancy. *Pediatrics International: Official Journal of the Japan Pediatric Society.* 2016;58(9):936–939.

73 Chhabra A, Kaushik R, Kaushik RM, Goel D. Extra-pontine myelinolysis secondary to hypernatremia induced by postpartum water restriction. *The Neuroradiology J.* 2017;30(1):84–87.

74 Hoorn EJ, Carlotti AP, Costa LA, et al. Preventing a drop in effective plasma osmolality to minimize the likelihood of cerebral edema during treatment of children with diabetic ketoacidosis. *J Pediatr.* 2007;150(5):467–473.

75 Haringhuizen A, Tjan DH, Grool A, van Vugt R, van Zante AR. Fatal cerebral oedema in adult diabetic ketoacidosis. *Nether J Med.* 2010;68(1):35–37.

76 Hannon MJ, Sherlock M, Thompson CJ. Pituitary dysfunction following traumatic brain injury or subarachnoid haemorrhage. In: "Endocrine Management in the Intensive Care Unit." *Best Pract Res Clin Endocrinol Metab.* 2011;25(5): 783–798.

77 Thompson CJ. Polyuric states in man. *Baillieres Clin Endocrinol Metab.* 1989;3(2):473–497.

78 Singer I, Oster JR, Fishman LM. The management of diabetes insipidus in adults. *Arch Intern Med.* 1997;157(12):1293–1301.

79 Robertson GL. Diabetes insipidus. *Endocrinol Metab Clin North Am.* 1995;24(3):549–572.

80 Chung HM, Kluge R, Schrier RW, Anderson RJ. Clinical assessment of extracellular fluid volume in hyponatremia. *Am J Med.* 1987;83(5):905–908.

81 Verbalis JG, Goldsmith SR, Greenberg A, et al. Diagnosis, evaluation, and treatment of hyponatremia: expert panel recommendations. *Am J Med.* 2013;126(10 Suppl 1):S1–42.

Part XI

Obesity and Clinical Lipidology

Introduction

Emergency Management Related to Obesity and Clinical Lipidology

Robert H. Eckel

Key Points

- Obesity is an excess of adipose tissue defined by a body mass index (BMI) of $\geq$30 kg/m2. Severe obesity defined as a BMI $\geq$40 kg/m^2 is now present in 7% of Americans.

- In India, SE Asia, and many other nations, the prevalence of obesity has increased less but the distribution of excess adipose tissue is more abdominal (often visceral), a location that contributes to insulin resistance and a higher risk of type 2 diabetes and cardiovascular disease (CVD).

- Obesity is associated with a plethora of other sequelae, including cancer, hypertension, obstructive sleep apnea, pulmonary thromboembolism, pulmonary hypertension, non-alcoholic fatty liver disease, cholelithiasis, degenerative joint disease, oligomenorrhea/infertility, erectile dysfunction, and cognitive impairment.

- The best treatment of obesity is prevention and an increased effort in pediatrics and primary care is needed. Lifestyle changes are important to lose and maintain weight loss.

- For severe obesity or a BMI $\geq$ 35 kg/m^2 with co-morbidities, a surgical procedure may be best. Presently metabolic surgery is the only obesity therapy proven to prolong life, a

benefit attributable to reductions in cancer as well as CVD-related mortality.

- Increasing evidence also indicates the value of metabolic surgery in treating patients with type 2 diabetes, with many patients free of diabetes medications and some postoperative patients rendered non-diabetic (i.e. in diabetes remission).

- Tremendous progress in understanding the relationship between lipoproteins and CVD has occurred during the past three decades, including major advances in the prevention and treatment of CVD. By far the most successful of the therapeutic strategies has been the use of statins. However, despite their widespread use and current cost-effectiveness, CVD remains the leading cause of death in the United States, and considerable residual risk remains, much of which is attributable to lipids and lipoproteins.

- Emerging therapeutics are aimed at reducing the poststatin residual risk of CVD by even more aggressive lowering of low-density lipoprotein (LDL) cholesterol (LDL-C); as well as targeting hypertriglyceridemia, low levels of high-density lipoprotein (HDL) cholesterol (HDL-C), and elevated lipoprotein (a).

Endocrine and Metabolic Medical Emergencies: A Clinician's Guide, Second Edition. Edited by Glenn Matfin.
© 2018 John Wiley & Sons Ltd. Published 2018 by John Wiley & Sons Ltd.

Obesity

Obesity is an excess of adipose tissue defined by a body mass index (BMI) of $\geq 30\,kg/m2$. Severe obesity, defined as a BMI $\geq 40\,kg/m^2$, is now present in 7% of Americans. Over the past 30 years, an obesity 'epidemic' has occurred that has affected not only the developed world but the developing world as well. In the recent Global Burden of Disease study, data from more than 195 countries have shown that the prevalence of obesity has more than doubled worldwide since 1980 and is now 5% in children and 12% in adults (1). Moreover in India, SE Asia and other nations, the prevalence of obesity has increased less but the distribution of excess adipose tissue is more abdominal (often visceral), a location that contributes to insulin resistance and a higher risk of type 2 diabetes and cardiovascular disease (CVD). Obesity is associated with a plethora of other sequelae, including cancer (e.g., breast, uterus, cervix, colon, esophagus, pancreas, kidney, prostate, thyroid), hypertension, obstructive sleep apnea, pulmonary thromboembolism, pulmonary hypertension, non-alcoholic fatty liver disease, cholelithiasis, degenerative joint disease, oligomenorrhea/infertility, erectile dysfunction, and cognitive impairment.

The best treatment of obesity is prevention and an increased effort in pediatrics and primary care is needed. The 2013 American Heart Association/American College of Cardiology Task Force on Practice Guidelines and The Obesity Society (AHA/ACC/TOS) Guideline for the Management of Overweight and Obesity in Adults (2) indicates that: (a) overweight (BMI $\geq 25 < 30\,kg/m^2$) and obese patients need to be counseled about CVD risk factors (high blood pressure, dyslipidemia, hyperglycemia); and (b) lifestyle changes that produce even modest, sustained weight loss of 3–5% produce clinically meaningful health benefits; and (c) greater weight loss produces greater benefits. With dietary intervention techniques aimed at reducing daily energy intake by at least 500 kCal daily, a range of 4–12 kg at 6 months is typical with a slow weight regain to follow. In general, there is no ideal diet for weight loss and no superiority for any particular diet. Thus, choosing a diet composition based on the patient's preferences and health status is best, with the assistance of a dietician when possible. For weight loss maintenance, face-to-face or telephone-delivered weight loss-maintenance programs that provide regular contact (monthly or more frequent) with a trained interventionist are evidence-based, and a high level of physical activity (i.e., 3–5 hours/week) is recommended. In this setting, an obsessive/compulsive behavior with frequent weighing predicts a more successful outcome.

For severe obesity or a BMI $\geq 35\,kg/m^2$ with co-morbidities, a surgical procedure may be best. Presently metabolic surgery is the only obesity therapy proven to prolong life, a benefit attributable to reductions in cancer as well as CVD-related mortality. Increasing evidence also indicates the value of metabolic surgery in treating patients with type 2 diabetes, with many patients free of diabetes medications and some postoperative patients with normal levels of glycosylated hemoglobin A1c rendered non-diabetic. In experienced hands, surgical mortality is now <0.3%.

Clinical Lipidology

Dyslipidemia is defined as an increase in low-density lipoprotein (LDL) cholesterol (LDL-C), triglycerides and/or reductions in high-density lipoprotein (HDL) cholesterol (HDL-C). An increase in the pro-atherogenic particle lipoprotein (a) could be included but presently this risk factor has been omitted from CVD risk screening because specific therapies are not yet available to document the value of lipoprotein (a) lowering. Nevertheless, when atherosclerotic CVD occurs in the absence of other risk factors and the family history is positive, elevations in lipoprotein (a) could be informative.

Evidence for reducing triglycerides is equivocal at best. Most randomized clinical trials in which triglyceride-lowering drugs have been used with statins in high-risk patients have not shown added benefit. Yet, most of these trials have suffered from design and adequate power. Nevertheless support for a fibrate such as fenofibrate in addition to a statin has been suggested when fasting triglycerides are >200 but <500 mg/dL (>2.3 but <5.6 mmol/L), but not when given to patients with triglycerides <200 mg/dL (<2.3 mmol/L). Two trials with treatment of patients who exhibit this same range of triglycerides with omega-3 fatty acids are ongoing. For patients with atherosclerotic CVD (ASCVD) or high risk with lower levels of HDL-C, extended release niacin and the cholesteryl ester transfer protein (CETP) inhibitor dalcetrapib added to existing statin therapy have failed to reduce CVD events. One additional CETP inhibitor trial (anacetrapib) has recently reported and, despite positive findings, (a modest 9% reduction in major coronary events), the sponsors have decided that further commercial development of the drug was not warranted.

The 2013 ACC/AHA Guideline on the Treatment of Blood Cholesterol to Reduce Atherosclerotic Cardiovascular Risk in Adults provides updated evidence for the benefit of LDL-C reductions and CVD outcomes (3). In addition to counseling patients about a heart-healthy lifestyle that includes a dietary pattern of fruits, vegetables, whole grains, low fat dairy, chicken, fish, legumes and nuts (reduced in saturated and *trans* fats) and 30–40 minutes of moderately vigorous physical activity four times a week, four benefit groups and indications for statin therapy have evolved, for adults at any age: (a) patients with known ASCVD or (b) patients with LDL-C >190 mg/dL (4.9 mmol/L). For these groups, high intensity statins, e.g., atorvastatin at 40–80 mg daily or rosuvastatin at 20–40 mg daily should be used; (c) patients with diabetes between the ages of 40–75 should be treated with at least a moderate intensity statin; and as should (d) patients with a calculated 10-year ASCVD event risk of ≥ 7.5%. This risk utilizes a risk estimator that now includes assessments for African-Americans in addition to Caucasians. For patients with a 5.0–7.5% 10-year risk, other factors such as a strong positive family history of premature ASCVD, an LDL-C ≥160 mg/dL (4.1 mmol/L), hs-CRP ≥ 2.0 mg/L, and/or subclinical atherosclerosis defined as a coronary artery calcification score ≥300 or >75%tile for age, gender, ethnicity, or an ankle brachial index (ABI) of <0.9 can be helpful in deciding to put patients on a statin. For this group, individualization of statin therapy needs important consideration and adverse effects need to be carefully discussed. Since the publication of the 2013 ACC/AHA Cholesterol Guideline, two trials have been completed: (a) Ezetimibe + simvastatin vs. simvastatin prescribed within 30 days of an acute coronary syndrome reduced the 4-point primary outcome of CVD death, myocardial infarction, unstable angina requiring hospitalization or stroke (IMPROVE-IT) (4); and (b) Evolocumab, one of two PCSK9 inhibitors, in addition to ongoing statin therapy reduced similar endpoints + coronary revascularization (5). These trials generate enthusiasm for more aggressive lowering of LDL-C.

Other important topics covered in Part XI include the emergency management of statin-induced myositis and rhabdomyolysis (6), and the role of severe hypertriglyceridemia in acute and chronic pancreatitis (7).

References

1 The GBD 2015 Obesity Collaborators. Health effects of overweight and obesity in 195 countries over 25 years. *N Eng J Med.* 2017 June 12. DOI: 10.1056/ NEJMoa1614362.

2 Jensen MD, Ryan DH, Apovian CM, et al. 2013 AHA/ACC/TOS Guideline for the Management of Overweight and Obesity in Adults: A Report of the American College of Cardiology/American Heart Association

Task Force on Practice Guidelines and The Obesity Society. *J Am Coll Cardiol.* 2014;63(25 Pt B):2985–3023.

3 Stone NJ, Robinson J, Lichtenstein AH, et al. 2013 ACC/AHA Guideline on the Treatment of Blood Cholesterol to Reduce Atherosclerotic Cardiovascular Risk in Adults: A Report of the American College of Cardiology/American Heart Association Task Force on Practice Guidelines. *Circulation.* 2014;129(25 Suppl 2):S1–S45.

4 Cannon CP, Blazing Mam Giugliano RP, et al. Ezetimibe added to statin therapy after acute coronary syndromes, *N Eng J Med.* 2015;372:2387–3297.

5 Sabatine MS, Giugliano RP, Keech AC, et al. Evolocumab and clinical outcomes in patients with cardiovascular disease. *N Eng J Med.* 2017;376:1713–1722.

6 Saxon DR, Eckel RH. Statin intolerance: a literature review and management strategies. *Prog Cardiovasc Dis.* 2016;59:153–164.

7 Brown WV, Brunzell JD, Eckel RH, Stone NJ. Severe hypertriglyceridemia. *J Clin Lipidol.* 2012;6:397–408.

43

Acute Emergencies Related to Bariatric Surgery

Michael A. Via and Jeffrey I. Mechanick

Key Points

- Overweight and obesity are characterized by an excess of body fat. Obesity is usually defined by body mass index (BMI) $\geq 30\,kg/m^2$ (although lesser cut-off values are used in Asians). The prevalence of overweight/obesity has increased considerably over the past decades in all parts of the world.

- Overweight and obesity are important modifiable risk factors for numerous associated disorders (e.g., type 2 diabetes (T2D), hypertension (HTN), hyperlipidemia, non-alcoholic fatty liver disease, cancers, musculoskeletal, and obstructive sleep apnea).

- Bariatric surgery (also termed "metabolic" surgery) has become recognized as the most definitive and successful means for the treatment of obesity and obesity-associated medical conditions.

- Bariatric surgery alters the anatomy of the gastrointestinal tract to restrict caloric intake (i.e., "restrictive") and/or reduce absorption (i.e., "malabsorptive"). In addition, many other mechanisms of weight loss are also involved.

- Several bariatric procedures are currently available, including laparoscopic adjustable gastric banding (LAGB), laparoscopic sleeve gastrectomy (LSG), and Roux-en-Y gastric bypass (RYGB).

- Over the past decade, both the establishment of high-volume metabolic surgical centers and the use of laparoscopic technique have led to dramatic improvements in surgical outcomes following bariatric procedures.

- Perioperative mortality as low as 0.04–0.5% has been consistently reported in case series.

- Benefits of surgery include weight loss and either significant improvement or complete amelioration of metabolic derangements, which must be balanced against the risks of each procedure.

- When considering bariatric surgery for patients with obesity, clinicians should be aware of potential adverse events that may develop following each type of surgery, as well as the marked improvement of associated diseases, such as T2D, HTN, and hyperlipidemia, among many other metabolic conditions.

- Many of the acute emergencies that commonly occur as a result of bariatric surgery are metabolic in nature, and are related to either hormonal changes or malabsorption induced by the procedure.

- Postoperatively, patients will need lifelong follow-up that should include recognition of common acute emergencies as well as the adjustment of medical therapies as comorbid conditions improve/evolve.

Endocrine and Metabolic Medical Emergencies: A Clinician's Guide, Second Edition. Edited by Glenn Matfin.
© 2018 John Wiley & Sons Ltd. Published 2018 by John Wiley & Sons Ltd.

Introduction

Overweight and obesity are characterized by an excess of body fat. Obesity is usually defined by body mass index (BMI) $\geq 30\,\text{kg/m}^2$ (lesser cut-off values are used in Asians), although as an anthropometric measure it can underperform as a predictor of health and sole guide for clinical decision-making. The prevalence of overweight and obesity has increased considerably over the past decades in all parts of the world. Overweight and obesity are important modifiable risk factors for numerous associated disorders (e.g., type 2 diabetes [T2D], hypertension [HTN], hyperlipidemia, non-alcoholic fatty liver disease, cancers, musculoskeletal, and obstructive sleep apnea [OSA]).

Bariatric Procedures

Bariatric surgery (also termed "metabolic" surgery) has become recognized as the most definitive and successful means for the treatment of obesity and obesity-associated medical conditions (1–3). Bariatric surgery alters the anatomy of the gastrointestinal (GI) tract to restrict caloric intake (i.e., "restrictive") and/or reduce absorption (i.e., "malabsorptive"). In addition, many other mechanisms of weight loss are also involved. Several bariatric procedures are currently available (Figure 43-1), including laparoscopic adjustable gastric banding (LAGB), laparoscopic sleeve gastrectomy (LSG), Roux-en-Y gastric bypass (RYGB), biliopancreatic diversion (BPD), and biliopancreatic diversion with duodenal switch (BPDDS).

RYGB is still the most frequently performed bariatric surgery worldwide, and the second most common bariatric procedure performed in the USA, accounting for 38% of all bariatric surgery cases (4). In this procedure, the stomach is divided into a small pouch that is anastomosed with a portion of distal ileum to restrict gastric volume and to induce malabsorption. The stomach remnant is allowed to drain through the bypassed portion of the small intestine until it reconnects with the distal ileum.

The LSG was initially intended as a restrictive procedure, however, the surgical creation of a gastric sleeve through resection of a large portion of the gastric antrum and fundus also induces malabsorption. This may be through reduced gastric acid production, as well as a host of other beneficial hormonal and metabolic effects. The LSG has become the most commonly performed bariatric procedure in the USA accounting for 58% of all bariatric surgery cases (4).

The BPD involves the creation of a small gastric pouch that is anastomosed to a short portion of ileum. In the BPDDS, the lesser curvature, antrum and pylorus are used to create a gastric pouch leaving the anterior portion of the duodenum in place. This is anastomosed distally to a short portion of ileum. BPD and BPDDS account for less than 1% of bariatric surgery in the USA, owing to higher rates of complications and malnutrition (4).

The LAGB is a purely restrictive procedure that involves the placement of an inflatable band around the stomach, reducing gastric volume. A subcutaneous reservoir can be accessed to inflate or deflate the band, as needed based on clinical response. Though previously common, recent trends show only 3% of bariatric surgeries performed in the USA are LAGB procedures (4).

Benefits of surgery include weight loss and either significant improvement or complete amelioration of metabolic derangements, which must be weighed against the risks of each procedure. When considering bariatric surgery for patients with obesity, clinicians should be aware of potential adverse events that may develop following each type of surgery, as well as the marked improvement of associated disease, such as T2D, HTN, and hyperlipidemia, among many other metabolic conditions. Postoperatively, patients will need lifelong follow-up that should include recognition of common acute emergencies as well as the adjustment of medical therapies as comorbid conditions improve/evolve.

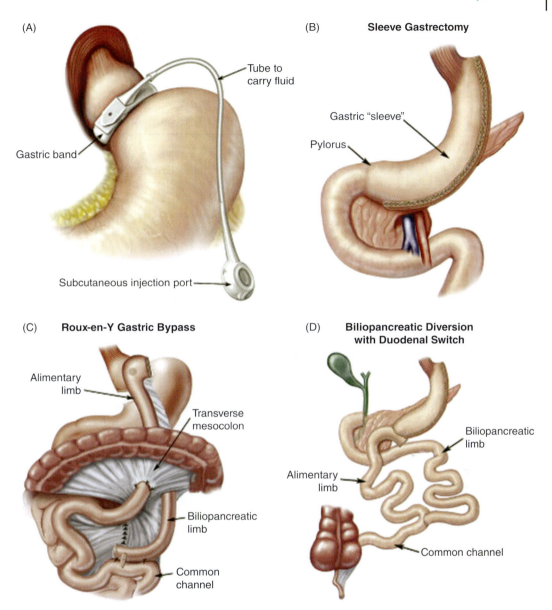

(A)

Tube to
carry fluid

Gastric band

Subcutaneous injection port

(B) **Sleeve Gastrectomy**

Gastric "sleeve"

Pylorus

(C) **Roux-en-Y Gastric Bypass**

Alimentary
limb

Transverse
mesocolon

Biliopancreatic
limb

Common
channel

(D) **Biliopancreatic Diversion
with Duodenal Switch**

Biliopancreatic
limb

Alimentary
limb

Common channel

Figure 43-1 Common types of bariatric surgery procedures. (A) Adjustable gastric band; (B) sleeve gastrectomy; (C) Roux-en-Y gastric bypass; (D) biliopancreatic diversion with duodenal switch. Reproduced with permission from John Wiley & Sons, Ltd.

Bariatric Surgery-Related Issues

Surgical Emergencies

Over the past decade, both the establishment of high-volume metabolic surgical centers and the use of laparoscopic technique have led to dramatic improvements in surgical outcomes following bariatric procedures (5). Adverse outcomes and observed benefits also depend on the type of bariatric procedure undertaken. Overall perioperative mortality as low as 0.04–0.5% has been consistently

Table 43-1 Acute surgical morbidity rates following bariatric surgery performed at dedicated bariatric surgical centers (%) (8,9)

	LAGB	LSG	RYGB*
Stricture formation and obstruction	0.13	0.42	1.4
Intestinal obstruction without stricture	0.03	0	0.2–0.9
Infection	0.14	0.64	0.3
Bleeding	0.05	0.64	1.0
Anastamotic leak	0	0.74	0.78

*Includes data from patients with RYGB performed laparoscopically.

reported in case series (6,7). The need for re-operation or surgical revision following bariatric surgery is 5% for RYGB, 1% for LAGB, and 3% for LSG. Rates of hospital readmission following bariatric surgery are 6% for RYGB, 2% for LAGB, and 5% for LSG (8). The most common reasons for hospital readmission after surgery are summarized in Table 43-1 and include intestinal obstruction, infection, bleeding, and anastomotic leak (8.9). While uncommon, clinical evaluation for these conditions should be undertaken in appropriate patients.

Nausea and Vomiting

Due to anatomic changes, patients may experience a significant amount of nausea and vomiting following bariatric surgery. Patients are at risk for dehydration, which can be mitigated with intravenous (IV) fluid administration, and slow transition to oral fluid intake. Appropriate use of anti-emetics is also warranted.

Venous Thromboembolism

Patients who undergo bariatric surgery are at increased risk for venous thromboembolism (VTE), including deep vein thrombosis (DVT) and pulmonary embolism (PE) events. This is due, in part, to the increased systemic inflammation, reduced rates of venous flow, and activation of coagulation pathways, including a two-fold increase of circulating fibrinogen levels with obesity, coupled with the general increased risk of VTE following surgery (10). Additionally, the laparoscopic approach increases intra-abdominal pressure during each procedure, which may increase risk of thrombus formation (10). Following laparoscopic bariatric surgery, rates of DVT have been reported in 3%, while PE has been reported in 1% of patients. Cases of portal or mesenteric venous thrombosis have also been reported, which most often present between postoperative days 3 and 30 (11). Symptoms include vague abdominal pain, and can manifest as liver cirrhosis or bowel ischemia. Computerized tomography (CT) with IV contrast is oftentimes diagnostic, with an accuracy rate of 90% (12).

There is no consensus for the optimal means of VTE prevention following bariatric surgery. The routine administration of low-molecular weight heparin and the use of compressive stockings have been suggested to reduce risk postoperatively (10).

Diarrhea and Dumping Syndrome

Obesity-related pelvic floor dysfunction results in fecal incontinence in as high as 20–35% of patients with obesity (13). Following bariatric surgery, the prevalence of fecal incontinence is reduced by approximately 10–15% (14).

Aside from this improvement, the surgical alteration of the GI tract can lead to an increase in frequency of bowel movements. In extreme cases, dumping syndrome may develop following RYGB, BPD, BPDDS, or LSG as a result of impaired stomach relaxation (15). Meals containing high amounts of carbohydrates can exacerbate this condition.

Patients with dumping syndrome experience sudden and large volume diarrhea secondary to rapid passage of chyme from the stomach to the small intestine (16). Delivery of incompletely digested food from the stomach can contribute to the associated symptoms, which include abdominal pain

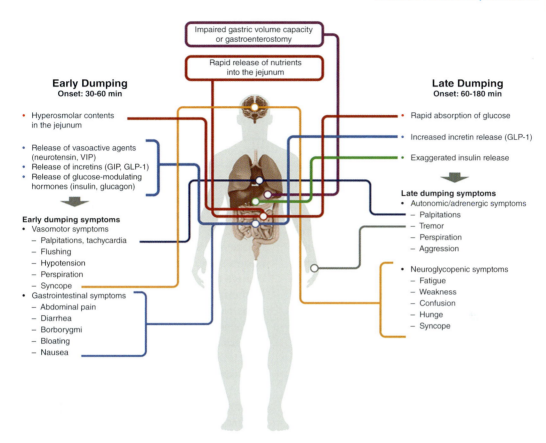

Figure 43-2 Pathophysiology of dumping syndrome (16)
GIP = gastric inhibitory peptide; GLP-1 = Glucagon-like peptide-1; VIP = Vasoactive inhibitory peptide.
Reproduced with permission from John Wiley & Sons, Ltd.

and cramping, nausea, flushing, diaphoresis, and lightheadedness ("early" dumping syndrome). Hypoglycemia may develop approximately 3 hours after meals, due to an exaggerated incretin response ("late" dumping syndrome) (Figure 43-2) (16,17).

Treatment of dumping syndrome includes dietary restriction of carbohydrates, especially simple sugars (e.g., sugar-containing beverages and sweets) (18). Separation of liquid and solid foods during a meal may also be beneficial (18). These dietary interventions may be all that is necessary to control dumping syndrome, justifying a detailed and thorough evaluation by a Registered Dietitian. If symptoms persist, the administration of acarbose with meals may provide symptomatic relief (19). In severe cases, the therapeutic use of somatostatin analogs (octreotide, lanreotide, or pasireotide) delay stomach emptying and improve the condition (16,20).

Hypoglycemia

Patients who undergo bariatric surgery may develop postprandial hypoglycemia without any of the other related GI symptoms that are typical of dumping syndrome. This phenomenon may also be associated with a sudden significant increase in incretin activity (21). The anatomic alterations resulting from RYGB, LSG, or BPD procedures yield significant increases in insulin sensitivity and pancreatic β-cell insulin production (16).

In some cases, the pancreatic β-cell response is exaggerated after bariatric surgery, leading to increased number of β-cells and/or overactive β-cell function in a condition known as nesidioblastosis (21,22). In these cases, patients experience hypoglycemia approximately 1–3 hours following meals, especially after the ingestion of a high carbohydrate load. Hypoglycemia events may be severe: blood glucose levels of 15–40 mg/dL (0.8–2.2 mmol/L) have been reported, and can cause seizures, altered mental status, or loss of consciousness. Following either a mixed meal test, or oral glucose tolerance test, measured serum insulin and C-peptide levels are inappropriately elevated during these hypoglycemic periods.

The use of somatostatin scanning or CT can help to rule out other causes of hyperinsulinemia, such as insulin-secreting tumors, as a cause of hypoglycemia. Calcium-stimulated selective mesenteric venous sampling can also confirm diffuse hyperactivity of pancreatic β-cells in this condition (22).

Nesidioblastosis has been reported following RYGB and BPD procedures (21). In most cases, strict adherence to a low carbohydrate diet mitigates the exaggerated insulin response in nesidioblastosis. For refractory cases, the use of α-glucosidase inhibitors such as acarbose or miglitol, or calcium channel blockers, can reduce the rate of hypoglycemia (23). Several published cases of post-bariatric surgery nesidioblastosis describe successful treatment and prevention of hypoglycemia with the use of either diazoxide, or somotostatin analogues (24–26). For patients with persistent hypoglycemia despite dietary and medical optimization, distal pancreatectomy may be considered although many patients experience repeat hypoglycemia post procedure, likely due to diffuse β-cell changes throughout the pancreas.

Management of Metabolic Disease

The anatomic changes that are introduced in RYGB, BPD, BPDDS, and LSG induce a rapid reduction in insulin resistance that occurs immediately following surgery. The molecular mechanisms for this have not been fully elucidated, but may include increased incretin response, increased circulating bile salt and fibroblast growth factor (FGF)-19 concentrations, rapid changes in individual dietary choices, reduced systemic inflammation, a changing GI microbiome profile, and likely several other pathways that have yet to be described or sufficiently validated (27).

As a consequence, the severity of metabolic disease changes rapidly following surgery. Treatment regimens for individual conditions, such as hypertension, hypercholesterolemia, obstructive sleep apnea, and T2D should be adapted to anticipated changes. In the weeks and months prior to surgery, patients are prescribed an intensive lifestyle change that may also require the adjustment of their medication regimen. Recommendations to the approach for obesity-associated medical conditions in relation to bariatric surgery are provided in Table 43-2.

In all cases, the severity of metabolic disease should be used to guide recommendations for prescribed postoperative medications. For example, a patient with T2D that is easily controlled with one or two oral anti-hyperglycemic agents is likely to achieve excellent glycemic control following LSG, RYGB, BPD, or BPDDS without the need for any medication. However, a patient with poorly controlled advanced T2D, who requires large doses of insulin is likely to continue to require some glucose-lowering medications postoperatively, albeit at a reduced dose.

Obstructive Sleep Apnea (OSA)

OSA is highly prevalent among patients with obesity and has been reported in approximately 60–90% of those undergoing bariatric surgery (28,29). Published guidelines recommend screening all patients for OSA prior to bariatric surgery (1,30). The administration of continuous positive airway pressure (CPAP) can significantly reduce daytime drowsiness and other complications of OSA (28). In the perioperative phase following bariatric surgery, the continued implementation of CPAP among patients with OSA has

Table 43-2 Suggested adaptation of medical treatment regimens for obesity-associated conditions in the preoperative and postoperative time courses of bariatric procedures

Obesity-associated condition	Preoperative	Immediate postoperative (up to 4 weeks)	Short-term postoperative (1-12 months)	Long-term postoperative
Type 2 diabetes	Intensify efforts for targeted glycemic control	Hold usual regimen, treat with insulin as required	Reintroduce individual medications as needed, favoring insulin-sensitizing medications over sulfonylureas or meglitinides, which can induce hypoglycemia. Patients who were severely uncontrolled or required insulin preoperatively are at risk for continued need for medical therapy.	Glycemic control may worsen with time, especially in patients with significant weight regain
Hypertension	Targeted blood pressure control	Resume home regimen	Reduce regimen/withdraw individual medications in a stepwise fashion every 1–2 months and monitor for improvement	Continue to reduce regimen and adjust as needed
Hypercholesterolemia	Continued use of cholesterol lowering regimen	Hold medications	Re-assess serum cholesterol levels at 3–6 months postoperatively	Monitor cholesterol levels regularly
Polycystic ovary syndrome	No specific changes	Hold medications, including oral contraceptives - risk for VTE	Depending on severity of PCOS, can resume preoperative regimen vs. observation for improvement without medications	Reduce regimen/withdraw individual medications and monitor for improvement
Obesity-related hypogonadism (male)	No specific changes	Hold medication regimen	Continue to withhold testosterone therapy to induce endogenous testosterone production. Reassess testosterone at 3–6 month intervals	Continue to evaluate, re-introduce testosterone therapy if necessary
Obstructive sleep apnea	Continued use of positive airway pressure devices	Continued use of positive airway pressure devices	Re-evaluate need for continued use of positive airway pressure devices every 3–6 months	Re-evaluate need for continued use of positive airway pressure devices every 3-6 months

VTE = venous thromboembolic event.

been shown to reduce both pulmonary surgical complications by 5-fold, and overall surgical complications by nearly 2-fold (31).

The rapid improvement in metabolic function following malabsorptive bariatric surgery is also associated with improvement in severity of OSA (32,33). As with many other metabolic conditions, OSA improves early and disproportionately to the weight loss following LSG or RYGB (32,33). In one prospective study of patients with OSA, the apnea-hypopnea index improved by 60% at 3 weeks following LSG or RYGB, while only a 5% reduction in weight was observed by that time (32).

Malabsorption

In RYGB, BPD, and BPDDS procedures, effective weight loss is achieved, in part, by intentionally creating a malabsorptive state. In some cases, the surgically created reduction in active small intestinal absorptive surface area yields clinically significant deficiencies in micronutrient or macronutrient absorption. Severe protein-calorie malnutrition necessitating nutritional support has been observed in approximately 1% of patients undergoing RYGB annually, with a 5% lifetime risk (34). The risk of severe protein-calorie malnutrition is greater following BPD, and is reported in approximately 20–30% of patients, highlighting the significant malabsorption that is induced by this procedure (35).

For typical patients undergoing bariatric surgical procedures, the greatest amount of weight loss is achieved in the first 18 months in the postoperative period (36). Protein-calorie malnutrition should be suspected in patients who continue to lose weight for 2 or more years after surgery. Other clinical signs that should raise suspicion include fatigue, weakness, muscle wasting, and persistent micronutrient deficiencies. The diagnosis of protein-calorie malnutrition should be made on a clinical basis and may be supported (though not diagnosed) through measurement of serum markers of protein

synthesis, such as albumin, prealbumin, or retinol binding protein.

Treatment options for protein-calorie malnutrition may include the use of high-calorie oral supplements, the placement of enteral feeding tubes, the use of parenteral nutrition (PN), or surgical revision or reversal (1). In the largest published series of 77 patients who underwent bariatric surgery and required PN, 38 had severe protein-calorie malnutrition (37). The remaining 39 subjects sustained surgical complications. Among the whole cohort, BMI declined from an average of $44.4 \pm 6.0\,\mathrm{kg/m^2}$ at the time of surgery to $23.2 \pm 6.4\,\mathrm{kg/m^2}$ at initiation of PN. Hypoalbuminemia and edema were present in 31 of the 38 with protein-calorie malnutrition. Eventually, 29 patients were weaned off PN, including 17 who underwent surgical revision.

Micronutrient Malabsorption

The reduction of the intestinal absorptive surface area following RYGB, BPD, and BPDDS procedures increases the risk of micronutrient malabsorption and deficiency. The reduction in gastric acid production in LSG may affect the liberation and dissolution of vitamins and essential trace metals. Contrary to initial belief, even though the intestinal surface area is intact following LSG, similar rates of micronutrient deficiency are noted in patients after this procedure when compared to RYGB (Table 43-3).

One effect of bariatric surgery is to induce changes in personal dietary choice. For example, in a cohort of 43 obese patients who underwent RYGB, food choice changed dramatically throughout their postoperative course (38). At 6 weeks postoperative, measured calorie density of each food item consumed was 30% less than preoperative dietary intake. These trends persisted for the 1-year duration of the study, and contributed to micronutrient deficiencies. Other factors related to nutrient intake after bariatric surgery included changes in taste perception and intensity, reduced vagal tone, and potential for surgically induced changes in

Table 43-3 Prevalence rates (%) of micronutrient deficiencies following bariatric surgery (40,50,51,55)

	LAGB	LSG	RYGB	BPD/BPDDS
Thiamin (B_1)	0	0	10–15	10–15
Folate (B_9)	10	10–20	15	15
Pyridoxine (B_6)	0	0–15	0	10
Cobalamin (B_{12})	10	10–20	30–50	22
Vitamin A	10	10–20	10–50	60–70
Vitamin D (<30 ng/dL)	30	30–70	30–50	40–100
Vitamin E	0	0–5	10	10
Vitamin K	0	0	0	60–70
Iron	0–32	15–45	25–50	25
Copper	–	10	10	70
Zinc	–	30	37	25

– data not available.

the intestinal microbiome affecting appetite and metabolism (39).

Dietary nutrient intake before bariatric surgery also plays a role in the development of deficiency states. High rates of micronutrient deficiencies such as vitamin D, vitamin B_{12}, vitamin C, and zinc, are common in the preoperative obese population, which is generally attributed to poor dietary choices and reduced intake (40). As a result of these combined risks, patients are universally advised to take vitamin supplements after both purely restrictive and malabsorptive bariatric surgery procedures, and are periodically monitored for deficiency (1). Despite these measures, micronutrient deficiency is common and can lead to clinically significant morbidity (41).

After bariatric surgery, common micronutrient deficiencies include iron, thiamin (vitamin B_1), folate, copper, and cobalamin (vitamin B_{12}). High rates of vitamin D insufficiency are also observed (42). Lipid-soluble vitamin deficiencies are common after BPD and BPDDS procedures (43).

Iron

Dietary iron is present either within a heme group or chelated within a non-heme structure. The acid environment of the stomach maintains ingested iron moieties in the ferric (3+) state in both these forms, for improved solubility. After transit to the duodenum, ferroreductase activity reduces iron to the ferrous state, which is required for absorption (44,45).

Following all types of bariatric surgery, diminished gastric acid production reduces the efficiency of iron absorption (41). Additionally, the bypassed duodenum in RYGB and BPD procedures limits the exposure of ingested iron to ferroreductase, which contributes to reduced iron absorption. Consequently, relatively high rates of iron deficiency are reported following bariatric procedures (Table 43-3).

Patients with clinically significant iron deficiency experience fatigue, microcytic anemia, hair loss, brittle nails, and angular cheilosis, which appears as wrinkled or crusted erythematous fissures at the corners of the mouth (45). Iron deficiency can lead to significant morbidity following malabsorptive bariatric procedures, especially in patients with underlying cardiovascular or pulmonary disease. Regular testing for serum iron levels at 6-month intervals and appropriate supplementation (oral or parenteral) are recommended (1).

Thiamin

Thiamin (vitamin B_1) is a water-soluble vitamin that serves as an important co-factor for several steps in glucose metabolism, amino acid synthesis, and the pentose phosphate shunt pathway. The majority of thiamin is obtained through dietary sources, while a small amount may be synthesized by enterocolonic bacteria (46). Deficiency states of thiamin include "wet" and "dry" beri beri, as well as Wernicke encephalopathy, which may develop if less than adequate amounts of thiamin are consumed or absorbed. Mild cases of thiamin deficiency may lead to symptoms of intractable nausea, vomiting, or neuropathy.

Dietary thiamin generally exists in a phosphorylated form that must be hydrolyzed prior to absorption. The majority of intestinal phosphatases that act on thiamin phosphate and thiamin pyrophosphate are located in the proximal intestine, which is bypassed in RYGB and BPD procedures (46). As a result of decreased hydrolysis and diminished intestinal absorptive surface area, thiamin deficiency may develop after these procedures and has been reported in 10–15% of patients following RYGB (47). Patients should be screened regularly and provided with a vitamin supplementation regimen that includes thiamin. Thiamin deficiency should be suspected in patients with symptoms of Wernicke encephalopathy, beri beri, unexplained vomiting or neuropathy (48). Treatment should include thiamine supplementation with 500 mg thiamin given IV daily for 3–5 days, followed by 250 mg daily until resolution of symptoms and eventually reducing to 100 mg daily (1).

Folate

Intestinal malabsoprtion following RYGB, BPD, and BPDDS procedures commonly leads to folate deficiency. This water-soluble vitamin is essential in one-carbon metabolism, DNA synthesis, and amino acid metabolism (46). Folate deficiency is reported in approximately 10% of patients undergoing RYGB, 5–10% of patients undergoing BPD, and 10% of patients undergoing LSG (40). Symptoms of anemia, fatigue, and risk for congenital neural tube defects may be seen in patients with folate deficiency. Thus, supplementation with folic acid 400 µg daily and regular monitoring of folate status is recommended in patients who have undergone malabsorptive bariatric procedures (1).

Copper

Copper functions at the active site of enzymes that catalyze redox reactions among diverse biochemical pathways that include neurotransmitter synthesis, superoxide synthesis, respiratory oxidation, and iron metabolism (49). GI absorption of copper takes place mainly in the duodenum, which is bypassed in the malabsorptive bariatric procedures. Copper deficiency has been reported in up to 70% of patients undergoing BPD. Lower rates of copper deficiency are also noted following LSG and RYGB (40).

Patients with copper deficiency may experience painful neuropathy, anemia, fatigue, and iron deficiency. Regular surveillance for copper deficiency is not currently recommended following malabsorptive bariatric surgery, however, patients who develop symptoms of copper deficiency or those with other signs of severe malabsorption may benefit from measurement of serum copper and ceruloplasmin levels, which is elevated in states of copper deficiency (1). Supplementation with copper 2 mg daily, either orally or parenterally should be administered in copper-deficient patients (1).

Cobalamin

Deficiency of cobalamin (vitamin B_{12}) is common following bariatric surgical procedures (40,50,51). This is partly due to the complex absorptive process of B_{12} that depends on the functional physiology of the GI tract. Dietary cobalamin is bound to the intrinsic factor, a peptide released from parietal cells located in the gastric antrum and fundus, for protection during the digestive processes. As gastric chyme progresses through the intestinal tract, dietary B_{12} is liberated from the intrinsic factor for absorption in the distal ileum. Alteration in stomach anatomy in RYGB, LSG, BPD, and BPDDS procedures reduces gastric parietal cell mass, potentially leading to B_{12} malabsorption and deficiency. Symptoms of B_{12} deficiency may range from subtle in nature to severe, and include neuropathy, muscle weakness, fatigue, anemia, and mood disorders. Rates of B_{12} deficiency are reported to be approximately 20% following LSG, 30–60% following RYGB, 20–40% following BPD, and 5–15% following LAGB.

Empiric supplementation with multiple vitamins that contain B_{12} is recommended. Screening for B_{12} deficiency at regular intervals and supplementing with high dose oral B_{12} preparations (1000 µg daily) or parenteral B_{12} injections are also recommended following malabsorptive bariatric procedures (1). Toxicity of B_{12} is not observed in humans (52).

Case Study

A 42-year-old female patient, with a history of obesity by BMI of 38 kg/m², hypertension, and poorly controlled type 2 diabetes, underwent RYGB. Prior to surgery she had been prescribed multiple daily injections of insulin, but was only able to maintain her glycosylated hemoglobin (HbA1c) at levels of approximately 9–10% (75–86 mmol/mol). Postoperatively, she had lost 90 lbs over 18 months, which reduced her BMI to 27 kg/m² and she no longer required any pharmacologic treatments for hypertension or T2D diabetes. Her recent HbA1c was measured to be 5.7% (38 mmol/mol). She was continued on calcium citrate, vitamin D, and multivitamin supplements. For the past 5 months, her weight has been stable.

She now complains of sensations of "pins and needles" and at times burning in her toes and feet bilaterally that is worse at night. These have been worsening over the last 4 months. During this time, she has also been experiencing episodic symptoms of shakiness, sweating, and extreme hunger that are similar to hypoglycemia episodes she had while taking insulin before her surgery. She reports these symptoms only occur during the day, and resolve with eating something sweet. Fingerstick measurement reveals capillary blood glucose levels of 54 mg/dL (3.0 mmol/L) during one such episode.

What Would Be Your Approach to the Patient's Management?

The multiple metabolic effects following bariatric surgery, especially RYGB, have the potential to cause more than one clinically significant medical condition. The patient presents with symptoms of neuropathy. It is unlikely to be diabetic neuropathy considering she did not have this prior to her surgery, and her diabetes improved significantly with the bariatric procedure. She is at risk for micronutrient deficiency. Serum levels of thiamine were found to be 5 nmol/L (normal 8–30 nmol/L), and B12 levels were 192 pg/mL (normal 200–900 pg/mL). Serum concentration of copper, zinc, folate, 25-hydroxyvitamin D, and iron were also assessed, and were at target levels. Supplementation with thiamine 500 mg daily was added to her daily regimen for 3 days, which was subsequently reduced to 250 mg daily for 5 days, and then reduced to 100 mg daily. In addition, weekly intramuscular injections of B12 1000 mcg were administered for 6 weeks followed by a reduced schedule of 1000 mcg B12 every 3 months. With these interventions, the symptoms of neuropathy resolved.

As for her hypoglycemia symptoms, she was instructed to follow a low carbohydrate diet, and to consume smaller meals. With this dietary intervention, her symptoms resolved, supporting clinical suspicion of the diagnosis of pancreatic nesidioblastosis. Had the symptoms persisted, further work-up with a mixed meal test, and consideration for pharmacologic therapy with an α-glucosidase inhibitor initially would be warranted.

Osteoporosis and Bone Fractures

Several factors contribute to the high rates of bone turnover that is observed following bariatric surgery. Reduced calcium absorption is observed following malabsorptive bariatric procedures and commonly causes secondary hyperparathyroidism (53,54). Moreover, vitamin D insufficiency is reported in 50–60% of patients after bariatric surgery, despite supplementation, which contributes directly to bone loss and worsens secondary hyperparathyroidism (55). The post-surgical secondary hyperparathyroidism that develops often does not fully resolve with calcium and vitamin D supplementation (53,54). This typically normal serum calcium level can distinguish this phenomenon from primary hyperparathyroidism, in which both parathyroid hormone and serum calcium are elevated.

Following bariatric procedures, the mechanical load on musculature and bones declines as patients lose weight, leading to decreased bone density and bone strength. This is analogous, though not as severe, to the bone loss that is observed in patients who are bed-bound, or among astronauts who sustain bone loss during the time spent in the near weightless space environment (56).

A rise in circulating serotonin following RYGB may also contribute to bone loss (57). Additionally, the malabsorption of other micronutrients (e.g., B$_{12}$) as well as protein malabsorption may contribute to bone loss following bariatric surgery.

The result of the above factors is a significant loss in bone density and bone strength. The greatest decline in bone density has been observed during the first year following surgery, with continued slower rates of decline subsequently (58). Following RYGB, a 10% reduction in bone mineral density is observed at the hip 1 year postoperatively (58).

Treatment for bone loss associated with bariatric surgery is preventive in nature. Postoperative supplementation with calcium is currently recommended for all patients (1). Calcium citrate is the preferred form of calcium for supplementation, owing to its superior absorption in conditions of reduced stomach acid production, including surgical alteration of the stomach following LSG, RYGB, LAGB, BPD, and BPDDS (59).

Vitamin D supplementation is also recommended, targeting a circulating 25-hydroxyvitamin D level of 30 ng/dL (80 nmol/L) or greater (1). The typical dose requirement for vitamin D supplements is 1000–2000 international units (IU) daily (42). Patients who have undergone malabsorptive procedures, including RYGB, BPD, and BPDDS, may require increasing doses of vitamin D supplementation (as high as 100,000 IU or more; with or without addition of calcitriol) to achieve target levels. If fat malabsorption is severe, intravenous calcitriol can be administered at a starting dose of 0.25–0.5 µg daily.

The typical pattern for decline in bone density is greatest in the first year postoperatively, with approximately a 10% loss of bone mineral density at the hip. This is followed by a period of slower decline. Bone density at the spine and forearm are minimally affected.

Several case-control and cohort studies demonstrate a 2- to 3-fold increase in fracture risk has been reported after bariatric surgery (60–62). However, other studies fail to demonstrate a change in fracture risk (63). Consequently, the use of bone antiresorptive agents, such as bisphosphonates, to prevent bone loss is not currently recommended. On an individual basis, use of antiresorptive agents can be considered in patients who sustain fractures, or among those who have continued bone loss after 2–3 years postoperatively (1). Adequate supplementation with calcium and vitamin D are required to prevent potential hypocalcemia if antiresorptive agents are given following bariatric surgery (64).

Oxalate Nephrolithiasis

Patients who undergo RYGB, BPD, and BPDDS bariatric procedures are at increased risk for the development of calcium oxalate nephrolithiasis (65–67). In one matched comparison study, a 7.6% incidence of nephrolithiasis was noted in 4636 subjects after undergoing RYGB with 5 years of follow-up, in contrast to an incidence of only 4.5% in controls who were obese (67,68). Both plasma and urine oxalate levels are increased in patients who have undergone RYGB and BPD, consistent with these findings (67,68). Increased rates of nephrolithiasis have not been described following LABG or LSG (69,70). An increase in intestinal oxalate absorption may result indirectly from fat malabsorption. The excess of unconjugated fatty acids in the intestinal lumen leads to increased luminal calcium-fatty acid salt formation. This diminishes the sequestration of luminal oxalate by ingested calcium, leading to greater oxalate absorption (65).

Generally, there is no modification for the clinical presentation and treatment of nephrolithiasis in patients who have undergone malabsorptive bariatric procedures. Hydration, stone collection for analysis, and urologic intervention are employed as necessary.

Prevention of stone formation with oral calcium supplementation reduces oxalate absorption in patients who have undergone RYGB, BPD, or BPDDS, and is currently recommended in these patients (1,71). Additionally, the measurement of 24-hour urinary calcium levels can aid in the titration of calcium supplements to avoid excessive calcium dosing while minimizing oxalate absorption. In the case of reduced urinary citrate excretion, supplementation with potassium citrate can also diminish renal stone formation (72).

Intestinal Adaptation and Pharmacology

In response to malabsorption by any etiology, including following malabsorptive bariatric surgery, the intestinal epithelium adapts to increase the absorptive surface area and to upregulate the expression and function of channel proteins responsible for the absorption of nutrients. This phenomenon of intestinal adaptation may be partly responsible for weight re-gain following malabsorptive bariatric surgery (73).

Another consequence of intestinal adaptation is to alter the intestinal absorption of pharmacologic agents and alcohol, which can change significantly in the postoperative period of malabsorptive procedures (74).

Several mechanisms are responsible for these changes that occur after malabsorptive surgery. In many cases the decrease in intestinal absorptive surface area reduces bioavailability of orally ingested drugs. For example, absorption of levothyroxine and of sertraline following RYGB, BPD, or BPDDS is greatly reduced. Patients may require higher doses to achieve normal circulating levels (75,76). An oral liquid formulation of levothyroxine may improve bioavailability following malabsorptive surgery (77).

Following RYGB, BPD, and BPDDS there is a decreased transit time to the distal ileum, which reduces the time to peak serum levels of medications that are absorbed in this region, including opiates (78). Intestinal cytochrome P450 activity serves as an important step in the first pass metabolism of some pharmacologic agents, such as atorvastatin. As a result of decreased intestinal cytochrome P450 activity following these procedures, circulating atorvastatin levels may increase (79). Over time, circulating levels of metformin and acetaminophen have been observed to increase following malabsorptive surgery, likely due to intestinal adaptation (78).

These few examples demonstrate the diverse set of changes in pharmacokinetics that occur after malabsorptive bariatric surgery. Prescribers must carefully monitor medication use in patients who have undergone these procedures to avoid both toxicity and insufficient medication dosing.

Alcohol

The absorption of ethyl alcohol increases following RYGB surgery. After a consumption of a 5 oz. glass of red wine, peak breath alcohol levels are approximately 2- to 3-fold higher at 3 and 6 months after RYGB compared to the same patients preoperatively (80). No changes in peak breath alcohol are noted following LSG or LAGB (81), suggesting that the enhancement in absorptive physiology following RYGB may be related to the specific anatomic changes of this procedure. Consequently, the risk for alcohol use disorders is increased following RYGB surgery. One study demonstrated a near doubling of the prevalence of alcohol use disorders during a 2 year period following RYGB surgery (82).

A reduction in activation of central reward pathways following RYGB may also contribute to the observed increase rate of alcohol use disorders, as well as to the 2- to 3-fold increase in substance abuse disorders and suicide attempts that have been observed following RYGB (83,84). In contrast, neither alcohol absorption nor central reward pathways are affected following LAGB or LSG surgery. Increased rates of alcohol or other substance use disorders have not been observed following these procedures (83.84).

Pregnancy and Reproduction

The weight loss and improved metabolic profile following bariatric surgery can increase fertility among obese women, especially in women with polycystic ovary syndrome (85). Contraception is encouraged for the first 2 years following bariatric surgery (1,85), however, several retrospective studies found no difference in outcomes among women who became pregnant within the first year of bariatric surgery in comparison to those who became pregnant in subsequent years (86,87). With the exception of the risk of prematurity and the risk of infants who are small for gestational age that are both increased following bariatric surgery, the rates for many other specific pregnancy complications are reduced, including gestational diabetes, hypertension of pregnancy, and macrosomia (88). To address the risk of micronutrient deficiency affecting pregnancy, published guidelines recommend generous micronutrient supplementation and careful monitoring among pregnant women who have previously undergone bariatric surgery.

Conclusions

The significant changes in GI physiology following bariatric surgery greatly impact patients who have undergone these procedures. Increased expertise with laparoscopic techniques and the emergence of high volume surgical centers have diminished rates of surgery-related morbidity in the immediate postoperative period. Care to diagnose and address OSA, which is highly prevalent in the obese population, contributes to a reduction in perioperative morbidity.

Many of the acute emergencies that commonly occur as a result of bariatric surgery are metabolic in nature and are related to either hormonal changes or malabsorption induced by the procedure. Clinical follow-up of patients who have undergone bariatric surgery includes measures for prevention, as well as recognition and treatment of dumping syndrome, nesidioblastosis, protein-calorie malnutrition, micronutrient deficiency, osteoporosis, nephrolithiasis, altered pharmacokinetic profiles of various medications, as well as alcohol, and other substance use disorders (89). The risk of these conditions remains high, necessitating lifelong follow-up.

References

1 Mechanick JI, Youdim A, Jones DB, et al. Clinical practice guidelines for the perioperative nutritional, metabolic, and nonsurgical support of the bariatric surgery patient–2013 update: cosponsored by American Association of Clinical Endocrinologists, the Obesity Society, and American Society for Metabolic & Bariatric Surgery. *Endocr Pract.* 2013;19(2): 337–372.

2 Schauer PR, Bhatt DL, Kirwan JP, et al. Bariatric surgery versus intensive medical

therapy for diabetes: 5-year outcomes. *N Engl J Med*. 2017;376(7):641–651.

3 Sjostrom L, Narbro K, Sjostrom CD, et al. Effects of bariatric surgery on mortality in Swedish obese subjects. *N Engl J Med*. 2007;357(8):741–752.

4 Khorgami Z, Shoar S, Andalib A, Aminian A, Brethauer SA, Schauer PR. Trends in utilization of bariatric surgery, 2010–2014: sleeve gastrectomy dominates. *Surg Obes Relat Dis*. 2017.

5 Bae J, Shade J, Abraham A, et al. Effect of mandatory centers of excellence designation on demographic characteristics of patients who undergo bariatric surgery. *JAMA Surg*. 2015;150(7): 644–648.

6 Buchwald H, Estok R, Fahrbach K, Banel D, Sledge I. Trends in mortality in bariatric surgery: a systematic review and meta-analysis. *Surgery*. 2007;142(4):621–632; discussion 632–625.

7 Gribsholt SB, Thomsen RW, Svensson E, Richelsen B: Overall and cause-specific mortality after Roux-en-Y gastric bypass surgery: a nationwide cohort study. *Surg Obes Relat Dis*. 2017.

8 Hutter MM, Schirmer BD, Jones DB, Ko CY, et al. First report from the American College of Surgeons Bariatric Surgery Center Network: laparoscopic sleeve gastrectomy has morbidity and effectiveness positioned between the band and the bypass. *Ann Surg*. 2011;254(3): 410–420; discussion 420–412.

9 Gribsholt SB, Svensson E, Richelsen B, Raundahl U, Sorensen HT, Thomsen RW: Rate of acute hospital admissions before and after Roux-en-y gastric bypass surgery: a population-based cohort study. *Ann Surg*. 2016;Dec.16.

10 Ruiz-Tovar J, Llavero C: Thromboembolic prophylaxis for morbidly obese patients undergoing bariatric surgery. *Adv Exp Med Biol*. 2017;906:9–13.

11 Stroh C, Birk D, Flade-Kuthe R, et al. Evidence of thromboembolism prophylaxis in bariatric surgery-results of a quality assurance trial in bariatric surgery in Germany from 2005 to 2007 and review of

the literature. *Obes Surg*. 2009;19(7): 928–936.

12 Goitein D, Matter I, Raziel A, Keidar A, et al. Portomesenteric thrombosis following laparoscopic bariatric surgery: incidence, patterns of clinical presentation, and etiology in a bariatric patient population. *JAMA Surg*. 2013;148(4):340–346.

13 Bharucha AE, Dunivan G, Goode PS, et al. Epidemiology, pathophysiology, and classification of fecal incontinence: state of the science summary for the National Institute of Diabetes and Digestive and Kidney Diseases (NIDDK) workshop. *Am J Gastroenterol*. 2015;110(1): 127–136.

14 Foster A, Laws HL, Gonzalez QH, Clements RH. Gastrointestinal symptomatic outcome after laparoscopic Roux-en-Y gastric bypass. *J Gastrointest Surg*. 2003;7(6):750–753.

15 Tack J, Piessevaux H, Coulie B, Caenepeel P, Janssens J. Role of impaired gastric accommodation to a meal in functional dyspepsia. *Gastroenterol*. 1998;115(6): 1346–1352.

16 van Beek AP, Emous M, Laville M, Tack J. Dumping syndrome after esophageal, gastric or bariatric surgery: pathophysiology, diagnosis, and management. *Obes Rev*. 2017;18(1): 68–85.

17 Toft-Nielsen M, Madsbad S, Holst JJ. Exaggerated secretion of glucagon-like peptide-1 (GLP-1) could cause reactive hypoglycaemia. *Diabetologia*. 1998;41(10): 1180–1186.

18 Rohof WO, Bisschops R, Tack J, Boeckxstaens GE. Postoperative problems 2011: fundoplication and obesity surgery. *Gastroenterol Clin N Am*. 2011;40(4): 809–821.

19 van der Kleij FG, Vecht J, Lamers CB, Masclee AA. Diagnostic value of dumping provocation in patients after gastric surgery. *Scand J Gastroenterol*. 1996; 31(12):1162–1166.

20 Deloose E, Bisschops R, Holvoet L, et al. A pilot study of the effects of the somatostatin analog pasireotide in postoperative

dumping syndrome. *Neurogastroenterol Motil.* 2014;26(6):803–809.

21 Ceppa EP, Ceppa DP, Omotosho PA, Dickerson JA, 2nd, Park CW, Portenier DD. Algorithm to diagnose etiology of hypoglycemia after Roux-en-Y gastric bypass for morbid obesity: case series and review of the literature. *Surg Obes Relat Dis.* 2012;8(5):641–647.

22 Emous M, Ubels FL, van Beek AP. Diagnostic tools for post-gastric bypass hypoglycaemia. *Obes Rev.* 2015;16(10):843–856.

23 Moreira RO, Moreira RB, Machado NA, Goncalves TB, Coutinho WF. Post-prandial hypoglycemia after bariatric surgery: pharmacological treatment with verapamil and acarbose. *Obes Surg.* 2008;18(12):1618–1621.

24 Myint KS, Greenfield JR, Farooqi IS, Henning E, Holst JJ, Finer N. Prolonged successful therapy for hyperinsulinaemic hypoglycaemia after gastric bypass: the pathophysiological role of GLP1 and its response to a somatostatin analogue. *Eur J Endocrinol.* 2012;166(5):951–955.

25 Arao T, Okada Y, Hirose A, Tanaka Y. A rare case of adult-onset nesidioblastosis treated successfully with diazoxide. *Endocr J.* 2006;53(1):95–100.

26 Schwetz V, Horvath K, Kump P, et al. Successful medical treatment of adult nesidioblastosis with pasireotide over 3 years: a case report. *Medicine (Baltimore).* 2016;95(14):e3272.

27 Batterham RL, Cummings DE. Mechanisms of diabetes improvement following bariatric/metabolic surgery. *Diabetes Care.* 2016;39(6):893–901.

28 Hallowell PT, Stellato TA, Schuster M, et al. Potentially life-threatening sleep apnea is unrecognized without aggressive evaluation. *Am J Surg.* 2007;193(3):364–367; discussion 367.

29 Frey WC, Pilcher J. Obstructive sleep-related breathing disorders in patients evaluated for bariatric surgery. *Obes Surg.* 2003;13(5):676–683.

30 Garvey WT, Mechanick JI, Brett EM, et al. American Association of Clinical Endocrinologists and American College of Endocrinology Comprehensive Clinical Practice Guidelines for Medical Care of Patients with Obesity. *Endocr Pract.* 2016;22 Suppl 3:1–203.

31 Kong WT, Chopra S, Kopf M, et al. Perioperative risks of untreated obstructive sleep apnea in the bariatric surgery patient: a retrospective study. *Obes Surg.* 2016;26(12):2886–2890.

32 Amin R, Simakajornboon N, Szczesniak R, Inge T. Early improvement in obstructive sleep apnea and increase in orexin levels after bariatric surgery in adolescents and young adults. *Surg Obes Relat Dis.* 2017;13(1):95–100.

33 Xu H, Zhang P, Han X, et al. Sex effect on obesity indices and metabolic outcomes in patients with obese obstructive sleep apnea and type 2 diabetes after laparoscopic Roux-en-Y gastric bypass surgery: a preliminary study. *Obes Surg.* 2016;26(11):2629–2639.

34 Santarpia L, Grandone I, Alfonsi L, Sodo M, Contaldo F, Pasanisi F. Long-term medical complications after malabsorptive procedures: effects of a late clinical nutritional intervention. *Nutrition.* 2014;30(11–12):1301–1305.

35 Fox SR. The use of the biliopancreatic diversion as a treatment for failed gastric partitioning in the morbidly obese. *Obes Surg.* 1991;1(1):89–93.

36 Sjostrom L, Lindroos AK, Peltonen M, et al. Lifestyle, diabetes, and cardiovascular risk factors 10 years after bariatric surgery. *N Engl J Med.* 2004;351(26):2683–2693.

37 Van Gossum A, Pironi L, Chambrier C, et al. Home parenteral nutrition (HPN) in patients with post-bariatric surgery complications. *Clin Nutr.* 2016;28(4):467–479.

38 Laurenius A, Larsson I, Melanson KJ, et al. Decreased energy density and changes in food selection following Roux-en-Y gastric bypass. *Eur J Clin Nutr.* 2013;67(2):168–173.

39 Zerrweck C, Zurita L, Alvarez G, et al. Taste and olfactory changes following laparoscopic gastric bypass and sleeve

gastrectomy. *Obes Surg.* 2016;26(6): 1296–1302.

40 Coupaye M, Riviere P, Breuil MC, et al. Comparison of nutritional status during the first year after sleeve gastrectomy and Roux-en-Y gastric bypass. *Obes Surg.* 2014;24(2):276–283.

41 Coupaye M, Puchaux K, Bogard C, et al. Nutritional consequences of adjustable gastric banding and gastric bypass: a 1-year prospective study. *Obes Surg.* 2009;19(1): 56–65.

42 Lanzarini E, Nogues X, Goday A, et al. High-dose vitamin D supplementation is necessary after bariatric surgery: a prospective 2-year follow-up study. *Obes Surg.* 2015;25(9):1633–1638.

43 Marinari GM, Murelli F, Camerini G, et al. A 15-year evaluation of biliopancreatic diversion according to the Bariatric Analysis Reporting Outcome System (BAROS). *Obes Surg.* 2004;14(3): 325–328.

44 Conrad ME, Cortell S, Williams HL, Foy AL. Polymerization and intraluminal factors in the absorption of hemoglobin-iron. *J Lab Clin Med.* 1966;68(4):659–668.

45 Han O. Molecular mechanism of intestinal iron absorption. *Metallomics.* 2011;3(2): 103–109.

46 Said HM. Intestinal absorption of water-soluble vitamins in health and disease. *Biochem J.* 2011;437(3):357–372.

47 Matrana MR, Vasireddy S, Davis WE. The skinny on a growing problem: dry beriberi after bariatric surgery. *Ann Intern Med.* 2008;149(11):842–844.

48 Bhardwaj A, Watanabe M, Shah JR. A 46-yr-old woman with ataxia and blurred vision 3 months after bariatric surgery. *Am J Gastroenterol.* 2008;103(6):1575–1577.

49 van den Berghe PV, Klomp LW. New developments in the regulation of intestinal copper absorption. *Nutr Rev.* 2009;67(11): 658–672.

50 Pellitero S, Martinez E, Puig R, et al. Evaluation of vitamin and trace element requirements after sleeve gastrectomy at long term. *Obes Surg.* 2017.

51 Homan J, Betzel B, Aarts EO, et al. Vitamin and mineral deficiencies after biliopancreatic diversion and biliopancreatic diversion with duodenal switch–the rule rather than the exception. *Obes Surg.* 2015;25(9):1626–1632.

52 Baltaci D, Deler MH, Turker Y, Ermis F, Iliev D, Velioglu U. Evaluation of serum Vitamin B12 level and related nutritional status among apparently healthy obese female individuals. *Niger J Clin Pract.* 2017;20(1):99–105.

53 Jin J, Robinson AV, Hallowell PT, Jasper JJ, Stellato TA, Wilhem SM. Increases in parathyroid hormone (PTH) after gastric bypass surgery appear to be of a secondary nature. *Surgery.* 2007;142(6):914–920; discussion 914–920.

54 Youssef Y, Richards WO, Sekhar N, et al. Risk of secondary hyperparathyroidism after laparoscopic gastric bypass surgery in obese women. *Surg Endosc.* 2007;21(8): 1393–1396.

55 Aarts E, van Groningen L, Horst R, et al. Vitamin D absorption: consequences of gastric bypass surgery. *Eur J Endocrinol.* 2011;164(5):827–832.

56 Orwoll ES, Adler RA, Amin S, et al. Skeletal health in long-duration astronauts: nature, assessment, and management recommendations from the NASA Bone Summit. *J Bone Miner Res.* 2013;28(6): 1243–1255.

57 Karsenty G, Yadav VK. Regulation of bone mass by serotonin: molecular biology and therapeutic implications. *Annual Rev Med.* 2011;62:323–331.

58 Vilarrasa N, Gomez JM, Elio I, et al. Evaluation of bone disease in morbidly obese women after gastric bypass and risk factors implicated in bone loss. *Obes Surg.* 2009;19(7):860–866.

59 Afshan S, Farah Musa AR, Echols V, Lerant AA, Fulop T. Persisting hypocalcemia after surgical parathyroidectomy: the differential effectiveness of calcium citrate versus calcium carbonate with acid suppression. *Am J Med Sci.* 2017;353(1):82–86.

60 Nakamura KM, Haglind EG, Clowes JA, et al. Fracture risk following bariatric surgery:

a population-based study. *Osteoporos Int.* 2014;25(1):151–158.

61 Rousseau C, Jean S, Gamache P, et al. Change in fracture risk and fracture pattern after bariatric surgery: nested case-control study. *BMJ.* 2016;354:i3794.

62 Lu CW, Chang YK, Chang HH, et al. Fracture risk after bariatric surgery: a 12-year nationwide cohort study. *Medicine (Baltimore).* 2015;94(48):e2087.

63 Lalmohamed A, de Vries F, Bazelier MT, et al. Risk of fracture after bariatric surgery in the United Kingdom: population based, retrospective cohort study. *BMJ.* 2012; 345:e5085.

64 Baptista Lopes V, Robbrecht D, van Thiel S, van Guldener C. Symptomatic hypocalcaemia on denosumab use. *Ned Tijdschr Geneeskd.* 2013;157(29):A6159.

65 Lieske JC, Kumar R, Collazo-Clavell ML. Nephrolithiasis after bariatric surgery for obesity. *Semin Nephrol.* 2008;28(2): 163–173.

66 Matlaga BR, Shore AD, Magnuson T, Clark JM, Johns R, Makary MA. Effect of gastric bypass surgery on kidney stone disease. *J Urol.* 2009;181(6):2573–2577.

67 Nelson WK, Houghton SG, Milliner DS, Lieske JC, Sarr MG. Enteric hyperoxaluria, nephrolithiasis, and oxalate nephropathy: potentially serious and unappreciated complications of Roux-en-Y gastric bypass. *Surg Obes Relat Dis.* 2005;1(5): 481–485.

68 Kumar R, Lieske JC, Collazo-Clavell ML, et al. Fat malabsorption and increased intestinal oxalate absorption are common after Roux-en-Y gastric bypass surgery. *Surgery.* 2011;149(5):654–661.

69 Lieske JC, Mehta RA, Milliner DS, Rule AD, Bergstralh EJ, Sarr MG. Kidney stones are common after bariatric surgery. *Kidney Int.* 2015;87(4):839–845.

70 Semins MJ, Matlaga BR, Shore AD, et al. The effect of gastric banding on kidney stone disease. *Urology.* 2009;74(4):746–749.

71 Mechanick JI, Kushner RF, Sugerman HJ, et al. American Association of Clinical Endocrinologists, The Obesity Society, and American Society for Metabolic &

Bariatric Surgery Medical guidelines for clinical practice for the perioperative nutritional, metabolic, and nonsurgical support of the bariatric surgery patient. *Endocr Pract.* 2008;14 Suppl 1:1–83.

72 Agrawal V, Liu XJ, Campfield T, Romanelli J, Enrique Silva J, Braden GL. Calcium oxalate supersaturation increases early after Roux-en-Y gastric bypass. *Surg Obes Relat Dis.* 2014;10(1):88–94.

73 Norholk LM, Holst JJ, Jeppesen PB. Treatment of adult short bowel syndrome patients with teduglutide. *Expert Opin Pharmacother.* 2012;13(2):235–243.

74 Sawaya RA, Jaffe J, Friedenberg L, Friedenberg FK. Vitamin, mineral, and drug absorption following bariatric surgery. *Curr Drug Metab.* 2012;13(9): 1345–1355.

75 Rubio IG, Galrao AL, Santo MA, Zanini AC, Medeiros-Neto G. Levothyroxine absorption in morbidly obese patients before and after Roux-En-Y gastric bypass (RYGB) surgery. *Obes Surg.* 2012;22(2):253–258.

76 Roerig JL, Steffen K, Zimmerman C, Mitchell JE, Crosby RD, Cao L. Preliminary comparison of sertraline levels in postbariatric surgery patients versus matched nonsurgical cohort. *Surg Obes Relat Dis.* 2010;8(1):62–66.

77 Pirola I, Formenti AM, Gandossi E, et al. Oral liquid L-thyroxine (L-t4) may be better absorbed compared to L-T4 tablets following bariatric surgery. *Obes Surg.* 2013;23(9):1493–1496.

78 Edwards A, Ensom MH. Pharmacokinetic effects of bariatric surgery. *Ann Pharmacother.* 2012;46(1):130–136.

79 Skottheim IB, Stormark K, Christensen H, et al. Significantly altered systemic exposure to atorvastatin acid following gastric bypass surgery in morbidly obese patients. *Clin Pharmacol Ther.* 2009; 86(3):311–318.

80 Woodard GA, Downey J, Hernandez-Boussard T, Morton JM. Impaired alcohol metabolism after gastric bypass surgery: a case-crossover trial. *J Am Coll Surg.* 2011;212(2):209–214.

81 Changchien EM, Woodard GA, Hernandez-Boussard T, Morton JM. Normal alcohol metabolism after gastric banding and sleeve gastrectomy: a case-cross-over trial. *J Am Coll Surg.* 2012;215(4):475–479.

82 King WC, Chen JY, Mitchell JE, et al. Prevalence of alcohol use disorders before and after bariatric surgery. *JAMA.* 2012;307(23):2516–2525.

83 Scholtz S, Goldstone AP, le Roux CW. Changes in reward after gastric bypass: the advantages and disadvantages. *Curr Atheroscler Rep.* 2015;17(10):61.

84 Backman O, Stockeld D, Rasmussen F, Naslund E, Marsk R. Alcohol and substance abuse, depression and suicide attempts after Roux-en-Y gastric bypass surgery. *Br J Surg.* 2016;103(10):1336–1342.

85 Kominiarek MA, Jungheim ES, Hoeger KM, Rogers AM, Kahan S, Kim JJ. American Society for Metabolic and Bariatric Surgery position statement on the impact of obesity and obesity treatment on fertility and fertility therapy Endorsed by the American College of Obstetricians and Gynecologists and the Obesity Society. *Surg Obes Relat Dis.* 2017.

86 Roos N, Neovius M, Cnattingius S, et al. Perinatal outcomes after bariatric surgery: nationwide population based matched cohort study. *BMJ.* 2013;347:f6460.

87 Dixon JB, Dixon ME, O'Brien PE. Birth outcomes in obese women after laparoscopic adjustable gastric banding. *Obstet Gynecol.* 2005;106(5 Pt 1):965–972.

88 Willis K, Lieberman N, Sheiner E. Pregnancy and neonatal outcome after bariatric surgery. *Best Pract Res Clin Obstet Gynaecol.* 2014;29(1):133–144.

89 Busetto L, Dicker D, Azran C, et al. Practical Recommendations of the Obesity Management Task Force of the European Association for the Study of Obesity for the Post-Bariatric Surgery Medical Management. *Obes Facts* 2017;10:597–632.

44

Chylomicronemia Syndrome

Very Severe Hypertriglyceridemia and Acute Pancreatitis

Anthony S. Wierzbicki

Key Points

- Acute complications of hyperlipidemia are few.
- Severe hypertriglyceridemia with excess chylomicrons is one of the causes of pancreatitis. Moreover, pancreatitis often is recurrent if hypertriglyceridemia is not appreciated as the cause of pancreatitis and if triglyceride levels are not adequately treated.
- The risk of pancreatitis is exponentially associated with triglyceride level with a 200-fold risk with concentrations above 20 mmol/L (or >2000 mg/dL; 22.4 mmol/L) though most cases occur above 34 mmol/L (3000 mg/dL). Given high variances, a cut-off 20 mmol/L (~2000 mg/dL) is often used as an indication for urgent referral for investigation and treatment.
- A particularly high-risk group of cases is associated with the physiological triglyceride elevation of pregnancy.
- The real cause of pancreatitis is chylomicrons which are pro-inflammatory, prone to coagulate, and cause damage to pancreatic cells.
- Hypertriglyceridemia-associated pancreatitis is often associated with normal amylase and lipase levels due to chylomicron-interference with spectrophotometric assays.
- The genetic basis of chylomicron-associated pancreatitis consists of both polygenic forms (i.e., multifactorial chylomicronemia syndrome, MFCS) and a rarer group of monogenic causes (i.e., familial chylomicronemia syndrome, FCS).
- Secondary causes of hypertriglyceridemia need to be identified and treated.
- Treatment is through a mix of dietary interventions to reduce chylomicron production by control of saturated fat and sugar intake; pharmacological interventions to reduce chylomicron formation and increase clearance of triglyceride-rich lipoproteins by the use of fibrates, omega-3 fatty acids and statins; and if necessary physical removal by plasmapheresis.
- Therapeutic options in development include antisense therapies to apolipoprotein C3 (excess apoC3 causes triglyceride accumulation by inhibiting lipoprotein lipase [LPL]) and gene therapy for LPL deficiency.

Introduction

Cholesterol and triglycerides are the major circulating lipids. Triglycerides are an energy source that can be stored as fat in adipose tissue or used as fuel by muscle and other tissues. Extreme triglyceride levels can be associated with acute complications (e.g., pancreatitis) but moderate chronic elevations are associated with premature risk of cardiovascular disease (CVD) complications. Cholesterol and triglyceride are not water-soluble and thus cannot be transported through the circulation as individual molecules. Lipoproteins are large spherical particles that transport cholesterol and triglycerides from one part of the body to another. Beta-lipoproteins (i.e., lipoproteins containing apolipoprotein B molecules) include chylomicrons, very low-density lipoprotein (VLDL), intermediate density lipoprotein (IDL), and low-density lipoprotein (LDL). Apolipoproteins (apos) are located on the surfaces of lipoproteins and function as ligands for binding to lipoprotein receptors (Figure 44-1). Chylomicrons contain apolipoprotein B_{48}. Apolipoprotein E is the ligand for hepatic receptors for remnant particles. Apolipoprotein B_{100} is the ligand for LDL (apolipoprotein B_{100}/E) receptors. It is found on the surface of VLDL, IDL, and LDL. Chylomicrons are cleared by the liver via the apoE ligand because they contain apoB_{48} and not apoB_{100} and thus are not cleared by an apoB_{100} mediated LDL receptor but also through a specific apoB_{48} receptor. Thus the liver LDL receptors internalize chylomicrons by attaching to apoE and apoB_{48}; they internalize VLDLs by attaching to apoB_{100} or apoE; and they internalize LDLs by attaching to apoB_{100}. In addition, apolipoproteins can act as cofactors for metabolic enzymes (e.g., apoC2 is the activating co-factor for lipoprotein lipase [LPL] while apoC3 inhibits LPL).

Food and hepatic synthesis are the major sources of triglycerides. They are transported by chylomicrons (dietary triglycerides) and VLDL (endogenous triglycerides) to adipose tissue and muscle, where LPL breaks down triglycerides derived from the chylomicrons and VLDL resulting in fatty acid and monoglyceride release which can then be stored as fat in adipose cells or used as fuel in muscle cells (Figure 44-1). The chylomicron and VLDL remnant particles return to the

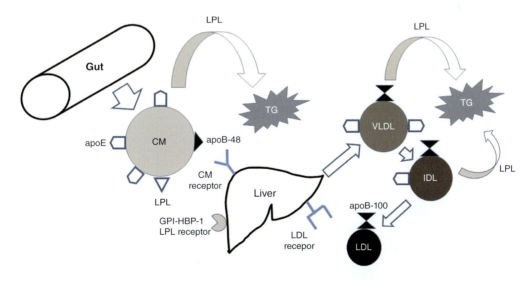

Figure 44-1 Schematic diagram of lipid metabolism.
CM = chylomicron; GPI-HBP1 = glycophosphoinisotol-HDL-binding protein-1; IDL = intermediate density lipoprotein; HDL = high-density lipoprotein; LDL = low-density lipoprotein; VLDL = very low-density lipoprotein.

liver, where hepatic lipase removes additional triglycerides from remnant particles converting them eventually into LDL. The LDL can then be cleared by the liver or used elsewhere within the body.

History

The first description of milky plasma (lipemia) was in 1799 and skin manifestations of high triglycerides (eruptive xanthomata) were reported in 1851 (1,2). These xanthomata were also termed xanthomata *diabetocorum* in the early 1900s because of their appearance in persons with untreated diabetes and concurrent milky plasma. Severe hypertriglyceridemia associated with acute pancreatitis was first reported by Speck in 1865 (2). The familial form of the human disease, familial chylomicronemia, was described in 1932 by Burger and Grutz (1) and identified to be caused by LPL deficiency in 1960 (3). Animal models include cats and mink (4). Interest in hypertriglyceridemia-associated pancreatitis was renewed in the 1970s by Cameron and associates (5) with identification of additional genes involved in the 1990s.

The development of the ultracentrifuge paralleling the use of electrophoresis allowed the separation of lipoproteins. Unlike lipoproteins associated with fasting plasma which migrate in an electric field, chylomicrons stay at the origin. Lipoprotein patterns were classified by Fredrickson, Levy. and Lees using paper electrophoresis (6). The presence or absence of VLDL and chylomicrons in fasting plasma defines type V (VLDL and chylomicronemia) versus type 1 hyperlipoproteinemia (chylomicronemia alone). Types IV and V hyperlipoproteinemia had increased VLDL levels while Types 1 and V were distinguished by the presence of chylomicrons. They recognized that acute pancreatitis and eruptive xanthomata occurred in the presence of chylomicronemia as in both types I and V hyperlipoproteinemia. Later separation techniques included the ultracentrifuge based on salt (later iodixanol) gradient solutions. Chylomicrons are a feature of post-prandial lipid metabolism and are usually cleared within 2–3 hours (7). Chylomicrons are usually present in fasting plasma with triglyceride levels above 10 mmol/L (~1000 mg/dL; 11.2 mmol/L) (8).

The risk of pancreatitis is exponentially associated with triglyceride concentrations. Significant risk occurs above 10 mmol/L (~1000 mg/dL) though case series are few and most data are retrospective. In a prospective study of patients admitted with acute pancreatitis, the peak plasma triglyceride distribution was bimodal (Figure 44-2) (8). Triglyceride levels less than 10 mmol/L (~1000 mg/dL) were associated with gall bladder disease and chronic alcoholism, while those above 20 mmol/L (~2000 mg/dL) were associated with the

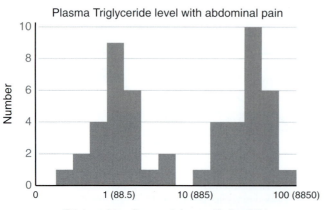

Figure 44-2 Association of triglyceride concentrations in patients with acute pancreatitis. Note bimodal distribution of triglyceride levels (8).
Reproduced with permission from Elsevier.

simultaneous presence of a familial form of hypertriglyceridemia with secondary forms of hypertriglyceridemia (9). In a case series of 129 patients with triglyceride-associated pancreatitis, presentation was rare with triglycerides <35 mmol/L (3000 mg/dL) (10). Hypertriglyceridemia-associated pancreatitis occurs with triglyceride levels <20 mmol/L (~2000 mg/dL) if chylomicronemia is present, but measured levels are dependent on the duration of fasting (i.e., the longer the fast, which may be voluntary due to patient not feeling well or therapeutic due to diagnosis of pancreatitis, this will lead to lower levels of chylomicrons when measured) (10,11). In a retrospective series of 354 patients with hypertriglyceridemia and pancreatitis, the odds ratio for developing pancreatitis was 15.9 for triglycerides 5-9 mmol/L (~440-800 mg/dL) but 359 for patients with genetically proven LPL deficiency (Figure 44-3) (12).

The clinical syndrome termed chylomicronemia syndrome was described in 1981 as a constellation of clinical findings including pancreatitis and eruptive xanthomata associated with very high triglyceride levels (13). Chylomicronemia syndrome is divided into an autosomal recessive lipid disorder of the LPL complex: familial chylomicronemia

syndrome (FCS) associated with five principal genes: LPL; apolipoprotein C2 (LPL co-factor); apolipoprotein A5 (expression factor which enhances triglyceride hydrolysis and remnant lipoprotein clearance); lipid-maturation factor-1 (LMF-1, required for the post-translational activation of LPL); and the LPL anchor, glycerophosphoinositol-HDL-binding protein-1 (GPIHBP1), which binds LPL to the endothelial surface; and a multifactorial chylomicronemia syndrome (MFCS) associated with single gene polymorphisms and rare variants associated with triglyceride elevation (14,15). MFCS subjects usually have secondary causes exacerbating the genetic predisposition to hypertriglyceridemia. The relationship of fasting triglyceride levels to clinical and (by inference) genetic classifications is given in Table 44-1 (16,17).

Epidemiology

Overall, the prevalence of severe hypertriglyceridemia in the general population is very low. The prevalence of very severe hypertriglyceridemia with triglyceride levels above 2000 mg/dL (22.4 mmol/L) was 7/39,090 individuals (1.8/10,000) in the

Figure 44-3 The risk of developing pancreatitis in patients with increased triglycerides (TG) and with lipoprotein lipase deficiency (LPLD) (12). Reproduced with permission from Elsevier.

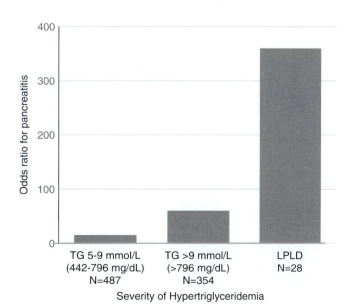

Table 44-1 Criteria proposed for clinical diagnosis of elevated triglyceride levels under fasting conditions (16)

US NCEP-ATP III and AACE 2017			US Endocrine Society Guidelines		
	mg/dL	mmol/L		mg/dL	mmol/L
Normal	<150	<1.7	Normal	<150	<1.7
Borderline-high triglycerides	150–199	1.7–2.3	Mild hypertriglyceridemia	150–199	1.7–2.3
High triglycerides	200–499	2.3–5.6	Moderate hypertriglyceridemia	200–999	2.3–11.2
Very high triglycerides	≥500	≥5.6	Severe hypertriglyceridemia	1000–1999	11.2–22.4
			Very severe hypertriglyceridemia	≥2000	≥22.4

The criteria developed for the US Endocrine Society Guidelines (16) focused on the ability to assess risk for premature cardiovascular disease (CVD) vs risk for pancreatitis. The designation of mild and moderate hypertriglyceridemia corresponded to the range of levels predominant in risk assessment for premature CVD, and this range contains the vast majority of patients with hypertriglyceridemia. Severe hypertriglyceridemia carries susceptibility for intermittent increases in levels about 2000 mg/dL (22.4 mmol/L) and subsequent risk of pancreatitis; very severe hypertriglyceridemia is indicative of high risk for pancreatitis. In addition, these levels suggest different etiologies. Presence of mild or moderate hypertriglyceridemia is commonly due to a dominant underlying cause in each patient, whereas severe or very severe hypertriglyceridemia is more likely due to several contributing factors. In comparison, NCEP-ATP III and American Association of Clinical Endocrinology (AACE) 2017 lipid guidelines are focused on premature CVD risk (17).

Lipid Research Clinics population based prevalence study in 1980 (1). In the National Health and Nutrition Examination Survey (NHANES), 2001–2006, the prevalence was similar at 3/5680 individuals (5.3/10,000) (18). Pancreatitis does occur at lower rates in patients with mild-moderate hypertriglyceridemia with the risk being increased 8.7-fold (95% confidence interval 3.7-20.0) (12/10,000 patient-years) in 116550 patients followed up for 6.7 years (19). The increase in risk was 1.17-fold per 1 mmol/L (88.5 mg/dL) triglycerides. This compares with a CVD risk in the same population of 3.4 (2.4–4.7)-fold or 78 CVD events/10000 patient-years. FCS makes up a small portion of very severe hypertriglyceridemia with a population prevalence of about 1/million in the United States and Europe. MFCS would then be estimated to be several hundred times more prevalent than FCS. Extreme hypertriglyceridemia has been reported in 12–20% of patients with acute pancreatitis (5,20). Referral and reporting bias likely do exist, but in the absence of gallstone disease and chronic alcoholism, very severe hypertriglyceridemia is a common cause of acute and especially recurrent pancreatitis if triglyceride levels are not adequately treated.

Pathophysiology

In FCS, the severe defect in plasma chylomicron and VLDL triglyceride hydrolysis leads to the accumulation of dietary fat as chylomicrons, even after an overnight fast (7). Chylomicron particles are pro-inflammatory and are initially confined to the lymphatic system. In FCS, excess particles overflow in significant quantities into venous and arterial systems due to inadequate clearance by the chylomicron, $apoB_{100}$/E (LDL) and scavenger receptors, which clear chylomicrons, triglyceride-rich VLDL and chemically modified (oxidized or glycated) lipoprotein particles respectively. Chylomicron particles act to transport bacterial lipopolysaccharides which are pro-inflammatory (21) and are also toxic to the endothelium (22). Hydrolysis of triglycerides by neutrophil-associated lipases leads to release of free fatty acids which induce amylasemia and pancreatic cell damage (23) and lyso-phospholipids which have pro-inflammatory actions on macrophages (24). In FCS hepatic triglyceride production is suppressed, so little VLDL is made. If increased triglyceride production occurs, then the secreted VLDL competes with the remaining plasma triglyceride removal mechanisms at the $apoB_{100}$/E receptor and aggravates the underling chylomicronemia.

In MFCS, mild to moderate hypertriglyceridemia can be due to hepatic over-secretion of triglyceride into plasma, often due to excess non-esterified fatty acid (NEFA) production from adipose tissue, or to defects in LPL-related triglyceride hydrolysis or both. Since the removal system is saturable (25), drugs or conditions that affect either triglyceride appearance or clearance lead to chylomicronemia.

In both FCS and MFCS, the pancreatitis may be related to the pro-inflammatory nature of chylomicrons, apoptosis of cells promoted by NEFA and microvascular damage with induction of pancreatic lipase and amylase (22,23).

Etiology

- *FCS*: Most FCS patients are homozygous or compound heterozygous for two defective LPL alleles. Over 100 gene variants have been described that lead to LPL deficiency (26–28). The most severe cases are due to null mutations due to insertions/deletions and premature stop-codons but most patients have missense variants, sometimes in catalytically important sites (exon 5-6) and sometime in regions that predispose to instability in the homo-dimeric structure of LPL required for enzyme activity or receptor binding (29). Other common LPL gene variants have no obvious clinical effects (30). About 10% of FCS is due to major gene defects in other proteins associated with LPL function, such as its co-factor apolipoprotein C2 (LPL activator); a hepatic co-secretory factor apolipoprotein A5; and in lipid-maturation factor-1 (LMF1, involved in the post-translation activation LPL). Some more severe cases are due to defects in the LPL anchor - GPIHBP1 (26). Homozygous or mixed mutations in these related proteins can lead to very severe hypertriglyceridemia and pancreatitis. In some severe cases only one mutation may be found, suggesting other factors may contribute to the FCS phenotype (31). A few non-genetic mimics of FCS exist, caused by circulating inhibitors (32) or autoantibodies to LPL or its co-factors (33,34).

- *MFCS*: MFCS is much more common than FCS (1). Most, if not all, patients with MFCS have a genetic form of moderate hypertriglyceridemia in their families caused by alleles at 134 loci associated with lipid metabolism, of which about 30 have significant effects on triglycerides (9,14,15) (see below). Following treatment of the secondary form of hypertriglyceridemia in MFCS, triglyceride levels usually decrease to levels seen in their moderately hypertriglyceridemic relatives (Figure 44-4) (9).

Clinical Features

Moderate dyslipidemia is asymptomatic but is exacerbated by secondary causes of hypertriglyceridemia. Both physiological and pharmacological factors exacerbate hypertriglyceridemia (Table 44-2) (16,17).

Cohort studies identify acute excess alcohol (54%) and diabetes (30%) as common secondary causes followed by medications including glucocorticoids, anti-oncologics (L-asparginase; anti-hormone therapies for breast cancer) and anti-depressants (35,36). Retinoid therapy for severe acne raises triglyceride levels and is contraindicated in patients with baseline triglyceride levels above 500 mg/dL (5.6 mmol/L) (37). Similarly rexinoid therapy such as the retinoid-X

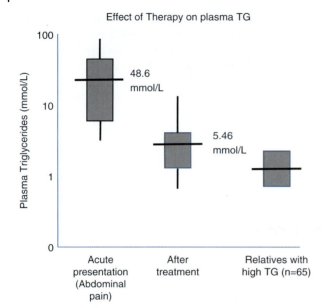

Figure 44-4 Plasma triglycerides in patients with MFCS before and after removal of secondary causes of hypertriglyceridemia, compared with their relatives with hypertriglyceridemia (9).
Reproduced with permission from Elsevier.

receptor agonist bexarotene used in the treatment of cutaneous T-cell lymphoma (mycosis fungoides) can severely exacerbate hypertriglyceridemia (38). Rarer causes include estrogen-based oral contraceptives, parenteral nutrition therapies such as intralipid (39), and the anesthetic propofol

Table 44-2 Causes of hypertriglyceridemia

Primary hypertriglyceridemia
- Familial combined hyperlipidemia (FCHL)
- Familial hypertriglyceridemia (FHTG)
- Familial Type III (remnant removal disease)
- Familial hypoalphalipoproteinemia (FHA)
- Familial chylomicronemia and related disorders

Primary genetic susceptibility
- Metabolic syndrome
- Treated type 2 diabetes

Secondary hypertriglyceridemia
- Excess alcohol intake
- Drug-induced (e.g., estrogens, retinoids, rexinoids, glucocorticoids, bile acid sequestrants, antiretroviral drugs, immunosuppressants, anti-psychotics)
- Untreated or poorly controlled diabetes mellitus
- Endocrine diseases (e.g., hypothyroidism)
- Renal disease
- Liver disease
- Pregnancy
- Autoimmune disorders

which is emulsified in 10% fat (40), and older antiretroviral drugs (41). There are far fewer issues with modern anti-retroviral therapies.

Pancreatitis is a potentially life-threatening complication of very severe hypertriglyceridemia. Patients with this complication often present with similar symptoms and signs as patients with other etiologies. However, there may be additional features in the history and physical examination that suggest the diagnosis of hypertriglyceridemia-associated pancreatitis.

A diagnostic algorithm for familial chylomicronemia has recently been devised (Figure 44-5) (42).

FCS

FCS often presents in early childhood. A history of consanguinity may be present, particularly in inbred populations. The diagnosis is often made in infancy because of the presence of severe colic or failure to thrive, accompanied by lipemic plasma. Other findings include pallor, hepatosplenomegaly and occasionally neurological presentations (43). Later in childhood, the detection of eruptive xanthomata or lipemic plasma in an asymptomatic child can be the initial presentation (44). Acute, recurrent pancreatitis is

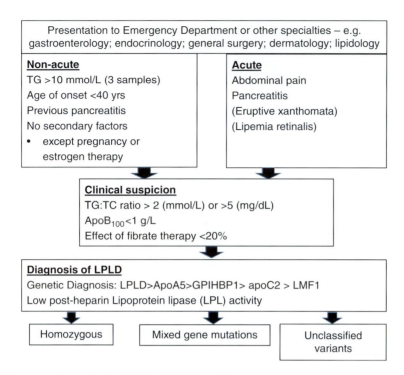

Figure 44-5 Diagnostic algorithm for FCS. Modified after (42).

a severe manifestation of the FCS at all ages. The trigger for acute pancreatitis is often an acute respiratory tract infection often viral and associated with mild hepatitis (e.g., coxsackie) (45). FCS caused by LPL, apoA5 or GPIHBP1 deficiency often presents with abdominal pain and pancreatitis in childhood, but apolipoprotein C2 deficiency is less severe and presents at an older age. As with many inherited errors, a large degree of heterogeneity exists. Some cases of FCS present in adolescence secondary to estrogen-based oral contraceptives or alcohol that increase hepatic VLDL triglyceride production (25). The obligate heterozygote parents often present with mild to moderate hypertriglyceridemia (46).

In children, gross lipemia has a variety of causes (47) including diabetes, but also rarer potentially treatable inherited causes such glycogen storage diseases (48), mitochondrial myopathy (49) or lipodystrophy syndromes (50,51).

The most critical presentation of FCS occurs in pregnancy. In the third trimester of pregnancy, triglyceride levels physiologically increase to 5–7.5 mmol/L (440–664 mg/dL) due to the effects of placental lactogen, estrogen and progesterone (52). In patients with LPL mutations, these changes are exaggerated. The spectrum of available medications is also substantially reduced in pregnancy. Pancreatitis in pregnancy is associated with a high risk of fetal and maternal mortality that can approach 5%.

MFCS

MFCS often initially presents with acute abdominal pain typical of pancreatitis. This form of acute pancreatitis is often associated with normal amylase and lipase levels (4), even in patients with hemorrhagic pancreatitis at laparoscopy or by computer tomography (CT) scan or magnetic resonance imaging (MRI). The pancreatitis often is recurrent, but does not become relapsing. With long-term multiple episodes of acute, recurrent pancreatitis, exocrine pancreatic insufficiency or secondary diabetes (i.e., type 3c or pancreatogenic diabetes)

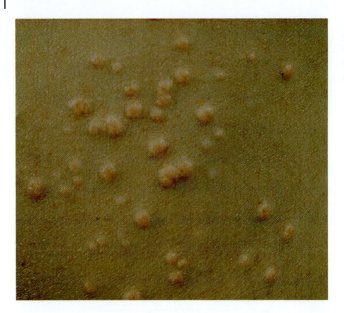

Figure 44-6 Photograph of cutaneous eruptive xanthomata. These often occur on the buttocks as this is a common pressure point for their development or along old scars (Koebner phenomenon).

may occur. The other most common presentation is through a laboratory report of lipemic plasma or severe hypertriglyceridemia (>2000 mg/dL; >20 mmol/L). Rarer presentations occur with the recognition of lipemia retinalis by ophthalmologists, eruptive xanthomata (Figure 44-6) by dermatologists, or acute recent memory loss (caused by a hyperviscosity-like syndrome) (13). These patients almost always have relatives with primary hypertriglyceridemia (Table 44-2), such as familial combined hyperlipidemia, monogenic familial hypertriglyceridemia, familial low HDL syndrome with hypertriglyceridemia and remnant removal disease (Type III) (53).

Investigations

In the emergency setting of acute pancreatitis work-up, non-fasting triglyceride levels are appropriate (42,54). However, in other settings the diagnosis and degree of hypertriglyceridemia are suggested to be based on fasting levels after a 12-h fast (16). Intake of liquids without caloric or caffeine content is acceptable during fasting. Once hypertriglyceridemia is diagnosed, secondary causes should be excluded (Table 44-2).

Genetic diagnosis is useful to establish the likely response to treatment. If available, post-heparin plasma LPL activity or mass may be measured but large molecular weight heparin should be used cautiously as it can exacerbate hypertriglyceridemia and should be avoided if proliferative retinopathy exists (55). Hypertriglyceridemia-associated pancreatitis is often associated with normal amylase and lipase levels due to chylomicron-interference with spectrophotometric assays (5). Acute pancreatitis is staged by standard clinical modified Atlanta criteria (56). Abdominal imaging, including ultrasound and CT (Balthazar grade >4), is the definitive test for pancreatitis in these circumstances (57). It is important to monitor serum or capillary blood glucose levels regularly (i.e., 4–6 hourly) in all patients with acute pancreatitis because of transient or permanent beta-cell failure/destruction.

Treatment

General Supportive Care

General supportive acute care for the patient admitted for hypertriglyceridemia-associated pancreatitis is initially identical

Table 44-3 Principal interventions for the treatment of acute and chronic asymptomatic presentations of severe hypertriglyceridemia and chylomicronemia.

	General	Lipid management	Glucose management
Acute pancreatitis	Resuscitation Oxygen Fluids Analgesia	Fibrate Statin MCT	Insulin (usually CII [VRIII])
		When recovering;- Omega-3 fatty acids	
Chronic treatment	Low carbohydrate; low fat diet	Fibrate Statin Omega-3 fatty acids Orlistat	Metformin Sitagliptin (although DPP-4 inhibitors do have a warning about pancreatitis although not proven) Pioglitazone (PPAR-alpha-gamma agonist)
			Add insulin Avoid GLP-1 agonist
Future chronic treatment		ApoC3 antisense (volanesorsen) Alipogene tiparvovec DGAT-1 inhibitor (pradigastat) Combined PPAR-alpha-delta agonists	

MCT = medium chain triglycerides; apoC3 = apolipoprotein C3; DGAT = diacyl glycerol acyl transferase; GLP-1 = Glucagon-like peptide-1; PPAR = peroxisomal proliferator activating receptor; CII = continuous insulin infusion; VRIII = variable rate intravenous insulin infusion.

to that for other causes of acute pancreatitis (e.g., analgesia, intravenous [IV] fluids, nil by mouth [NPM]) (Table 44-3). Secondary causes should be addressed and precipitating drugs should be stopped. In the absence of oral fat ingestion triglyceride concentrations halve approximately every 48 hours. Insulin therapy (generally given intravenously via continuous insulin infusion [CII], also known as variable rate intravenous insulin infusion [VRIII] using an effective and safe protocol), often combined with heparin, is also used if hyperglycemia is present (58). Insulin and heparin can both suppress hypertriglyceridemia. However, as the patient begins oral intake (usually after pain is controlled), chylomicronemia syndrome patients need to avoid oral fat intake. In addition, IV hyperalimentation with fat emulsions is also contraindicated.

Dietary Interventions

In FCS infants presenting with abdominal pain or failure to thrive, discontinuation of breast feeding with replacement by very low fat formula feeding will cause a marked decrease in triglyceride levels and decrease in symptoms. Later in childhood, dietary fat calories (especially saturated fatty acids) should be restricted to the extent that is required for control of the very severe hypertriglyceridemia and abdominal pain. Diets supplemented in omega-3 fatty acids show a better triglyceride response (59). As a result, dietary fat may only provide ~5–15% of total daily calories. Children quickly learn which foods to avoid and how to avoid acute pancreatitis by immediately decreasing fat and calorie intake for a day of two after the onset of abdominal pain. Dietary indiscretion is more common during adolescence. Long-chain fatty acids may be replaced by medium-chain triglycerides (MCT). MCT are a source of calories that do not enter the thoracic duct as chylomicrons, but act directly as mitochondrial energy source after uptake into liver and muscle (60).

Lipid-Lowering Drug Therapies

Most other drugs for LPL deficiency act through a peroxisomal lipid metabolism, though this is closely linked to mitochondrial metabolism. Fibrates which are peroxisomal proliferator activating receptor (PPAR)-alpha agonists have a variable response profile, depending on residual LPL enzyme and receptor activity through their actions to maximize LPL expression and reduce apolipoprotein C3 expression (excess apoC3 causes triglyceride accumulation by inhibiting LPL) (61). They have been shown to reduce post-prandial lipids in patients with mild hypertriglyceridemia and diabetes by 23% but usually reduce triglycerides 50–70% in MFCS and about 30–50% in FCS based on case series (36). They do not work in null LPL deficiency (1).

Omega-3 fatty acids lower plasma triglyceride levels in hypertriglyceridemia in a dose-proportional manner acting through the GP120 receptor, PPAR-gamma and anti-inflammation pathways. Their use in MFCS is well established (62), but case reports in FCS are conflicting with some suggesting they may aggravate the severe hypertriglyceridemia of FCS (60). This may reflect the age of the literature as earlier omega-3 fatty acid preparations were only partly purified (MaxEPA). More modern formulations of mixed docosahexaenoic acid (DHA)-eicosapentaenoic acid (EPA) (Omacor; Lovaza) or pure eicosapentaeonic acid (VascEPA; EPAnova) contain far less saturated fatty acids and have less effect in

raising LDL-cholesterol (LDL-C). In fact, a rise in LDL-C is to be expected as chylomicrons are cleared by the liver re-secreted as VLDL and these are metabolized to LDL particles.

Statins are used to increase the clearance of triglyceride-rich lipoproteins through their action using apolipoprotein E as a ligand for the LDL (apoB$_{100}$/E) receptor. There is evidence from meta-analysis of CVD prevention trials that the mild anti-inflammatory action of statins (63) may also reduce the incidence of pancreatitis (64).

Orlistat inhibits gastric lipase and hence free fatty acid production which is used as the basis of chylomicron synthesis in the enterocyte. It can be used to reduce intestinal chylomicron formation and reduces triglycerides by 25% in FCS or MFCS (65).

Hypoglycemic Therapies

Hypoglycemic therapies are used aggressively in the treatment of FCS even when only insulin resistance is present (66). Metformin can reduce triglycerides and enhance chylomicron clearance in this situation and may clear hepatic steatosis (67). Similarly there is some data for the use of the PPAR-gamma (and mild PPAR-alpha) agonist pioglitazone to clear hepatic steatosis, reduce both triglycerides and glucose (68). The data on other agents is more limited. Dipeptidyl-peptidase-4 (DPP-4) inhibitors improve hyperglycemia. Sitagliptin specifically may reduce enterocyte chylomicron production (69) but there are reports that DPP-4 inhibitors may be associated with excess pancreatitis (70). Glucagon-like peptide-1 agonists (GLP-1) reduce glucose and triglycerides (71) but show a stronger association with pancreatitis.

The use of oral estrogen contraceptives and alcohol intake can precipitate very severe hypertriglyceridemia and acute pancreatitis. With dietary fat restriction accompanied by high dose omega-3 fatty acid treatment (first two trimesters) and off-label fibrate treatment with drugs such as bezafibrate or fenofibrate, allied with tight glycemic control with metformin or insulin, successful pregnancies have become more common (52,72).

Lipid Extraction Treatments

Physical removal of lipoproteins is necessary in severe cases (73). Apheresis can be used but problems may arise from hyperviscosity and coagulability of chylomicrons clogging columns. Plasmapheresis is more successful and extracts triglyceride-rich lipoproteins, however, regular plasmapheresis is not indicated in FCS because it has no advantage over total dietary fat restriction.

Other Interventions

- *FCS*: Isolated case reports exist of metabolic surgical interventions in patients with FCS refractory to standard interventions (74,75). These have not been systematically evaluated.
- *MFCS*: The primary goal of treatment of MFCS is to prevent the development of acute pancreatitis. The initial presentation of MFCS often is severe, requiring hospitalization in an intensive care unit. The diagnosis of hypertriglyceridemia-induced pancreatitis is strongly suggested by plasma triglyceride levels above 2000 mg/dL (22.4 mmol/L) on admission. Values sometimes can be as high as 30,000 mg/dL (340 mmol/L). Acute therapy is the same as for pancreatitis due to other diseases,

although lipid emulsions should not be used for parenteral feeding, since their use will exacerbate the hypertriglyceridemia.

Patients with MFCS usually have multiple causes of hypertriglyceridemia, including a common familial form of moderate hypertriglyceridemia and a secondary cause. With therapy for the hyperglycemia and moderate dietary fat restriction, plasma triglyceride levels can decrease significantly in these patients. However, the diabetes-related defect in adipose tissue LPL that occurs in these very hyperglycemic patients may persist for 3 months, leading to continuing severe hypertriglyceridemia (76). Dietary fat restriction can be eased after 3 months and the need for fibrates reassessed but usually they are continued to prevent relapses of hypertriglyceridemia. If fasting plasma triglyceride levels remain above 1000 mg/dL (11.2 mmol/L) after treating or removing the precipitating cause of the very severe hypertriglyceridemia fibrate, omega-3 fatty acid and statin therapy are indicated (Table 44-4) (54).

A secondary goal of therapy is the prevention of CVD in some MFCS patients (16,17). This may relate to overlap of chylomicronemia with other genetic primary hypertriglyceridemia syndromes (Table 44-2), such as familial combined hyperlipidemia where

---

Table 44-4 Major points in the treatment of very severe hypertriglyceridemia

1. Familial chylomicronemia, for example, LPL deficiency, is very rare but is associated with very severe hypertriglyceridemia onset in early childhood.
   - It should be treated with strict dietary fat restriction to decrease triglyceride levels to those at which abdominal pain does not occur.
2. All patients are at increased risk of developing acute, recurrent pancreatitis with triglyceride level above 1000 mg/dL (11.2 mmol/L).
   - Although pancreatitis usually ensues only with values >2000 mg/dL (22.4 mmol/L), levels can rapidly exceed this level in patients with values >1000 mg/dL (11.2 mmol/L).
3. MFCS patients have underlying heterozygous or polygenic form of familial hypertriglyceridemia as well as secondary exacerbating cause(s) of hypertriglyceridemia (Table 44-2).
4. In MFCS the secondary causes of hypertriglyceridemia need to be identified and treated (Table 44-2).
5. Certain drugs are known to be the cause of very severe hypertriglyceridemia and pancreatitis and should ideally be avoided or discontinued.
6. Fibrate, omega-3 fatty acid and statin therapy are indicated for long-term therapy in patients with MFCS who have persistent hypertriglyceridemia above 1000 mg/dL (11.2 mmol/L).

strong family histories of premature CVD coexist with protean lipid abnormalities (77). However a more direct link exists now that the apoA5 gene also associated with severe hypertriglyceridemia has been linked with CVD (78).

Emerging Therapies

Newer therapies are on the horizon for FCS (79) including novel derivatives of omega-3 fatty acids, inhibitors of diacyclglyceryl-acyl-transferase-1 (DGAT-1; pradigastat) (80), novel PPAR agonists as well as antisense therapeutics (81).

A gene therapy for LPL deficiency, alipogene tiparvovec, has been approved for adults in Europe with proven homozygous LPL deficiency allied with the presence of immunodetectable LPL and recurrent pancreatitis (82,83). Another promising innovation is antisense therapies to apolipoprotein C3 (volanesorsen) that reduce triglycerides by 60–80% in severe hypertriglyceridemia (84) and have been added to LPL gene therapy (85). Another approach is the use of an antisense oligonucleotide therapy AGPTL3 that reduces triglycerides and cholesterol subfractions (LDL and high density lipoprotein [HDL]) (86) but this has not yet been investigated in patients with FCS.

Case Study

A 23-year-old woman was admitted by the surgical team with a diagnosis of central abdominal pain caused by pancreatitis. She had a previous history of chronic non-specific abdominal pain. Ultrasound imaging followed by CT imaging showed fluid accumulation around the pancreas. The provisional diagnosis was idiopathic pancreatitis – possibly viral. The ward rang the laboratory to complain that no relevant clinical biochemistry results were available due to lipemia. An updated set of results was issued with total cholesterol 8.3 mmol/L (321 mg/dL), triglycerides 45 mmol/L (3986 mg/dL), and HDL-cholesterol 0.3 mmol/L (11.6 mg/dL). The plasma sodium

---

was 129 mmol/L, potassium 4.0 mmol/L, creatinine 70 μmol/L (0.79 mg/dL), estimated glomerular filtration rate (eGFR) 90 mls/min; calcium 2.20 mmol/L (8.8 mg/dL); albumin 40 g/L; phosphate 0.8 mmol/L (2.48 mg/dL), bilirubin 14 μmol/L (0.82 mg/dL); alanine transaminase (ALT) – lipemic; alkaline phosphatase 200 iu/L (44–147 iu/L); amylase 200 iu/L (<100 iu/L); C-reactive protein 4500 iu/L (<3 iu/L); glucose 9 mmol/L (162 mg/dL); HbA$_{1c}$ 37 mmol/mol (5.5%).

The diagnosis was changed to lipemia-induced pancreatitis. After 48 hours supportive management on fluids and nil by mouth, the triglycerides were 10 mmol/L (885 mg/dL); total cholesterol 4.5 mmol/L (175 mg/dL); amylase 200 iu/L with other biochemical assays within the normal range and on discharge 2 days later triglycerides 5.6 mmol/L (496 mg/dL) with total cholesterol 4.2 mmol/L (162 mg/dL), amylase 125 iu/L. The patient was discharged on fenofibrate therapy with a referral to the Lipid clinic for diagnosis and further investigation.

Do You Agree with This Assessment and Recommendation?

The presentation is typical with severe lipemia and TG:TC ratio >2 (mmol/L) or >5 (mg/dL) (Figure 44-4). There is often a previous history of mild pancreatitis usually ascribed to non-specific causes and an acute viral illness as a precipitant for admission. Laboratory results are compromised due to severe lipemia giving a factitious hyponatremia (i.e., 'pseudo-hyponatremia' due to interference with indirect sodium-potassium electrode present on standard biochemical analysers though normal on blood gas machine); calcium only measurable using a direct electrode (blood gas machine); liver enzymes especially ALT and AST unreportable due to interference from chylomicrons and an amylase (once clear of interference range) only just outside the reference range. The triglyceride elevation mostly resolves with a half-life of 24 hours though often a residual hypertriglyceridemia persists. Acutely drug therapy is often not required though in more severe cases fibrate therapy is used. Patients are prescribed a fibrate to upregulate triglyceride clearance and reduce the rate of recurrence of pancreatitis. All such patients should be referred to a specialist Lipid service for further investigation including genetic diagnosis and advice on concomitant drug therapies (e.g., oral contraception) and consequences of the condition for future pregnancy.

Conclusions

Severe hypertriglyceridemia remains an under-diagnosed cause of pancreatitis (see Case study). The complexities of treating FCS are also not well understood outside of specialist units, given its lesser response to standard available therapies (Table 44-4). The emergence of novel therapeutics such as antisense therapies to apolipoprotein C3 (apoC3 is an LPL inhibitor) and a direct gene therapy intervention for LPL deficiency (alipogene tiparvovec) mean that it should be possible to manage this orphan disorder successfully in the future.

Acknowledgments

The current author wishes to acknowledge the contributions to the previous edition by the late John Brunzell and Alan Chait, upon which portions of this chapter are based.

References

1 Brunzell JD, Deeb SS. Familial lipoprotein lipase deficiency, Apo C-II deficiency, and hepatic lipase deficiency In: Valle D, Beaudet AL, Vogelstein B, et al., eds. *The Online Metabolic and Molecular Bases of Inherited Disease*. New York: McGraw-Hill; 2001:2789–2816.

2 Yadav D, Pitchumoni CS. Issues in hyperlipidemic pancreatitis. *J Clin Gastroenterol*. 2003;36: 54–62.

3 Havel RJ, Gordon RS, Jr. Idiopathic hyperlipemia: metabolic studies in an affected family. *J Clin Invest*. 1960;39: 1777–1790.

4 Savonen R, Nordstoga K, Christophersen B, et al. Chylomicron metabolism in an animal model for hyperlipoproteinemia type I. *J Lipid Res*. 1999;40: 1336–1346.

5 Cameron JL, Capuzzi DM, Zuidema GD, Margolis S. Acute pancreatitis with hyperlipemia: the incidence of lipid abnormalities in acute pancreatitis. *Ann Surg*. 1973;177:483–489.

6 Fredrickson DS, Lees RS. A system for phenotyping hyperlipoproteinemia. *Circulation*. 1965;31:321–327.

7 Julve J, Martin-Campos JM, Escola-Gil JC, Blanco-Vaca F. Chylomicrons: advances in biology, pathology, laboratory testing, and therapeutics. *Clin Chim Acta*. 2016;455: 134–148.

8 Brunzell JD, Bierman EL. Chylomicronemia syndrome: interaction of genetic and acquired hypertriglyceridemia. *Med Clin North Am*. 1982;66:455–468.

9 Brunzell JD, Schrott HG. The interaction of familial and secondary causes of hypertriglyceridemia: role in pancreatitis. *J Clin Lipidol*. 2012;6:409–412.

10 Lloret Linares C, Pelletier AL, Czernichow S, et al. Acute pancreatitis in a cohort of 129 patients referred for severe hypertriglyceridemia. *Pancreas*. 2008;37: 13–18.

11 Tremblay K, Methot J, Brisson D, Gaudet D. Etiology and risk of lactescent plasma and severe hypertriglyceridemia. *J Clin Lipidol*. 2011;5:37–44.

12 Gaudet D, de Wal J, Tremblay K, et al. Review of the clinical development of alipogene tiparvovec gene therapy for lipoprotein lipase deficiency. *AtherosclerSuppl*. 2010;11:55–60.

13 Chait A, Robertson HT, Brunzell JD. Chylomicronemia syndrome in diabetes mellitus. *Diabetes Care*. 1981;4:343–348.

14 Hegele RA, Ban MR, Hsueh N, et al. A polygenic basis for four classical Fredrickson hyperlipoproteinemia phenotypes that are characterized by hypertriglyceridemia. *Hum Mol Genet*. 2009;18:4189–4294.

15 Johansen CT, Wang J, Lanktree MB, et al. An increased burden of common and rare lipid-associated risk alleles contributes to the phenotypic spectrum of hypertriglyceridemia. *Arterioscler Thromb Vasc Biol*. 2011;31:1916–1926.

16 Berglund L, Brunzell JD, Goldberg AC et al. Evaluation and treatment of hypertriglyceridemia: an Endocrine Society Clinical Practice Guideline. *J Clin Endocrinol Metab*. 2012;97:2969–2989.

17 Jellinger PS, Handelsman Y, Rosenblit PD, et al. AACE/ACE 2017 guidelines for the management of dyslipidemia and prevention of atherosclerosis (in press). doi:10.4158/EP17164.GL

18 Christian JB, Bourgeois N, Snipes R, Lowe KA. Prevalence of severe (500 to 2,000 mg/dl) hypertriglyceridemia in United States adults. *Am J Cardiol*. 2011;107:891–897.

19 Pedersen SB, Langsted A, Nordestgaard BG. Nonfasting mild-to-moderate hypertriglyceridemia and risk of acute pancreatitis. *JAMA Intern Med*. 2016;176:1834–1842.

20 Farmer RG, Winkelman EI, Brown HB, Lewis LA. Hyperlipoproteinemia and pancreatitis. *Am J Med*. 1973;54:161–165.

21 de Vries MA, Klop B, Alipour A, et al. In vivo evidence for chylomicrons as mediators of postprandial inflammation. *Atherosclerosis*. 2015;243:540–545.

22 Dumnicka P, Maduzia D, Ceranowicz P, et al. The interplay between inflammation, coagulation and endothelial injury in the early phase of acute pancreatitis: clinical implications. *Int J Mol Sci*. 2017;18.

23 Yang F, Wang Y, Sternfeld L, et al. The role of free fatty acids, pancreatic lipase and Ca+ signalling in injury of isolated acinar cells and pancreatitis model in lipoprotein lipase-deficient mice. *Acta Physiol (Oxf)*. 2009;195:13–28.

24 Bentley C, Hathaway N, Widdows J, et al. Influence of chylomicron remnants on human monocyte activation in vitro. *Nutr Metab Cardiovasc Dis*. 2011;21:871–878.

25 Brunzell JD, Hazzard WR, Porte D, Jr., Bierman EL. Evidence for a common, saturable, triglyceride removal mechanism for chylomicrons and very low density lipoproteins in man. *J Clin Invest*. 1973;52:1578–1585.

26 Surendran RP, Visser ME, Heemelaar S, et al. Mutations in LPL, APOC2, APOA5, GPIHBP1 and LMF1 in patients with severe hypertriglyceridaemia. *J Intern Med*. 2012;272:185–196.

27 Gotoda T, Shirai K, Ohta T, et al. Diagnosis and management of type I and type V hyperlipoproteinemia. *J Atheroscler Thromb*. 2012;19:1–12.

28 Rahalkar AR, Giffen F, Har B, et al. Novel LPL mutations associated with lipoprotein lipase deficiency: two case reports and a literature review. *Can J Physiol Pharmacol*. 2009;87:151–160.

29 Peterson J, Ayyobi AF, Ma Y, et al. Structural and functional consequences of missense mutations in exon 5 of the lipoprotein lipase gene. *J Lipid Res*. 2002;43:398–406.

30 Nickerson DA, Taylor SL, Weiss KM, et al. DNA sequence diversity in a 9.7-kb region of the human lipoprotein lipase gene. *Nat Genet*. 1998;19:233–240.

31 Chokshi N, Blumenschein SD, Ahmad Z, Garg A. Genotype-phenotype relationships in patients with type I hyperlipoproteinemia. *J Clin Lipidol*. 2014;8:287–295.

32 Brunzell JD, Miller NE, Alaupovic P, et al. Familial chylomicronemia due to a circulating inhibitor of lipoprotein lipase activity. *J Lipid Res*. 1983;24:12–19.

33 Pruneta-Deloche V, Marcais C, Perrot L, et al. Combination of circulating antilipoprotein lipase (Anti-LPL) antibody

and heterozygous S172 fsX179 mutation of LPL gene leading to chronic hyperchylomicronemia. *J Clin Endocrinol Metab*. 2005;90:3995–3998.

34 Yamamoto H, Tanaka M, Yoshiga S, et al. Autoimmune severe hypertriglyceridemia induced by anti-apolipoprotein C-II antibody. *J Clin Endocrinol Metab*. 2014;99:1525–1530.

35 Tada H, Kawashiri MA, Nakahashi T, et al. Clinical characteristics of Japanese patients with severe hypertriglyceridemia. *J Clin Lipidol*. 2015;9:519–524.

36 Sandhu S, Al-Sarraf A, Taraboanta C, et al. Incidence of pancreatitis, secondary causes, and treatment of patients referred to a specialty lipid clinic with severe hypertriglyceridemia: a retrospective cohort study. *Lipids Health Dis*. 2011; 10:157.

37 Lilley JS, Linton MF, Fazio S. Oral retinoids and plasma lipids. *Dermatol Ther*. 2013;26:404–410.

38 Scarisbrick JJ, Morris S, Azurdia R, et al. U.K. consensus statement on safe clinical prescribing of bexarotene for patients with cutaneous T-cell lymphoma. *BrJ Dermatol*. 2013;168:192–200.

39 Mirtallo JM, Dasta JF, Kleinschmidt KC, Varon J. State of the art review: intravenous fat emulsions: Current applications, safety profile, and clinical implications. *Ann Pharmacother*. 2010;44:688–700.

40 Devaud JC, Berger MM, Pannatier A, et al. Hypertriglyceridemia: a potential side effect of propofol sedation in critical illness. *Intensive Care Med*. 2012;38:1990–1998.

41 Dave JA, Levitt NS, Ross IL, et al. Anti-retroviral therapy increases the prevalence of dyslipidemia in South African HIV-infected patients. *PLoS One*. 2016;11:e0151911.

42 Stroes E, Moulin P, Parhofer KG, et al. Diagnostic algorithm for familial chylomicronemia syndrome. *Atheroscler Suppl*. 2017;23:1–7.

43 Feoli-Fonseca JC, Levy E, Godard M, Lambert M. Familial lipoprotein lipase deficiency in infancy: clinical, biochemical,

and molecular study. *J Pediatr*. 1998;133: 417–423.

44 Pouwels ED, Blom DJ, Firth JC, et al. Severe hypertriglyceridaemia as a result of familial chylomicronaemia: the Cape Town experience. *S Afr Med J*. 2008;98: 105–108.

45 Parenti DM, Steinberg W, Kang P. Infectious causes of acute pancreatitis. *Pancreas*. 1996;13:356–371.

46 Hokanson JE, Brunzell JD, Jarvik GP, et al. Linkage of low-density lipoprotein size to the lipoprotein lipase gene in heterozygous lipoprotein lipase deficiency. *Am J Hum Genet*. 1999;64:608–618.

47 Blackett PR, Wilson DP, McNeal CJ. Secondary hypertriglyceridemia in children and adolescents. *J Clin Lipidol*. 2015;9:S29–S40.

48 Derks TG, van Rijn M. Lipids in hepatic glycogen storage diseases: pathophysiology, monitoring of dietary management and future directions. *J Inherit Metab Dis*. 2015;38:537–543.

49 Laforet P, Vianey-Saban C. Disorders of muscle lipid metabolism: diagnostic and therapeutic challenges. *Neuromuscul Disord*. 2010;20:693–700.

50 Ajluni N, Meral R, Neidert AH, et al. Spectrum of disease associated with partial Lipodystrophy (PL): lessons from a trial cohort. *Clin Endocrinol (Oxf)*. 2017.

51 Gupta N, Asi N, Farah W, et al. Clinical features and management of non-HIV related lipodystrophy in children: a systematic review. *J Clin Endocrinol Metab*. 2016:jc20162271.

52 Goldberg AS, Hegele RA. Severe hypertriglyceridemia in pregnancy. *J Clin Endocrinol Metab*. 2012;97:2589–2596.

53 Chait A, Brunzell JD. Severe hypertriglyceridemia: role of familial and acquired disorders. *Metabolism*. 1983; 32:209–214.

54 Viljoen A, Wierzbicki AS. Diagnosis and treatment of severe hypertriglyceridemia. *Expert Rev Cardiovasc Ther*. 2012;10: 505–514.

55 Kobayashi J, Nohara A, Kawashiri MA, et al. Serum lipoprotein lipase mass:

clinical significance of its measurement. *Clin Chim Acta*. 2007;378:7–12.

56 Banks PA, Bollen TL, Dervenis C, et al. Classification of acute pancreatitis–2012: revision of the Atlanta classification and definitions by international consensus. *Gut*. 2013;62:102–111.

57 Balthazar EJ, Robinson DL, Megibow AJ, Ranson JH. Acute pancreatitis: value of CT in establishing prognosis. *Radiology*. 1990;174:331–336.

58 Kuchay MS, Farooqui KJ, Bano T, et al. Heparin and insulin in the management of hypertriglyceridemia-associated pancreatitis: case series and literature review. *Arch Endocrinol Metab*. 2017:0.

59 Helk O, Schreiber R, Widhalm K. Effects of two therapeutic dietary regimens on primary chylomicronemia in paediatric age: a retrospective data analysis. *Eur J Clin Nutr*. 2016;70:1127–1131.

60 Rouis M, Dugi KA, Previato L, et al. Therapeutic response to medium-chain triglycerides and omega-3 fatty acids in a patient with the familial chylomicronemia syndrome. *Arterioscler Thromb Vasc Biol*. 1997;17:1400–1406.

61 Wierzbicki AS, Reynolds TM. Familial hyperchylomicronaemia. *Lancet*. 1996;348:1524–1525.

62 Bays HE, Ballantyne CM, Kastelein JJ, et al. Eicosapentaenoic acid ethyl ester (AMR101) therapy in patients with very high triglyceride levels (from the Multi-center, plAcebo-controlled, Randomized, double-blINd, 12-week study with an open-label Extension [MARINE] trial). *Am J Cardiol*. 2011;108:682–690.

63 Wierzbicki AS, Poston R, Ferro A. The lipid and non-lipid effects of statins. *Pharmacol Ther*. 2003;99:95–112.

64 Preiss D, Tikkanen MJ, Welsh P, et al. Lipid-modifying therapies and risk of pancreatitis: a meta-analysis. *JAMA*. 2012;308:804–811.

65 Wierzbicki AS, Reynolds TM, Crook MA. Usefulness of Orlistat in the treatment of severe hypertriglyceridemia. *Am J Cardiol*. 2002;89:229–231.

66 Eleftheriadou I, Grigoropoulou P, Katsilambros N, Tentolouris N. The effects of medications used for the management of diabetes and obesity on postprandial lipid metabolism. *Curr Diabetes Rev*. 2008; 4:340–356.

67 Grosskopf I, Ringel Y, Charach G, et al. Metformin enhances clearance of chylomicrons and chylomicron remnants in nondiabetic mildly overweight glucose-intolerant subjects. *Diabetes Care*. 1997;20:1598–1602.

68 Al Majali K, Cooper MB, Staels B, et al. The effect of sensitisation to insulin with pioglitazone on fasting and postprandial lipid metabolism, lipoprotein modification by lipases, and lipid transfer activities in type 2 diabetic patients. *Diabetologia*. 2006;49:527–537.

69 Xiao C, Dash S, Morgantini C, et al. Sitagliptin, a DPP-4 inhibitor, acutely inhibits intestinal lipoprotein particle secretion in healthy humans. *Diabetes*. 2014;63:2394–2401.

70 Tkac I, Raz I. Combined analysis of three large interventional trials with gliptins indicates increased incidence of acute pancreatitis in patients with type 2 diabetes. *Diabetes Care*. 2017;40:284–286.

71 Zhong J, Maiseyeu A, Rajagopalan S. Lipoprotein effects of incretin analogs and dipeptidyl peptidase 4 inhibitors. *Clin Lipidol*. 2015;10:103–112.

72 Ewald N, Hardt PD, Kloer HU. Severe hypertriglyceridemia and pancreatitis: presentation and management. *Curr Opin Lipidol*. 2009;20:497–504.

73 Stefanutti C, Julius U. Treatment of primary hypertriglyceridemia states: general approach and the role of extracorporeal methods. *Atheroscler Suppl*. 2015;18:85–94.

74 Gasbarrini G, Mingrone G, Greco AV, Castagneto M. An 18-year-old woman with familial chylomicronaemia who would not stick to a diet. *Lancet*. 1996;348: 794.

75 Hsu SY, Lee WJ, Chong K, et al. Laparoscopic bariatric surgery for the treatment of severe hypertriglyceridemia. *Asian J Surg*. 2015;38:96–101.

76 Brunzell JD, Porte D, Jr., Bierman EL. Abnormal lipoprotein-lipase-mediated plasma triglyceride removal in untreated diabetes mellitus associated with hypertriglyceridemia. *Metabolism*. 1979; 28:901–907.

77 Wierzbicki AS, Graham CA, Young IS, Nicholls DP. Familial combined hyperlipidaemia: under-defined and under-diagnosed? *Curr Vasc Pharmacol*. 2008;6:13–22.

78 Do R, Stitziel NO, Won HH, et al. Exome sequencing identifies rare LDLR and APOA5 alleles conferring risk for myocardial infarction. *Nature*. 2015;518:102–106.

79 Hajhosseiny R, Sabir I, Khavandi K, Wierzbicki AS. The ebbs and flows in the development of cholesterol-lowering drugs: prospects for the future. *Clin Pharmacology Therapeutics*. 2014;96: 64–73.

80 Meyers CD, Tremblay K, Amer A, et al. Effect of the DGAT1 inhibitor pradigastat on triglyceride and apoB48 levels in patients with familial chylomicronemia syndrome. *Lipids Health Dis*. 2015; 14:8.

81 Wierzbicki AS, Viljoen A. Anti-sense oligonucleotide therapies for the treatment of hyperlipidemia. *Expert Opin Biol Ther*. 2016;9:1–10.

82 Wierzbicki AS, Viljoen A. Alipogene tiparvovec: gene therapy for lipoprotein lipase deficiency. *Expert Opin Biol Ther*. 2013;13: 7–10.

83 Gaudet D, Methot J, Dery S, et al. Efficacy and long-term safety of alipogene tiparvovec (AAV1-LPLS447X) gene therapy for lipoprotein lipase deficiency: an open-label trial. *Gene Therapy*. 2013;20: 361–369.

84 Gaudet D, Alexander VJ, Baker BF, et al. Antisense inhibition of apolipoprotein C-III in patients with hypertriglyceridemia. *N Engl J Med*. 2015;373:438–447.

85 Gaudet D, Brisson D, Tremblay K, et al. Targeting APOC3 in the familial chylomicronemia syndrome. *N Engl J Med*. 2014;371:2200–2206.

86 Gaudet D, Gipe DA, Pordy R, et al. Safety and efficacy of evinacumab, a monoclonal antibody to ANGPTL3, in patients with homozygous familial hypercholesterolemia receiving concomitant lipid-lowering therapies. *J Clin Lipidol*. 2016;10:715.

45

Statin-Related Myopathy and Rhabdomyolysis

Connie B. Newman and Jonathan A. Tobert

Key Points

- Statin-induced myopathy (incidence <0.1%) is defined as unexplained muscle pain or weakness and creatine kinase (CK) elevations >10 × upper limit of normal (ULN), taking into account that women have lower reference ranges for CK compared to men.
- Statin-induced rhabdomyolysis is an extreme form of myopathy with no agreed definition, although it is characterized by CK >40 × ULN, possible myoglobinuria, and possible acute kidney injury (AKI).
- Statins are one of many causes of rhabdomyolysis and statin-related rhabdomyolysis is less frequent than many other etiologies. Statin-induced rhabdomyolysis is often associated with concomitant use of interacting medications.
- Patients with rhabdomyolysis who appear healthy and do not have elevations in serum creatinine may be managed by discontinuation of the statin, oral hydration, and careful monitoring, without hospitalization.
- Patients with rhabdomyolysis who are clearly ill, elderly, weak, or have severe muscle weakness and/or evidence of AKI should

- be treated with intensive intravenous hydration using normal (0.9%) saline at a rate of 250–500 mL per hour in the in-hospital setting. Use of bicarbonate and mannitol are not recommended.
- Patients may be restarted on a statin if a precipitating cause (such as an interacting medication or excessive physical activity) was found and can be avoided in the future. The chosen statin should be one with fewer drug interactions. If there was no precipitating cause, restarting another statin at a low dose can be considered. Patients who are restarted on a statin should be carefully monitored for muscle symptoms and CK levels. In all these cases, the health care provider should have a conversation with the patient about the benefits and risks of statin therapy.
- Alternatively, other lipid-lowering drugs with lower risk of myopathy may be considered (e.g., ezetimibe, bile acid sequestrants, or the proprotein convertase subtilisin/kexin type 9 [PCSK9] inhibitors).

Introduction

3-Hydroxy-3-methyl-glutaryl coenzyme A (HMG-CoA) reductase inhibitors (statins) are by far the most commonly prescribed medications used to lower low-density lipoprotein cholesterol (LDL-C) levels. In the United States, more than 25 million adults over the age of 40 take a statin (1) to reduce LDL-C and the risk of myocardial infarction (MI), ischemic stroke, and other atherosclerotic cardiovascular events.

Endocrine and Metabolic Medical Emergencies: A Clinician's Guide, Second Edition. Edited by Glenn Matfin.
© 2018 John Wiley & Sons Ltd. Published 2018 by John Wiley & Sons Ltd.

Multiple randomized controlled trials (RCTs) have demonstrated that statins reduce atherosclerotic cardiovascular events, including cardiovascular death (2–4). Serious adverse effects of statins are rare: myopathy/rhabdomyolysis occurs in less than 0.1% of patients (5); severe liver disease in 0.001% (6); and new onset diabetes mellitus in 0.2% (7,8). Of these, rhabdomyolysis, which is a severe form of myopathy (see below), is associated with extremely high levels of creatine kinase (CK), exceeding 40 times the upper limit of normal (ULN), skeletal muscle necrosis, and potentially acute kidney injury (AKI), and can be a medical emergency.

This chapter will define the terminology used to describe muscle symptoms and disease associated with statins, and describe the evaluation and management of patients with myopathy, including those with rhabdomyolysis.

Definition of Terms

Although there is some variability in the literature, in this chapter we use the original definition of myopathy (9), which has been accepted by the U.S. Food and Drug Administration (FDA) and is used in the USA prescribing information of all statins that provide a definition. Myopathy is defined as unexplained muscle pain or weakness accompanied by elevations in CK >10 times ULN. All statins may rarely cause myopathy, and its more serious form, rhabdomyolysis. There is no consensus on the definition of statin-induced rhabdomyolysis, although it is generally agreed that a minimum requirement is CK >40 × ULN, and that is the definition used here. Some authors require in addition evidence of AKI (10). When diagnosing myopathy and rhabdomyolysis, the clinician should be aware of sex and ethnic differences in normal levels of CK. For example, in a cohort of 1016 Swedish people all aged 70, Carlsson et al. (11) found that the ULN of CK for men was 4.98 µkat/l (298 U/L), but much lower for women, 3.01 µkat/l (180 U/L). The difference is most likely attributable to the smaller muscle mass of women. In addition, the ULN is substantially higher in people of African origin (12). Laboratory reference values do not always take sex and ethnic differences into account.

Historical Background

Rhabdomyolysis caused by a statin was first reported (13,14) in 1988 in five cardiac transplant patients taking cyclosporine and lovastatin, the first statin available for prescription use. Renal failure developed in two of the five patients (15). Muscle biopsies in two patients showed either necrosis (13) or nonspecific abnormalities (14), with no evidence of inflammation. At about the same time, myopathy was reported in a single patient taking lovastatin in a phase 3 trial (16). Because of these and other cases, the risk of myopathy with lovastatin and the increased risk due to drug-drug interactions were recognized and included in the *Warnings* section of the prescribing information for lovastatin (15).

Thirty years later the mechanism of myopathy with statins remains unclear. The adverse effect is confined to skeletal muscle; cardiomyopathy has never been associated with any statin. The risk of myopathy is related to the concentration of HMG-CoA reductase inhibitory activity in plasma (i.e., the concentration of the statin and/or its active metabolites). Beyond this, little has been established.

Myopathy and rhabdomyolysis have been reported with all statins. The risk is dose-related, and attempts to expand the dosage range have led to an unacceptable risk with some statins. The first instance was cerivastatin, which was withdrawn from the market in 2001 (5,17). A few years later, SEARCH (10), which randomized over 12,000 patients to simvastatin 80 mg or 20 mg, found that the incidence of myopathy with simvastatin 80 mg was 0.9%, compared to 0.02% with simvastatin 20 mg. Consequently, simvastatin 80 mg is not recommended for therapy unless the individual has been on treatment

Table 45-1 Principal drug interactions of statins associated with increased risk of myopathy/rhabdomyolysis. From USA prescribing information as of January 2018.

Interacting drug	Statins (normal dose range, mg) and daily dose limitations in mg*						
	Lova (10–80)	Simva (5–80#)	Atorva (10–80)	Prava (10–80)	Fluva (20–80)	Rosuva (5–40)	Pitava (2–4)
Gemfibrozil	Avoid	Avoid	Avoid	Avoid	Avoid	Avoid	Avoid
Calcium channel blockers			NDL	NDL	NDL	NDL	NDL
verapamil	20	10					
diltiazem	20	10					
amlodipine	NDL	20					
Antiarrhythmics			NDL	NDL	NDL	NDL	NDL
amiodarone	40	20					
dronedarone	20	10					
Macrolide antibiotics						NDL	
clarithromycin	Avoid	Avoid	20	40	20		NDL
erythromycin	Avoid	Avoid	NDL	*Caution*	NDL		1
telithromycin	Avoid	Avoid	NDL	*Caution*	NDL		NDL
Antifungal azoles				NDL		NDL	NDL
itraconazole	Avoid	Avoid	20		NDL		
ketoconazole	Avoid	Avoid	NDL		NDL		
posaconazole	Avoid	Avoid	NDL		NDL		
voriconazole	Avoid	Avoid	NDL		NDL		
fluconazole	NDL	NDL	NDL		20 b.i.d		
Immunosupressants							
cyclosporine	Avoid	Avoid	Avoid	20	20 b.i.d	5	Avoid
Miscellaneous							
nefazodone	Avoid	Avoid	NDL	NDL	NDL	NDL	NDL
danazol	20	Avoid	NDL	NDL	NDL	NDL	NDL
ranolazine	NDL	20	NDL	NDL	NDL	NDL	NDL
colchicine	*Caution*	*Caution*	*Caution*	*Caution*	*Caution*	*Caution*	*Caution*
HIV protease inhibitors and other antiretroviral drugs, hepatitis C protease inhibitors	Numerous interactions, see prescribing information						

NDL = No dose limitation; *Doses (mg) are the maximum statin dose recommended if the interacting drug must be given concomitantly. # Simvastatin 80 mg dose not approved for therapy unless the individual has been on treatment at that dose for more than one year without myopathy.

with that dose for more than one year without myopathy.

Cyclosporine interacts with all statins via multiple mechanisms to increase the plasma concentration of the statin and/or active metabolites (18) (Table 45-1). In addition to cyclosporine, two of the original five transplant patients were also taking gemfibrozil, and a third erythromycin. Gemfibrozil is now known to have a pharmacokinetic (PK) interaction with all statins, significantly raising the plasma levels of the statin and/or active metabolites, and thus increasing the risk of myopathy/rhabdomyolysis. Erythromycin has been shown to be a potent inhibitor of CYP3A4, the enzyme that metabolizes simvastatin, lovastatin, and atorvastatin (19).

Risk Factors and Prevention of Myopathy/Rhabdomyolysis

Suspected risk factors for statin-induced myopathy/rhabdomyolysis include older age, female sex, diabetes, and Chinese ancestry (20). Risk increases with statin dose, because larger doses produce higher levels of HMG-CoA reductase activity in plasma. Although all statins can cause myopathy and rhabdomyolysis, the risk differs among statins due to intrinsic properties of the drug, and the susceptibility of the statin to drug interactions, as noted below. Pre-existing muscle disease and hypothyroidism are also possible risk factors, and starting an interacting drug is a well-established precipitant. In patients with renal impairment, the prescribing information for several statins recommends lower doses in order to decrease the risk of myopathy. Based on data from several placebo-controlled CV outcome trials in patients with chronic kidney disease (CKD) (21–23), impaired renal function does not appear to be a risk factor for statin-induced myopathy, providing they are used at the doses recommended for patients with renal insufficiency.

All patients starting treatment with a statin should be told that there is a very low (<1 in 1000) risk of myopathy, and advised to report new unexplained muscle symptoms promptly, so that CK can be measured to diagnose, or much more commonly, rule out myopathy. Some clinicians also measure CK before starting a statin, in order to obtain a baseline value. Attention to potential drug interactions is important when selecting the initial statin and during follow-up. There is considerable variation in the PK characteristics of members of the statin class

(18,24), and hence substantial differences in the vulnerability to drug interactions that increase the risk of myopathy. Because they are CYP3A4 substrates and also subject to considerable first-pass metabolism, simvastatin and lovastatin are the most vulnerable. Atorvastatin is also a CYP3A4 substrate but first-pass metabolism is less (24), so it is less vulnerable. The other four statins are not CYP3A4 substrates, but can be the "victim" of other drug interactions via different mechanisms. The principal drug interactions affecting the risk of myopathy and rhabdomyolysis are shown in Table 45-1.

Statin-Associated Muscle Symptoms (SAMS)

Myalgia or other muscle symptoms during statin treatment without significant elevations in CK (<3 × ULN) are referred to as SAMS (25), a term that does not imply causality. SAMS do not constitute a serious adverse event requiring emergency management, but are a common complaint in patients taking statins and therefore should be understood. These non-serious muscle symptoms account for about half of the cases of statin intolerance, a term describing discontinuation of statin therapy because of symptoms that are perceived to be caused by the statin (25–27). Despite claims that these non-serious muscle symptoms are caused by statins, it is now recognized that in the vast majority of cases the symptoms are not pharmacologically related to statin use, and result from the nocebo effect, a term used to describe symptoms caused by perception of harm from a medication, chemical or other potentially toxic agent. The nocebo effect is a normal neuropsychological phenomenon that can cause patients to attribute background muscle symptoms to the statin (7,26,28,29).

Muscle Symptoms with CK ≥ 5 to 10 × ULN

Management of patients with sex-specific CK levels in this range and unexplained muscle symptoms depends upon clinical judgment. These patients may be close to developing myopathy. Management should be individualized for each patient, taking into account age, gender, other diseases, medications, and CV risk. In all cases medications should be reviewed and any interacting medicines discontinued if possible.

In patients who appear healthy and do not have malaise or severe muscle pain, the statin can be continued and the CK repeated within 5 days. If the repeat CK is rising, then the statin should be discontinued and CK and muscle symptoms monitored.

After CK returns to normal, consideration should be given to restarting a statin, especially in those patients at high CV disease risk. The statin could be the same one, if an interacting medication was identified and discontinued, or a different statin which does not have that interaction. If the interacting drug cannot be discontinued, then a different statin should be started, using a lower dose. However, if all statins have this drug interaction, and the interacting medication is essential, a lower dose of a statin could be tried initially. Ezetimibe, bile acid sequestrants, or a proprotein convertase subtilisin/kexin type 9 (PCSK9) inhibitor can be added if additional LDL-C reduction is needed. In all these scenarios, CK and muscle symptoms should be carefully monitored.

If the CK elevation persists after statin discontinuation, and hypothyroidism and other etiologies are ruled out, muscle disease may be the underlying cause and a consultation with a neuromuscular specialist is appropriate before considering restarting a statin.

Myopathy

Definition and Clinical Characteristics

Statin-induced myopathy should be considered in any patient taking a statin who develops muscle pain or weakness that cannot be explained by other causes (see Table 45-2), and that is accompanied by CK elevations above $10 \times$ ULN (using gender-specific ULN). Statin myopathy causes bilateral muscle pain or weakness, usually in the proximal muscles of the legs, and sometimes the back and shoulders.

Statin myopathy can occur as early as a few days after starting the statin or after a dose increase, but more typically within a few months. However, the onset can be years later, and such cases are often the result

Table 45-2 Etiology of muscle symptoms. Adapted from (30).

CK normal	CK possibly increased
Viral illness	Physical activity
Vitamin D deficiency	Trauma
Hyperthyroidism	Hypothyroidism
Cushing's syndrome	Metabolic, inflammatory myopathies
Adrenal insufficiency	Seizure
Hypoparathyroidism	Severe chills
Medications-glucocorticoids, anti retrovirals	Illicit drug overdoses
Fibromyalgia	
Polymyalgia rheumatica	
Systemic lupus	
Tendon or joint problem	
Peripheral arterial disease	

of starting an interacting drug. Myopathy occurs with all statins and is dose-related, with the possible exception of atorvastatin (31,32).

Evaluation

Interacting medications are a common cause of myopathy and must be looked for. Strenuous unaccustomed exercise and trauma can greatly increase CK, whether a patient is taking a statin or not. Physical examination should include evaluation of muscle strength, function, and tenderness. Laboratory tests include CK, thyroid-stimulating hormone (TSH), BUN, creatinine and electrolytes. Risk factors for myopathy (and rhabdomyolysis) are discussed earlier.

Management

When statin myopathy is diagnosed, the statin should be immediately discontinued, and CK, BUN and creatinine measured. If rhabdomyolysis is not suspected, management includes monitoring of CK and symptoms. CK levels usually fall within a few days, returning to normal within two weeks.

After the symptoms have resolved and the CK is within the normal range, statin therapy could be considered and discussed with the patient, taking into account CV risk, and precipitating factors. Consideration may be given to the same statin, perhaps at a lower dose, if an interacting medication has been identified and discontinued, or a different statin at a low dose if no interacting drugs were involved. CK and muscle symptoms should be carefully monitored, with a repeat CK in 1 to 2 weeks.

Rhabdomyolysis

Definition

Although rhabdomyolysis is a rare adverse effect of statins (incidence about 0.01%), it remains a major clinical challenge and medical emergency because it often leads to acute renal failure, which can be fatal if not promptly managed. There is no uniform definition for rhabdomyolysis. The main feature is skeletal muscle necrosis which causes the release of muscle components into the circulation (33,34). CK is markedly elevated to levels above 40 × ULN. Myoglobinuria (due to myoglobin release from muscle tissue) can cause AKI. Myoglobin in sufficient concentration may cause "brown" or "tea-colored" urine, but neither myoglobinuria nor elevated blood levels of myoglobin are necessary for the diagnosis. (34,35). Myoglobinuria may be absent because myoglobin has a short half-life of 2–4 h, and its detection depends upon muscle mass, urinary concentration, and assay sensitivity (35). If myoglobinuria is present, a urine dipstick will typically be positive for hemoglobin because it cannot distinguish between hemoglobin and myoglobin (33). Patients with rhabdomyolysis of any etiology may develop AKI because of hypovolemia, which reduces renal blood flow, and/or myoglobinuria, which may cause renal tubular obstruction or capillary damage, leading to leakage and edema, and metabolic acidosis (36,37).

Etiology

Trauma is the commonest cause of rhabdomyolysis, and its importance has long been appreciated. During the Battle of Britain in World War II, bombing of London (the Blitz) resulted in crush injuries that led to muscle necrosis, renal failure, and death. Several cases of rhabdomyolysis were described in detail by Bywaters and Beall (38). As shown in Table 45-3, in addition to physical trauma, there are many causes of rhabdomyolysis, including toxins, infections, and endocrine disorders. Case reports suggest that rhabdomyolysis is associated with a variety of medications, although the causality is not clear. Drug overdoses that lead to prolonged stupor and immobility can cause rhabdomyolysis due to compression of a limb beneath the body, with resulting ischemia. In a retrospective study of 2371 patients admitted to two Boston medical centers between January

Table 45-3 Causes of rhabdomyolysis other than medications (although anesthetics included)

Causes	Examples
Physical/metabolic	
Trauma	Crush injury, severe burn, electrical injury, vascular or orthopedic surgery, anti-shock garments, immobility
Physical Exertion	Excessive exertion/exercise, seizures, delirium tremens, sickle cell crisis
Temperature extremes	Malignant hyperthermia, severe hypothermia, heatstroke
Metabolic	Hyponatremia, hypokalemia, hypocalcemia, hyperosmotic conditions
Muscle ischemia	Thrombosis, embolism, compression
Diseases	
Infections	Potentially any severe infection.
Inflammatory myopathies	Polymyositis, dermatomyositis
Endocrine disorders	Hypo- and hyperthyroidism, diabetic ketoacidosis, hyperglycemic hyperosmolar state, adrenal insufficiency, hyperaldosteronism
Anesthetics, alcohol, illicit drugs, toxins	
Anesthetics, neuromuscular blockers	Barbiturates, benzodiazepines, propofol, succinylcholine in Duchenne/Becker muscular dystrophy
Alcohol and illicit drugs	Overdose leading to unconsciousness and resulting prolonged pressure on a limb beneath the body
Toxins	Carbon monoxide, snake bites, insect stings
Genetic[‡]	Inborn errors of metabolism, muscular dystrophies, carnitine palmitoyltransferase (CPTII) deficiency, McArdles disease (myophosphorylase deficiency), LPIN1 gene deficiency, idiopathic recurrent rhabdomyolysis (Meyer-Betz syndrome)

[‡]For additional genetic causes, see (33).

2000 and March 2011, the most common causes were trauma (26%), surgery (21%), immobilization (18%), and sepsis (10%) (39). Statins were causal in 2.7% of this cohort. In many patients, including those with statin-induced rhabdomyolysis, there may be more than one cause.

Clinical Characteristics

There are several reviews of rhabdomyolysis due to any cause (33,34,40,41) and a case report series of statin-induced rhabdomyolysis (42). The most frequent symptoms in statin-induced rhabdomyolysis are muscle pain and/or weakness, sometimes with inability to walk (42). Muscle symptoms are generally bilateral and affect the proximal

muscles of the legs more than the arms. Fever, nausea, vomiting, confusion, agitation, and delirium may be present (42). As noted earlier, CK is markedly elevated due to its release from skeletal muscle, and the urine is often dark due to myoglobinuria. AKI, with elevated BUN and creatinine, and diminished urine output may be noted at presentation or develop later. Similarly, hyperkalemia due to potassium release from muscle and decreased renal clearance may be present at diagnosis or later, and can cause cardiac arrhythmias if severe.

Other laboratory abnormalities include hyperphosphatemia (due to breakdown of muscle tissue), hypocalcemia, hyperuricemia, hyponatremia, elevation in hepatic transaminases, metabolic acidosis, and possibly hypercalcemia in the late phase due to calcium efflux from injured muscle (33,41,43). Compartment syndrome in the extremities is usually seen with trauma or post-surgery, and the pooling of fluid may lead to hypotension and shock (44). There is a risk of disseminated intravascular coagulation (DIC) because of thromboplastin release and thrombosis of capillaries and arterioles.

In a case report series of 112 published reports of statin-related rhabdomyolysis (42), including 79 men and 33 women, 53% of the men and 42% of the women were older than age 65. Weakness or muscle pain was the most common symptoms. Interacting medications were reported in most cases: 98% for simvastatin (n = 51); 21% for atorvastatin (n = 19); 50% for cerivastatin, rosuvastatin, pravastatin, fluvastatin combined (n = 42). Use of fibrates was reported in 24 cases. In 39 cases reporting creatinine, baseline renal insufficiency was present in 29% of men and 50% of women, with mean creatinine 3.5 mg/dL. In those cases reporting urinalysis, myoglobinuria was present in 28, and no myoglobinuria in 2.

It is difficult to estimate the mortality rate for statin-induced rhabdomyolysis because the cases are rare, and the total number of patients with rhabdomyolysis due to statins is not known. In the case report series described above, the mortality rate was 15% (17 cases); with more deaths in people of age 56–75 years (42). Most of the fatal cases reported baseline CV disease and diabetes (13 and 10 cases, respectively). In a series including 65 patients with statin-induced rhabdomyolysis, the rate of AKI requiring renal replacement therapy and/or mortality was about 8–9%, which was much lower than the rate for most of the other causes (39). However, the data from both studies are derived from a small sample of patients with statin-induced rhabdomyolysis. A much lower mortality rate was found in a retrospective analysis of the FDA database (1997–2000) which reported death from rhabdomyolysis in 0.15 per million prescriptions (45).

Evaluation of the Patient with Suspected Statin-Induced Rhabdomyolysis

The most important test in the initial evaluation is CK, which by definition is >40 × sex-specific ULN, although somewhat lower levels would generally be considered rhabdomyolysis if accompanied by myoglobinuria. CK has a half-life of 1.5 days, and usually returns to normal within 4 weeks of stopping the statin (33). Evaluation includes history and physical examination to determine other causes and potential precipitating factors, such as concomitant interacting medications, excessive exercise, and genetic predisposition (Table 45-3). The physical examination should include assessment of muscle tenderness, strength and function, mental status, and signs of abnormal coagulation such as ecchymoses, petechiae, bleeding, and venous thromboembolism. Serum creatinine and urine output are measured to assess kidney function. AKI has been defined by the Acute Kidney Injury Network as a rapid deterioration of kidney function (within 48 hours) as determined by increase in serum creatinine (≥0.3 mg/dL or ≥1.5 fold from baseline), or urine output less than 0.5 ml/kg/hour for 6 or more hours (http://www.akinet.org/akinstudies.php) (46). Blood tests that require monitoring include CK, BUN, creatinine, electrolytes (with attention to potassium), hepatic transaminases, bilirubin, uric acid, calcium and phosphorus (33,44). Other tests include TSH, to assess hypothyroidism and an arterial or venous blood gas to evaluate acid-base balance.

If electrolytes are abnormal, particularly if serum potassium is high, an electrocardiogram (ECG) should be obtained. The patient must be carefully monitored for mental status, muscle symptoms, and urine output. In addition, examination for signs of abnormal coagulation may reveal DIC, which is more common in patients with renal deterioration.

Clinical Management

Management of a patient with rhabdomyolysis (Table 45-4) focuses on intensive

Table 45-4 Management of rhabdomyolysis and its complications. Adapted from (36).

Complication	Management
Volume depletion with or without deterioration in renal function	Immediate (within 6 h) aggressive IV hydration with 0.9% normal saline, beginning with a bolus followed by 250–500 mL or more per hour, targeting urine output 3 ml/kg or 200–300 ml/hour; continue for at least 24 h. Continue hydration until CK has decreased to <1000 U/L. Monitor for CHF and pulmonary edema. Mannitol not recommended.
Acute kidney injury	Hemodialysis; No evidence that CRRT is more beneficial than intermittent hemodialysis
Hyperkalemia [K^+] >5.5 mmol/L	Slow IV push of insulin (10–14 U) and 25–50 ml 50% glucose (insulin alone if the serum glucose is ≥250 mg/dL [13.9 mmol/L]) decreases [K^+] 10–30 minutes after, lasting 2–4 h. May add nebulizer over 10 min of albuterol 10–20 mg in 4 ml normal saline. Add bicarbonate if metabolic acidosis. Long-term: cation exchange resin (sodium polystyrene sulfonate) orally or as retention enema (avoid sorbitol and avoid after surgery) Hemodialysis if above not effective or [K^+] rapidly rising Loop diuretics only after patient is no longer hypovolemic with care to avoid hypokalemia, hypocalcemia
Metabolic acidosis, urine pH < 6.5, serum pH < 7.2	Aggressive IV hydration. No good evidence that bicarbonate improves outcomes.
Hypocalcemia	Special treatment not recommended. IV hydration as above; Avoid administration of calcium chloride or gluconate unless dangerous cardiac arrhythmia or other features of severe hypocalcemia (e.g., tetany)
Hyperphosphatemia	Oral phosphate binders
Hepatic inflammation, increased AST, ALT, bilirubin	Hydration as above
Compartment syndrome	Monitor pressure by Doppler ultrasound or invasively with catheter. If pressure >40 mmHg (or as clinically indicated), direct decompression by fasciotomy.
Disseminated intravascular coagulation (DIC)	Supportive therapy. If significant hemorrhaging, fresh frozen plasma and emergency hematology consult.

CRRT = continuous renal replacement therapy.

hydration, in order to prevent further muscle damage and renal dysfunction, and correction of serious electrolyte disturbances. In addition, it is critical to identify life-threatening complications such as renal failure, compartment syndrome, and DIC (Table 45-4) (41).

Treatment of statin-induced rhabdomyolysis is similar to treatment of rhabdomyolysis due to other causes. However, hospitalization depends upon clinical judgment, as some patients with statin-induced rhabdomyolysis who appear healthy and have no signs of renal deterioration may recover without hospitalization. The immediate first step when statin-related rhabdomyolysis is suspected is to discontinue the statin and other interacting medications. Patients who are very ill or extremely weak, especially if elderly, or those with increased creatinine or "brown" urine should be hospitalized, and IV hydration started as soon as possible. Hydration requires an hourly infusion of 250–500 mL or more of normal (0.9%) saline, to achieve urine output of 300 ml/hour (33–35), while avoiding fluid overload, which could lead to congestive heart failure and pulmonary edema. The rate of infusion has not been properly studied (41). Normal saline is commonly used (33,43,47,48), although there are no RCTs showing that it is superior to other fluids (33,36). Intravenous hydration should be continued, with adjustment of the rate to avoid fluid overload, until the rhabdomyolysis resolves, or the patient develops AKI requiring dialysis.

Bicarbonate has been used to alkalinize the urine with the hope of reducing the precipitation of myoglobin in renal tubules (41) and to treat metabolic acidosis with urine pH < 6.5 (35,36). However, in 2010, an international consensus conference on "Prevention and Management of Acute Renal Failure in the ICU Patient" concluded that there is no evidence that the use of sodium bicarbonate is superior to normal saline for increasing urine pH (46). Alkalinization of the plasma may cause hypocalcemia. The routine use of mannitol is also not recommended (46,49).

High serum potassium levels should be treated in order to avoid arrhythmias (Table 45-4) (33,36). Hypocalcemia usually corrects with hydration, and should not be treated with calcium gluconate or other forms of calcium, unless the patient has hyperkalemia, hypocalcemia-related ECG changes, and physical signs (e.g., tetany). Loop diuretics have been used to help correct high potassium levels but only after the patient is no longer hypovolemic (with care to avoid hypokalemia and hypocalcemia) but experience is limited and a general recommendation for their use cannot be made. Oral phosphate binders may be taken for hyperphosphatemia.

If AKI develops, or does not improve with IV hydration, renal replacement therapy may be necessary to treat hyperkalemia, metabolic acidosis, fluid overload, and azotemia (36,46). There are no data showing that continuous renal replacement therapy (CRRT) is superior to intermittent hemodialysis (50). Although CRRT has been found to remove myoglobin, it is not known whether removal of myoglobin prevents AKI or

decreases its progression (51). AKI usually resolves in patients with statin-induced rhabdomyolysis.

Follow-up

Restarting statin therapy after an episode of rhabdomyolysis should be discussed with the patient, and depends upon the individual's CV risk, and controllable associated factors that have contributed to rhabdomyolysis, especially interacting medications. If an interacting drug has been identified, and there is no other precipitating factor for rhabdomyolysis, consideration should be given to permanently discontinuing the interacting medication if another replacement can be found. A different statin less susceptible to drug interactions should be considered, along with frequent monitoring of muscle symptoms and CK. If no controllable factors are present and the decision is made to restart statin therapy, the statin chosen should be used at a lower equivalent dose than the statin causing the rhabdomyolysis. Pravastatin up to 40 mg daily is often a suitable choice; at this dose, pravastatin lowers LDL cholesterol by only 35% on average, but has few drug interactions and very rarely causes rhabdomyolysis. Ezetimibe, bile acid sequestrants, or PCSK9 inhibitors may be used to compensate for reduced reduction of LDL-C (52). If rhabdomyolysis was caused by a low potency statin dose without a drug interaction or other controllable factor, which is the situation in only a minority of cases, statin therapy should not be restarted.

In individuals who are not candidates for statin therapy after myopathy or rhabdomyolysis, or in those who refuse to restart statin therapy, alternate lipid-lowering treatments should be considered. These also include ezetimibe, bile acid sequestrants, and/or PCSK9 inhibitors. Ezetimibe rarely if ever causes myopathy or rhabdomyolysis, but lowers LDL-C by only 18% on average, which is not sufficient for many people. Adding a bile acid sequestrant to ezetimibe may reduce LDL-C further by about another 18%. Bile acid sequestrants are not absorbed and do not cause myopathy.

Monoclonal antibodies to PCSK9, alirocumab and evolocumab, also known as PCSK9 inhibitors, were approved in the United States in 2015, where they are indicated for lowering LDL-C as an adjunct to diet and maximally tolerated statin therapy in people with clinical CV disease and/or familial hypercholesterolemia. Alirocumab is administered subcutaneously twice a month, and evolocumab may be given twice a month or once a month, depending upon the dose. PCSK9 binds to LDL receptors on hepatocytes and causes LDL receptor degradation, resulting in higher blood levels of LDL-C. Monoclonal antibodies to PCSK9 inhibit the binding of PCSK9 to LDL receptors, thus increasing the number of LDL receptors that can clear LDL, and decreasing LDL-C levels in the blood. PCSK9 inhibitors reduce LDL-C by about 60% either as monotherapy or when added to statins (53). One 78-week study in 2341 patients at high risk for CV events (53) found a significant difference between alirocumab and placebo in the incidence of myalgia (5.4% versus 2.9%, respectively, $p = 0.006$), but this difference does not appear to have been replicated to date. In particular, a CV outcome trial (54) comparing evolocumab and placebo in over 27,000 statin-treated patients with atherosclerotic disease over a median follow-up period of 2.2 years found no significant difference between the treatment groups in the incidence of muscle-related adverse events, or of rhabdomyolysis.

In people with clinical CV disease or familial hypercholesterolemia who have had myopathy or rhabdomyolysis and are not candidates for statins, and for whom oral non-statin lipid lowering therapies such as ezetimibe and bile acid sequestrants cannot provide adequate LDL-C reduction, treatment with alirocumab or evolocumab may be considered. Cost is a major barrier, however; all statins except pitavastatin are available in generic form, whereas alirocumab and evolocumab are branded biologics costing about 100 times more than generic statins.

Case Study

A 63-year-old woman with type 2 diabetes, hypercholesterolemia and hypertension returned from a vacation in South Africa, and a few days later developed a dry cough and mild shortness of breath, which persisted for 3 weeks. Medications were metformin 1000 mg twice daily, simvastatin 40 mg (which she had taken for 5 years), amlodipine 5 mg, and vitamin D 2000 IU daily. Physical examination was unremarkable. Her temperature was 99.5°F (37.2°C). Chest X-ray showed bilateral infiltrates, and the diagnosis of atypical pneumonia (likely mycoplasma) was made. Erythromycin 500 mg orally four times daily for 2 weeks was prescribed. About 9 days later, she noted severe muscle pain in both thighs, and had difficulty walking. She presented to the emergency room. BP 130/80, HR 80, and body temperature unchanged. On physical examination, the patient had muscle tenderness and weakness in both thighs. Serum CK was 10,560 U/L (normal range 38–176 U/L) which was 60 times ULN, and her urine was dark.

What Do You Think the Diagnosis Is?

She was admitted with a suspected diagnosis of rhabdomyolysis. All medications were discontinued and she was immediately treated with IV normal saline at a rate of 250 ml/hour; blood glucose was managed by small doses of insulin. Other laboratory tests on admission were BUN 26 mg/dL (3–20 mg/dL), creatinine 1.8 mg/dL (0.5–1.1 mg/dL), AST 1400 U/L (15–45 U/L), ALT 430 U/L (10–70 U/L), LDH 750 U/L (140–280), myoglobin 320 µg/L (15–80), Thyroid function tests normal, and hemoglobin A1C 7.3% (56 mmol/mol). Bilirubin was normal. Electrolytes were normal with the exception of potassium 5.6 mmol/L (3.5–5.2 mmol/L). Arterial blood gas showed pH 7.4. ECG was normal. IV hydration was continued, maintaining urine output of 250–300 ml/hour, until BUN and creatinine were normal on day 5. CK peaked on day 3 at 12,000 U/L and subsequently declined, reaching a level of 150 IU/L on day 14. Muscle symptoms gradually improved, and on day 14 she had no muscle pain or weakness. AST and ALT peaked on day 3, and slowly returned to normal over 2 weeks.

What Do You Think Is the Cause of the Rhabdomyolysis?

This case illustrates the presentation and clinical course of rhabdomyolysis in a patient taking simvastatin and an interacting medication. The patient is a woman with type 2 diabetes, hypertension, and increased CV risk, managed by blood pressure control and simvastatin 40 mg. She developed atypical pneumonia, treated with erythromycin, and 9 days later severe muscle symptoms were noted, along with CK elevation above 60 times ULN, confirming the diagnosis of rhabdomyolysis. The rhabdomyolysis was precipitated by the interaction between erythromycin, a potent inhibitor of CYP3A4 (19), and simvastatin, which is metabolized by CYP3A4 (see Table 45-1). This interaction causes a 4-fold increase in plasma levels of simvastatin acid, the principal active metabolite. The patient was also taking amlodipine, which is a weak inhibitor of CYP3A4 that can raise the plasma total HMG-CoA reductase inhibitory activity derived from simvastatin by 30% (55). Another sign of muscle necrosis was the dark urine, caused by myoglobin, which can lead to AKI. Creatinine was mildly elevated, and hyperkalemia was present (serum potassium 5.6 mmol/L). Liver transaminases and LDH were also elevated, consistent with the diagnosis of rhabdomyolysis. Aggressive hydration with normal saline was appropriately initiated as soon as possible, and all medications were discontinued. CK peaked on day 3 of hospitalization, and then slowly declined to normal. All laboratory abnormalities returned to normal after hydration and discontinuation of all medications. The muscle symptoms slowly improved and were resolved by day 14. She was discharged from the hospital on amlodipine 5 mg without a statin.

Subsequently treatment with a different statin, rosuvastatin 10 mg was started 3 weeks after discharge, because the rhabdomyolysis was caused primarily by the drug-drug interaction with erythromycin, and the patient had increased CV risk requiring statin treatment. Rosuvastatin is not metabolized by CYP3A4 and is therefore less susceptible to drug interactions. CK and muscle symptoms were closely monitored for 3 months. The patient remained free of muscle symptoms and CK remained normal.

Conclusions

Myopathy, defined as unexplained muscle pain or weakness and CK elevations >10 times ULN, and its severe form, rhabdomyolysis, with CK increases >40 times ULN, and possible AKI, are caused by statins, with an incidence of less than 0.1% for myopathy, and about 0.01% for rhabdomyolysis. Rhabdomyolysis, a medical emergency, is characterized by muscle cell necrosis, and potential AKI, which can be fatal. Statin-induced rhabdomyolysis is more common at high doses and is often precipitated by drug-drug interactions that increase the plasma concentration of the statin and/or active metabolites. Treatment involves immediate discontinuation of the statin, and hydration. Renal function and electrolytes should be carefully monitored. After stopping the statin, CK typically returns to near normal within 4 weeks. Muscle symptoms resolve in most cases. AKI may take months to resolve.

The decision to restart statin therapy is based upon multiple factors such as the degree of CV risk, age, interacting medications, potency of the statin, and the severity of the rhabdomyolysis. If the rhabdomyolysis was caused by a low potency statin at a low dose, without involvement of other factors, statin therapy should not be restarted and alternative lipid-lowering agents (e.g., ezetimibe, bile acid sequestrants, or PCSK9 inhibitors) should be considered. However, for other patients, especially those who had been taking interacting medications which have been discontinued, careful assessment of benefit/risk and a discussion with the patient may lead to the decision to treat with a different statin, preferably one with few drug interactions either as monotherapy or in combination with alternative lipid-lowering agents if additional LDL-C reduction is needed (52).

References

1 Gu Q, Paulose-Ram R, Burt VL, Kit BK. Prescription cholesterol-lowering medication use in adults aged 40 and over: United States, 2003–2012. *NCHS Data Brief*. 2014.177:1–8.

2 Scandinavian Simvastatin Survival Study Group. Randomised trial of cholesterol lowering in 4444 patients with coronary heart disease: the Scandinavian Simvastatin Survival Study (4S). *Lancet*. 1994;344:1383–1389.

3 Heart Protection Study Collaborative Group. Effects of cholesterol-lowering with simvastatin on stroke and other major vascular events in 20,536 people with cerebrovascular disease or other high-risk conditions. *Lancet*. 2004;363: 757–767.

4 Cholesterol Treatment Trialists' (CTT) Collaboration. Efficacy and safety of more intensive lowering of LDL cholesterol: a meta-analysis of data from 170,000 participants in 26 randomised trials. *Lancet*. 2010;376:1670–1681.

5 Graham DJ, Staffa JA, Shatin D, et al. Incidence of hospitalized rhabdomyolysis in patients treated with lipid-lowering drugs. *JAMA*. 2004;292(21):2585–2590.

6 Björnsson E, Jacobsen EI, Kalaitzakis E. Hepatotoxicity associated with statins: reports of idiosyncratic liver injury post-marketing. *J Hepatology*. 2012;56(2): 374–380.

7 Collins R, Reith C, Emberson J, et al. Interpretation of the evidence for the efficacy and safety of statin therapy. *Lancet*. 2016;388(10059):2532–2561.

8 Preiss D, Sattar N. Statins and the risk of new-onset diabetes: a review of recent evidence. *Curr Opin Lipidology*. 2011;22(6): 460–466.

9 Tobert JA. Efficacy and long-term adverse effect pattern of lovastatin. *Am J Cardiol*. 1988;62(15):28j–34j.

10 Study of the Effectiveness of Additional Reductions in Cholesterol and Homocysteine (SEARCH) Collaborative Group. Intensive lowering of LDL cholesterol with 80 mg versus 20 mg simvastatin daily in 12,064 survivors of myocardial infarction: a double-blind randomised trial. *Lancet*. 2010;376:1658–1669.

11 Carlsson L, Lind L, Larsson A. Reference values for 27 clinical chemistry tests in 70-year-old males and females. *Gerontology*. 2010;56(3):259–265.

12 Neal RC, Ferdinand KC, Ycas J, Miller E. Relationship of ethnic origin, gender, and age to blood creatine kinase levels. *Am J Med*. 2009;122(1):73–78.

13 Norman DJ, Illingworth DR, Munson J, Hosenpud J. Myolysis and acute renal failure in a heart-transplant recipient receiving lovastatin [letter]. *N Eng J Med*. 1988;318(1):46–47.

14 East C, Alivizatos PA, Grundy SM, Jones PH, Farmer JA. Rhabdomyolysis in patients receiving lovastatin after cardiac transplantation [letter]. *N Engl J Med*. 1988;318(1):47–48.

15 Tobert JA. Reply to Norman et al. and East et al. *N Engl J Med*. 1988;318(1):48.

16 Lovastatin Study Group III. A multicenter comparison of lovastatin and cholestyramine therapy for severe primary hypercholesterolemia. *JAMA*. 1988; 260(3):359–366.

17 Staffa JA, Chang J, Green L. Cerivastatin and reports of fatal rhabdomyolysis [letter]. *N Engl J Med*. 2002;346:539–540.

18 Kellick KA, Bottorff M, Toth PP, The National Lipid Association's Safety Task F.

A clinician's guide to statin drug-drug interactions. *J Clin Lipidol*. 2014;8(3 Suppl):S30–S46.

19 Kantola T, Kivisto KT, Neuvonen PJ. Erythromycin and verapamil considerably increase serum simvastatin and simvastatin acid concentrations. *Clin Pharmacol Ther*. 1998;64(2):177–182.

20 Link E, Parish S, Armitage J, et al. SLCO1B1 variants and statin-induced myopathy: a genomewide study. *N Engl J Med*. 2008;359(8):789–799.

21 Wanner C, Krane V, Marz W, et al. Atorvastatin in patients with type 2 diabetes mellitus undergoing hemodialysis. *N Engl J Med*. 2005;353(3):238–248.

22 Fellstrom BC, Jardine AG, Schmieder RE, et al. Rosuvastatin and cardiovascular events in patients undergoing hemodialysis. *N Engl J Med*. 2009;360(14):1395–1407.

23 SHARP Collaborative Group. Study of Heart and Renal Protection (SHARP): randomized trial to assess the effects of lowering low-density lipoprotein cholesterol among 9,438 patients with chronic kidney disease. *Am Heart J*. 2010;160(5):785–794 e10.

24 Neuvonen PJ, Niemi M, Backman JT. Drug interactions with lipid-lowering drugs: mechanisms and clinical relevance. *Clin Pharmacol Ther*. 2006;80(6):565–581.

25 Stroes ES, Thompson PD, Corsini A, et al. Statin-associated muscle symptoms: impact on statin therapy: European Atherosclerosis Society Consensus Panel Statement on Assessment, Aetiology and Management. *European Heart J*. 2015; 36(17):1012–1022.

26 Newman CB, Tobert JA. Statin intolerance: reconciling clinical trials and clinical experience. *JAMA*. 2015;313(10): 1011–1012.

27 Tobert JA, Newman CB. Statin tolerability: in defence of placebo-controlled trials. *Euro J Prev Card*. 2016;23(8):891–896.

28 Finegold JA, Manisty CH, Goldacre B, Barron AJ, Francis DP. What proportion of symptomatic side effects in patients taking statins are genuinely caused by the drug?

Systematic review of randomized placebo-controlled trials to aid individual patient choice. *Euro J Prev Card*. 2014; 21(4):464–474.

29 Tobert JA, Newman CB. The nocebo effect in the context of statin intolerance. *J Clin Lipidology*. 2016;10(4):739–747.

30 Joy TR, Hegele RA. Narrative review: statin-related myopathy. *Ann Intern Med*. 2009;150(12):858–868.

31 Newman C, Tsai J, Szarek M, Luo D, Gibson E. Comparative safety of atorvastatin 80 mg versus 10 mg derived from analysis of 49 completed trials in 14,236 patients. *Am J Cardiol*. 2006;97(1):61–67.

32 LaRosa JC, Grundy SM, Waters DD, et al. Intensive lipid lowering with atorvastatin in patients with stable coronary disease. *N Engl J Med*. 2005;352(14):1425–1435.

33 Zutt R, van der Kooi AJ, Linthorst GE, Wanders RJ, de Visser M. Rhabdomyolysis: review of the literature. *Neuromuscul Disord*. 2014;24(8):651–669.

34 Chavez LO, Leon M, Einav S, Varon J. Beyond muscle destruction: a systematic review of rhabdomyolysis for clinical practice. *Crit Care*. 2016;20(1):135.

35 Scharman EJ, Troutman WG. Prevention of kidney injury following rhabdomyolysis: a systematic review. *Ann Pharmacother*. 2013;47(1):90–105.

36 Bosch X, Poch E, Grau JM. Rhabdomyolysis and acute kidney injury. *N Engl J Med*. 2009;361(1):62–72.

37 Prendergast BD, George CF. Drug-induced rhabdomyolysis: mechanisms and management. *Postgrad Med J*. 1993; 69(811):333–336.

38 Bywaters EG, Beall D. Crush injuries with impairment of renal function. *BMJ*. 1941;1(4185):427–432.

39 McMahon GM, Zeng X, Waikar SS. A risk prediction score for kidney failure or mortality in rhabdomyolysis. *JAMA Intern Med*. 2013;173(19):1821–1828.

40 Huerta-Alardin AL, Varon J, Marik PE. Bench-to-bedside review: rhabdomyolysis – an overview for clinicians. *Crit Care*. 2005;9(2):158–169.

41 Zimmerman JL, Shen MC. Rhabdomyolysis. *Chest*. 2013;144(3): 1058–1065.

42 Mendes P, Robles PG, Mathur S. Statin-induced rhabdomyolysis: a comprehensive review of case reports. *Physiother Can*. 2014;66(2):124–132.

43 Cervellin G, Comelli I, Lippi G. Rhabdomyolysis: historical background, clinical, diagnostic and therapeutic features. *Clin Chem Lab Med*. 2010;48(6): 749–756.

44 Petejova N, Martinek A. Acute kidney injury due to rhabdomyolysis and renal replacement therapy: a critical review. *Crit Care*. 2014;18(3):224.

45 Omar MA, Wilson JP. FDA adverse event reports on statin-associated rhabdomyolysis. *Ann Pharmacother*. 2002;36(2):288–295.

46 Brochard L, Abroug F, Brenner M, et al. An Official ATS/ERS/ESICM/SCCM/SRLF statement: prevention and management of acute renal failure in the ICU patient: an international consensus conference in intensive care medicine. *Am J Respir Crit Care Med*. 2010;181(10):1128–1155.

47 Gunal AI, Celiker H, Dogukan A, et al. Early and vigorous fluid resuscitation prevents acute renal failure in the crush victims of catastrophic earthquakes. *J Am Soc Nephrol*. 2004;15(7):1862–1867.

48 Sinert R, Kohl L, Rainone T, Scalea T. Exercise-induced rhabdomyolysis. *Ann Emerg Med*. 1994;23(6):1301–1306.

49 Brown CV, Rhee P, Chan L, Evans K, Demetriades D, Velmahos GC. Preventing renal failure in patients with rhabdomyolysis: do bicarbonate and mannitol make a difference? *J Trauma*. 2004;56(6):1191–1196.

50 Zeng X ZL, Wu T, Fu P. Continuous renal replacement therapy (CRRT) for rhabdomyolysis (Review). *Cochrane Database Syst Rev*. 2014(6).

51 Chatzizisis YS, Misirli G, Hatzitolios AI, Giannoglou GD. The syndrome of rhabdomyolysis: complications and treatment. *Eur J Intern Med*. 2008; 19(8):568–574.

52 Jellinger PS, Handelsman Y, Rosenblit PD, et al. AACE/ACE 2017 guidelines for the management of dyslipidemia and prevention of atherosclerosis. *Endocrine Prac*. 23 (Suppl 2) 1–87.

53 Robinson JG, Farnier M, Krempf M, et al. Efficacy and safety of alirocumab in reducing lipids and cardiovascular events. *New Engl J Med*. 2015;372(16):1489–1499.

54 Sabatine MS, Giugliano RP, Keech AC, et al. Evolocumab and clinical outcomes in patients with cardiovascular disease. *N Engl J Med*. 2017 376:1713–1722.

55 Nishio S, Watanabe H, Kosuge K, Uchida S, Hayashi H, Ohashi K. Interaction between amlodipine and simvastatin in patients with hypercholesterolemia and hypertension. *Hypertens Res*. 2005;28(3): 223–227.

Index

Note: Page numbers in *italics* refer to Figures; Page numbers in **bold** refer to Tables

Endocrine and Metabolic Medical Emergencies: A Clinician's Guide, Second Edition. Edited by Glenn Matfin.
© 2018 John Wiley & Sons Ltd. Published 2018 by John Wiley & Sons Ltd.

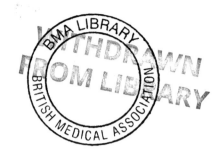